Estimated Safe and Adequate Daily Dietary Intakes of Additional Selected Vitamins and Minerals (United States)[a]

Age (years)	Vitamins: Biotin (μg)	Vitamins: Pantothenic Acid (mg)
Infants		
0–0.5	10	2
0.5–1	15	3
Children		
1–3	20	3
4–6	25	3–4
7–10	30	4–5
11 +	30–100	4–7
Adults	30–100	4–7

Age (years)	Trace Elements[b]				
	Chromium (μg)	Molybdenum (μg)	Copper (mg)	Manganese (mg)	Fluoride (mg)
Infants					
0–0.5	10–40	15–30	0.4–0.6	0.3–0.6	0.1–0.5
0.5–1	20–60	20–40	0.6–0.7	0.6–1.0	0.2–1.0
Children					
1–3	20–80	25–50	0.7–1.0	1.0–1.5	0.5–1.5
4–6	30–120	30–75	1.0–1.5	1.5–2.0	1.0–2.5
7–10	50–200	50–150	1.0–2.0	2.0–3.0	1.5–2.5
11 +	50–200	75–250	1.5–2.5	2.0–5.0	1.5–2.5
Adults	50–200	75–250	1.5–3.0	2.0–5.0	1.5–4.0

[a]Because there is less information on which to base allowances, these figures are not given in the main table of the RDA and are provided here in the form of ranges of recommended intakes.
[b]Because the toxic levels for many trace elements may be only several times usual intakes, the upper levels for the trace elements given in this table should not be habitually exceeded.

Source: *Recommended Dietary Allowances*, © 1989 by the National Academy of Sciences, National Academy Press, Washington, D.C.

Estimated Minimum Requirements of Sodium, Chloride, and Potassium

Age (years)	Sodium[a] (mg)	Chloride (mg)	Potassium[b] (mg)
Infants			
0.0–0.5	120	180	500
0.5–1.0	200	300	700
Children			
1	225	350	1000
2–5	300	500	1400
6–9	400	600	1600
Adolescents	500	750	2000
Adults	500	750	2000

[a]Sodium requirements are based on estimates of needs for growth and for replacement of obligatory losses. They cover a wide variation of physical activity patterns and climatic exposure but do not provide for large, prolonged losses from the skin through sweat.
[b]Dietary potassium may benefit the prevention and treatment of hypertension and recommendations to include many servings of fruits and vegetables would raise potassium intakes to about 3500 mg/day.

Source: *Recommended Dietary Allowances*, © 1989 by the National Academy of Sciences, National Academy Press, Washington, D.C.

Median Heights and Weights and Recommended Energy Intakes (United States)

Age	Weight		Height		Average Energy Allowance			
(years)	(kg)	(lb)	(cm)	(inches)	REE[a] (cal/day)	Multiples of REE[b]	cal per kg	cal per day[c]
Infants								
0.0–0.5	6	13	60	24	320		108	650
0.5–1.0	9	20	71	28	500		98	850
Children								
1–3	13	29	90	35	740		102	1300
4–6	20	44	112	44	950		90	1800
7–10	28	62	132	52	1130		70	2000
Males								
11–14	45	99	157	62	1440	1.70	55	2500
15–18	66	145	176	69	1760	1.67	45	3000
19–24	72	160	177	70	1780	1.67	40	2900
25–50	79	174	176	70	1800	1.60	37	2900
51 +	77	170	173	68	1530	1.50	30	2300
Females								
11–14	46	101	157	62	1310	1.67	47	2200
15–18	55	120	163	64	1370	1.60	40	2200
19–24	58	128	164	65	1350	1.60	38	2200
25–50	63	138	163	64	1380	1.55	36	2200
51 +	65	143	160	63	1280	1.50	30	1900
Pregnant (2nd and 3rd trimesters)								+300
Lactating								+500

[a]REE (resting energy expenditure) represents the energy expended by a person at rest under normal conditions.
[b]Recommended energy allowances assume light to moderate activity and were calculated by multiplying the REE by an activity factor.
[c]Average energy allowances have been rounded.

Source: *Recommended Dietary Allowances*, © 1989 by the National Academy of Sciences, National Academy Press, Washington, D.C.

Daily Values (used on food labels)

Daily Reference Values (DRVs)[a]

Food Component	DRV
fat	65 g[d]
saturated fatty acids	20 g
cholesterol	300 mg[e]
total carbohydrate	300 g
fiber	25 g
sodium	2,400 mg
potassium	3,500 mg
protein[b]	50 g

Reference Daily Intakes (RDIs)[c]

Nutrient	Amount	Nutrient	Amount
vitamin A	5,000 International Units (IU)	vitamin B_6	2.0 mg
		folic acid	0.4 mg
vitamin C	60 mg	vitamin B_{12}	6 μg[f]
thiamin	1.5 mg	phosphorus	1.0 g
riboflavin	1.7 mg	iodine	150 μg
niacin	20 mg	magnesium	400 mg
calcium	1.0 g	zinc	15 mg
iron	18 mg	copper	2 mg
vitamin D	400 IU	biotin	0.3 mg
vitamin E	30 IU	pantothenic acid	10 mg

[a]Based on 2,000 calories a day for adults and children over 4 only.
[b]DRV for protein does not apply to certain populations; Reference Daily Intake (RDI) for protein has been established for these groups: children 1 to 4 years: 16 g; infants under 1 year: 14 g; pregnant women: 60 g; nursing mothers: 65 g.
[c]Formerly the U.S. RDA, based on National Academy of Sciences' 1968 Recommended Dietary Allowances.
[d](g) grams
[e](mg) milligrams
[f](μg) micrograms

Source: R. Kurtzweil, 'Daily Values' encourage healthy diet, *FDA Consumer*, May 1993, pp. 40–45.

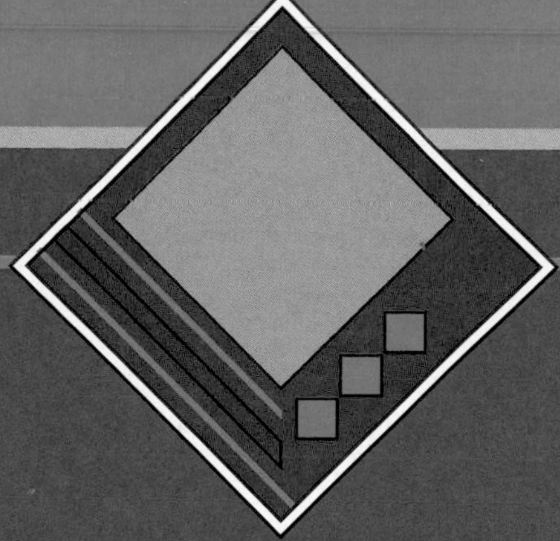

Hamilton/Whitney's

Nutrition

CONCEPTS AND CONTROVERSIES

SIXTH EDITION

Frances Sienkiewicz Sizer

Eleanor Noss Whitney

WEST PUBLISHING COMPANY

Minneapolis/St. Paul New York Los Angeles San Francisco

West's Commitment to the Environment

In 1906, West Publishing Company began recycling materials left over from the production of books. This began a tradition of efficient and responsible use of resources. Today, up to 95 percent of our legal books and 70 percent of our college and school texts are printed on recycled, acid-free stock. West also recycles nearly 22 million pounds of scrap paper annually—the equivalent of 181,717 trees. Since the 1960s, West has devised ways to capture and recycle waste inks, solvents, oils, and vapors created in the printing process. We also recycle plastics of all kinds, wood, glass, corrugated cardboard, and batteries, and have eliminated the use of Styrofoam book packaging. We at West are proud of the longevity and the scope of our commitment to the environment.

Production, Prepress, Printing and Binding by West Publishing Company.

610 Opperman Drive
P.O. Box 64526
St. Paul, MN 55164-0526

Printed in the United States of America

01 00 99 98 97 96 95 94 8 7 6 5 4 3 2

Library of Congress Cataloging-in-Publication Data

Sizer, Frances Sienkiewicz.
Nutrition: concepts and controversies/Frances Sienkiewicz Sizer, Eleanor Noss Whitney. — 6th ed.
p. cm.
Rev. ed. of: Nutrition/Eva May Nunnelley Hamilton. 5th ed. © 1991.
Includes bibliographical references and index.
ISBN 0-314-02692-4 (Student Version)
ISBN 0-314-02890-0 (Annotated Instructor's Edition)
1. Nutrition. 2. Food. I. Whitney, Eleanor Noss. II. Hamilton, Eva May Nunnelley. Nutrition. III. Title.
QP141.H34 1994
613.2—dc20

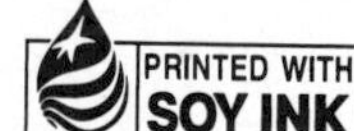

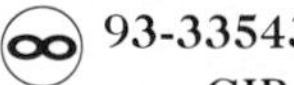

93-33543
CIP

Production Credits

Cartoonist: Gary Carroll
Composition: Parkwood Composition
Copyediting: June Gomez
Cover and Text Design: Janet Bollow
Cover Image: *Fruit in Glass Compote* by Emma Jane Cady, Abby Aldrich Rockefeller Folk Art Center, Williamsburg, VA
Dummy Artist: David Farr, Imagesmythe, Inc.
Illustrations: J/B Woolsey Associates, with select figures from Sandra McMahon
Index: Jo-Anne Naples, Naples Editing Services

Photo Credits

3 Henry Church, Still Life, The Collection of Frances O. Stem-Babinsky; **6** © Roy Morsch/The Stock Market; **7** © Stacy Pick/Stock Boston; **8** © Ray Stanyard; **8** © David Young-Wolf/PhotoEdit; **15** © David R. Frazier; **15** Thomas Harm and Tom Peterson/Quest Photographic Inc.; **21** © Ray Stanyard; **24** © Tom McCarthy/PhotoEdit; **29** Marilyn Herbert; **40, 41** Thomas Harm and Tom Peterson/Quest Photographic Inc.; **44** © Felicia Martinez/PhotoEdit; **46, 47** Thomas Harm and Tom Peterson/Quest Photographic Inc.; **49** © Stephen McBrady/PhotoEdit; **56, 57** Thomas Harm and Tom Peterson/Quest Photographic Inc.; **59** © John Burwell, Burwell/Burwell Photography; **60** © Merritt Vincent/PhotoEdit; **64** © Lawrence Migdale/Photo Researchers; **65** © John Burwell, Burwell/Burwell Photography; **68** © Michael Newman/PhotoEdit; **76** © David Young-Wolf/PhotoEdit; **88** © Michael Newman/PhotoEdit; **89** From D. W. Fawcett, The Cell, 2nd ed. (Philadelphia: Saunders, 1981); color by Kidd & Company; **110** © Steven Rothfeld/Tony Stone Worldwide; **121, 124** Thomas Harm and Tom Peterson/Quest Photographic Inc.; **130** © Tony Freeman/PhotoEdit; **142** © David R. Frazier; **144, 147, 149** Thomas Harm and Tom Peterson/Quest Photographic Inc.; **164, 165** © Ray Stanyard; **167** Thomas Harm and Tom Peterson/Quest Photographic Inc.; **176** © Robert Brenner/PhotoEdit; **180** © Martin Chaffer/Tony Stone Worldwide; **184** © Irving Geis/Science Photo Researchers; **186** From D. W. Fawcett, The Cell, 2nd ed. (Philadelphia: Saunders, 1981); color by Kidd & Company; **195** Thomas Harm and Tom Peterson/Quest Photographic Inc.; **200** © Alan Oddie/PhotoEdit; **201** © Steve Maines/Stock Boston; **203** © Ray Stanyard; **208** © Williams & Edwards/The Image Bank; **209, 210** Thomas Harm and Tom Peterson/Quest Photographic Inc.; **216** © David R. Frazier; **217** David J. Farr/ImageSmythe; **218** Nutrition Today, H. Stanstead, J. Carter, and W. Darby, Nutritional Deficiencies, Nutrition Today Aid #5 (Nutrition Today: Annapolis, MD) 1975; **219** Thomas Harm

(continued following index)

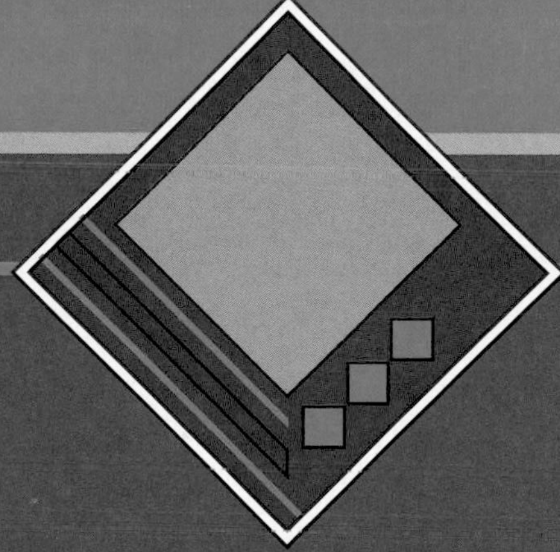

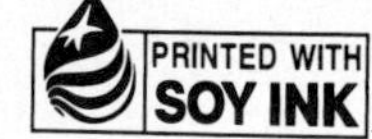

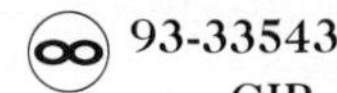

To the memory of May Hamilton, whose loving touch has been evident in these pages ever since she coauthored the first edition.

Ellie and Fran

ABOUT THE AUTHORS

Eleanor Noss Whitney, Ph.D., R.D., received her B.A. in Biology from Radcliffe College in 1960 and her Ph.D. in Biology from Washington University, St. Louis, in 1970. Formerly on the faculty at the Florida State University, she now devotes full time to research, writing, and consulting in nutrition, health, and environmental issues. Her earlier publications include articles in *Science*, *Genetics*, and other journals. Her textbooks include *Understanding Nutrition*, *Understanding Normal and Clinical Nutrition*, *Nutrition and Diet Therapy*, and *Essential Life Choices*, among others.

Frances Sienkiewicz Sizer, M.S., R.D., attended Florida State University where, in 1980, she received her B.S., and in 1982, her M.S. in nutrition. She is a founding member and vice president of Nutrition and Health Associates, an information resource center in Tallahassee, Florida which maintains an ongoing bibliographic data base that tracks research in over 1,000 topic areas of nutrition. Her textbooks include *Life Choices: Health Concepts and Strategies*, *Making Life Choices*, *The Fitness Triad: Motivation, Training, and Nutrition*, and others. In addition to writing, she has served as a nutrition consultant to schools and alcoholism programs in Florida, and she lectures at universities in the southeast. She maintains a professional membership in the American Dietetic Association.

Contents in Brief

Contents

CHAPTER 15

APPENDIXES

Preface

With this sixth edition, *Nutrition: Concepts and Controversies* celebrates its 15th anniversary of publication. These years of service to students and professors in the classrooms across the nation have brought us welcomed comments about our book. We have learned that our perspectives on established nutrition knowledge are exceptionally valuable, that our glimpses into areas of rapid change keep interest high, and that our personal writing style and clear figures appeal to both verbal and visual learners. We have also learned that today's students appreciate colorful pages, and this edition presents thoroughly updated fundamentals with an upbeat new design.

This sixth edition also sports some new practical features that carry the science of nutrition into the grocery store. Beginning in Chapter 2, each of six chapters presents a "Checking Out Food Labels" feature that illuminates the important new information found on food labels. The chapters on vitamins and minerals feature "Snapshots," capsules of information that depict food sources and teach some salient facts about each nutrient.

We hope that you will enjoy using this sixth edition as we have enjoyed creating it for you. Along with its new topics come amenities such as new art and photos that we feel complement the pages and assist in learning.

Chapter 1 of this edition begins with a personal challenge to nutrition science. It asks the question so many people ask of nutrition scientists: "What should I do, when scientists keep changing their minds?" We answer with a lesson in sound scientific thinking and the context in which study results may be rightly viewed. We then introduce the nutrients and explore the concept of nutrient density. Finally, the important role of cuisine in a person's heritage helps to spotlight and honor this country's multicultural nature.

Chapter 2 brings together the concepts of diet planning through food grouping systems and exchange systems, and features the new Daily Food Guide with its Pyramid of food choices. Chapter 3 presents a thorough, but brief, introduction to the workings of the human body with major emphasis on the digestive system.

The next five chapters offer details on the nutrients. Chapters 4 through 6 are devoted to the energy-yielding nutrients—carbohydrates, lipids, and proteins. Chapters 7 and 8 present the vitamins, minerals, and water, with special emphasis on the emerging importance of the antioxidant nutrients.

A series of five chapters then applies nutrition knowledge to specific life situations. Chapter 9 relates energy balance to body composition, obesity, and underweight, and presents weight maintenance as a life-long effort. Chapter 10 presents the relationships between fitness, physical activity, and nutrition—relationships that are of interest to the casual exerciser and athlete alike. Chapter 11 applies the essence of the previous chapters to two broad and rapidly changing areas within nutrition: immunity and disease prevention. Chapters 12 and 13 point out the importance of nutrition throughout the lifespan, from gestation through old age.

Chapter 14 focuses on foods. It considers the problems and advantages of food technology, with a special emphasis on food safety for consumers. Chapter 15 touches on the vast problems of the global food supply—world hunger, environmental pollution, overpopulation—and shows how everyday food choices link each person with the meaningful whole.

The Controversies of this book's title are optional readings printed with colored borders. Many are new to this edition and others have been updated. One that deserves special mention is Controversy 6, which compares the advantages and drawbacks of vegetarian and nonvegetarian foodways, leaving it to the reader to answer its title question, "Whose diet is best?" Controversy 9 tackles some pressing questions surrounding the issues of safety and effectiveness of weight-loss diets, diet profiteers, and attitudes toward overweight people in this country. Controversy 10 presents current thinking about eating disorders, along with the new diagnostic criteria for 1994. Controversy 13 offers a basic understanding of the roles nutrition plays in the regulation of the brain and applies scientific evidence to the currently popular question of whether nutrient supplements might improve brain functioning. Controversy 14 evaluates new food technologies and welcomes the reader to ponder the future. The final Controversy of this book outlines ways in which agriculture can ensure a high-quality food supply into the next century.

The Food Feature sections that appear in most chapters act as bridges between theory and practice; they are personal applications of the concepts in the chapters. Consumer Cautions present information on juicing, supplements, and other nutrition-related marketplace choices to empower students to make informed decisions.

New or major terms in chapters are defined in the margins of the pages where they are introduced. Terms in Controversy sections are grouped together and defined in tables within the sections. The reader who wishes to locate any definition can do so by consulting the index, which lists their page numbers in boldface type.

The appendixes have been updated. Notice especially Appendix A, which now presents the most complete listings ever of nutrient contents of over 1,700 foods. Appendix B supplies the RNI, Guidelines, and the Food Guide for our Canadian readers. Appendix C presents aids to calculations, with special emphasis on calculating percentages of calories from energy nutrients. Appendix D provides both the U.S. and Canadian Exchange Systems. Appendix E offers an invaluable list of current addresses and telephone numbers for those interested in additional information.

Our lists of source notes have grown longer in this edition, partly because nutrition information in scientific journals has increased exponentially in the recent past, and partly in response to requests from readers who wish to develop bibliographies on our topics. To make space, we have removed many older source notes, but anyone who wishes to obtain our older sources can do so easily by consulting an older edition of this book, or by contacting the publisher.

Our purpose in writing this book is to enhance the understanding of nutrition science in ways that apply to everyday life and thereby to enhance the quality of life for our readers. We hope you find this book enlightening and useful, and that you will enjoy it. And to all our long-time readers, happy anniversary.

Acknowledgments

We are grateful to our associates, Linda DeBruyne and Sharon Rolfes for their valued assistance in our work. We thank Linda DeBruyne especially for Chapters 7 and 8 of this edition and for her work on the Food Diary and Activity Manual. Thanks to Sharon Rolfes and Stephanie Johnson for the creation of the video disk that accompanies this edition. Thanks also to Caroline Ann Sizer for her unflagging effort and joyful assistance at each stage of this writing, and for her encouragement, which made heavy tasks seem lighter. Thanks, too, to our associate Lori Turner for much of the *Instructor's Manual;* thanks to Margaret Hedley, University of Guelph, who prepared the Canadian material for the manual; and to Linda Hahn, California State University, Los Angeles, who prepared the section on Teaching Strategies for the manual. For the special Instructor's Edition of the text, we thank Judy Kaufman of Monroe Community College for preparing all margin references to the multi-media resources and Lori Turner, Tallahassee Community College, for preparing the Lecture Outlines that open the instructor's version of the text. Many thanks also to Louise Little of the University of Delaware for her content review of our food label features. Special thanks to Simin Bolourchi Vaghefi, University of North Florida, and to Geoffrey Webb, University of East London, for inviting us to their classes at the University of North Florida and for their many good ideas. Thanks to John Woolsey and associates for bringing our figures to their full potential. To Tom Peterson and Tom Harm of Quest Photographic, our thanks for creating the attractive photographs of food throughout the book. Our thanks also to Gary Carroll for his charming cartoons.

Special thanks to our editors, Peter Marshall, Becky Tollerson, Stacy Lenzen, and Chris Hurney, and to their staff, for their tireless efforts to ensure the highest quality of all facets of this book. Thanks also to Jana Kicklighter of Georgia State University for preparing the *Student Study Guide* and the *Test Bank*. Thanks also to Bob Geltz, Betty Hands, Nancy Belleque and their staff at ESHA research for the table of food composition (Appendix A), and for the computerized diet analysis program that accompanies this book. Thanks, too, to Janet Bollow for our appealing new design. To our reviewers, many heartfelt thanks for their many thoughtful ideas and suggestions.

Reviewer List

Elizabeth Applegate
University of California—Davis

Garry Auld
Colorado State University

Elaine Blyler
California State University—Northridge

Ann Bock
New Mexico State University

Joanne Caid
California State University—Fresno

Wen Chiu
Shoreline Community College

Mary Capra
University of Northern Colorado

A. J. Clark
Auburn University

Paula Cook
University of Maryland

Dorothy DeLessio
Johnson and Wales University

Kathy Engelbert-Fenton
University of Utah

Amelia Finan
Anne Arundel Community College

Joyce Gilbert
Sante Fe Community College

James Golick
College of DuPage

Deloy Hendricks
Utah State University

Ann Hertzler
Virginia Polytechnic Institute and State University

Jayanthi Kandiah
Ball State University

Judy Kaufman
Monroe Community College

Billie Lane
Chattanooga State Technical Community College

Patricia Mogan
Orange Coast Community College

Marsha Read
University of Nevada

Chris Rosenbloom
Georgia State University

Anne Smith
The Ohio State University

Samuel Smith
University of New Hampshire

Danielle Torisky
James Madison University

Simin Bolourchi Vaghefi
University of North Florida

Elise West
Cornell University

Julian Williford, Jr.
Bowling Green State University

Loyanne Wilson
Eastern Kentucky University

Roberta Wilson
University of Puget Sound

Ione Wood
Clovis Community College

Lisa Young
New York University

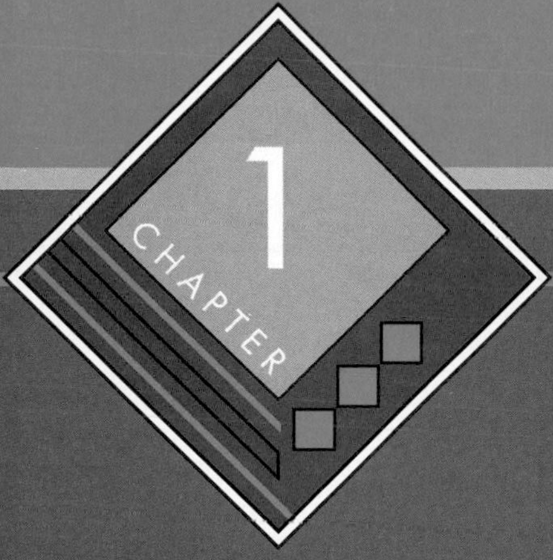

Food Choices and Human Health

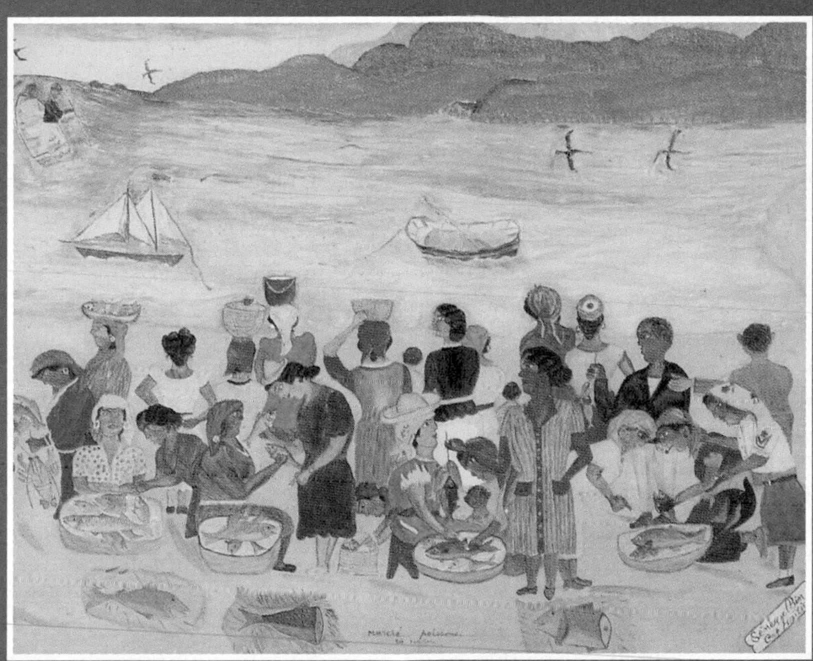

Sènéque Obin 1893–1977, *Marché* Poissons before 1957 (Fish Market), Collection of Siri von Reis, New York, New York

Contents

food medically, any substance that the body can take in and assimilate that will enable it to stay alive, and to grow; the carrier of nourishment; socially, a more limited number of such substances defined as acceptable by each culture.

nutrition the study of the nutrients in foods and in the body; sometimes also the study of human behaviors related to food.

diet the foods (including beverages) a person usually eats and drinks.

1

If you care about your body, and if you have strong feelings about **food,** then you have much to gain from learning about **nutrition**—the study of how food nourishes the body. It is a fascinating, much talked-about subject. Each day, newspapers, radio, and television broadcast stories of new findings on nutrition and heart health, nutrition and cancer avoidance. Daily, magazine advertisements and television commercials bombard you with multicolored pictures of delicious foods to tempt you—pizza, burgers, cakes, sweet drinks, alcoholic beverages, and many more. Several times a day you get hungry and turn from your other activities to eat a meal. And if you are like most people, you wonder, "Is this food good for me?" or you berate yourself, "I probably shouldn't be eating this."

The study of nutrition can benefit both your physical and emotional health. When you learn which foods serve you best, you can work out ways of choosing foods, planning meals, and designing your **diet** wisely. This benefits your physical health. In addition, food facts can dispel food fears. Knowing the facts can relieve you of feeling guilty or worried that you aren't eating well. Thus, you can enhance your enjoyment of eating, and this benefits your emotional health.

Nutrition is a science—a field of knowledge composed of facts. Scientists have obtained these facts by systematically observing what people eat and noting how healthy they are, and also by experimenting to see how various foods and diets affect animals' and people's health. From these observations and experiments, they have assembled many findings and have drawn conclusions, such as "A diet high in fat presents a risk of heart disease and cancer," or "Up to a certain point, sugar in the diet presents no harm to health," or "Certain minimum amounts of vitamin A and the mineral zinc are indispensable to maintain the health of the eyes."

Further scientific investigation then goes on to answer further questions, such as "Just how high in fat can the diet be without harming health?" "How does fat relate to heart disease and cancer?" "Just how much sugar is OK?" "What does excess sugar do to health?" "Just how much vitamin A and zinc are needed to maintain vision?" "What, exactly, do these nutrients do in the body?"

Unlike some other areas of science, such as astronomy and physics, nutrition is a relatively young science. Most nutrition research has been conducted within the past century, that is, since 1900. The first vitamin was identified in 1897, and the first protein structure was not fully described until 1945. Much remains to be learned about foods' and nutrients' effects on the body. Because nutrition science is an active, changing, growing body of knowledge, you often hear reports of scientific findings that seem to contradict other findings and of interpretations of those findings that conflict with one another.

For this reason, people who don't understand how science operates may despair as they try to understand from current reports what is really going on. They may even become distrustful: "The scientists themselves don't even know what is true; how am I supposed to know?" To help consumers make correct judgments regarding their food choices and diets, the first section of this chapter is devoted to the apparent scientific contradictions in nutrition science.

Other than the points just now being investigated, many facts in nutrition are known with great certainty—enough to fill this book and many more. And where there are conflicts and contradictions, researchers today are energetically attempting to resolve them. Everyone wants to know how food affects health—naturally, because we love food and we care about our health.

This book devotes many chapters to the science of nutrition. This chapter provides background on the human level by offering answers to the following questions:

1. What does food do for the body and its owner?
2. What sorts of foods should Americans eat today to best support their health?

◆ If the Scientists Don't Know, How Can I?

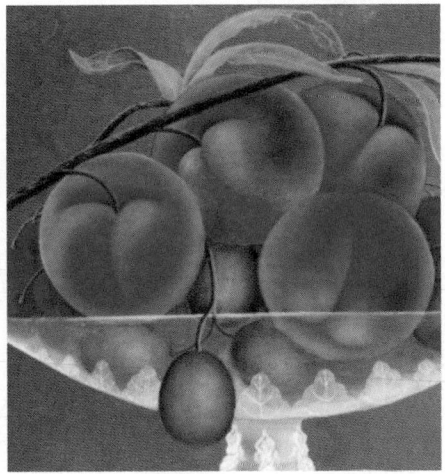

Everyone stampedes for oat bran, red wine, or fish oil based on today's news that these products are good for health. Then tomorrow's news reports, "it isn't true after all," and everyone drops oat bran, red wine, and fish oil and takes up the next latest craze. Meanwhile, they complain with frustration, "Those scientists don't know anything."

In truth, though, it is a scientist's business not to know. Scientists ask questions—that's their job. Then they design experiments designed to test for various possible answers. When they have ruled out some possibilities and found evidence for others, they submit their findings, not to the news media, but to boards of reviewers composed of other scientists who will try to pick them apart. If the reviewers consider the conclusions to be well supported by the evidence, they endorse the work for publication, not in the news media, but in scientific journals where still other scientists can read it.

Once a new finding is published, it is still only preliminary. The next step is for other scientists to attempt to duplicate what the first ones have done or to challenge the findings by designing experiments to disprove them.

Only when a finding has stood up to rigorous, repeated testing in several kinds of experiments performed by several different researchers is it finally considered confirmed. Even then, to be strict about it, no such thing as a *fact* exists in science. Science consists of *hypotheses* that can always be challenged and revised. Some, though, like the hypothesis that the earth revolves about the sun, are so well supported by so many observations and experimental findings that they are generally accepted as facts. What we "know" in nutrition is confirmed in the same way: it results from years of replicating study findings.

The news media are hungry for new findings, though, and reporters often latch onto ideas from the scientific labs before they have been fully tested. To tell the truth, sometimes scientists get excited about their findings, too, and leak them to the press before they have been through a rigorous review conducted by their peers. As a result, the public often is exposed to late-breaking news stories from scientific labs before the findings are fully confirmed. Then when the hypothesis being tested fails to hold up to a later challenge, consumers feel betrayed by what is simply the normal course of science at work.

It follows that if you act on new science news that is hot off the press, you do so at your own risk. Applying a new nutrition finding is not like buying a new appliance: there is no warranty; it is not backed by consumer testing; and it is not a crime for the finding to be invalidated.

It also follows that people who take action based on single studies are almost always acting impulsively, not scientifically. The real scientists are trend watchers. They evaluate the methods used in each study, assess each study in light of all the evidence gleaned from other studies, and little by little, modify their picture of what is true. As evidence accumulates, they become more and more confident about being able to make recommendations that apply to people's health and lives. Single studies are interesting, perhaps even exciting, but learn to withhold judgment about how to apply the findings until they have been repeated and confirmed.

Media sensationalism may even overrate the importance of true, replicated findings. This happened when oat bran hit the news. Oat bran has been shown to lower blood cholesterol, a lipid indicative of heart-disease risk, but bran is one of several hundred factors that affect blood cholesterol. A news report on oat bran may fail to mention that cutting fat intake is still the major blood cholesterol-lowering step to take. Science is constantly building on an already-existing foundation of knowledge, but journalists and television reporters often pick single news items and blow them up out of proportion to the whole.[1]

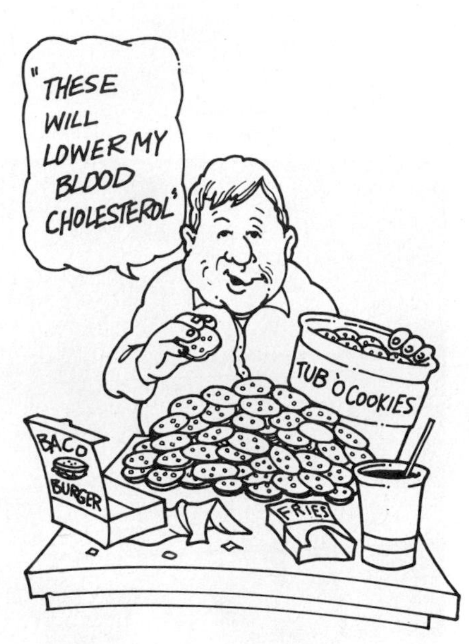
"THESE WILL LOWER MY BLOOD CHOLESTEROL"
TUB 'O COOKIES
BACO BURGER
FRIES

Also, new findings need definition. Oat bran is truly a cholesterol reducer; but how much bran does it take to produce the desired effects? Do little oat-bran pills or powders meet the need? Do oat-bran cookies? How many? Does everyone respond the same way to them? How much of a dietary indiscretion can a person commit and still rectify it with oat-bran cookies? One reviewer dealing with a report on this very topic observed, "To get the equivalent of the oat fiber in one bowl of oatmeal, it would [be] necessary to eat 90 cookies."[2] An oat bran muffin eaten after a high-fat, fast-food lunch and steak dinner cannot undo all the damage that the meal did.

People who know how science works do not let reports of single findings throw them. After one study found no cholesterol-lowering effect of oat bran on a particular population under a particular set of conditions, many people abandoned oats as a cholesterol fighter. This was a mistake because the bulk of available evidence still supports the original finding. Today, oat bran's cholesterol-lowering effect is considered to be established.[3] The whole process of discovery, challenge, and vindication took almost ten years of research; some take many years longer.

In science, single findings almost never make a crucial difference to the whole picture, but like single frames in a movie, they contribute a little to it. It takes many such frames to tell the whole story.

Because science is a step-by-step, information-gathering and testing process, some of the older reports are among the most valuable. A hypothesis first advanced in 1960 that stands up to many kinds of testing for several decades has real strength. Naturally, though, when it is reported today, it is the researchers who reported the original finding who are properly given the credit for it. Scientific information is not like new cars or this year's hemlines; "new" does not usually mean "improved." In fact, any science report based on "all new references" is suspect, for truly strong facts are based on years of strong, original work. This is why, even in science books published just this year, you'll see references to older reports. In science, some of the oldies are the real goodies; they not only were exciting and new when they first appeared, but they have stood up to the test of time.

KEY POINT Scientists uncover nutrition facts by experimenting. Single findings must be replicated before they can be considered valid. New nutrition news is not always to be believed; old news has stood up to the test of time.

Table 1-1
Elements in the Six Classes of Nutrients

The nutrients listed in the colored area contain carbon and are organic.

	Carbon	Oxygen	Hydrogen	Nitrogen[a]	Minerals[b]
Water		X	X		
Carbohydrate	X	X	X		
Fat	X	X	X		
Protein	X	X	X	X	
Vitamins	X	X	X	X	
Minerals					X

[a]All of the B vitamins contain nitrogen, *amine* means nitrogen.
[b]Protein and some vitamins contain the mineral sulfur; vitamin B_{12} contains the mineral cobalt.

The Human Body and Its Food

As your body lives each day, it moves and works, and to move or work, it must use **energy.** The energy that fuels the body's work comes indirectly from the sun by way of plants. Plants capture and store the sun's energy in their tissues as they grow. When you eat plant-derived foods such as fruits, grains, or vegetables, you obtain and use the solar energy they have stored. Animals obtain their energy in the same way, and when you eat animal tissues you are eating compounds containing energy originally from the sun. Solar energy is first stored in plants, and then eaten by animals and stored in their tissues in turn.

The body also requires six kinds of **nutrients**—families of molecules indispensable to its functioning—and foods deliver these. Table 1-1 lists the six classes of nutrients. Four of these six are **organic,** that is, the nutrients are derived from living things that have captured solar energy, either directly or indirectly, and converted the energy into compounds containing the element carbon. The human body is made of the same materials as foods are, arranged in different ways (Figure 1-1).

energy the capacity to do work. The energy in food is chemical energy: it can be converted to mechanical, electrical, heat, or other forms of energy in the body. Food energy is measured in calories, defined on page 12.

nutrients components of food that help to nourish the body, that is, to provide energy, to serve as building material, to help maintain or repair body parts, or for growth. The nutrients include water, carbohydrate, fat, protein, vitamins, and minerals.

organic carbon containing. Four of the six classes of nutrients are organic: carbohydrate, fat, protein, and vitamins. (Strictly speaking, organic compounds include only those made by living things and do not include carbon dioxide and a few carbon salts.)

energy-yielding nutrients the nutrients the body can use for energy. (They may also supply building blocks for body structures.)

The Nutrients in Foods

Foremost among the six classes of nutrients in foods is *water,* which is constantly lost from the body and must constantly be replaced. Among the four organic nutrients, three are **energy-yielding nutrients,** meaning that the body can use the energy they contain. The *carbohydrates* and *fats* (formally called *lipids*) are especially important energy-yielding nutrients. As for *protein,* it does double duty: it can yield energy, but it also provides materials that form structures and working parts of body tissues. (Alcohol yields energy, too, but it is not a nutrient; see Table 1-4's note, page 13.)

The fifth and sixth classes of nutrients are the *vitamins* and the *minerals.* These provide no energy to the body. A few minerals serve as parts of body structures (calcium and phosphorus, for example, are major constituents of bone), but all vitamins and minerals serve as regulators. As regulators, the vitamins and minerals assist in all body processes: digesting food; moving muscles; disposing of wastes; growing new tissue; healing wounds; obtaining energy from carbohydrate, fat, and protein; and every other process necessary to maintain life. Later chapters are devoted to each

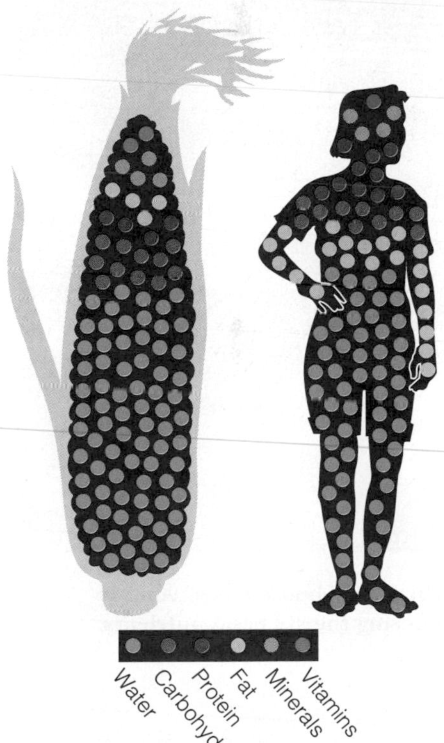

Figure 1-1

MATERIALS OF FOOD AND THE HUMAN BODY

Foods and the human body are made of the same materials.

essential nutrients the nutrients the body cannot make for itself (or cannot make fast enough) from other raw materials—nutrients that are obtained in food and needed by the body.

supplements pills, liquids, or powders that contain purified nutrients; or foods that contain purified nutrients added in amounts per serving greater than 50% above a standard considered sufficient for all healthy human beings.

elemental diets diets composed of purified ingredients of known chemical composition, intended to supply all essential nutrients to people who cannot eat foods.

of these six classes of nutrients in the order just named (except for water, which is treated with the minerals).

When you eat food, then, you are not just engaging in a pleasurable activity; you are providing your body with energy and nutrients. Furthermore, some of the nutrients are **essential nutrients,** meaning that if you do not receive them from food, you will develop deficiencies; the body cannot make them for itself. Essential nutrients are found in all six classes of nutrients. Water is essential; so is carbohydrate; so are some lipids, some parts of protein, the vitamins, and so are all of the minerals important in human nutrition, too.

Scientists have worked out ways to measure the energy and nutrient contents of foods. They have also narrowed down the amounts of energy and nutrients various types of people need—people of both sexes, of different ages, and of different walks of life. Thus after studying human nutritional requirements (the subject of Chapter 2 of this book), you can state with some accuracy just what your own body needs—this much water, that much carbohydrate and fat, so much protein, and so forth. Might it be possible, then, to simply take pills or **supplements** in place of food? No, because as it turns out, food offers more than just the six basic nutrients.

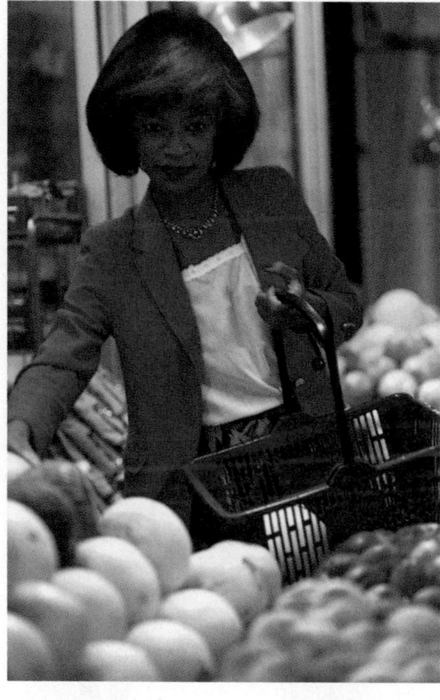

When you choose foods, you are choosing the six basic nutrients.

KEY POINT Food supplies energy and nutrients. The most vital nutrient is water. The energy-yielding nutrients are carbohydrates, fats (lipids), and protein. The helper nutrients are vitamins and minerals.

Food: More Than Just Nutrients

Nutrition science has achieved the ability to state what nutrients human beings need to *survive*—at least for a time. The 1970s and 1980s saw an explosion of interest and skill in the making of **elemental diets**—diets that are totally chemically defined, used for people in the hospital who cannot eat ordinary food. These formulas, administered to severely ill people for days and weeks at a time, support not only continued life but recovery from malnutrition and infection and the healing of wounds.

However, these diets are not sufficient to enable people to *thrive*. Elemental diets support life but not optimal growth and health; and they often lead to nutrient deficiencies. Although each time this happens the nutrient deficiency can be detected and corrected, it shows that the definition of these diets is not yet perfect for all people in all settings.

Even if a person's basic nutrient needs are perfectly understood and met, concoctions of nutrients still lack something that foods provide. The story of a girl who could not eat illustrates this point. She had a severe intestinal disorder: her digestive tract was almost completely nonfunctional. She had to be fed nutrient mixtures through a vein. Deficiencies developed and were recognized and remedied, but still something was missing—she wanted to eat food. Her health care providers therefore occasionally allowed her to eat whatever she wanted, even though everything she ate had to be collected into a bag through an opening in her abdominal wall after only a few minutes in her intestines. Clearly real food did something important for her emotional health:

> *Her psychological outlook was completely changed. She was happy. The tastes, sounds, sights, and smells of the food gave her great gratification. But, most especially, it was interesting to note that the condition of her skin and hair improved, and the pink on her cheeks and the look of 'wellness' returned.*[4]

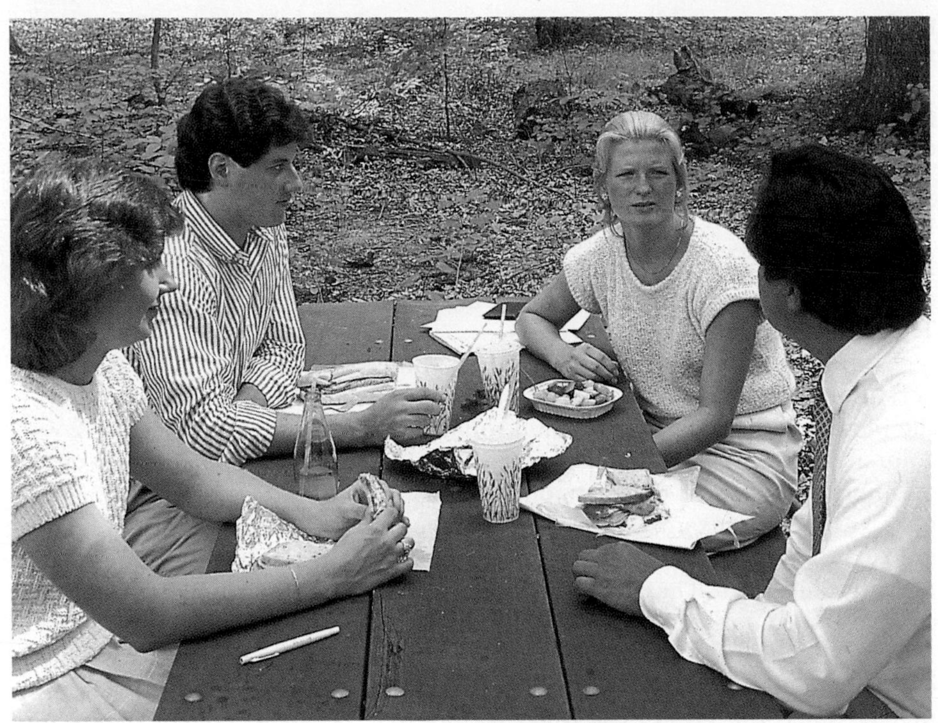

When you eat foods, you are receiving more than just nutrients.

Whether this effect of real food was physical or psychological remains unknown. According to the physician caring for the girl, "It was just something . . . we were not able to give through a needle."[5] This physician has abundant knowledge and years of experience and is not likely to ascribe mysterious powers to food without justification.

satiety (sat-EYE-uh-tee) the feeling of fullness or satisfaction that food conveys.

Science demands explanations, though: what is this mysterious "something" food offers that cannot be provided through a needle? Part of the answer may lie in the reaction of the digestive tract to food. The stomach and intestines are dynamic living organs, and they constantly change in reaction to the foods they receive. When a person is fed through a vein, the digestive organs, like unused muscles, weaken and grow smaller. Experiments have shown that when the intestine receives food, it releases hormones, chemical messengers that regulate the body's maintenance; when not fed, it fails to receive stimulation and so withers. In light of this knowledge, medical wisdom now dictates that when a hospital client has to be fed through a vein, the duration should be as short as possible, and real food, taken into the intestine, should be reintroduced as early as possible.[6]

The hormones that the intestines release in response to food also affect the brain. The messages they deliver seem to have something to do with **satiety**—the sense of satisfaction that makes a person feel, "There, that was good. Now I'm full." Both physical and emotional comfort accompany satiety: after a good meal you can relax, enjoy entertainment, rest, or sleep. One writer says, "One cannot think well, love well, sleep well, if one has not dined well."[7]

Food does still more than maintain the intestine and convey messages of comfort to the brain. Foods are chemically complex. Even an ordinary potato contains hundreds of different compounds. People are complex, too, and the relationship between people and food is ancient. In view of all this,

nonnutrients a term used in this book to mean compounds other than the six nutrients that are present in foods.

ethnic foods foods associated with particular cultural subgroups within a population.

perhaps the fact that food gives more to us than just nutrients is not surprising; it would be surprising if it were otherwise.

KEY POINT In addition to nutrients, food conveys emotional satisfaction, and possibly hormonal stimuli that contribute to health.

Nonnutrients in Foods

In addition to the many nutrients foods contain, to which many of the chapters to come are devoted, foods also contain many other compounds. This book calls them **nonnutrients.**

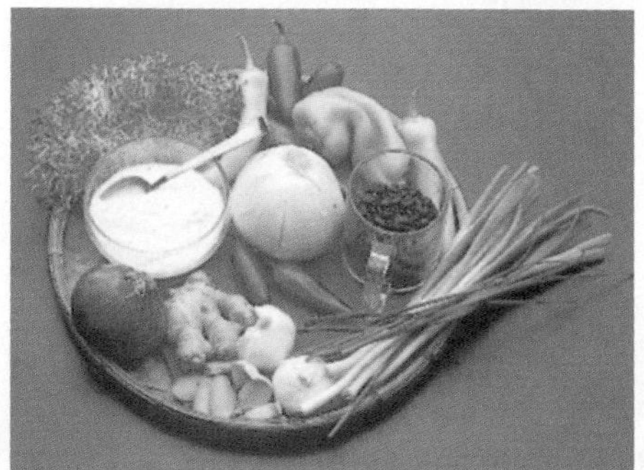

Some foods offer beneficial nonnutrients.

Among the nonnutrients in foods are the compound that gives hot peppers their burning taste; the compound that gives garlic its pungent flavor; the pigments that give spinach and tomatoes their dark green and dark red colors; the yeast cells that make bread rise; and thousands upon thousands of others. Some foods contain nonnutrients that have drug effects—there is one in grapes, for example, that seems to help kill viruses.[8] Some substances are toxic: there is one in cabbage, for example, that in excess can damage the thyroid gland. That doesn't mean that cabbage is a harmful food, of course; it also contains nonnutrients that have an anticancer effect.

Many medical drugs also come from plants. The drug effects of plants, including foods, have been known to human beings for over 20,000 years, that is, since the Stone Age when people first began to collect plants for their medicinal properties. For all that time, and no doubt for thousands of years before that, people were developing a relationship with plants that involved much more than a mere dependency for nutrients. They learned to turn to food for comfort, for relief of pain, for pleasure, and even for the cure of some ailments. Ever since then, food has meant many things to people, and many cultural and social traditions have been attached to the preparing, serving, eating, and sharing of food.

KEY POINT Foods contain compounds other than nutrients that give them their tastes, aromas, colors, and other characteristics.

Cultural and Social Meanings Attached to Food

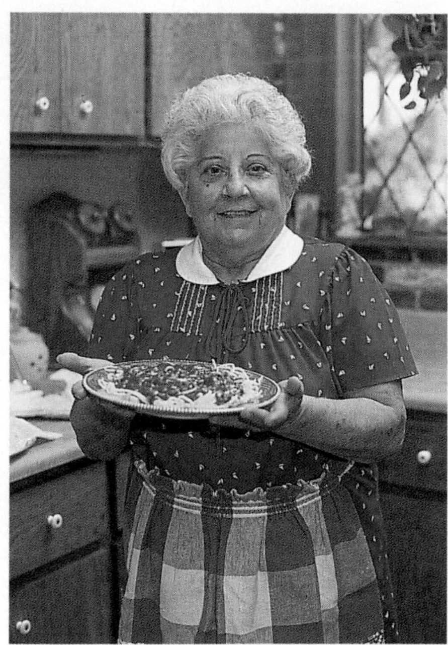

Sharing ethnic food is a way of sharing culture.

Besides conveying comfort, satiety, nutrients, and nonnutrients, foods express our cultures, our philosophies, and our beliefs. People from every country enjoy special foods that represent their own histories. As a result, the sharing of food can be symbolic: people offering foods that represent their heritages are expressing a willingness to share cherished values with others. People accepting those foods are symbolically accepting not only the person doing the offering but the person's culture. This is why meetings of heads of states worldwide most often take place surrounding a meal and why couples entering into cross-cultural marriages invite each other to share traditional holiday meals.

The same is true within a nation of mixed cultures such as the United States. Years ago, sociologists believed the United States to be a "melting pot," a single, "American" culture. In reality, though, our nation resembles a mosaic more than a melting pot because people of similar heritages tend to coalesce into district cultural communities. This arrangement provides a wealth of unique cultural experiences for those who choose to seek them. One of the most enjoyable ways to sample other cultures is to try some of the **ethnic foods** they have to offer.

Those who work toward harmony and understanding among people recommend experiences that include sampling cuisines.[9] Luckily, this is easy to do for most people living in the United States, since ethnic restaurants and food festivals here are as common as hamburger places. A menu in an "American-style" restaurant might list spaghetti (Italian), nachos (Mexican), hot dogs with sauerkraut (German), croissants (French), stewed okra (African), baked squash (Native American), and egg rolls (Chinese). These traditional everyday foods, now adapted to locally available ingredients, have all become an integral part of the "American diet."

omnivores people who eat foods of all kinds, foods of both plant and animal origin, including animal flesh.

vegetarians people who exclude from their diets animal flesh and possibly animal products such as milk, cheese, and eggs. See Table 1-2, the Glossary of Vegetarian Terms.

Cultures attach special, though sometimes inaccurate, meanings to particular foods. Common among several subcultures in our society are the beliefs that meat gives strength and is therefore especially important for men to eat, whereas fruits confer beauty and are suitable for women. Later chapters reveal that meats and fruits are of equal importance in the nutrition of both men and women and that meat can equally safely be omitted from the diets of both, provided that other foods are suitably chosen.

Cultural traditions regarding food are not inflexible; they keep evolving as people move about, learn new things, and teach each other. Today, some people are ceasing to be **omnivores** and are becoming **vegetarians,** as they discover the advantages associated with low-meat and no-meat diets.

People choose vegetarianism for a multitude of reasons. Some believe that we should not kill animals to eat their meat. Some believe that we should not even partake of animal products such as milk, cheese, and eggs. Today, on learning that the human population is straining the earth's resources of land and water and that raising grains for direct consumption by people requires less land and water than does raising grains to feed animals, some believe we should eat less meat for environmental reasons.

A small glossary of terms related to vegetarianism appears in Table 1-2. The nutrition implications of these traditions are discussed often in the chapters to come.

All of these considerations—physical, psychological, cultural, social, and philosophical—make up the framework within which people choose the foods they eat. Still other considerations bear more immediately on a person's day-to-day food choices. Among factors people cite to explain daily food choices are:

Personal preference: You like them.

Habit: They are familiar; you always eat them.

Ethnic heritage or tradition: They are the foods of your ethnic group.

Social pressure: They are offered; you feel you can't refuse them.

Availability: There are no others to choose from.

Convenience: They are quick and easy to prepare.

Economy: They are within your means.

Positive associations: They are eaten by people you admire, or they indicate status, or they remind you of fun.

Emotional needs: Foods can make you feel better for awhile.

Values or beliefs: They fit your religious tradition, square with your political views, or honor the environmental ethic.

Nutritional value: You think they are good for you.

Only the last of these reasons for choosing foods reflects that you are conscious of their importance to your nutritional health. Similarly, the choice

Table 1-2
Glossary of Vegetarian Terms

- **lacto-vegetarians** vegetarians who use milk and milk products in their diets.
- **lacto-ovo vegetarians** vegetarians who use milk, milk products, and also eggs in their diets.
- **vegans** (VAY-guns, VEJ-uns) vegetarians who include no animal-derived products in their diets. These people are also called **strict vegetarians.**

malnutrition any condition caused by excess or deficient food energy or nutrient intake or by an imbalance of nutrients. Nutrient or energy deficiencies are classed as forms of *undernutrition;* nutrient or energy excesses are classed as forms of *overnutrition.*

of where, as well as of what, to eat is often based more on social needs than on nutrition judgments. College students often choose to eat out and especially often choose to eat at fast-food restaurants. Their intent is to socialize, to get out, to save time, and to date; they are not always conscious of the need to obtain healthful food.[10]

In conclusion, then, food does many things for people. One of them, though—and the one that is most crucial to physical health—is that it nourishes the body. That function of food is the focus of this book.

KEY POINT Cultural traditions and social values revolve around food. Some values are expressed through foodways.

Food as Nourishment

If you live for 65 years or longer, you will have consumed more than 70,000 meals, and your remarkable body will have disposed of 50 tons of food. The effects on your body of the foods you choose accumulate. At 65 years of age you will see and feel those effects, if you know what to look for.

Your body renews its structures continuously, and each day it builds a little muscle, bone, skin, and blood, replacing old tissues with new. In this way some of the food you eat today becomes part of "you" tomorrow. The best food for you, then, is the kind that supports the growth and maintenance of strong muscles, sound bones, healthy skin, and sufficient blood to cleanse and nourish all parts of your body. This means you need food that provides not only energy but also sufficient nutrients in all of the classes named earlier: water, carbohydrates, fats, protein, vitamins, and minerals. If the foods you eat provide too little of any of these, then your health will suffer a little. If the foods you eat provide too little of one or more nutrients every day for years, then by the time you are old, you may well suffer severe disease effects.

The point of this is that a well-chosen array of foods supplies enough energy and enough of each nutrient to prevent **malnutrition.** The forms of malnutrition such a diet prevents include both deficiencies of nutrients and imbalances and excesses, which can also take a toll on health over time.

KEY POINT The nutrients in food support growth, maintenance, and repair of the body. Deficiencies, excesses, and imbalances of nutrients bring on the diseases of malnutrition.

Nutrition and Disease Prevention

A former surgeon general remarked that your choice of diet profoundly influences your long-term health prospects. (Only two lifestyle habits are more influential: smoking and other tobacco use; and excessive drinking.)[11] Many older people suffer from debilitating conditions that could have been largely prevented had they known the nutrition principles that we know today and applied those principles throughout their lives.

The poor health conveyed by a poor diet consists not only of the various forms of malnutrition just described, but also of other diseases, especially the so-called diseases of old age: heart disease, diabetes, some kinds of cancer, dental disease, adult bone loss, and others. We should hasten to say that these diseases cannot be prevented just by a good diet; they are to some extent determined by people's genetic constitutions, activities, and lifestyles. However, within the range set by your inheritance, the likelihood that you will develop these diseases is strongly influenced by your food choices.

Some people overestimate and some underestimate the influence of diet in preventing diseases and poor health. It is difficult to get diet's exact role in perspective—not only difficult for individual people, but also difficult for research scientists who are spending their working lives trying to figure out exactly how diet relates to health and various diseases. Three different views of the relationship may help to show the connections.

First, remember the role of genetics. Different diseases are differently influenced by genetics and nutrition, as shown in Figure 1-2. A disease such as sickle-cell anemia, for example, is *purely* hereditary—nothing a person eats affects the likelihood of the person's contracting this anemia. Sickle-cell anemia is shown at left in the figure as a nutrition-unresponsive, genetic disease. In contrast, a condition such as "low birthweight," listed at right in the figure, is often a nutrition-responsive condition. An infant's low birthweight is usually not genetic, but is caused by the mother's poor nutrition during pregnancy; and it can lead to severe illness and death of the infant. Diseases and conditions of poor health are arrayed all along the spectrum from purely genetic to purely nutritional; the more nutrition-responsive a disease or health condition is, the more successfully sound nutrition can prevent it.

Second, remember that some diseases, such as heart disease and cancer, are not one disease but many. Two people may both have heart disease, but not the same form of it. People differ genetically from each other in thousands of ways. One person's heart disease may be nutrition-responsive, another may not be. No simple statement can be made about the extent to which diet can help a given person avoid or slow the course of a disease, yet clearly in some cases it helps a lot.

Third, remember that other lifestyle choices people make, besides their choices of what foods to eat, also affect their health. Tobacco and alcohol use were already mentioned and other substance abuse can be equally destructive of health. Other major health determinants include physical activity, sleep, stress, and home and job conditions, including environmental quality.

In the context of all of these frameworks, healthful nutrition can help prevent some diseases, sometimes with great impact. Table 1-3 shows some of the relationships, and later chapters return to examine these relationships in detail.

KEY POINT Choice of diet influences long-term health, within the range set by genetic inheritance. Nutrition has no influence on some diseases but is tightly linked to others.

Figure 1-2

NUTRITION AND DISEASE

Not all diseases are equally influenced by diet. Some are purely hereditary, like sickle-cell anemia. Some may be inherited (or the tendency to develop them may be inherited) but may be influenced by diet, like some forms of diabetes. Some are purely dietary, like the vitamin and mineral deficiency diseases.

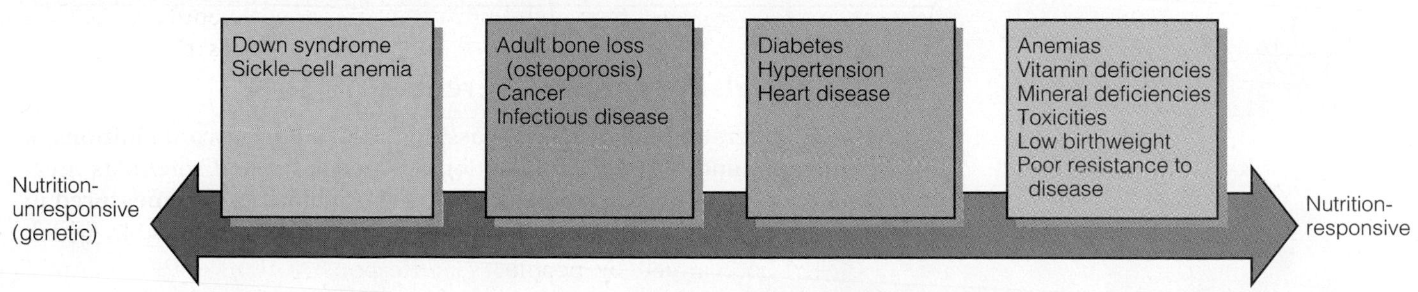

calories units of energy. A kilocalorie (*kcalorie*, abbreviated *kcal*) is, strictly speaking, the unit used to measure the energy in food: it is the amount of heat energy necessary to raise the temperature of a kilogram (a liter) of water 1 degree Celsius. This book follows the common practice of using the lowercase term *calorie* (abbreviated **cal**) to mean the same thing.

grams units of weight. A gram (g) is the weight of a cubic centimeter (cc) or milliliter (ml) of water under defined conditions of temperature and pressure.

Table 1-3
Nutrition Measures to Prevent Diseases

Adequate Intake of Essential Nutrients, Especially *Protein*, and *Energy* from Food Helps Prevent

- *In Pregnancy*
  - Low birthweight
  - Poor resistance to disease
  - Some forms of birth defects
  - Some forms of mental/physical retardation
- *In Infancy and Childhood*
  - Growth deficits
  - Poor resistance to disease
- *In Adulthood and Old Age*
  - Poor resistance to infectious diseases
  - Susceptibility to some forms of cancer

Moderation in Intake of *Energy* from Food Helps Prevent

- Obesity and related diseases, such as diabetes and hypertension

Moderation in *Fat* Intake Helps Prevent

- Susceptibility to obesity, some cancers, and atherosclerosis

Adequate *Fiber* Intake Helps Prevent

- Digestive malfunctions such as constipation and diverticulosis and possibly colon or other cancers
- Possibly heart disease

Moderation in *Sugar* Intake Helps Prevent

- Dental caries

Moderation in *Alcohol* Intake Helps Prevent

- Liver disease
- Malnutrition

Adequate Intake of *Any Essential Nutrient* Prevents

- Deficiency diseases such as cretinism, scurvy, and folate-deficiency anemia

Moderation in Intake of *Essential Nutrients* Prevents

- Toxicity states

Adequate *Calcium* Intake Helps Prevent

- Adult bone loss

Adequate *Iron* Intake Helps Prevent

- Anemia

Adequate *Fluoride* Intake Helps Prevent

- Dental caries

Moderation in *Sodium* Intake Helps Prevent

- Hypertension and related diseases of the heart and kidney

Adequate *Vitamin* Intake Helps Prevent

- Susceptibility to certain cancers

Nutrition Goals for Disease Prevention

To support understanding of the discussions that follow, two definitions, a set of numbers, and a sample calculation are needed. Food scientists measure food energy in **calories,** units of heat. Food quantities are measured in **grams,** units of weight. The most energy-rich of the nutrients is fat, which contains 9 calories in one gram. Carbohydrate and protein each contain only 4 calories in a gram (see Table 1-4).

Table 1-4
Calorie Values of Energy Nutrients

Energy Nutrient	Energy
Carbohydrate	4 cal/g
Fat (lipid)	9 cal/g
Protein	4 cal/g

Note: Alcohol contributes 7 cal/g that the human body can use for energy. Alcohol is not classed as a nutrient, however, because it cannot be used to promote growth, maintenance, or repair. It is a toxin. When alcohol contributes a substantial portion of the energy in a person's diet, it damages body organs.

The content of fat in food is often expressed as "percent of calories," and "30 percent of calories from fat" is a key limit to keep in mind. A food whose fat contents are higher than 30 percent is considered undesirably high in fat, unless eaten with low-fat foods to bring the average down. Suppose a food contains 5 grams of fat and a total of 120 calories of energy. You can calculate what percentage of the calories in that food are from fat, because 5 grams of fat at 9 calories per each gram of fat totals 45 calories. Out of 120 calories, 45 calories represent 45/120, or 37.5 percent of the total. Appendix C spells out such calculations.

On September 5, 1990, the U.S. Department of Health and Human Services (U.S. DHHS) released *Healthy People 2000*, a set of health objectives for the nation.[12] The objectives numbered 297 in all, in 22 different priority areas, of which nutrition was one. The objectives listed under "Nutrition" provide a quick scan of the health goals that the Department thought were within the province of nutritional science (see Table 1-5 on the next page).

The first four U.S. DHHS objectives indicate that nutrition can influence four health conditions for better or worse. These conditions are heart disease, cancer, overweight, and growth retardation in infants.

The next eight objectives identify the factors in the diet best known to influence the risks of contracting these conditions. According to the U.S. DHHS, we need less fat and more complex carbohydrate and fiber in our diets. We need to balance our energy intakes and exercise better to control our weight. Many people need more calcium and iron, and many need less salt. Women should breastfeed their babies more and longer; and parents need to learn infant-feeding practices that will minimize the chances of tooth decay.

The last nine U.S. DHHS objectives related to nutrition are intended to improve delivery of nutrition services. Food labels have been improved, but people need to learn to use them properly, and the labels need still more improvements. The selections of foods in restaurants and schools should be nutritious. School and preschool children and the elderly should have nutritious foods available to them, and sound nutrition education and information should be available through schools, workplaces, and health care providers. These lists provide a summary of what the nation's top health agency thinks is most important in the nutrition picture.

In 1991, a year after the U.S. DHHS objectives were published, some progress was apparent in some areas. Heart disease deaths had fallen slightly. More people were using nutrition labels to make food choices, and more restaurants were offering low-fat, low-calorie items on their menus.[13]

Nutrition monitoring of the U.S. population is ongoing. To make it easier than it has been in the past, the agencies involved agreed in 1990 to cooperate, rather than to compete. According to a ten-year plan embodied in the National Nutrition Monitoring Act of 1990, the principal government agencies monitoring the nation's nutrition will use the same standards, units, and research designs so that they can compare and compile their results meaningfully. They will also share results, using computer links, so that each agency can easily access what the others have done.

Among the agency names you may hear in connection with these efforts are three: the U.S. DHHS already mentioned, the U.S. Department of Agriculture (USDA), and the Centers for Disease Control (CDC). You are also

Table 1-5
Nutrition-Related Health Objectives for the Nation, Year 2000

Disease-Related Objectives
1. Reduce *heart disease* deaths. 2. Reverse the rise in *cancer* deaths. 3. Reduce the prevalence of *overweight.* 4. Reduce *growth retardation* among low-income children.
Nutrient and Food Objectives
5. Reduce dietary *fat* intake.[a] 6. Increase intakes of complex *carbohydrate* and *fiber*-containing foods.[b] 7. Increase the proportion of *overweight* people taking effective steps to control their weight. 8. Increase *calcium* intakes among teenagers, pregnant women, women who are breastfeeding their infants, and adults in general. 9. Reduce *salt* intakes and purchases of foods high in salt. 10. Remedy *iron* deficiencies in children and women. 11. Encourage *breastfeeding* of infants immediately after birth and the continuation of breastfeeding for at least six months after birth. 12. Teach parents *infant-feeding practices* that will minimize the chances of tooth decay.[c]
Nutrition Information and Service Objectives
13. Promote people's learning of how best to use *food labels* to correctly select nutritious foods. 14. Make food labels more informative and complete. 15. Make more low-fat, low-saturated fat foods available. 16. Encourage more restaurants and institutions to serve low-fat, low-calorie foods. 17. Improve the nutrition quality of school lunches and breakfasts and child-care foodservice meals. 18. Make sure as many elderly people as possible receive home food services. 19. Offer nutrition education in more schools from preschool through 12th grade. 20. Encourage workplaces to provide nutrition education and/or weight-management programs for their employees. 21. Support health care providers in offering nutrition assessment, nutrition counseling, and referrals to qualified nutrition experts as part of their services.

[a]The exact objective is to reduce fat intake to an average of 30 percent of calories or less, and saturated fat intake to less than 10 percent of calories. How to do this is described in Chapter 5.

[b]The objective is spelled out: increase these intakes in the diets of adults to five or more daily servings of vegetables (including legumes) and fruits and to six or more daily servings of grain products.

[c]The objective emphasizes *nursing-bottle syndrome,* discussed in Chapter 12.

Source: Healthy People 2000: National Health Promotion and Disease Prevention Objectives (Washington, D.C.: U.S. Department of Health and Human Services, 1990).

likely to hear of two research projects. The Health and Nutrition Examination Surveys (HANES) involve:

- Asking people what they have eaten.
- Recording measures of their health status.

The National Food Consumption Surveys (NFCS) involve:

- Recording what people have actually eaten on a certain day.
- Evaluating the foods they have chosen against recommended food selections.

So much for what the experts say they would like to accomplish in terms of improved health and nutritious food choices. How, in fact, should we go about choosing foods to accomplish these objectives?

KEY POINT The U.S. Department of Health and Human Services has published a set of health objectives for the nation. The goals are to reduce the incidence of heart disease, cancer, overweight, and growth retardation, to improve nutritional health, and to improve delivery of nutrition services.

The Challenge of Choosing Foods

The foods you choose should fit your tastes, personality, family and cultural traditions, lifestyle, and budget. At their best, well-planned meals convey pleasure, too, and they should also be nutritious, or at least the diet you build from them should be. Foods today, however, come in astounding numbers and varieties. Consumers can lose track of what they contain and how they can best be put together into health-promoting diets.

The Variety of Foods to Choose From

If someone had listed the variety of foods available several hundred years ago, the list might have been relatively short. The basic foods—foods that have been around for a long time such as vegetables, fruits, meats, and grains—would have been on that list. (At various times, these foods may be called *unprocessed, natural, whole,* or *farm* foods.) An easy way to obtain a nutritious diet is to consume a variety of selections from among these foods each day, but data from a recent HANES Survey show that on a given day as many as 45 percent of our people consume no fruits or fruit juices and 22 percent eat no vegetables. Many more eat some of these foods, but not as many servings as recommended.[14]

The variety of foods available to us today, ironically, may make it more difficult, rather than easier, to plan nutritious diets. The food industry offers

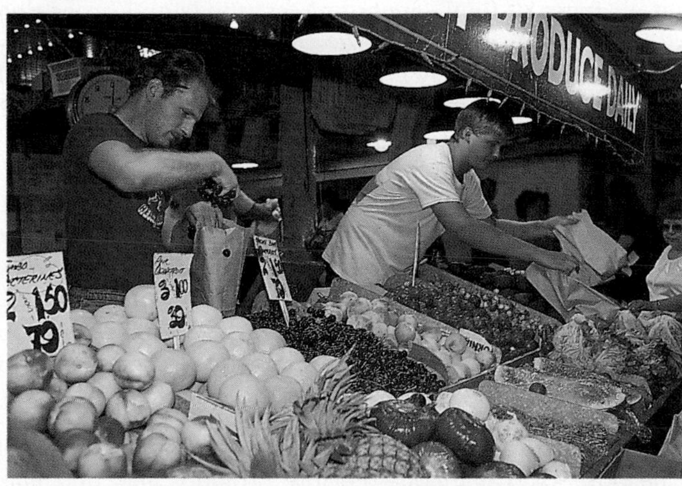

Foods once looked like this . . .

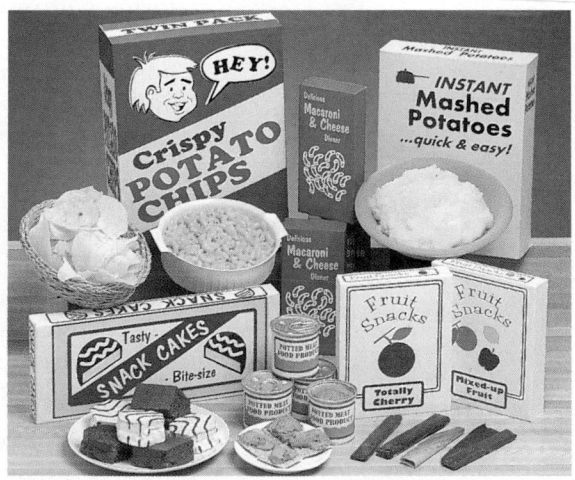

. . . but now foods often look like this.

Table 1-6
Glossary of Food Types

The purpose of this little glossary is to reveal that good-sounding food names don't necessarily signify that foods are nutritious. Read the comment at the end of each definition.

- **basic foods** milk and milk products; meats and similar foods such as fish and poultry; vegetables, including dried beans and peas; fruits; and grains. These foods are generally considered to form the basis of a nutritious diet. Also called *whole foods.*
- **enriched (fortified) foods** foods to which nutrients have been added. If the starting material is a whole, basic food such as milk or whole grain, the result may be highly nutritious. If the starting material is a partitioned food such as sugar or salt, the result may be a nutrient-empty food.
- **fast foods** restaurant foods that are available within minutes after customers order them—traditionally, hamburgers, french fries, and milkshakes; more recently salads and other vegetable dishes as well. These foods may or may not meet people's nutrient needs well, depending on the selections made and on the energy allowances and nutrient needs of the eater.
- **natural foods** a term that has no legal definition. To convey the sense that a food is nutritious, this book uses the term *basic food* or *food of high nutrient density* instead. Some so-called natural foods, such as raw sugar, are partitioned foods, and so are not nutritious.
- **partitioned foods** foods composed of parts of whole foods, such as butter (from milk), sugar (from beets or cane), or corn oil (from corn). Partitioned foods are usually empty of nutrients and are not nutritious.
- **processed foods** foods subjected to any process, such as enrichment, milling, alteration of texture, addition of additives, cooking, or others. Depending on the starting material and the process, a processed food may or may not be nutritious.
- **staple foods** foods used frequently or daily, for example, rice (in the Far East) or potatoes (in Ireland). If well chosen, these foods are nutritious; certainly, they should be.

thousands of foods, many of which are mixtures of the basic ones, and many of which are even constructed from artificial ingredients.

Table 1-6 presents a glossary of terms related to foods. A reading of the terms will reveal that all types of food—including fast foods and processed foods—can be nutritious or nonnutritious. How nutritious foods are depends on the nutrients and calories they contain.[15] In short, to select well among foods, as among people, you need to know more than just their names; you need to know the foods' inner qualities.

Even more importantly, you need to know how to combine foods into nutritious diets. Foods are not nutritious by themselves; each is of value only in so far as it contributes to a nutritious diet.[16] A key to wise diet planning is to make sure that the foods you eat daily, your staple foods, are especially nutritious.

Are juices especially nutritious? You might be led to think so, if you encountered certain books making claims that juices offer special health benefits. The following Consumer Caution inspects this claim.

KEY POINT Foods come in a bewildering variety in the marketplace, but the foods that form the basis of a nutritious diet are ordinary milk and milk products; meats, fish, and poultry; vegetables and dried peas and beans; and fruits and grains.

Claims Made for Juices and Raw Foods

CONSUMER CAUTION Many books have appeared on the market that proclaim juice as a therapeutic wonder. Often these books are located conveniently near housewares departments that stock juice-making machines. The books would have you believe that juices can cure all the ills people commonly experience, from acne and age spots to obesity and varicose veins. Some even promise cancer cures or help for AIDS victims, if ill people will purchase and use the three- to four-hundred-dollar juice machines being promoted. The person who is suffering from an incurable disease might well suspect that the claims are fake, but be unable to turn down any glimmer of hope, no matter how high the price or faint the hope. When false claims are published in books, not on labels, the authors can say anything, and rest secure in knowing that the constitutional right of freedom of the press protects them.

To answer the question of what nutritional benefits one can expect from juice, here are some facts. Juice is a liquid extract of fruits or vegetables, separated from the solids. Juices that are not diluted with water or sweetened with sugar contain approximately the same nutrients, in the same proportions, as the fresh produce from which they were made. Unlike the original produce, though, juices are concentrated—that is, ounce for ounce, juices contain more calories, carbohydrates (including sugars), vitamins, and minerals than do fruits and vegetables. The examples in Table 1-7 on the next page help make this clear. As you can see, when you convert a whole food into a juice you gain little or nothing in nutrient density. The nutrients per spoonful go up, but the calories per spoonful go up, too—in proportion.

An unfortunate side effect of juicing, from the digestive tract's point of view, is the loss of fiber from the original food. In fact, the main effect of juicing is to separate the liquid from the pulp in fruits and vegetables, and the pulp contains most of the fiber. The digestive tract depends on fiber from food to keep its contents moving, to provide nutrients for its colonies of bacteria, and to hold water that eases elimination of feces. Low-fiber diets also carry implications for disease states, as Chapter 4 will show. Unfortunately, most people obtain too many calories and far too little fiber in their diets. If juice is the only fruit or vegetable product available, it is certainly more nutritious than sugary soft drinks or "punches" that bear little resemblance to food. A juice contains more vitamins and minerals per calorie than a sugar-sweetened punch, and usually presents fewer calories per swallow. Still, the body benefits most from eating whole foods with the natural fiber intact. For thirst, it requires water. Juice provides no special benefits.

A related claim runs like this: Since the human body is a living system, only foods that contain "living" cells can support the body's own live cells. Therefore, freshly picked raw fruits and vegetables and their juices must contain the most power to support life. Some claim that people should eat nothing but raw fruits and vegetables, to the

(continued on next page)

Claims Made for Juices and Raw Foods *continued*

Table 1-7
Juices vs Whole Foods—Calories, Carbohydrate, and Fiber

	Calories	Carbohydrate (g)	Fiber (g)
1 c fresh pineapple chunks	76	19	2
1 c unsweetened pineapple juice	140	34	1
1 c fresh orange segments	85	21	4
1 c fresh orange juice	111	26	1
1 c apple (raw, peeled, slices)	65	16	3
1 c apple juice (clear)	116	29	<1
1 c cooked carrots	70	16	6
1 c carrot juice	98	22	4
1 c tomatoes (raw, chopped)	38	8	3
1 c tomato juice	42	10	2
1 c canned vegetable juice cocktail	46	11	2

omission of meats, grains, and milk products. The mystery of the idea is appealing, but scientific flaws abound in this reasoning.

First, cells in a raw food such as a whole tomato or a peach are not technically alive. After they are plucked from a plant, some enzymatic activity does continue within their cells, but this activity is generally of one sort—the sort that destroys molecules. Once a fruit or vegetable loses its connection to the living plant on which it grew, it ceases to build new molecules because building reactions require energy. The source of energy for plants, photosynthesis in the green plant, has been cut off in picked fruits or vegetables. In a tomato or a peach, post-harvest reactions soften the cell walls and other fibrous structures as the fruit ages. Cell walls break down and liberate the cell's juices. Large molecules break apart to create fragments that enrich the fruit's color, aroma, and flavor—a process known as ripening. Technically, the only living part of a harvested fruit or vegetable is the seed, because it alone has the power, if given fresh energy from sunlight, to grow and synthesize new molecules.

Another problem with the "living food" theory is that chewing and digesting would immediately snuff the life out of any living thing, anyway. Chewing bursts cells open, liberating their contents and making nutrients accessible to digestive enzymes. The digestive system breaks down all large molecules except its own enzymes, which are specially protected from the digestive chemicals. A plant's enzymes, along with other molecules, simply yield basic nutrients. By the time the mouth, stomach, and small intestine are done with a food, it bears no resemblance to the original "living" substance.

Many people experience indigestion, too, when they try to eat too many raw foods. For one thing, any fiber not broken down before reaching the colon readily becomes available to the bacteria of the colon, which use it for energy that allows them to multiply; the whole process creates gas and other waste products. (There is no harm in this, but enough is enough, of course.) For another thing, an abrupt change from a mostly cooked diet to a mostly raw-food diet can cause digestive problems until the system has a chance to adapt. Cooked foods are easier to digest because cooking bursts cell walls open and changes the forms of certain nutrients, making them more digestible.[17]

In summary, juices are fine as part of a balanced diet, and so are raw foods in moderation, but neither offers any miraculous benefit. The body thrives when presented with ordinary foods that contain the nutrients it needs, in whatever form they are served.

The Construction of Nutritious Diets from Foods

A nutritious diet has five characteristics. One is **adequacy:** the foods provide enough of each essential nutrient, fiber, and energy. Another is **balance:** the choices do not overemphasize one nutrient or food type at the expense of another. The third is **calorie control:** the foods provide the amount of energy you need to maintain appropriate weight—not more, not less. The fourth is **moderation:** the foods do not provide excess fat, salt, sugar, or other constituents. The fifth is **variety:** the foods chosen differ from one day to the next.

Any nutrient could be used to demonstrate the importance of dietary *adequacy.* Iron provides a familiar example. It is an essential nutrient; you lose some every day, so you have to keep replacing it; and you can get it into your body only by eating foods that contain it.* If you eat too few of the iron-containing foods, you can develop iron-deficiency anemia: with anemia you can feel weak, tired, and unenthusiastic; may have frequent headaches; and can do very little muscular work without disabling fatigue. If you add iron-rich foods to your diet, you soon feel more energetic. Some foods are rich in iron; others are notoriously poor. Meat, fish, poultry, and legumes are in the iron-rich category, and an easy way to obtain the needed iron is to include these foods in your diet regularly.

adequacy the description of a diet that provides all of the essential nutrients, fiber, and energy in amounts sufficient to maintain health and body weight.

balance the description of a diet that provides foods of a number of types in proportion to each other, such that foods rich in some nutrients do not crowd out of the diet foods that are rich in other nutrients. Also called *proportionality.*

calorie control control of energy intake, a feature of a sound diet plan.

moderation the description of a diet that provides no constituent in excess.

variety the description of a diet in which different foods are used for the same purposes on different occasions—the opposite of *monotony.*

*A person can also take supplements containing iron, but later discussions demonstrate that this is not as effective as eating iron-rich foods.

nutrient density a measure of nutrients provided per calorie of food.

To appreciate the importance of dietary *balance*, consider a second essential nutrient, calcium. Most foods that are rich in iron are poor in calcium. Calcium's best food sources are milk and milk products, which happen to be extraordinarily poor iron sources. A diet lacking calcium causes poor bone development during the growing years and increases a person's susceptibility to disabling bone loss in adult life. Children and adults are advised to consume enough milk, milk products, or other calcium-rich foods each day to meet their calcium needs—but not so much as to crowd iron-rich foods out of the diet.

Clearly, to obtain enough of both iron and calcium, which seldom appear together in the same foods, one has to balance one's food choices. Balancing the whole diet to provide enough but not too much of every one of the 40-odd nutrients the body needs for health is a juggling act that requires considerable skill. As you will see in Chapter 2, food group plans can help you achieve dietary adequacy and balance because they recommend specific amounts of foods of each type.

Energy intakes should not exceed energy needs. Nicknamed *calorie control*, the technique of balancing energy intakes from food with energy expenditures in activity achieves control of body fat content and weight. The many strategies that promote this goal appear in Chapter 9.

Intakes of certain food constituents such as fat, cholesterol, sugar, and salt should be limited for health's sake (more on health effects in later chapters). A major guideline already mentioned is to keep fat intake below 30 percent of total calories. Some people take this to mean that they must never indulge in a delicious beefsteak or hot-fudge sundae, but they are misinformed, since *moderation*, not total abstinence, is the key. A steady diet of steak and ice cream might be harmful, but once a week as part of an otherwise moderate diet plan, these foods might have little impact; and a once-a-month treat of these foods would have practically no effect at all. Moderation also means that limits, even for desirable food constituents, are necessary. For example, while a certain amount of fiber in foods contributes to the health of the digestive system, too much fiber leads to nutrient losses.

As for *variety*, it is generally agreed that people should not eat the same foods day after day, for two reasons. One reason is that some less-known nutrients and some nonnutrient food components could be important to health; some foods may be better sources of these than others. Another reason is that a monotonous diet may deliver large amounts of unwanted plant toxins or chemical contaminants. Each such undesirable item in a food is diluted by all the other foods eaten with it and is even further diluted if several days are skipped before it is eaten again. Last, variety adds interest—trying new foods can be a source of pleasure.

According to the experts, it is not easy for adults in the United States to meet these objectives. In particular, people seem to be able to make their diets either adequate or moderate, but find it hard to do both. It is as if they had a choice—either get all your nutrients and overconsume fat calories or keep your fat in line and risk running short on nutrients.[18] Those who managed to do both numbered only 2 percent of several thousand adults who were surveyed. That finding defines the challenge for the health-conscious eater: try to achieve adequacy and moderation at the same time.

Because this challenge is the key to good nutrition, this chapter's Food Feature is devoted to the skill required to meet it. The Food Feature offers a tool to help make it easy—the concept of **nutrient density.**

All of this discussion, though, points to the principle that is central to achieving nutritional health. It is not the individual foods you choose, but the ways you combine them into meals and the ways you arrange meals to follow one another over days and weeks that determines how well you are nourishing yourself.

KEY POINT A well-planned diet is adequate in nutrients, is balanced with regard to food types, offers food energy that matches energy expended for activity, is moderate in unwanted constituents, and offers variety. Foods of high nutrient density form the foundation of such a diet.

FOOD FEATURE

Getting the Most Nutrients for Your Calories

To help with calorie control while attempting to balance the diet and to make it adequate, the planner is bound to find certain foods especially useful. These are foods that are rich in nutrients relative to their energy contents, that is, foods with high nutrient density. Consider calcium sources, for example. Ice cream and nonfat milk both supply calcium, but the milk is "denser" in calcium per calorie. A cup of ice cream contributes about 200 calories, a cup of nonfat milk only 90—and with a little more calcium. Or consider iron. A 3-ounce serving of high-fat beef pot roast offers about the same amount of iron as a 3-ounce serving of water-packed tuna, but the beef contains over 300 calories, the tuna about 100.* Most people cannot, for their health's sake, afford to choose foods without regard to their energy contents. Those who do very often fill up their caloric allowances while leaving nutrient needs unmet.

For the person who plans and prepares the meals for a family, consciousness of nutrient density is especially important. In fact, the family food-preparer is well advised to *center* the meal on foods of high nutrient density. The foods that present the most nutrients per calorie are the vegetables, especially the nonstarchy vegetables such as onions, peppers, tomatoes, and mushrooms. These take time to prepare, but time invested this way pays off in nutritional health. Twenty minutes spent peeling and slicing vegetables for a stir-fry is a better investment in nutrition than 20 minutes spent fixing a fancy, high-fat, high-sugar dessert.

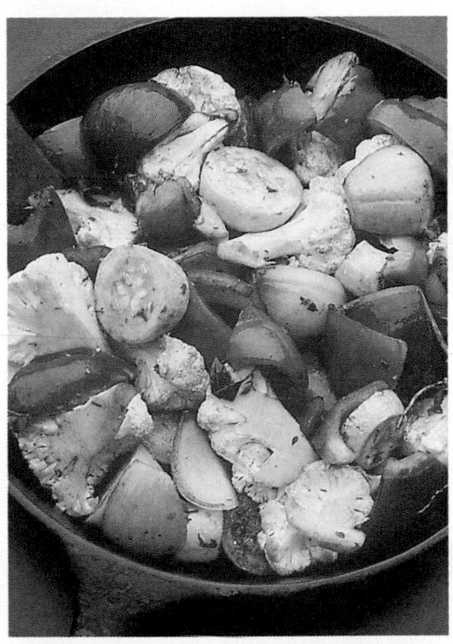
Would it take more time to prepare this dish than to prepare a batch of cookies? No, less time and less cleanup too.

Investing meal-preparation time in nutritious foods is especially important if time is limited. In today's households, although both men and women spend equal amounts of their time, some 71 hours a week, sleeping and taking care of personal needs, women still do most of the cooking and food shopping. Since more women are employed today than earlier, they can spend only a very little time on food preparation—most spend less than 30 minutes preparing the evening meal, and 20 percent spend less than 15 minutes.[19]

Nutrient density is such a useful concept in diet planning that experts recommend it be used on food labels. That is, food labels should express

*These are approximate numbers; the actual values for these foods are listed in Appendix A.

Figure 1-3

HOW THE EXPERTS JUDGE WHICH FOODS ARE MOST NUTRITIOUS

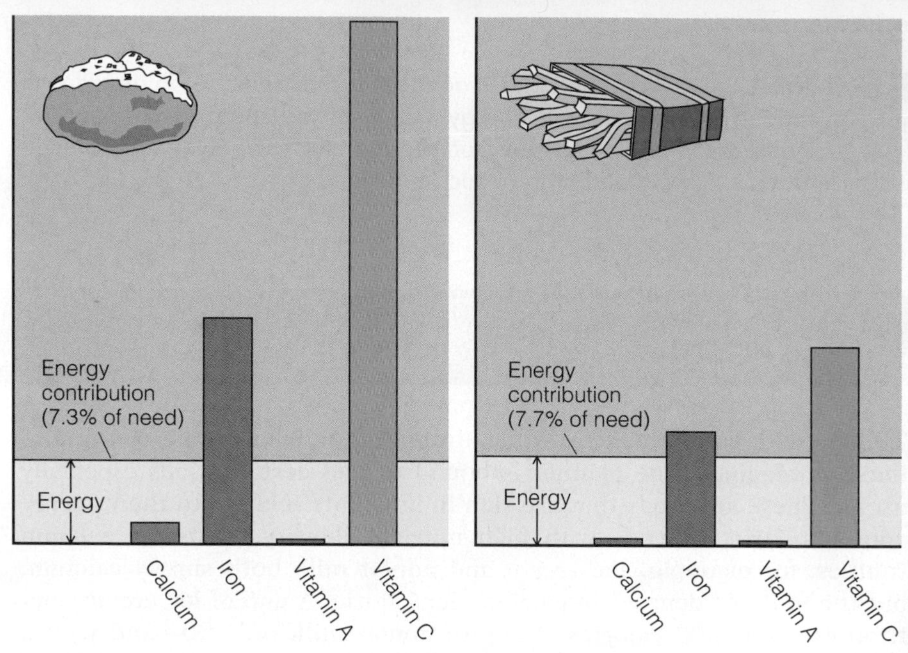

their nutrient contents "per calorie" in the food.[20] While labels have not yet evolved to this stage, this book encourages you to think in those terms. Watch for the tables and figures in later chapters that show the best buys among foods, not in nutrients per dollar, but in nutrients per calorie. Figure 1-3 offers a preview of the way this viewpoint can help you distinguish among more and less nutritious foods.

To help with diet planning, a person can refer to lists of foods grouped so that all the foods on one list supply approximately equal amounts of nutrients and calories per portion. Such lists of interchangeable foods appear in Chapter 2, with a special section, Checking Out Food Labels, the first in a series showing how to read food labels.

Notes

1. J. Anderson, Making nutrition sense from nutrition headlines, *Food Insight Reports* from the International Food Information Council Foundation, 1100 Connecticut Avenue NW, Suite 430, Washington, DC 20036, 1992.
2. J. P. Goldberg, Nutrition and health communication: The message and the media over half a century, *Nutrition Reviews* 50 (1992): 71–77.
3. C. M. Ripsin and coauthors, Oat products and lipid lowering: a meta-analysis, *Journal of the American Medical Association* 267 (1992): 3317–3325.
4. F. D. Moore, Current thoughts on malabsorption: Parenteral, enteral, and oral feeding (commentary), *Journal of the American Dietetic Association* 86 (1986): 1169–1170.
5. Moore, 1986.
6. C. W. Lo and W. A. Walker, Changes in the gastrointestinal tract during enteral or parenteral feeding, *Nutrition Reviews*, July 1989, pp. 193–198.
7. V. Woolf, *A Room of One's Own* (New York: Harcourt, Brace, 1929), p. 30.
8. J. Konowalchuk and J. I. Speirs, Virus inactivation by grapes and wines, *Applied and Environmental Microbiology*, December 1976, pp. 757–763.

9. *Teaching Tolerance*, Southern Poverty Law Center, 400 Washington Avenue, Montgomery, AL 36104. This is a free journal for those interested in ways to promote cultural harmony.
10. A. A. Hertzler and R. Frary, Dietary status and eating out practices of college students, *Journal of the American Dietetic Association* 92 (1992): 867–869.
11. *The Surgeon General's Report on Nutrition and Health, Summary and Recommendations* (Washington, D.C.: DHHS [PHS] publication no. 88–50211, 1988).
12. *Healthy People 2000: National Health Promotion and Disease Prevention Objectives* (Washington, D.C.: U.S. Department of Health and Human Services, 1990).
13. Little progress reported toward nutrition objectives of Healthy People 2000, *Journal of the American Dietetic Association* 92 (1992): 1465.
14. B. H. Patterson, G. Block, W. F. Rosenberger, D. Pee, and L. L. Kahle, Fruit and vegetables in the American diet: Data from the NHANES II Survey, *American Journal of Public Health* 80 (1990): 1443–1449.
15. Fast food and the American diet, Chapter 7 in *Issues in Nutrition* (New York: American Council on Science and Health, 1991): 26–29.
16. The single food fallacy, Chapter 2 in *Issues in Nutrition* (New York: American Council on Science and Health, 1991), pp. 46–47.
17. M. A. Eastwood, The physiological effect of dietary fiber: An update, *Annual Review of Nutrition* 12 (1992): 19–35.
18. S. P. Murphy, D. Rose, M. Hudes, and F. E. Viteri, Demographic and economic factors associated with dietary quality for adults in the 1987-88 Nationwide Food Consumption Survey, *Journal of the American Dietetic Association* 92 (1992): 1352–1357.
19. Convenient food and the new household economics, *Journal of the American Dietetic Association* 92 (1992): p. 981.
20. R. G. Hansen, Why calories count: Communicating moderation and a balanced diet, *Food Technology*, October 1991, pp. 86–93.

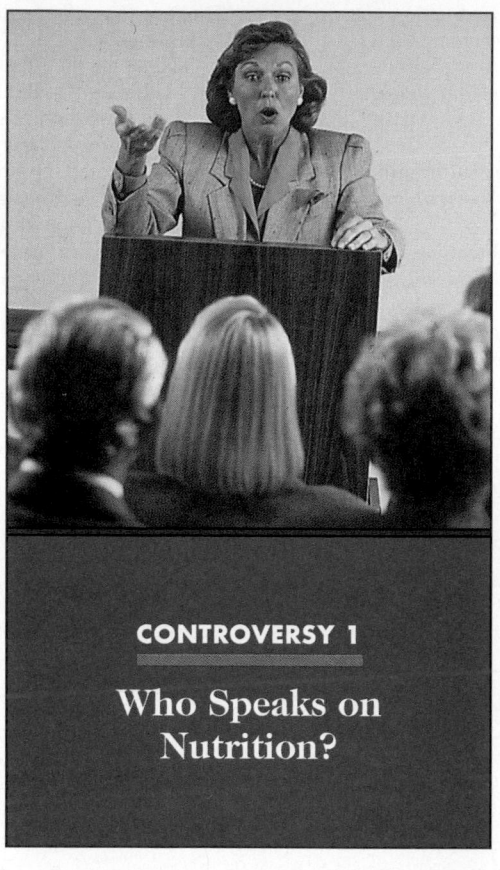

CONTROVERSY 1

Who Speaks on Nutrition?

Nutrition news surrounds people as they read newspapers, turn the pages of magazines, talk with friends, and watch television. Today more than ever before, people want to know what nutrition news they can believe and safely use. They want to know how best to take care of themselves. Some people seek miracles, too: supplements for weight loss without effort, nutrients to forestall aging or to prevent baldness or to increase sexual potency. People's heightened interest in nutrition and health care translates into a deluge of dollars spent on services and products peddled by both legitimate and fraudulent businesses. Consumers who obtain legitimate care can improve their health. Those enticed into scams, however, may lose their health, their savings, or both. Unfortunately, nutrition **fraud (quackery,** defined in Table C1-1) rings cash registers to the tune of $25 billion annually. Ironically, quacks spread useless or even dangerous advice, **placebo** products, and unproven procedures that not only rob people of the very health they are seeking by stealing their resources, but also delay legitimate strategies that could truly improve health.

How can people distinguish valid nutrition information from **misinformation?** One excellent approach is to notice who is purveying the information: quacks or qualified sources. At the extremes, science and quackery may be easy to tell apart, but between the extremes lies an abundance of less easily recognized nutrition information and misinformation. An instructor at a gym, a physician, a health-store clerk, an author of a book (and seller of juice machines) all recommend nutrition regimens. Can you believe these people? What qualifies them to give nutrition advice? Would following their advice be helpful or harmful? In short, when you are confused or need sound dietary advice, how can you tell whom to ask?

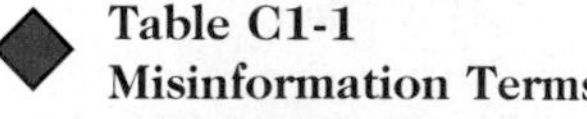

Table C1-1
Misinformation Terms

- **fraud** or **quackery** the promotion, for financial gain, of devices, treatments, services, plans, or products (including diets and supplements) that alter or claim to alter a human condition without proof of safety or effectiveness. (The word *quackery* comes from the term *quacksalver,* meaning a person who quacks loudly about a miracle product—a lotion or a salve.)
- **misinformation** false or misleading information.
- **placebo** (plah-SEE-bo) a sham treatment; an inert harmless medication. The *placebo effect* is the healing effect that the act of treatment, rather than the treatment itself, often has.

IDENTIFYING QUACKS There would be little problem identifying nutrition quacks if they still rode into town in wooden wagons hawking snake oil to "cure what ails you" for 50 cents a bottle. But those days are gone. Today's quacks manipulate consumers in less obvious ways. Fraudulent claims *sound* logical, but they lack the research support found in nutrition science. In fact, you can learn to identify fraud by the unscientific characteristics shown in Figure C1-1.

The makers of fraudulent claims are usually not credentialed professionals. Usually their only qualifications are just words on pretty paper. Occasionally, though, a person with all the earmarks of the real thing turns out to be just plain dishonest.

The scope of the problem of nutrition misinformation almost defies description. Fraud in weight loss alone often claims the attention of Congress, whose members struggle to control it. At a subcommittee meeting on the problem of deception and fraud, the chairman said this about nutrition fraud:

> *This subcommittee has found the medical field is riddled with hucksters who ply their dubious wares and their miracle cures, while Government regulators sit snoozing on the sidelines.*[1]

In short, quackery respects neither science nor honesty in its pursuit of money. Each of this book's chapters includes a Consumer Caution section to alert you to nutrition frauds.

Figure C1-1 **EARMARKS OF NUTRITION QUACKERY** The more of these claims you hear about nutrition information, the less likely it is to be valid.

Bent truth
The claim is based on true scientific findings, but misstates them or states them incompletely.

Logic without proof
The claim seems to be based on sound reasoning, but hasn't been scientifically tested and shown to hold up.

Too good to be true
The claim presents enticingly simple answers to complex problems. It says what most people want to hear. It sounds magical.

Persecution claims
The person or institution pushing the product or service claims to be persecuted by the medical establishment or tries to convince you that physicians "want to keep you ill so that you will continue to pay for office visits."

Suspicions about food supply
The person or institution pushing the product or service urges distrust of the current methods of medicine or suspicion of the regular food supply, with "alternatives" for sale (providing profit to the seller) under the guise that people should have freedom of choice.

Authority not cited
The studies cited sound valid, but are not referenced, so that it is impossible to check and see if they were conducted scientifically.

Motive: personal gain
The person or institution making the claim stands to make a profit if it is believed.

Testimonials
The evidence presented to support the claim is in the form of praise by people who have been "healed," "made younger," and the like by the product or treatment.

Advertisement
The claim is being made by an advertiser who is paid to make claims for the product or procedure. (Look for the word "Advertisement," probably in tiny print somewhere on the page.)

Fake credentials
The person or institution making the claim is titled "doctor," "university," or the like, but has simply created or bought the title and is not legitimate.

Unreliable publication
The studies cited are published, but in a newsletter, magazine, or journal that publishes misinformation.

Unpublished studies
Scientific studies are cited, but are nowhere published and so cannot be critically examined.

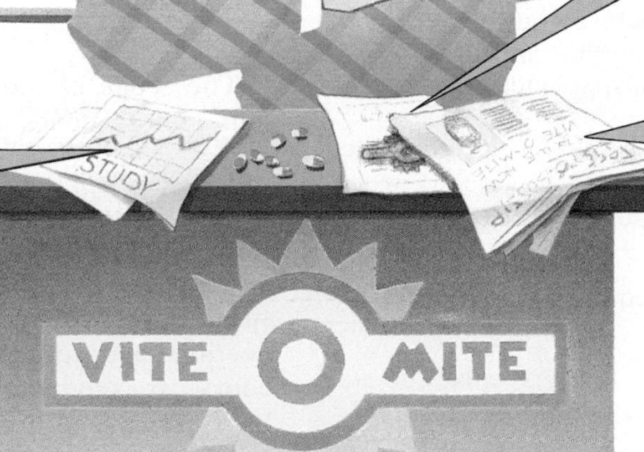
STEP RIGHT UP! VITE-O-MITE WILL MAKE YOU AS HEALTHY AS A HORSE-GUARANTEED! FEEL STRONGER, LOSE WEIGHT. IMPROVE YOUR MEMORY ALL WITH THE HELP OF VITE-O-MITE! OH SURE. YOU MAY HAVE HEARD THAT VITE-O-MITE IS NOT ALL THAT WE SAY IT IS. BUT THAT'S WHAT THE FDA WANTS YOU TO THINK! OUR DOCTORS AND SCIENTISTS SAY IT'S THE ULTIMATE VITAMIN SUPPLEMENT. SAY NO! TO THE WEAKENED VITAMINS IN TODAY'S FOODS. VITE-O-MITE INCLUDES POTENT SECRET INGREDIENTS THAT YOU CANNOT GET WITH ANY OTHER PRODUCT! YESSIREE FOLKS. STEP RIGHT UP!
BEFORE
AFTER
280lbs.
160lbs.
STUDY
VITE O MITE

Table C1-2
Credible Sources of Nutrition Information

Government health agencies, volunteer health agencies, consumer groups, and professional health organizations provide consumers with reliable health and nutrition information. Credible sources of nutrition information include:

- Government health agencies such as the Federal Trade Commission (FTC), the U.S. Department of Health and Human Services (U.S. DHHS), the Food and Drug Administration (FDA), and the U.S. Department of Agriculture (USDA).
- Volunteer health agencies such as the American Cancer Society, the American Diabetes Association, and the American Heart Association.
- Reputable consumer groups such as the Better Business Bureau, the Consumers Union, the American Council on Science and Health, and the National Council Against Health Fraud.
- Professional health organizations such as the American Dietetic Association, the Society for Nutrition Education, and the American Medical Association.

Appendix E provides addresses for these and other organizations.

Source: Data from J. M. Ashley and R. Alfin-Slater, Position of the American Dietetic Association: Identifying food and nutrition misinformation, *Journal of the American Dietetic Association* 88 (1988): 1589–1591.

IDENTIFYING VALID NUTRITION INFORMATION As Chapter 1 explained, nutrition is a science. That is, it derives information from scientific research. Scientists must systematically conduct research studies and cautiously interpret the findings before they can provide practical nutrition information. The following techniques are characteristic of scientific research:

- Scientists test their ideas by conducting controlled experiments. They report their methods and procedures in detail so that other scientists can verify the findings through replication.
- Scientists recognize the inadequacy of anecdotal evidence or testimonials.
- Scientists who use animals in their research do not apply their findings directly to human beings.
- Scientists may use specific segments of the population in their research. When they do, they are careful not to generalize the findings to all people.
- Scientists report their findings in reputable scientific journals. Their work must survive screening by their peers before it is accepted for publication.

With each report from scientists, the field of nutrition changes a little—each finding contributes another piece to the whole body of knowledge. Table C1-2 lists some sources of credible nutrition information.

WHO ARE THE TRUE NUTRITION EXPERTS? Most people turn to their physicians for dietary advice. Physicians are expected to know all about health-related matters and to be able to translate ideas into guidelines for health-promoting behavior.[2] But are physicians the best sources of accurate and current information on nutrition? Only about half of all medical schools in the United States require students to take even one nutrition course.[3] Students attending these classes receive an average of 20 hours of nutrition instruction—an amount most graduates consider inadequate.[4] While many experts call for a greatly expanded role of nutrition in the medical curriculum, they acknowledge that the curriculum carries a heavy burden already.[5] Many see it as a challenge to integrate adequate, meaningful nutrition into already-existing courses.[6]

In 1990, Congress passed a law mandating that:

> *"students enrolled in United States medical schools and physicians practicing in the United States [must] have access to adequate training in the field of nutrition and its relationship to human health."*[7]

Plans are now in the works to make nutrition education a standard course in medical schools. Enlarging on this idea, the American Dietetic Association (ADA) asserts that standardized nutrition education should be made part of the curricula for all sorts of health care professionals: physician's assistants, dental hygienists, physical and occupational therapists, social workers, and all others who provide services directly to clients.[8] This way more people would have access to reliable nutrition information.

Even though most physicians are not schooled adequately in nutrition, some are superbly qualified to speak on nutrition. All physicians appreciate the connections between health and nutrition because of their course work in biochemistry and physiology. Those who have specialized in the area called clinical nutrition in medical schools that offer that specialty are especially well qualified. Membership in the American Society for Clinical Nutrition, whose journal is cited many times throughout this text, is another sign of knowledge of nutrition. Still, few physicians have the time or experience to develop diet plans and provide detailed diet instruction for clients. Often physicians wisely refer their clients to nutrition specialists for diet advice.

To what specialists should physicians refer their clients for nutrition advice? Table C1-3 presents a glossary of terms associated with reliable nutrition advice.

Fortunately the credential that indicates a qualified nutrition expert is easy to spot—you can confidently call on a **registered dietitian (RD).** A registered dietitian has the educational background necessary to deliver reliable nutrition advice and care. To become an RD, a person must earn an undergraduate degree requiring some 60 or so semester hours in nutrition and food science; complete a year's clinical internship or the equivalent; pass a national examination administered over five competency areas by the **American Dietetic Association (ADA)***; and maintain up-to-date knowledge by participating in required continuing education activities (attending seminars, taking courses, or writing professional papers). Meeting these established criteria certifies that a dietitian is the genuine article.

Dietitians are easy to find in most communities because they perform a multitude of duties in a variety of settings. They work in foodservice operations, in pharmaceutical companies, in the food industry, in home health agencies, in long-term care institutions, in private clinics, in public health departments, in research centers, in education settings, in some fitness centers, and in hospitals.

Dietitians can assume a number of different responsibilities depending on their work settings and positions.[9] Dietitians in hospitals have many subspecialties. Administrative dietitians manage the foodservice system; clinical dietitians provide client care (see Table C1-4); and nutrition support team dietitians coordinate nutrition care with the efforts of other health care professionals. In the food industry, dietitians conduct

Table C1-4
Responsibilities of a Clinical Dietitian

- Assesses clients' nutrition status.
- Determines clients' nutrient requirements.
- Monitors clients' nutrient intakes.
- Develops, implements, and evaluates clients' nutrition care plans.
- Counsels clients to cope with unique diet plans.
- Teaches clients and their families about nutrition and diet plans.
- Provides training for other dietitians, nurses, interns, and dietetics students.
- Serves as liaison between clients and the foodservice department.
- Communicates with physicians, nurses, pharmacists, and other health care professionals about clients' progress, needs, and treatments.
- Participates in professional activities to enhance knowledge and skill.

Table C1-3
Glossary Terms of Identifying Valid Nutrition Advice

- **American Dietetic Association (ADA)** the professional organization of dietitians in the United States. The Canadian equivalent is the Canadian Dietetic Association (CDA), which operates similarly.
- **dietitian** a person trained in nutrition, food science, and diet planning. See also *registered dietitian.*
- **public health nutritionist** a dietitian who specializes in public health nutrition. (A *nutritionist* is just someone who engages in the study of nutrition. Some nutritionists are RDs, whereas others are self-described experts whose training is questionable and who are not qualified to give advice. In states with responsible legislation, the term applies only to people who have master of science (MS) or doctor of philosophy (PhD) degrees from properly accredited institutions.)
- **registered dietitian (RD)** a dietitian who has graduated from a university or college after completing a program of dietetics. The program must be accredited by the American Dietetic Association (or Canadian Dietetic Association). The dietitian must serve in an internship or coordinated program to practice the necessary skills, pass the association's *registration* examination, and maintain competency through continuing education. Many states also require licensing for practicing dietitians.
- **registration** listing. With respect to health professionals, listing with a professional organization that requires specific course work, experience, and passing of an examination.

*The five content areas included on the registration examination for dietitians are nutrition services; foodservice systems; management; education and communication; and evaluation and standards. L. C. Webb and J. O. Maillet, The development of test specifications for the registration examinations, *Journal of the American Dietetic Association* 90 (1990): 1134–1135.

Table C1-5
Terms Describing Institutions of Higher Learning, Legitimate and Fraudulent

- **accredited** approved; in the case of medical centers or universities, certified by an agency recognized by the U.S. Department of Education.
- **correspondence school** a school that offers courses and degrees by mail. Some correspondence schools are accredited; others are *diploma mills.*
- **diploma mill** an organization that awards meaningless degrees without requiring its students to meet educational standards.
- **license to practice** permission under state or federal law, granted on meeting specified criteria, to use a certain title (such as *dietitian*) and to offer certain services. Licensed dietitians may use the initials LD after their names.

research, develop products, and market services. Dietitians who specialize in public health nutrition work in government-funded agencies to provide nutrition services to populations. Among their many roles, public health nutritionists help plan, coordinate, and evaluate programs; act as consultants to other agencies; manage finances; and much more.[10] Those with advanced degrees of coursework in public health are well placed for employment in this vast field.

DETECTING FAKE CREDENTIALS In contrast to RDs, thousands of people possess fake nutrition degrees and claim to be nutrition counselors, nutritionists, or "dietists." These and other such titles may sound meaningful, but most of these people lack the established credentials of the ADA-sanctioned dietitian. If you look closely, you can see signs that their expertise is fake.

Take, for example, a nutrition expert's educational background. The minimal standards of education for a dietitian specify a bachelor of science (BS) degree in food science and human nutrition (or related fields) from an **accredited** college or university (Table C1-5 defines this and related terms). Such a degree generally requires four to five years of study. In contrast, a fake nutrition expert may display a degree from a six-month correspondence course; such a degree is simply not the same.[†] In some cases, schools posing as legitimate **correspondence schools** offer even less—they are actually **diploma mills,** fraudulent businesses that sell certificates of competency to anyone who pays the fees, from under a thousand dollars for a bachelor's degree to several thousands for a doctorate. Buyers ordering multiple degrees are even given discounts. To obtain these "degrees," a candidate need not read any books or pass any examinations.

Lack of proper accreditation is the identifying sign of a fake educational institution. To guard educational quality, an accrediting agency recognized by the U.S. Department of Education (DOE) certifies that certain schools meet the criteria defining a complete and accurate schooling, but in the case of nutrition, quack accrediting agencies cloud the picture. Fake nutrition degrees are available from schools "accredited" by more than 30 phony accrediting agencies.[‡]

To dramatize the ease with which anyone can obtain a fake nutrition degree, one writer enrolled for $82 in a nutrition diploma mill that billed itself as a correspondence school. She made every attempt to fail. She intentionally answered all the examination questions incorrectly. Even so, she received a "nutritionist" certificate at the end of the course, together with a letter from the "school" explaining that they were sure she must have just misread the test.

In a similar stunt, Ms. Sassafras Herbert was named a "professional member" of a nutrition association. For her efforts, Sassafras has received a wallet card and is listed in a sort of fake *Who's Who* in nutrition that is distributed at health fairs and trade shows nationwide. Sassafras is a poodle. Her master, Victor Herbert, MD, paid $50 to prove that she could be awarded these honors merely by sending in her name. Mr. Charlie Herbert also is a professional member of such an organization; Charlie is a cat.

State laws don't necessarily help consumers distinguish experts from fakes; some states allow anyone to use the titles *dietitian* or *nutritionist.* But some states are beginning to respond to the need by allowing only RDs or people with certain graduate degrees to call themselves dietitians. Many states now provide a

[†]To find out whether a correspondence school is accredited, write the National Home Study Council, Accrediting Commission, 1601 Eighteenth Street NW, Washington, DC 20009, or call (202) 234-5100.

[‡]The American Council on Education publishes a directory of accredited institutions, professionally accredited programs, and candidates for accreditation in *Accredited Institutions of Postsecondary Education Programs Candidates* (available from many libraries). For additional information, write the Council on Postsecondary Accreditation, One Dupont Circle, Suite 305, Washington, DC 20036, or call (202) 452-1433.

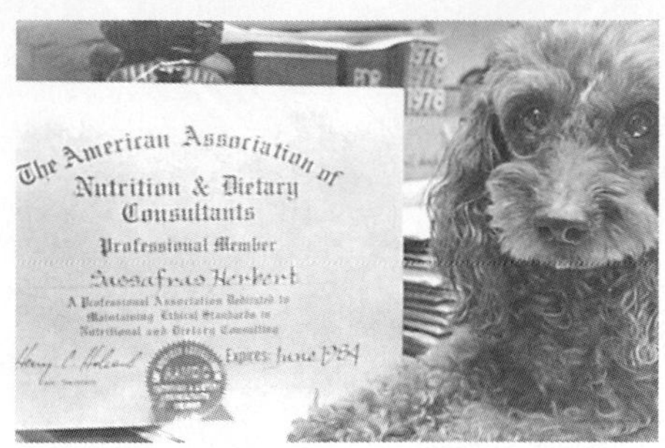

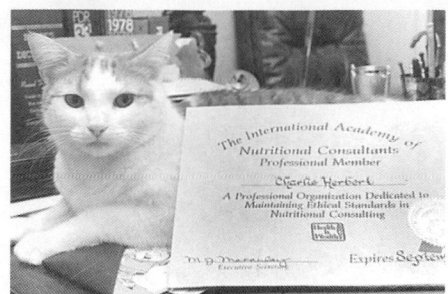

Sassafras and Charlie display their professional credentials.

further guarantee: the license to practice.[11] Licensing provides a way to identify people who have met minimal standards of education and experience.

By knowing who is qualified to speak on nutrition, consumers are one step ahead of the nutrition quacks. Does the instructor at the spa have a degree in nutrition from an accredited university? No? Better check the instructor's advice with someone who does. Is the author of the magazine article an RD or otherwise qualified to write on nutrition? No credentials means you cannot know whether to believe what you've read. Have you seen the health-store clerk's license to practice as a dietitian? If not, seek a qualified source—an RD or a person with an advanced degree in nutrition.

In summary, to check a provider's qualifications, first look for the degrees and credentials listed by the person's name (such as MD, RD, MS, PhD, or LD). Then find out what you can about the reputations of the institutions that awarded the degrees. Then call and ask your state's health-licensing agency if dietitians are licensed in your state and (if so) if the person giving you dietary advice has met licensing criteria. If not, find someone better qualified, since your health is your most precious asset.

Notes

1. R. Wyden, *Deception and Fraud in the Diet Industry*, part I, serial no. 101–50 (Washington, D.C.: Government Printing Office, 1990): p. 1.
2. E. A. Young, National Dairy Council award for excellence in medical/dental nutrition education lecture, 1992: Perspectives on nutrition in medical education, *American Journal of Clinical Nutrition* 56 (1992): 745–751.
3. Young, 1992.
4. A. G. Swanson, 1990 ASCN Nutrition educators' symposium and information exchange: Nutrition sciences in medical-student education, *American Journal of Clinical Nutrition* 53 (1991): 587–588.
5. Young, 1992.
6. R. F. Kushner and coauthors, Implementing nutrition into the medical curriculum: A user's guide, *American Journal of Clinical Nutrition* 52 (1990): 401–403; R. L. Weinsier and coauthors, Priorities for nutrition content in a medical school curriculum: A national consensus of medical educators, *American Journal of Clinical Nutrition* 50 (1989): 707–712; A. Lopez, M. S. Read, and E. B. Feldman, 1987 ASCN Workshop on Nutrition Education for Medical/Dental Students and Residents—Integration of nutrition and medical education: Strategies and techniques, *American Journal of Clinical Nutrition* 47 (1988): 534–550.
7. National Nutrition Monitoring and Related Research Act of 1990, public law 101–445, as quoted in C. H. Halstead, Toward standardized training of physicians in clinical nutrition, *American Journal of Clinical Nutrition* 56 (1992): 1–3.
8. Position of the American Dietetic Association: Nutrition education of health professionals, *Journal of the American Dietetic Association* 91 (1991): 611–613.
9. M. T. Kane and coauthors, Role delineation for dietetic practitioners: Empirical results, *Journal of the American Dietetic Association* 90 (1990): 1124–1133.
10. B. Haughton and J. Shaw, Functional roles of today's public health nutritionist, *Journal of the American Dietetic Association* 92 (1992): 1218–1222.
11. D. A. Dougherty and J. Garey, President's page: ADA support for licensing, *Journal of the American Dietetic Association* 89 (1989): 1508–1510.

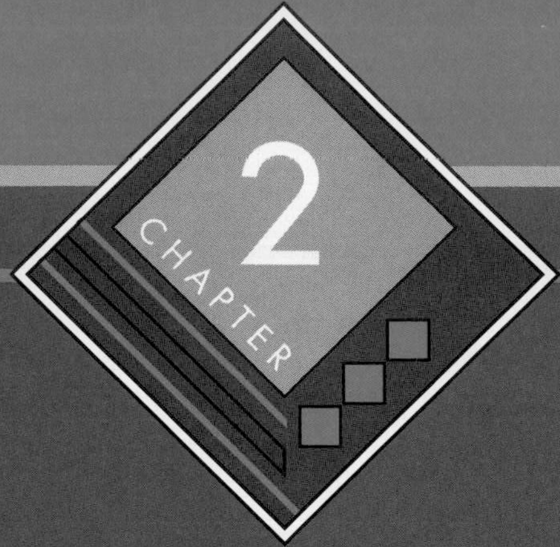

Nutrition Standards and Guidelines

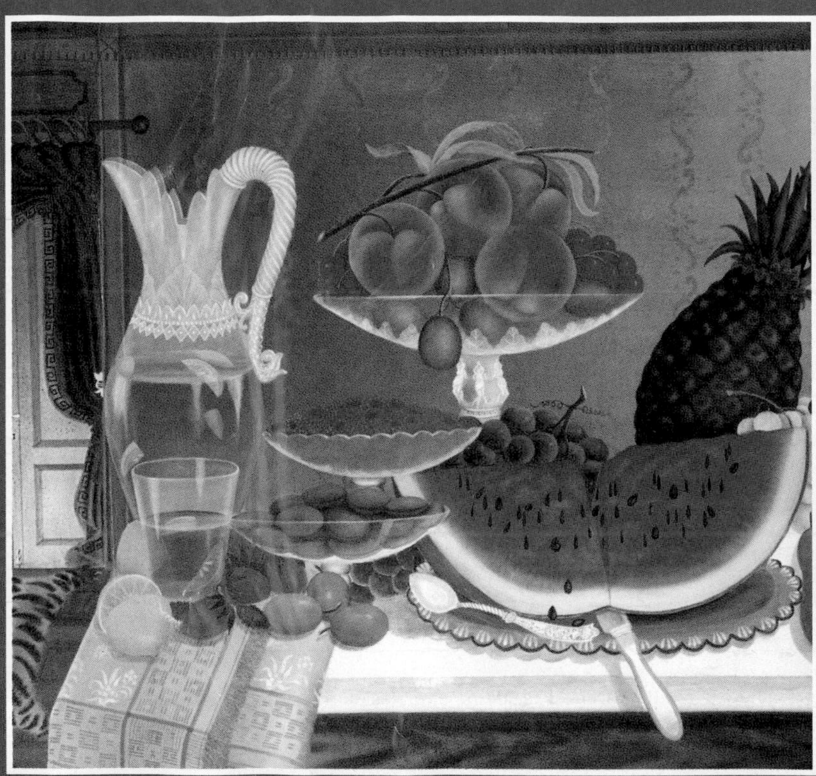

Contents

Henry Church, *Still Life,* The Collection of Frances O. Stem Babinsky.

2

Eating well is easy, in principle. All you have to do is choose a selection of foods that supplies appropriate amounts of the essential nutrients, fiber, and energy without excess intakes of fat, sugar, and salt. A few people do this automatically, but most do not. Many people are overweight, undernourished, or suffer from nutrient excesses or deficiencies that impair their health—that is, they suffer from malnutrition. You may not think that this applies to you, but you may already be suffering ill effects from less-than-optimal nutrient intakes without knowing it. Accumulated over years, the effects of malnutrition can seriously impair the quality of your life. Putting it positively, you can enjoy the best of vim, vigor, and vitality if you learn now to nourish yourself optimally.

To master the task of meeting your nutrition needs, you may find it useful to learn the answers to several questions. How much energy and how much of each nutrient do you need? Which types of foods supply which nutrients? How much of each type of food do you have to eat to get enough? And how can you eat all these foods without gaining weight and without getting too much fat, sugar, or salt? This chapter begins by identifying some ideals for nutrient intakes and ends by showing how to achieve them.

Recommended Dietary Allowances (RDA) average daily consumption levels of energy and selected nutrients suggested for the maintenance of health for the United States population.

Nutrient Recommendations

The **Recommended Dietary Allowances (RDA)** are used in the United States as a standard for healthy people's energy and nutrient intakes. The Canadian equivalent is the Recommended Nutrient Intakes for Canadians (RNI); it is presented in Appendix B. (The Daily Values are standards used on food labels and are described later.)

RDA

A committee of qualified nutrition experts appointed by the government publishes *recommendations* concerning appropriate nutrient intakes for the general population of this country.* These are the Recommended Dietary Allowances (RDA), and they are used and referred to so often that they are presented on pages A through C of the inside front cover of this book. As you can see, the main RDA table includes recommendations for protein, 11 vitamins, and 7 minerals, while the additional tables include 2 more vitamins and 8 more minerals as well as energy (calories). Periodically the committee on the RDA meets to reexamine and to revise these recommendations on the basis of new research regarding people's nutrient needs. It then publishes an updated set of RDA.[1]

The RDA have been much misunderstood. One young woman, on first learning of their existence, was outraged: "You mean Uncle Sam tells me that I must eat exactly 46 grams of protein every day?" This is not the committee's intention, and the RDA are recommendations, not commandments. The following facts will help put the RDA in perspective:

- The ongoing creation of the RDA is *funded* by the government, but the committee that determines the RDA is composed of scientists representing a variety of specialties.

RDA are set for:

- Energy.
- Protein.
- Vitamins:
  A, C, D, E, K, thiamin, riboflavin, niacin, B_6, B_{12}, folate.
- Minerals:
  Calcium, phosphorus, magnesium, iron, zinc, iodine, selenium.

Estimated safe and adequate intakes are given in ranges for:

- Vitamins:
  Biotin, pantothenic acid.
- Minerals (trace elements):
  Copper, manganese, fluoride, chromium, molybdenum.

Estimated minimum requirements of healthy persons are given for:

- Sodium, potassium, chloride.

See inside front cover.

*This is a committee of the Food and Nutrition Board (FNB) of the National Academy of Sciences/National Research Council (NAS/NRC).

balance study a laboratory study in which a person is fed a controlled diet and the intake and excretion of a nutrient are measured. Balance studies are valid only for nutrients like calcium (chemical elements) that don't change while they are in the body.

requirement that amount of a nutrient that will just prevent the development of specific deficiency signs; distinguished from the RDA, which is a generous allowance with a margin of safety.

- The RDA are based on reviews of available scientific research to the greatest extent possible and are revised periodically to keep them up to date.
- Except for sodium, potassium, and chloride, the RDA are not minimum requirements nor are they optimal intakes. They are safe and adequate intakes that include a generous margin of safety.
- The RDA are recommended *average* daily intakes. They are set high enough to ensure that body nutrient stores are kept full to meet needs during periods of inadequate intakes lasting a day or two for some nutrients and up to a month or two for others.
- The RDA are most appropriately used to plan diets for population groups such as school children or military personnel, but people like to use them to estimate the adequacy of their own individual intakes. They can be used this way if compared with intakes over a significant period of time.
- The RDA are estimates of the needs of healthy persons only. Medical problems alter nutrient needs.

Separate recommendations are made for different sets of people: men, women, pregnant women, children, and other groups. They are also separated by age. Children aged 4 to 6 years, for example, have their own RDA. Each individual can look up the recommendations for his or her own age and sex group.

No RDA is set for carbohydrate or fat. The assumption is that you will use a certain portion of your daily energy allowance meeting your protein RDA and then will distribute the remaining calories among carbohydrate and fat to meet your energy RDA. Later, this chapter will show how to balance energy sources to best support health. The next two sections describe the processes the committee goes through in selecting the RDA values, first for nutrients, then for energy.

KEY POINT The RDA used in the United States and the RNI used in Canada represent suggested average daily intakes of energy and selected nutrients for healthy people in the population.

RDA for Nutrients

If you use the RDA to estimate the adequacy of your own diet, you need to be aware that individuals' nutrient needs vary and that the allowances are designed primarily for use with whole populations. A theoretical discussion will illustrate these points.

Suppose we were the committee members, and we had the task of setting an RDA for nutrient X (any essential nutrient). Ideally our first step would be to try to find out how much of that nutrient given individuals need. We would review studies of deficiency states, of nutrient stores and their depletion, and of the factors influencing them. We would try to select the most valid data for use in our work. Among the experiments we might review or conduct would be measures of the body's intake and excretion (in the case of nutrients that aren't changed before they are excreted) to find out how much of an intake is required to balance excretion (this is called a **balance study**). For each individual subject, we could determine a **requirement** to achieve balance for nutrient X. With an intake below the requirement, a person would slip into negative balance or experience declining stores that could, over time, lead to deficiency of the nutrient.

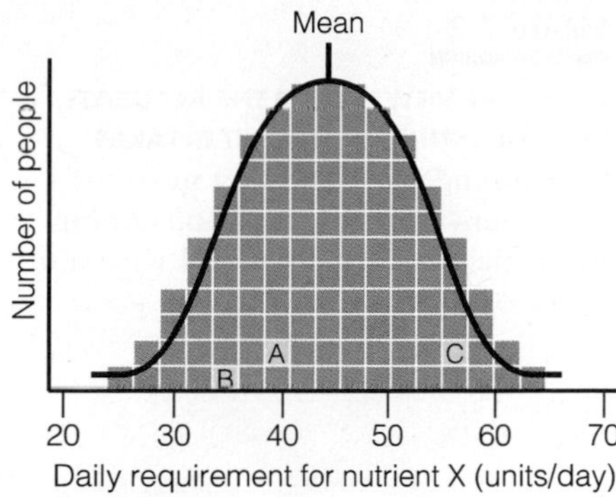

Figure 2-1

INDIVIDUALITY OF NUTRIENT REQUIREMENTS

Each square represents a person. A, B, and C are Mr A, Mr B, and Mr C. Each person has a different requirement.

With sufficient study, we would find that different individuals have different requirements. Mr A might need 40 units of the nutrient each day to maintain balance; Mr B might need 35; Mr C, 65. If we looked at enough individuals, we might find that their requirements were distributed as shown in Figure 2-1—with most requirements near the midpoint (here, 45), and only a few at the extremes.

To set the RDA, we would then have to decide what intake to recommend for everybody. Should we set it at the mean (shown in Figure 2-1 at 45 units)? This is the average requirement for nutrient X; it is probably the closest to everyone's need, assuming the distribution shown in Figure 2-1. (Actually the data for most nutrients other than protein indicate a distribution that is much less symmetrical.) But if people took us literally and consumed exactly this amount of nutrient X each day, half the population would begin to develop internal deficiencies and even possibly observable symptoms of deficiency diseases. Mr C (at 65) would be one of those people.

Perhaps we should set the RDA for nutrient X at or above the extreme, say at 70 units a day, so that everyone would be covered. (Actually we didn't study everyone, so some individual we didn't happen to test might have a still higher requirement.) This might be a good idea in theory, but what about a person like Mr B, who requires only 35 units a day? The recommendation would be twice his requirement, and to follow it, he might spend money needlessly on foods containing nutrient X to the exclusion of foods containing other nutrients he needs.

The choice we would finally make, with some reservations, would be to set the RDA at a reasonably high point so that the bulk of the population would be covered but not so high as to be excessive. In this example a reasonable choice might be to set it at 63 units a day. By moving the RDA further toward the extreme, we would pick up few additional people but inflate the recommendation for most people (including Mr A and Mr B).

The committee makes judgments of this kind when setting the RDA for nutrients. The RDA for nutrients are set well above the mean or average requirement as the committee can best determine from available information. In theory, relatively few healthy people's individual requirements, then, are not covered by the RDA.

For these reasons the RDA cannot be taken personally by any individual, that is, you can't know exactly what your own personal requirement may be. The committee makes several assumptions that may not apply to you at all. For example, they assume that you are eating a diet that includes adequate energy, protein, and all the other nutrients. They also assume that you receive your nutrients in the form of foods, not supplements, because food components affect nutrient absorption. This may describe you exactly; then again, it may not. On the other hand, except as noted earlier, the RDA are not minimum requirements. *R* stands for "recommended," not for "required." The RDA are allowances, and they are generous. Even so, they do not necessarily cover each individual for every nutrient. On average, one should probably try to get 100 percent or more of the RDA for every nutrient to ensure an adequate intake over time.

Beyond a certain point, though, it is unwise to consume large amounts of any nutrient. It is naive to think of the RDA simply as a minimum with more being better. A more accurate view is to see your nutrient needs as falling within a range, with danger zones both below and above the range. Figure 2-2 illustrates this point. The RDA reflect this consideration especially clearly in the tables for the trace minerals (inside front cover), which are stated in terms of "safe and adequate" ranges of intakes.

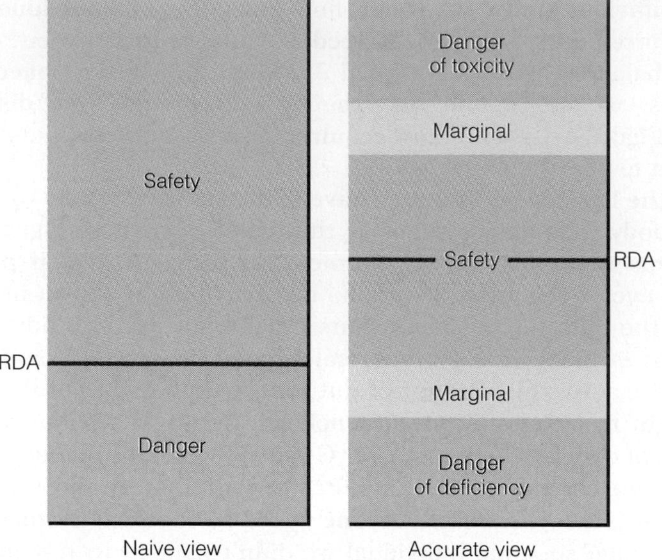

Figure 2-2

THE NAIVE VIEW VERSUS THE ACCURATE VIEW OF OPTIMAL NUTRIENT INTAKES
Consuming too much of a nutrient endangers health, just as consuming too little does. The RDA fall within a range of safe intake levels.

The RDA committee decided to estimate minimum requirements for sodium, potassium, and chloride. For sodium and its partner, chloride, there is danger in calling a high end of the intake scale "safe" because people differ in their sensitivities to salt. A level that may be harmless in one person could easily worsen high blood pressure in another. A range for potassium proved difficult to justify, so the committee also provided a minimum for potassium. For each of these three minerals, the committee estimated the amount needed for growth and for replacement of normal daily losses, and then set the minimum requirement at that level.

The RDA and other such recommendations are for the maintenance, not the restoration, of health. Under the stress of serious illness or malnutrition, a person may require a much higher intake of certain nutrients or may not be able to handle even the RDA amount. Therapeutic diets adjust the RDA upward to account for increased needs from medical conditions, such as recovery from surgery, burns, fractures, illnesses, or addictions.

With the understanding that they are approximate, flexible, and generous, we can use the RDA as a set of yardsticks to measure the adequacy of diets in whole populations, such as those of the United States.[2]

KEY POINT The RDA are a set of yardsticks for measuring the adequacy of nutrient intakes of groups of people and can also be used as a tool for evaluating people's individual intakes.

RDA for Energy

In setting allowances for food energy intakes, the committee took a different approach than for the nutrients. The committee had set generous allowances for protein, vitamins, and minerals, believing that a little bit extra, for a nutrient, would fill body stores enough to last through brief periods of deficient intakes. However, extra energy, even a little bit extra, on a daily basis would be harmful because it would lead to obesity. The committee therefore centered the energy RDA around the mean requirements for each age and sex group. The committee defined an acceptable variation of

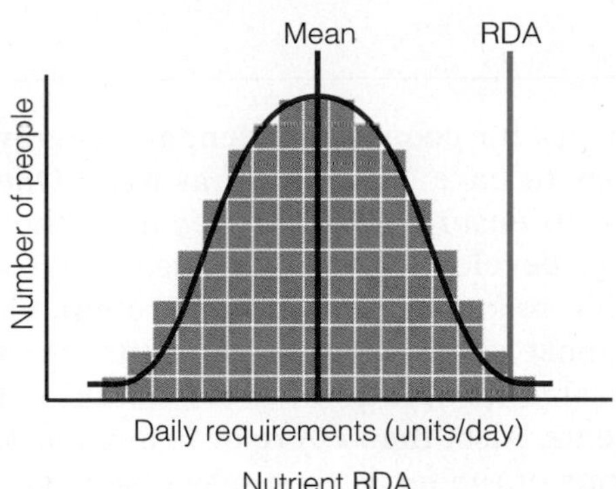

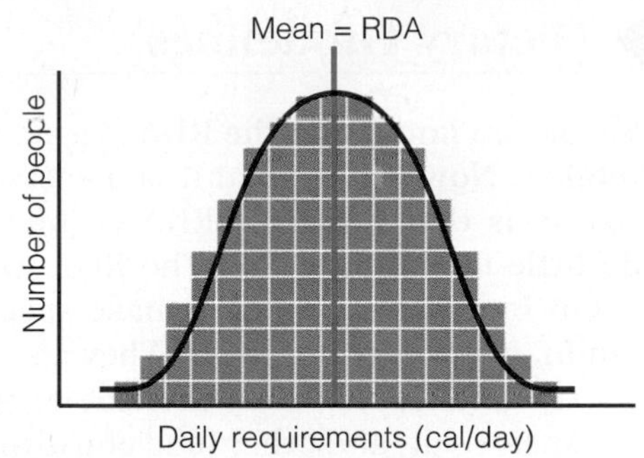

Figure 2-3

THE DIFFERENCES BETWEEN THE NUTRIENT RDA AND THE ENERGY RDA
The nutrient RDA are set so that nearly all people's requirements will be met by them (boxes represent people). The energy RDA are set at the average, or mean, so that half the population's requirements will fall below and half above them.

20 percent above this amount to accommodate growth, large body size, or physical activity (these require more energy), and of 20 percent below this amount for most aging people or those of small body size (these require less energy). Figure 2-3 illustrates the differences between the nutrient RDA and the energy RDA set by the committee.

The energy RDA listed on the inside front cover are thus recommendations for **average** persons within groups of particular age, sex, height, weight, and activity levels according to data from extensive surveys of the U.S. population. For example, the **reference woman** aged 19 to 24 years stands 5 feet 5 inches tall and weighs 128 pounds. The **reference man** of the same age stands 5 feet 10 inches tall and weighs 160 pounds. Very few people exactly fit the average for their groups, but as Figure 2-3 showed, most people's needs fall close to those shown. The best way to ensure that your food energy intake actually fits your own particular requirement is to monitor your weight compared to your food energy intake over a period of time. Chapter 9 revisits the energy RDA and shows how to control your energy intake to meet your needs.

As mentioned previously, no RDA is set for carbohydrate or fat. The committee expects that you will use the energy RDA as a guide for deciding how much carbohydrate and fat to include in your diet.

average a mathematical point halfway between two values; also called the *mean.*

reference woman and man actual median figures for heights and weights of people of each age-sex group in the U.S. population.

KEY POINT The energy RDA was set at the mean of people's needs so as to discourage overconsumption of food energy.

Other Nutrient Standards

Different nations and international groups have published different sets of standards similar to the RDA. The RNI for Canadians are shown in Appendix B; they differ from the RDA in some respects, partly because of differences in interpretation of the data they were derived from and partly because people's food intakes and daily lives in Canada differ somewhat from those in the United States.

The Canadian RNI are in Appendix B.

Countries other than the United States and Canada use other standards. Many countries use recommendations developed by two international groups: the World Health Organization (WHO) and the Food and Agriculture Organization (FAO). The WHO/FAO recommendations are considered sufficient for the maintenance of health in nearly all healthy people worldwide.

Appendix E provides addresses for WHO, FAO, and other agencies.

KEY POINT Many nations and groups issue recommendations for nutrient intakes appropriate for specific groups of people.

Table 2-1
Dietary Guidelines for Americans

- Eat a variety of foods.
- Maintain healthy weight.
- Choose a diet low in fat, saturated fat, and cholesterol.
- Choose a diet with plenty of vegetables, fruits, and grain products.
- Use sugars only in moderation.
- Use salt and sodium in moderation.
- If you drink alcoholic beverages, do so in moderation.

Note: Dietary Guidelines for Americans is a government document developed by the U.S. Department of Agriculture and the U.S. Department of Health and Human Services. These guidelines derive from *The Surgeon General's Report on Nutrition and Health,* DHHS (PHS) publication no. 88–50211 (Washington, D.C.: Government Printing Office, 1988); *Diet and Health: Implications for Reducing Chronic Disease Risk* (Washington, D.C.: National Academy Press, 1989); and the *Recommended Dietary Allowances,* 10th ed. (Washington, D.C.: National Academy Press, 1989).

Dietary Guidelines

So far you know that the RDA is a standard for people's nutrient and energy intakes. Now why should it be necessary to have "guidelines" as well? One reason is that while the RDA do much to ensure nutrient *adequacy,* they do little for *moderation.* The RDA were developed to ensure adequate nutrient intakes, and so they make specific recommendations for protein, vitamin, and mineral intakes. They also make some general statements about energy intakes, but they do little to protect people from excess intakes of fat, sugar, salt, and other food constituents. Also, the RDA refer to nutrients, not foods. People need guidance in terms of the foods they select each day.

To ensure dietary moderation where needed, the governments of many of the developed countries have published separate sets of recommendations. Among them are two from the United States, one from Canada, and one intended for all the people of the world. These sets of standards are, respectively, the *Dietary Guidelines for Americans* (Table 2-1), the *Diet and Health Recommendations* (Table 2-2), the *Nutrition Recommendations for Canadians* (Table 2-3), and the *World Health Organization's (WHO) Population Nutrient Goals* (Table 2-4 on page 38). The WHO Goals alone set both upper and lower limits for nutrients, and they have been proposed as an international set of guidelines. Many other sets of recom-

Table 2-2
Diet and Health Recommendations

- Reduce total *fat* intake to 30 percent or less of calories. Reduce saturated fatty acid intake to less than 10 percent of calories and the intake of cholesterol to less than 300 milligrams daily.[a]
- Increase intake of starches and other *complex carbohydrates.*[b]
- Maintain *protein* intake at moderate levels.[c]
- Balance food intake and physical activity to maintain appropriate *body weight.*
- For those who drink *alcoholic beverages,* limit consumption to the equivalent of less than 1 ounce of pure alcohol in a single day.[d] Pregnant women should avoid alcoholic beverages.
- Limit total daily intake of *salt* (sodium chloride) to 6 grams or less.[e]
- Maintain adequate *calcium* intake.
- Avoid taking dietary *supplements* in excess of the RDA in any one day.
- Maintain an optimal intake of *fluoride,* particularly during the years of primary and secondary tooth formation and growth.

Note: Italics added to highlight the areas of concern.

[a]The intake of fat and cholesterol can be reduced by substituting fish, poultry without skin, lean meats, and low-fat or nonfat dairy products for fatty meats and whole-milk products; by choosing more vegetables, fruits, cereals, and legumes; and by limiting oils, fats, egg yolks, and fried and other fatty foods.

[b]Every day eat five or more servings of a combination of vegetables and fruits, especially green and yellow vegetables and citrus fruits, and six or more daily servings of a combination of breads, cereals, and legumes.

[c]Meet at least the RDA for protein; do not exceed twice the RDA.

[d]The committee does not recommend alcohol consumption. One ounce of pure alcohol is the equivalent of two cans of beer, two small glasses of wine, or two average cocktails.

[e]Limit the use of salt in cooking; avoid adding it to food at the table. Consume salty, highly processed salty, salt-preserved, and salt-pickled foods sparingly. Six grams of salt are the equivalent of 2.4 grams of sodium.

Source: Adapted from the National Academy of Sciences report, *Diet and Health: Implications for Reducing Chronic Disease Risk* (Washington, D.C.: National Academy Press, 1989).

Table 2-3
Nutrition Recommendations for Canadians

The Canadian Diet Should:
1. Provide energy consistent with the maintenance of body weight within the recommended range.
2. Include essential nutrients in amounts recommended in the RNI (see Appendix B).
3. Include no more than 30% of energy as fat and no more than 10% as saturated fat.
4. Provide 55% of energy as carbohydrate from a variety of sources.
5. Reduce sodium contents.
6. Include no more than 5% of total energy as alcohol, or two drinks daily, whichever is less.
7. Contain no more caffeine than the equivalent of four regular cups of coffee per day.
8. Provide 1 milligram fluoride per liter of water.
Source: Adapted from Scientific Review Committee and the Communications/Implementation Committee, *Nutrition Recommendations . . . A Call for Action* (Ottawa: Canadian Government Publishing Centre, 1989).

mendations have been published, and all are similar with respect to advice on which nutrients to emphasize and which to control.

Notice that these guidelines do not require that you give up your favorite foods or eat strange, unappealing foods. Many studies show that almost anyone's diet, with minor adjustments, can fit most of these recommendations.[3] The secret seems to be to modify the diet in four ways. First, cultivate the willingness to watch portion sizes, especially of fat-rich foods such as meat and dairy products. Second, omit or limit a few foods, especially pure fats, such as margarine. Third, make substitutions, such as nonfat for high-fat dairy products. Finally, eat more of some foods, such as grains, fruits, and vegetables. These four tactics together can change a potentially harmful diet into one that supports nutrition and health superbly. You will see them again wherever diet changes are discussed.

If the experts who develop such documents were to ask us, we would add one more recommendation to their lists: choose foods that you enjoy. While it is of prime importance to choose foods that meet nutrient needs, it is equally important to seek out delicious foods that meet the needs for pleasure and fun. The joys of eating are physically beneficial to the body because they trigger health-promoting changes in the nervous, hormonal, and immune systems. They ensure that people will eat and thus obtain the nutrients needed for healthy body systems, along with healthy skin, glossy hair, and the natural good looks that accompany health. People tend to repeat what brings them pleasure, and so they are most likely to stay with foods they like. Remember to enjoy your foods.

Dietary recommendations encourage health of individuals and are also best for the earth itself. Chapter and Controversy 15 explore the relationships between people, their food choices, and the planet's well-being.

KEY POINT The Dietary Guidelines, the Nutrition Recommendations for Canadians, and the WHO Population Nutrient Goals along with other similar recommendations address the problems of overnutrition and undernutrition. They recommend weight control, controlled consumption of fat, and generous intakes of carbohydrate-rich foods. To implement the recommendations requires controlling portions, limiting fat intakes, substituting nutrient-dense for fat-rich foods, and amplifying servings of low-fat grains, fruits, and vegetables.

Table 2-4
The WHO Population Nutrient Goals

	Limits for Population Average Intakes	
	LOWER LIMIT	UPPER LIMIT
Total fat	15% of energy	30% of energy[a]
Saturated fatty acids	0% energy	10% of energy
Polyunsaturated fatty acids	3% energy	7% of energy
Dietary cholesterol	0 mg/day	300 mg/day
Total carbohydrate	55% of energy	75% of energy
Complex carbohydrates[b]	50% of energy	75% of energy
Dietary fiber[c]	27 g/day	40 g/day
Sugars[d]	0% of energy	10% of energy
Protein	10% of energy	15% of energy
Salt	—	6 g/day[c]

Note: The lower limit defines the minimum intake needed to prevent deficiency diseases, while the upper limit expresses the maximum intake compatible with the prevention of chronic diseases. This set of guidelines is proposed by WHO for acceptance as a set of international standards.

[a]An interim goal for nations with high fat intakes; further benefits would be expected by reducing fat intake towards 15% of total energy.

[b]A daily minimum intake of about 2 cups vegetables and fruits, including about a half cup of legumes, nuts, and seeds.

[c]From mixed food sources.

[d]Added refined sugars, not the sugars found naturally in fruits, vegetables, and milk.

Source: Reproduced, by permission, from: *Diet, Nutrition and the Prevention of Chronic Diseases. Report of a WHO Study Group.* Geneva, World Health Organization, 1990, p. 108 (WHO Technical Report Series, No. 797).

Diet Planning with Food Groups and Other Tools

food group plans diet planning tools that sort foods of similar origin and nutrient content into groups and then specify that people eat certain minimum numbers of servings of foods from each group.

exchange lists diet planning tools that organize foods with respect to their nutrient contents and calorie amounts. Foods on any single list can be used interchangeably.

Diet planning connects nutrition theory with the food on the table. To help people plan menus, two kinds of guides are available: **food group plans,** which describe food groups and dictate numbers of servings to choose each day, and **exchange lists,** which identify the particular foods to choose, specify portion sizes, and provide estimates of the amounts of carbohydrate, fat, and protein that each type of food contains.

Food Group Plans

In the past decades, school children learned about the Four Food Group Plan, which taught generations of people to recognize key nutrients provided by certain related groups of foods. Recently, scientists updated this bedrock of nutrition wisdom to better support the needs of people in the 1990s. Now called the Daily Food Guide (see Figure 2-4 on pages 40 and 41), the plan offers five groups instead of four, but many of the original concepts still apply.

The Daily Food Guide replaced the old Four Food Group Plan.

The foods in each group are notable contributors of certain key nutrients (see the figure), but you can count on them to supply many other nutrients as well. If you design your diet around this plan, it is assumed that you will obtain adequate amounts not only of the nutrients named in Figure 2-4 but also of the other two dozen or so essential nutrients because they are distributed among the same groups of foods. This is true in theory, but in practice diet planners using this plan must be sure to choose mostly *nutrient-dense* foods in each group because some processes strip foods of some nutrients and add calories from fat. With this caution, the Daily Food Guide can provide a reasonable foundation for diet planning. Figure 2-4 provides a key to indicate a few foods within each group with high, moderate, and low nutrient densities to give you an idea of which are which.

To use the plan, most adults must choose at least six servings from the breads-and-cereals group; three from the vegetables group; two from the fruits group; two from the meat, poultry, fish, and alternates group; and two from the milk, cheese, and yogurt group. Many people use shorthand to remember the pattern: six, three, two, two, and two. These are the minimum numbers of servings. The plan's makers suggest that to meet additional energy needs, a person should choose more servings of foods from these very same groups.

Some foods—such as butter, margarine, cream, sour cream, salad dressing, mayonnaise, potato chips, jelly, broth, coffee, tea, alcoholic beverages, and others—don't fit into any of the food groups. Some of these contribute a few nutrients, but most primarily contribute energy. Their nutrient contents have been greatly diluted by fat, sugar, alcohol, or water. They are grouped together into a miscellaneous category of extras that the plan's originators suggest should be used sparingly.

The food groups are represented in the pyramid-shaped diagram at the bottom of Figure 2-4. The pyramid shape with grains at the bottom is intended to convey the idea that you should eat more grain foods than anything else: grains form the foundation of a good diet. Fruits and vegetables appear next in volume. Meats and milks, while important, must be limited in number of servings because although they are dense in nutrients such as protein and are important sources of vitamins and minerals, they can also be high in fat and calories. Fats, oils, and sweets occupy only a tiny triangle at the top of the pyramid, indicating that they should be used sparingly. Alcoholic beverages are excluded from the pyramid. So are items such as spices, coffee, tea, and diet soft drinks. These provide few, if any, nutrients, but used judiciously, they can add flavor and pleasure to meals.

The beauty of the Daily Food Guide lies in its simplicity. Also, although it may appear rigid, it can actually be very flexible once its intent is understood. For example, the user can substitute cheese for milk because both supply the key nutrients for the milk group. The user can choose legumes (beans) and nuts as alternatives to meats. One can adapt the plan to mixed dishes such as casseroles as well as to national and cultural cuisines.

As mentioned, the way the Pyramid displays the Daily Food Guide tends to deemphasize meats and animal products such as milk, cheese, and eggs and to emphasize grains, fruits, and vegetables. This scheme can assist vegetarians in their food choices, while encouraging others to choose foods from plants most often. The food group that includes the meats also includes *meat alternates*—foods such as legumes and nuts. As for the food group that includes milk and milk products, people who choose not to use dairy foods can substitute soy "milk"—a product made from soybeans that fills the same nutrient needs, provided that it is fortified with calcium and vitamin B_{12}. In short, people who choose to eat no meats or products taken from animals can still use the Daily Food Guide to make their diets adequate.

Vegetarians will find more tips about choosing the right foods to supply the nutrients they need in the chapters to come.

Figure 2-4

THE DAILY FOOD GUIDE AND THE FOOD GUIDE PYRAMID

KEY: Nutrient Density
- ■ Foods generally highest in nutrient density (good first choice).
- ■ Foods moderate in nutrient density (reasonable second choice).
- ■ Foods lowest in nutrient density (limit selections).

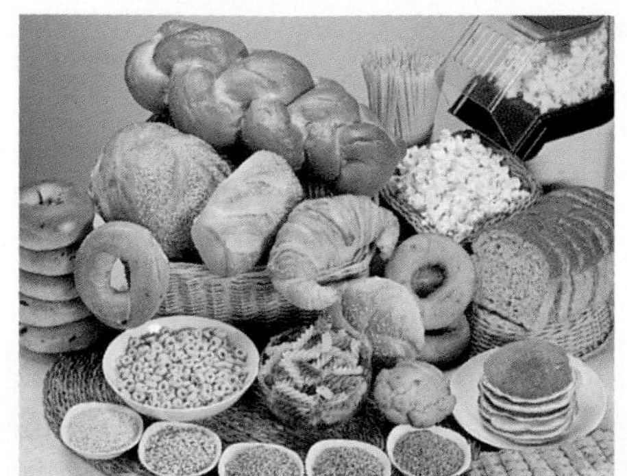

BREADS, CEREALS, AND OTHER GRAIN PRODUCTS

These foods are notable for their contributions of complex carbohydrates, riboflavin, thiamin, niacin, iron, protein, magnesium, and fiber.
6 to 11 servings per day.
Serving = 1 slice bread; ½ c cooked cereal, rice, or pasta; 1 oz ready-to-eat cereal; ½ bun, bagel, or English muffin; 1 small roll, biscuit, or muffin; 3 to 4 small or 2 large crackers.

- ■ Whole grains (wheat, oats, barley, millet, rye, bulgur), enriched breads, rolls, tortillas, cereals, bagels, rice, pastas (macaroni, spaghetti), air-popped corn.
- ■ Pancakes, muffins, cornbread, crackers, low-fat cookies, biscuits, presweetened cereals.
- ■ Croissants, fried rice, granola.

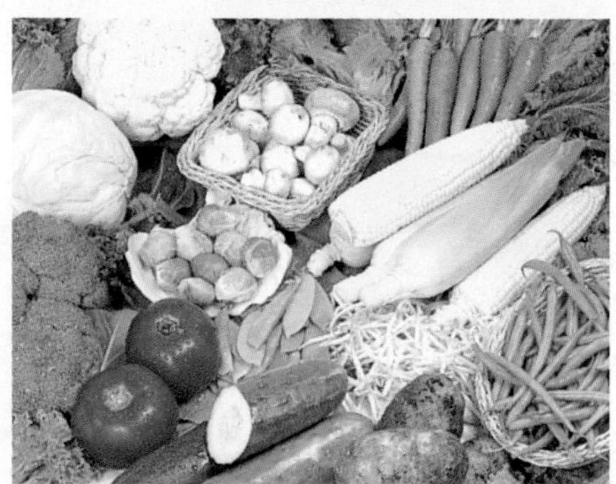

VEGETABLES

These foods are notable for their contributions of vitamin A, vitamin C, folate, potassium, magnesium, and fiber, and for their lack of fat and cholesterol.
3 to 5 servings per day (use dark green, leafy vegetables and legumes several times a week).
Serving = ½ c cooked or raw vegetables; 1 c leafy raw vegetables; ½ c cooked legumes; ¾ c vegetable juice.

- ■ Bean sprouts, broccoli, brussels sprouts, cabbage, carrots, cauliflower, cucumbers, green beans, green peas, leafy greens (spinach, mustard, and collard greens), legumes, lettuce, mushrooms, tomatoes, winter squash.
- ■ Corn, potatoes, sweet potatoes.
- ■ Avocados, french fries, olives, tempura vegetables.

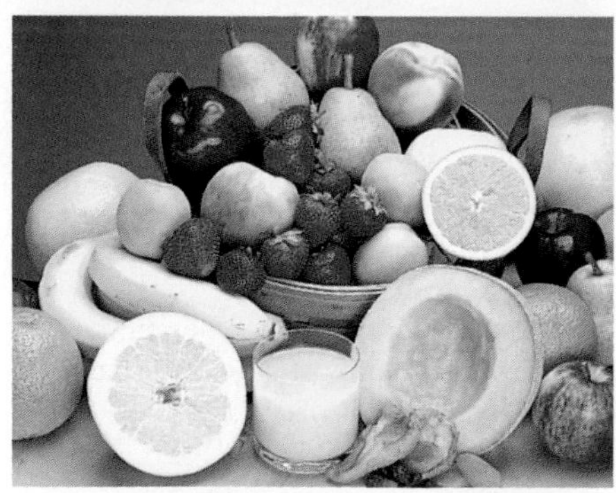

FRUITS

These foods are notable for their contributions of vitamin A, vitamin C, potassium, and fiber, and for their lack of sodium, fat, and cholesterol.
2 to 4 servings per day.
Serving = typical portion (such as 1 medium apple, banana, or orange, ½ grapefruit, 1 melon wedge); ¾ c juice; ½ c berries; ½ c diced, cooked, or canned fruit; ¼ c dried fruit.

- ■ Apricots, cantaloupe, grapefruit, oranges, orange juice, peaches, strawberries, apples, bananas, pears.
- ■ Canned or frozen fruit.
- ■ Dried fruit, coconut.

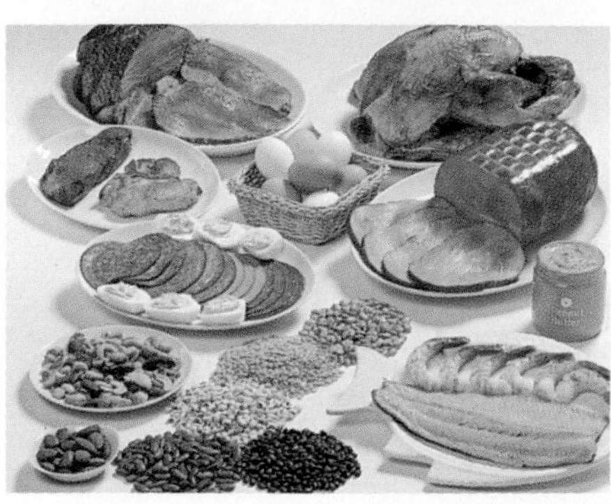

MEAT, POULTRY, FISH, AND ALTERNATES

These foods are notable for their contributions of protein, phosphorus, vitamin B_6, vitamin B_{12}, zinc, magnesium, iron, niacin, and thiamin.
2 to 3 servings per day.
Serving = 2 to 3 oz lean, cooked meat, poultry, or fish (total 5 to 7 oz per day); count 1 egg, ½ c cooked legumes, or 2 tbs peanut butter as 1 oz meat (or about ⅓ serving).

- ■ Poultry, fish, lean meat (beef, lamb, pork, veal), legumes, egg whites.
- ■ Fat-trimmed beef, lamb, pork; refried beans; egg yolks, tofu, tempeh.
- ■ Hot dogs, luncheon meats, peanut butter, nuts, sausage, bacon, fried fish or poultry, duck.

Figure 2-4

THE DAILY FOOD GUIDE AND THE FOOD GUIDE PYRAMID (continued)

MILK, CHEESE, AND YOGURT

These foods are notable for their contributions of calcium, riboflavin, protein, vitamin B_{12}, and, when fortified, vitamin D and vitamin A.
2 servings per day.
3 servings per day for teenagers and young adults, pregnant/lactating women, women past menopause.
4 servings per day for pregnant/lactating teenagers.
Serving = 1 c milk or yogurt; 2 oz process cheese food; 1½ oz cheese.

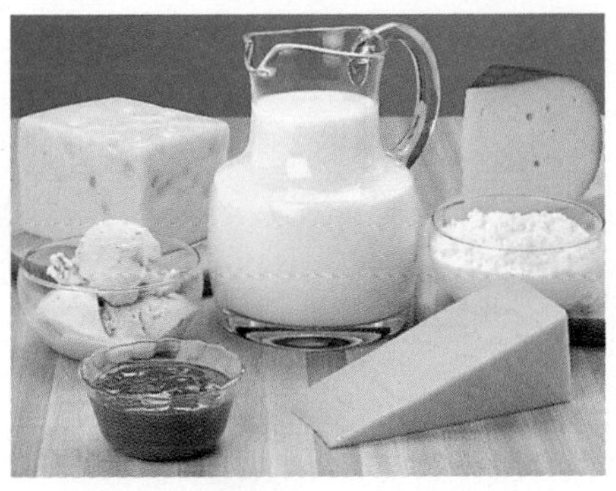

- Nonfat and 1% low-fat milk (and nonfat products such as buttermilk, cottage cheese, cheese, yogurt); fortified soy milk.
- 2% low-fat milk (and low-fat products such as yogurt, cheese, cottage cheese); sherbet; ice milk.
- Whole milk (and whole-milk products such as cheese, yogurt, cottage cheese); cream; sour cream; cream cheese; custard; milk shakes; pudding; ice cream.

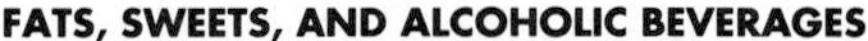

FATS, SWEETS, AND ALCOHOLIC BEVERAGES

These foods are notable for their contributions of sugar, fat, alcohol, and food energy. No servings are suggested because these foods provide few nutrients. Note that some of the following items, for example doughnuts, are high in both sugar and fat. Alcoholic beverages are not classed as foods; they contribute few nutrients but they do contribute calories, and so are mentioned here.

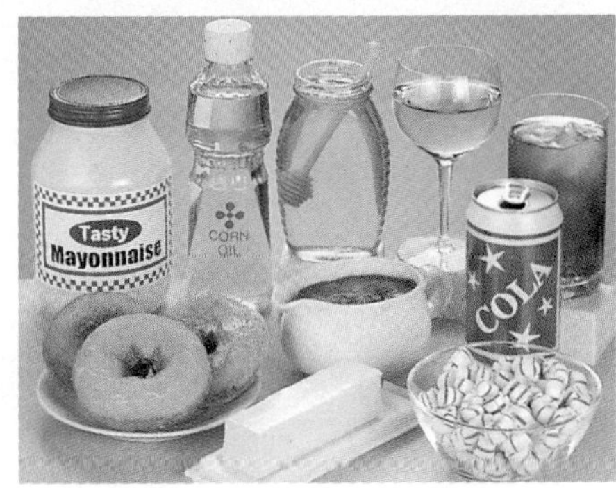

- Foods high in fat include margarine, salad dressings, oils, mayonnaise, cream, cream cheese, butter, gravy, and sauces.
- Foods high in sugar include cake, pie, cookies, doughnuts, sweet rolls, candy, soft drinks, fruit drinks, jelly, syrup, gelatin, desserts, sugar, and honey.
- Alcoholic beverages include wine, beer, and liquor.

Note: Serve children at least the lower number of servings from each group, but in smaller amounts (for example, ¼ to ⅓ cup rice). Children should receive the equivalent of 2 cups of milk each day, but in smaller quantities per serving (for example, 4 half-cup portions). Pregnant women may require additional servings of fruits, vegetables, meats, and breads to meet their higher needs for energy, vitamins, and minerals.

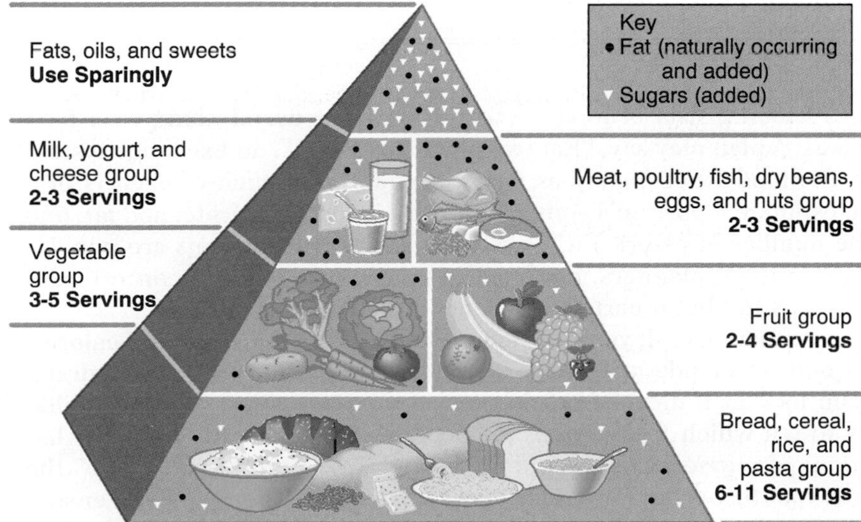

FOOD GUIDE PYRAMID: A GUIDE TO DAILY FOOD CHOICES

The breadth of the base shows that grains (breads, cereals, rice, and pasta) deserve most emphasis in the diet. The tip is smallest: use fats, oils, and sweets sparingly.

The Daily Food Guide does have drawbacks, however. It does not limit food choices to foods low in calories. People who select the minimum number of servings from among the most nutrient-dense foods in each group and who strictly limit foods from the fats, sweets, and alcoholic beverages group can keep their energy intakes as low as 1,600 calories a day, but people who use the higher-calorie foods in each group and who eat large servings, even without extra fats, sweets, or alcohol added in, can easily obtain too many calories. In the cheese-for-milk substitution just mentioned, an amount of cheddar cheese sufficient to meet a day's calcium requirement would carry with it almost 700 calories, over 70 percent of them from fat. A day's calcium from nonfat milk brings fewer than 350 calories, with hardly any fat. Less obvious but significant over time are energy differences between sliced bread and biscuits, fish and hotdogs, or even green beans and sweet potatoes—all proper substitutions according to the Daily Food Guide. High-calorie choices may be just what some people, such as athletes, need to meet their high energy requirements, but for others such choices can dramatically boost energy intakes and, over time, add to body weight.

The Pyramid attempts to caution consumers about fats and added sugars in food groups by sprinkling symbols for those two constituents across the pictures of the groups most likely to contain them. This scheme may be difficult to put into practical use. For example, the bread group is sprinkled with both the symbols for fat and added sugar because baked goods often contain a lot of added fat and sugar. Consumers wishing to avoid those products may find it impossible to identify individual high-fat or high-sugar foods within a group just by using the Pyramid alone.

Another criticism of the Daily Food Guide can be that a person who chooses the right number of servings from each group may make consistently nutrient-poor choices, and so fail to meet the day's needs for some nutrients. A diet can easily lack vitamin E, for example, because this vitamin is easily destroyed in processing or refined out of foods. Other plans have been developed from time to time and may serve some people's needs in other ways. Canada has developed such a plan, and its outline is given in Table 2-5. Appendix B provides the details of the Canadian plan.

Details of Canada's Food Guide to Healthy Eating are found in Appendix B.

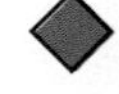

Table 2-5
Canada's Food Guide to Healthy Eating

Food Group	Servings/day
Grain products	5–12
Vegetables and fruit	5–10
Milk products	Children 4–9 years: 2–3 Youth 10–16 years: 3–4 Adults: 2–4 Pregnant & Breast-feeding Women: 3–4
Meat and alternatives	2–3

KEY POINT Food group plans divide and organize foods by their nutrients and origins to provide patterns of intake that cover nutrient needs.

Exchange Lists

Exchange lists are lists of food portions. They are useful along with food group plans. A plan may say, "Eat two portions of fruit"; an exchange system will list the foods that qualify as fruits; specify how much of each is in a portion; estimate a portion's contents of protein, carbohydrate, and fat; and state the number of calories it contributes. Exchange systems are popular among careful diet planners, particularly people who wish to control calories as well as to obtain certain nutrients in desired quantities.

Recommendations ask you to take in no more than 30 percent of calories from fat and to include at least 55 percent of calories from carbohydrate. When you look at a meal of salad, mashed potatoes, meat loaf, and milk, it's easy to tell which *food groups* are represented. How can you tell what proportions of *nutrients* foods contain, though? You can learn to "see" the nutrients, too, through a few tricks of memorization. Then, you can ensure that your diet is up to standards set not only for adequacy as food group plans are, but also for moderation and calorie control, the special advantages of exchange systems.

The user of an exchange system develops a "feel" for what is in foods and a sense of which foods are similar to each other in energy and selected nutrient contents. The exchange system was developed originally for use by people with diabetes but is now widely recognized as an excellent diet-planning tool for healthy people. It organizes foods into six lists according to their energy in calories, and their carbohydrate, fat, and protein contents in grams. It facilitates weight control; it also helps people to estimate their intakes of fat, saturated fat, fiber, and salt.

Appendix D gives complete details of the U.S. and Canadian exchange systems.

A convenient way to remember or "see" the foods, portion sizes, and energy values of the six exchange lists is to keep in mind one typical member of each list. For example:

- Milk—1 cup nonfat milk (90 calories)
- Vegetables—½ cup cooked carrots (25 calories)
- Fruits—1 small orange (60 calories)
- Starch/bread—1 small potato/1 slice bread (80 calories)
- Meat—1 ounce lean beef (55 calories)
- Fat—1 teaspoon butter (45 calories)

The number of calories assigned to a portion of food on a list is an average for the entire list. Individual foods on a list differ slightly in exact energy amounts but are close enough so that you can use the average values for them. Table 2-6 shows the carbohydrate, fat, and protein in grams, and the average calorie values that pertain to each list.

Table 2-6
The Six Exchange Lists

List	Portion Size	Carbohydrate (g)	Protein (g)	Fat (g)	Energy (cal)[d]
Starch/bread[a]	1 slice	15	3	Trace	80
Meat[b]	1 oz				
Lean		—	7	3	55
Medium-fat		—	7	5	75
High-fat		—	7	8	100
Vegetable[c]	½ c	5	2	—	25
Fruit	1 portion	15	—	—	60
Milk	1 c				
Nonfat		12	8	Trace	90
Low fat		12	8	5	120
Whole		12	8	8	150
Fat	1 tsp	—	—	5	45

Note: This is the U.S. exchange system. The complete details, and those of the Canadian system, are shown in Appendix D.

[a]This list includes starchy vegetables such as lima beans, potatoes, and corn, as well as cereal, bread, pasta, and other grain products. For portion sizes see Appendix D.

[b]This list includes cheese and peanut butter as well as meat.

[c]This list includes low-calorie vegetables only.

[d]These are approximate, rounded values assigned to each exchange for ease in remembering.

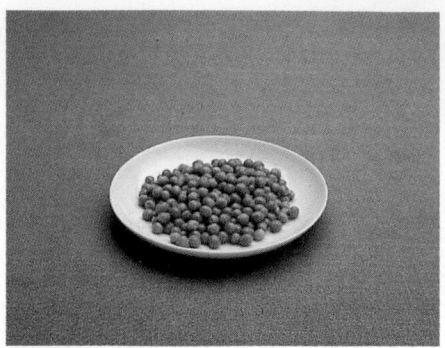
100 grams peas (about ½ cup).

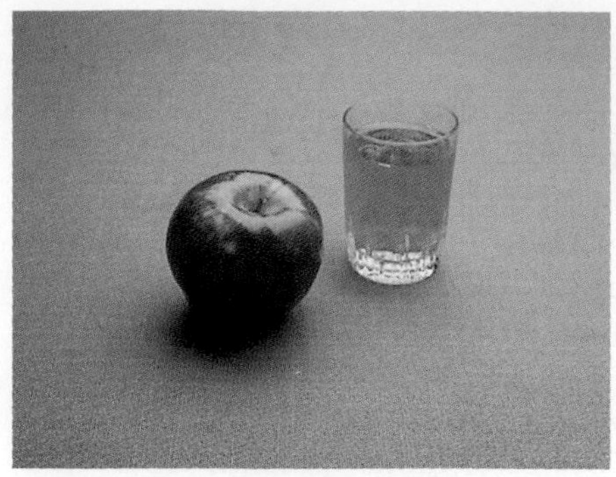
100 ml juice (about ½ cup).

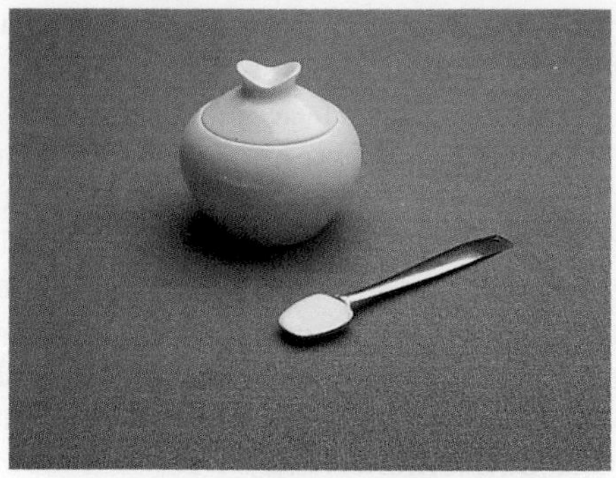
5 grams sugar (about 1 teaspoon).

Figure 2-5

STANDARD PORTION SIZES

Portions in the exchange system are specific. Shown here are three typical portions: 100 grams of a food (which is about the same as ½ cup), 100 milliliters of a juice (which is also about the same as ½ cup), and 5 grams of a powder, sugar (which is about the same as a teaspoon). Cooks who like to switch back and forth between the British and metric systems have learned to use these values interchangeably.

Potatoes are listed with starch/breads in the exchange system; the Daily Food Guide lists them with the starchy vegetables.

The exchange system pays strict attention to portion sizes. Only if you measure a portion correctly do you obtain the number of calories and amounts of energy nutrients intended. To use the system meaningfully, you must therefore become familiar with portion sizes, even if it means measuring your foods for awhile. Figure 2-5 shows what some typical portions look like, and Figure 2-6 (on pages 46 and 47) shows the foods that belong together in the exchange lists. The last figure of this chapter shows how to determine the carbohydrate, protein, and fat grams and calorie content of a whole day's worth of meals using the exchange system.

Some surprises await the newcomer to the exchange system. For example, cheese is classed as a meat because its protein and fat contents are similar to those of meat. (In the Daily Food Guide cheese is listed with milk because of its calcium content.) Although most people think of corn as a vegetable, the exchange system lists it with starch/breads as a "starchy vegetable." Lima beans, potatoes, and other starchy vegetables are also listed with the breads, not the vegetables as in the Daily Food Guide, because they are similar to the other starch/breads list foods in calorie and carbohydrate content. Similarly, olives are not classed as a "fruit," as a botanist would claim; they are a "fat" because they are more like butter than like berries in fat content. Bacon is also a member of the fat list because its nutrient content is more like that of fat than of meat.

To help control fat intakes, the user of the exchange system is taught to become very conscious of the fats in foods. The vegetable list includes only low-calorie vegetables prepared without added fat, so a half cup of any cooked vegetable or a cup of raw vegetable will provide about 25 calories. The system's standard milk is nonfat milk. Whole-milk and low-fat items are treated as milk with fat added, and so are listed separately. Not only milks but also meats and cheeses are separated into three categories by their fat contents. Milks are classed as nonfat, low-fat, and whole milk products; meats and cheeses as lean, medium-fat, and high-fat items. To further help you keep track of your fat intakes, the fat list includes items such as cream, cream cheese, nuts, coconut, coffee whitener, and avocados, high-fat foods that you might not recognize as such.

Sugar is also extra. The fruit list specifies "unsweetened"; if you eat sugar, you have to keep track of its extra calories. One-half cup canned peaches or one-half a small banana counts as one fruit, but a piece of cherry pie is not a fruit. It includes a fruit if it contains ten large cherries, but it also includes bread and fat exchanges and added sugar. (Thus it might be counted as one fruit, two starch/breads, and three fats, with two tablespoons added sugar.) The starch/bread list also makes clear which starchy foods contain added fat, such as muffins, rolls, taco shells, biscuits, and cookies.

A warning: a *portion* in the exchange system is not the same as a *serving* in the Daily Food Guide, especially when it comes to meats. Portions of meats and most cheeses in the exchange system are single ounces, much smaller than a suggested 2–3 ounce serving. This is not to recommend that you eat only one ounce of meat at a given meal but that you note carefully the number of ounces in your meat servings—again, for the sake of controlling fat intakes.

Repeat: one meat exchange is 1 ounce; a recommended serving (2–3 ounces) equals 3 meat exchanges.

Nutritionists designed the exchange system to simplify, not to complicate, their analysis of foods. It is not precise, so there is no point in struggling to calculate calories and grams to several decimal places. Don't let the system get in the way of your approach to foods. Don't try to break down complicated dishes to the last crouton or pinch of parsley. Use the system to make estimates easy. For example, treat a typical sandwich or one-cup serving of a casserole as: 1 fat, 2 starch/breads, and 2 medium-fat meat exchanges.[4]

The sandwich described by these values is the kind people make at home, consisting of two slices of bread, a teaspoon of mayonnaise, a slice of ham and a slice of cheese, and various adornments such as mustard, pickles, lettuce, and tomato. If your sandwich looks more like an 8- or 10-inch hoagie, assign it double the shortcut values given for the homemade type. As for casseroles, most starch, meat, cheese, and sauce casseroles fit this description well. For other types, check Table D-8 of Appendix D and pick values for a dish that resembles the one you've eaten.

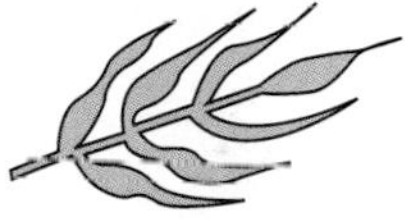

Fiber symbol

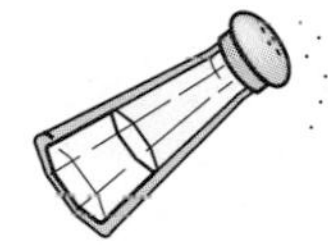

Sodium symbol

The exchange system booklets identify foods high in fiber and sodium with these symbols, so that users can choose foods wisely. In Appendix D these foods are identified using miniature versions of the same symbols. To obtain the original booklet, which is handy to carry around, write to the American Dietetic Association (ADA) at the address given in Appendix E.

The exchange lists point out fiber and sodium, too, wherever they are present in significant quantities. In Appendix D, foods high in fiber can be picked out by the wheat symbol they bear (choose them often). The saltshaker symbol identifies foods high in sodium, so that people who must avoid them can do so.

KEY POINT Unlike the Daily Food Guide, the exchange system facilitates calorie control because the foods on each list provide approximately equal amounts of carbohydrate, fat, and protein, and therefore energy. It is an excellent tool for balancing these nutrient intakes in diet planning.

Using the Daily Food Guide with Exchange Lists

The Daily Food Guide guides you to plan a day's meals consisting of all the servings you need from each class of nutritious foods. Once the plan is made, the exchange lists enable you to pick the exact foods to put in it. By using the two together, you can easily achieve the goals of a good diet mentioned in Chapter 1: *a*dequacy, *b*alance, *c*alorie control, *m*oderation, and *v*ariety.

Table 2-7 (page 48) shows that when you use the Daily Food Guide as a pattern and the exchange lists as guides for choosing the items to eat, you can meet the plan's requirements and still eat fewer than 1,600 calories. Even if you are only moderately active, you can probably still eat an additional 600 to 1,200 calories without gaining weight. The more active you are, the higher the energy allowance you "earn." A wise choice is to invest

Figure 2-6

THE EXCHANGE SYSTEM: PORTION SIZES, EXAMPLE FOODS, AND NUTRIENT AND ENERGY CONTENTS

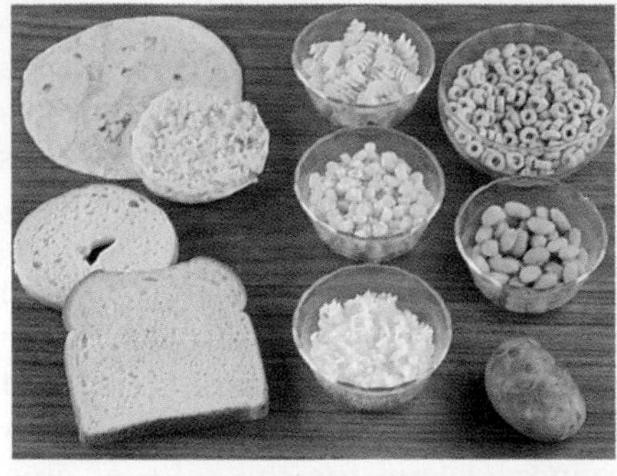

STARCH/BREADS

1 slice bread (1 portion) is like:
¾ c ready-to-eat cereal.
½ c cooked pasta.
⅓ c cooked rice.
⅓ c cooked beans.
½ c corn.
1 small (3-oz) potato.
½ bagel or English muffin.
1 tortilla
(1 bread = 15 g carbohydrate, 3 g protein, trace of fat, and 80 cal.)

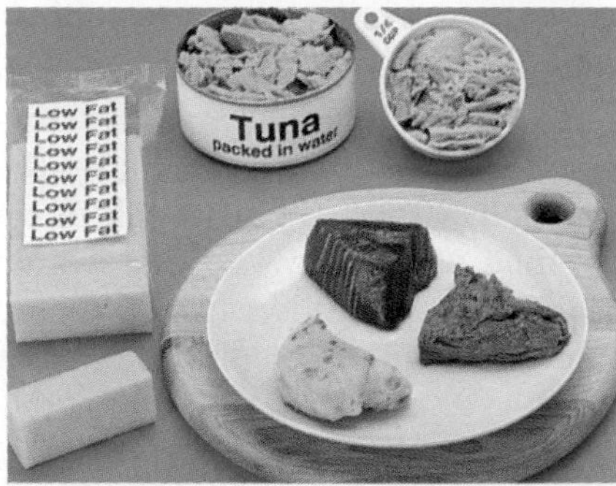

MEATS (LEAN)

1 oz lean meat (1 portion) is like:
1 oz beef or pork tenderloin.
1 oz chicken (without skin).
1 oz fresh fish.
¼ c tuna (canned in water).
1 oz low-fat cheese.
(1 lean meat = 7 g protein, 3 g fat, and 55 cal.)

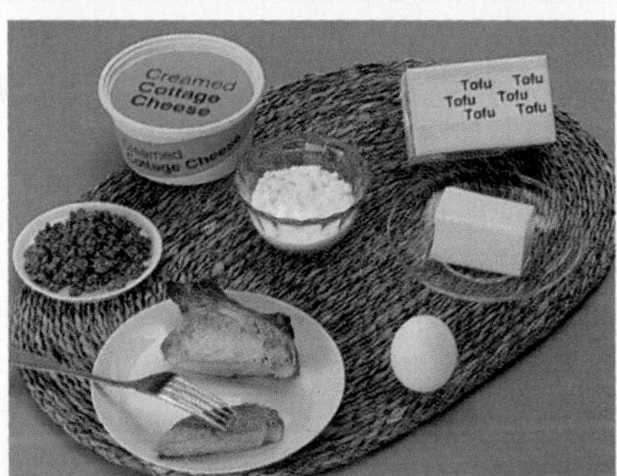

MEATS (MEDIUM-FAT)

1 oz medium-fat meat has the protein content of 1 oz lean meat, but with 5 g fat (2 g more fat than lean meat).
Examples:
1 oz ground beef.
1 oz pork chop.
1 egg.
¼ c creamed cottage cheese or ricotta.
4 oz tofu.
(1 medium-fat meat = 7 g protein, 5 g fat, and about 75 cal.)

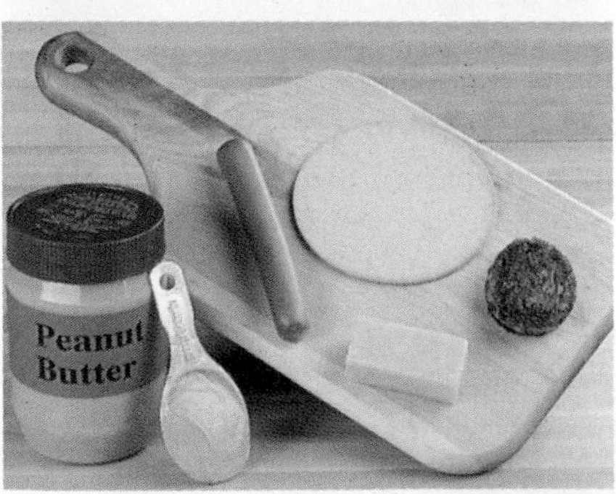

MEATS (HIGH-FAT)

1 oz high-fat meat has the protein content of 1 oz lean meat, but with an estimated **extra "1 fat"**—that is, the 3 g fat of a lean meat plus 5 g additional fat.
Examples:
1 oz pork sausage.
1 oz luncheon meat (such as bologna).
1 oz cheddar cheese.
1 small hot dog (frankfurter).[a]
1 tbs peanut butter.[b]
(1 high-fat meat = 7 g protein, 8 g fat, and 100 cal.)

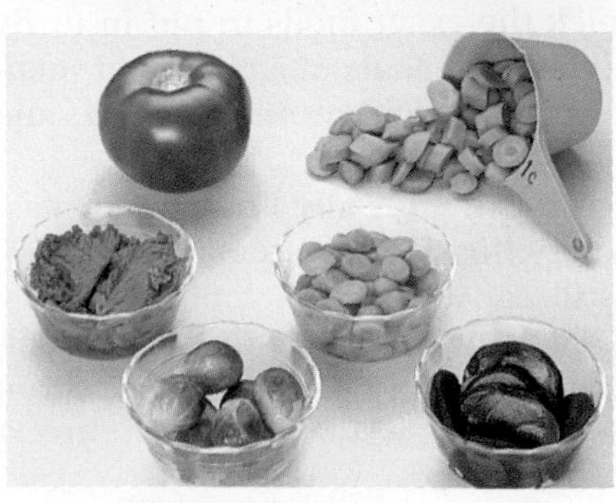

VEGETABLES

½ c cooked carrots (1 portion) is like:
½ c cooked greens.
½ c cooked brussels sprouts.
½ c cooked beets.
1 c raw carrots.
1 lg tomato.
(1 vegetable = 5 g carbohydrate, 2 g protein, and 25 cal.)[c]

[a]A regular frankfurter counts as 1 high-fat meat exchange plus 1 fat exchange.

[b](Don't stop reading now, and don't swear off peanut butter, necessarily. You'll need to read about the polyunsaturated character of its fat in Chapter 5, and the B vitamin contributions it makes in Chapter 7 before deciding how much of a place it should have in your diet.)

[c]Some vegetables such as lettuce, celery, cucumbers, and mushrooms can be eaten freely because their energy value is less than 20 calories per serving.

Figure 2-6

THE EXCHANGE SYSTEM: PORTION SIZES, EXAMPLE FOODS, AND NUTRIENT AND ENERGY CONTENTS (continued)

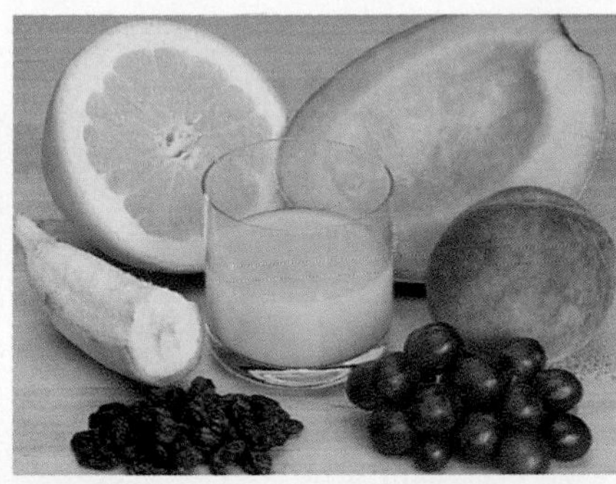

FRUITS

½ small banana (1 portion) is like:
1 small apple, peach, orange, or pear.
½ grapefruit.
½ c orange, apple, or grapefruit juice.
15 small grapes.
⅓ cantaloupe.
2 tbs raisins.
(1 fruit = 15 g carbohydrate and 60 cal.)

MILKS (NONFAT AND VERY-LOW-FAT)

1 c nonfat milk (1 portion) is like:
1 c nonfat yogurt, plain.
1 c lowfat buttermilk.
½ c evaporated nonfat milk.
⅓ c dry nonfat milk.
(1 nonfat milk = 12 g carbohydrate, 8 g protein, trace of fat, and 90 cal.)

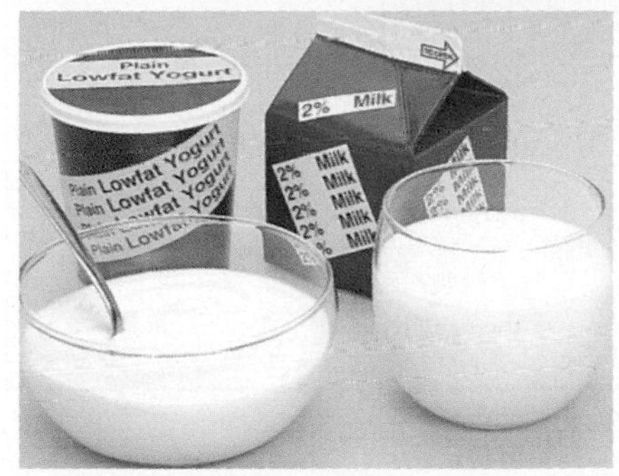

MILKS (LOW-FAT)

1 c low-fat milk has the protein and carbohydrate content of 1 c nonfat milk, but with 5 g fat.
Examples:
1 c 2% milk.
1 c low-fat yogurt, plain.
(1 low-fat milk = 12 g carbohydrate, 8 g protein, 5 g fat, and 120 cal.)

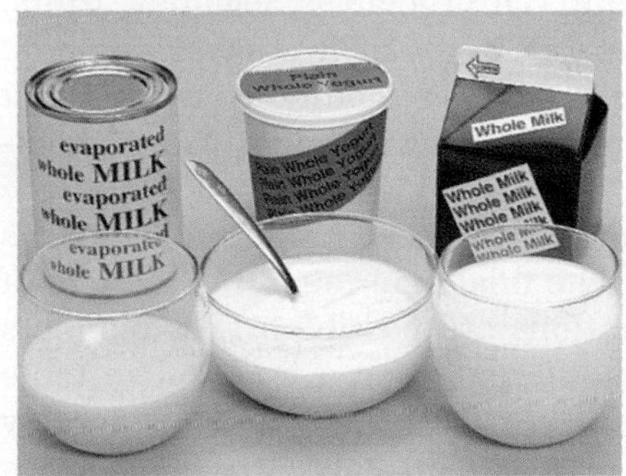

MILKS (WHOLE)

1 c whole milk has the protein and carbohydrate content of 1 c nonfat milk, but with 8 g fat.
Examples:
1 c whole milk.
½ c evaporated whole milk.
1 c whole yogurt, plain.
(1 whole milk = 12 g carbohydrate, 8 g protein, 8 g fat, and 150 cal.)

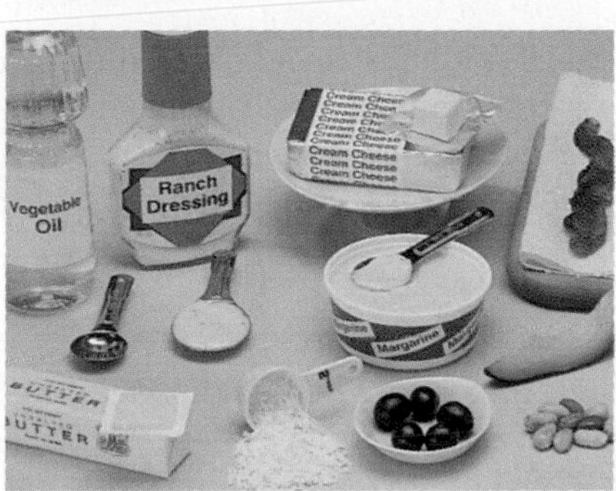

FATS

1 tsp butter (1 portion) is like:
1 tsp margarine.
1 tsp any oil.
1 tbs salad dressing.
5 large olives.
10 large peanuts.
⅛ medium avocado.
1 slice bacon.
2 tbs shredded coconut.
1 tbs cream cheese.
(1 fat = 5 g fat and 45 cal.)

Table 2-7
Diet Planning Using the Daily Food Guide and the Exchange System

Pattern from the Daily Food Guide	Selections Made from the Exchange Lists	Example	Energy Cost (cal)
Grains—6 servings	Starch/breads—select 6 exchanges[a]	3 breads 2 pasta 1 cereal	480
Meat—2 servings (2 to 3 oz each)	Meat list—select 6 exchanges[b]	6 oz lean meat	330
Fruits—2 servings	Fruit list—select 2 items	2 fruits	120
Vegetables—3 servings	Vegetable list—select 2 exchanges starch/bread select 1 exchange	2 vegetables 1 starchy vegetable	130
Milk—2 c	Milk list—select 2 exchanges	2 c nonfat milk	180
Added fat—4 tsp	Fat list—select 4 exchanges	4 fats	180
Added sugar—6 tsp	Add sugar (30 g) from all sources	8 oz cola	120
		Total:	1540

[a]Because the starchy vegetables are on the same list with the grains, some of them can be substituted for grains according to the exchange system.

[b]Caution: In the Daily Food Guide 1 serving is 2 to 3 oz. On the exchange lists a portion equals 1 oz. Therefore 2 servings according to the Food Guide equal 4 to 6 exchanges.

many of those additional calories in additional vegetables, legumes, fruits, and whole-grain foods and only a few in luxury items such as sweet desserts, butter, margarine, oil, or alcohol. If you make these additions, make them by conscious choice rather than through the unintentional use of high-calorie foods.

With judicious selections the diet can meet the need for all the nutrients and provide some luxury items as well. The final plan might be like one of those outlined in Table 2-8 (many variations are possible). Diet planners use different patterns of exchanges for different energy levels. The table shows that a person eating 3,000 calories per day could use considerably more bread portions, for example, than a person eating 1,500 calories per day.

Remember the goals of a good diet: ABCMV.

Wise diners read labels of packaged foods to help them determine the foods' nutrient contents and to decide how the foods may fit into their total eating plan. The next section begins a series of special features that also appear in Chapters 4, 5, 6, 8, and 14. These features explain how to gain insight from the information on food labels.

KEY POINT Food group plans and exchange lists, used together, ease diet planning. Food group plans provide the framework that ensures adequacy and balance; exchange lists supply the items to go in the frame, achieving calorie control, moderation, and variety.

Table 2-8
Diet Plans for Different Energy Intakes[a]

	Energy Level (cal)						
Exchanges	1,200	1,500[b]	1,800	2,000	2,200	2,600	3,000
Starch/breads	4	6	8	10	11	13	15
Vegetables	3	4	4	4	6	6	6
Fruits	3	4	5	5	5	5	6
Milks	2	2	2	2	2	3	3
Meats[c]	5	5	5	6	6	7	8
Fats	4	5	7	7	8	10	12

[a]These patterns of exchanges supply about 30% of the calories as fat, in accordance with the view that a moderate fat intake is desirable. For higher-energy patterns, such as athletes might need, see Chapter 10.

[b]Diets providing fewer than about 1,500 calories may not provide adequate nutrients.

[c]Meat exchanges consist of lean meats. To include higher fat meats, deduct fat exchanges as appropriate.

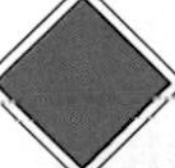

CHECKING OUT FOOD LABELS

First Facts

A package of potato chips is potato, fat, and salt, and it must bear a label to tell you its nutrient composition. In contrast, a potato is a potato, and it bears no label to tell you what nutrients it contains. So how can you assign fresh foods useful roles in your diet? In regard to the potato, you may be able to read about it on a sign or handout near the potato bin at the grocery store. Grocers often voluntarily post placards in fresh-food departments of groceries to provide consumers with nutrition information for the 20 most popular types of fruits, vegetables, and seafoods.

As for most packaged foods, you can use them artfully in diet planning if you can interpret their labels. The Nutrition Education and Labeling Act of 1990 brought sweeping changes in the requirements for label information. Most food labels must conform with all the new requirements.[5] Exceptions include plain coffee, tea, spices, and other foods contributing few nutrients; foods produced by small businesses; and those prepared and sold in the same establishment.* An easy way to recognize a new label is to look for the words "Nutrition Facts" on the new label's information panel. The old label says, "Nutrition Information."

According to law, every food label must state the following:

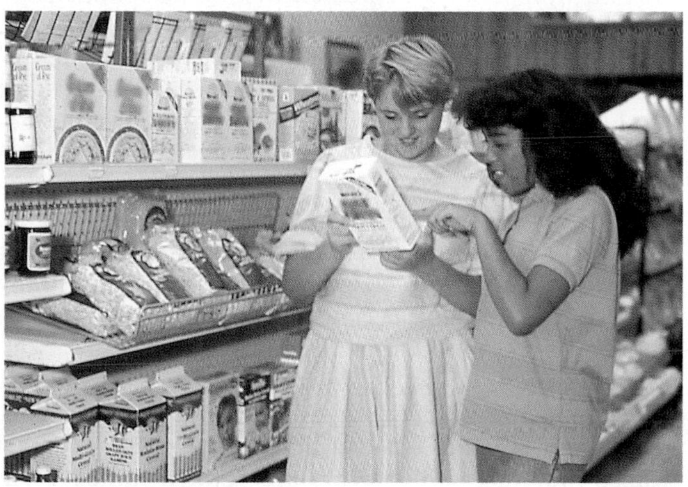

Modern-day entertainment: Reading food labels.

- The common or usual name of the product
- The name and address of the manufacturer, packer, or distributor

(continued on next page)

*Restaurants making "heart healthy" claims for menu items may be required to provide nutrient information for consumers.

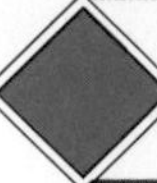

CHECKING OUT FOOD LABELS

First Facts *continued*

- The net contents in terms of weight, measure, or count

Then, the label must list in ordinary language the following:

- The ingredients, in descending order of predominance by weight

In the past, a few foods, such as mayonnaise and ice cream, were exempt from the requirement to list their ingredients. Manufacturers, instead, were held to strict standards called standards of identity that described the exact proportions of ingredients allowed in the products. Now all foods, including those with standards of identity, must list their ingredients on their labels.[6]

INGREDIENT LIST

Knowing how to read an ingredient list puts you many steps ahead of the naive buyer. Whatever is listed first is the ingredient that predominates by weight. Compare the ingredient list on an orange powder whose first three ingredients are "sugar, citric acid, orange flavor." You can tell that sugar is the chief ingredient. Now look at a canned juice whose ingredient list begins with "water, orange juice concentrate, pineapple juice concentrate." This product is clearly made of reconstituted juice. Water is first on the label because it is the main constituent of juice. Sugar is nowhere to be found among the ingredients because sugar has not been added to the product. (Sugar does occur naturally in juice, though, so the label *does* specify sugar grams; details in Chapter 4.)

Now look at a cereal whose entire list contains just one item: "100 percent shredded wheat." No question, this is a whole-grain food. Finally, compare a cereal whose first three ingredients are "puffed milled corn, sweeteners (sugars: corn syrup, sucrose, honey, dextrose), salt." If you can recognize that sugar, corn syrup, honey, and dextrose are all different versions of sugar (and you will, after Chapter 4), you'll know that this product may contain close to half its weight as sugar.

DAILY VALUES

The **Daily Values** reflect the RDA and other health recommendations and were designed solely for listing nutrients on food labels. Students who learn about the RDA ask why experts deemed it necessary to develop a whole new set of standards for food labels. Why not just use the RDA? The answer is that the RDA values vary from group to group, whereas on a label, one set of values must apply to everyone. For example, a team from a food firm trying to choose an RDA value for iron would be stopped cold on seeing five RDA values for iron. To which RDA should they compare their product? The one for young women? For 6-year-old boys? What single value would be most useful? The Daily Values solve this dilemma.

On the way to developing the Daily Values, the Food and Drug Administration (FDA) first developed two other sets of standards. One set contains the old labeling values, the U.S. RDA for vitamins and minerals.* The FDA calls these the **Reference Daily Intakes (RDI).**

The other set covers nutrients, such as fat and fiber, not included in the RDI. These nutrients have substantial impacts on health. To account for these nutrients, the FDA consulted the National Research Council's book, *Diet and Health,* and generated another set of standards they called **Daily Reference Values (DRV).** Together these two sets of standards bear the combined name of *Daily Values* (see Figure 2-7), and they meet the needs of industry and consumers. The Daily Values are intended to be simple and easy to interpret. Only students of nutrition ever need know that they are, in reality, two separate sets of values meticulously developed and combined to meet the nation's nutrition information needs. The Daily Values are listed on the inside front cover, page C.

NUTRITION FACTS

Food labels must provide the following nutrient information on the "Nutrition Facts" panel:

- Standard serving size expressed in both common household and metric measures to allow comparison of foods within a food category.
- Number of servings or portions per box, can, package, or other unit
- Total food energy (calories) per serving
- Food energy (calories) from fat per serving
- Fat (grams) per serving with breakdown for saturated fat (grams) and cholesterol (milligrams)

*The U.S. RDA has been the labeling standard since 1975. Some day, the U.S. RDA values may be replaced with a more current set that reflects 1989 RDA standards.

CHECKING OUT FOOD LABELS

First Facts *continued*

DAILY VALUES are made up of:

REFERENCE DAILY INTAKES
—the labeling standards
for vitamins and minerals,
formerly called the U.S. RDA.
They cover adults with
high nutrient needs.

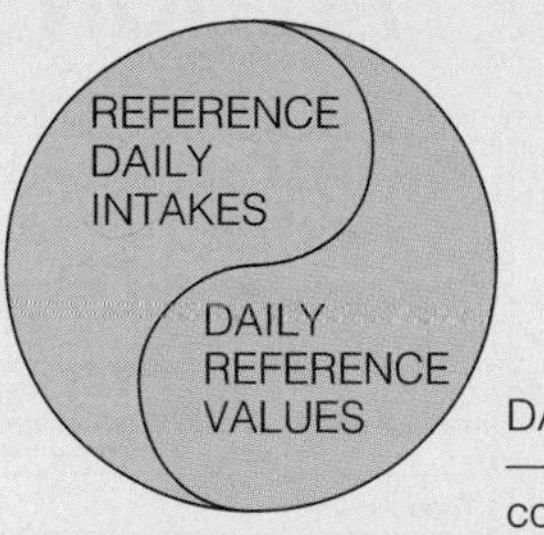

DAILY REFERENCE VALUES
— a set of values developed to
cover nutrients not addressed
by the RDA, such as fat and
fiber.

Figure 2-7

HOW THE *REFERENCE DAILY INTAKES* AND THE *DAILY REFERENCE VALUES* ARE COMBINED TO CREATE THE *DAILY VALUES*

Daily Values a combination of two sets of nutrient intake standards, the Reference Daily Intakes derived from the RDA and the Daily Reference Values derived from the NRC report on *Diet and Health*, intended for use on food labels.

Reference Daily Intakes a set of nutrient intake standards reflecting the 1968 RDA values for an adult with high nutrient needs; on food labels, part of the Daily Values. Previously known as the U.S. RDA.

Daily Reference Values intake values based on NRC's *Diet and Health* values for nutrients for which no RDA exist; used on food labels as part of the Daily Values.

- Sodium (milligrams) per serving
- Carbohydrate (grams) per serving
- Fiber and sugars (grams) per serving
- Protein (grams) per serving

In addition, for each of the nutrients just named plus vitamins A and C, calcium, and iron, amounts in a serving of the food must be stated as percentages of the Daily Values for a person requiring 2,000 calories per day.

A package's size helps to determine how much information it must deliver. Small packages of less than 40 square inches, such as a tuna can, must deliver the information listed above but can stop there. Tiny packages, with less than 12 square inches, such as a roll of mints, may provide only a phone number for consumers to call to obtain nutrient information. Large labels of 40 or more square inches, however, must include all of the above information and must also list the Daily Values for two people: one who consumes 2,000 calories per day and one who consumes 2,500 calories per day. The label may also provide a reminder of the calories in a gram of carbohydrate, fat, and protein.

One more factor helps to determine requirements for a label—the nutrient value of the food. A food that contains insignificant amounts of more than half of the nutrients listed above may bear a simplified label that provides information only on the nutrients the food does contain. The side panel of the box of cereal in Figure 2-8 provides all this information. The chicken label shows a condensed format, and the candy package provides only a phone number, as required.

HEALTH MESSAGES ON LABELS

At one time, a food manufacturer who hoped to promote a food as having special health-promoting powers labeled it as a "health food." Today, that term is banned from use because it implies that to gain health, the consumer need only choose and eat that food. Some claims about health are allowed, however, as long as they meet a strict set of guidelines set forth by the FDA.

Seven claims linking nutrients and food constituents to disease states are allowable under FDA guidelines. The following list describes them, and the terms in bold are defined in Table 2-9 (page 53). A statement on a label is permitted to refer to the following:

1. Calcium as related to osteoporosis. Foods making this claim must be **high** in calcium.

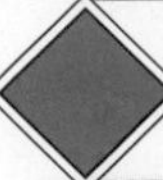

CHECKING OUT FOOD LABELS
First Facts *continued*

Figure 2-8

INTRODUCING A FOOD LABEL

What's on a Label

The package must always state the product name, the name and address of the manufacturer, and the weight or measure.

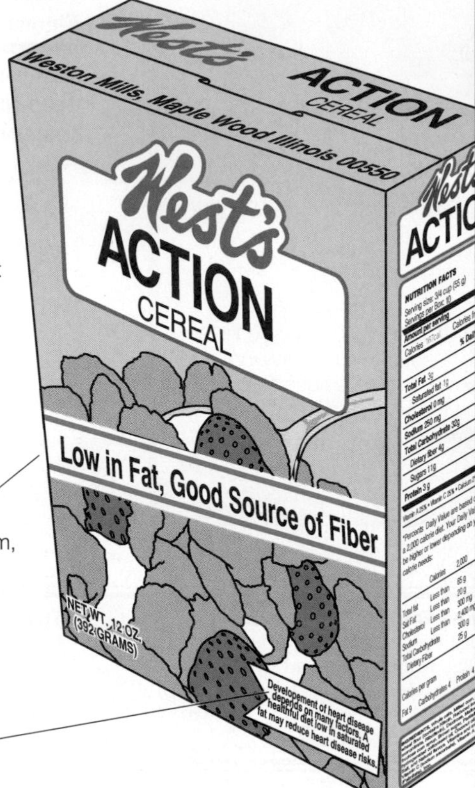

The label may state information about sodium, calories, fat, or other constituents.

Approved health claims may be made, but only in terms of total diet.

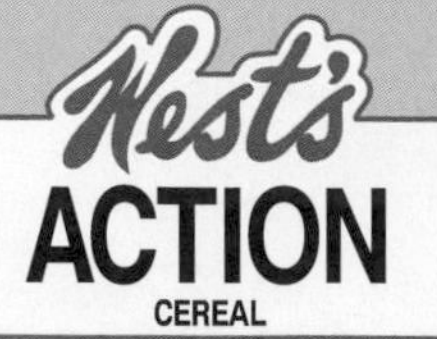

Nutrition Facts

Serving size 3/4 cup (55g)
Servings per Box 10

Amount per serving	
Calories 167	Calories from Fat 27
	% Daily Value*
Total Fat 3g	5%
Saturated Fat 1g	5%
Cholesterol 0mg	0%
Sodium 250mg	10%
Total Carbohydrate 32g	11%
Dietary fiber 4g	16%
Sugars 11g	
Protein 3g	
Vitamin A 25% •	Vitamin C 25%
Calcium 2% •	Iron 25%

*Percent Daily Values are based on a 2,000 calorie diet. Your daily values may be higher or lower depending on your calorie needs.

	Calories	2,000	2,500
Total Fat	Less than	65g	80g
Sat Fat	Less than	20g	25g
Cholesterol	Less than	300mg	300mg
Sodium	Less than	2,400mg	2,400mg
Total Carbohydrate		300g	375g
Dietary Fiber		25g	30g

Calories per gram
Fat 9 • Carbohydrate 4 • Protein 4

INGREDIENTS, Whole oats, Milled corn, Enriched wheat flour (contains Niacin, Reduced iron, Thiamin mononitrate, Riboflavin), Dextrose, Maltose, High-fructose corn syrup, Brown sugar, Partially hydrogenated cottonseed oil, Coconut oil, Walnuts, Salt, and Natural flavors. Vitamins and minerals: Vitamin C (sodium ascorbate), Vitamin A (Palmitate), Iron.

Serving size and calorie information

Percentage of Daily Value for nutrients

Reference values

This allows comparison of some values for nutrients in a serving of the food with the needs of a person requiring 2,000 or 2,500 calories per day to show how the product fits into the daily diet.

Calorie/gram reminder

Ingredients in descending order of predominance

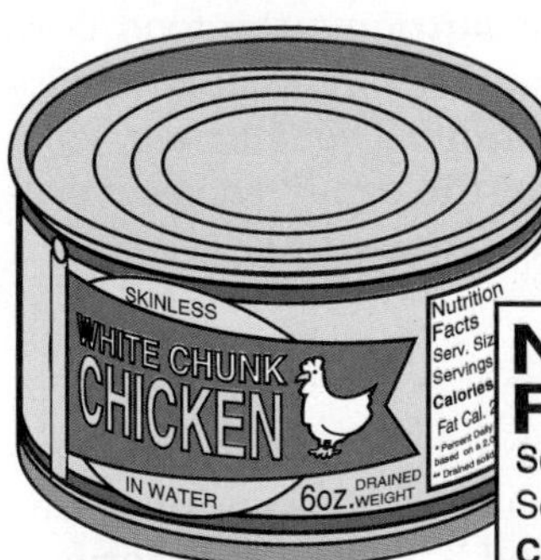

A container with fewer than 40 square inches of surface area can present fewer facts in this format.

Nutrition Facts

Serv. Size 1/3 cup (85g)**
Servings 2
Calories 111
Fat Cal. 23

*Percent Daily Values (DV) are based on a 2,000 calorie diet.
** Drained solids only

Amount/serving		%DV*	Amount/serving		%DV*
Total Fat	3g	5%	**Total Carb.**	0g	0%
Sat. Fat	1g	5%	Dietary Fiber	0g	0%
Cholest.	60mg	20%	Sugars	0g	
Sodium	200mg	8%	**Protein**	21g	

Vitamin A 0% • Vitamin C 0% • Calcium 0% • Iron 2%

Serving sizes in household and metric measures		
1 tsp	=	5 ml
1 tbsp	=	15 ml
1 cup	=	240 ml
1 fl. oz.	=	30 ml
1 oz.	=	28 g

Key		
tsp	=	teaspoon
tbsp	=	tablespoon
fl. oz.	=	fluid ounce
oz.	=	ounce
ml	=	milliliter
g	=	gram

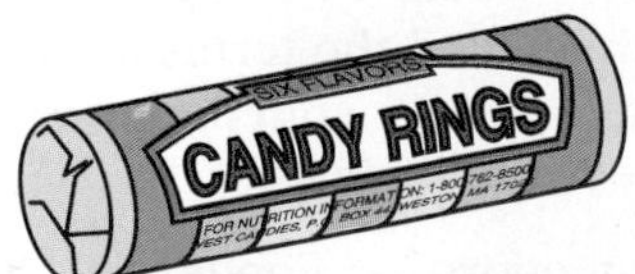

Packages with fewer than 12 square inches of surface area need not carry nutrition information, but they must provide an address or telephone number for obtaining more information.

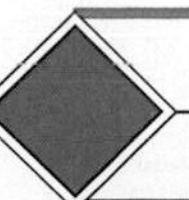

CHECKING OUT FOOD LABELS

First Facts *continued*

Table 2-9
Terms Used on Food Labels

Energy Terms

- **diet, dietetic** terms used to indicate that a food is either a *low-calorie* or a *reduced-calorie* food.
- **low calorie** containing no more than 40 cal per serving.
- **reduced calorie** containing 25 percent fewer calories per serving than a "regular" product.

Fat Terms (meat and poultry products)

- **extra lean** contains:
  - not more than 5 g of fat
  - not more than 2 g of saturated fat
  - not more than 95 mg of cholesterol per serving.
- **lean**[a] contains:
  - not more than 10 g of fat
  - not more than 4.5 g of saturated fat
  - and less than 95 mg cholesterol per serving.

Fat and Cholesterol Terms (all products)

- **fat free** containing 0.5 g or less of fat per serving.
- **low cholesterol** containing fewer than 20 mg of cholesterol per serving *and* fewer than 2 g saturated fat per serving.
- **low fat** containing 3 g or less fat per serving.
- **low saturated fat** containing 1 g or less saturated fat per serving.
- **percent fat free** may be used only if the product meets the definition of *low fat* or *fat free.* Requires disclosure of g fat per 100 g food.
- **reduced saturated fat** containing 25 percent or less of the saturated fat in the comparison food *and* reduced by more than 1 gram per serving.
- **saturated fat free** containing 0.5 g or less of saturated fat and 0.5 g or less of *trans*-fatty acids.

Other Terms

- **free, without, no, zero** containing no amount or a trivial amount. *Calorie-free* means containing fewer than 5 calories per serving; *sugar-free* or *fat-free* means containing less than half a gram per serving.
- **fresh** raw, unprocessed or minimally processed with no added preservatives.
- **good source** provides 10 to 19 percent of the Daily Value per serving.
- **healthy** a term allowable in food names, so long as the food is low in fat, saturated fat, cholesterol, and sodium.
- **high** provides 20 percent or more of the Daily Value per serving.
- **imitation food** this term must be used to describe a food intended to replace a standard food, if the replacement food lacks one or more nutrients provided by the original food. For example, imitation cheese for pizza lacks the calcium of real mozzarella cheese.
- **less, fewer** provides 25 percent less of a nutrient or calories than a reference food. This may occur naturally or as a result of altering the food. For example, pretzels, which are usually low in fat, can claim to provide less fat than potato chips, a comparable food.
- **light** this descriptor has three meanings on labels:
  1. a serving provides one-third fewer calories or half the fat of the regular product.
  2. a serving of a low-calorie, low-fat food provides half the sodium normally present.
  3. the product is light in color and texture, so long as the label makes this intent clear, as in "light brown sugar."
- **more** contains 10 percent more of the Daily Value than a comparable food. The nutrient may be added or may occur naturally.
- **reduced** altered to provide 25 percent less of a nutrient or calories than a "regular" product.

Sodium Terms

- **low sodium** containing 140 mg or fewer sodium per serving.
- **very low sodium** containing 35 mg or less sodium per serving.

[a]The word *lean* as part of the brand name (as in "Lean Supreme") indicates that the product contains fewer than 10 grams of fat per serving.

Source: The new food label, *FDA Backgrounder,* 10 December 1992; Nutrition labeling of meat and poultry products, *FSIS Backgrounder,* January 1993.

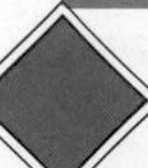

CHECKING OUT FOOD LABELS
First Facts *continued*

2. Sodium as related to hypertension (high blood pressure). Food must be **low sodium.**
3. Dietary fat and cancer. Food must be **low fat.**
4. Dietary saturated fat and cholesterol as related to coronary heart disease. Food must be **low saturated fat, low cholesterol,** and low fat.
5. Fiber-containing grain products, fruits, and vegetables and cancer. The food must be low fat, and, without added fiber, it must be a **good source** of dietary fiber.
6. Fruits, vegetables, and grain products that contain fiber, particularly soluble fiber, and risk of coronary heart disease. Foods must be low saturated fat, low fat, and low cholesterol. They must also contain at least 0.6 grams of soluble fiber (explained in Chapter 4) per serving.
7. Fruits and vegetables and cancer. Food must be low fat and, without added nutrients, it must be a good source of fiber, vitamin A, or vitamin C.[7]

These claims are permitted on food labels because they are well supported by the available scientific evidence.

The only foods permitted by law to bear health claims are ones that live up to their implied connection to health. When choosing a food that makes a health claim, you can therefore rely on some basic assumptions. Such a food cannot contain any nutrient or food constituent in an amount that increases disease risks. Specifically, a serving of the product may contain no more than 20 percent of the Daily Value for the following:

- Total fat
- Saturated fat
- Cholesterol
- Sodium

This means that whole milk, even though it is a rich source of calcium, may not make a claim about osteoporosis because it contains too much saturated fat to qualify. Low-fat and nonfat milks, however, do qualify to bear the calcium and osteoporosis claim.

Those who design labels must proceed carefully. For example, use of the word ***healthy*** in a name such as "Healthy Start" or the use of a heart-shaped logo may imply that a food is health promoting. Foods bearing such words or logos must not exceed limits set for fat, saturated fat, cholesterol, and sodium contents. An obvious exception would be a heart-shaped Valentine's Day candy box, which all but the most wishful of thinkers would know contained *un*healthy food.

A food label may say only that a substance "may" or "might" reduce disease risks. This tentative wording reflects that science is still accumulating evidence concerning the roles of diet in diseases. Also, claims must state that the development of a disease rests on many factors. A permissible health claim might look like this:

> *Development of heart disease depends on many factors. A healthful diet low in saturated fat and cholesterol may lower blood cholesterol levels and may reduce the risk of heart disease.*

Health claims on labels are so carefully controlled that they can be a great asset to consumers who would rather not worry about grams, percentages, and other mathematical speed bumps that would slow them down in grocery store aisles. Much of the math previously required of nutrition-conscious shoppers has already been performed by food manufacturers and their results are printed on the labels. Between the honest and accurate numbers, and the carefully defined words on labels, shoppers who take the time to use them can learn a lot about the foods they are buying.

FOOD FEATURE

Getting a Feel for the Nutrients in Foods

Figure 2-9 illustrates a playful contrast between two days' meals. One, labeled "Monday's Meals," shows the result of following the recommendations of this chapter. The other set of choices, "Tuesday's Meals," were chosen less for concern with nutrition and more for convenience and familiarity. The two sets of meals were made similar in energy (calories) so that other differences would stand out.

Now, how can a person compare these sets of meals with regard to their calories and energy-yielding nutrients? These days, people often use computers to perform nutrient calculations with lightning speed. This convenience may make working with paper, pencils, and erasers seem a bit old-fashioned, but for the person who puts some effort into just a few hand calculations, the benefits last a lifetime. The person soon develops a "feel" for the energy-yielding nutrients in meals and learns to size up the nutrients on plates of food just by looking at them.

Using the exchange system, you estimate the grams of carbohydrate, fat, and protein in the meals. Once you know the gram amounts of these nutrients, a few simple calculations can lead you to meaningful comparisons with dietary recommendations.

A Look Behind the Scenes: The Making of Figure 2-9 The list below explains how we used the exchange system to determine the total calories and the percentages of calories from carbohydrate, fat, and protein, in the two days' meals.

1. We assigned each food an *exchange value.*
   - Example: Each shredded wheat biscuit in Monday's meals constitutes one starch/bread exchange. Therefore, two biscuits constitute two exchanges.
2. We consulted the exchange lists in Appendix D to determine the grams of carbohydrate, protein, and fat in each type of exchange.
   - Example: Each starch/bread exchange offers 15 grams of carbohydrate/ 0 grams of fat/ 3 grams protein.
3. We summed each column of gram amounts to obtain estimates of the total grams of carbohydrate, fat, and protein for the whole day.
   - Example: 224 total grams of carbohydrate.
4. We multiplied each gram total by the appropriate number of calories per gram. The appropriate number here is 4 because each gram of carbohydrate yields 4 calories.
   - Example: 224 × 4 = 896 calories from carbohydrate.
5. We summed up all three calorie amounts to find the total calories in all the day's foods.
   - Example: 896 cal carbohydrate + 486 cal fat + 372 cal protein = 1,754 calories total.
6. Finally we used these numbers to determine percentages of calories from each of the energy-yielding nutrients. Details of percentage calculations are in Appendix C, but here is the general formula.
   - General formula: (calories from a nutrient ÷ total calories) × 100 = the percentage of calories from that nutrient.

Reminder:
carbohydrate and protein = 4 cal/g,
fat = 9 cal/g.

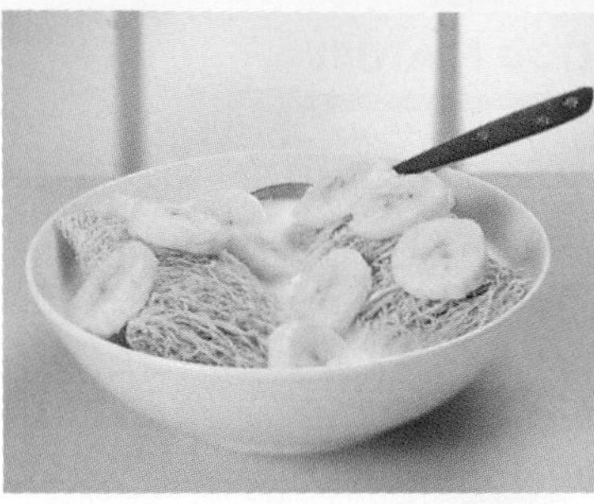

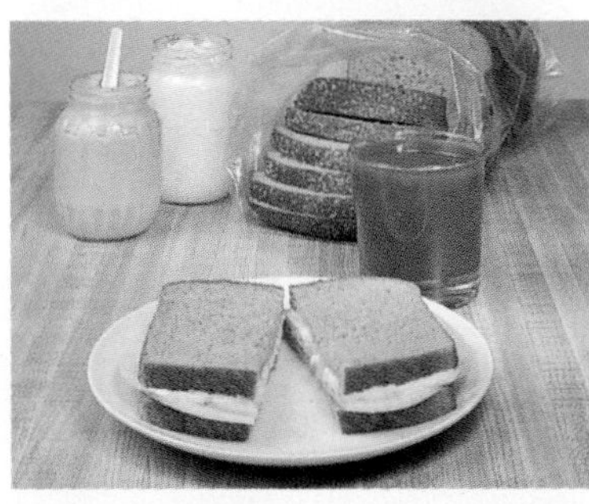

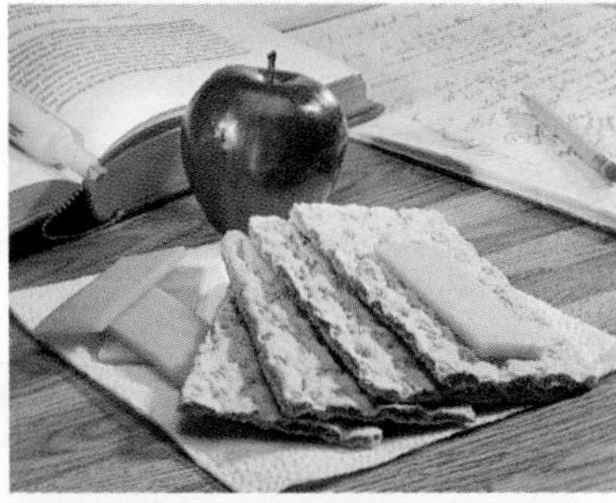

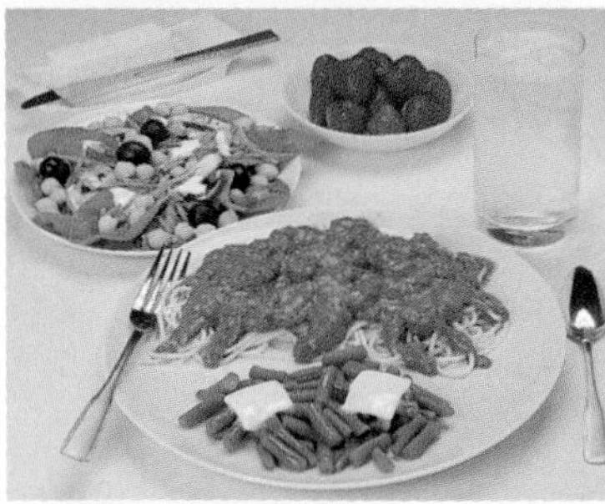

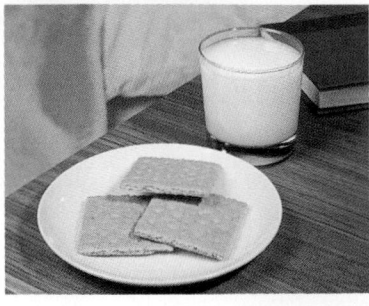

Figure 2-9

TWO DAYS' MEALS COMPARED

MONDAY'S MEALS

Monday's meals were based on nutrient dense choices from the Daily Food Guide.

Foods	**Exchanges**	**Grams Carb/Fat/Pro**
Before heading off to classes, a student eats breakfast:		
2 shredded wheat biscuits	2 starch/bread	30/0/6
1 c 1% low-fat milk	1 nonfat milk	12/0/8
½ banana (sliced)	1 fruit	15/0/0
Then goes home for a quick lunch:		
1 turkey sandwich on whole-wheat bread	[2 starch/bread	30/0/6
with mayonnaise and mustard	2 lean meat	0/6/14
	1 fat]	0/5/0
1 c vegetable juice (canned)	2 vegetable	10/0/4
While studying that afternoon, the student eats a snack:		
4 whole-wheat crackers	1starch/bread	15/0/3
1 oz cheddar cheese	1 high-fat meat	0/8/7
1 apple	1 fruit	15/0/0
That night, the student makes dinner:		
A salad made with:		
1 c raw spinach leaves, shredded carrots, and sliced mushrooms	[free	0/0/0
⅓ c garbanzo beans	1 starch/bread	15/0/3
5 lg olives and 1 tbs ranch salad dressing	2 fat]	0/10/0
A dinner of:		
1 c spaghetti with meat sauce	[2 starch/bread	30/0/6
	1 vegetable	5/0/2
	3 medium-fat meat]	0/15/21
½ c green beans	1 vegetable	5/0/2
2 tsp butter	2 fat	0/10/0
And, for dessert:		
1¼ c strawberries (fresh)	1 fruit	15/0/0
Later that evening, the student enjoys a bedtime snack:		
3 graham crackers	1 starch/bread	15/0/3
1 c 1% low-fat milk	1 nonfat milk	12/0/8

		Carb	Fat	Pro
Total calories: 1,754	**gram totals:**	224	54	93
51% cal from carbohydrate*	× cal/g	× 4	× 9	× 4
28% cal from fat*	= calories	896	486	372
21% cal from protein*	from carbohydrate, fat, and protein			

*Rounded values.

Figure 2-9

TWO DAYS' MEALS COMPARED (continued)

TUESDAY'S MEALS

Tuesday's meals are lower on the nutrient density scale.

Foods	**Exchanges**	**Grams Carb/Fat/Pro**
Today, the student starts the day with a fast-food breakfast:		
1 c coffee	free	0/0/0
1 English muffin with an egg, cheese, and bacon	[2 starch/bread	30/0/6
	1 med-fat meat	0/5/7
	1 high-fat meat	0/8/7
	1 fat]	0/5/0
Between classes, the student returns home for a quick lunch:		
1 peanut butter and jelly sandwich on white bread	[2 starch/bread	30/0/6
	1 high fat meat]	0/8/7
1 c whole milk	1 whole milk	12/8/8
While studying, the student drinks:		
12 oz diet cola	free	0/0/0
Bag of chips (14 chips)	[1 starch/bread	15/0/3
	2 fat]	0/10/0
That night for dinner, the student eats:		
A salad made with:		
1 c lettuce	free	0/0/0
1 tbs blue cheese dressing	1 fat	0/5/0
A dinner of:		
6 oz steak	6 lean meat	0/18/42
½ baked potato (large) with 1 tbs butter	[1 starch/bread	15/0/3
and 1 tbs sour cream	3½ fat]	0/18/0
12 oz diet cola	free	0/0/0
And, for dessert:		30/0/6
4 sandwich-type cookies	[2 starch/bread	0/10/0
	2 fat]	

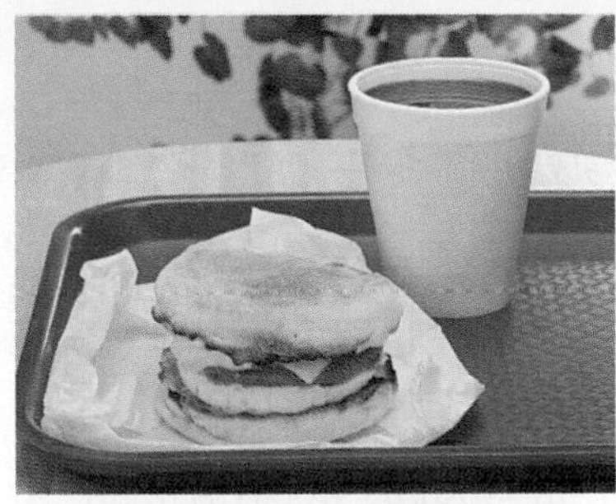

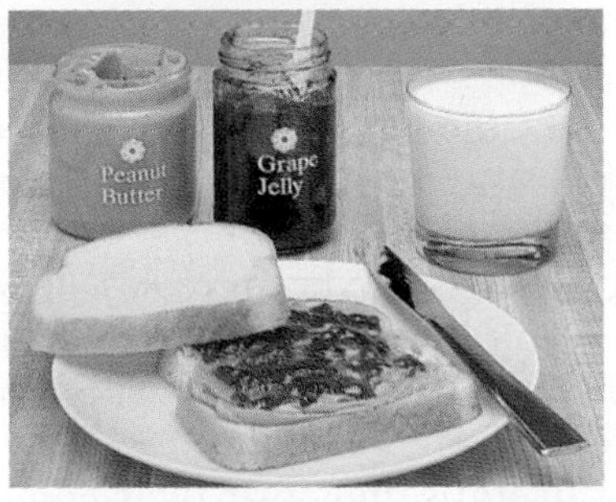

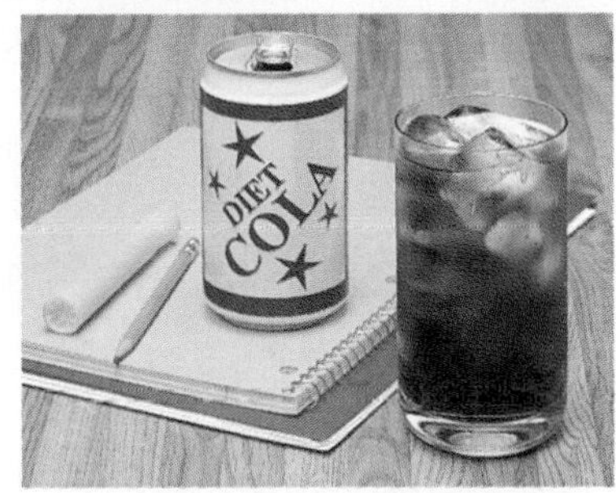

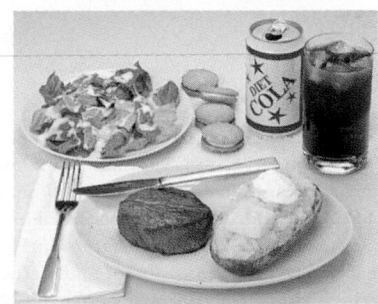

		Carb	Fat	Pro
Total calories: 1,763	**gram totals:**	132	95	95
30% cal from carbohydrate*	**× cal/g**	× 4	× 9	× 4
49% cal from fat*	**= calories**	528	855	380
22% cal from protein*	**from carbohydrate, fat, and protein**			

*Rounded values.

- Example: (896 calories from carbohydrate ÷ 1,754 total calories) × 100 = 51% of calories from carbohydrate.

7. We compared the percentages of nutrients from these meals with the recommendations made in Table 2-2 earlier.

To see how fat and protein percentages work out, check example 4 in Appendix C.

Compared with recommendations to obtain 55 percent of calories from carbohydrate, the meals listed for Monday came close, with 51 percent. Tuesday's meals, however, fell far short, providing just 30 percent of calories from carbohydrate. Table 2-2 also makes the recommendation to hold fat intakes to 30 percent of calories. Tuesday's meals, with 49 percent of calories from fat, exceeded this recommendation by far. Future chapters will clarify the health significance of these figures. Also notice that the person choosing Monday's meals is able to consume more food, and so more nutrients, for fewer calories. Monday's meals are more nutrient dense.

Five steps to finding the percentages of calories from carbohydrate, fat, and protein in a meal:

1. Apply the exchange system to estimate the grams of carbohydrate, fat, and protein.
2. Total the grams of each energy nutrient in the day's meals.
3. Multiply the grams of each nutrient by calories per gram.
4. Add to obtain total calories.
5. Apply the percentage formula once for each nutrient:
(one nutrient's cal ÷ total cal) × 100 = % of cal from that nutrient.

Computers may be miracles of ease and speed, but they are rarely available on line with diners in cafeterias or fast food counters where real-life decisions must be made. Those who can "see" the nutrients in their foods can make informed choices before eating meals, while others must wait until they visit their computers to find out how well they did in choosing.

◆ Notes

1. Food and Nutrition Board, *Recommended Dietary Allowances*, 10th ed. (Washington, D.C.: National Academy of Sciences, 1989).
2. R. K. Johnson and coauthors, Maternal employment and the quality of young children's diets: Empirical evidence based on the 1987–1988 Nationwide Food Consumption Survey, *Pediatrics* 90 (1992): 245–249. This is but one of many studies using RDA values to draw conclusions concerning adequacy of the diet.
3. J. Hallfrisch and coauthors, Acceptability of a 7-day higher-carbohydrate, lower-fat menu: The Beltsville Diet Study, *Journal of the American Dietetic Association* 88 (1988): 163–168.
4. M. J. Franz, Diabetes and nutrition: State of the science and the art, *Topics in Clinical Nutrition* 3 (1988): 1–16.
5. J. E. Foulke, Cooking up the new food label, *FDA Consumer*, May 1993, pp. 33–38.
6. M. Segal, What's in a food? *FDA Consumer*, April 1993, 14–18.
7. D. Farley, Claim specifics, *FDA Consumer*, May 1993, pp. 20–21.

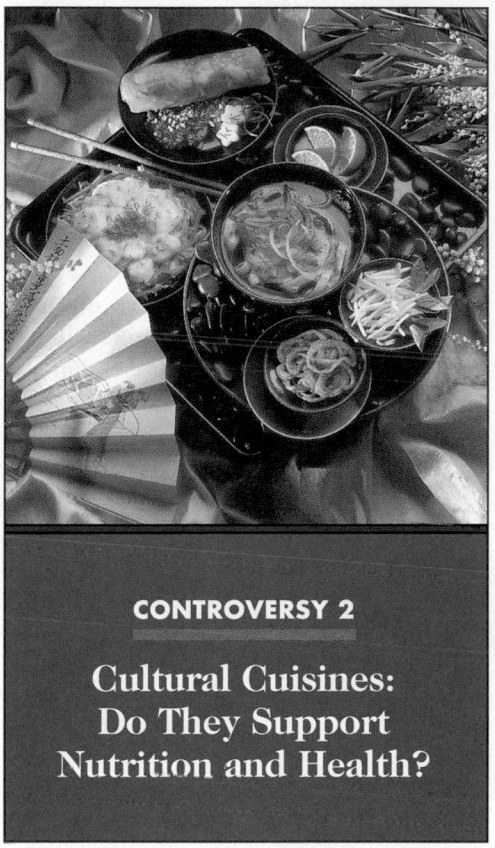

CONTROVERSY 2

Cultural Cuisines: Do They Support Nutrition and Health?

Do some foodways support health better than others? This section presents a few of the many ethnic foodways to show how basic diet-planning principles can apply to all sorts of cuisines. A study of food-ways is especially important to anyone who counsels another in nutrition. To be useful, the advice must honor the learner's own preferences among the many possible eating patterns of human beings on earth, and it must take into account the built-in health benefits of many ethnic ways of eating.

Ethnic foods have all become an integral part of the "American diet," and can be held to the same diet principles described in the preceding chapter. The variety provided by ethnic foods can help ensure adequacy, but only moderation helps to control energy and fat intakes. How then can people choose ethnic meals that will benefit them? Keep this question in mind as you read the following sections.

NORTHERN EUROPEAN INFLUENCE Immigrants from northern Europe vastly influenced traditional American home cooking. For example, an evening meal of a hearty portion of roasted meat; side dishes of mashed potatoes or boiled cabbage, and bread; and fruit pie for dessert characterizes the cuisines of Germany, England, and Ireland. Immigrants from those countries brought this meal plan with them to the New World, and it typifies evening meals across the United States. Variations on the plan are numerous: a New England boiled dinner includes corned (spiced and cured) beef boiled together with potatoes, carrots, and cabbage; Brunswick stew simmers game, pork, or poultry along with corn, tomatoes, and onions. Even a Thanksgiving turkey dinner with all the trimmings follows the scheme. Traditionally, people have filled their plates with meat and served starches and vegetables on the side. Today's health advice, however, would be to load each plate with tasty vegetables and grains and limit the meat to a 2 to 3-ounce portion.

Another familiar meal of northern European derivation is the "American" breakfast of eggs with bacon and biscuits. While the English serve baked beans with breakfast, Americans may choose potatoes or grits. The English choice here might hold an advantage: including legumes at breakfast provides a needed fiber boost. More fruit, less protein and fat, and a lower-fat choice of bread would improve it further.

Every eating style has advantages and drawbacks. The Northern European style of eating provides abundant protein and ensures adequacy of all the nutrients associated with meat. It delivers a lot of fat, though, and is short on fiber and the vitamins and minerals associated with fruits and vegetables. People who eat as the northern Europeans do can improve their nutrition by reducing meat portion sizes, by cutting down on added fats, and by choosing more whole grains, fruits, and vegetables.

The famed cuisines of France have influenced the cuisines of neighboring Italy, the British Isles, and Ireland and are among the world's most popular foodways. The French expertly combine butter, cream, eggs, and wine into classic sauces. Meats and vegetables, fragrant with herbs, often provide carriers for the sauces. A party spread (pâté) is made with chopped liver, seasonings, and fat. Pastry crusts hold meats in rich sauces for main dishes, or pastry may wrap sweetened fruits for dessert. "A la mode" is the French way of asking for a topper of ice cream on a dessert.

All the choices just named make for extraordinarily high-fat meals, but the considerable pleasures of eating French food can be enjoyed without harm to health. A suggestion to "keep it simple" can lead you to discover a wonderful, lesser-known side to country French cuisine: elegant clear soups (with no toasted cheese on top); steamed and poached seafood (hold the buttery or creamy sauces); many foods prepared in wine sauces; layered "gratins" of vegetables (not cheese);

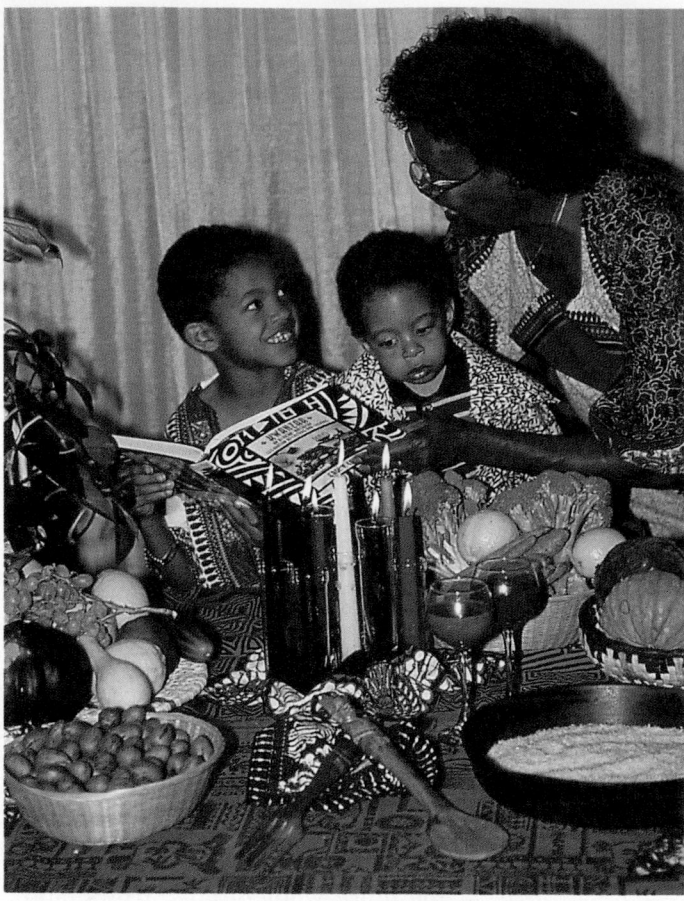

Ethnic meals and family gatherings help maintain ethnic traditions.

herb-seasoned baked vegetables (with no added butter); mixtures of fruit (without pastry crusts); stews of beans or vegetables flavored with lean meat and surprise nonfat seasonings such as oranges; and huge loaves of french bread—fluffy on the inside with crispy crust just right for soaking up light sauces.

The popular notion that daily consumption of red wine protects the French and other peoples of the Mediterranean region against heart disease, while not proved, may have some validity. Studies do show low rates of heart disease in populations that use moderate amounts of wine (red or white) as a beverage with meals. Other correlations have not been ruled out, though, and correlations are not causes. Small doses of alcohol seem to provide some cardiovascular protection (see Controversy 11), but a person considering using wine for the heart must also consider the other ways that alcohol impacts on the body. French people are much more likely to contract cancer of the stomach and esophagus than are those in the United States, and they suffer many times the cases of cirrhosis of the liver as a direct result of high alcohol intakes. Additionally, high intakes of alcohol can *damage* the heart.[1] Still, the French have heart disease rates lower than U.S. rates, despite a similar intake of fat. Some alternative explanations are suggested by insights into other Mediterranean diets (section below).

French influence on cuisines of the United States can be seen clearly in the bayou regions of Louisiana. The French Acadians from Canada who settled in southern Louisiana preserved their French country-cooking heritage and easily adapted it to the local Louisiana food supply. Today their descendants have made Cajun food popular with people across the nation.

Along with Acadian French influence, African-American culture also steered the evolution of Cajun culture, where high value is placed on traditional parties and festivals centered on food. Cajun dishes include spicy stews (gumbo, jambalaya) thickened with a roux (flour mixed with oil and heated until toasty brown), sausages, hot red pepper sauce, red beans and rice, seafood, and dirty rice (rice made brown with chopped chicken livers and seasonings). These dishes are celebrations in their own right. Cajun coffee brewed with chicory root often accompanies puffed and sugared doughnuts known as beignets (pronounced ben-YAY).

Many Cajun foods perfectly meet the recommendations presented in Chapter 2. Nutritionists agree with enthusiastic diners that red beans and rice is a classic dish—full of flavor from expert use of spice and abundant in carbohydrate, protein, and fiber, while low in fat. A jambalaya (stew) of seafood (crawfish, shrimp, froglegs, or redfish), tomatoes, vegetables, and rice seasoned with a little strong-flavored sausage is packed with vitamins and minerals, adequate in protein, rich in carbohydrate, and usually low in fat. By limiting such choices as deep-fried seafoods and beignets, Cajun food enthusiasts can easily achieve the goals embodied in the Dietary Guidelines.

MEDITERRANEAN DIETS AND THE HEART Coastal populations that share the bounty found in Mediterranean waters may also share some important health advantages. Mediterranean peoples die less frequently of heart disease and certain cancers than do people of northern Europe and North America.[2] While popular sources report marvels of "the Mediterranean diet," scientists who have attempted to precisely define that diet or to state conclusively what effects one can expect from eating it have run into problems.[3] One problem is that diets of the Mediterranean region are those of Italy, Spain, Portugal, France, and Greece, and all differ substantially from each other. Also, some of the data backing claims about causes of death in those countries were collected in the 1960s, a time when the majority of people there still consumed traditional diets uninfluenced by Western trends. Still, even with limitations, the links between Mediterranean diets and health are worth pondering.

Today's Greek and Italian cuisines, for example, stem from among the most ancient human foodways on earth.[4] Ancient Greeks and Romans ate mostly grain foods such as breads and cakes, along with seeds including lentils and beans, fish and other seafoods, goat cheese, vegetables, and fruits (especially grapes and figs). They ate meat on special occasions only, and drank wine diluted half-and-half with water. The favored cooking fat in those days was oil pressed from olives; butter was shunned as a "food of barbarians." In modern U.S. terms, the ancient Greek and Roman diets fit fairly well into the pattern put forth by our own Daily Food Guide. Unfortunately, no one knows much about the causes of death in those days, but it is believed that the people lived only to the age of 40 years or so, dying in war, in childbirth, or from infectious diseases. Few lived long enough to develop heart disease or cancer.

Today, Greeks are known for a robust cuisine that includes whole broiled fish and other seafoods; roasts and stews of vegetables such as eggplant with lamb, chicken, or beef; and the flavors of fresh lemons, garlic, and herbs (dill, mint, and parsley); and, always, olives and their oil, which lavishly season many dishes.[5] Traditional Greek salads lack lettuce but combine chunks of tomato, peppers, cucumbers, onions, a salty cheese (feta), anchovies, and cured ripe olives with a tangy olive oil and lemon dressing. A famous Greek soup of eggs and lemon juice may also top stuffed grape leaves or other leaves. Gyros (pronounced YEE-roce, meaning "a circle" in Greek) is a large cone of high-fat, highly seasoned ground meat that slowly turns as it roasts over open flames. When cooked, the gyros is thinly sliced, dressed with yogurt and cucumber, and served in a pita (pocket) bread as the original lunchmeat sandwich. As for Greek desserts, small wedges of honey-soaked pastry (baklava) and other nutty pastries are traditional at celebrations. Because of their intense sweetness, small servings of these desserts usually satisfy the eaters.

At first glance, the Greek diet seems startlingly high in fat. It contains up to 42 percent of its calories as fat, mostly from olive oil and olives.[6] According to U.S. guidelines, the Greek population would be urged to eat less fat and to lose weight to protect their hearts. Yet Greeks living in Greece enjoy one of the longest life expectancies worldwide (1986 data) and less often die from cardiovascular disease than Westerners, despite the tendency of many Greeks to carry excess body fat.[7] These facts have led to the suggestion that a diet similar to that of Greece might be better and easier to follow than the very-low-fat diet traditionally prescribed in the United States for improving the health of the heart.[8]

Like Greece, Italy also relies on the Mediterranean Sea for seafoods, but the cuisine of Italy is perhaps best known here for its pastas and pizza. Almost everybody in the United States likes Italian foods. What teenager would turn down a slice of pizza, a food native to Naples? Who wouldn't like spumone—ice cream with fruits, nuts, and flavorings?

The cuisines of Italy differ from north to south of the so-called pasta line. Generally people living in the northern regions of that country consume abundant meat, butter, cheese, eggs, and cream to accompany pasta and baked cornmeal (polenta). In the southern regions, the diet is more "Mediterranean" in character; wheat pastas are most often served with vegetables such as artichokes, eggplants, peppers, and tomatoes. Beans appear on the table more often than meat, and all dishes are seasoned with olive oil, not butter. Northern pastas are egg based and usually ribbon shaped or stuffed like dumplings (tortellini), while southern varieties are made without eggs and are shaped more like macaroni.

Many Italian dishes receive high marks in nutritional balance and adequacy. The abundant vegetables and pasta, eggplant and tomatoes, and bean and pasta soups are high in nutrients. Unlike the Greeks, Southern Italians also keep total fat intakes low.[9] Heart disease death rates are low among natives of Italy (and neighboring Spain), so advisors of those countries are reluctant to suggest "improvements" for their diets.[10]

Some questions surrounding Mediterranean diets remain unanswered. For example, while heart disease rates may be low in Mediterranean countries, no one can explain why the incidence of stroke is almost double that of the United States. If a diet can receive the credit for heart health, should it also be blamed for increased incidence of stroke?

Also, while the link between diet and heart disease overall is strong, no one knows for sure what part of the diet might be beneficial in this regard. Many think using olive oil instead of butter or shortening is the key factor affecting the heart, but others point to the protective effects of both nutrients and nonnutrients found in vegetables, seafoods, or seasonings.[11] They say that while fat may play a role, an antioxidant effect from constituents of plant foods is probably more important in defending the heart. (More about antioxidants appears in Chapters 7 and 11.) Active lifestyles may play a role, as may differences in tobacco use; exercise reduces heart disease risk and smoking greatly increases it.

WEST AFRICAN FOODS IN THE DEEP SOUTH When you spread peanut butter on your bread, do you know you are eating an African food? Actually peanut *butter* is considered an American food, invented by George Washington Carver, an agricultural scientist. However, peanuts and peanut paste have always been staple foods of Africans and were brought to U.S. soil by African slaves. If you have ever eaten boiled peanuts, today a southern specialty, you have partaken of a dish that emerged with the origins of humankind in Africa. Similarly, okra and blackeye (cow) peas are of African origin.

African crops tended on Southern agricultural plantations were eaten by everyone living there. Often African foods accompanied native American greens, sweet potatoes, and wild fish and game. Today's rural southern cuisine varies little between African Americans and people of European descent.

Southern food provides ample vitamins and minerals from collards and other greens, okra, tomatoes, meats, and corn. Sweet potatoes are a rich source of vitamin A, starch, and fiber and are naturally low in fat. Cajun seafood gumbo (similar to an African dish of the same name) was already mentioned as a nutritious mixture of low-fat foods.

Unfortunately, many southern meals are perilously rich in fat: salted pork, smoked bacon and its fat, or lard flavor some traditional dishes, and others are fried in fats. A favored southern treat, fried green tomatoes, gains its tangy taste from unripe (green) tomatoes that are dipped in spicy cornmeal batter and deep fried. Biscuits, a bread of choice, are made with almost as much shortening as flour and are often served with butter or fat-rich gravy. Recipes for buttery, nut-filled pecan pie are a source of family pride. For people choosing these treats, moderation is a worthy goal.

Southerners also like large servings of high-fat, high-salt meats, such as fried chicken, fatty pork cuts or sausages, and spareribs, greatly overemphasizing protein and fat in the diet while shorting whole grains, fruits, and vegetables. Southerners of rural areas often suffer the ills associated with too much fat and salt: heart disease, hypertension, obesity, and diabetes. The trick to choosing health-promoting rural southern food is to choose plain baked sweet potatoes and other vegetables, braised meats and stews, beans and rice, cooked greens, and cornbread; and to avoid the fatty, salty fried meats and vegetables, biscuits, and gravies.

NATIVE AMERICAN DIETS Within 200 years, Native Americans have seen unprecedented changes in their foodways. Hunter-gatherer and agricultural lifestyles of history have given way to a modern culture relying on fast foods, alcohol, abundant high-fat meats, and dairy products. Figure C2-1 shows how some of these changes affect nutrient intakes. Researchers conclude that for Native Americans, the effects of the changes on health have been overwhelmingly negative.

A well-studied example of a group that suffers the effects of a "modernized" diet are the Pima Indian tribe of central Arizona. For thousands of years up to 1930, the Pima diet consisted of wild and cultivated desert legumes, cactus leaves and fruit, fish, venison (deer meat), small seeds, mesquite pods, acorns, and corn.[12] In 1930, a change began. The tribe largely replaced their traditional wild foods, which had become scarce, with modern ones such as wheat flour, lard, sugar, coffee, and ready-to-eat cereals that were easily obtained. The result has been tragic—the Pima now suffer the highest per capita rate of diabetes known among any people in the world.[13] Likewise, the Sioux Indians rarely ever suffered heart disease when consuming their traditional diets, but now suffer one of the highest known rates of heart and artery disease.

Both the Pima and Sioux tribes changed not only their diets, but also their highly active lifestyles. Modern-day Pima and Sioux no longer hunt game on the windswept plains, toil in the fields, or cook over stone fireplaces as their ancestors once did. They now drive to supermarkets to purchase convenience foods to cook in microwave ovens. The Sioux also traded their occasional ceremonial pipes for daily cigarette smoking, a new habit that is especially damaging to the heart.

While changed diets and lifestyles almost certainly contributed to the changes in Native American health, a researcher points out that, "we've seen very large differences in risk factors and also fairly sizable differences in disease rates" between tribes, despite a universal adoption of modern foods and television watching.[14] Native diets are not perfect, either. They may not provide adequate amounts of some nutrients, and availability of foods depends on such unpredictable factors as weather changes and herd movements. While modern foods are usually safe and sanitary, Native Alaskans eating traditional foods suffer more botulism (a deadly food poisoning) than any other group worldwide. Modern descen-

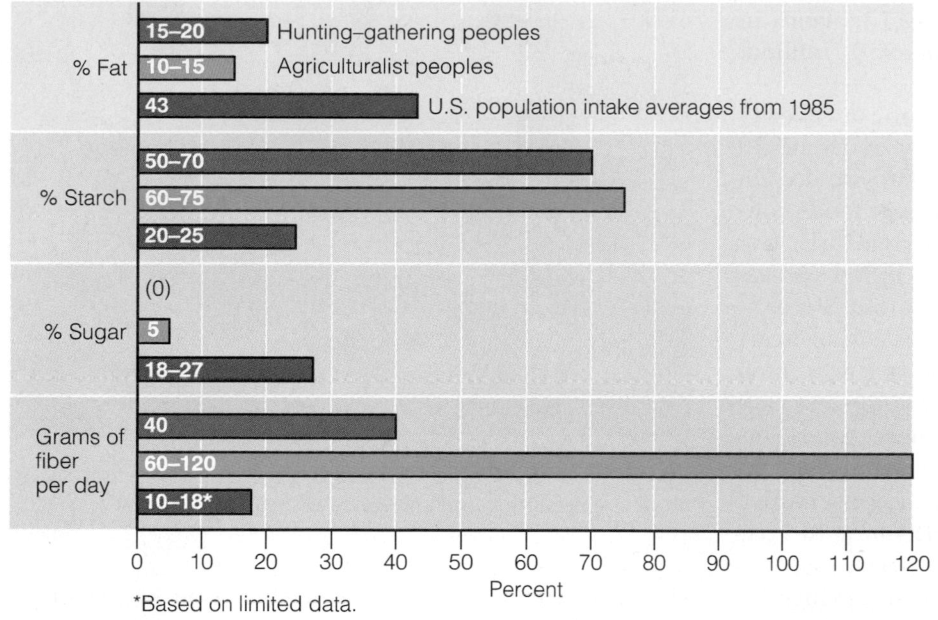

Figure C2-1

SOME DIFFERENCES BETWEEN NATIVE DIETS AND AFFLUENT DIETS

The percentages referred to here are the percent of total daily caloric intake.

Source: Data for hunter-gatherers and agriculturists from WHO Study Group, Diet, nutrition, and the prevention of chronic diseases, World Health Organization Technical Report Series 797 (Geneva: WHO, 1990): 43; Data for U.S. population averages from *Diet and Health: Implications for Reducing Chronic Disease Risk* (Washington, D.C.: National Academy Press, 1989), pp. 41–84.

dants changed the ancient methods of preserving meat, fish, and blubber (fat) in slight but critical ways that encourage the growth of the bacteria that cause botulism.[15] The point is that all diets, even those that have supported human beings through many centuries, have drawbacks. Still, by studying them, scientists are beginning to believe that when Native Americans consumed their original high-fiber, low-fat native foods, their hearts and bodies benefited.

MEXICAN ETHNIC FOODS In a Mexican restaurant you can order beautiful plates of complex food mixtures—tortillas filled with meats and cheeses, some fried and crisp and others baked and soft, along with flavored rice, refried beans, sour cream, guacamole (avocado sauce), and salsa (tomato sauce). These foods are of Mexican origin, but they are not the day-to-day fare of Mexican families, although they are typical of festive foods prepared for special occasions. A normal Mexican lunch or supper is simple, perhaps offering a stew of beans, meat, rice, and potatoes served with tortillas or bread, tomato salsa, and lettuce salad or cooked vegetable.[16] A Mexican breakfast might include tortillas and eggs.

As familiar as the hamburger place, taco stands sell fast food to millions of U.S. diners each day. Fancier Mexican places have also caught on. If carefully chosen, these foods can make valuable contributions to the diet. Many traditional Mexican dishes (even the fast-food type) provide beans in abundance. Beans are high in nutrient density and fiber while low in fat, although the refried variety may be cooked with lard. Soft corn tortillas filled with beans, lettuce, and salsa with a side order of rice are a nutritious choice. Slightly different choices bring an extraordinarily high-fat meal, such as a fried tortilla shell filled with commercial-grade, high-fat ground beef and topped with cheese and sour cream.

Mexican cuisine presents choices that determine whether meals benefit the diner's health or harm it. For the special occasion meal described earlier, the wise diner avoids adding sour cream and skips the fried varieties of stuffed tortillas. A dish called fajita—lean meats, marinated and sizzled on a grill, wrapped in soft tortillas with chili salsa toppings—is low in fat. Salsa (a spicy sauce, usually of tomatoes) is rich in vitamins and zest but adds no fat burden to the meal. As for high-fat guacamole, you needn't avoid this avocado mixture altogether. The type of fat avocados contain is not thought to contribute to disease risk; they are fattening, however, and should be limited by people who tend to gain weight.

THE CHINESE ADVANTAGE Tried and true, the diet of China has supported the health of people there for thousands of years. The foodways of China reflect that economy is essential in a land crowded with more than 1000 people per acre and where only 10 percent of the land can be used to grow food. China has over a billion people, of whom 75 percent are involved in agriculture. Contrast these figures with the United States:

population density—people per acre—113; land in farms—about 50 percent; population—250 million; farmers—1 to 2 percent.

There seems to be little malnutrition or obesity among Chinese people, even though they consume 20 percent more calories of food each day than we do. On the whole, Chinese people eating traditional foods consume a diet nutritionally similar to the agriculturist diet depicted in Figure C2-1, and they have blood cholesterol values about half of those in the United States.[17] Only four of each 100,000 Chinese males die of heart disease each year, while 67 of each 100,000 U.S. men do so. Chinese living in China also suffer much less cancer of the colon and rectum than do Chinese Americans who have adopted a Western diet.[18] It seems worthwhile to study the fine points of a diet so conservative of resources yet so supportive of health—not to convince you to eat all Chinese meals but perhaps to encourage you to adopt some of its governing principles and to apply them to foods of all origins.

Chinese meals do not follow the separate meat-vegetable-starch pattern of northern European origin. The vegetables and meats are cooked together, each flavor complementing the other. The total amount of meat (or fish or egg) in a Chinese dish is very small by Western standards; instead, there is abundant rice at almost every meal. The Chinese also usually partake of soup or tea throughout each meal. Meals center on a staple starch food (every diner has a personal rice dish), with other foods chosen according to each person's appetite (from family-style serving dishes).

Vegetables and fruits provide variety, and subtle flavors in main dishes come largely from fat-free seasonings and sauces such as ginger root, scallions, rice wine, garlic, hoisin sauce, oyster sauce, bean sauce, and plum sauce. In traditional recipes, most sauces add tasty flavors but no fat, unlike our gravies, butter, or sour cream. Just a tablespoon or two of peanut oil cooks an entire dish.

Cooking foods the Chinese way preserves nutrients. The water in which rice is cooked may dissolve nutrients, but then it soaks back into the rice rather than being drained away, so the nutrients are retained. All food is cut into bite-sized pieces before cooking so that it will be easy to eat with chopsticks; cooking finely cut-up food requires only short times and so destroys few nutrients. No extra water is used, and none is thrown away, so nutrients are not lost that way either.

The Chinese diet and cooking techniques are also land efficient, as they must be in view of the scarcity of agricultural land and fuels. Nearly all of the calories come from plants rather than animals. A million calories in wheat or rice can be produced on less than an acre of land; a million calories in beef require 17 acres. In a world in which fuel and land are becoming increasingly scarce, the Chinese way of eating offers a model to other nations.

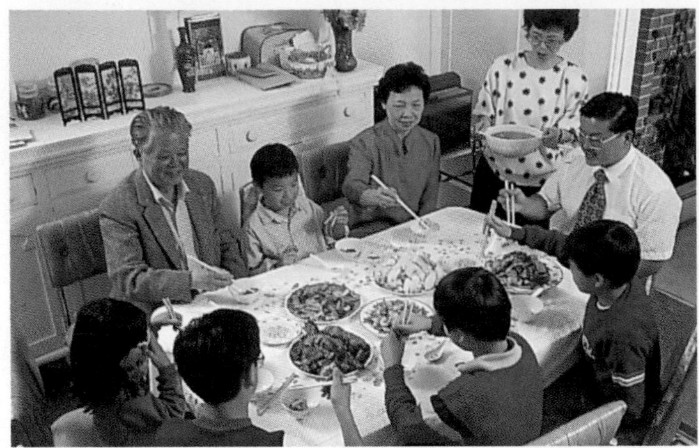

Sharing and enjoying traditional foodways is one way to show appreciation and tolerance of others.

Some Chinese dishes do have nutrition drawbacks, though. Some recipes are high in sodium, and deep-fried dishes are very high in fats. In China, deep-fried foods are eaten only seldom, but Chinese restaurants in this country feature them often and the cooks often prepare foods with extra fats and meats to appeal to U.S. appetites. Another drawback to traditional Chinese diets is the inclusion of many salted, fermented pickles. Diets high in such foods have been linked to a high incidence of digestive tract cancers. Dishes served in Chinese restaurants rarely include these fermented items because they are not suited to Western tastes.

THE CHANGING JAPANESE DIET Traditional Japanese cuisine bears similarities to the Chinese diet. Grains such as rice or millet form the bulk of most traditional Japanese meals. Vegetables and fruits are next in prominence, and seafood, eggs, poultry, and meats play supporting roles. For a favored traditional snack, a Japanese commuter might stop by a "noodle house" for a bowl of noodles in a clear, seasoned broth—a dish of Chinese origin. A Japanese delicacy popular in the United States is sushi—vinegar-flavored rice holding bits of colorful vegetables and seafood, wrapped in a seaweed wrapper and served with horseradish or seasoned soy sauce. In the United States, the word *sushi* has come to mean "raw fish" because the dish sometimes contains raw fish, but sushi actually refers to vinegared rice, and many types of sushi are made with cooked ingredients. Sushi delights diners visually, as do most traditional Japanese foods in Japan. The visual imagery created on the plate is at least as important as the taste of the food.

Since the 1950s, Japan has undergone astounding social and economic changes from a rural developing country struggling to feed its population to an industrial and economic world leader. Today, Japan's cuisine reflects the "hurry-up" lifestyle of a nation buzzing with mass communications media, high incomes, and high expenses. Time-consuming, home-cooked traditional dishes, while still favored in restaurants, have proved impractical for the two-income family of the 1990s.

In a land where rice once occupied center stage at every meal, meats, bread, and milk products now dominate. Meat consumption in Japan has jumped more than tenfold over that of the 1940s.[19] Egg intakes have risen more than sixfold in the same period. Vegetable intakes have fallen precipitously, and margarine intakes have more than doubled. Japanese families choose microwaveable frozen entrees, instant noodle and curry mixes, precooked hamburgers, and fried shrimp. Ice cream has replaced fruit as the preferred dessert, and instant coffee is replacing tea. High-fat snacks from hamburger places, southern-fried chicken restaurants, and doughnut shops have shoved low-fat noodles into the background. In fact, the new Japanese consumer delights in imported foods: kiwi from New Zealand, prepared foods from Thailand, and mangoes and avocados from the tropics are gaining in popularity.[20]

The health implications of such changes are turning out to be two sided. On one side, deaths in Japan had been declining steadily through the last decade as modern sanitation and immunizations brought infectious diseases under control. In the last two years, however, this trend may have begun a reversal due to the numbers of heart attacks and strokes edging upward. Japanese men who grew up consuming a "Western" diet are more likely to suffer from diabetes than are men who grew up on traditional Japanese diets, and diabetes is a risk factor for heart disease.[21] On the other side, the new diet provides much more protein than a traditional rice-based diet, and extra protein during the growing years has allowed the younger generation to grow taller and stronger than any generation before them.[22] In general, Japan still enjoys a lower overall rate of heart disease than many other nations, but new choices present new risks.[23]

People in the United States who wish to dine in the Japanese style can freely choose from traditional dishes, wary only of a few battered and deep-fried meats and vegetables (tempuras). A traditional Japanese chef may

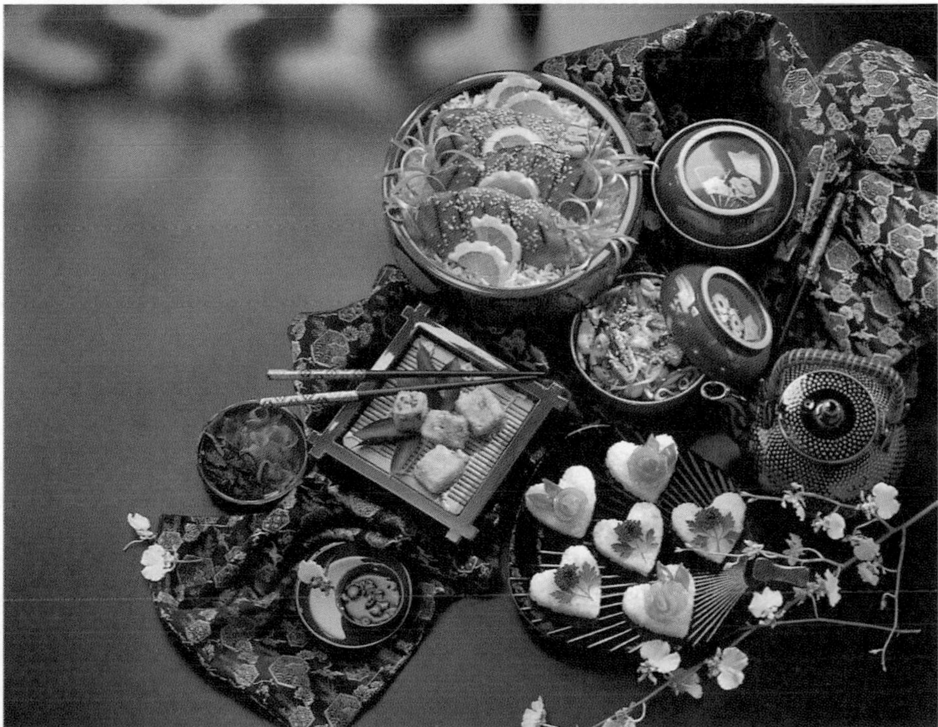

The visual imagery of Japanese food is at least as important as its taste.

Table C2-1
Characteristics of Selected Ethnic Diets

Staple Foods	Strengths of the Diet	Weaknesses of the Diet
Hispanic Americans from Cuba, Haiti, Puerto Rico		
Include: ■ steamed rice; wheat breads. ■ starchy vegetables (beans, cassavas, yams, pumpkins, yuccas); mangoes; bananas; bread; fruit; guavas; pineapples; papaya; plantains; green peppers; tomatoes; garlic. ■ dried, salted fish; goat, chicken, pork. ■ milk custard; cheeses; ice cream. ■ lard; olive oil; sugar; jams and jellies; sweet pastries; sugared fruit juices; coffee. *Exclude:* ■ green, leafy vegetables; milk as a beverage for adults; fish other than dried and salted.	Provides adequate protein, many other nutrients, and fiber	May provide too much fat, especially animal fat; may lack calcium
Hispanic Americans from Mexico, Central America		
Include: ■ steamed rice, corn and flour tortillas; hominy ■ many varieties of beans; chili peppers; tomatoes; mangoes; prickly pear fruit; cactus leaves and fruit; squashes. ■ meat and sausages; fish; poultry; eggs; seeds and nuts. ■ milk cheeses; milk custards and bread puddings. ■ lard; chocolate and coffee drinks; cakes; pastries. *Exclude:* ■ green, leafy vegetables; yellow vegetables; milk as a beverage for adults.	Most nutrients can be obtained	Is high in calories and fat, especially saturated fat, and high in sugar

toss together a mixture of mushrooms, carrots, and bamboo shoots with bits of seafood or meat; season it with fat-free (but salty) soy sauce; add sesame seeds; and serve it with a large portion of rice. Shrimp in rice-cake soup presents a clear broth, mushrooms, shrimp, and spinach and is served with mochi (rice cakes). A fish-and-noodle casserole might contain a lean fish fillet, broth seasoned with sugar, soy sauce, and mirin (a syrupy rice wine) with a big bowl of thick noodles. Beware of any restaurant that claims to serve traditional Japanese meals but then focuses the meals on large portions of meat. Such meals may be consumed by today's Japanese diners, but they are not traditional cuisine, and they carry the same drawbacks that accompany northern European-style foodways.

Many other cuisines and foodways are of interest. Table C2-1 lists some of them, with brief descriptions of some foods that characterize each.

RELIGIOUS DIETARY TRADITIONS A discussion of ethnic foodways would not be complete without mention of foodways practiced by some of the world's major religious groups. Special food rituals and ceremonies help give religious groups, like national groups, their distinct identity.

The Jewish laws set forth an extensive set of dietary rules obeyed by Orthodox Jews worldwide: they eat only foods that are fit to eat according to the Jewish bible, the *Torah*, which sets the laws. These foods are called *kosher*, a term that does not mean types of foods

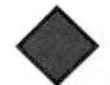

Table C2-1
Characteristics of Selected Ethnic Diets (continued)

Staple Foods	Strengths of the Diet	Weaknesses of the Diet
African Americans from West Indies, Central or South America and Recent African Immigrants		
Include: ■ millet, corn, wheat, rice, or barley. ■ starchy roots such as cassavas, yams; plantains; bananas; coconuts; peanuts; fresh fruits; hot peppers; tomatoes; onions; okra. ■ palm oil; fruit wine; tea; coffee; honey; molasses. *Exclude:* ■ milk and milk products; meat and fish limited use.	Is low in fat and salt; is high in fiber	Is low in calcium, iron, and vitamin B_{12}; is potentially low in protein, depending on availability of foods
Korean Americans from South Korea		
Include: ■ rice; noodles. ■ leafy vegetables; kimchi (hot pickled cabbage); sea vegetables; hot peppers; seasonal fruits; mushrooms. ■ small fish with bones; grilled beef; chicken; squid, octopus, and lobster; mussels; eggs. ■ fermented milk beverage (kefir). ■ tea; lard and vegetable fat for frying; sesame oil; nuts and seeds; ginger; sugar as seasoning. *Exclude:* ■ cheeses, fresh milk, butter.	Is adequate in protein	Is high in fat; is monotonous in winter (kimchi is served at each meal, to the exclusion of other vegetables); without the traditional small fish with bones, calcium can be lacking
Vietnamese Americans from Vietnam		
Include: ■ rice, rice noodles; french bread and croissants. ■ hot peppers; curries of asparagus and potatoes; salads; tropical fruits and vegetables; lemons and limes. ■ small portions of poultry; eggs; fish pâtés; nuoc nam (a strong, fermented fish sauce). ■ sweets, candies, sweetened drinks; coffee; tea; butter. *Exclude:* ■ milk and milk products.		Can be low in iron or calcium

such as pickles, bagels, lox, or corned beef, but foods prepared according to the laws of the *Torah*. Kosher laws restrict the selection and preparation of animal-derived foods. Cuisines vary among Jews from Eastern Europe, Germany, the Soviet Union, the Middle East, and India, for example, but the kosher laws apply to all.[24]

The laws of kosher permit some foods and exclude others—beef but not pork, fin fish but not shellfish—and they dictate handling methods for permitted foods. For example, blood is forbidden as food, and thus meats must be specially prepared to remove the blood. Processed foods made according to kosher laws are identified by an insignia "U" or "K" on the label, meaning

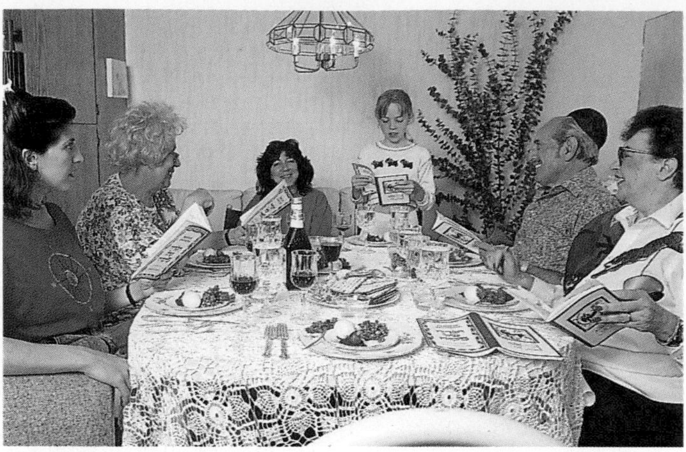

To honor cultural and religious foodways honors the people who share them.

that the food has been deemed kosher by a rabbi. Kosher law prohibits Jews from combining milk and meat in the same meal. This leads some kosher cooks to replace milk with nondairy creamer in meals that include meat. Nutritionally, however, creamers do not replace milk, and they may carry more of the type of fat implicated in heart disease. A better choice is to use soy "milk" products that are formulated to resemble the nutrient and cooking qualities of milk products.

Just as with other cuisines, Jewish cuisines and kosher foods can be evaluated according to dietary standards. A Jewish meal of European origin might be improved by reducing schmaltz (chicken fat) used in cooking or by frying latke (potato pancakes) in nonstick pans, not in oil. Bagels with lox or low fat or nonfat cream cheese are an excellent breakfast choice—bagels are naturally low in fat, and lox is thinly sliced salmon. A person dining on European Jewish cuisine would do well to limit meat servings (usually beef) to the 2- to 3-ounce serving sizes recommended by the Daily Food Guide, and to fill the plate with grains such as noodles and with fruits and vegetables.

Occasionally someone suggests that the laws of kosher originated for reasons of health, that kosher food was "clean" and therefore kept people safe from foodborne illnesses. However, religious commitment is the sole intent of those who keep kosher, and few of the rules of kosher offer special benefits to health.

Food symbolism abounds in most other religions as well. Among Christians, a revered expression of faith is the sacrament of eating a bite of bread or bread wafer and taking a sip of grape juice or wine, symbolizing the last supper of Jesus Christ. During certain days of Lent, the period prior to Easter, many Christians eat only vegetarian dishes, giving up meat until Easter dinner. Eastern Orthodox Christians observe many fast days on which they consume no animal products at all. The Mormon faith allows no alcohol, coffee, or tea. Many Seventh-day Adventists consume no meat but include eggs and milk products; they also shun alcohol, coffee, and tea. In addition, Seventh-day Adventist doctrine advises followers to avoid strong spices such as mustard or pepper and discourages between-meal snacks.

Other faiths, such as Islam, Muslim, Hinduism, and Buddhism, prohibit some dietary practices while promoting others. Informed diet planners know that to honor a person's cultural or religious foodways honors the person. Sometimes respecting a person's foodways can provide nourishment of self-esteem, and this can be as important to health as nourishment for the body.

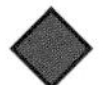

Notes

1. I. Diamond, Alcoholic myopathy and cardiomyopathy, *New England Journal of Medicine* 320 (1989): 458–460.
2. F. Berrino and P. Muti, Mediterranean diet and cancer, *European Journal of Clinical Nutrition* 43 (1989): 49–55.
3. A. Ferro-Luzzi and S. Sette, The Mediterranean diet: An attempt to define its present and past composition, *European Journal of Clinical Nutrition* 43 (1989): 13–29.
4. J. C. Waterlow, Diet of the classical period of Greece and Rome, *European Journal of Clinical Nutrition* 43 (1989): 3–12.
5. D. Kromhout and coauthors, Food consumption patterns in the 1960s in seven countries, *American Journal of Clinical Nutrition* 49 (1989): 889–894.
6. A. Trichopoulou, Correspondence, *New England Journal of Medicine* 327 (1992): 53.
7. World Health Organization, Life expectancy, number of survivors, and chances per 1000 of eventually dying from specified causes, at selected ages, by sex, latest available year in *World Health Statistics Annual* (Geneva: World Health Organization, 1989): 158–163.
8. F. M. Sacks and W. W. Willet, More on chewing the fat, *New England Journal of Medicine* 325 (1991): 1740–1742.
9. The Mediterranean diet and food culture—a symposium, *European Journal of Clinical Nutrition* (Supplement) 43 (1989).
10. L. Masana and coauthors, The Mediterranean-type diet: Is there a need for further modification? *American Journal of Clinical Nutrition* 53 (1991): 886–889.
11. W. P. T. James, G. G. Duthie, and K. W. J. Whale, The Mediterranean diet: Protective or simply nontoxic? *European*

Journal of Clinical Nutrition 43 (1989): 31–41.
12. J. C. Brand and coauthors, Plasma glucose and insulin responses to traditional Pima Indian meals, *American Journal of Clinical Nutrition* 51 (1990): 416–420.
13. B. A. Swinburn, Deterioration in carbohydrate metabolism and lipoprotein changes induced by modern, high-fat diet in Pima Indians and Caucasians, *Journal of Clinical Endocrinology and Metabolism* 73 (1991): 156–165.
14. R. Fabsitz, Administrator of the Strong Heart Study, as quoted by K. A. Fackelmann, *Science News* 142 (1992): 168–170.
15. M. Segal, Native food preparation fosters botulism, *FDA Consumer*, January-February 1992, pp. 23–26.
16. S. J. Algert and T. H. Ellison, Mexican American food practices, customs, and holidays, *Ethnic and Regional Food Practices* (series) (Chicago and Alexandria, Va.: American Dietetic Association and American Diabetes Association, 1989).
17. L. Roberts, Diet and health in China, *Science* 240 (1988): 27.
18. A. S. Whittemore and coauthors, Diet, physical activity, and colorectal cancer among Chinese in North America and China, *Journal of the National Cancer Institute* 82 (1990): 915–926.
19. M. Motoko, Eating is a solitary pastime, *Japan Quarterly* 36 (1989): 207–210.
20. B. Cutler, Move over, miso, *American Demographics*, May 1988, pp. 56–57.
21. E. H. Tsunehara, D. L. Leonetti, and W. Y. Fujimoto, Diet of second-generation Japanese-American men with and without noninsulin-dependent diabetes, *American Journal of Clinical Nutrition* 52 (1990): 731–738.
22. E. A. Martin and V. A. Beal, *Roberts' Nutrition Work with Children*, 4th ed. (Chicago: University of Chicago Press, 1978); M. Stepanek, Tall tales from Tokyo, *Far Eastern Economic Review*, 9 January 1993, pp. 30–31.
23. T. Matsuzaki, Longevity, diet, and nutrition in Japan: Epidemiological studies, *Nutrition Reviews* 50 (1992): 355–359.
24. C. Higgins and H. S. Warshaw, Jewish food practices, customs, and holidays, *Ethnic and Regional Food Practices* (series) (Chicago and Alexandria, Va.: American Dietetic Association and American Diabetes Association, 1989).

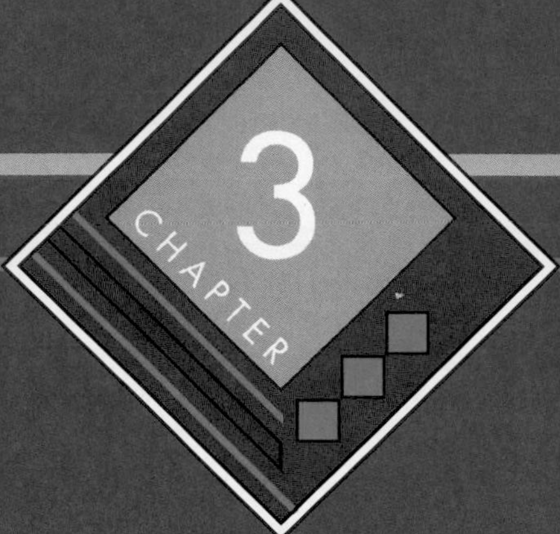

The Remarkable Body

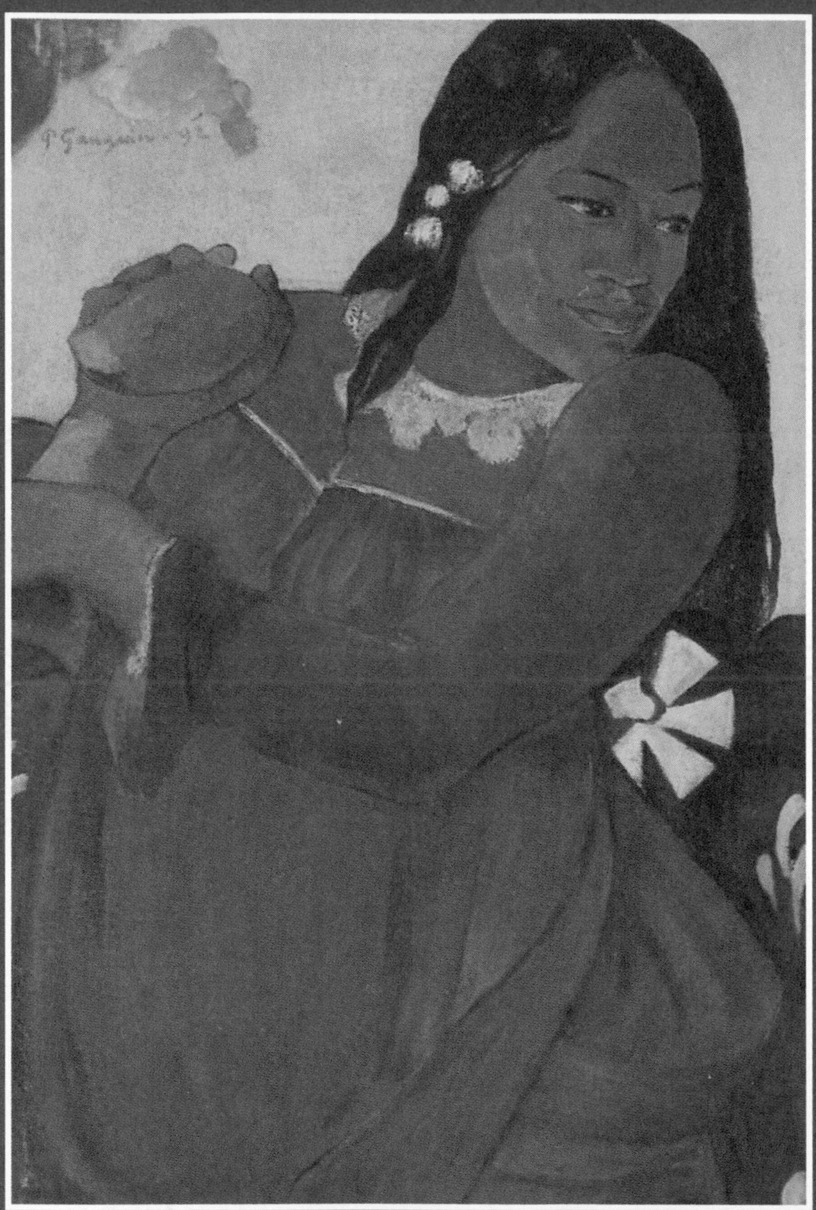

Paul Gauguin, *Woman of the Mango,* 1892, The Baltimore Museum of Art; The Cone Collection, formed by Dr. Claribel Cone and Miss Etta Cone of Baltimore, Maryland, BMA 1950, 213.

Contents

At the moment of conception, you received from your mother and father the genes that determine how your body works. Many of these genes are thousands of centuries old and have not changed since the Stone Age, when your ancestors walked the earth coated with fur and carrying clubs. You are living with the food, the luxuries, the smog, the additives, and all the other problems and pleasures of the 20th century, and in this country's melting pot of cultures and traditions, you may not have learned any time-tested and proven way of patterning your food intake. There is no guarantee that your diet, haphazardly chosen, will meet the needs of your Stone-Age body. Unlike your ancestors, you have to learn how your body works and what it needs from food to serve it best. Hence the study of nutrition, so that you can bring your mind into the act of nourishing your body.

cells the smallest units in which independent life can exist. All living things are single cells or organisms made of cells.

The Body's Cells

The human body is composed of billions of **cells,** and none of them knows anything about food. *You* may get hungry for fruit, milk, or bread, but each cell of your body needs nutrients—the vital components of foods. How the body's cells cooperate to obtain and use nutrients are the subjects of this chapter.

Each of the body's cells is a self-contained, living entity (see Figure 3-1), although each depends on the rest of the body to supply its needs. Among the cells' most basic needs are the needs for energy and the oxygen with which to burn it. Cells also need water to maintain the environment in which they live. They need building blocks and control systems to maintain themselves. They especially need the nutrients they cannot make for them-

A membrane encloses each cell's contents.

These finger-like projections are typical of cells that absorb nutrients in the intestines.

A separate, inner membrane encloses the cell's nucleus.

Inside the nucleus is the hereditary material, which contains the genes. The genes control the inheritance of the cell's characteristics and its day to day workings. They are faithfully copied each time the cell duplicates itself.

On these membranes, instructions from the genes are translated into proteins that perform functions in the body.

Many other structures are present. This is a mitochondrion, a structure that takes in nutrients and releases energy from them.

Figure 3-1

A TYPICAL CELL (SIMPLIFIED DIAGRAM)

genes units of a cell's inheritance, made of a chemical, DNA (deoxyribonucleic acid). Each gene directs the making of a protein to do the body's work. (Proteins are described fully in Chapter 6.)

enzyme a protein catalyst. A catalyst is an agent that promotes a chemical reaction without itself being altered in the process.

tissues systems of cells working together to perform specialized tasks. Examples are muscles, nerves, blood, and bone.

organs discrete structural units made of tissues that perform specific jobs, such as the heart, the liver, and the brain.

body system a group of related organs that work together to perform a function. Examples are the circulatory system, the respiratory system, and the nervous system.

blood the fluid of the cardiovascular system, composed of water, red and white blood cells, other formed particles, nutrients, oxygen, and other constituents.

lymph (LIMF) the fluid that moves from the bloodstream into tissue spaces and then travels in its own vessels, which eventually drain back into the bloodstream.

arteries blood vessels that carry blood containing fresh oxygen supplies from the heart to the tissues (see Figure 3-2).

veins blood vessels that carry used blood from the tissues back to the heart (Figure 3-2).

capillaries minute, weblike blood vessels that connect arteries to veins and permit transfer of materials between blood and tissues (see Figures 3-2 and 3-3).

selves, the essential nutrients, which must be supplied from food. The first principle of diet planning is that the foods we choose must provide energy, water, and the essential nutrients.

In the human body every cell works in cooperation with every other to support the whole. The cell's **genes** determine the nature of that work. Each gene is a blueprint that directs the production of a piece of protein machinery, most often an **enzyme,** that helps to do the cell's work. Each cell contains a complete set of genes, but different ones are active in different types of cells. For example, in some intestinal cells, the genes for making digestive enzymes are active; in some of the body's fat cells, the genes for making enzymes that metabolize fat are active.

Cells are organized into **tissues** that perform specialized tasks. For example, individual muscle cells are joined together to form muscle tissue, which can contract. Tissues, in turn, are grouped together to form whole **organs.** In the organ we call the heart, for example, muscle tissues, nerve tissues, connective tissues, and other types all work together to pump blood. Some body functions require several related organs to perform them. The organs that work together to perform functions are parts of **body systems.** For example, the heart, lungs, and blood vessels cooperate as parts of the cardiovascular system to deliver oxygen to all the body tissues. The next few sections present the body systems with special significance to nutrition.

KEY POINT The body's cells need energy, oxygen, water, and nutrients to remain healthy and to do their work. Genes direct the making of each cell's machinery, including enzymes. Specialized cells are grouped together to form tissues and organs; organs work together in body systems.

The Body Fluids and the Cardiovascular System

Body fluids supply the tissues continuously with energy, oxygen, water, and building materials. The fluids constantly circulate to pick up fresh supplies and to deliver wastes to points of disposal. Every cell continuously draws oxygen and nutrients from those fluids, and releases carbon dioxide and other waste products into them.

The body's main fluids are the **blood** and **lymph.** Blood travels within the **arteries, veins,** and **capillaries,** as well as within the heart's chambers (Figure 3-2). Lymph travels in separate vessels of its own. Other fluids circulate around the cells, such as the plasma of the blood or the fluid surrounding muscle cells (Figure 3-3, page 74). Fluid surrounding cells is derived from the blood in the capillaries; it squeezes out through capillary walls and flows around the outsides of cells, permitting exchange of materials. Some of the extracellular fluid returns to the blood by reentering the capillaries. The fluid remaining outside the capillaries forms lymph which travels around the body by way of its own vessels. The lymph eventually returns to the bloodstream where large lymph and blood vessels join. In this way, all cells are served by the cardiovascular system.

The fluid inside cells provides a medium in which all cell reactions take place. Its pressure also helps cells hold their shape. Intracellular fluid is formed from water drawn from the extracellular fluid.

As the blood travels through the cardiovascular system, it delivers materials cells need and picks up their wastes. The blood picks up oxygen in

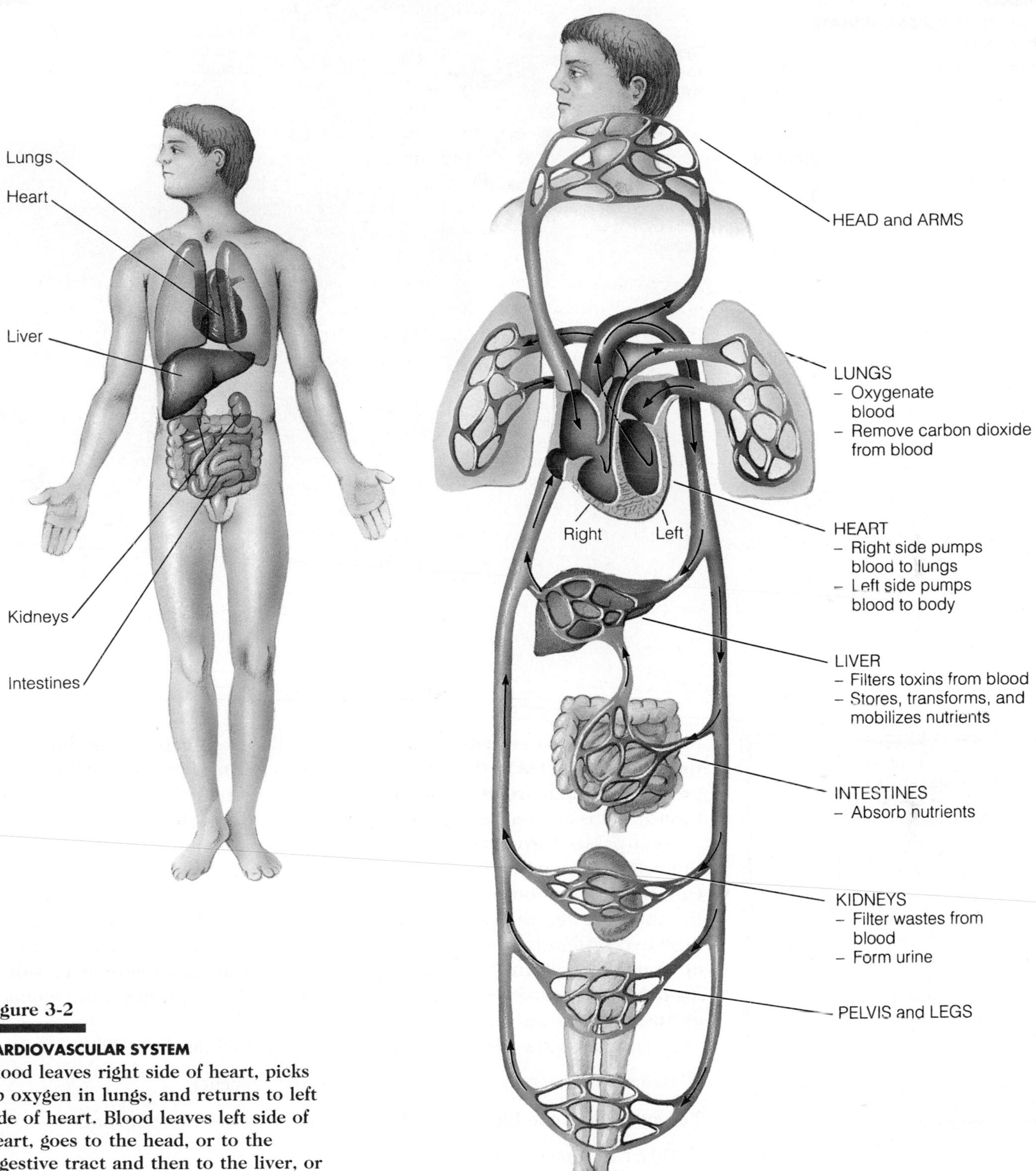

Figure 3-2

CARDIOVASCULAR SYSTEM

Blood leaves right side of heart, picks up oxygen in lungs, and returns to left side of heart. Blood leaves left side of heart, goes to the head, or to the digestive tract and then to the liver, or to the lower body, and then returns to right side of heart.

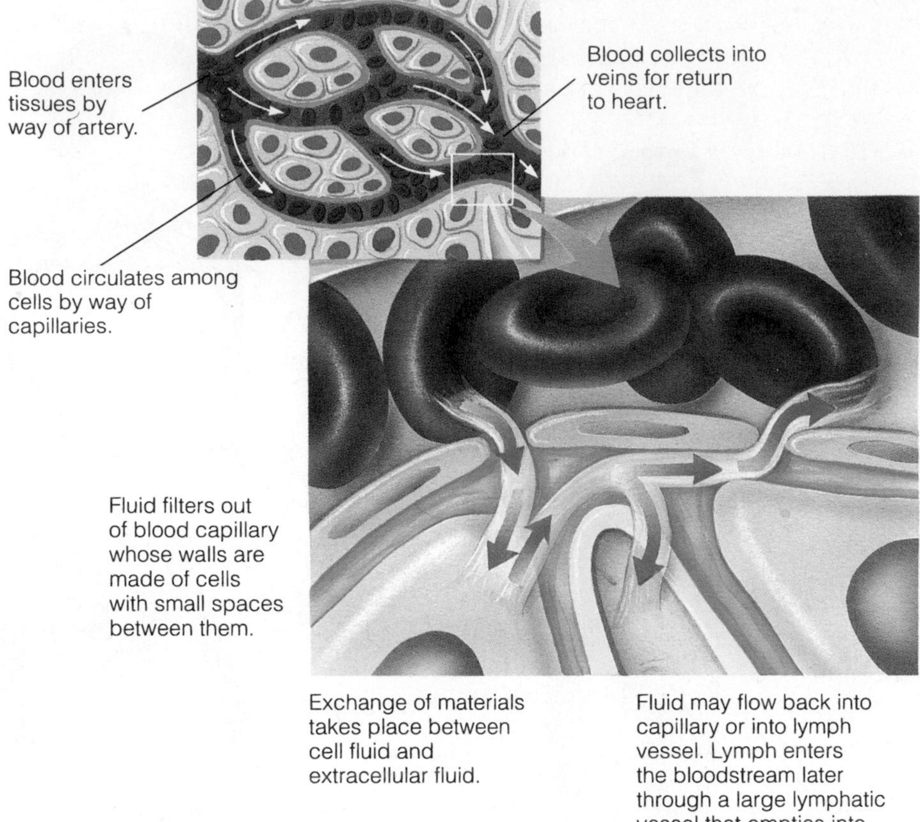
Blood enters tissues by way of artery.
Blood collects into veins for return to heart.
Blood circulates among cells by way of capillaries.
Fluid filters out of blood capillary whose walls are made of cells with small spaces between them.
Exchange of materials takes place between cell fluid and extracellular fluid.
Fluid may flow back into capillary or into lymph vessel. Lymph enters the bloodstream later through a large lymphatic vessel that empties into a large vein.

Figure 3-3

HOW THE BODY FLUIDS CIRCULATE AROUND CELLS

The upper left-hand box shows a tiny portion of tissue with blood flowing through its network of capillaries (greatly enlarged). The bottom right-hand box illustrates the movement of the extracellular fluid.

lungs the organs of gas exchange. Blood circulating through the lungs releases its carbon dioxide and picks up fresh oxygen to carry to the tissues.

intestine a long, tubular organ of digestion and the site of nutrient absorption.

liver a large, lobed organ that lies just under the ribs. It filters the blood, removes and processes nutrients, manufactures materials for export to other parts of the body, and destroys toxins or stores them to keep them out of the circulation.

kidneys a pair of bean-shaped organs that filter the blood of its wastes, make urine, and release urine to the bladder for excretion from the body.

the **lungs** and also releases carbon dioxide there, as Figure 3-4 shows. All the blood circulates to the lungs, then returns to the heart, where it receives powerful impetus from the pumping heartbeats that push it out to all body tissues. Thus all tissues receive oxygenated blood fresh from the lungs.

As it passes through the digestive system, the blood delivers oxygen to the cells there and picks up most nutrients other than fats from the **intestine** for distribution elsewhere. Lymphatic vessels pick up most fats from the intestine and then transport the fats to the blood. All blood leaving the digestive system is routed directly to the **liver,** which has the special task of chemically altering the absorbed materials to make them better suited for use by other tissues. Later, in passing through the **kidneys,** the blood is cleansed of wastes.

In summary, the blood is routed as follows (look again at Figure 3-2):

- Heart to tissues to heart to lungs to heart (repeat).

The portion of the blood that flows by the intestine travels from:

- Heart to intestine to liver to heart.

To ensure efficient circulation of fluid to all your cells, you need an ample fluid intake. This means drinking sufficient water to replace the water lost each day. Cardiovascular fitness is essential, too, and constitutes an ongoing project that requires attention to both nutrition and physical activity. Healthy red blood cells also play a role, for they carry oxygen to all the other cells, enabling them to use fuels for energy. Since red blood cells arise, live, and die within about four months, your body replaces them constantly, a manufacturing process that requires many essential nutrients from food. Many kinds of blood disorders are caused by dietary deficiencies of vitamins or minerals; the blood is very sensitive to malnutrition.

microbes bacteria, viruses, or other organisms invisible to the naked eye; some cause diseases; also called *microorganisms.*

 **KEY POINT** Blood and lymph deliver oxygen and nutrients to all the body's cells and carry waste materials away from them. The cardiovascular system ensures that these fluids circulate properly among all organs.

The Immune System

Many of the body's cells cooperate to maintain their defenses against infection. The skin presents a physical barrier, while the body's cavities (lungs, digestive tract, and others) are lined with membranes that resist penetration by invading **microbes** or unwanted substances. The body's linings are easily damaged by vitamin and other nutrient deficiencies, and health care providers inspect both the skin and the inside of the mouth to detect signs of malnutrition. (The chapters on protein, vitamins, and minerals present details of the signs of deficiencies.)

When microbial infection penetrates these first lines of defense (the skin and linings), the lymph and blood present internal defenses. White blood

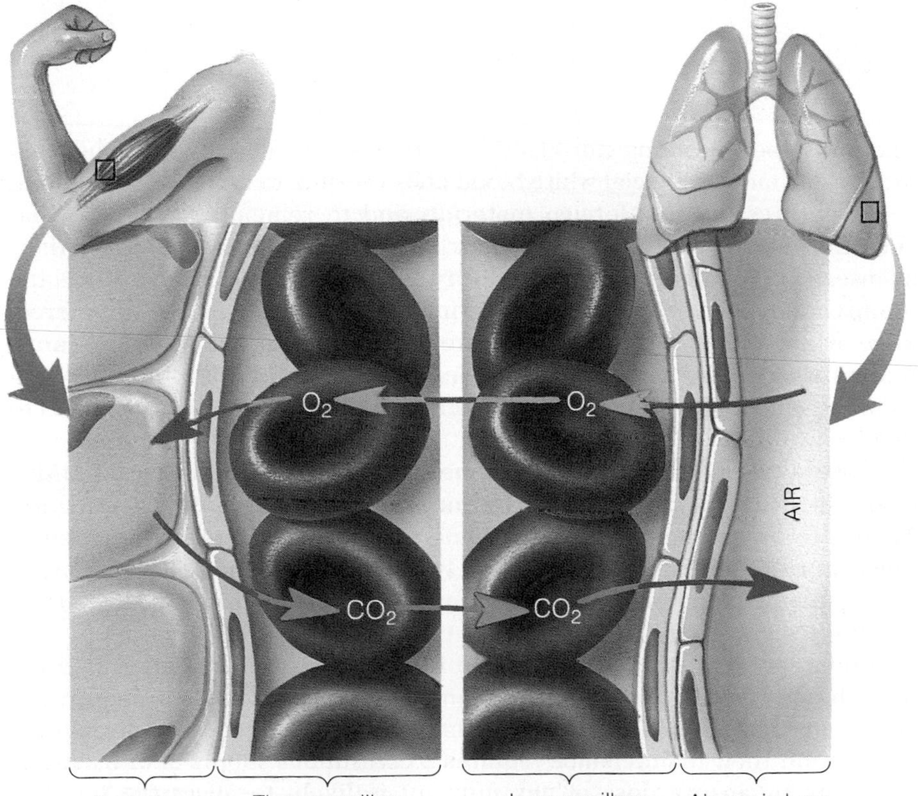
O2
O2
AIR
CO2
CO2
Body tissue
Tissue capillary
Lung capillary
Air sac in lung
In body tissues, red blood cells give up their oxygen (O_2) and absorb carbon dioxide (CO_2).
In the air sacs of the lungs, the red blood cells give up their load of carbon dioxide (CO_2) and absorb oxygen (O_2) from air to supply to body tissues.

Figure 3-4

OXYGEN-CARBON DIOXIDE EXCHANGE IN THE LUNGS

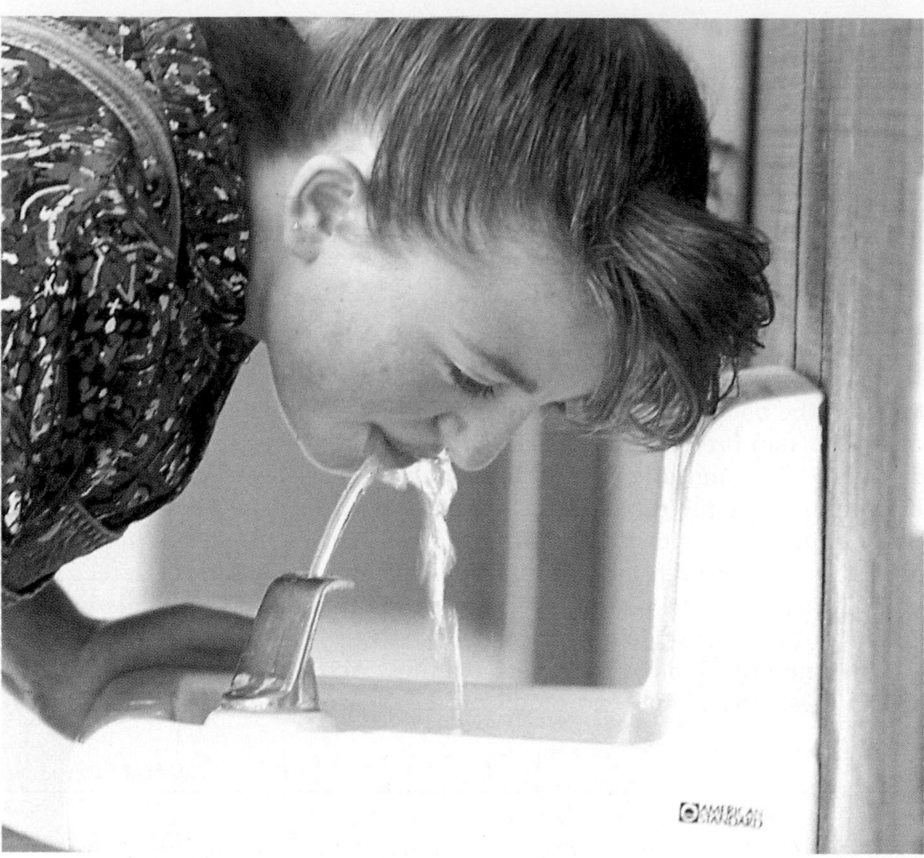

All the body's cells live in water.

immunity the body's ability to resist or eliminate potentially harmful foreign materials or abnormal cells.

antibodies proteins made by cells of the immune system, expressly designed to combine with and to inactivate specific antigens.

antigens microbes or substances that are foreign to the body.

cells and blood proteins can inactivate, remove, or destroy microbes and foreign substances. Special white blood cells are able to recognize the chemical structures of some foreign materials and to remember them, so that when they again encounter the invader, the cells can quickly mobilize their defenses. This ability provides **immunity** against many diseases, such as the mumps and chickenpox, that the body has previously fought and conquered. Some white blood cells produce proteins that act as ammunition **(antibodies)** designed to destroy specific targets **(antigens).** Still other cells can gobble up and digest the injured invaders—to clean up the battlefield, so to speak.

In some cases, the immune response may also cause harm. Some diseases, such as rheumatoid arthritis and a severe form of diabetes, are thought to be caused when the immune system is somehow stimulated to attack normal body parts, progressively destroying them. Likewise, organ transplant recipients must take immunity-suppressing drugs to prevent an attack on their foreign new organs by the immune system.

Immune system components reside in the bones, in the digestive tract, in the blood vessels, in the lymph organs, and in glands of their own. White blood cells and antibodies are in constant flux, being made and dismantled rapidly, and their maintenance requires a continuous supply of nutrients. A deficiency or an overdose of any nutrient is likely to affect the immune system adversely, and a deficiency of nutrients early in an infant's development can weaken immune defenses for life.

Chapter 11 offers more on nutrition's contributions to the body's defense systems.

 **KEY POINT** The immune system enables the body to resist disease. Its successful functioning depends to a great degree on an adequate nutrient supply.

◆ The Hormonal and Nervous Systems

In addition to nutrients, oxygen, wastes, immune cells, and proteins, the blood also carries chemical messengers, **hormones,** from one system of cells to another. These communicate changing conditions that demand responses. Hormones are secreted and released directly into the blood by organs known as glands. For example, when the **pancreas** (a gland) detects a high concentration of the blood's sugar, glucose, it releases **insulin,** a hormone. Insulin stimulates the muscle and other cells to remove glucose from the blood and to store it. When the blood glucose level falls, the pancreas secretes another hormone, **glucagon,** to which the liver responds by releasing into the blood some of the glucose it stored earlier. Thus, blood glucose levels are maintained.

Glands and hormones abound in the body. Each gland monitors a condition and produces one or more hormones to regulate it. Each hormone acts as a messenger that stimulates various organs to take appropriate actions.

Nutrition affects the hormonal system. Fasting, feeding, and exercise alter hormonal balances. People who become very thin have an altered hormonal balance that may make them unable to maintain their bones. People who eat high-fat diets have hormone levels that may make them susceptible to certain cancers.

Hormones also affect nutrition. Along with the nervous system, they regulate hunger and affect appetite. They carry messages to regulate the digestive system, telling the digestive organs what kinds of foods have been eaten and how much of each digestive juice to secrete. Hormones also regulate the menstrual cycle in women, and they affect the appetite changes many women experience during the cycle and in pregnancy. An altered hormonal state is thought to be at least partly responsible, too, for the loss of appetite that sick people experience. Hormones also regulate the body's reaction to stress, suppressing hunger and the digestion and absorption of nutrients. When questions about a person's nutrition are asked, the state of that person's hormonal system is often part of the answer.

The body's other major communication system is, of course, the nervous system. With the brain and spinal cord as central controllers, the nervous system receives and integrates information from sensory receptors all over the body—sight, hearing, touch, smell, taste, and others—which all communicate to the brain the state of both the outer and inner worlds, including the availability of food and the need to eat. The nervous system also sends instructions to the muscles and glands, telling them what to do.

The nervous system's role in hunger regulation is coordinated by the brain. The sensations of hunger and appetite are perceived by the brain's **cortex,** the thinking, outer layer. However, much of the brain's regulatory work goes on in the deep brain centers without the person's (or the cortex's) awareness. Deep inside the brain, the **hypothalamus** (Figure 3-5) monitors many body conditions, including the availability of nutrients and

hormones chemicals that are secreted by glands into the blood in response to conditions in the body that require regulation. These chemicals serve as messengers, acting on other organs to maintain constant conditions.

pancreas an organ with two main functions. One is an *endocrine* function—the making of hormones such as insulin, which it releases directly into the blood (*endo* means "into" the blood). The other is an *exocrine* function—the making of digestive enzymes, which it releases through a duct into the small intestine to assist in digestion (*exo* means "out" into a body cavity or onto the skin surface).

insulin a hormone from the pancreas that helps glucose enter cells from the blood.

glucagon a hormone from the pancreas that stimulates the release of glucose from the liver.

cortex the outermost layer of something. The brain's cortex is that part of the brain in which conscious thought takes place.

hypothalamus (high-poh-THAL-uh-mus) a part of the brain that senses a variety of conditions in the blood, such as temperature, glucose content, salt content, and others. It signals other parts of the brain or body to change those conditions when necessary.

Chapter 4 describes the regulation of blood glucose in greater detail.

Hormones and the bones are topics of Controversy 8; hormones and appetite are discussed in Chapter 13.

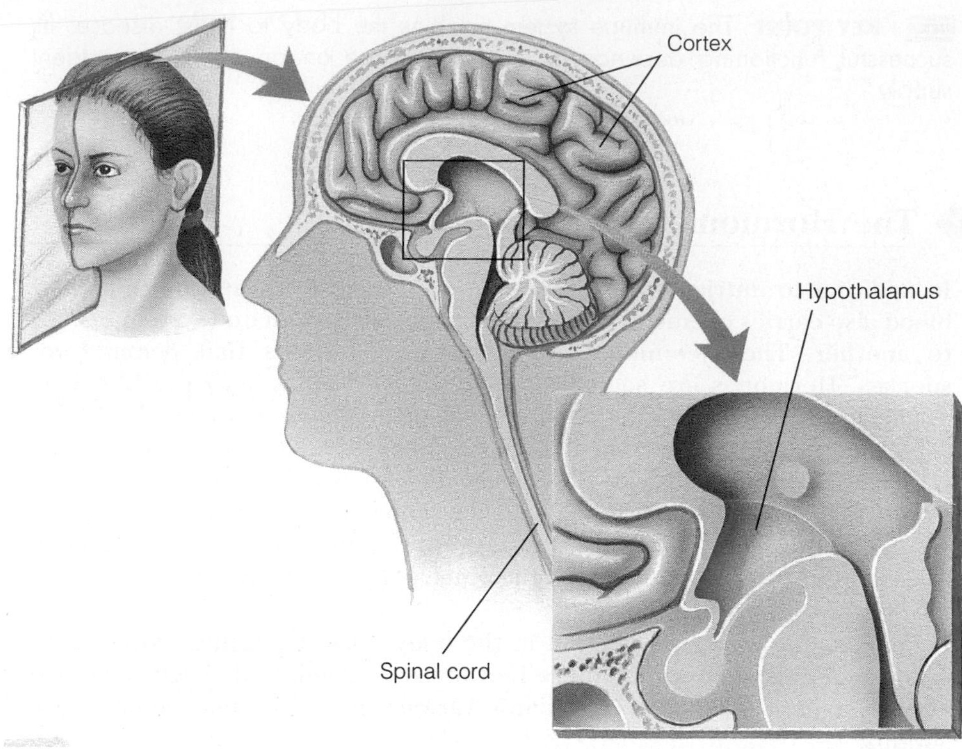

Figure 3-5

CUTAWAY SIDE VIEW OF THE BRAIN SHOWING THE HYPOTHALAMUS AND CORTEX

The hypothalamus monitors the body's conditions and sends signals to the brain's thinking portion, the cortex, which decides on actions.

fight-or-flight reaction the body's instinctive, hormone- and nerve-mediated reaction to danger, also known as the *stress response.*

epinephrine the major hormone that elicits the stress response.

norepinephrine a compound related to epinephrine that helps to elicit the stress response.

water. The digestive tract sends messengers to the hypothalamus by way of hormones and nerves signaling hunger, the physiological need for food. The signals also stimulate the stomach to intensify its contractions and secretions, causing hunger pangs (and gurgling sounds). When your cerebral cortex becomes conscious of hunger, you eat. The conscious mind of the cortex, however, can override such signals, and can allow a person to choose to delay eating despite hunger, or to eat when hunger is absent.

A marvelous adaptation of the human body, the ability to respond to physical danger, involves the workings of both the hormonal and nervous systems. Known as the **fight-or-flight reaction** or as the *stress response,* this adaptation is present with only minor variations in all animals, showing how universally important it is to survival. It is a magnificently well-coordinated response. When danger is detected, nerves fire and glands supply the compounds **epinephrine** and **norepinephrine.*** Every organ of the body responds. The pupils of the eyes widen so that you can see better; the muscles tense up so that you can jump, run, or struggle with maximum strength; breathing quickens and deepens to provide more oxygen. The heart races to rush the oxygen to the muscles, and the blood pressure rises to deliver efficiently the fuel the muscles need for energy. The liver pours forth glucose from its stores, while the fat cells release fat. The digestive system shuts down to permit all the body's systems to serve the muscles and nerves. With all action systems at peak efficiency, the body can respond with amazing speed and strength to whatever threatens it.

In ancient times, stress was usually physical danger, and the response to it was violent physical exertion. In the modern world, stress is seldom physical, but the body's reaction to it is still the same. What stresses you today

*Strictly speaking, norepinephrine is a neurotransmitter.

may be a checkbook out of control or a teacher who suddenly announces a pop quiz. Under these stresses, you are not supposed to fight or run as your Stone-Age ancestor did. You smile at the "enemy" and suppress your fear. But your heart races, you feel it pounding, and hormones still flood your bloodstream with glucose and fat. When the fat isn't used for fuel by your muscles it ends up clinging to the walls of your arteries, which harden and so bring on cardiovascular disease.

Your number-one enemy today is not a man-eating tiger who prowls around your cave, but a disease of modern civilization: atherosclerosis. Years of fat accumulation in the arteries and stresses that strain the heart lead to heart attacks, not from overexertion but from chronic underexertion paired with sudden high blood pressure. It would be better to include daily exercise as part of a healthy lifestyle. And, whenever you feel threatened or upset, it would be best to run, shout, or punch a pillow to use up the fuel and to exercise the heart and muscles that have geared up for action.

digestive system the body system composed of organs that break down complex food particles into smaller absorbable products. The *digestive tract*, or *alimentary canal* are names for the tubular organs that extend from the mouth to the anus.

digest to break apart to smaller pieces, a main function of the digestive tract with respect to food.

absorb to take in, as nutrients are taken into the intestinal cells after digestion, the main function of the digestive tract with respect to nutrients.

KEY POINT The hormonal and nervous systems coordinate and help regulate body processes through communication among all the organs. They respond to the need for food, govern the act of eating, regulate digestion, and call for the stress response.

◆ The Digestive System

When your body needs food, your brain and hormones alert your conscious mind to the sensation of hunger. Then when you eat, your taste buds guide you in judging whether foods are acceptable (see Figure 3-6).

Sweet and salty tastes seem to be universally desirable, but most people have aversions to bitter and sour tastes alone (see Figure 3-7). The enjoyment of sweetness encourages people to consume ample energy, especially from foods containing sugars, the energy fuel for the brain. The pleasure of a salty taste prompts them to consume sufficient amounts of two very important minerals—sodium and chloride.

The instinctive liking for sugar and salt can lead to drastic overeating of these substances. Sugar has become available in pure form only in the last hundred years, so is relatively new to the human diet. While salt is somewhat older, both are being added liberally, today, to foods by manufacturers to tempt us to eat their products.

Once you have eaten, your brain and hormones then direct the many organs of the **digestive system** to **digest** and to **absorb** the complex mixture of chewed and swallowed food that you have delivered to them. A diagram showing the digestive tract and its associated organs appears in Figure 3-8. The tract itself is a flexible, muscular tube measuring about 26 feet in length from the mouth through the throat, esophagus, stomach, small intestine, large intestine, and rectum to the anus. In a sense the human body is itself a tube that surrounds this series of digestive organs. When you have swallowed something, it still is not inside the body; it is only inside the inner bore of this tube. Only when a nutrient or other substance passes through the cells forming the digestive tract wall does it actually enter the body's tissues. Many things pass into the body and out again, unabsorbed. A baby playing with beads may swallow one, but the bead will not really enter the body. It will reappear in the feces within a day or two.

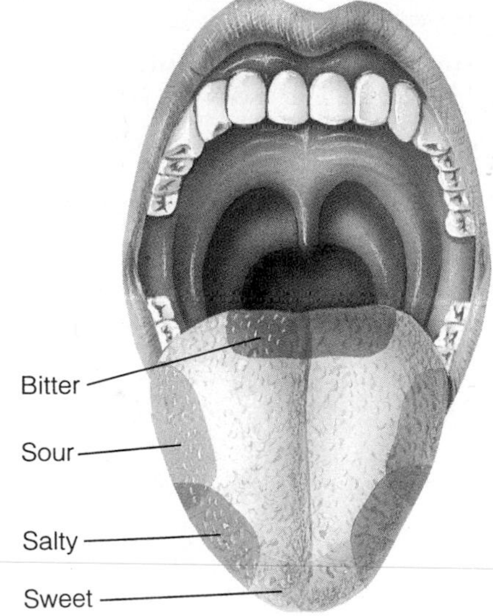

Figure 3-6

THE TASTE BUDS
Four basic kinds of taste buds are located on specific areas of the tongue. Each senses a single taste sensation: sweet, sour, bitter, or salty. Other factors that affect a food's flavor are aroma, texture, and temperature. In fact, the detection of a food's aroma is thousands of times more sensitive than detection of taste. The nose can detect just a few molecules responsible for the aroma of frying bacon, for example, even if they are diluted in several rooms full of air.

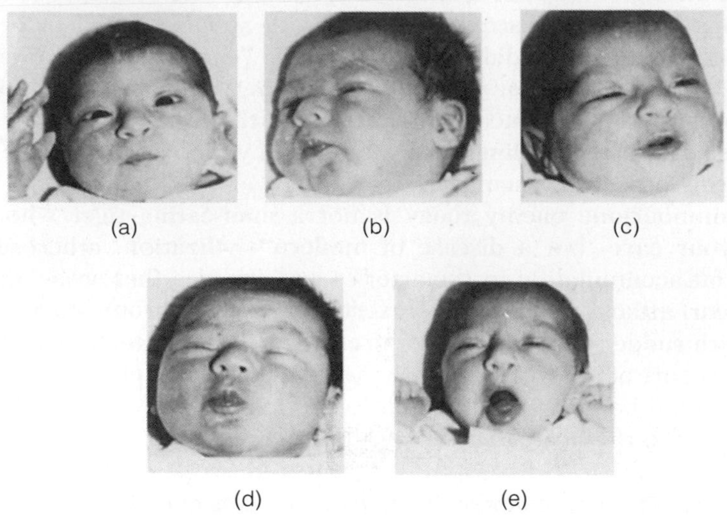

Figure 3-7

THE INNATE PREFERENCE FOR SWEET TASTE
This newborn baby is (a) resting and (b) tasting distilled water, (c) tasting sugar, (d) tasting something sour, and (e) tasting something bitter.

Source: Taste-induced facial expressions of neonate infants from the classic studies of J. E. Steiner, in *Taste and Development: The Genesis of Sweet Preference*, ed. J. M. Weiffenbach, HHS publication no. NIH 77-1068 (Bethesda, Md.: U.S. Department of Health and Human Services, 1977), pp. 173–189, with permission of the author.

peristalsis (perri-STALL-sis) the wavelike muscular squeezing of the esophagus, stomach, and small intestine that pushes their contents along.

stomach a muscular, elastic, pouchlike organ of the digestive tract that grinds and churns swallowed food and mixes it with acid and enzymes, forming chyme.

The digestive system's job is to digest food to its component nutrients and then to absorb those nutrients, leaving behind the substances, such as fiber, that are appropriate to excrete. To do this the system works at two levels: one, mechanical; the other, chemical.

The Mechanical Aspect of Digestion

The mechanical job of digestion is to chew and to crush foods and to add sufficient water to them so that the digestive enzymes can gain access to all of the component molecules. This job begins in the mouth, where large solid food pieces such as bites of meat are torn into shreds that can be swallowed without choking. Chewing also softens rough or sharp foods, such as fried tortilla chips, to prevent their tearing the esophagus. Nutrients trapped inside indigestible skins, such as seeds, must be liberated by breaking these skins before they can be digested. Chewing bursts open kernels of corn, for example, which would otherwise traverse the tract and exit undigested.

Once food has been mashed and moistened for comfortable swallowing, longer chewing times provide no additional advantages to digestion. In fact, for digestion's sake, a relaxed, peaceful attitude during a meal aids digestion much more than does an extended chewing time.[1]

Sometimes, swallowing does not go smoothly and the person chokes (Figure 3-9, page 82). To prevent choking, cut food into small pieces, chew until food is crushed and moistened, refrain from talking or laughing while food is present in the mouth, and do not attempt to eat while breathing hard. Should choking occur, the victim can be helped by application of the Heimlich Maneuver, as demonstrated in Figure 3-10.

Other organs take up the task of liquefying foods through the various mashing and squeezing actions of the stomach and intestines. The best known of these actions is **peristalsis,** a series of squeezing waves that start with the tongue's movement during a swallow and pass all the way down the esophagus. The stomach and the intestines also push food through the tract by waves of peristalsis. Figure 3-11 shows a peristaltic wave moving down the esophagus. Besides these actions, the **stomach** holds swallowed

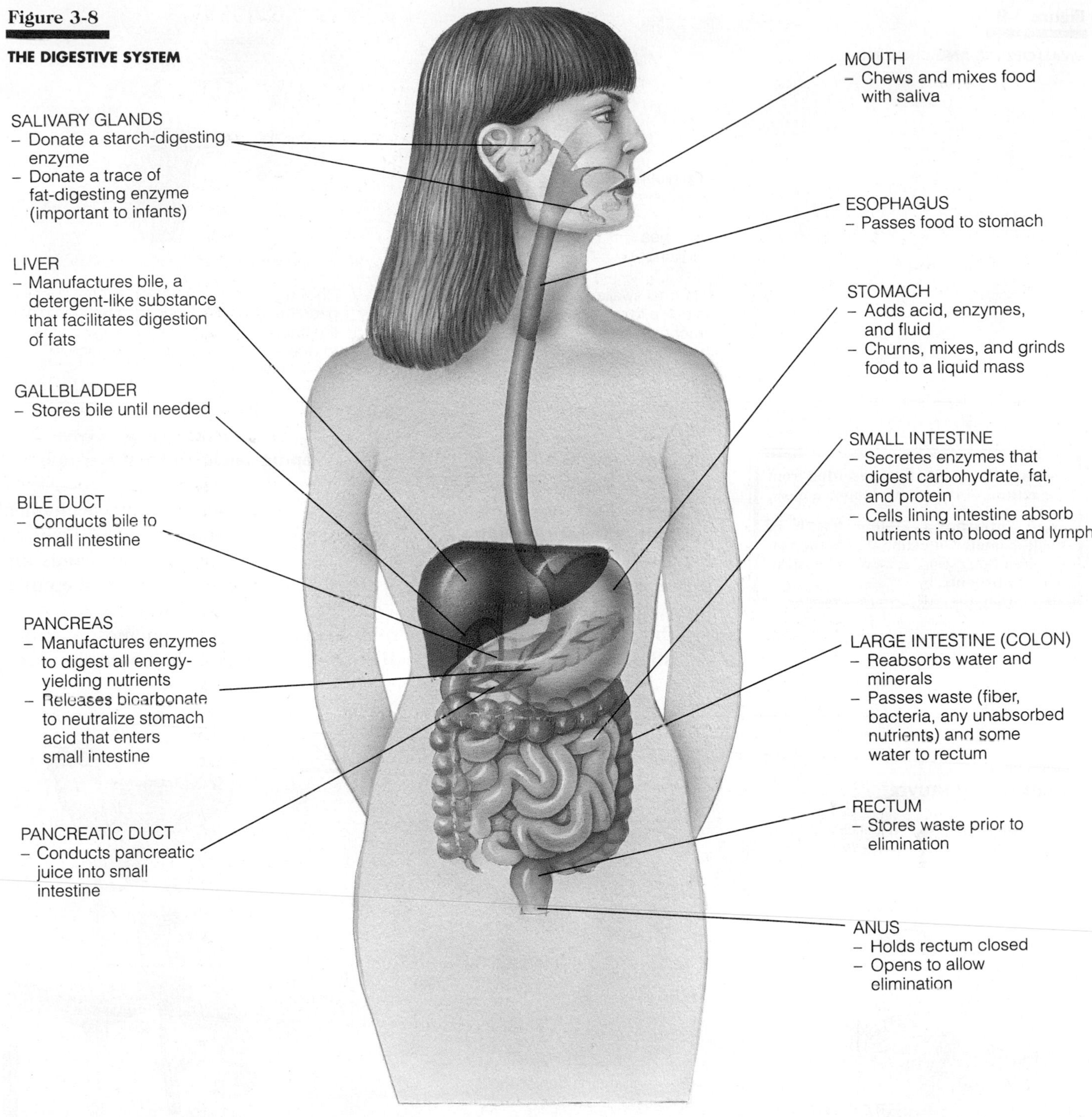
SALIVARY GLANDS
– Donate a starch-digesting enzyme
– Donate a trace of fat-digesting enzyme (important to infants)
LIVER
– Manufactures bile, a detergent-like substance that facilitates digestion of fats
GALLBLADDER
– Stores bile until needed
BILE DUCT
– Conducts bile to small intestine
PANCREAS
– Manufactures enzymes to digest all energy-yielding nutrients
– Releases bicarbonate to neutralize stomach acid that enters small intestine
PANCREATIC DUCT
– Conducts pancreatic juice into small intestine
MOUTH
– Chews and mixes food with saliva
ESOPHAGUS
– Passes food to stomach
STOMACH
– Adds acid, enzymes, and fluid
– Churns, mixes, and grinds food to a liquid mass
SMALL INTESTINE
– Secretes enzymes that digest carbohydrate, fat, and protein
– Cells lining intestine absorb nutrients into blood and lymph
LARGE INTESTINE (COLON)
– Reabsorbs water and minerals
– Passes waste (fiber, bacteria, any unabsorbed nutrients) and some water to rectum
RECTUM
– Stores waste prior to elimination
ANUS
– Holds rectum closed
– Opens to allow elimination

Figure 3-8

THE DIGESTIVE SYSTEM

food for a while and mashes it into a fine paste; the stomach and intestines also add water, so that the paste becomes more fluid as it moves along.

When a bite of food passes through the circular muscle at the base of the esophagus, it enters the stomach. The circular muscle squeezes the opening between the esophagus and stomach to narrow it. This action ordinarily

Figure 3-9

SWALLOWING AND CHOKING

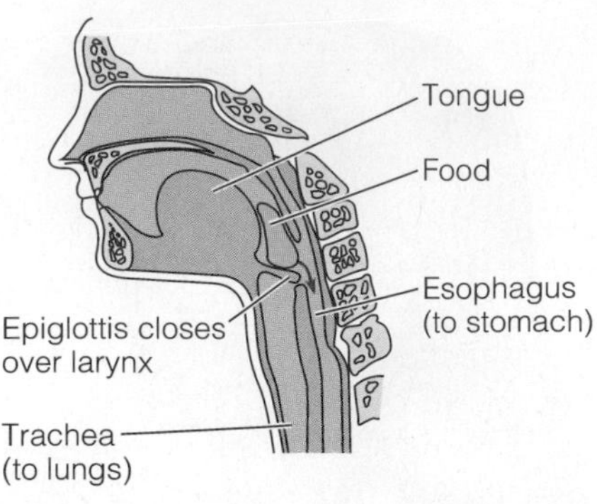

A normal swallow. The epiglottis acts as a flap to seal the entrance to the lungs (trachea) and direct food to the stomach via the esophagus.

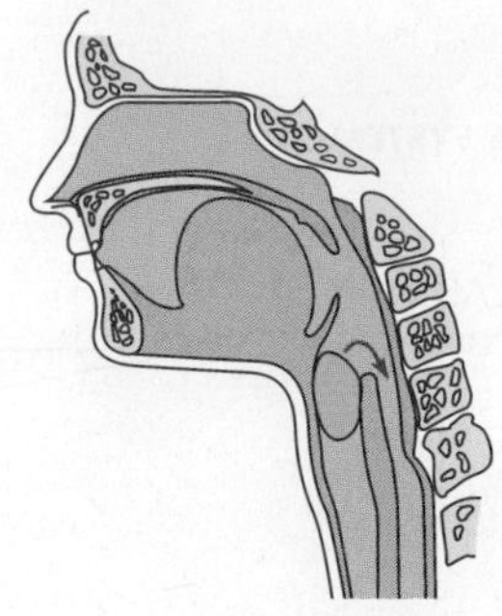

Choking. A choking person cannot speak or gasp because food lodged in trachea blocks the passage of air. The red arrow points to where the food should have gone to prevent choking.

---

chyme (KIME) the fluid resulting from the actions of the stomach upon a meal.

small intestine a 20-foot length of small-diameter intestine that is the major site of digestion of food and absorption of nutrients.

prevents the stomach contents from creeping back up in the esophagus when the stomach contracts.

Figure 3-12 shows the muscular stomach. The stomach's first mechanical action is to store swallowed food in a lump in its upper portion. Little by little the stomach transfers the food to its lower portion that grinds and mixes it thoroughly, ensuring that digestive chemicals mix with the entire mass, now called **chyme.**

While the stomach plays some roles in chemical digestion, most chemical digestion takes place in the **small intestine,** beyond the stomach, as de-

---

Figure 3-10

THE HEIMLICH MANEUVER

Source: Adapted from H. J. Heimlich and M. H. Uhley, The Heimlich maneuver, *Clinical Symposia* 31 (1979): 1–32.

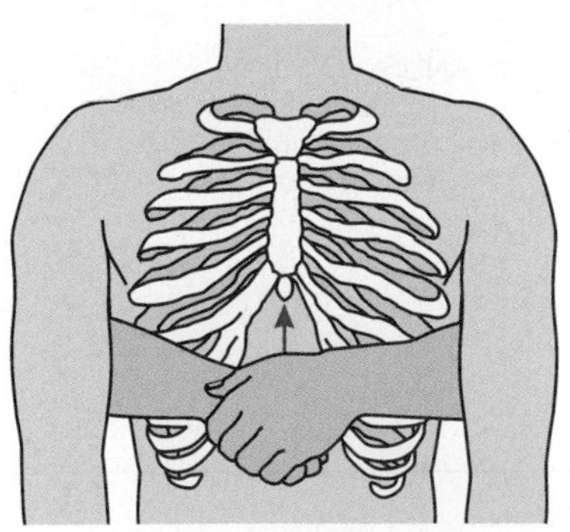

Rescuer positions fist directly against victim's abdomen as shown.

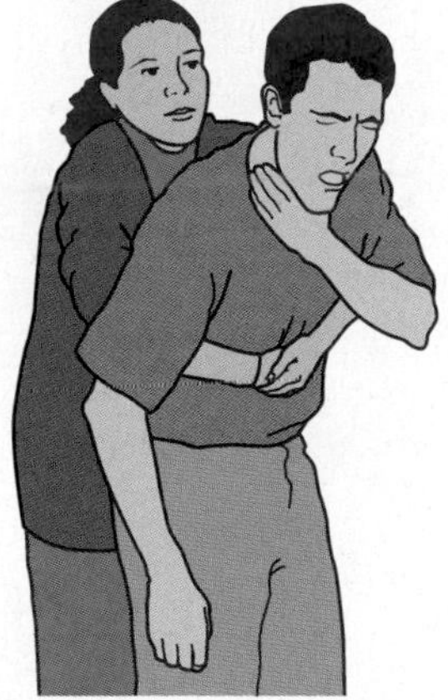

1. Rescuer stands behind victim and wraps her arms around victim's waist.
2. Rescuer makes a fist with one hand and places the thumb side of the fist against the victim's abdomen, slightly above the navel and below the rib cage.
3. Rescuer grasps fist with other hand and rapidly squeezes it inward and upward three or four times in rapid succession.
4. Rescuer repeats the process if necessary.

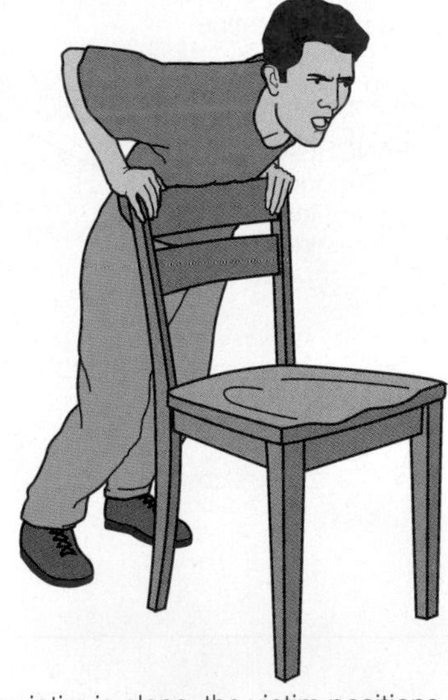

If the victim is alone, the victim positions himself or herself over edge of fixed horizontal object, such as a chair back, railing, or table edge, and presses abdomen into edge with quick movement.

scribed in the next section. The process is complicated, and only small amounts of food are processed at one time while the stomach acts as a holding tank. The muscular **pyloric valve,** at the stomach's lower end (Figure 3-12, on the next page) controls the exit of the chyme, allowing only a little at a time to be squirted forcefully into the small intestine. Within a few hours after a meal, the stomach empties itself by means of these powerful squirts.

By the time the intestinal contents have arrived in the **large intestine** (also called the **colon**), digestion and absorption are nearly complete. The colon's task is mostly to absorb water and minerals, leaving a paste of fiber and other undigested materials, the **feces,** suitable for excretion. The fiber provides bulk against which the muscles of the colon can work. The rectum stores this fecal material to be excreted at intervals. From mouth to rectum, the transit of a meal is accomplished in as short a time as a single day or as long as three days.[2]

Some people wonder whether the digestive tract works best at some hours in the day, and whether the timing of meals can affect how a person feels. Timing of meals is important to feeling well, not because the digestive tract is unable to digest food at certain times, but because the body requires nutrients to be replenished every few hours. Digestion is virtually continuous, limited only during sleep and exercise. Most people sleep most soundly after an early supper; eating late may interfere with normal sleep. One study found that a midnight meal altered conditions in the stomach throughout the next day.[3] As for exercise, it is best pursued a few hours after eating because digestion can inhibit physical work (see Chapter 10).

pyloric (pye-LORE-ick) **valve** the circular muscle of the lower stomach that regulates the flow of partly digested food into the small intestine.

large intestine (colon) the portion of the intestine that completes the absorption process.

colon the large intestine.

feces waste material remaining after digestion and absorption are complete, eventually discharged from the body.

KEY POINT The digestive tract renders *food* into absorbable *nutrients* and undigested wastes by mechanical and chemical means. The mechanical actions include chewing, mixing by the stomach, and moving of the tract's contents by peristalsis. After digestion and absorption, wastes are excreted.

The Chemical Aspect of Digestion

Several organs of the digestive system secrete special digestive juices that perform the complex chemical processes of digestion. Digestive juices con-

Figure 3-11

PERISTALTIC WAVE PASSING DOWN THE ESOPHAGUS

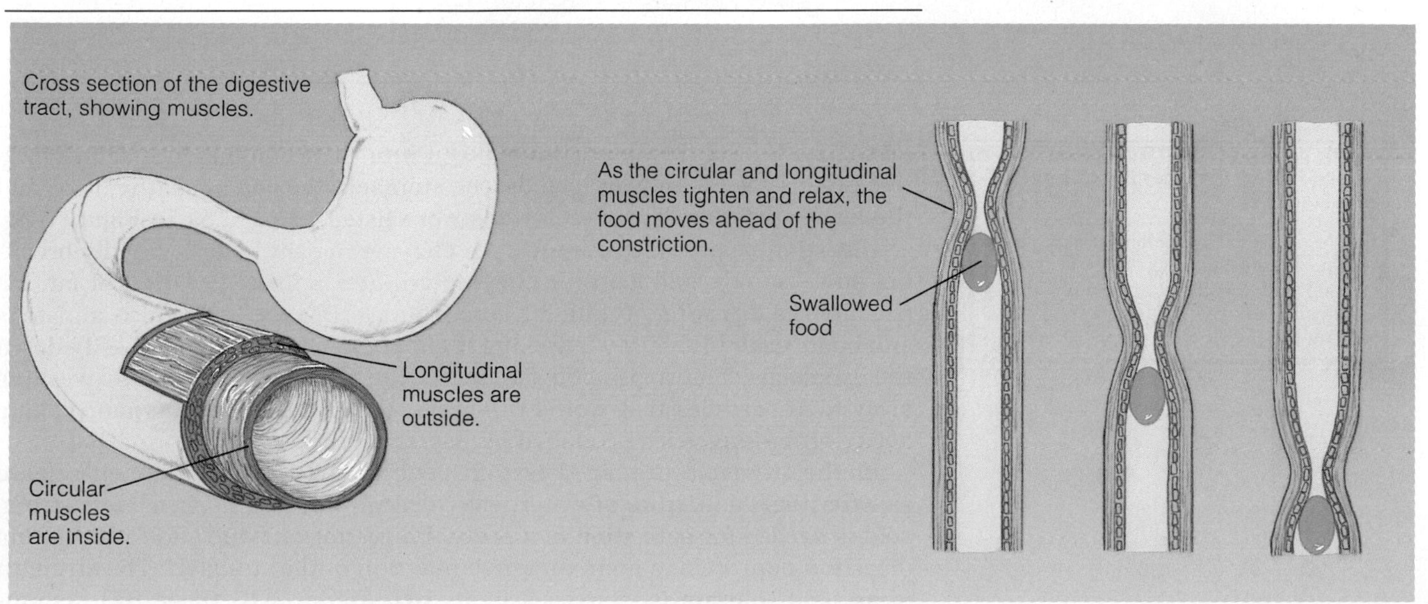
Cross section of the digestive tract, showing muscles.
Longitudinal muscles are outside.
Circular muscles are inside.
As the circular and longitudinal muscles tighten and relax, the food moves ahead of the constriction.
Swallowed food

Figure 3-12

THE MUSCULAR STOMACH

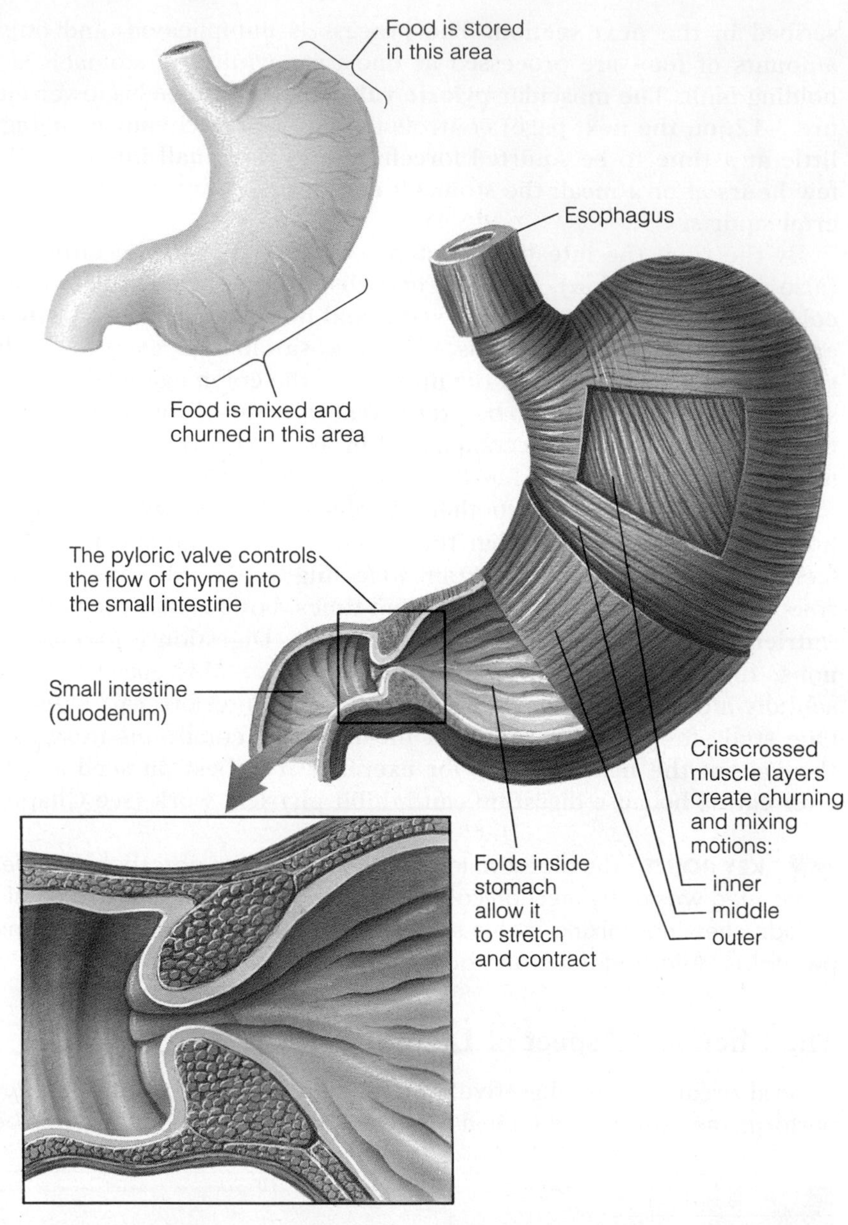

gastric juice the digestive secretion of the stomach.

pH a measure of acidity on a point scale. A solution with a pH of 1 is a strong acid; a solution with a pH of 7 is neutral; a solution with a pH of 14 is a strong base.

tain enzymes that break nutrients down into their component parts. Digestive organs are the salivary glands, the stomach, the pancreas, the liver, and the small intestine. Their secretions were listed on page 81 in Figure 3-8.

Digestion begins in the mouth. An enzyme in saliva starts rapidly breaking down starch, and another enzyme initiates a little digestion of fat, especially the digestion of milk fat, important in infants. Saliva also moistens and coats each bite of food, making it slippery and able to pass easily down the esophagus. Saliva also helps maintain the health of the teeth by washing away food particles that would otherwise foster decay and by neutralizing decay-promoting acids produced by bacteria in the mouth.

In the stomach, protein digestion begins. Cells in the stomach release **gastric juice,** a mixture of water, enzymes, and hydrochloric acid. A strong acid is needed for activation of a protein-digesting enzyme and for initiating digestion of protein, a main digestive function of the stomach. The strength of an acid solution is expressed as its **pH.** Figure 3-13 (page 87) demonstrates that saliva is only weakly acidic, while the stomach's gastric juice is much more strongly acidic.

Sometimes, instead of traveling down the digestive tract, acidic gastric juice backs up from the stomach into the esophagus causing **heartburn.** This can happen after a person eats or drinks excessively, so that the overfull stomach squeezes some of its contents back up through the muscular closure that normally prevents backflow. Just leaning over or lying down after a meal can cause it because the muscular closure between the esophagus and stomach is not as tight as, say, the seal made by the pyloric valve at the entrance to the small intestine. A person who experiences heartburn can try eating smaller meals, drinking liquids an hour before or after, but not during, meals, relaxing in a sitting position (not lying down) after meals, and avoiding irritating foods. Specifically, chemical irritants in foods, such as acid or the "hot" component of hot peppers make heartburn feel worse. Substances in coffee, fat, chocolate syrup, and alcoholic liquors may increase acidity in the stomach and trigger reflexes to relax the muscular closure of the stomach.[4] One other preventable factor that causes heartburn is smoking. The obvious action to take, of course, is to quit smoking. An easier, but not the best, route to temporary relief is to take antacid medication. Antacids do relieve heartburn for a while but they place a demand on the stomach to secrete more acid to counteract them. Antacids are designed to treat symptoms of conditions such as **ulcers** to provide relief while they heal. Those who would take them daily to relieve heartburn should seek medical help. The cause may be simply overeating, but it may be serious—a **hernia** or obstruction. Also, the ingredients in antacids interfere with the body's handling of many nutrients; future chapters point out these effects.

Students often wonder, upon learning of the powerful digestive juices and enzymes within the digestive tract, how the tract's own cellular lining escapes being digested along with the food. Indeed, if it were not for specialized cells that secrete a thick, viscous substance known as **mucus,** the structures of the tract lining would be exposed to chemical attack. Mucus coats and protects the digestive tract lining.

In the small intestine, the digestive process gets under way in earnest. The small intestine is "the" organ of digestion and absorption, and it finishes what the mouth and stomach have started. The small intestine works with the precision of a laboratory chemist. As the thoroughly liquefied and partially digested nutrient mixture arrives there, hormonal messengers signal the gallbladder to contract and to squirt the right amount of the **emulsifier, bile,** into the intestine. Other hormones notify the pancreas to release **pancreatic juice** containing the alkaline compound **bicarbonate** in amounts precisely adjusted to neutralize the stomach acid that has reached the small intestine.

Meanwhile the pancreatic and intestinal enzymes act on the chemical bonds that hold the large nutrients together so that smaller and smaller pieces are released into the intestinal fluids. The cells of the intestinal wall also hold some digestive enzymes on their surfaces, which perform last-minute breakdown reactions necessary before nutrients can be absorbed. Finally, the digestive process releases pieces small enough for the cells to absorb and use. Digestion and absorption of carbohydrate, fat, and protein are essentially complete by the time the intestinal contents enter the colon. However, water, fiber, and some minerals remain in the tract. Table 3-1 provides a summary of all the processes involved.

The digestive system can adjust to whatever mixture of foods is presented to it. People sometimes wonder if the digestive tract has trouble digesting

heartburn a burning sensation in the chest (heart) area caused by backflow of stomach acid into the esophagus.

ulcers erosions in the topmost, and sometimes underlying, layers of cells that form linings. Ulcers of the digestive tract commonly form in the esophagus, stomach, or upper small intestine.

hernia a protrusion of an organ or part of an organ through the wall of the body chamber that normally contains the organ. An example is a *hiatal* (high-AY-tal) *hernia* in which part of the stomach protrudes through the diaphragm into the space normally occupied by the esophagus, heart, and lungs.

mucus (MYOO-cus) a slippery coating of the intestinal tract lining (and other body linings) that protects the cells from exposure to digestive juices (and other destructive agents). The adjective form is *mucous* (same pronunciation). The digestive tract lining is a *mucous membrane.*

emulsifier (ee-MULL-sih-fire) a compound with both water-soluble and fat-soluble portions that can attract fats and oils into water, to form an emulsion.

bile a compound made by the liver, stored in the gallbladder, and released into the small intestine when needed. It emulsifies fats and oils to ready them for enzymatic digestion.

pancreatic juice fluid secreted by the pancreas that contains enzymes to digest carbohydrate, fat, and protein as well as sodium bicarbonate, a neutralizing agent.

bicarbonate a common alkaline chemical; a secretion of the pancreas; also, the active ingredient of baking soda.

Table 3-1
Summary of Chemical Digestion

	Mouth	Stomach	Small Intestine, Pancreas, Liver, and Gallbladder	Large Intestine (Colon)
Sugar and Starch	The salivary glands secrete saliva to moisten and lubricate food; chewing crushes and mixes it with a salivary enzyme that initiates starch digestion.	Digestion of starch continues while food remains in the upper storage area of the stomach. In the lower digesting area of the stomach, hydrochloric acid and an enzyme of the stomach's juices halt starch digestion.	The pancreas produces an enzyme that digests starch and releases it into the small intestine. Intestinal cell walls possess enzymes to break sugars and starch fragments to simple sugars, which then are absorbed.	Undigested carbohydrates reach the colon and are partly broken down by intestinal bacteria.
Fiber	The teeth crush fiber and mix it with saliva to moisten it for swallowing.	No action.	Fiber binds cholesterol and some minerals.	Most fiber excreted with feces; some fiber digested by bacteria in colon.
Fat	Fat-rich foods are mixed with saliva. The tongue produces traces of a fat-digesting enzyme that accomplishes some breakdown, especially of fats in milk. The enzyme is stable at low pH and is especially important to digestion in nursing infants.	Fat tends to rise from the watery stomach fluid and foods and float on top of the mixture. Only a small amount of fat is digested. Fat is last to leave the stomach.	The liver secretes bile; the gallbladder stores it and releases it into the small intestine. Bile emulsifies the fat and readies it for enzyme action. The pancreas produces fat-digesting enzymes and releases them into the small intestine to split fats into their component parts (primarily fatty acids).	Some fatty materials escape absorption and are carried out of the body with other wastes.
Protein	In the mouth, chewing crushes and softens protein-rich foods and mixes them with saliva.	Stomach acid works to uncoil protein strands and to activate the stomach's protein-digesting enzyme. Then the enzyme breaks the protein strands into smaller fragments.	Enzymes of the small intestine and pancreas split protein fragments into smaller fragments or free amino acids. Enzymes on the intestinal cell wall break some protein fragments into free amino acids for absorption. Some protein fragments are also absorbed.	The large intestine carries undigested protein residue out of the body. Normally, almost all food protein is digested and absorbed.
Water	Mouth donates watery, enzyme-containing saliva.	Stomach donates acidic, watery, enzyme-containing gastric juice.	Small intestine, pancreas, and liver donate watery, enzyme-containing juices; pancreatic juice is alkaline.	Large intestine reabsorbs water and some minerals.

certain foods in combination—for example, fruit and meat. Proponents of the fad of "food combining" claim that the digestive tract cannot perform certain digestive tasks at the same time, but this is a gross underestimation of the tract's capabilities. The truth is that all foods, regardless of identity, are broken down by enzymes into the basic molecules that make them up. In fact, scientists who study digestion suggest that the tract analyzes the diet's nutrient contents and delivers juice and enzymes appropriate for digesting those nutrients.[5] The pancreas is especially sensitive in this regard, and has been observed to adjust its output of enzymes to digest carbohydrate, fat, or protein to an amazing degree. The pancreas of a person who suddenly consumes a meal unusually high in carbohydrate, for example, would begin increasing its output of carbohydrate-digesting enzymes within 24 hours, while reducing outputs of other types.[6] This sensitive mechanism ensures that foods of all types are well used by the body.

The next section reviews the major processes of digestion by showing how the nutrients in a mixture of foods are handled. The foods used to illustrate the digestive process are those in a peanut butter and banana sandwich. But whether the nutrients in the digestive tract occurred originally in this meal or in a chili dog makes little difference to the digestive tract, which can promptly polish off either or both.

KEY POINT Chemical digestion begins in the mouth, where food is mixed with an enzyme in saliva that acts on carbohydrates. Digestion continues in the stomach, where stomach enzymes and acid break down protein. Digestion continues in the small intestine, where the liver and gallbladder contribute bile that emulsifies fat, and where the pancreas and small intestine donate enzymes that continue digestion so that absorption can occur.

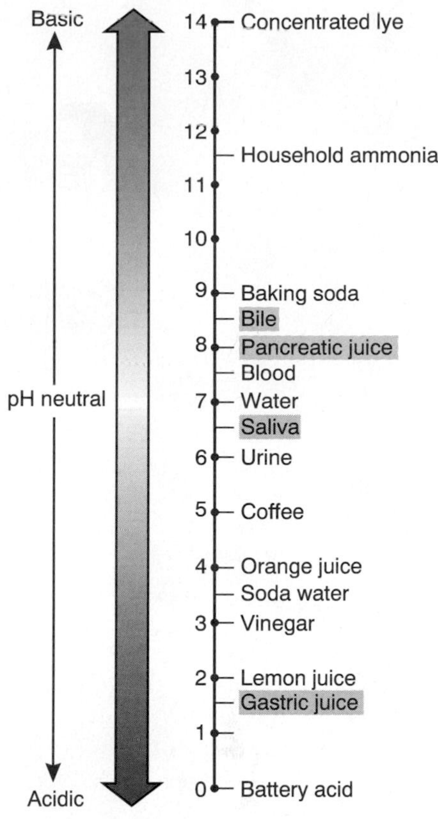

Figure 3-13

pH VALUES OF DIGESTIVE JUICES AND OTHER COMMON FLUIDS

A substance's acidity or alkalinity is measured in pH units. Each step down the scale indicates a tenfold increase in concentration of hydrogen particles. For example, a pH of 2 is 1,000 times stronger than a pH of 5.

The Digestive Fate of a Sandwich

The process of rendering foods into nutrients and absorbing them into the body fluids is remarkably efficient. In a healthy body, about 90 percent of the carbohydrate, fat, and protein that pass through the intestinal tract are digested to their component parts in time to be absorbed. Here, we follow a peanut butter and banana sandwich on whole wheat, sesame seed bread through the tract for the purpose of reviewing digestive processes in order of their occurrence in the body.

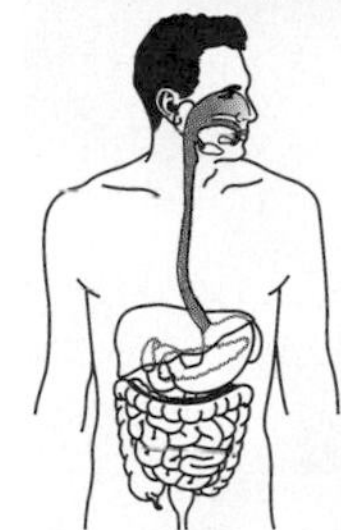

In the Mouth In each bite, food components are crushed, mashed, and mixed with saliva by the teeth and the tongue. The sesame seeds are crushed and torn open by the teeth to break through the indigestible fiber coating so that digestive enzymes can reach the nutrients inside the seeds. The peanut butter is the "extra crunchy" type, but the teeth grind the chunks to a paste before the bite is swallowed. The carbohydrate-digesting enzyme of saliva begins to break down the starches of the bread, banana, and peanut butter to sugars. Each swallow triggers a peristaltic wave that travels the length of the esophagus and carries one bite of food to the stomach.

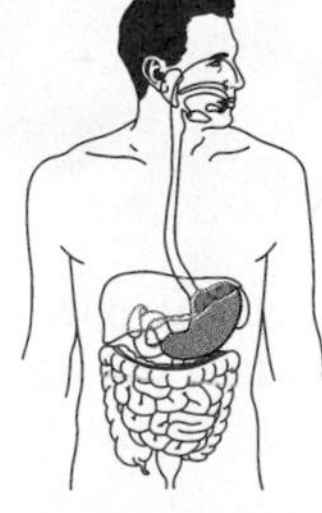

In the Stomach The stomach collects bite after swallowed bite in its upper storage area. Starch continues to be digested until the mass has been mixed with gastric juice. Small portions of the mashed sandwich are pushed into the digesting area of the stomach. Acid in gastric juice unwinds proteins and an enzyme clips into pieces the protein strands from the bread, seeds, and peanut butter. The sandwich has now become a thick liquid mass called chyme, and it enters the small intestine. It bears no resemblance to the original food. The starches have been partly split, proteins have been uncoiled and clipped, and the fat is forming a separate layer.

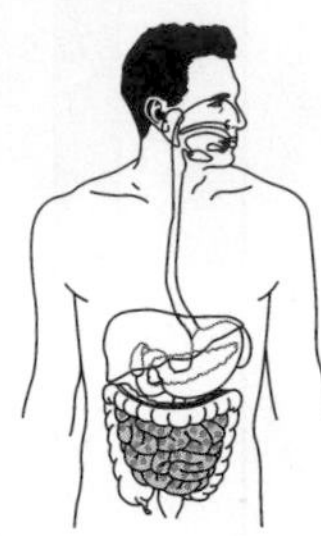

In the Small Intestine Some of the sweet sugars in the banana require so little processing that they begin to traverse the linings of the digestive tract immediately on contact. The nearby liver donates bile through a duct into the small intestine. The bile blends the fat from the peanut butter and seeds with the watery enzyme-containing digestive fluids. The nearby pancreas contracts and squirts enzymes into the small intestine to break down the fat, protein, and starch in the chemical soup that just an hour ago was a sandwich. The cells of the small intestine itself produce enzymes to complete these processes. As the enzymes do their work, smaller and smaller chemical fragments are liberated from the chemical soup and are absorbed into the blood and lymph through the cells of the small intestine's wall. Vitamins and minerals are absorbed here, too. They all eventually enter the bloodstream to nourish the tissues.

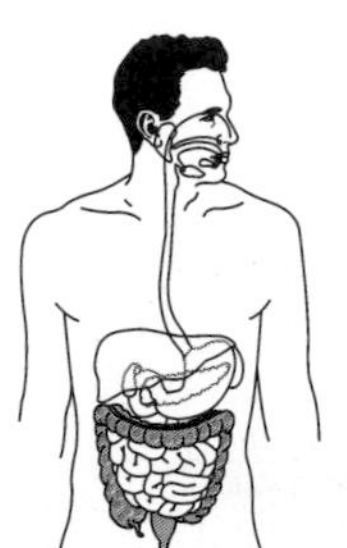

In the Large Intestine (Colon) The fibers from the seeds, whole wheat bread, peanut butter, and banana are partly digested by the bacteria living in the colon and some of the products are absorbed. Most fiber passes through the large intestine unabsorbed. In the large intestine, fiber fragments, fluid, and some minerals are absorbed, while the undigested fiber and some other components pass out of the colon, excreted as feces.

KEY POINT The mechanical and chemical actions of the digestive tract break food down to nutrients with remarkable efficiency.

Absorption and Transport of Nutrients

Once the digestive system has broken food down to its nutrient components, the rest of the body awaits their delivery. The cells of the intestinal lining absorb nutrients from the mixture within the intestine and deposit them in the blood and lymph. Every molecule of nutrient must traverse one of these cells if it is to enter the body fluids. The cells are selective: they recognize some of the nutrients that may be in short supply in the body. The mineral calcium is an example. The less calcium in the body, the more calcium the intestinal cells absorb. The cells are also extraordinarily efficient: they absorb enough nutrients to nourish all the body's other cells.

The intestinal tract lining is composed of layered sheets of cells, and the sheets poke out into millions of finger-shaped projections **(villi).** Every cell on every villus has a brushlike covering of tiny hairs **(microvilli)** that can trap the nutrient particles. Each villus (projection) has its own capillary network and a lymph vessel so that as nutrients move across the cells, they can immediately mingle into the body fluids. Figure 3-14 provides a close look at these details.

The small intestine's lining, villi and all, is wrinkled into thousands of folds, so that its absorbing surface is enormous. If the folds, and the villi that cover them, were spread out flat, the total area would equal a third of a football field in size. The billions of cells of that surface, although they weigh only 4 to 5 pounds, absorb enough nutrients to nourish the other 150 or so pounds of body tissues.

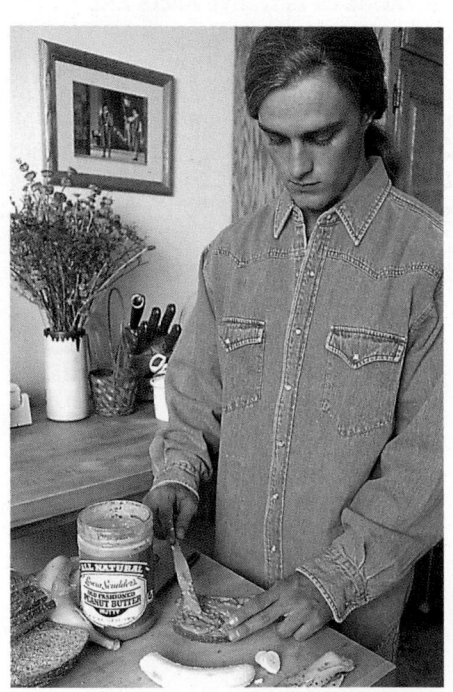

To become part of your body, food must first be digested and absorbed.

Figure 3-14

DETAILS OF THE SMALL INTESTINAL LINING

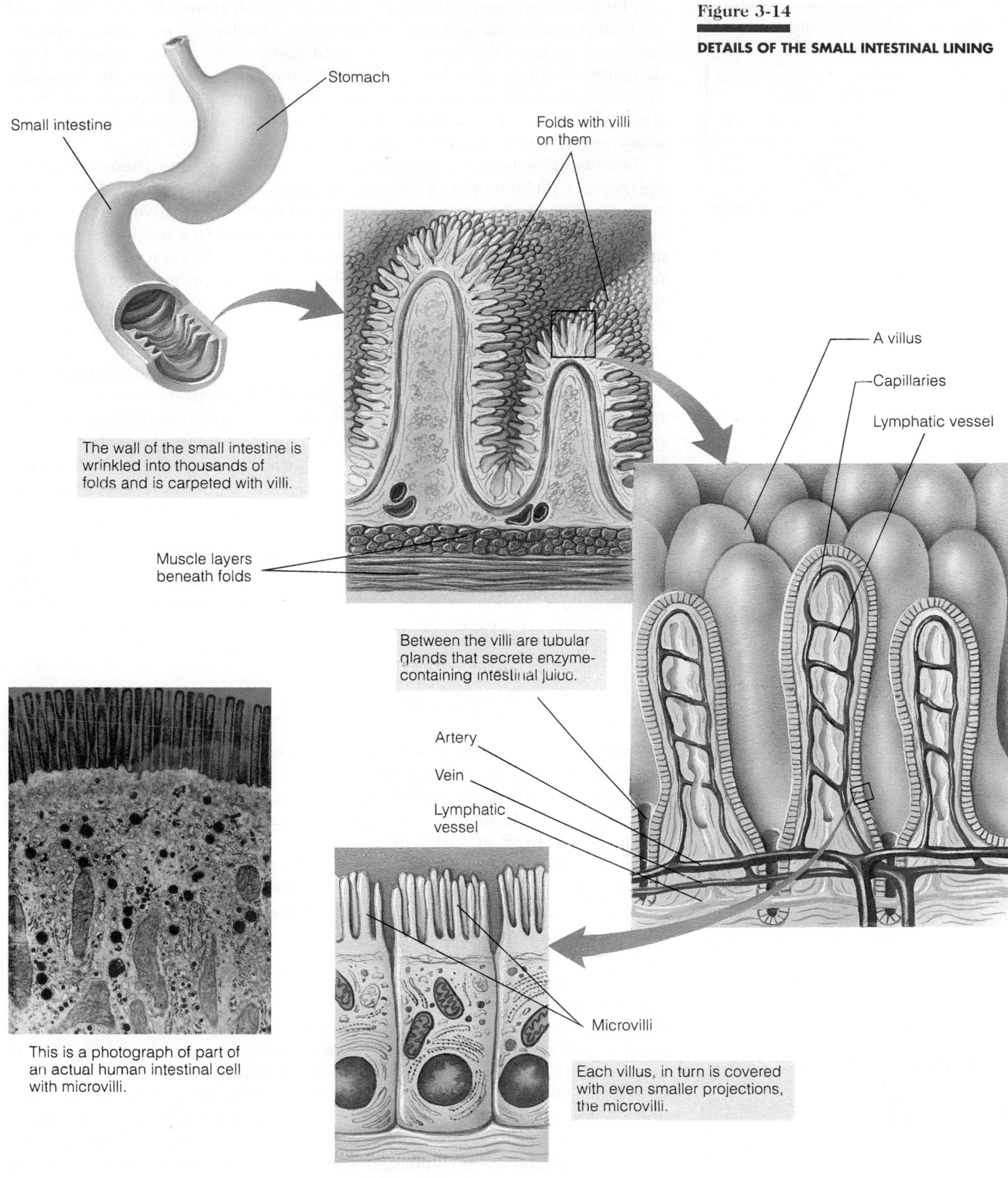
Stomach
Small intestine
Folds with villi on them
A villus
Capillaries
Lymphatic vessel
The wall of the small intestine is wrinkled into thousands of folds and is carpeted with villi.
Muscle layers beneath folds
Between the villi are tubular glands that secrete enzyme-containing intestinal juice.
Artery
Vein
Lymphatic vessel
Microvilli
This is a photograph of part of an actual human intestinal cell with microvilli.
Each villus, in turn is covered with even smaller projections, the microvilli.

villi (VILL-ee, VILL-eye) fingerlike projections of the sheet of cells that line the intestinal tract; the villi make the surface area much greater than it would otherwise be (singular: *villus*).

microvilli (MY-croh-VILL-ee, MY-croh-VILL-eye) tiny, hairlike projections on each cell of every villus that can trap nutrient particles and transport them into the cells (singular: *microvillus*).

The blood and lymph then take over the job of transporting nutrients to their ultimate consumers, the body's cells. The lymphatic vessels initially transport most of the products of fat digestion and a few vitamins, later delivering them to the bloodstream. The blood vessels carry the products of carbohydrate and protein digestion, most vitamins, and the minerals from the digestive tract to the liver. Thanks to these two transportation systems, every nutrient soon arrives at the place where it is needed.

The digestive system's millions of specialized cells are themselves sensitive to an undersupply of energy, nutrients, or dietary fiber. In cases of severe undernutrition of energy and nutrients, the absorptive surface of the small intestine shrinks. The surface may be reduced to a tenth of its normal area, making it impossible to obtain what few nutrients a limited food supply may provide. Without sufficient fiber to provide an undigested bulk for the tract's muscles to push against, the muscles become weak from lack of exercise. Malnutrition that impairs digestion is self-perpetuating because impaired digestion makes malnutrition worse.

So far, this chapter has shown that all the cells of the body's organs and systems rely on the digestive tract to provide the nutrients and water they need to remain alive and perform their life-sustaining functions. It has also mentioned that cells generate wastes. The next section introduces the body's primary organs of waste removal, the kidneys, and describes how these marvelous organs monitor and adjust the contents of dissolved substances in the blood.

KEY POINT The digestive system feeds the rest of the body and is itself sensitive to malnutrition. The folds and villi of the small intestine enlarge its surface area to facilitate nutrient absorption through uncountable microvilli on individual cell surfaces. Blood and lymph deliver nutrients to body cells.

◆ The Excretory System

Cells generate a number of wastes, and each must be eliminated. Many of the body's organs play roles in removing body wastes. Carbon dioxide waste from the cells travels in the blood to the lungs, where it is exchanged for oxygen, as already mentioned. Other wastes are pulled out of the bloodstream by the liver. The liver processes these wastes and either tosses them out into the digestive tract with bile, to leave the body with the feces, or prepares them to be sent to the kidneys for disposal in the urine. Organ systems work together to dispose of the body's wastes, but the kidneys are waste-removal specialists.

The kidneys straddle the cardiovascular system and filter the passing blood. Waste materials, dissolved in water, are collected by the kidney's working units, the **nephrons.** These wastes become urine, which travels in tubes that deliver urine to the urinary **bladder.** The bladder empties periodically, removing the wastes from the body. Thus the blood is purified continuously throughout the day, and dissolved materials are excreted as necessary. One dissolved mineral, sodium, helps to regulate blood pressure, and its excretion or retention by the kidney is a vital part of the body's blood pressure controlling mechanism. As you might expect, the kidneys' work is regulated by hormones secreted by glands that respond to conditions in the blood (such as the sodium concentration).

nephrons the working units in the kidney, consisting of intermeshed blood vessels and tubules.

bladder the sac that holds urine until time for elimination.

Because the kidneys remove toxins that could otherwise damage body tissues, whatever supports the health of the kidneys supports the health of the whole body. A strong cardiovascular system and an abundant supply of water are important to keep blood flushing swiftly through the kidneys. In addition, the kidneys need sufficient energy to do their complex sifting and sorting job, and many vitamins and minerals serve as the cogs in their machinery. Exercise and nutrition are vital to healthy kidney function.

 **KEY POINT** The kidneys adjust the blood's composition in response to the body's needs, disposing of everyday wastes and helping remove toxins. Nutrients, including water, and exercise help keep them healthy.

Storage Systems

The human body is designed to eat at intervals of about four to six hours, but cells need nutrients around the clock. Providing them with a constant flow of the needed nutrients requires the cooperation of many body systems. These systems store and release nutrients to meet the cells' needs between meals. Among the major storage places are the liver and muscles, which store carbohydrate; and the fat cells, which store fat as well as other things.

Nutrients collected from the digestive system sooner or later all move through a vast network of capillaries that weave among the liver cells. This arrangement ensures that liver cells have access to the newly arriving nutrients for processing. While later chapters provide the details, it is important to know now that the liver converts excess energy-containing nutrients into two forms. It makes some into **glycogen** (a carbohydrate) and some into fat. The liver stores the glycogen to meet the body's ongoing glucose needs. Liver glycogen can sustain cell activities when the intervals between meals become long; muscle cells make and store glycogen, too. Without glucose absorbed from food, the body (including the muscle cells) draws on liver glycogen. Should no food be available, the liver's glycogen supply dwindles; it can be effectively depleted within as few as three to six hours. Muscles store glycogen, too, but selfishly reserve it for their own use.

glycogen a storage form of carbohydrate energy (glucose), described more fully in Chapter 4.

fat cells cells that specialize in the storage of fat and that form the fat tissue.

Whereas the liver stores glycogen, it ships out fat in packages (see Chapter 5) to be picked up by cells that need it. All body cells may withdraw fat from these packages, and the fat that remains is stored in the **fat cells,** which hold fat to meet long-term energy needs. Fat tissue stores the body's reserve supply of fat, but unlike the liver, fat tissue has virtually infinite storage capacity. It can continue to supply the body's cells with fat for days, weeks, or possibly even months when no food is eaten.

These storage systems for glucose and fat ensure that the body's cells will not go without energy even if the body is hungry for food. Body stores also exist for many other nutrients, each with a characteristic capacity. For example, liver and fat cells store many vitamins, and bones provide reserves of calcium, sodium, and other minerals. Stores of nutrients are available to keep the blood levels constant and to meet cellular demands.

Some nutrients are stored in the body in much larger quantities than are others. For example, certain vitamins are stored without limit, even if they reach toxic levels within the body. Other nutrients are stored in only small amounts, regardless of the amount taken in, and these can readily be depleted. As you learn how the body handles various nutrients, pay particular attention to their storage so that you can know your tolerance limits. For example, you needn't eat fat at every meal, since fat is stored abundantly. On the other hand, you normally do need to have a source of carbohydrate at intervals throughout the day because the liver stores less than one day's supply of glycogen.

KEY POINT The body's energy stores are of two principal kinds: fat in fat cells (in potentially large quantities) and glycogen in liver cells (in smaller quantities). Other tissues store other nutrients.

Other Systems

In addition to the systems described above, the body has many more: bones, muscles, reproductive organs, and others. All of these cooperate, enabling each cell to carry on its own life. Each system ensures, through hormonal or nerve-mediated messengers, that its needs will be met by the others, and each contributes to the welfare of the whole by doing its own specialized work. Each system needs a continuous supply of many specific nutrients to maintain itself and to carry out its work. Calcium is particularly important for bones, for example; iron for muscles; glucose for the brain. But all systems need all nutrients, and every system is impaired by an undersupply or oversupply of them.

While external events clamor and vie for attention, the body remains quiet in its life-sustaining work. Of the billions of cells in the body, only a small percentage make up the cortex of the brain, where the conscious mind resides. When the cells of the cortex receive messages from other cells, the person "becomes conscious" of a need for decision and action. In modern life the need may be complex, as, for example, when a person feels anxious and decides to consult an advisor; or the need may be simple, as when a person feels hungry and decides, "I'd better eat."

Most of the body's work is directed automatically by the unconscious portions of the brain and nervous system, and this work is finely regulated to achieve a state of well-being. But you need to involve your cerebral cortex, your consciousness, so as to cultivate an understanding and appreciation of your body's needs. In doing so, attend to nutrition first. The rewards are liberating—ample energy to tackle life's tasks, a robust attitude, and the glowing appearance that comes from the best of health. Indulge yourself in the foods that best meet your body's needs and support its health. Read on, and learn to let nutrition principles guide your choices.

KEY POINT To achieve optimal function, the body's systems require nutrients from outside, and these have to be supplied through a human being's conscious food choices.

◆ Notes

1. D. R. Morse and coauthors, Oral digestion of a complex-carbohydrate cereal: Effects of stress and relaxation on physiological and salivary measures, *American Journal of Clinical Nutrition* 49 (1989): 97–105.
2. An enjoyable, accurate book that answers many questions about digestion and absorption is D. F. Magee and A. F. Dalley II, *Digestion and the Structure and Function of the Gut,* Karger Continuing Education Series, Volume 8 (Basel, Switzerland: Karger, 1986).
3. S. Lanzon-Miller and coauthors, The timing of the evening meal affects the pattern of 24-hour intragastric acidity, *Alimentary Pharmacology and Therapeutics* 4 (1990): 547–557.
4. J. H. Meyer, The stomach and nutrition in M. E. Shils, J. A. Olson, and M. Shike, eds., *Modern Nutrition in Health and Disease* (Philadelphia: Lea & Febiger, 1994) pp. 1029–1035.
5. J. A. Deutsch, The role of the stomach in eating, *American Journal of Clinical Nutrition* 42 (1985): 1040–1043; P. M. Brannon, Adaptation of the exocrine pancreas to diet, *Annual Reviews of Nutrition* 10 (1990): 85–105.
6. Brannon, 1990.

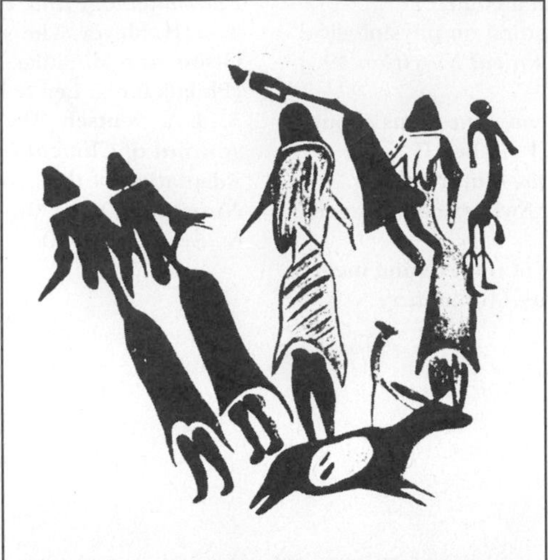

CONTROVERSY 3

Should We Be Eating "Natural," "Cave-Person" Foods?

Some people are unwilling to follow the food group plans advocated by traditional nutrition teaching. They'd rather have simpler rules to follow. One popular notion is that you can "just eat the way our cave-dwelling ancestors did—they were healthy." This Controversy looks at that proposition and applies some scientific criticism to it.

According to the cave-person diet advocates, you may be clothed in the latest fashions, and your car may be the maker's latest model, but your body is of prehistoric design—it is a cave-person body. Actually, our earliest ancestors were not cave dwellers and are properly called the people of the Stone Age, but never mind; the idea still is worth examining. You have come a long way from the Stone Age in many ways: in language skills, in the arts, in medicine, and especially in the use of machinery. But it is true that your body handles food and physical activity in virtually the same way as your ancestors' bodies did, 20,000 and more years ago. The muscles, heart, and lungs have hardly changed at all, and the brain, too, responds in the same ways to what the body sees, smells, and tastes.

The world, however, has changed vastly, especially in the last hundred years. The earth is far more crowded than it used to be. Our ancestors roamed the wilderness; today, more than half of the world's people live in cities. Extremes contrast with each other: poverty and death from malnutrition and related causes are common in the developing world; problems caused by overabundance are common in the developed countries. In the United States and Canada, excesses of food, and especially of processed foods, even cause health problems. Processed foods are often much higher in fat, salt, and sugar and lower in fiber, vitamins, and minerals than the wild foods eaten by our ancestors. Too, most people's lifestyles offer much less physical activity than did the lives of their ancestors. Many people face new technological byproducts in their environments, too, such as smog and water pollution. Your Stone-Age body is stressed by contending with these new problems. Naturally, people are inclined to wonder whether we should live and eat more nearly as our ancestors did.

THE TIME AND WORLD OF OUR ANCESTORS Before arriving at any conclusions, it is necessary to know what our ancestors ate and how healthy they were. We have to begin by deciding which ancestors to study—our farmer forebears and the early agricultural people who preceded them, or the hunter-gatherer people who lived still longer ago.

People have farmed the land for 10,000 years or more, 50 times longer than the period since the beginning of the industrial era, about 1800 A.D. Ten thousand years may seem long, but try a second comparison. Imagine all of human existence on earth to have occurred within the last 24 hours. Then the agricultural era would have begun only 3½ minutes ago, and the industrial era would have begun 4 *seconds* ago.[1] People who grow their own food have thus occupied the earth for only a few *hundred* generations, while people who hunted for their food roamed the earth for *thousands* of generations. Figure C3-1 depicts the magnitude of the differences between the earlier people's times on earth and our time.

The people we should study are therefore the earliest ones, the hunter-gatherers, before agriculture. They were the people of the Stone Age, the paleolithic period, from 10,000 to about 500,000 years ago (*paleo* means "ancient"; *lith* means "stone," referring to the stone tools they used). The Stone-Age people's way of life and diet persisted for close to half a million years. Enough time elapsed during those years to permit natural selection of genes for traits that favored survival in the life, and with the diet, of the time, generation after generation. Many of the genes for these traits persist in our inheritance today. Thousands of years old, those genes still support physical characteristics in us that favored survival in the conditions of those early times.

The more we know about the Stone-Age people, then, the better we can understand our bodies' needs today.

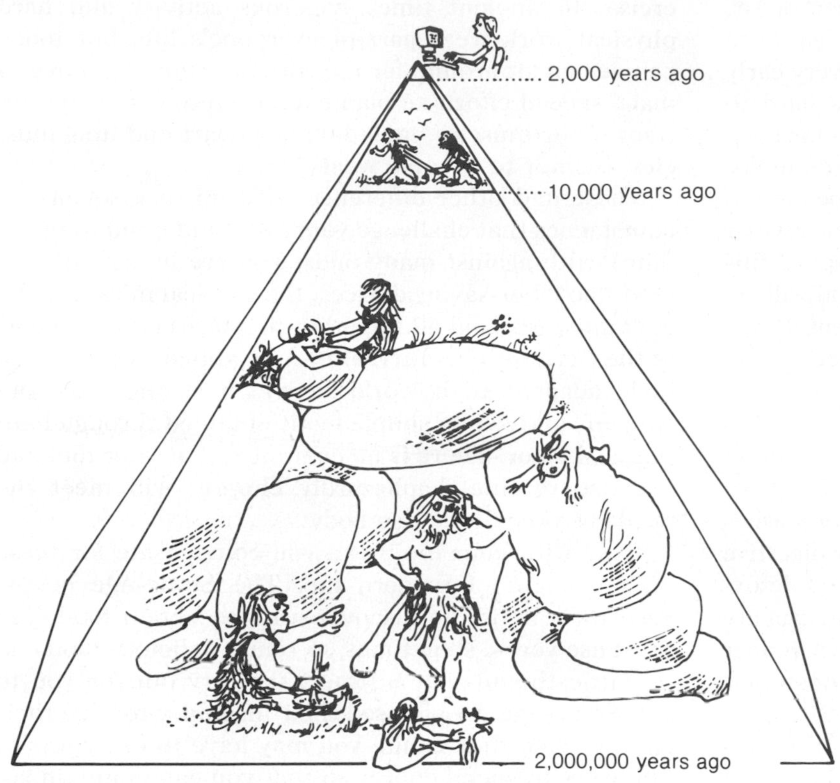

Figure C3-1

A PERSPECTIVE ON MODERN HUMAN BEINGS' TIME ON EARTH
The *space* occupied in the pyramid is proportional to the *time* spent on earth.

The publication of several popular novels in the *Earth's Children* series by Jean Auel has made it possible for people to learn informally not only about food and activities of those times but also about what the culture, traditions, and daily experiences of those people may have been like.* The stories in the novels are fictional, but the descriptions are based on facts.

THE ANCIENT BODY IN THE MODERN WORLD Food was not available all the time for the Stone-Age people. Times of plenty alternated with times of famine. The human body adapted well to this state of affairs. It was omnivorous—able to digest and to use the nutrients from both plants and animals. This made wide food choices possible and presented the least likelihood of starvation in the face of a food supply that depended on place and season. The body could also store excess energy in its fat tissue when food was plentiful. Then people could draw on that fuel supply during famine or illness.

*The first of the series was *Clan of the Cave Bear.*

Our bodies can do the same things today. We too can eat many kinds of food. We too efficiently store surplus energy in body fat. Today, though, these abilities confer less of an advantage. Not all the foods available to us today benefit our health, and in food-abundant societies, times of famine never come. Our overeating and storage of excess fat often now produce conditions that shorten life. Excess body fatness precipitates diabetes in susceptible people, it aggravates high blood pressure, it renders certain cancers more likely, and it worsens arthritis, among other things.

The body feels hungry at approximately four- to six-hour intervals, even though it may have sufficient fat stores to last for many days. This adaptation served the Stone-Age people well, for it drove them to continue stocking fuel within their bodies as often as their digestive systems could perform the task. They ate whenever food was available, even when they had sufficient body fat and nutrient stores for temporary needs. As a result, they never had to dip deeply into those stores until the food supply ran out.

Furthermore, the Stone-Age people's appetites were especially stimulated whenever they encountered foods that were rich in food energy—those with the taste of oils or fats or the sweetness of concentrated sugar. Foods that tasted of salt also appealed to their taste buds, for pure salt was rarely available in the very early times and the essential nutrient sodium was hard to come by. Novel foods also appealed to them—for good reasons. For long periods their diets were monotonous; their eagerness to try new foods probably helped to ensure that they would obtain the nutrients their regular diet might have lacked. Today, people still respond this way to foods. We prefer tasty, high-fat foods and will eat even when full if new delicious foods present themselves. This is why the dessert cart can entice you to stuff yourself, even after you've eaten a large meal.

The sense of taste is also the front line of the body's defense against poisons: people refuse foods that don't taste "right." The second line of defense is the stomach's rejection response; the body vomits up or washes out via diarrhea whatever "disagrees" with the digestive system. The third line is the liver's filtering and detoxifying systems. Toxins that get into the bloodstream are removed from it by the liver cells, which then render them harmless and put them away in permanent storage or release them for excretion in the urine.

For example, protection against the harmful effects of one ancient and familiar substance—alcohol—is built into the body's genes. One of those genes, expressed in the liver, codes for an enzyme that converts alcohol into substances the body can use or excrete. So long as the liver is not overwhelmed with alcohol, the system works efficiently.

The same is not true of all poisons. Alcohol has been around ever since the first fruit ripened and fermented, so there have been millions of years for natural selection to mold a detoxifying system for it. On the other hand, most of the additives intentionally put into foods and the pollutants and toxins that get in by mistake are new to the body. If it can't excrete them, it may accumulate harmful quantities or convert them to odd, unfamiliar substances that can interfere with metabolism or cause cancer or birth defects. An important new area of study in nutrition is the study of the body's handling of these substances.

In other ways, too, the body is adapted to the conditions of earlier times. Heredity has given each human being a body that can *develop* to run after prey, to fight enemies, or to carry heavy burdens long distances; it responds to physical exertion by becoming stronger and swifter. Among the muscles that become stronger in response to exercise are the heart and lung muscles, and they also (like all muscles) become weaker without exercise. In ancient times, vigorous activity and hard physical work were part of everyone's life, but today people can sit around for months at a time. We have to make special efforts to plan exercise into our daily routines if our muscles, including our heart and lung muscles, are not to become weak.

These and other differences add up to a set of circumstances that challenge your body and mind to maintain health against many odds. You are living with the food, the labor-saving devices, the medical miracles, the contaminants, and all the other pleasures and problems of the twentieth century. However, you are housed in a body adapted to a world in which strong men and women survived on simple foods obtained through hard physical labor. There is no guarantee that your diet and exercise routine, haphazardly chosen, will meet the needs of your Stone-Age body.

Only with your brain can you compensate for these disadvantages of modern life. The Stone-Age people used their brains to discover ways to obtain food; you must use yours, sometimes, to refuse delicious food and to battle the ancient instincts that cry out for you to eat. Stone-Age people used their ingenuity to save their energy when they could; you may have to use yours to find ways to spend energy so that you can maintain appropriate weight and keep your heart and muscles fit. You have an advantage, though. Unlike your ancestors, you can learn more about how your body works and what it needs from food.

THE STONE-AGE DIET Researchers have studied what the Stone-Age people actually ate. Analysis of their probable diet from fossilized remains of their meals and excretions has produced a picture of what foods they ate and how much of each nutrient they received. The figures are undoubtedly not exact, but it is interesting to compare them with those of today. Early people probably consumed 3,000 calories per day and apparently were never obese. (Today we consume fewer than 2,000 calories a day and still many of us are obese because we get so little exercise.)

Given their large energy allowances, and the exclusively nutrient-dense food options from which they were forced to choose, the Stone-Age people probably met all of their nutrient needs well. For example, although they drank no milk and made no cheese, their intakes of calcium were probably close to 1,500 milligrams a day, thanks to the fruits and vegetables they consumed. Today we fall short of 800 milligrams, although recommendations state that many people (and especially young people) need more than 1,000 milligrams to preserve the integrity of their bones. Stone-Age people probably consumed close to 400 milligrams a day of vitamin C, whereas we take in less than 100 milligrams. They ingested much more fiber than we do today, 45 grams or so, as compared with our 20 grams or less. Counterbalancing these pluses, they also ate more dirt, and even gravel![2]

The Stone-Age people achieved their abundant nutrient intakes using only two of the four groups of foods we think of as important: meat and fruits/vegetables. Their intakes of meat, and therefore of protein, were two to five times higher than ours are today, but most of their meats were lean, whereas many of ours are high in fat. The fats in their meats included a type thought to be preventive against heart disease and cancer, and known to be lacking from our meats today, the so-called omega-3 fatty acids described in Chapter 5. They apparently consumed cereal grains rarely, if at all, and they had no dairy foods whatsoever.[3] (Remember, they lived before the dawn of agriculture.)

Although their total energy intakes were higher than ours, the people of the Stone Age had lower intakes of two no-no's that plague modern eaters: fat and sodium. Their cholesterol intakes were similar to ours, however, because even lean meat contains cholesterol. Also, their diet seldom contained concentrated sweets such as honey, and there was no such thing as table sugar.

Were the earlier people healthier, then, than we are today? Not necessarily. Many died of starvation during times of climatic extremes. Many must have suffered vitamin deficiencies and food-borne diseases.[4] Stone-Age people died younger than we do, and this is one reason why the so-called degenerative "diseases of old age" were less common then than they are today.

Our longer lives are not the only reason for today's prevalence of cancer and heart disease, though; our diets share the blame.[5] This has been learned from the evidence available on primitive people living today: tribes in Africa and other places whose diets and ways of life resemble those of the Stone-Age people. These people's lifestyles enable them to attain the age of 60 years relatively free of degenerative diseases.[6]

Breast cancer, for example, was practically unheard of in Stone-Age women but is a major killer of relatively young women today.[7] Some believe that our diet evokes a surprisingly strong estrogen response, and estrogen has been linked to breast cancer. The Stone-Age diet is believed to have been less estrogenic.

Does this mean we should abandon the use of grains and dairy products and eat only meat and fruits/vegetables? No—even if we did, we would not be eating like the Stone-Age people or today's few remaining primitive tribes. Our foods are different. Our meats differ in the amounts and types of fat they contain. Our fruits and vegetables are totally different. And the Stone-Age people's environment, with its vast, city-less open spaces no longer exists for us.

Still, even if we cannot eat the same foods they did, we can attempt to duplicate their activity and nutrient intake levels using the foods available to us. Clearly we should emulate them in incorporating more physical activity into our days. If we exercise more, we can eat more without getting fat; if we eat more, we can obtain more nutrients; and if we obtain more nutrients, we are better protected against deficiencies.

In conclusion, no one can go back to the days of the Stone-Age people and live as they did. We can learn from them, though, the importance of getting more exercise and of eating wholesome foods that will support our health as well as, or even better than, theirs did.

◆ Notes

1. A. E. Harper, 1990 Atwater lecture: The science and the practice of nutrition: Reflections and directions, *American Journal of Clinical Nutrition* 53 (1991): 413–420.
2. S. M. Garn and W. R. Leonard, What did our ancestors eat? *Nutrition Reviews* 47 (1989): 337–345.
3. S. B. Eaton and M. Konner, Paleolithic nutrition, a consideration of its nature and current implications, *New England Journal of Medicine* 312 (1985): 283–289.
4. Garn and Leonard, 1989.
5. A. Leaf and P. C. Weber, A new era for science in nutrition, *American Journal of Clinical Nutrition* 45 (1987): 1048–1053.
6. Eaton and Konner, 1985.
7. S. B. Eaton, Women's reproductive cancers in evolutionary context (abstract) in *AAAS Annual Meeting Abstracts of Papers* (Washington, D.C.: American Association for the Advancement of Science, 1993) p. 181.

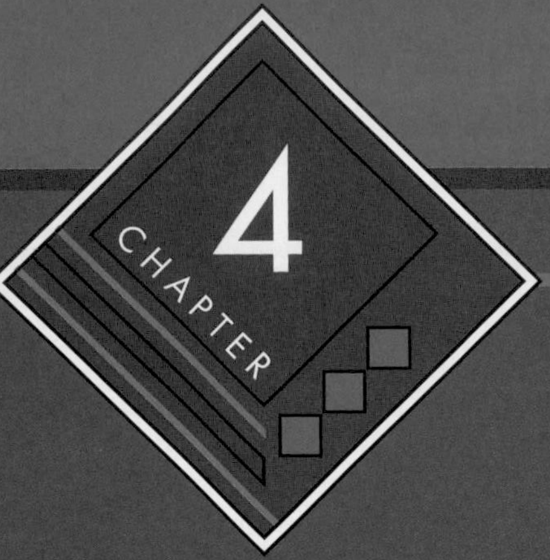

The Carbohydrates: Sugars, Starch, Glycogen, and Fibers

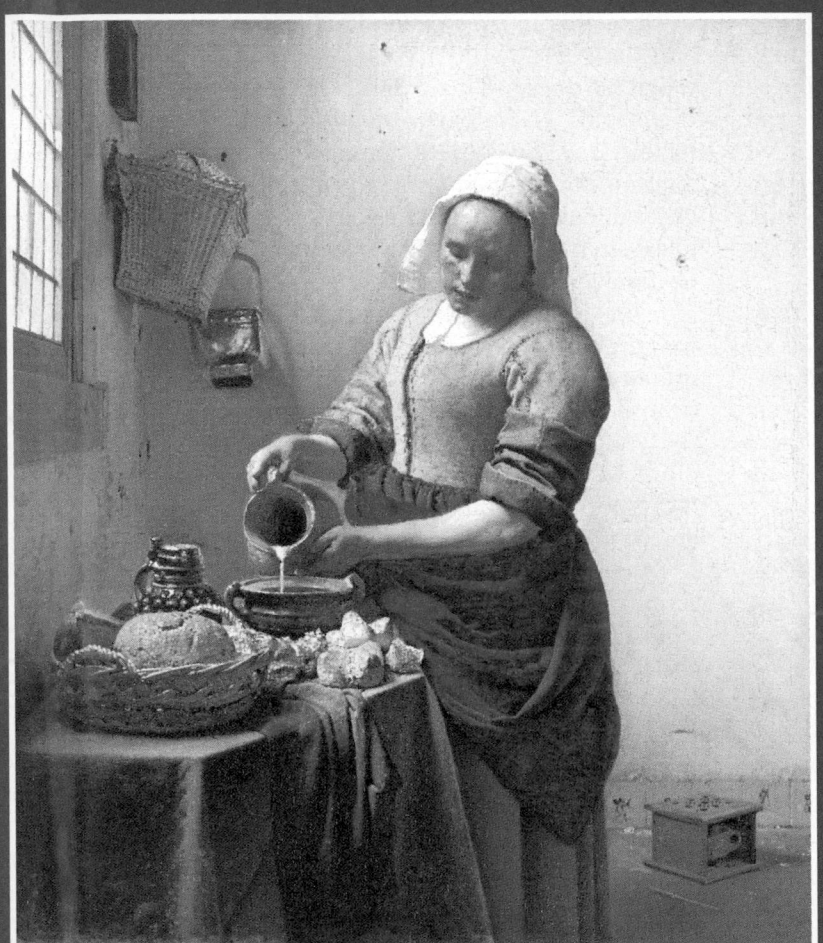

Jan Vermeer, *The Kitchenmaid*, Rijkmuseum, Amsterdam (A2344).

Contents

4

It is impossible to single out the most important nutrient. Nutrients work together in harmony, each affecting the functions of many others. However, **carbohydrates** are ideal to meet your body's energy needs, to keep your digestive system fit, to feed your brain and nervous system, and (perhaps surprisingly) to help keep your body lean. Years of false propaganda about the evils of carbohydrate's supposed "fattening powers" have misled millions of weight-conscious people to avoid carbohydrate-rich foods, a counterproductive tactic. People who wish to lose fat and to maintain lean tissue can do no better than to design their diets around low-fat foods that supply carbohydrates in abundance. Digestible carbohydrates, together with fats and protein, give bulk to foods and provide energy for the body. Fiber, made mostly of indigestible carbohydrates, yields little or no energy but provides other important benefits.

All carbohydrates are not equal as far as nutrition is concerned. This chapter invites you to learn to distinguish between the **complex carbohydrates** (starch and fiber), which are put to good use in the body, and the **simple carbohydrates** (sugars), some of which are less valuable to most people's health. The Controversy then asks whether the sugar added to foods harms health and whether the alternative sweeteners designed to replace sugar are preferable.

This chapter on the carbohydrates is the first of three on the energy-yielding nutrients. Chapter 5 deals with the fats and Chapter 6 with protein.

carbohydrates compounds composed of single sugars or multiples of them. The name means "carbon and water" and a chemical shorthand for carbohydrate is CHO, signifying carbon (C) and water (H_2O).

complex carbohydrates long chains of sugar units arranged to form starch or fiber. Also called *polysaccharides.*

simple carbohydrates sugars, including both single sugar units and linked pairs of sugar units. The basic sugar unit is a molecule containing six carbon atoms, together with oxygen and hydrogen atoms.

A Close Look at Carbohydrates

Carbohydrates contain the sun's radiant energy, captured in a form that living things can use to drive the processes of life. Thus they form the first link in the food chain that supports all life on earth. Carbohydrate-rich foods come almost exclusively from plants; milk is the only animal-derived food that contains significant amounts of carbohydrate.

Green plants make carbohydrate through **photosynthesis** in the presence of **chlorophyll** and sunlight. In this process water (H_2O), absorbed by the plant's roots, donates hydrogen and oxygen, while carbon dioxide gas (CO_2), absorbed into its leaves, donates carbon and oxygen. Water and carbon dioxide combine to yield the most common of the **sugars,** the single sugar **glucose.** Scientists know the reaction in the minutest detail, and yet it has never been reproduced from scratch; it requires green plants to make it happen (see Figure 4-1).

Energy from the sun drives the photosynthesis reaction. The energy becomes trapped in the chemical bonds that hold six atoms of carbon together in the sugar glucose. Glucose provides energy for the work of all cells of the stem, roots, flowers, and fruits of the plant. For example, in the roots, far from the energy-giving rays of the sun, each cell takes some of the glucose made in the leaves, breaks it down (to carbon dioxide and water), and uses the energy thus released to fuel its own growth and water-gathering activities.

Some energy remains in the sugars stored in plants. This is the part of photosynthesis that is important to our survival. The next few sections describe the forms that carbohydrates take, with their treasures of stored energy awaiting use in the human body.

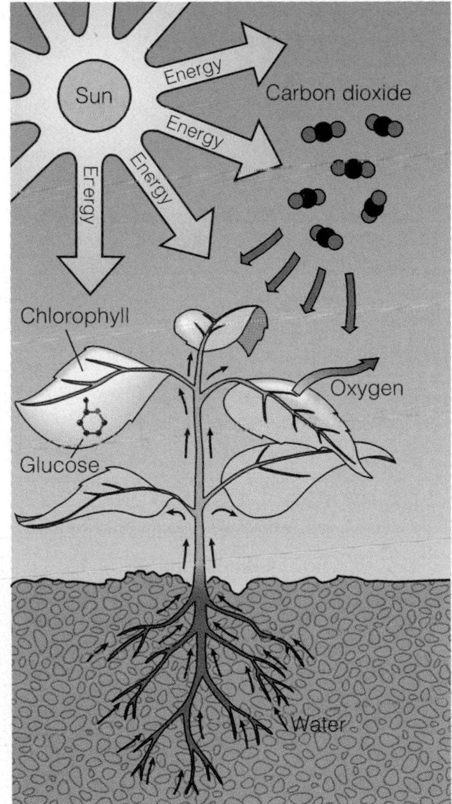

Figure 4-1

CARBOHYDRATE—MAINLY GLUCOSE—IS MADE BY PHOTOSYNTHESIS

The sun's energy becomes part of the glucose molecule—its calories, in a sense. In the molecule of glucose on the leaf here, dots represent the carbon atoms; bars represent the chemical bonds that contain energy.

photosynthesis the synthesis of carbohydrates by green plants from carbon dioxide and water using the green pigment chlorophyll to trap the sun's energy (*photo* means "light"; *synthesis* means "making").

chlorophyll the green pigment of plants, which traps energy from sunlight for use in photosynthesis.

sugars *simple carbohydrates*, that is, molecules of either single sugar units or pairs of those sugar units bonded together.

glucose (GLOO-cose) a single sugar used in both plant and animal tissues for quick energy; sometimes known as blood sugar; also called *dextrose*.

monosaccharides single sugar units (*mono* means "one" and *saccharide* means "sugar unit").

disaccharides pairs of single sugars linked together (*di* means "two").

fructose (FROOK-toce) a monosaccharide, sometimes known as fruit sugar (*fruct* means "fruit"; *ose* means "sugar").

galactose (ga-LACK-toce) a monosaccharide; part of the disaccharide lactose (milk sugar).

lactose a disaccharide composed of glucose and galactose—milk sugar (*lact* means "milk"; *ose* means "sugar").

maltose a disaccharide composed of two glucose units—malt sugar.

sucrose (SOO-crose) a disaccharide composed of glucose and fructose—table, beet, or cane sugar.

Single sugars are monosaccharides.

Pairs of sugars are disaccharides.

KEY POINT Through photosynthesis, plants combine carbon dioxide, water, and the sun's energy to form glucose. Carbohydrates are made of carbon, hydrogen, and oxygen held together by energy-containing bonds: *carbo* means "carbon"; *hydrate* means "water."

Sugars

Altogether, six sugar molecules are important in nutrition. Three are single sugars, or **monosaccharides.** The other three are the double sugars, or **disaccharides.** All of their chemical names end in *ose*, which means *sugar*, and while they all sound alike to the newcomer, they take on distinct characteristics to the nutrition enthusiast who quickly gets to know each individually.

The three monosaccharides are glucose, already described, **fructose,** and **galactose.** Fructose, or fruit sugar, the intensely sweet sugar of fruit, is made by rearranging the atoms in glucose molecules. Fructose occurs mostly in fruits; in honey; and as part of table sugar. Glucose and fructose are the most common monosaccharides in nature.

The other monosaccharide, galactose, has the same numbers and kinds of atoms, but they are arranged still differently. Galactose is one of the two single sugars bound together to form the pair that make up the sugar of milk. It does not occur free in nature; it is instead tied up in milk sugar until it is freed during digestion.

The three other sugars important in nutrition are disaccharides, linked pairs of single sugars. All three contain glucose. In **lactose,** the sugar of milk just mentioned, glucose is linked to galactose.

In malt sugar, or **maltose,** there are two glucose units. Maltose appears wherever starch is being broken down. It occurs in germinating seeds and arises during the fermentation process that yields alcohol. It also arises during the digestion of starch in the human body.

The last of the six sugars, **sucrose,** is the most familiar. It is table sugar, the product most people think of when they use the term *sugar*. In sucrose, fructose and glucose are bonded together. Table sugar is obtained by refining the juice from sugar beets or sugar cane, but sucrose also occurs naturally in many vegetables and fruits. It is as sweet as fruit sugar, because it too contains the sweet monosaccharide, fructose. It is of major importance in human nutrition, and research about its effects on the human body is a topic of Controversy 4.

When you eat a food containing single sugars, you can absorb them directly into your blood. When you eat disaccharides, though, you must digest them first. Enzymes in your intestine must split the disaccharides into separate monosaccharides; then they can enter the bloodstream. The blood delivers all products of digestion first to the liver, which possesses enzymes to modify nutrients, making them useful to the body. Glucose is the most-used monosaccharide inside the body, so the liver quickly converts fructose or galactose to glucose, or to smaller pieces that can serve as building blocks for either glucose or fat.

When people learn that the energy of fruit comes from sugars, they may think that eating fruit is the same as eating concentrated sweets such as candy or cola beverages. Not so. Fruits differ from concentrated sweets in nutrient density. The sugars of fruits arrive in the body diluted in large volumes of water, packaged in fiber, and mixed with many vitamins and needed minerals. In contrast, all types of refined sugars, even honey, arrive in the body in concentrated form, practically devoid of nutrients. From the body's point of view, fruits are vastly different from purified sugars, except that both provide glucose in abundance.

Starch

Glucose occurs in foods not only in sugars but also in long strands, in which thousands of glucose units are strung together. These are the **polysaccharides.** Starch is one of these; glycogen is another; some of the fibers are others.

Starch is a plant's storage form of glucose. As a plant matures, it not only provides energy for its own needs but also stores energy in its seeds for the next generation to use. For example, after a corn plant reaches its full growth and has many leaves manufacturing glucose, it begins to store **starch** in its seeds for the growth of new plants next season. Glucose is soluble in water and would be washed away by rains while the seed lay in the soil. Starch is an insoluble substance that will stay with the seed and nourish it until it forms shoots with leaves that can catch the sun's rays. A kernel of corn, then, is really a seed with its germ embedded in this nutritive material. The starch of corn and other foods is nutritive for human beings also, because they can digest the starch to glucose and extract the sun's energy stored in its chemical bonds. A later section describes starch digestion in greater detail.

polysaccharides another term for complex carbohydrates, compounds of long strands of glucose units linked together (*poly* means "many").

starch a plant polysaccharide composed of glucose, digestible by human beings.

glycogen (GLY-co-gen) a polysaccharide composed of glucose, made and stored by liver and muscle tissues of human beings and animals as a storage form of glucose. Glycogen is not a significant food source of carbohydrate and is not counted as one of the complex carbohydrates in foods.

Strands of many sugar units are polysaccharides.

Glycogen

Just as plants store glucose in long chains of starch, so do animal bodies store glucose in long chains of **glycogen** (sometimes called *animal starch*). Glycogen resembles starch in that it consists of glucose molecules linked together to form chains, but its chains are longer and are more highly branched. A later section describes the body's handling of these packages of stored glucose. The relationships between the monosaccharides, disaccharides, and polysaccharides are summed up in Figures 4-2 and 4-3.

Carbohydrate plays a prominant role in the global carbon cycle. Carbon dioxide, water, and energy are combined in plants to form glucose; the

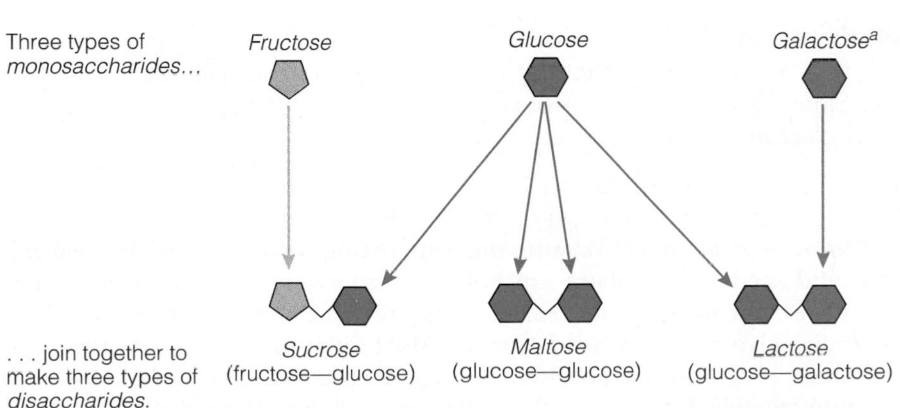

[a]Galactose does not occur in foods singly but as part of lactose.

Figure 4-2

HOW MONOSACCHARIDES JOIN TO FORM DISACCHARIDES

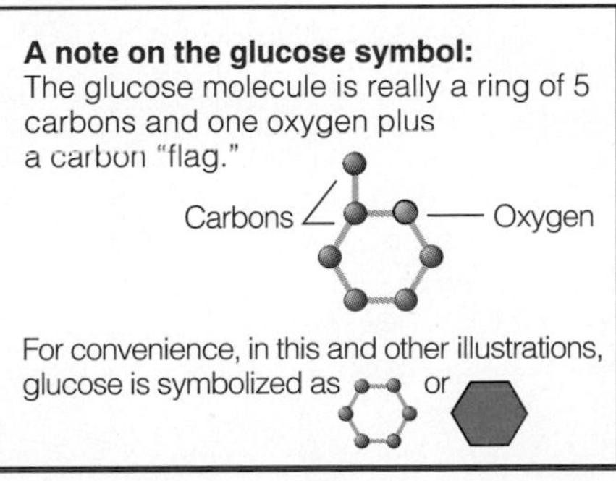

A note on the glucose symbol:
The glucose molecule is really a ring of 5 carbons and one oxygen plus a carbon "flag."
Carbons
Oxygen
For convenience, in this and other illustrations, glucose is symbolized as or

Figure 4-3

HOW GLUCOSE MOLECULES JOIN TO FORM POLYSACCHARIDES

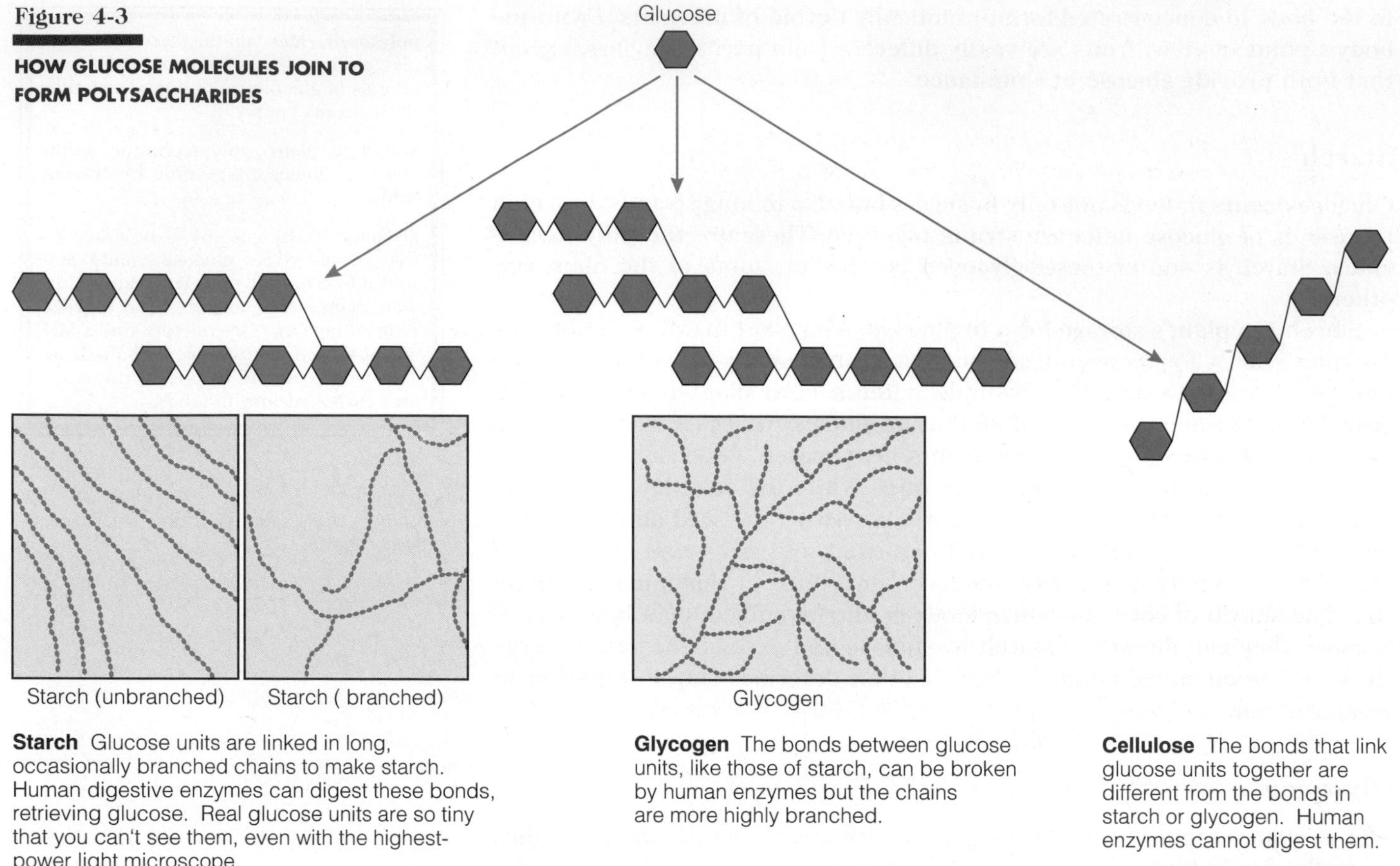

Starch Glucose units are linked in long, occasionally branched chains to make starch. Human digestive enzymes can digest these bonds, retrieving glucose. Real glucose units are so tiny that you can't see them, even with the highest-power light microscope.

Glycogen The bonds between glucose units, like those of starch, can be broken by human enzymes but the chains are more highly branched.

Cellulose The bonds that link glucose units together are different from the bonds in starch or glycogen. Human enzymes cannot digest them.

fibers the indigestible polysaccharides in food, comprised mostly of *cellulose, hemicellulose,* and *pectin.* Also called *nonstarch polysaccharides.*

plants may store the glucose in the polysaccharide starch. Then animals or people eat the plants. In the body the liver and muscles may store the glucose as the polysaccharide glycogen, but ultimately it becomes glucose again. The glucose delivers the sun's energy to fuel the body's activities. In the process, glucose breaks down to waste products, carbon dioxide and water, which are excreted. Later, these compounds are used again by plants as raw materials to make carbohydrate. Chapter 15 comes back to humankind's relationship with the earth's food chain.

KEY POINT Glucose is the most important monosaccharide in the human body. Most other monosaccharides and disaccharides become glucose in the body. Starch is a storage form of glucose in plants. Glycogen is the storage form of glucose in animals, including human beings.

Fibers

The **fibers** of a plant contribute the supporting structures of its leaves, stems, and seeds. Most fibers are polysaccharides—chains of sugars—just as starch is, but in fibers the sugar units are held together by bonds that human digestive enzymes cannot break. Most fibers therefore pass through the human body without providing energy for its use. The best known of these polysaccharides are *cellulose* (shown in Figure 4-3), *hemicellulose,* and *pectin.* (Other fibers are *gums, mucilages,* and *lignins.*) The first two are found in the familiar strings of celery, the skins of corn kernels, and the membranes surrounding kernels of wheat. In the body these two provide

roughage, which aids in digestion and elimination. Pectin, isolated from plants such as apples or citrus fruits, may be used as a food additive to thicken jelly, to keep salad dressing from separating, and to otherwise alter texture and consistency of processed foods.

The term *dietary fiber* describes substances that cannot be broken down by *human* digestive enzymes. They are, however, vulnerable to breakdown by the enzymes of bacteria that reside in the digestive tracts of human beings. Some of these substances are changed by intestinal bacteria into products that are absorbed and contribute a few calories' worth of energy to the body.

Some animals, such as cattle, depend heavily on their intestinal bacteria to make available the energy of glucose derived from the abundant fiber cellulose in their fodder. When we eat beef, we receive indirectly some of the sun's energy that was originally stored in the fiber of the plants the cattle ate. Beef, of course, contains no fiber itself; no meats or dairy products contain fiber. The human body derives just small amounts of energy from fiber breakdown in its own digestive tract, as a later section on digestion shows.

Fibers are classified by chemists according to how readily they dissolve in water. Some fibers are **insoluble fibers,** some, **soluble fibers.** Each type of fiber exerts important effects on people's health, described later.

roughage (RUFF-idge) the rough parts of food, an imprecise term that has largely been replaced by the term fiber.

insoluble fibers the tough, fibrous structures of fruits, vegetables, and grains; indigestible food components that do not dissolve in water.

soluble fibers indigestible food components that readily dissolve in water and often impart gummy or gel-like characteristics to foods. An example is pectin from fruit used to thicken jellies.

KEY POINT Little fiber is digested by the human enzymes in the digestive tract. Most fiber passes through the digestive tract unchanged.

The Need for Carbohydrates

Glucose from carbohydrate is the preferred fuel for most body functions. Only two other nutrients provide energy to the body: protein and fats. Protein-rich foods are usually expensive and provide no advantage over carbohydrates when used to make fuel for the body. In fact, their overuse has disadvantages, as explained in Chapter 6. Fats are not normally used as fuel by the brain and central nervous system, and diets high in fats are associated with many disease states. Thus, of the possible alternatives, glucose is the preferred energy source. It is especially important as the chief fuel of nerve cells, including those of the brain, which depends almost exclusively on glucose for its energy. And starchy foods, or complex carbohydrates, are the preferred source of glucose.

A myth about complex carbohydrates wrongly accuses them of being "fattening" ingredients of foods. Some people are still startled to hear that we need to consume more starchy foods rather than less. Yet much evidence supports this assertion. Gram for gram, carbohydrates donate fewer calories than do dietary fats, so a diet of high-carbohydrate foods is likely to be *lower* in calories than a diet of high-fat foods. Also, to convert glucose to fat in the body requires chemical conversions that cost many of the glucose's original calories, making glucose even less fattening. Government agencies in many countries, recognizing the value of complex carbohydrates, urge their citizens to consume abundant foods that contain them. Table 4-1 reviews the U.S. recommendations first presented in Chapter 2 as well as the World Health Organization's recommended upper and lower limits for carbohydrate intakes.

Table 4-1
Recommendations Concerning Intakes of Carbohydrates

1. Recommendations for Complex Carbohydrates

Dietary Guidelines

- Every day eat 5 to 9 servings[a] of a combination of vegetables and fruits. Also, increase intake of starches and other complex carbohydrates by eating 6 to 11 daily servings of a combination of breads, cereals, and legumes.

World Health Organization

- Lower limit: 50 percent of total calories from complex carbohydrates
- Upper limit: 75 percent of total calories from complex carbohydrates

2. Recommendations for Refined Sugars

Dietary Guidelines

- Use sugars only in moderation.

World Health Organization

- Lower limit: 0 percent of total calories from refined sugars
- Upper limit: 10 percent of total calories from refined sugars

3. Recommendations for Dietary Fiber

Dietary Guidelines

- Increase your fiber intake by eating more of a variety of foods that contain fiber naturally.

Recommended Dietary Allowances (RDA)

- A desirable fiber intake [should] be achieved not by adding fiber concentrates to the diet, but by consumption of fruits, vegetables, legumes, and whole-grain cereals, which also provide minerals and vitamins.

World Health Organization

- Lower limit: 27 grams of dietary fiber a day
- Upper limit: 40 grams of dietary fiber a day

[a]Serving sizes were presented in Figure 2-4 of Chapter 2.

Unlike complex carbohydrates, pure sugars displace nutrient-dense foods from the diet. Purified, refined sugar (sucrose) contains no other nutrients—protein, vitamins, minerals, or fiber—and so can be termed an empty-calorie food. If you choose 400 calories of sugar in place of 400 calories of starchy food such as whole-grain bread, you lose not only the starch but also the vitamins, minerals, and fiber of the bread. You can afford to do this only if you have already met your nutrient needs for the day and still have calories to spend. A word for teenaged girls and others who have limited calorie budgets and who often obtain too few nutrients: high-sugar, empty-calorie foods contribute to malnutrition. This chapter's Food Feature offers more about the sugars in foods.

Foods containing starch offer additional benefits if fibers come with the starch, as they usually do. Fibers benefit health in all these ways:

- Promote feelings of fullness because they absorb water and swell. Soluble fibers in a meal also slow the movement of food through the upper digestive tract, so that you feel fuller longer.

- Reduce energy consumption by displacing calorie-dense concentrated fats and sweets from the diet while donating little energy. Fibers therefore can help in weight control.
- Prevent **constipation, hemorrhoids,** and other intestinal problems by keeping the contents of the intestine moist and easy to eliminate.
- Help prevent bacterial infection of the appendix **(appendicitis)** by the same mechanism.
- Are associated with reduced incidence of colon cancer (see Chapter 11). This is possibly because insoluble fibers speed transit of cancer-causing materials through the colon, or prevent their contact with the living cells lining the tract, or both.
- Stimulate the muscles of the digestive tract so that they retain their health and tone. This prevents **diverticulosis,** in which the intestinal walls become weak and bulge out in places.
- Reduce the risks of heart and artery disease by lowering blood cholesterol.[1] Soluble fibers bind the cholesterol in bile and carry it out of the body, preventing it from being recycled into the bloodstream. This reduces the whole body content of cholesterol (Figure 4-4). Also, some soluble fibers are digested by intestinal bacteria to yield small, fat-like products that are absorbed. These products are thought to inhibit the liver's production of cholesterol.[2] High-fiber foods may also lower blood cholesterol by displacing fatty, cholesterol-raising foods from the diet.[3]
- Improve the body's handling of glucose, even in people with **diabetes,** perhaps by slowing the digestion or absorption of carbohydrate. A high-

constipation hardness and dryness of bowel movements, associated with discomfort in passing them from the body.

hemorrhoids (HEM-or-oids) swollen, hardened (varicose) veins in the rectum, usually caused by the pressure resulting from constipation.

appendicitis inflammation and/or infection of the appendix; a sac protruding from the intestine.

diverticulosis (dye-ver-tic-you-LOH-sis) outpocketing or ballooning out of areas of the intestinal wall, caused by weakening of the muscle layers that encase the intestine.

diabetes (dye-uh-BEET-eez) a hereditary disease (technically termed *diabetes mellitus*) characterized by inadequate or ineffective insulin, which renders a person unable to regulate blood glucose normally. (A later section gives details.)

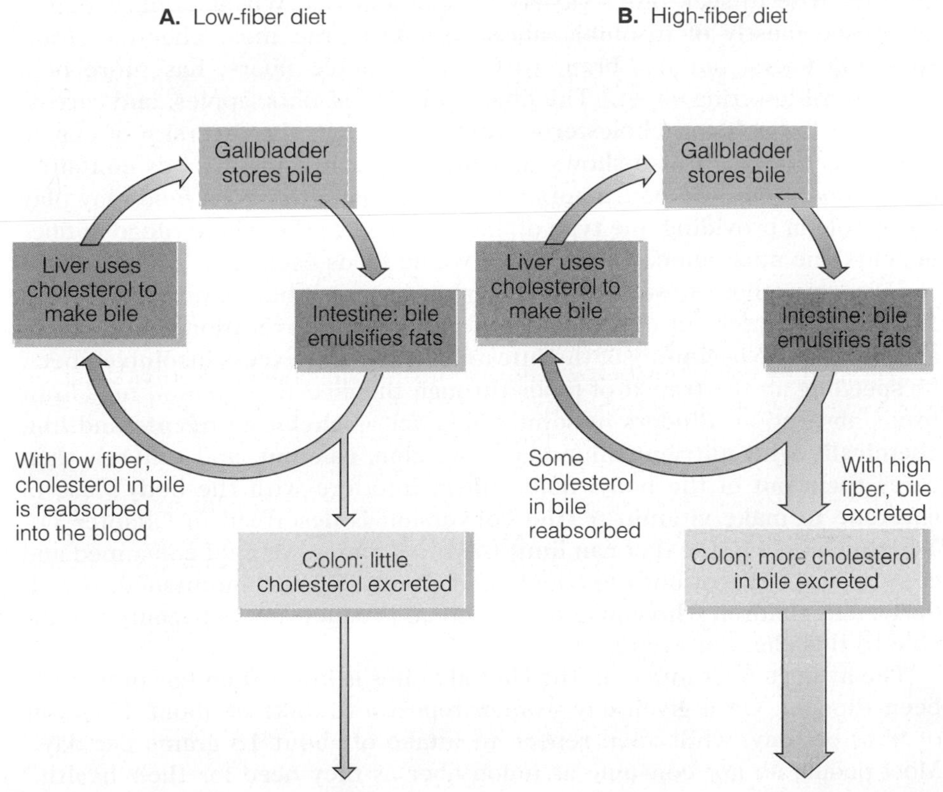

Figure 4-4

ONE WAY FIBER IN THE INTESTINE MAY LOWER CHOLESTEROL IN THE BLOOD

Table 4-2
Characteristics, Sources, and Health Effects of Fiber

Fiber Type	Major Food Sources	Possible Health Effects
Water Soluble[a] Pectins	Barley Fruits Legumes Oats, oat bran Rye Seeds Vegetables	Lowers blood cholesterol; slows glucose absorption; slows transit of food through upper digestive tract.
Water Insoluble Cellulose Hemicellulose	Brown rice Fruits Legumes Seeds Vegetables Wheat bran Whole grains, such as wheat	Softens stools; regulates bowel movements; speeds transit of fecal material through colon; reduces colon cancer risk; reduces risks of diverticulosis and appendicitis.

[a]Gums and mucilages are also among the water-soluble fibers. Psyllium, a fiber laxative and a cereal additive under study for safety by the FDA, has both soluble and insoluble properties.

chelating (KEE-late-ing) **agents** molecules that surround other molecules and are therefore useful in either preventing or promoting movement of substances from place to place.

fiber meal eaten for breakfast continues to exert regulatory effects on blood glucose after lunch.[4]

People choosing high-fiber foods in hopes of receiving some of these benefits are wise to seek out a variety of fiber sources. Wheat bran, which is composed mostly of insoluble fibers, is one of the most effective stool-softening fibers, but oat bran, with more soluble fibers, has more of a cholesterol-lowering effect.[5] The fibers of legumes, oats, apples, and carrots may also lower blood cholesterol. Table 4-2 shows the diversity of effects of different fibers; it also shows that most unrefined plant foods contain a mix of fiber types. To consumers this means that although a food may play a star role in providing one type of fiber, to receive the whole range of fiber benefits one must choose a variety of whole foods each day.

Like any other substances, if taken in excess, fibers can cause harm. Fibers carry water out of the body and can cause dehydration. Most iron is absorbed at the beginning of the intestinal tract, and excess insoluble fibers, by speeding up the transit of foods through the digestive system, may limit iron's absorption. Binders in some fibers act as **chelating agents** and link chemically with nutrient minerals (iron, zinc, calcium, and others), then carry them out of the body. Some fibers interfere with the body's use of carotene to make vitamin A (the conversion is described in Chapter 7).[6] Too much bulk in the diet can limit the total amount of food consumed and cause deficiencies of both nutrients and energy. The malnourished, the elderly, and children who consume no animal products are especially vulnerable to this chain of events.

Chelating agents are often sold by supplement vendors to "remove poisons" from the body. Some valid medical uses such as treatment of lead poisoning exist, but most of the chelating agents sold over-the-counter are promoted based on unproven claims.

The average fiber intake in the United States is lower than has previously been thought. On a given day women report an intake of about 12 grams of fiber per day, while men report an intake of about 18 grams per day.[7] Most people do not consume as much fiber as they need for their health.[8]

There is no Recommended Dietary Allowance (RDA) for fiber, but the Committee on RDA acknowledges the need for fiber and specifies that the need should be met by eating unprocessed, fiber-containing foods and *not* by eating refined fiber sources such as bran.[9] The World Health Organization recommends a daily intake of 27 to 40 grams of dietary fiber.[10]

The addition of purified fibers, such as oat or wheat bran, to foods is easily taken to extreme. One report tells of a man who required emergency intestinal surgery for the removal of a blockage formed by too many oat bran muffins; the bran had rendered his digestive system unable to work.[11] This doesn't mean that people should avoid bran-containing foods, but just that they should use bran, separated from its original food product, with moderation. A less extreme concern lies in what purified fiber might displace from the diet. Purified fibers are, in one way, like refined sugars: the nutrients that may have accompanied them originally have been lost. Furthermore, a purified fiber such as cellulose may not affect the body the same way as the cellulose in whole grains.[12] This chapter's Consumer Caution provides information about choosing wisely among grain foods, and the Food Feature shows where carbohydrates and fibers are found in foods.

KEY POINT Complex carbohydrates are the preferred energy source for the body. Fibers help maintain the health of the digestive tract and help to prevent or control certain diseases. Most people probably need 27 to 40 grams of fiber each day. Fiber needs are best met with whole foods. Purified fiber in large doses can have undesirable effects.

Refined, Enriched, and Whole-Grain Bread

CONSUMER CAUTION For many people, bread supplies much of the carbohydrate, or at least most of the starch, in a day's meals. Any food used in such abundance in the diet should be scrutinized closely, and if it doesn't measure up to high nutrition standards, it should be replaced with a food that does. For people who eat bread, the meanings of the words associated with the wheat flour that makes up the bread—**refined, enriched,** and **whole grain**—hold the key to understanding this product, in which they invest many calories per day (see Table 4-3).

The part of the wheat plant that is made into flour and then into bread and other baked goods is the seed or kernel. The wheat kernel (a whole grain) has four main parts: the **germ,** the **endosperm,** the **bran,** and the **husk,** as shown in Figure 4-5. The germ is the part that grows into a wheat plant, and so it carries with it concentrated food to support the new life. It is especially rich in vitamins and minerals. The endosperm is the soft, white, inside portion of the kernel, containing starch and proteins that help nourish the seed as it sprouts. The bran, a protective coating around the kernel, similar in function to the shell of a nut, is also rich in nutrients and fiber. The husk, commonly called chaff, is the dry outermost layer and is unusable for most purposes except for animal feed.

(continued on next page)

Table 4-3
Terms that Describe Grain Foods

- **bran** the protective fibrous coating around a grain; the chief fiber donator of a grain.
- **endosperm** the bulk of the edible part of a grain, the starchy part.
- **enriched** refers to addition of nutrients to a refined food product. As originally defined by law, this term means that thiamin, riboflavin, niacin, and iron have been added to refined grains and grain products at specified levels. After enrichment, a grain product has approximately the same amount of thiamin, niacin, and iron and about twice as much riboflavin as the original whole-grain product. The term *enriched* can refer to addition of more nutrients than just these four; read the label.
- **germ** the nutrient-rich inner part of a grain.
- **husk** the outer, inedible part of a grain.
- **refined** refers to the process by which the coarse parts of food products are removed. For example, the refining of wheat into flour involves removing three of the four parts of the kernel—the chaff, the bran, and the germ—leaving only the endosperm, composed mainly of starch and a little protein.
- **unbleached flour** a tan-colored endosperm flour with texture and nutritive qualities that approximate those of regular white flour.
- **wheat flour** any flour made from wheat, including white flour.
- **white flour** an endosperm flour that has been refined and bleached for maximum softness and whiteness.
- **whole grain** refers to a grain milled in its entirety (all but the husk), not refined.
- **whole-wheat flour** flour made from whole-wheat kernels; a whole-grain flour.

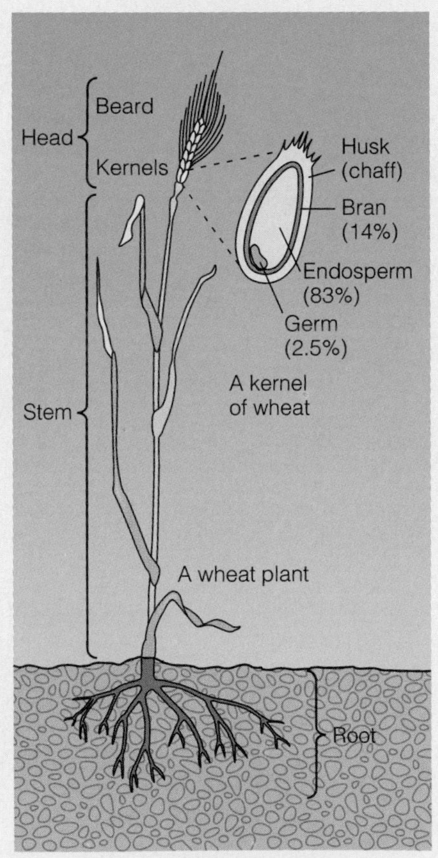

Figure 4-5

A WHOLE WHEAT PLANT AND A SINGLE KERNEL

In earlier times people milled wheat by grinding it between two stones, blowing or sifting out the inedible chaff, and retaining the nutrient-rich bran and germ as well as the endosperm. Then milling machinery was "improved," or so the makers thought, and it became possible to remove the dark, heavy germ and bran as well, leaving a whiter, smoother-textured flour. People came to look on this flour as more desirable than the crunchy, dark-brown, "old-fashioned" flour.

Bread eaters suffered a tragic loss of needed nutrients in turning to white bread. Many people developed deficiencies of iron, thiamin, riboflavin, and niacin—nutrients that they had formerly received from whole-grain bread. Finally the problem was recognized, and the Enrichment Act was passed stating that iron, niacin, thiamin, and riboflavin must be added to refined grain products before they were sold. (The Enrichment Act of 1942 is still in effect today.) This doesn't make a single slice of refined bread "rich" in these nutrients, but people who eat several or many slices of bread a day obtain significantly more of them than they would from unenriched white bread, as Figure 4-6 shows. Today you can almost take for granted that all breads; grain products such as rice, macaroni, and spaghetti; and all types of cereals have been enriched with at least these four nutrients.

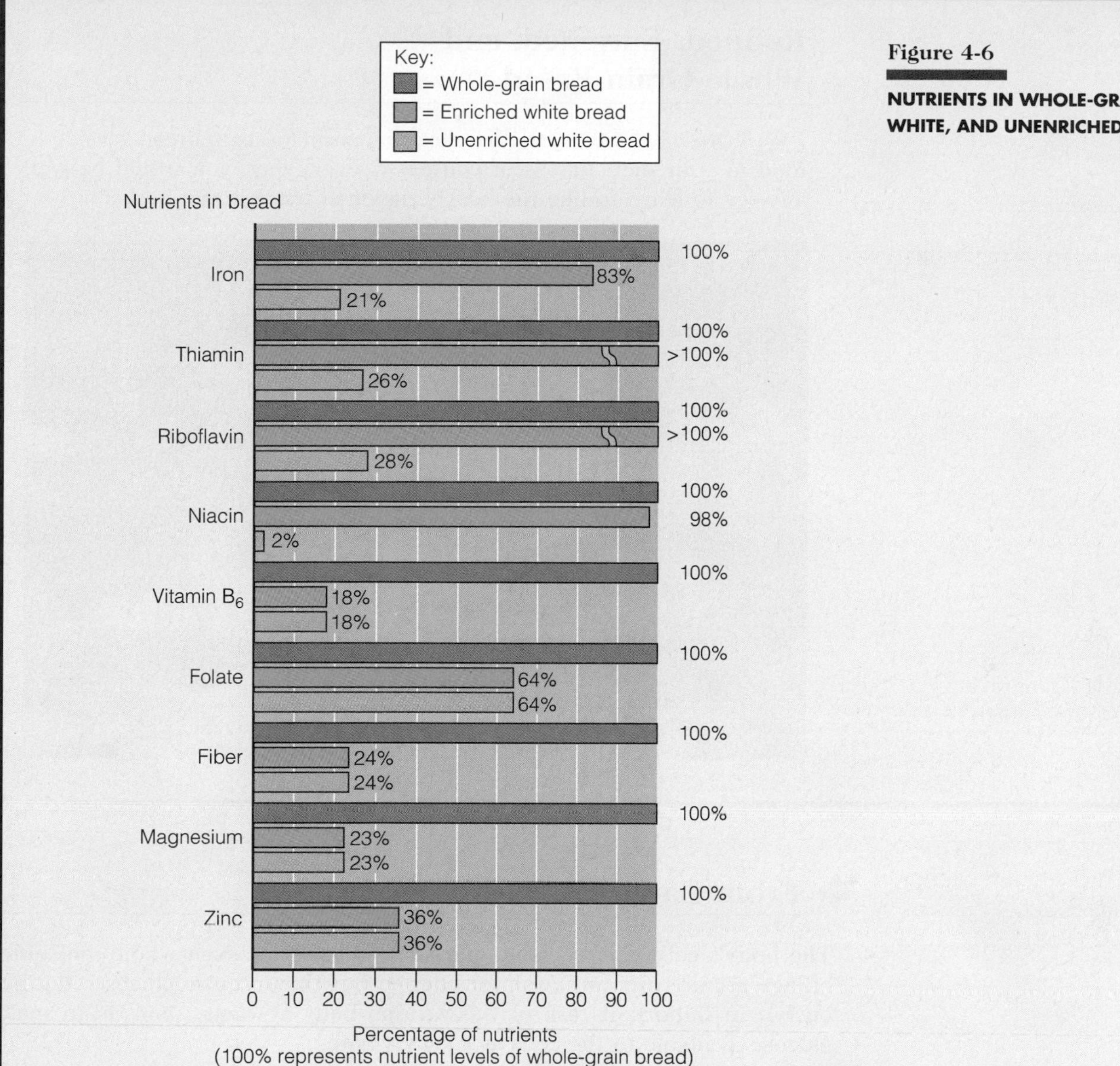

Figure 4-6

NUTRIENTS IN WHOLE-GRAIN, ENRICHED WHITE, AND UNENRICHED WHITE BREADS

To a great extent the enrichment of grain products eliminated these four known deficiency problems, but many other deficiencies went undetected for many more years. The trouble with *enriched* flour is that it is comparable to whole grain only with respect to these four nutrients and not with respect to others. Enriched products still contain less magnesium, zinc, folate, vitamin B_6, vitamin E, and chromium than whole-grain products do. When a grain is refined, fiber is lost, too. Bread sold for weight-reduction dieting may be fortified with pure cellulose, but adding cellulose alone is not enough; the bread still lacks other vitamins and minerals.

Only *whole-grain* flour contains all nutritive portions of the grain. Notice, too, the distinctions between **wheat flour** and **whole-wheat flour,** and between **white flour** and **unbleached flour** among the terms

(continued on next page)

Refined, Enriched, and Whole-Grain Bread *continued*

CONSUMER CAUTION that describe grain foods. If bread is a staple food in your diet, that is, if you eat it every day, you would be well advised to learn to like the hearty flavor of whole-grain bread.

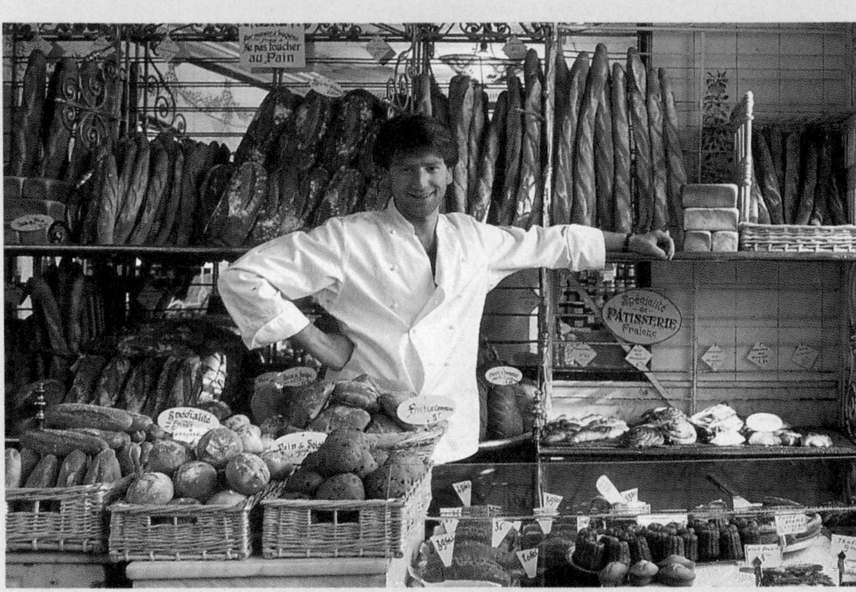

In Western societies, bread is the staff of life.

◆ From Carbohydrates to Glucose

The body's cells cannot use foods such as bread or even whole molecules of lactose, sucrose, or starch for energy, but they require glucose continuously. An important task of the various body systems, then, is to make glucose available to the cells at a steady rate.

Digestion and Absorption of Carbohydrate

To obtain glucose from newly-eaten food, the digestive system must first render the starch and disaccharides from the food into monosaccharides that can be absorbed through the cells lining the small intestine. The largest of the digestible carbohydrate molecules, starch, requires the most extensive breakdown. Disaccharides, on the other hand, must be split only once before they can be absorbed.

As Chapter 3 described, digestion of starch begins in the mouth, where a salivary enzyme mixes with food and begins to split starch into maltose. While chewing a bite of bread, you may have noticed that a slightly sweet taste develops. This is because maltose is being liberated from starch by the enzyme. The salivary enzyme continues to act on the starch in the swallowed bite of bread while it remains tucked in the stomach's storage area together with other swallowed bites. Slowly, each chewed lump is pushed downward to the lower stomach, to be thoroughly mixed with the stomach's acid, enzymes, and other juices. Enzyme molecules are made of protein, and as such, they eventually succumb to deactivation by the stomach's protein-digesting secretions. Starch digestion therefore ceases in the stomach, but it resumes at full speed in the small intestine, where another starch-splitting enzyme is delivered by the pancreas. This enzyme breaks starch down entirely into disaccharides and small polysaccharides.

Sucrose and lactose from food, and maltose and small polysaccharides freed from starch, undergo one more split to yield free monosaccharides before they are absorbed. This split is accomplished by enzymes that are attached to the cells of the small intestinal lining. The conversion of a bite of bread to nutrients for the body is completed when monosaccharides cross these cells and are washed away in a rush of circulating blood that carries them to the waiting liver. Figure 4-7 presents a quick review of the events of carbohydrate digestion.

Once in the body, the absorbed carbohydrates follow any of several paths to the cells and may be used in any of several ways. The liver converts fructose and galactose to glucose or products of glucose metabolism (such as fats). The circulatory system transports the glucose and fats to the cells. Liver and muscle cells may store circulating glucose as glycogen; all cells

Figure 4-7

HOW CARBOHYDRATE IN FOOD BECOMES GLUCOSE IN THE BODY

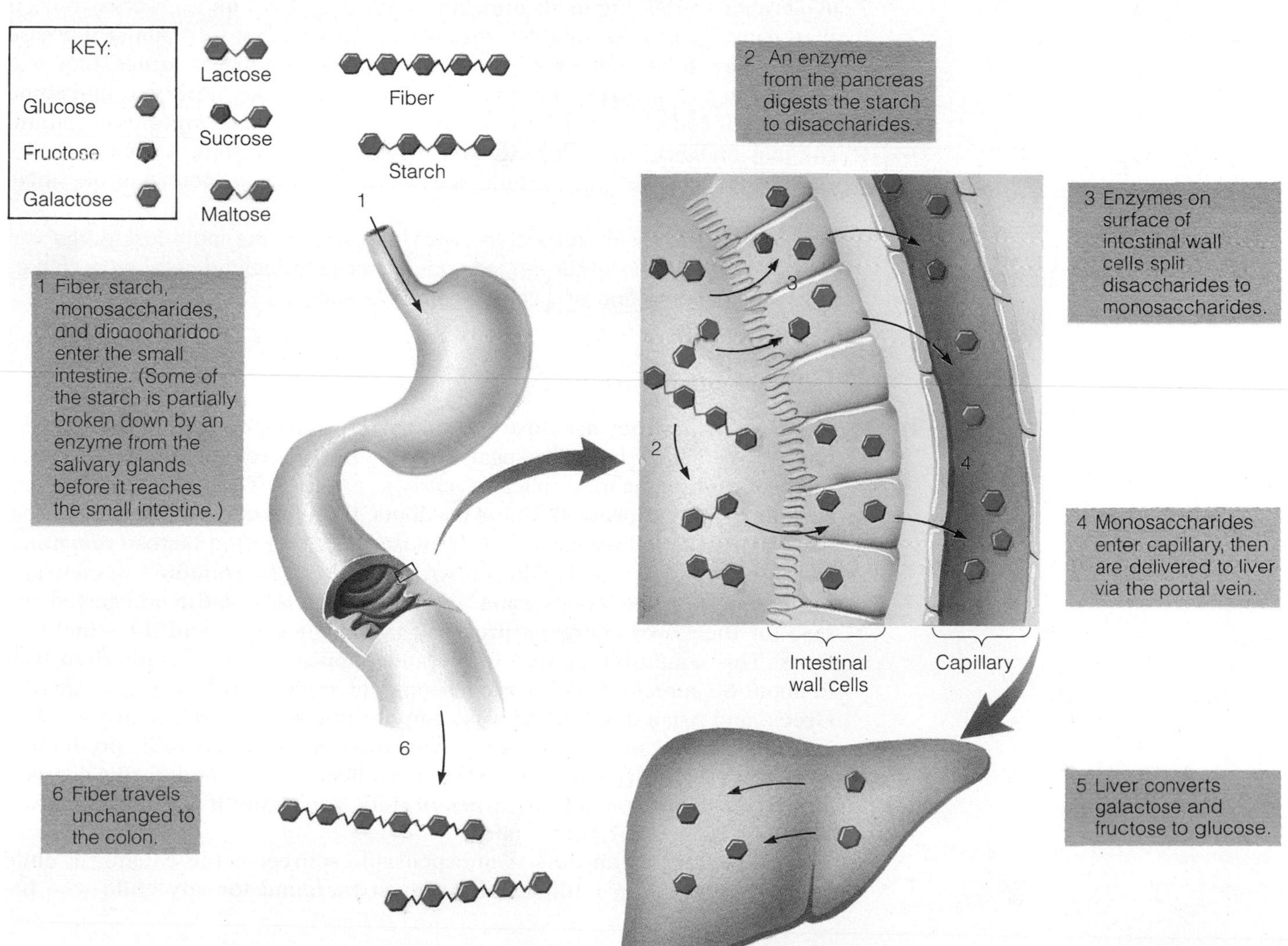

lactase the intestinal enzyme that splits the disaccharide lactose to monosaccharides during digestion.

lactose intolerance inability to digest lactose due to a lack of the enzyme lactase.

may split it for energy.

Other carbohydrates are digested, but fibers remain in the tract to help regulate digestive activities. Fibers:

- *Moderate nutrient absorption* rates by entrapping nutrient molecules and preventing their contact with absorptive surfaces.
- *Delay cholesterol and other sterol absorption*, probably by the same mechanism.
- *Stimulate bacterial fermentation* in the colon (described below).
- *Increase stool weight* by holding water within the feces.

These four actions underlie the many health benefits of fibers listed earlier in this chapter.[13]

As mentioned, molecules of fiber are not changed by human digestive enzymes. Some dietary fibers can, however, be digested by the billions of living inhabitants of the human digestive tract, the resident bacteria. So active are these inhabitants in breaking down substances from food that one expert claims they constitute "an organ of intense metabolic activity that is involved in nutrient salvage."[14] Digestion of fibers by resident bacteria yields waste products, mainly small fat fragments that the body absorbs and can use to provide a tiny bit of energy.[15] A by-product of this process is any of several odorous gases, which may make people want to avoid fiber-containing foods altogether. Don't give up on high-fiber foods if they cause gas. Instead, start with small amounts and gradually increase them; chew foods thoroughly to break up hard-to-digest lumps that can ferment in the intestine; and try many fiber-rich foods until you find some that do not cause the problem. In some instances, such symptoms as painful gas may indicate that the digestive tract has undergone a change in its ability to digest the sugar in milk, a condition known as lactose intolerance.

KEY POINT With respect to starch and sugars, the main task of the various body systems is to convert them into glucose to fuel the cells' work. Fibers help regulate digestion and contribute a little energy.

Lactose Intolerance

Many people, as they age, lose the ability to produce enough of the enzyme **lactase** to digest the milk sugar lactose. In children of nonwhite races, **lactose intolerance** may appear as early as age four. Thereafter, on drinking milk or eating lactose-containing products, these people experience nausea, pain, diarrhea, and excessive gas because the undigested lactose remaining in the intestine demands dilution with fluid from surrounding tissues, and ultimately from the bloodstream. Intestinal bacteria use the undigested lactose for their own energy, a process that produces gas and intestinal irritants. This condition, lactose intolerance, appears to be an inherited trait in about 80 percent of the world's people, including most people of African, Greek, and Asian descent.[16] It also can develop temporarily in anyone who is malnourished or sick, making avoidance of milk and milk products a temporary necessity. Lactose intolerance affects people to differing degrees. Some can tolerate small quantities of milk, especially if the milk's lactose has been reduced by about half.[17]

Because milk is an almost indispensable source of the calcium a child needs for growth, a milk substitute must be found for any child who becomes lactose intolerant. Women who fail to consume enough calcium during youth may later develop weak bones, so women, too, must search for substitutes if they become unable to tolerate milk. Sometimes yogurt or cheese makes an acceptable substitute: the bacteria or molds that help create these products digest the lactose of milk as they convert the milk to the fermented product. Other yogurts have milk solids that contain lactose added; these are listed with the ingredients on the label. Alternatively, people can choose milk products that have undergone treatment with lactose-digesting enzymes. Enzyme pills or drops can be purchased over-the-counter. When taken with milk-containing meals, these products can help to digest lactose by replacing the missing natural enzymes. In all cases, the trick is to find ways of splitting lactose to glucose and galactose so that the body can absorb the products, rather than leaving the lactose undigested to feed the bacteria of the colon.

Sometimes sensitivity to milk is due not to lactose intolerance but to an allergic reaction to the protein in milk. Children and adults with this problem often cannot tolerate cheese or yogurt either, and they have to find nondairy calcium sources. Good choices are calcium-fortified orange juice or soy milk, or canned sardines or salmon with the bones. Controversy 8 examines the topic of milk in adult diets in relation to the adult bone disease, osteoporosis.

KEY POINT Lactose intolerance is a common condition in which the body fails to produce sufficient amounts of the enzyme needed to digest the sugar of milk. Uncomfortable symptoms result and can lead to milk avoidance. Lactose-intolerant people need milk substitutes that contain calcium.

The Body's Use of Glucose

Carbohydrates serve structural roles in the body, such as forming part of the internal organs' protective coatings of mucus; but their main role is to serve as an energy source. Glucose is not only the main original unit from which carbohydrate-rich foods are made, it is also the basic carbohydrate unit that each cell of the body uses for energy. The body handles its glucose judiciously. It maintains an internal supply for use in case of need, and it tightly controls its blood glucose concentration to ensure that glucose remains available for ongoing use.

Storing Glucose as Glycogen

After a meal, as blood glucose rises, the pancreas is the first organ to respond. It releases the hormone **insulin,** which signals the body's tissues to take up surplus glucose. From some of this excess glucose, muscle and liver cells build the polysaccharide glycogen. The muscles hoard two thirds of the body's total glycogen and use it just for themselves during exercise. The liver stores the other one third and is more generous with its glycogen: it makes it available as blood glucose for the brain or other organs when the supply runs low.

Glycogen is wondrously designed for its task of releasing glucose on demand. Instead of having long chains with occasional branches, as starch does, that are cleaved linearly during digestion, glycogen is many-branched, so that hundreds of ends stick out at each molecule's surface. When the

insulin a hormone secreted by the pancreas in response to a high blood-glucose concentration; it assists cells in drawing glucose from the blood.

glucagon a hormone of the pancreas that acts on the liver when blood-glucose concentration dips, stimulating the release of glucose into the blood.

protein-sparing action the action of carbohydrate and fat in providing energy that allows protein to be used for purposes it alone can serve.

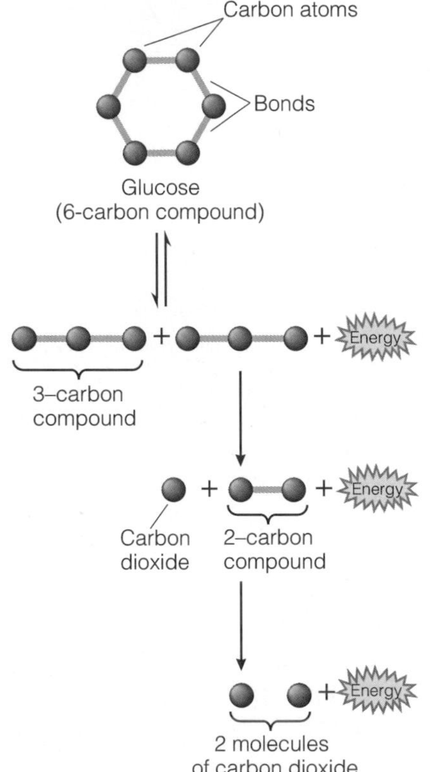

Figure 4-8

THE BREAKDOWN OF GLUCOSE YIELD ENERGY AND CARBON DIOXIDE

The bonds between the carbon atoms in glucose are split apart by human-cell enzymes, liberating the energy stored there for the cell's use. The first split yields two 3-carbon fragments. The two-way arrows mean that these fragments can also be rejoined to make glucose again. Should they instead be broken down further into 2-carbon fragments, they cannot rejoin to make glucose. The carbon atoms liberated when the bonds split are combined with oxygen and released into the air, via the lungs, as carbon dioxide. Although not shown here, water is also produced at each split.

blood glucose concentration drops and cells need energy, a pancreatic hormone, **glucagon,** floods the bloodstream. Thousands of enzymes within the liver cells respond by attacking a multitude of ends simultaneously, and they release a surge of glucose into the blood for use by all the other body cells. Another hormone, epinephrine, does the same thing as part of the body's defense mechanism in times of danger.

To a person living in the Stone Age, this internal source of quick energy was indispensable. Life was fraught with physical peril. The person who stopped and ate before running from a man-eating tiger did not survive to produce our ancestors. The quick-energy response in a stress situation works to our advantage today as well. (For example, it accounts for the energy you suddenly have to clean up your room when you learn that a special person is coming to visit.) To meet such emergencies, we are well advised to eat and to store carbohydrate every four to six waking hours.

You might rightly ask, "What kind of carbohydrate?" Candy bars and sugary beverages supply sugar energy quickly, but they are not the best choices. Starchy foods best sustain glycogen stores and the blood glucose that is the true source of "quick energy." Starchy foods also provide an assortment of other nutrients that help cells to use their glucose.

KEY POINT Glycogen is the body's form of stored glucose; the liver stores it for use by the whole body. Muscles have their own private glycogen stock for muscle use only. The hormone glucagon acts to liberate stored glucose from the liver.

Splitting Glucose for Energy

Glucose fuels the work of most of the body's cells. When a cell splits glucose for energy, it performs an intricate sequence of maneuvers that are of great interest to the biochemist—and of no interest whatever to most people who eat bread and potatoes. One fact that everybody needs to understand, though, is that there is no good substitute for carbohydrate. There is a point at which glucose is forever lost to the body, and this can have serious consequences. That is why carbohydrate was mentioned as *essential* on page 6 of Chapter 1. The following details are given for the purpose of making this point clear.

Inside a cell, the glucose is broken in half, releasing some energy. These halves have two pathways open to them. They can be put back together to make glucose, or they can be further broken apart into smaller fragments. If they are broken into smaller fragments, they can never again be reassembled to form glucose. The smaller fragments can yield still more energy and in the process break down completely to carbon dioxide and water; or they can be hitched together into units of body fat. Figure 4-8 shows how glucose is broken down to yield energy and carbon dioxide.

Although glucose can be converted into body fat, body fat can never be converted into glucose to feed the brain adequately. This is one reason why fasting and low-carbohydrate diets are dangerous. When there is a severe carbohydrate deficit, the body has two problems. Having no glucose, it has to turn to protein to make some (it has this ability), thus diverting protein from vitally important functions of its own such as maintaining the body's immune defenses. Protein's functions in the body are so indispensable that carbohydrate should be kept available precisely to prevent the use of protein for energy. This is called the **protein-sparing action** of carbohydrate.

Also, without sufficient carbohydrate, the body cannot use its fat in the normal way. (Carbohydrate has to combine with fat fragments before they can be used for energy.) Using fat without the help of carbohydrate causes the body to go into **ketosis,** a condition in which unusual products of fat breakdown **(ketone bodies)** accumulate in the blood. Ketosis during pregnancy can cause brain damage to the fetus with irreversible mental retardation after birth. In nonpregnant adults it disturbs the body's normal acid-base balance.

ketosis (kee-TOE-sis) an undesirably high concentration of ketone bodies, such as acetone, in the blood and urine.

ketone (KEE-tone) **bodies** acidic, fat-related compounds; they can arise from the incomplete breakdown of fat when carbohydrate is not available.

The minimum amount of carbohydrate needed to ensure complete sparing of body protein and avoidance of ketosis is around 100 grams a day in an average-sized person. This has to be digestible carbohydrate, and considerably more (three or four times more) than this minimum is recommended.[18] The servings of vegetables, fruits, and grains recommended in Table 4-1 (page 104) would deliver 125 grams at a minimum, and 200 to 400 grams on average. This chapter's Food Feature shows how to estimate grams of carbohydrate in foods.

KEY POINT Without glucose the body is forced to alter its uses of protein and fats. The body breaks down its own muscles and other protein tissues to make glucose and converts its fats into ketone bodies, incurring ketosis.

Returning Glucose to the Blood

Should your glucose supplies ever fall too low, you would feel dizzy and weak. Should blood glucose ever climb abnormally high, you might become confused or have difficulty breathing. Both conditions could be dangerous, but luckily the body normally guards against such occurrences.

The maintenance of a normal blood-glucose concentration depends on the two safeguards already mentioned. When blood glucose starts to fall too low, it is replenished by drawing on liver glycogen stores. When it starts to rise too high, the body siphons off the excess into the liver, to be converted to glycogen or fat, and into the muscle, to be converted to glycogen.

To replenish blood glucose, the hormone glucagon triggers the breakdown of liver glycogen to free glucose. Other hormones also act in this manner, including epinephrine (the stress hormone) and some that promote the conversion of protein into glucose. However, the liver's glycogen stores can be depleted within half a waking day. As for protein, only a little can be spared. When body protein is used, it is taken from blood, muscle, or organ proteins; no surplus of protein is stored specifically for emergencies. As for fat, it cannot regenerate enough glucose to make a difference.

Obviously, when blood glucose falls and stores are depleted, a meal or a snack can replenish the supply. The meal or snack you choose may, however, flood the blood with glucose, requiring the body to protect itself against too *high* a blood-glucose concentration.

Within limits, some foods elevate blood glucose and insulin concentrations higher than do others. The effect, called the **glycemic effect,** is worth a moment's attention. Scientists measure the glycemic effect by administering a food or a meal and then observing how fast and how high the blood glucose rises and how quickly the body responds by bringing it back to normal. Most people can quickly adjust, but people with abnormal carbohydrate metabolism may experience extreme blood-glucose levels. These people do well to choose most often foods with a low glycemic effect such

glycemic (gligh-SEEM-ic) **effect** a measure of the extent to which a food raises the blood-glucose concentration and elicits an insulin response as compared with pure glucose.

as dried beans, pasta, barley, bulgur (wheat), pumpernickel bread, the sugar fructose, and any food with the soluble fiber psyllium added. These foods produce a slow, sustained rise in blood glucose.[19]

Many factors work together to determine a food's glycemic effect, and the result is not always what a person might expect.[20] Ice cream, for example, produces less of a response than potatoes; baked potatoes produce less of a response than mashed; a sweet, juicy apple produces a low response (probably due to the apple's soluble fiber); dried beans of all kinds are notable for keeping blood glucose remarkably steady. Importantly, a food's glycemic effect differs when it is eaten alone or as part of a mixed meal. The foods in mixed meals tend to balance each other with regard to glycemic index. Most people eat a variety of foods in a meal and so need not worry at all about the glycemic index of the foods they choose. Most people's systems control their blood glucose perfectly, regardless of the glycemic index ratings of the foods they consume.

KEY POINT Blood-glucose regulation depends mainly on the hormones insulin and glucagon. Certain carbohydrate foods produce a greater rise and fall in blood glucose than do others. Most people have no problem regulating their blood-glucose levels, especially when they consume regular mixed meals.

Converting Glucose to Fat

When food is tempting, people may continue to eat beyond the amount they need. After meeting the body cells' immediate energy needs and filling glycogen stores to capacity, the body takes a third path for handling incoming carbohydrates. Say you have eaten and are now sitting, watching a ball game on television, eating pretzels, and drinking a cola. Your digestive tract is delivering molecules of glucose to your bloodstream, and your blood is carrying these molecules to your liver and other body cells. The body cells use what glucose they can for their energy needs of the moment. More glucose is linked together and stored as glycogen until the muscles and liver are full to capacity with glycogen. Still the glucose keeps coming, and the liver has no choice but to handle the excess. The liver breaks the extra glucose into small fragments and puts them together into more permanent energy-storage compounds—fats. (This would happen with excess protein or fat, too.) The fats are then released into the blood, carried to the fatty tissues of the body, and deposited there. Unlike the liver cells, which can store only about four to six hours' worth of glycogen, the fat cells can store unlimited quantities of fats. Moral: you had better play the game if you are going to eat the food.

Even though *excess* carbohydrate is converted to fat and stored, a balanced diet, high in complex carbohydrates helps control body weight and lean tissue. Researchers are beginning to understand this seeming paradox and the results of the work are fascinating; they are presented in full in Controversy 5. The current thrust seems to be that, calorie for calorie, carbohydrate-rich foods contribute much less to body fatness than do fat-rich foods. Had you chosen fatty potato chips instead of low-fat pretzels for your ballgame snack, your body would have stored even greater amounts of fat for the calories taken in. Thus, if you want to eat until full, never skip a meal, and yet remain lean, then you should make every effort to choose foods that, together, comprise a diet with 55 percent or more of its calories from carbohydrates and 30 percent or less from fats. The Food Feature of this chapter provides the first set of tools required for the job of designing such a diet. Once you have learned to identify the carbohydrates in foods, you must then learn where the fats come in (Chapter 5's Food Feature) and how to obtain adequate protein without overdoing it (Chapter 6).

KEY POINT The liver converts extra energy compounds into fat, a more permanent and unlimited energy-storage compound than glycogen.

diabetes (DYE-uh-BEET-eez) **mellitus** (MELL-ih-tus) a disorder of blood-glucose regulation usually caused by insufficiency or relative ineffectiveness of insulin.

Type I diabetes, or **insulin-dependent diabetes mellitus (IDDM)** the type of diabetes in which the person produces no insulin at all; also known as *juvenile-onset diabetes,* although some cases arise in adulthood.

Type II diabetes, or **noninsulin-dependent diabetes mellitus (NIDDM)** the type of diabetes in which the fat cells resist insulin, also called *adult-onset diabetes.*

Diabetes and Hypoglycemia

Some people have physical conditions that render their bodies unable to handle carbohydrates in the normal way. One of these, diabetes, is common in developed nations and can be detected by way of a timed blood test. Another, hypoglycemia, is rare as a true disease condition, but many people believe they experience its symptoms at times.

Diabetes

Diabetes can lead to or contribute to any of a number of other diseases and is itself among the top 10 killers of adults and the leading cause of blindness in the United States. Several diseases have been called diabetes, but by far the most common ones are the two main forms of **diabetes mellitus** described here. Both types are disorders of blood-glucose regulation.

In the first, less common type, **Type I diabetes** (about 20 percent of cases), the person's own immune system attacks the cells of the pancreas that normally synthesize the hormone insulin. Why this happens is unknown but is the subject of intense study. Soon the pancreas can no longer produce insulin, and after each meal, blood glucose remains elevated, even though body tissues are simultaneously starving for glucose. The person must receive insulin periodically to assist the cells in taking up the needed glucose from the blood; therefore this type of diabetes is called **insulin-dependent diabetes mellitus (IDDM).**

Insulin is made of protein, and if it were taken orally, the digestive system would digest it. Insulin must therefore be injected, either by daily shots or by an insulin pump that delivers insulin through an implanted needle. Medical researchers are working to learn how to transplant healthy tissue into the pancreas to get it working again, or to develop a vaccine or other drug that may prevent IDDM by preventing the body's attack on its own pancreas.

The second, predominant, type of diabetes mellitus, **Type II** (80 percent of cases), is characterized by insulin resistance of the body's cells, including fat cells.[21] Insulin may be present, often in abnormally large amounts, and it does stimulate cells to take up glucose, but more slowly than normal. Blood glucose rises too high, as in IDDM, but in this case insulin may also build up. This type of diabetes is therefore called **noninsulin-dependent diabetes mellitus (NIDDM).** Eventually the pancreas becomes less and less able to make insulin.[22] At this point, people with NIDDM may need to take insulin to supplement their own supply, especially late in the course of the disease. A preferred therapy, if drugs are necessary, is to take a drug that stimulates the person's own pancreas to secrete insulin.

glucose tolerance the ability of the body to respond to dietary carbohydrate by regulating its blood-glucose concentration promptly to a normal level.

hyperglycemia (HIGH-per-gligh-SEEM-ee-uh) an abnormally high blood-glucose concentration (*hyper* means "too much"; *glyce* means "glucose"; *emia* means "in the blood").

NIDDM tends to occur late in life. People with the disease often become obese because they overeat due to their cells' resistance to insulin—while they are waiting for their cells to be fed, so to speak. Figure 4-9 demonstrates one theory on how this may become a cycle—the larger the fat cells become, the more insulin resistant they become, and the obesity worsens insulin resistance just as insulin resistance worsens obesity.[23] Weight loss in overweight people with diabetes often helps control the disease. The incidence of this type of diabetes also increases with increasing age, for in all people, the pancreatic cells that produce insulin progressively lose their function with time.[24] In some people this age-related decline in cell function is more rapid or more severe than in others, and these people especially need to beware of excess weight gain and also to watch their alcohol intakes. Heavy use of alcohol may present a risk for NIDDM development.[25]

Diabetes can be diagnosed by means of a **glucose tolerance** test, in which the body is challenged to handle a sudden, large amount of glucose. After fasting overnight, the subject is fed a sugary drink. Four or six hours later, when blood glucose should be normal, the person's blood glucose will still be elevated **(hyperglycemia)** and possibly the blood insulin will be, too.[26] Table 4-4 lists symptoms that can warn a person of diabetes.

Although its symptoms are controllable for the most part, diabetes' effects can be severe and may progress even when blood glucose is controlled by drugs.[27] Problems may include impaired circulation leading to disease of the feet and legs often necessitating amputation; kidney disease sometimes requiring hospital care or kidney transplant; impaired vision or blindness due to cataracts and damaged retinas; nerve damage; skin damage; and strokes and heart attacks.[28] The root cause of all these conditions is probably the same. Diabetes causes fatty blockage or destruction of capillaries that feed the body organs, and tissues die from lack of nourishment.[29] The person is advised to control not only weight but also all possible risk factors that might contribute to heart and blood vessel disease (atherosclerosis and hypertension). These are discussed in Chapter 11.

The exchange system used throughout this book was originally developed for people with diabetes, to control calorie, carbohydrate, sugar, and fat intakes. Now, however, the system is often praised as the best possible system for people in perfect health to manage their diets. A diet constructed of a balanced pattern of foods from the exchange lists is best for weight control. Weight Watchers as well as other reputable weight control systems use it. Such a diet also has all the characteristics important in disease prevention and meets most dietary guidelines. The diet:

- Is adequate (deficiencies in trace minerals, especially chromium, may hasten diabetes onset).
- Has ample fiber (fiber helps regulate blood glucose concentration).
- Is low in concentrated sugar.
- Is high in complex carbohydrates (thought to assist in blood-glucose regulation).
- Is low in fat (helping to protect against cardiovascular disease).
- Is not too high in protein (to protect the kidneys).

A person at risk for diabetes can do no better than to adopt such a diet long before any symptoms appear.

Exercise is important too. It not only helps to maintain a desirable body weight, but it also heightens tissue sensitivity to insulin and is considered by some to help prevent or forestall NIDDM.[30]

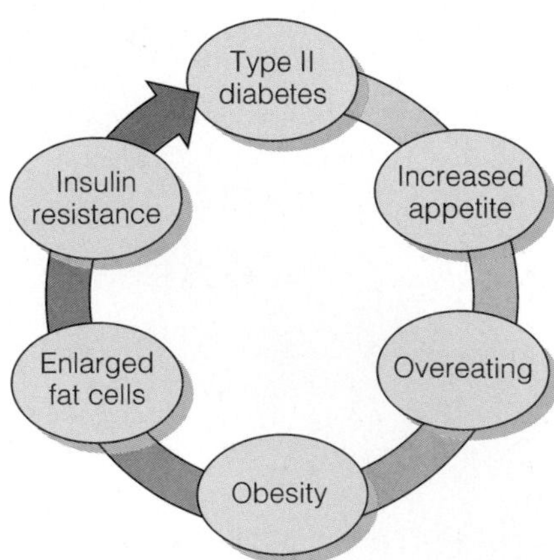

Figure 4-9

THE OBESITY-DIABETES CYCLE

KEY POINT Diabetes is an example of the body's abnormal handling of glucose. Inadequate or ineffective insulin leaves blood glucose high and cells undersupplied with glucose energy. This causes blood vessel and tissue damage. Weight control and exercise may be most effective in preventing the predominant form of diabetes (Type II) and the illnesses that accompany it.

hypoglycemia a blood-glucose concentration below normal, a symptom that may indicate any of several diseases, including impending diabetes (NIDDM).

postprandial hypoglycemia a drop in blood glucose that follows a meal and that is accompanied by symptoms of the stress response. Also called *reactive hypoglycemia.*

fasting hypoglycemia hypoglycemia that occurs after 8 to 14 hours of fasting.

Hypoglycemia

The term **hypoglycemia** refers both to a *symptom*, low blood glucose, and to a variety of conditions, including *disease conditions*, that cause that symptom. One such condition is **postprandial hypoglycemia,** literally, "low blood glucose after (or caused by) a meal." The symptoms are fatigue, weakness, irritability, a rapid heartbeat, anxiety, sweating, trembling, hunger, and headaches—symptoms common enough from many causes so that people easily misdiagnose themselves as having this meal-induced condition.

A different kind of hypoglycemia exists in a person who has symptoms while well advanced into the fasting state (for example, overnight). The symptoms of **fasting hypoglycemia** are different from those of postprandial hypoglycemia: headache, mental dullness, fatigue, confusion, amnesia, and even seizures and unconsciousness.

It takes more than guesswork to diagnose postprandial hypoglycemia, though. A diagnosis requires a test to detect low blood glucose while the symptoms are present to confirm that both occur simultaneously.[31] When they do, the diagnosis is confirmed.

Only a few people suffer from truly abnormal conditions that cause hypoglycemia. Many of the cases result from severe disease that endangers health and life. Conditions such as cancer, pancreatic damage, infection of the liver with accompanying damage (hepatitis), or advanced alcohol-induced liver disease can all produce hypoglycemia.[32]

In a very few other cases, symptoms occur together with a drop in blood glucose that cannot be explained by a disease state, and that can be relieved by eating.[33] In a study of people with postprandial hypoglycemia, researchers determined that a portion of hard-to-digest starch (raw cornstarch in this case) eaten along with sugar effectively prevented a drop in blood glucose together with the associated symptoms.[34] The authors of the study suggest what some people have suspected for a long time—that a sugary meal promotes symptoms in those few people who have postprandial hypoglycemia, but that certain starches and other nutrients taken with the sugar can prevent the problem.

Hypoglycemia can be experimentally produced in just about everyone, and with hypoglycemia come symptoms of impaired thought processes, memory, and psychomotor activity.[35] To produce even mild hypoglycemia and its symptoms in normal healthy people, however, requires administering drugs that work by overwhelming the body's sensitive glucose control team, insulin and glucagon. Without such intervention, those hormones rarely fail to keep blood glucose within normal limits, and symptoms that people ascribe to hypoglycemia hardly ever correlate to low blood glucose in blood tests.[36]

Medical science cannot fully explain why many people with normal glucose regulation report symptoms of hypoglycemia. There is no doubt that some people may be more sensitive than others to slight changes in their blood glucose. Perhaps these people experience symptoms even when their blood glucose remains within the range considered normal.[37]

Table 4-4
Warning Signs of Diabetes

- Excessive urination and thirst.
- Weight loss with nausea, easy tiring, weakness, or irritability.
- Cravings for food, especially for sweets.
- Frequent infections of the skin, gums, vagina, or urinary tract.
- Vision disturbances; blurred vision.
- Pain in the legs, feet, or fingers.
- Slow healing of cuts and bruises.
- Itching.
- Drowsiness.
- Abnormally high glucose tolerance test results.[a]

[a]In one type of test, value of >200 mg glucose/100 ml blood two hours after glucose administration.

For people who seem to experience reactive hypoglycemia after meals, it may help to avoid oscillating between low-carbohydrate dieting and sudden large sugar doses. Two findings suggest that these pointers may be on the mark:

1. A person with *normal* glucose regulation can develop the symptoms of hypoglycemia on taking a large dose of simple sugar after three days of following a low-carbohydrate diet.
2. A person who appears to have postprandial hypoglycemia by traditional testing may have it only after a simple-sugar load, and not after eating mixed meals.

If you experience symptoms between meals, try to eliminate them by eating regular mixed meals rather than sugary snacks. If you are *not* prone to such symptoms, you still might bring them on if you deprived your system of carbohydrate for days and then dumped in a large dose all at once. Eat regularly, and eat balanced meals.

Part of eating right is choosing wisely among the many foods available. Two features follow that can help with choices of carbohydrate-containing foods. First, the Food Feature explains how to integrate foods into a diet that meets the body's needs for carbohydrate. The Checking Out Food Labels section then provides information about reading carbohydrate information on labels of processed foods.

KEY POINT Postprandial hypoglycemia is a rare medical condition in which blood glucose falls too low. It can be a warning of organ damage or disease. Many people believe they experience symptoms of hypoglycemia, but their symptoms normally do not accompany below-normal blood glucose.

FOOD FEATURE

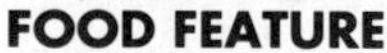

Meeting Carbohydrate Needs

For a review of how the exchange lists work, see Chapter 2.

This Food Feature illustrates how the exchange system can show you where the carbohydrates are in your meals and how much carbohydrate you are consuming. In the same way, it can reveal the fat and protein in meals, as the next two chapters will explain.

Breads, cereals, vegetables, fruits, and milk—these are the foods noted for their contributions of valuable energy-yielding carbohydrates: starches and dilute sugars. To learn how much starch and sugars these foods offer, consult the exchange lists (Appendix D). Remember that all of the foods on any one list are interchangeable with respect to carbohydrate, fat, and protein. Within a list you can trade one food for another without altering your carbohydrate intake. Carbohydrate-containing foods appear in four of the six lists; Figure 4-10 provides details.

The Starch/Bread List A slice of whole-wheat bread contains 15 grams of carbohydrate as starch. Equivalent foods are other breads, cereals, potatoes, rice, pasta, corn, peas, limas and other beans (legumes), and many other foods that are predominantly complex carbohydrate. Be aware that starchy vegetables such as corn and green peas actually resemble breads more closely than vegetables in their starch content. People who like breads and starchy vegetables are happy to learn that the guidelines encourage people to use them freely. They know that if calories are a problem, they should cut out some fat, not complex carbohydrate, from foods. Some foods in this group, especially baked goods such as biscuits, muffins, and snack crackers, do contain fat, however.

The Vegetable List In the exchange list, portions of vegetables are small, only a half cup. This small portion size is a vestige of the days when people thought that meat should be the center of a meal and that vegetables should only decorate the plate. The opposite now seems to be a healthier strategy, so you are encouraged to double your servings to 1-cup portions of vegetables.

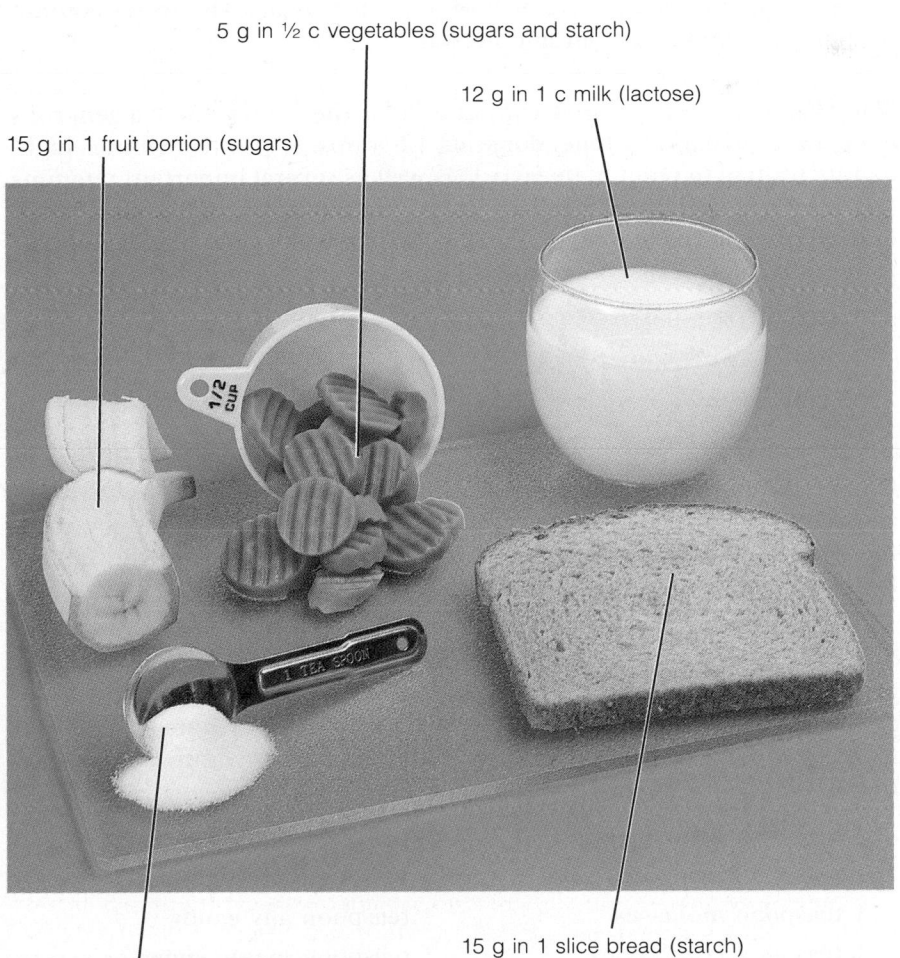

Figure 4-10

CARBOHYDRATES IN FOODS

Four of the six exchange lists contain carbohydrates, so you need only know four values and learn a value for concentrated sugar (which is not on the exchange lists). The lists identify with a logo a few items that are especially high in fiber, but all whole plant foods are valuable fiber contributors if you eat enough of them.

One Exchange	Carbohydrate (g)
Starches/grains	15
Vegetables	5
Fruits	15
Milks	12
Sugars (1 tsp)[a]	5
Meats	0
Fats	0

[a]Sugars are not officially part of the exchange system, but do have to be counted.

A half-cup portion of carrots or any other vegetable on this list contains 5 grams of carbohydrate as a mixture of starch and sugars. Such a portion is called a vegetable exchange. The vegetable exchanges include half-cup portions of tomatoes, cooked greens, okra, onions, summer squash, beets, and others. Each of these foods also contributes a little protein and no fat. Some vegetables are so low in carbohydrate and calories that the exchange system calls them "free foods." Among these are lettuce, parsley, and radishes.

For the lists of fruit exchanges and bread exchanges, see Appendix D.

The Fruit List A typical fruit portion, such as a half cup of orange juice, contains 15 grams of carbohydrate, mostly as sugars, including the fruit sugar fructose. Fruits vary greatly in their water and fiber contents, and therefore their sugar concentrations vary also. The portion sizes of different fruits are adjusted so that each contains 15 grams of carbohydrate. Thus in a diet plan they are interchangeable; you can "exchange" any fruit portion for any other without altering the amount of carbohydrate consumed. Among the fruit exchanges are one-third cup pineapple juice, one-half cup applesauce, and half of a small banana. The fruits contain insignificant amounts of fat and protein.

The Milk List A portion (1 cup) of milk or the equivalent is a generous contributor of carbohydrate, donating 12 grams. It also contributes high-quality protein (a point in its favor), as well as several important vitamins and minerals. Milk products vary in fat contents, an important consideration in choosing among them; Chapter 5 provides the details. Similar to milk in these respects are the other items on the milk list:

1 cup buttermilk
1 cup yogurt (plain)
⅓ cup dry milk powder
½ cup canned, evaporated milk, undiluted

Cream and butter, although dairy products, are *not* on the milk list because they contain little or no carbohydrate and insignificant amounts of the other nutrients important in milk. They are found on the fat list instead.

Sugar The exchange lists do not include concentrated sugar, not surprisingly, since the exchange system was originally designed for use by people with diabetes. But since sweets supply carbohydrate, it is useful to have a portion size, calorie amount, and carbohydrate amount for them:

1 teaspoon **brown sugar**
1 teaspoon **raw sugar**
1 teaspoon **molasses**
1 teaspoon **corn syrup**
1 teaspoon **honey**
1 teaspoon jam
1 teaspoon jelly
1 teaspoon any candy
1 teaspoon **maple sugar** or syrup

Each of these teaspoons is equivalent in sugar content to a teaspoon of white sugar and can be assumed to supply about 20 calories and 5 grams of carbohydrate. We repeated the *1 teaspoon* with each item to reemphasize that each is like white sugar, in spite of many people's belief that some are different or "better." See Table 4-5, which defines sugar terms.

For a person who uses ketchup liberally, it may help to remember that a tablespoon of it contains a teaspoon of sugar. And for the soft-drink

Table 4-5
Terms that Describe Sugar

Note: The term *sugars* here refers to all of the monosaccharides and disaccharides. On a food label the term *sugar* means sucrose. See Controversy 4 for terms concerning *artificial sweeteners* and *sugar alcohols.*

- **brown sugar** white sugar with molasses added, 95% pure sucrose.
- **concentrated fruit juice sweetener** a concentrated sugar syrup made from dehydrated, deflavored fruit juice, commonly grape juice, used to sweeten products that can then claim to be "all fruit."
- **confectioner's sugar** finely powdered sucrose, 99.9% pure.
- **corn sweeteners** corn syrup and sugar solutions derived from corn.
- **corn syrup** a syrup, mostly glucose, partly maltose, produced by the action of enzymes on cornstarch. *High-fructose corn syrup (HFCS)* is mostly fructose; glucose (dextrose) and maltose make up the balance.
- **dextrose** an older name for glucose.
- **fructose, galactose, glucose** the monosaccharides.
- **granulated sugar** common table sugar, crystalline sucrose, 99.9% pure.
- **honey** a concentrated solution primarily composed of glucose and fructose produced by enzymatic digestion, by bees, of the sucrose in nectar.
- **invert sugar** a mixture of glucose and fructose formed by the splitting of sucrose in an industrial process. Sold only in liquid form, sweeter than sucrose, invert sugar forms during certain cooking procedures and works to prevent crystallization of sucrose in soft candies and sweets.
- **lactose, maltose, sucrose** the disaccharides.
- **levulose** an older name for fructose.
- **maple sugar** a concentrated solution of sucrose derived from the sap of the sugar maple tree, mostly sucrose. This sugar was once common but is now usually replaced by sucrose and artificial maple flavoring.
- **molasses** a syrup left over from the refining of sucrose from sugar cane; a thick, brown syrup. The major nutrient in molasses is iron, a contaminant from the machinery used in processing it.
- **raw sugar** the first crop of crystals harvested during sugar processing. Raw sugar cannot be sold in the United States because it contains too much filth (dirt, insect fragments, and the like). Sugar sold as "raw sugar" domestically is not actually raw but has gone through over half of the refining steps.
- **turbinado** (ter-bih-NOD-oh) **sugar** raw sugar from which the filth has been washed; legal to sell in the United States.
- **white sugar** pure sucrose, produced by dissolving, concentrating, and recrystallizing raw sugar.

Processed foods contain surprisingly large amounts of sugar.

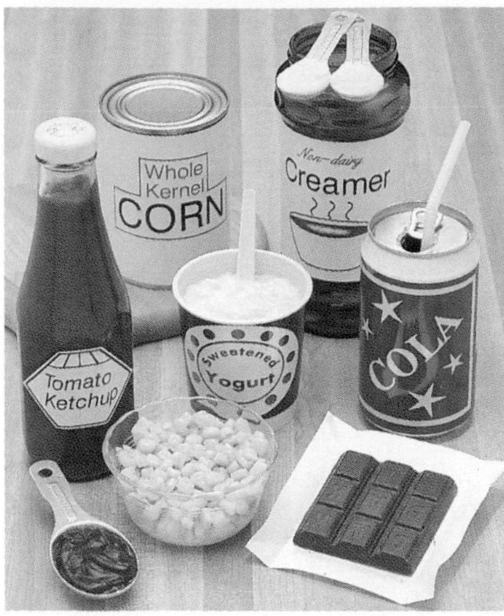

½ c canned corn = 3 tsp sugar (15 g sugar/60 cal from sugar)
12 oz cola = 8 tsp sugar (40 g sugar/160 cal from sugar)
1 tbsp ketchup = 1 tsp sugar (5 g sugar/20 cal from sugar)
1 tbsp creamer = 2 tsp sugar (10 g sugar/40 cal from sugar)
8 oz sweetened yogurt = 7 tsp sugar (35 g sugar/140 cal from sugar)
2 oz chocolate = 8 tsp sugar (40 g sugar/160 cal from sugar)

user, a 12-ounce can of a sugar-sweetened cola contains about 8 or more teaspoons of sugar. The margin photo shows the sugar contents of other processed foods.

What about the nutritional value of a product such as molasses or honey in place of white sugar? Molasses contains over 3 milligrams of iron per tablespoon and so if used frequently can contribute some of this important nutrient. However, it is less sweet than the other sweeteners, so it takes more molasses to provide the same sweetness as sugar. Also, its iron comes from the iron machinery in which the molasses is made, as an iron salt not easily absorbed by the body. And honey is no better for health than other sugars by virtue of being "natural." As a matter of fact, honey is chemically almost indistinguishable from sucrose. Honey contains the two monosaccharides glucose and fructose in approximately equal amounts. Sucrose contains the same monosaccharides but joined together in the disaccharide form. Spoon for spoon, however, sugar contains *fewer* calories than honey because the dry crystals of sugar take up more space than the sugars of honey dissolved in its water. No form of sugar is "more healthy" than white sugar, as Table 4-6 shows.

It would be absurd to rely on any sugar for nutrient contributions. A tablespoon of honey (64 calories) does offer 1/10 milligram of iron, but an adult would need to eat 150 tablespoons of honey a day—9,600 calories—to obtain the needed 15 milligrams of iron. The nutrients of honey just don't add up as fast as its calories. Thus if you choose molasses, brown sugar, or honey, choose them not for their nutrient contributions but for the pleasure they give. These tricks can help magnify the sweetness of foods without boosting their calories:

- Serve sweet food warm (heat enhances sweet tastes).
- Add sweet spices such as cinnamon, nutmeg, allspice, or cloves.
- Add a tiny pinch of salt; it will make food taste sweeter.
- Try reducing the sugar added to recipes by one third.
- Select fresh fruits, fruit juice, or fruits canned without sugar or in light syrup rather than heavy syrup.
- Use small amounts of sugar substitutes in place of sucrose. Sugar alcohols, discussed in this chapter's Controversy, help protect teeth from decay.
- Read food labels for clues on sugar content.

Finally, enjoy whatever sugar you do eat. Sweetness is one of life's great sensations, and you need not forego it completely. The person who cares about nutrition and loves sweets can artfully combine the two by using moderate amounts of sugar with creative imagination to enhance the flavors of nutritious foods.

Carbohydrates in a Day's Meals Chapter 2 introduced the basic tools to ensure that your diet provides adequate, balanced, and varied meals to meet your nutrient needs while not exceeding your limits. According

Table 4-6
The Empty Calories of Sugar

At first glance, honey, jelly, and brown sugar look more nutritious than plain sugar, but when compared with a person's nutrient needs, none contributes anything to speak of. The cola beverage is clearly an empty-calorie item, too.

Food	Energy (cal)	Protein (g)	Fiber (g)	Calcium (mg)	Iron (mg)	Magnesium (mg)	Potassium (mg)	Zinc (mg)	Vitamin A (RE)	Thiamin (mg)	Riboflavin (mg)	Niacin (mg)	Vitamin B_6 (mg)	Folacin (mg)	Vitamin C (mg)
Sugar (1 tbsp)	45	0	0	0	0.0	0	0	0.0	0	0	0	0.0	0	0	0
Honey (1 tbsp)	65	0	0	1	0.1	0	11	0.0	0	0	0	0.1	0	2	0
Jelly (1 tbsp)	49	0	0	1	0.0	1	11	0.0	0	0	0	0.0	0	0	1
Brown sugar (1 tbsp)	52	0	0	12	0.3	4	3	0.0	0	0	0	0.0	0	0	0
Cola beverage (12 fl oz)	151	0	0	9	0.1	3	4	0.1	0	0	0	0.0	0	0	0
Daily Values	2,000	56	25	1,000	18.0	400	—	15.0	1,000	1.5	1.7	20.0	2.0	400	60

to the dietary guidelines, more than 55 percent of daily energy should come from carbohydrate, mostly complex carbohydrate. The sample diet plans of Table 2-8 (page 49) provide amounts close to this recommended percentage, so they take care of the energy-yielding complex carbohydrate—starch. But what about the *other,* noncaloric, complex carbohydrate—fiber? Happily, fiber accompanies other carbohydrates in whole, natural foods. As long as the choices are made of foods such as whole grains, potatoes with skins, or apples with peels, no special effort need be spent on obtaining fiber, as Table 4-7 on the next page shows.

The choice of whole foods, including whole grains, is especially important for staple foods, as already emphasized. Does this mean that you should never eat refined white rolls, potato chips, or apple jelly? No. An occasional white roll, like an occasional candy bar, will not ruin a diet's adequacy. A few people, such as athletes, regularly need the extra energy provided by easy-to-eat refined grain products and concentrated sweets. For the bulk of the population's diet, though, the best daily choices are whole foods, partly because of their fiber contributions. Constructed of whole foods, the diet can easily supply 27 to 40 grams of dietary fiber daily. One slice of whole-grain bread, a cup of vegetables, another of legumes, and two portions of fruit together provide more than 25 grams. Appendix A lists the amounts of fiber in each of over 1,700 foods.

If high-fiber foods are new to you, your digestive system may need some time to adjust to them. Start slowly. Eat small amounts of salad and fresh cooked vegetables at first. Choose breads made with a mixture of white and whole-grain flours (these appear as light tan breads with flecks of brown). Try whole-grain crackers, cereals, bread sticks, or puffed grain cakes, which are especially easy to like. One trick to add fiber and the nutrients of whole grain to your day's foods, especially as a first step in switching to whole-grain products, is to use **wheat germ**

wheat germ the germ of the wheat grain.

Table 4-7
Fiber in Selected Foods[a]

Fruits (with skins): ≈2 g fiber
- apple, banana, 1 small
- strawberries, cherries, ¾ c
- cantaloupe, ½ melon

Grains and cereals: ≈2 g fiber[b]
- whole-wheat bread, 1 slice
- cracked-wheat bread, 2 slices
- shredded wheat, ½ biscuit
- oatmeal, cooked, 1 c
- popcorn, popped, 2 c

Vegetables (cooked): ≈2 g fiber
- broccoli, carrots, ½ c
- corn, ⅓ c; green beans, ⅔ c
- lettuce, raw, 2 c
- potato, 1 small; tomato, 1 large

Legumes (cooked): ≈8 g fiber
- dried beans, cooked/canned, ½ c
- dried lentils or peas, cooked, 1 c

Miscellaneous: ≈1 g fiber
- peanut butter, 2½ tsp
- walnuts, ¼ c
- pickle, 1 large
- strawberry jam, 1 tbsp

[a]App. A lists fiber grams for over 1,700 foods.
[b]Purified fibers and high-fiber cereals can be extremely fiber-rich, but whole-food sources of fiber are preferred.

liberally in toppings, coatings, and mixed dishes as well as on cereal. Wheat germ, unlike purified fiber, is rich in fiber and nutrients, but it also contains oil and so is high in calories; you might use it as a stepping stone to whole grains rather than as a permanent substitute.

Chapter 2 also introduced a set of meals that a hypothetical student ate (Figure 2-9, pages 56–57). Monday's meals were excellent choices nutritionally, partly because they contained abundant carbohydrate and fiber. The figure showed how to use exchange system estimates to determine carbohydrate amounts in a day's meals; if you were to look them up in Appendix A, you would obtain different, but similar, numbers. You have to become familiar with the exchange system before this technique saves time, but a few practice sessions are enough to make estimating carbohydrate grams easy. To estimate the fiber, use the symbols and notes in Appendix D, and remember that all vegetable list items donate between 2 and 3 grams per serving.

Carbohydrate is important, but it is only a part of the story. The Food Features of Chapters 5 and 6 will provide information on limiting fat and on obtaining enough, but not too much, protein.

CHECKING OUT FOOD LABELS
How to Read Carbohydrate Information on a Food Label

Chapter 2 introduced food labels as valuable tools for the shopper. This section is about using food labels to judge the carbohydrate contents of foods. Cereal, a food on which people rely for carbohydrate, serves as our example (see Figure 4-11).

CALORIES PER SERVING

The first number to look at on any label is the one given the top priority position—the number of calories in a serving of the food. Reading from the cereal label depicted here, one serving of the cereal contains 194 calories. If the shopper were the typical adult for whom food labels are designed, that is, a person who needs 2,000 calories per day, then this cereal would meet about 10 percent of the shopper's daily calorie need.

TOTAL CARBOHYDRATE

A few lines down from the calorie amount, the label lists "total carbohydrate" in grams per serving. This total includes the starch and also the fiber and sugars in a serving of the food. The total carbohydrate in our example cereal is 32 grams per serving. The fiber grams are also listed separately (4 g), as are the grams of sugars (11 g). FDA chose to use the plural term *sugars* to alert consumers that the grams listed reflect both added sugars and those that occur naturally in foods. Some manufacturers also elect to state separately the complex carbohydrate (termed "other carbohydrate" on labels) amounts in grams, but this detail is not required.

The "% Daily Value" column compares the total carbohydrates in a serving of the food with a person's daily need. The reference values are listed in the Daily Values

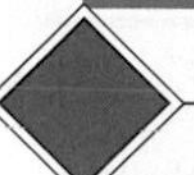

CHECKING OUT FOOD LABELS

How to Read Carbohydrate Information on a Food Label *continued*

chart at the bottom of the label. The shopper can therefore read that a serving of this cereal meets "11%" of the daily need for carbohydrate for a person requiring 2,000 calories a day.

Notice that the Daily Values chart lists the carbohydrate needs of two people, one requiring 2,000 calories a day and the other needing 2,500 calories a day—300 grams and 375 grams respectively. The "% Daily Value" column, however, applies only to the 2,000-calorie diet. People who require more or less than 2,000 calories and who are curious about how well a food meets their own probable daily needs must work out the calculations for themselves. In this discussion, we assume that the hypothetical label-reader's need is 2,000 calories, the same value that is used to determine percentages on labels.

The Daily Value standard for carbohydrate is based on the recommendation for health which states that 60 percent of the calories in the diet should derive from carbohydrate. The Daily Value ideal of 300 grams carbohydrate was calculated for consumers by determining the number of grams providing 60 percent of 2,000 calories.

As just mentioned, a serving of this cereal meets "11%" of the day's needed 300 grams of total carbohydrate. This means that, to meet the Daily Value recommendation, a person would need to eat about 10 servings of this or other foods providing about the same amounts of total carbohydrate per serving. This is reasonable, and it is in keeping with the Daily Food Guide of Chapter 2 that recommends 6 to 11 servings of high-carbohydrate foods, such as breads, cereals, and other grain products. Don't forget, too, that foods without labels, such as fresh fruits and vegetables, also contribute to carbohydrate intakes throughout the day.

Is this food a wise choice from the point of view of total carbohydrate contributed? To find out, compare the carbohydrate it provides with the calories it provides. It contributes about 10 percent of the daily need of calories, and about 10 percent of the carbohydrate needs, too, so it should fit well into the diet.

Rule of thumb for identifying high-carbohydrate foods: Look for 14 to 15 grams of carbohydrate for each 100 calories of product. These foods will provide 55 to 60 percent of calories as carbohydrate.

FIBER

Consumers can easily compare the fiber in a food to their fiber needs. This food lists "16%" of the Daily Value for fiber. To meet the entire day's need, then,

Figure 4-11

WEST'S ACTION CEREAL

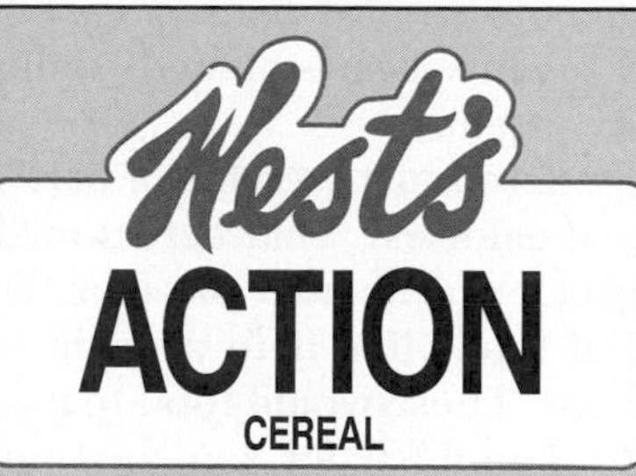

Nutrition Facts

Serving size 3/4 cup (55g)
Servings per Box 10

Amount per serving	
Calories 194	Calories from Fat 54
	% Daily Value*
Total Fat 6g	9%
Saturated Fat 4g	20%
Cholesterol 0mg	0%
Sodium 250mg	10%
Total Carbohydrate 32g	11%
Dietary fiber 4g	16%
Sugars 11g	
Protein 3g	

Vitamin A 25% •	Vitamin C 25%
Calcium 2% •	Iron 25%

*Percent Daily Values are based on a 2,000 calorie diet. Your Daily Values may be higher or lower depending on your calorie needs.

	Calories	2,000	2,500
Total Fat	Less than	65g	80g
Sat Fat	Less than	20g	25g
Cholesterol	Less than	300mg	300mg
Sodium	Less than	2,400mg	2,400mg
Total Carbohydrate		300g	375g
Dietary Fiber		25g	30g

Calories per gram
Fat 9 • Carbohydrate 4 • Protein 4

INGREDIENTS, Whole oats, Milled corn, Enriched wheat flour (contains Niacin, Reduced iron, Thiamin mononitrate, Riboflavin), Dextrose, Maltose, High-fructose corn syrup, Brown sugar, Partially hydrogenated cottonseed oil, Coconut oil, Walnuts, Salt, and Natural flavors. Vitamins and minerals: Vitamin C (sodium ascorbate), Vitamin A (Palmitate), Iron.

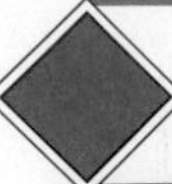

CHECKING OUT FOOD LABELS

How to Read Carbohydrate Information on a Food Label *continued*

would require only about seven servings of foods similar to this one in their fiber contents.

What if another cereal offered just 2 grams of fiber in a standard serving of equal calories? That cereal might be less desirable as a provider of fiber in the diet. You would need 14 servings of foods like it to provide the day's total fiber requirement. These would total to more than 2,700 calories, a hefty number for someone on a limited calorie budget. Nutrients and fiber in cereals can easily be compared from one brand to the next because manufacturers must use the standard serving sizes mandated by the Food and Drug Administration for each type of food.

SUGARS

◆ Notice that the label lists sugars only in grams, leaving a blank in the space to the right where the percent of Daily Value figures normally appear. This is because no Daily Value standard exists for sugars. Consumers who wish to evaluate a food's sugar content with regard to a health recommendation must choose their own standard and calculate the value for themselves.

Table 4-1 at the beginning of this chapter listed several recommendations for intakes of refined sugar, but none of those can be applied to the information provided about "sugars" on labels. This is because the sugars listed on labels reflect not only the refined sugars that people are urged to limit in the diet, but also the naturally occurring sugars of fruits, vegetables, milk products, and other wholesome foods. FDA made the decision to count the sugars from all sources together for the convenience of the chemist analyzing foods, because the fructose from fruit and the fructose from high-fructose corn sweeteners are indistinguishable in laboratory tests.

This leaves consumers guessing as to how many of the grams of sugars were added to their food by the manufacturers and how many were present in the original food. A committed consumer can make some intelligent guesses, however, by comparing one product to the next. For example, the cereal of Figure 4-11 lists 11 grams of sugars. A glance down at the ingredient list confirms that an unknown quantity of sugar in several forms has indeed been added to the product. Now, the consumer must find a cereal of similar grain composition, one made with oats, corn, and wheat flour but to which no sugar has been added. The grams of "sugars" listed on that label state "0" or "1" gram. This means that all or almost all of the grams of sugars listed on the label of the cereal in Figure 4-11 have been added by the manufacturer, because no sugars or just a trace occurred naturally in the grains.

Similarly, a can of apples packed in water might list 10 grams of "sugars" on the label because apples naturally contain sugars. Another can of apples, sweetened with sucrose, might list 15 grams of "sugars" on the label. The consumer who compares the two can tell that the difference between these two sugar values (5 grams per serving) is all added sucrose. Once consumers become accustomed to analyzing labels of similar products in this way, many such comparisons become possible.

INGREDIENTS

◆ The ingredients are listed in order of predominance by weight. This cereal is made mostly from whole oats blended with smaller amounts each of two refined grains (milled corn and wheat flour). Each refined grain individually comprises less of the weight of the cereal than does oats, but together, the refined grains may outweigh the whole grains in the cereal. The more whole grains, the better, so the comparison is worth making.

A clue to the proportion of whole grains to refined grains in this cereal is found in its fiber content. A serving of the cereal provides 4 grams of fiber, an amount found in a serving of many whole-grain cereals (one whole shredded wheat biscuit, for example). Since the ingredient list mentions no added fiber, you can deduce that whole grain provides a major portion of the weight of the cereal.

Four types of sugars listed among the ingredients in Figure 4-11 are accounted for in the total grams of sugars listed on the Nutrition Facts panel. The consumer can compare the grams of sugars (11 grams) to the grams of total carbohydrate (32 grams) and deduce that the cereal is two-thirds grain, and not mostly sugars. All in all, then, this cereal makes a reasonable contribution to a day's total carbohydrate and fiber needs without providing too much sugar.

Notes

1. C. M. Ripsin and coauthors, Oat products and lipid lowering: A meta-analysis, *Journal of the American Medical Association* 267 (1992): 3317-3325.
2 M. A. Eastwood, The physiological effects of dietary fiber: An update, *Annual Review of Nutrition* 12 (1992): 19–35.
3. J. F. Swain and coauthors, Comparison of the effects of oat bran and low-fiber wheat on serum lipoprotein levels and blood pressure, *New England Journal of Medicine* 322 (1990): 147–152.
4. S. M. Saheen and S. E. Fleming, High-fiber foods at breakfast: Influence on plasma glucose and insulin responses to lunch, *American Journal of Clinical Nutrition* 46 (1987): 804–811.
5. L. Cara and coauthors, Effects of oat bran, rice bran, wheat fiber, and wheat germ on postprandial lipemia in healthy adults, *American Journal of Clinical Nutrition* 55 (1992): 81–88.
6. Dietary fiber reduces B-carotene utilization, *Nutrition Reviews* 45 (1987): 350–352.
7. S. Welsh and J. F. Guthrie, Changing American diets in A. Bendich and C. E. Butterworth, Jr. (eds.), *Micronutrients in Health and in Disease Prevention* (New York: Marcel Dekker, 1991), pp. 381–408.
8. E. Lanza and coauthors, Dietary fiber intake in the U.S. population, *American Journal of Clinical Nutrition* 46 (1987): 790–797.
9. Food and Nutrition Board, *Recommended Dietary Allowances*, 10th ed. (Washington, D.C.: National Academy of Sciences, 1989), p. 42.
10. WHO Study Group on Diet, Nutrition and Prevention of Noncommunicable Diseases, Diet, nutrition, and the prevention of chronic diseases, *Nutrition Reviews* 49 (1991): 291–301.
11. S. G. Cooper and E. J. Tracey, Small-bowel obstruction caused by oat-bran bezoar, *New England Journal of Medicine* 320 (1989): 1148–1149.
12. J. L. Slavin, Dietary fiber: Classification, chemical analyses, and food sources, *Journal of the American Dietetic Association* 87 (1987): 1164–1171; D. M. Klurfeld, The role of dietary fiber in gastrointestinal disease, *Journal of the American Dietetic Association* 87 (1987): 1172–1177.
13. Dietary fibre: Importance of function as well as amount, *Lancet* 340 (1992): 1133–1134.
14. M. A. Eastwood, The physiological effect of dietary fiber: An update, *Annual Review of Nutrition* 12 (1992): 19–35.
15. M. I. McBurney and L. U. Thompson, Dietary fiber and energy balance: Integration of the human ileostomy and in vitro fermentation modes, *Animal Feed Science and Technology* 23 (1989): 261–275.
16. J. M. Saavedra and J. A. Perman, Current concepts in lactose malabsorption and intolerance, *Annual Review of Nutrition* 9 (1989): 475–502.
17. J. C. Brand and S. Holt, Relative effectiveness of milks with reduced amounts of lactose in alleviating milk intolerance, *American Journal of Clinical Nutrition* 54 (1991): 148–151.
18. Food and Nutrition Board, 1989, p. 41.
19. K. Indar-Brown, C. Noreberg, and Z. Madar, Glycemic and insulinemic responses after ingestion of ethnic foods by NIDDM and healthy subjects, *American Journal of Clinical Nutrition* 55 (1992): 89–95; T. M. Wolever and coauthors, The glycemic index: Methodology and clinical implications, *American Journal of Clinical Nutrition* 54 (1991): 846–854.
20. G. M. Reaven, Parma Symposium: Current controversies in nutrition, *American Journal of Clinical Nutrition* 47 (1988): 1078–1082.
21. M. F. Saad and coauthors, A two-step model for development of non-insulin-dependent diabetes, *American Journal of Medicine* 90 (1991): 229–235.
22. L. Ressetti, A. Giaccari, and R. A. DeFronzo, Glucose toxicity, *Diabetes Care* 13 (1990): 610–630.
23. S. Lillioja and coauthors, Impaired glucose tolerance as a disorder of insulin action, *New England Journal of Medicine* 318 (1988): 1217–1225.
24. H. Shimokata and coauthors, Age as independent determinant of glucose tolerance, *Diabetes* 40 (1991): 44–51; M. J. Busby, Glucose tolerance in women: the effects of age, body composition, and sex hormones, *Journal of the American Geriatric Society* 40 (1992): 497–502.
25. T. L. Holbrook, E. Barrett-Connor, and D. L. Wingard, A prospective population-based study of alcohol use and non-insulin-dependent diabetes mellitus, *American Journal of Epidemiology* 132 (1990): 902–909.
26. E. T. Skarfos, K. I. Selinus, and H. O. Lithell, Risk factors for developing non-insulin dependent diabetes: A 10 year follow-up of men in Uppsala, *British Medical Journal* 303 (September 21, 1991): 755–760.
27. J. Randal, Insulin key to diabetes but not a full cure, *FDA Consumer*, May 1992, pp. 15–19.
28. D. M. Nathan, Long-term complications of diabetes mellitus, *New England Journal of Medicine* 328 (1993): 1676–1685.
29. M. W. Steffes and S. M. Mauer, Toward a basic understanding of diabetic complications, *New England Journal of Medicine* 325 (1991): 883–884.
30. Susan P. Helmrich and coauthors, Physical activity and reduced occurrence of non-insulin-dependent diabetes mellitus, *New England Journal of Medicine* 325 (1991): 147–152; A dissenting view appears in a letter by R. S. Surwitt and J. D. Lane, Physical activity and non-insulin-dependent diabetes mellitus, *New England Journal of Medicine* 325 (1991): 1887.
31. F. J. Service, Hypoglycemia and the postprandial syndrome, *New England Journal of Medicine* 321 (1989): 1472–1474.
32. K. S. Polonsky, A practical approach to fasting hypoglycemia, *New England Journal of Medicine* 326 (1992): 1020–1021.
33. J. Palardy and coauthors, Blood glucose measurements during symptomatic episodes in patients with suspected postprandial hypoglycemia, *New England Journal of Medicine* 321 (1989): 1421–1425.
34. R. Lozano, S. A. Chalew, and A. A. Kowarski, Cornstarch ingestion after oral glucose loading: Effect on glucose concentrations, hormone response, and symptoms in patients with postprandial hypoglycemic syndrome, *American Journal of Clinical Nutrition* 52 (1990): 667–670.
35. A. B. Stevens and coauthors, Psychomotor performance and counterregulatory responses in healthy volunteers, *Diabetes Care* 12 (1989): 12–17.
36. V. Marks, Functional Hypoglycemia: Fact or fancy, *Hypoglycemia* (New York: Raven Press, 1987), pp. 1–17.
37. Palardy and coauthors, 1989.

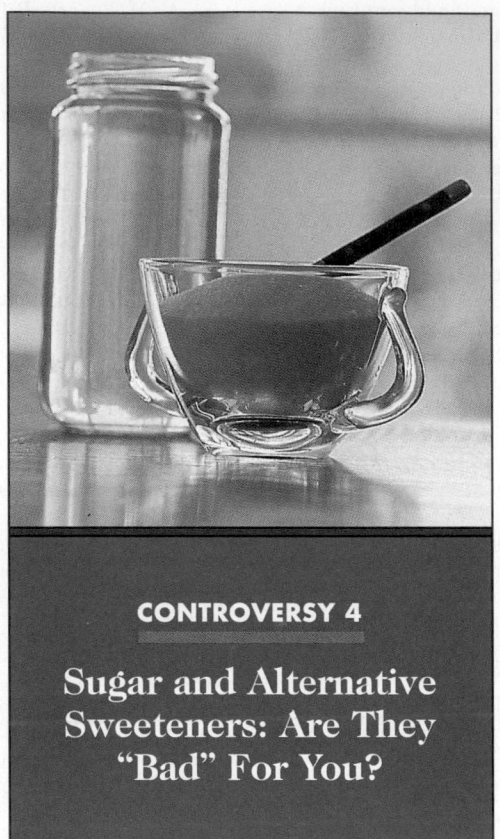

CONTROVERSY 4

Sugar and Alternative Sweeteners: Are They "Bad" For You?

For every person in the United States today, 136 pounds of sugar, about 25 percent of the total energy in the nation's diet, disappears from the marketplace annually. Of this 136 pounds, people probably consume about 80 to 90 pounds each, on average. This is dramatically more than a century ago, when purified sugar was almost unknown and people's sugar intakes amounted to only 20 pounds per year, all from whole-food sources. Since that time, the amount of sugar in the diet has crept upward. Over half of the sugar consumed today is added directly from the sugar bowl or during food preparation at home. The other half is added by food manufacturers, mostly as high-fructose corn syrup.

Figure C4-1 presents two ways of looking at sugar intakes. The top line traces the amounts of sugar used up each year—the 136 pounds per capita just mentioned. This figure includes sugar purchased and wasted, such as that in the brine of sweet pickles, in jam that spoils and is thrown away, in discarded stale bakery goods, and in sugar discarded by industry. It also includes sugar converted to gases and alcohol by fermentation. Yeast used to make bread and fermented alcoholic beverages use up large quantities of sugar each year. In contrast to the "sugar used up" line of Figure C4-1, the bottom dotted line represents one estimate of how much sugar a typical consumer actually eats in one year.[1] Other estimates exist, and figures somewhere between the two lines shown are probably close to the true average intake.

Figure C4-1 on the next page does not show that consumption of artificial sweeteners also rose dramatically within this same time period. People who choose artificial sweeteners to cut their sugar intakes might be surprised if they were to keep track of both. Even if they do add artificial sweeteners to their diets, people seem not to cut sugar intakes at all.

Do sugars harm people's health? Some people think so. And if they do, are sugar substitutes a better choice? This Controversy addresses these questions, and in the process, demonstrates how nutrition researchers pursue their answers, step by step, via scientific inquiry.

EVIDENCE CONCERNING SUGAR

Sugar is accused by some of causing nutritional problems. It is said to (1) promote and maintain obesity, (2) cause and aggravate diabetes, (3) increase the risk of heart disease, (4) disrupt behavior in children and adults, and (5) cause dental decay and gum disease. Is it guilty or innocent of these charges?

Obesity Does sugar cause obesity? In one experiment designed to answer part of this question, researchers conducted a laboratory study in which they measured the effect of a sucrose-rich diet on deposits of fat in rats.[2] These rats had brain lesions that caused insensitivity to appetite controls, so the animals became obese no matter what sort of chow they ate. The experiment showed an effect of sucrose, not on total body fat, but on its distribution. The diet high in sucrose caused deposits of more belly fat than did a diet of regular rat chow.

More direct evidence on obesity in people comes from population studies. In many countries incidence of obesity increases as sugar consumption rises. But this evidence does not all point to sugar as the sole cause. Wherever sugar intake has increased, usually fat and total calorie intakes have also risen. Simultaneously, physical activity has declined. On the other hand, obesity also occurs where sugar intakes are low, and obese people in many instances eat less sugar than thin people do.[3] Fat is more calorie dense than sugar and can easily contribute to obesity. Fat often occurs together with sugar in sweet treats and snacks. Studies of populations by themselves cannot separate the effects of eating sugar from those of eating too much fat or of exercising too little.

Concentrated sweets do make it easy for people to consume large amounts of calories quickly, however, and that is why most diet plans recommend avoiding them. Some people believe that eating even small amounts of sugar triggers binges; for them, conscientious sugar avoidance is an important part of weight-

Figure C4-1

U.S. SUGAR INTAKES

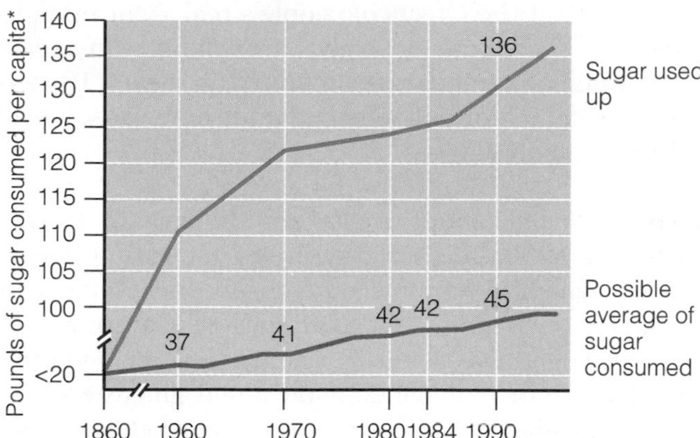

*Note: These amounts reflect both table sugar added at home and sugar sweeteners added in processing.

Source: Data through 1984 from C. Lecos, Our insatiable sweet tooth, *FDA Consumer*, October 1985, p. 25; data for 1990 from U.S. Dept. of Agriculture, *Sugar and Sweetener Situation and Outlook Report*, March 1991; Method used to extrapolate "possible average of sugar consumed" values from G. H. Anderson, Myths and facts about sugar, *Contemporary Nutrition*, 16 (1991): 1. (Extrapolation was based on actual data for 1977 to 1978 and so may not apply equally to other years but is presented here for contrast with sugar disappearance figures. From 1977 to 1978, per capita consumption at the 90th percentile was 84 lb per year.)

loss dieting.[4] For others the inclusion of small amounts of sugar in a weight-loss plan makes the plan easier to follow. In short, the effects of sugar on a person's eating style and body weight depend on the user.

Diabetes Does sugar cause or contribute to Type II diabetes? Recall from the chapter that in diabetes, insulin secretion or tissue responsiveness to it becomes abnormal. This, of course, affects the body's ability to manage sugar. At one time people thought that eating sugar caused diabetes by "overstraining the pancreas," but now we know that this is not the case. Body fatness is more closely related to diabetes than diet is. High rates of diabetes have not been reported in any society in which obesity is rare. Still, it can be asked whether people with the genetic tendency to develop this type of diabetes should avoid eating sugar. The evidence on this point is conflicting and interesting.

In populations around the world, a profound increase, by as much as tenfold, in the incidence of diabetes has occurred simultaneously with an increase in sugar consumption. This has been true for the Japanese, Israelis, Africans, Native Americans, Eskimos, Polynesians, and Micronesians. Yet in other populations, no relationship has been found between sugar intake and diabetes. Wherever starch, rather than sugar, is the major carbohydrate in the diet, diabetes is rare. But this does not prove that sugar causes diabetes or that starch prevents it. The apparent protective effect of starch might be due, for example, to the chromium or fiber that comes with it. Sugar is not thought to raise blood glucose levels any more than do starches.[5] The fairest conclusion that can be drawn is that obesity is a major causal factor but that sugar may share in the guilt as a contributor to Type II diabetes.

Once a person has diabetes, is it all right to use moderate amounts of sugar? It has been thought so, because sucrose-containing foods seem to exert no more of a glycemic effect (see page 115) than do starchy foods.[6] But the amount of sucrose in the standard U.S. diet is clearly too much for those with diabetes. Most authorities agree that, as part of the carbohydrate in a controlled diet, modest amounts of sucrose are acceptable for those with diabetes.[7] However, *other* body responses must also be considered. Researchers have shown that people with diabetes who eat a diet that contains more than just modest amounts of sucrose experience many undesirable metabolic effects, among them raised blood lipids, which suggest a high risk of heart disease (discussed next). Many health care professionals allow clients concentrated sweets in amounts equaling 5 to 10 percent of total calories consumed, but only as a planned part of the carbohydrate in meals or for reversal of diabetic hypoglycemia caused by too much insulin.

Heart Disease Does eating sugar raise the risk of heart disease? Logic says that sugar converted to fat and transported through the bloodstream might cause the sort of fat deposits in the arteries that are known to lead to heart disease. Again, a research study using rats provides some clues. When researchers fed rats a diet with sucrose as the only carbohydrate source, the rats sustained microscopic damage to their arteries, and their blood tested high for both triglycerides and cholesterol.[8] Rats fed starch instead of sugar did not develop the damage or the elevated blood lipids. Speculating that the essential trace mineral selenium might be present in the starch but absent from the sugar, the researchers then tried supplementing the diet of some sucrose-fed rats with the mineral selenium at a level of about twice the established minimum for rats. The rats eating high-sucrose diets plus selenium did not sustain artery damage as did rats fed sugar without selenium, but their blood lipids increased to just as high a level. Keep in mind that the rats consumed sucrose as their only source of carbohydrate; even people with a highly unusual craving for sweets wouldn't choose such a diet to live on. The protective effect of selenium seen in this study is interesting, but no one can yet guess what it might mean in terms of nutrition. (Quacks love these sorts of results, though, and use them to market expensive, unnecessary supplements.)

Fat is clearly the major *dietary* culprit in the heart disease susceptibility of most people, but there is a *hereditary* culprit, too, and some people may tend to develop raised blood lipid levels in response to carbohydrate and alcohol. If their heart disease risk is assessed as high, they are told to restrict their intakes of carbohydrate and alcohol.

Some research has appeared to indicate that the rise in blood lipids in response to sugar may be caused by fructose, and that sucrose causes the rise because it contains fructose.[9] High-fructose corn syrup sweetens many processed foods including beverages, pastries, and other products, and U.S. intakes of the sweetener have climbed in recent years.

The effect of sugar on blood lipids may depend not only on the diet's sugar content, but on its total carbohydrate content. In one study, people with diabetes were given two diets, both equal in grams of carbohydrate. One diet, however, contained more sucrose and the other more starch. Both groups responded about the same: their blood lipids did not seem to change much, even with high sucrose intakes. The researchers suggest the possibility that sucrose may affect blood lipids only when both total carbohydrate and sucrose intakes are high.[10]

Sucrose may also contribute to heart disease by aggravating high blood pressure. From studies of rats, it appears that animals with impaired kidney function retain sodium when they are fed sucrose.[11] (Sodium raises the blood pressure as Chapter 8 explains.) From studies of people, it is known that human beings initially excrete large amounts of sodium and water if they fast or restrict their carbohydrate intakes. When they resume eating carbohydrate (glucose, sucrose, or especially fructose), they regain both sodium and water. However, the hormonal regulation of fluid balance quickly adjusts to different carbohydrate intakes, and within a few days the effect on blood pressure is gone. Such transient fluctuations in blood pressure are different from the dangerous, sustained hypertension associated with heart disease. A high-sugar diet does not cause a significant sustained increase in blood pressure in healthy subjects.

Experiments implicating sugar in heart and artery disease have used diets so high in sugar that the results may not reflect the effects of people's real sugar intakes. No one has shown conclusively, throughout many years of research, that moderate amounts of sugar (10 percent of total calories) affect the disease process in healthy human beings.

Behavior What about sugar and behavior? In the 1970s and 1980s, claims appeared that eating sugary foods caused children to become unruly and adolescents and adults to exhibit antisocial and even criminal behavior.[12] Sugar was labeled a toxin and an addictive drug. The brain is dependent on blood glucose for its energy, and some proponents of the sugar-behavior idea believe that eating sucrose causes wide fluctuations in blood glucose level, with frequent hypoglycemia and resultant irrational and violent behavior. A criminal defense was even won on the argument that the defendant was in the habit of eating high-sugar "junk food," notably Twinkies, and therefore had become hypoglycemic, and therefore was not responsible for his actions.

A decade of research following those years yielded only mixed or negative results. Most experts agreed that the "sugar-behavior" theory had been put to rest. Some early reports were simply not based on valid research techniques (for example, using hair analysis to diagnose hypoglycemia). Still, many people clung to the idea that sugar affects behavior, especially the behavior of children. Teachers, parents, grandparents, and others believe that the children they know react to sugar, despite evidence to the contrary.

Today, research has once again become active on the idea that sugar may somehow influence behavior. There are many ways in which it might do so: by altering the levels of chemicals in the brain that affect mood, by inducing nutrient deficiencies, and others. One group of researchers studying children propose that behavior changes may be brought about by the series of hormones the body releases after consuming sugar.[13] It is known that blood glucose is not regulated by diet but by hormones, and one of those is the stress hormone, norepinephrine. The researchers fed a syrupy beverage to 9 adults and 14 children and then tested their blood norepinephrine levels three hours later, after insulin had time to store the sugar. The blood-*sugar* levels of both groups had dropped only slightly, but the blood *norepinephrine* was elevated. In the children it had shot up to double the level seen in the adults. The children also complained of symptoms such as weakness and nervousness during the test period. While it is tempting to declare as proven the idea that sugar elevates blood norepinephrine levels in children and that this leads to behavior changes, many more studies are needed before the theory can be confirmed as fact.

Another way sugar has been theorized to affect behavior is by providing energy. In a study of 13 children hospitalized for psychiatric disorders, researchers gave the children either plain orange juice or orange juice sweetened with sucrose or fructose. The children given the sugar-added drinks became more active and exhibited more inappropriate behavior than the children who had received the plain drinks. The researchers concluded that added calories from sugar permitted children to exert more energy (the so-called "Halloween effect"); they did not suggest that sugar, specifically, had a negative effect on behavior.[14]

A group of researchers set out to find out whether children diagnosed as hyperactive became more aggressive or less attentive after eating sugar.[15] These researchers tested sugar and two noncaloric sweeteners. When 17 children with hyperactivity and 9 children without the disorder were given a high-sugar breakfast, neither group behaved more aggressively. Those children with hyperactivity, however, became more distractible (paid less attention) than usual after the sugary breakfast. This effect was not seen after a breakfast sweetened with aspartame or saccharin. Perhaps some children with hyperactivity are especially sensitive to sugar's effects.

Several well-controlled studies have shown that sugar calms normal children, a finding consistent with convincing biochemical evidence. One such study using sucrose, cyclamate (an artificial sweetener), and aspartame in school-aged children, showed no differences in activity, social interactions, learning performance, or mood in response to the artificial sweeteners, but showed that sugar made the children less active.[16] In other studies, sugar has calmed juvenile delinquents with pronounced behavioral problems.[17] In older violent offenders, problems of blood glucose regulation has been reported to go hand in hand with severe behavioral disturbance.[18]

Other studies have failed to demonstrate any consistent effects of sucrose on behavior in either normal or hyperactive children.[19] In conclusion, occasional behavioral reactions to sugar may be possible, but until research proves otherwise, the idea that sugar alone directly affects behavior adversely in most healthy children or adults remains all but ruled out.

Dental Caries Does sugar cause **dental caries?** Caries are a serious public health problem. They afflict nearly everyone in the country, half by the time they are two years old. One of the most successful measures taken to reduce the incidence of dental decay is fluoridation of community water. But sugar has something to do with dental caries too.

Caries develop as acids produced by bacterial growth in the mouth eat into tooth enamel. Bacteria establish colonies known as **plaque** whenever they can get a foothold on tooth surfaces. Once established, they multiply and affix themselves more and more firmly unless they are brushed, flossed, or scraped away. Eventually the acid of plaque creates pits that deepen into cavities. Below the gum line, plaque works its way down until the acid erodes the roots of teeth and the jawbone in which they are embedded, loosening the teeth and leading to infections of the gums. Gum disease severe enough to threaten tooth loss afflicts 95 percent of our population by their later years.[20] Table C4-1 defines some terms related to caries.

Bacteria thrive on carbohydrate. Carbohydrate as sugar has been named as the main causative factor in forming cavities.[21] However, starch also supports bacterial growth if the bacteria are allowed sufficient time to work on it. Of prime importance is the length of time the food stays in the mouth, and this depends on the food's composition, how sticky it is, how often you eat it, and on whether you brush your teeth afterwards.[22]

Bacteria produce acid for 20 to 30 minutes after exposure to sugar. Thus if you were to eat three pieces of candy, one right after the other, your teeth would be exposed to approximately 30 minutes of acid demineralization. Should you eat the candy pieces at half-hour intervals, though, the acid exposure time would be 90 minutes. Likewise, slowly sipping a sugary soft drink may be more harmful than drinking quickly and emptying the mouth of sugar. Some forms of candy, such as milk chocolate and caramels, may be less harmful than once believed because the sugar dissolves completely and is washed away in saliva. Particles from breads, granola bars, sugary cereals, oatmeal cookies, raisins, salted crackers, and chips, on the other hand, may be worse than once thought, because they get stuck in the teeth and do not dissolve. These particles may remain in contact with tooth surfaces for hours, providing a feast for bacteria and greatly increasing the likelihood of caries.[23] A table in Chapter 13 lists foods of both high and low caries potential.

Table C4-1
Dental Terms

- **dental caries** decay of the teeth (*caries* means "rottenness").
- **plaque** (PLACK) a mass of microorganisms and their resultant deposits on the crowns and roots of the teeth, a forerunner of dental caries and gum disease. (The term *plaque* is used in another connection—arterial plaque in atherosclerosis. See Chapter 11.)

Total sugar intakes still play a major role in caries incidence, though, and populations with diets of more than 10 percent of calories from sugar are demonstrated to have an unacceptably high incidence of dental caries.[24] Worldwide, many governing agencies urge their citizens to consume no more than 10 percent of calories from sugar because of sugar's link with dental caries.

Mechanically disturbing bacteria by flossing every 24 hours may effectively prevent formation of cavities, regardless of the carbohydrate content of the diet. And some people may *never* get cavities because they have inherited resistance to them. It is clear, though, that sugar is an energy source for the bacteria that cause tooth decay and that when exposure is sufficient in susceptible people, it is guilty as charged.[25]

PERSONAL STRATEGY FOR USING SUGAR Evidence against sugar in harming health has been inconclusive.[26] Meanwhile, consumers must choose foods to eat each day. Should they avoid all sugar? The Dietary Guidelines suggest only that people "use moderation" concerning sugar, not that they avoid it altogether. The World Health Organization's recommendations are more specific and recommend that sugar should not contribute more than 10 percent of a person's total calorie intake.[27] A person who eats 2,000 calories of energy a day, then, is allowed 200 calories from sugar. Those 200 calories of sugar, 10 teaspoons or so, sound like quite a lot. But when you add up all the sugar teaspoons present in common foods, as the Food Feature of Chapter 4 did, 200 calories-worth may start to seem restrictive.

One way that people may attempt to limit their sugar intakes is by using artificial sweeteners or sugar substitutes. These do provide sweetness without sucrose, but many of them have been subjects of controversy concerning their safety. Still, in our sweet-toothed, overweight population, many people perceive sugar substitutes as a way to cheat the scales.

People who want to avoid sugar may choose from two sets of alternative sweeteners. One set is the sugar alcohols, which are energy-yielding sweeteners sometimes referred to as nutritive sweeteners. The other is the artificial sweeteners, which provide virtually no energy, also referred to as nonnutritive sweeteners.

EVIDENCE CONCERNING SUGAR ALCOHOLS The sugar alcohols are familiar to people who use special dietary products. Among them are **mannitol, sorbitol, xylitol,** and **maltitol.** All the sugar alcohols can be metabolized by human beings, and they all provide about as much energy as sucrose (4 calories per gram).

A proven benefit of sugar alcohols is that ordinary mouth bacteria cannot metabolize them as rapidly as they metabolize other carbohydrates. So sugar alcohols do not contribute as much to dental caries.

Mannitol is the least satisfactory of the sugar alcohols just named. It is less sweet than sucrose, so large amounts have to be used to obtain the same sweetness (see Table C4-2). It lingers unabsorbed in the intestine

Table C4-2
Sweetness of Sugar Alternates

Sugar Alternate	Relative Sweetness[a]
Sugars	
Sucrose	100
Fructose	170
Sugar Alcohols	
Sorbitol	45
Mannitol	70
Maltitol	90
Xylitol	100
Noncaloric Sweeteners	
Acesulfame-K	200
Cyclamate	4,500
Aspartame	20,000
Saccharin	30,000
Sucralose	60,000
Alitame	200,000

[a]The relative sweetness depends on the temperature, acidity, and other flavors of the foods in which the substance occurs. The sweetness of pure sucrose is the standard with which the approximate sweetness of sugar substitutes is compared.

Source: Data from W. L. Dills, Sugar alcohols as bulk sweeteners, *Annual Review of Nutrition* (1989): 161–186; S. A. Schlicker and C. Regan, Innovations in calorie-reduced foods: A review of fat and sugar replacement technologies, *Topics in Clinical Nutrition*, November 1990, pp. 50–60; V. M. Sardesai and T. H. Waldsham, Natural and synthetic intense sweeteners, *Journal of Nutritional Biochemistry* 2 (1991): 236–244.

for a long time, available to intestinal bacteria for their energy. As they consume the mannitol, the bacteria multiply, attract water, produce irritating waste, and cause diarrhea.

More practical than mannitol, sorbitol sweetens sugar-free gums and candies; but it, too, has drawbacks. At least two teaspoons as much sorbitol (with twice the calories) must be used to deliver the sweetness of one teaspoon of sucrose. Also, like mannitol, it can cause diarrhea when consumed in large quantities.

Xylitol is popular, especially in chewing gums, thanks to reports that it helps to prevent dental caries. It not only doesn't support caries-producing bacteria, it may actually inhibit their production of acid and prevent them from adhering to the teeth.[28] Xylitol occurs naturally in many fruits, and also arises in the body during normal metabolic processes. Most people can tolerate the small amounts present in food. Xylitol in large amounts slows down the emptying of the stomach but also stimulates release of a hormone (motilin) that speeds up intestinal activity and so causes diarrhea.[29]

Maltitol is used in some carbonated beverages and canned fruits, as well as in Japanese bakery products, and other sweets that are said not to cause tooth decay. At first thought to be unabsorbable from the gastrointestinal tract, maltitol was recommended for weight-loss dieters and for people with diabetes. Maltitol may donate somewhat fewer calories, gram for gram, than sucrose to the body because it is poorly absorbed and because some of it may be lost in diarrhea. Maltitol, however, is expensive to make, and costs limit its use.

The person who wishes to reduce energy intake should be aware that the sugar alcohols *do* provide energy. The body handles them differently from sugar, but they are not calorie free.

EVIDENCE CONCERNING ARTIFICIAL SWEETENERS

Like the sugar alcohols, artificial sweeteners make foods taste sweet without promoting dental decay. Unlike sugar alcohols, they have the added attraction of being calorie free. Also unlike sugar alcohols, the human taste buds perceive them as super-sweet. But are they safe? All substances are toxic if high enough doses are consumed. Artificial sweeteners, their components, and metabolic by-products are no exception. The Food and Drug Administration (FDA) has asked the question of whether artificial sweeteners are harmful to human beings at normal use and potential overuse levels. Based on the answers available to date, the FDA has set **acceptable daily intake (ADI)** levels for some of them. Table C4-3 defines some sugar substitute terms.

The big three synthetic sweeteners are **saccharin, cyclamate,** and **aspartame.** A sweetener called **acesulfame-K** has recently joined their ranks.

Saccharin Saccharin has had a rocky history of acceptance, although it is now consumed by millions of Americans primarily in prepared foods and beverages, secondarily as a tabletop sweetener. Questions about its safety surfaced in 1977, when experiments suggested that it caused bladder tumors in rats. As a result, the FDA proposed banning it. The public outcry in favor of retaining it was so loud, however, that Congress placed a moratorium on any action, and the ban proposal has since been withdrawn. Products containing saccharin are required to carry the warning label now familiar to all consumers of diet products: "Use of this product may be hazardous to your health. This product contains saccharin, which has been determined to cause cancer in laboratory animals."

Table C4-3
Sugar Substitute Terms

- **acceptable daily intake (ADI)** the estimated amount of sweetener that can be consumed daily over a person's lifetime without any adverse effects.
- **acesulfame** (AY-see-sul-fame) **potassium,** also called **acesulfame-K** a zero-calorie sweetener approved by the FDA.
- **alitame** a noncaloric sweetener formed from the amino acids L-aspartic acid and L-alanine. FDA is considering its approval.
- **aspartame** a compound of phenylalanine and aspartic acid that tastes like the sugar sucrose but is much sweeter. It is used in both the United States and Canada.
- **cyclamate** a zero-calorie sweetener under consideration for use in the United States and used restrictively in Canada.
- **maltitol, mannitol, sorbitol, xylitol** sugar alcohols that can be derived from fruits or commercially produced from dextrose; absorbed more slowly and metabolized differently than other sugars in the human body and not readily used by ordinary mouth bacteria.
- **saccharin** a zero-calorie sweetener used freely in the United States but restricted in Canada.
- **sucralose** a noncaloric sweetener derived from a chlorinated form of sugar that travels through the digestive tract unabsorbed. Canada has approved the sweetener; in the United States, the FDA is considering its approval.

Does saccharin cause cancer? The evidence that it does so in animals is as follows. Rats that had been fed diets containing saccharin from the time of weaning to adulthood were mated. The offspring of those rats were then fed saccharin throughout their lives, and were found to have a higher incidence of bladder tumors than comparable animals not fed saccharin. In Canada, on the basis of these findings, all uses of saccharin were banned except use as a tabletop sweetener to be sold in pharmacies with a warning label.

In the United States, a large-scale population study involving 9,000 people showed a distinctly greater risk of cancers in women who drank two or more saccharin-sweetened diet sodas a day and in people who both smoked heavily and used artificial sweeteners. Another study involving over 1,000 people showed little or no excess risk of bladder cancers.

A solid clue has emerged from the laboratory based on some physiological differences between the urinary systems of rats and human beings.[30] Rats excrete far less water in their urine than people do. As a result, rats can highly concentrate substances in just small amounts of water in their urine. Dissolved substances in such high concentrations are likely to crystallize. In safety tests, saccharin overdoses caused crystals to form in the rats' bladders, and the crystals probably caused the tumors. Human beings cannot concentrate urinary substances to such a degree, so they would never form saccharin crystals, even if they consumed larger-than-normal doses of saccharin. They would, however, lose large amounts of water as the kidneys struggled to free the blood of the overload.

It goes without saying that overloading on huge saccharin doses is probably not safe, but consuming moderate amounts almost certainly does not cause bladder cancer in human beings. Although no ADI has been set for saccharin, the amount of saccharin that can be commercially added to foods or drinks is limited to about 30 milligrams per serving. Additionally, the recommendation is made not to exceed total daily saccharin intakes of 1,000 milligrams for adults or 500 milligrams for children.[31]

Cyclamate Cyclamate has had a shorter commercial life than saccharin, dominating the artificial sweetener market for only 20 years. The 1970 ban on its use in the United States still stands but FDA is now considering repeal of the ban. Originally thought to be a safe additive, a cyclamate-saccharin blend was linked to cancer in rats. This led to a flurry of studies that have failed to prove cyclamate carcinogenic. In 1985 the National Academy of Sciences concluded that evidence to date did not indicate cyclamate as a cause of cancer in human beings, but warranted further studies and close monitoring of those populations that use it.[32] In Canada, cyclamate is restricted to use as a tabletop sweetener on the advice of a physician and as a sweetening additive in medicines.

Aspartame Aspartame is one of the most thoroughly studied substances ever to be approved for use in foods.[33] Within only a few years after aspartame received the FDA's approval, manufacturers began using it to sweeten dozens of products including diet drinks, candies, chewing gum, presweetened cereal, gelatins, baked goods and mixes, and pudding. Aspartame provides 4 calories per gram, as does protein, but because so little is used, it is virtually calorie free. Aspartame is also available as a powder to use at home in place of sugar, under the brand name *Equal.* In powdered form it is mixed with lactose, so a 1-gram packet contains 4 calories.

Aspartame sales have far surpassed sales of saccharin. Aspartame's amazing popularity is mostly due to its flavor, which is almost identical to that of sugar. Another lure drawing people to aspartame is the hope that it may be completely harmless, unlike the other sweeteners, whose laboratory records seem tarnished. Furthermore, aspartame is touted as safe for children, so families wishing to limit their children's sugar intakes are offering them Nutrasweet products instead.

Aspartame is a simple chemical compound: two protein fragments (the amino acids phenylalanine and aspartic acid) joined together. In the digestive tract the two fragments are split apart, absorbed, and metabolized just as they would be if they had come from protein in food. The flavors of the components give no clue to the combined effect; one of them tastes bitter, and the other is tasteless. But aspartame is 200 times sweeter than sucrose.

An inherited metabolic disease known as phenylketonuria (PKU) poses problems with respect to aspartame. People with PKU have the hereditary inability to dispose of phenylalanine eaten in excess of the need for building proteins. Unusual products made from phenylalanine build up and damage the tissues. PKU causes irreversible, progressive brain damage if untreated early. Newborns in the United States are tested for PKU; if they have it, the treatment is to limit dietary intake of phenylalanine.

Adults with PKU can use some aspartame, but there is a compelling reason why children with PKU should not get their phenylalanine from this source. Phenylalanine occurs in such protein-rich and nutrient-rich foods as milk and meat, and the PKU child is allowed only a limited amount of these foods. The child has difficulty obtaining the many essential nutrients, such as calcium, iron, and the B vitamins, found along with phenylalanine in these foods. To suggest that such a child squander any of the limited phenylalanine allowance on the purified phenylalanine of aspartame, with none of the associated nutrients to support normal growth, would be to invite nutritional disaster. People with PKU need to know which products contain aspartame and how to avoid them. Product labels offer a special warning for people with PKU.

Other concerns about aspartame's safety have had to do with compounds that arise briefly during its metabolism. These compounds (methyl alcohol, formaldehyde, and diketopiperazine, or DKP) are not toxic at the levels generated, and concerns about them have been laid to rest.

An important safety concern is what effects, if any, aspartame might have on the brain. While no experimental evidence has shown a connection, some 5,500 individual complaints have been received by the Centers for Disease Control (CDC), many of which claim that aspartame gives people headaches.[34]

Every day, millions of people use aspartame. Every day, millions of people have headaches. Anyone who claims, on this basis, that aspartame causes headaches is using personal experience to jump to conclusions. In the case of sweeteners and headaches, only casual reports of a link, no true connections, have been shown. Some of the headache sufferers might indeed be reacting to the artificial sweetener, but they might also be reacting to another substance such as caffeine in the same or other foods or to factors in their lives unrelated to foods.

Other complaints, about 250 in all, have linked aspartame intakes to seizures. People who experienced seizures reported to the FDA that they believed their seizures were related to ingesting aspartame. When the reports were scrutinized scientifically, though, the seizures were found unrelated to aspartame intake. The authors who analyzed the evidence suggested that the topic warranted no further research.[35] As is true for reports of headaches, any claims of a causal relationship between aspartame and seizures is not supported by science.

On approving aspartame, the FDA assumed that no one would consume more than the ADI of 50 milligrams per kilogram of body weight in a day. In Canada, the acceptable level is set at 40 milligrams per kilogram.[36] These seem to be reasonable numbers. Most adults in the United States and other countries consume less than 10 milligrams per kilogram, significantly less than the ADI level.[37] Still, the ADI amount is not impossible to exceed. For a 132-pound person, it adds up to 80 packets of Equal. About 15 soft drinks sweetened only with aspartame provide this maximum amount. A child who drinks a quart of Kool-Aid on a hot day and who also has pudding, chewing gum, cereal, and other products sweetened with aspartame can pack in more than the daily ADI limit. Infants or toddlers under two years old should probably not be fed artificially sweetened foods and drinks.

Acesulfame-K For 15 years of testing and use, the artificial sweetener **acesulfame potassium** (or acesulfame-K) has been used without reported health problems. An ADI of 15 milligrams per kilogram bodyweight was set for acesulfame-K on its approval. Marketed under the trade names Sunette and Sweet One, this sweetener is about as sweet as aspartame and is used in chewing gum, beverages, instant coffee and tea, gelatins, and puddings as well as for table use. Unlike aspartame, acesulfame-K holds up well during cooking, and since it contains no phenylalanine, it need bear no warnings to people with PKU. Further research concerning safety of acesulfame-K and consumer acceptance of products sweetened with it will determine its place on the grocery shelves.

Other Artificial Sweeteners Two other artificial sweeteners are awaiting FDA approval—**sucralose,** already approved in Canada, and **alitame.** Sucralose is a chlorinated form of sugar that travels through the digestive tract unabsorbed and therefore is noncaloric. Alitame resembles aspartame in being composed of two amino acids, but unlike aspartame it is stable when heated.

DO ARTIFICIAL SWEETENERS HELP OR HINDER WEIGHT LOSS EFFORTS? Lately, this assumption has been called into question. Artificial sweetener use has climbed dramatically, but sugar use also continues to rise. A study of the intakes of aspartame, saccharin, and sugar among college students confirmed what these trends seem to indicate.[38] Most students who reported using artificial sweeteners said they did not lower their intakes of sugars or reduce their total food intakes. Instead, they consumed artificial sweeteners in addition to sugars.

Some interesting clues concerning sweeteners and food intakes have come from rat studies. When saccharin is added experimentally to rats' drinking water, the rats consume more food than when plain water is offered.[39] It seems that something about saccharin makes rats eat more food.

It has been suggested that the same effect may occur in human beings. Human subjects given aspartame-sweetened beverages do seem to eat more food than normal.[40] Artificial sweeteners may turn out to be a blockade to weight loss rather than the facilitator dieters seek.[41]

The human study of aspartame and food intakes just mentioned has been criticized.[42] The researchers relied on self reporting of hunger by the subjects with no objective measure of food intake, and self-reporting is not a reliable research method. Another group of researchers followed up on this original observation with a study that was more convincing. This time, three sweeteners—aspartame, saccharin, and acesulfame-K—were tested for their effects on feelings of hunger, which were measured as objectively as possible during the testing. They found that all three sweeteners left subjects feeling hungrier than normal.[43] It could be that the perception of a supersweet taste on the tongue might trigger nervous and hormonal responses in the body that ready it to digest, absorb, and metabolize carbohydrate. When no carbohydrate is delivered, the systems are left in a ready state, a state that could be interpreted as hunger.[44] Researchers who tested this idea found that when subjects were given aspartame-sweetened gum to chew, their hunger increased.

A question the research has not yet addressed is whether the increased hunger brought on by noncaloric sweeteners actually leads to increased food consumption. When researchers tried to measure actual food intakes after consumption of sweeteners, they obtained mixed results. In one such study, subjects ate yogurt sweetened with saccharin, yogurt sweetened with glucose, yogurt sweetened with saccharin and with starch added, or plain yogurt. An hour later, the group that had eaten saccharin-sweetened yogurt without supplemental starch ate significantly more food than the other groups, not only at lunchtime but throughout the day.[45] The researchers proposed that this might have been due to a deficit of calories, or perhaps specifically of carbohydrate calories, in the group that ate more.

While many studies on saccharin seem to confirm that increased food intake follows its use, the bulk of research on aspartame has gone the other way. One group of researchers found consistently in five studies performed over two years that aspartame *reduced* appetite and had a small, negative effect on food intake.[46] The effect was seen using an amount of sweetener equivalent to that in one or two cans of aspartame-sweetened soft drinks.[47] The subjects who received fewer calories when their sugar was replaced with aspartame ate somewhat more food later on, but only enough to equalize their calorie intakes.[48]

Another sweetener, however, has shown a clear, strong ability to cut the appetite *and* to reduce food intake. That sweetener is sugar. When various sweeteners were given to 20 subjects in beverages an hour before lunchtime, none reported feeling hungrier and none ate more of a lunch salad after any of the alternative sweeteners than after plain water. Those who had consumed sugar, however, ate smaller amounts of the salad than the others.[49] The common belief that sugar "spoils the appetite" may have proved true. The effect on total calorie intake was seen. The subjects had displaced nutritious food calories with the empty calories of sugar.

PERSONAL STRATEGIES FOR USING ARTIFICIAL SWEETENERS Current evidence indicates that moderate intakes of artificial sweeteners pose no health risks.[50] However, consumers must wait for research to reveal the final word about whether artificial sweeteners are useful in weight loss efforts or whether they increase the appetite. The wisest course for those who wish to use artificial sweeteners to cut calories may be: Go ahead and use them in moderation, but keep track of feelings of hunger and of actual food intakes. If either increases when using artificial sweeteners, a switch to plain water or other unsweetened beverages may prove more helpful for weight loss. Small portions of sugar-sweetened foods may be worth considering, especially if their calories strongly curb the appetite.

◆ Notes

1. G. H. Anderson, Myths and facts about sugar, *Contemporary Nutrition* 16 (1991): 1.
2. Y. Keno and coauthors, High sucrose diet increases visceral fat accumulation in VMH-lesioned obese rats, *International Journal of Obesity* 15 (1991): 205–211.
3. C. J. Lewis and coauthors, Nutrient intakes and body weights of persons consuming high and moderate levels of added sugars, *Journal of the American Dietetic Association* 92 (1992): 708–713.
4. M. A. Gannon and J. E. Mitchell, Subjective evaluation of treatment methods by patients treated for bulimia, *Journal of the American Dietetic Association* 86 (1986): 520–521.
5. W. H. Glinsmann, H. Irausquin, and Y. K. Park, Evaluation of health aspects of sugars contained in carbohydrate sweeteners; Report of Sugars Task Force, *Journal of Nutrition*, 116 (1986): S1–S216.
6. A. L. Peters, M. B. Davidson, and K. Eisenberg, Effect of isocaloric substitution of chocolate cake for potato in type 1 diabetic patients, *Diabetes Care* 13 (1990): 888–892.
7. C. A. Beebe and coauthors, Nutrition management for individuals with noninsulin-dependent diabetes mellitus in the 1990s: a review by the diabetes care and education dietetic practice group, *Journal of the American Dietetic Association* 91 (1991): 196–202, 205–207; Nutrition Subcommittee of the British Diabetic Association's Professional Advisory Committee, Dietary recommendations for people with diabetes: an update for the 1990s, *Diabetes Medicine* 9 (1992): 189–202.
8. M. K. Lockwood and C. D. Eckhert, Sucrose-induced lipid, glucose, and insulin elevations, microvascular injury, and selenium, *American Journal of Physiology* 262 (1992): R144–R149.
9. J. E. Swanson, Metabolic effects of dietary fructose in healthy subjects, *American Journal of Clinical Nutrition* 55 (1992): 851–856.
10. C. Abraira and J. Derler, Constant carbohydrate diets in NIDDM: Variation in sucrose, *American Journal of Medicine* 84 (1988): 193–200.
11. G. M. Reaven and H. Ho, Sugar-induced hypertension in Sprague-Dawley rats, *American Journal of Hypertension* 4 (1991): 610–614; M. el Zein and coauthors, Development of sugar-induced blood pressure elevation after uninephrectomy in a resistant rat strain, *Journal of the American College of Nutrition* 10 (1991): 24–33.
12. S. Buchanan, The most ubiquitous toxin, *American Psychologist*, November 1984, pp. 1327–1328, as cited by R. Milich, S. Lindgren, and M. Wolraich, The behavioral effects of sugar: A comment on Buchanan, *American Psychologist*, February 1986, pp. 218–220.
13. T. W. Jones and coauthors, Oral glucose provokes excessive adrenomedullary and symptomatic responses in normal children, *Pediatric Notes* 14 (1990): 86.
14. R. J. Prinz and D. B. Riddle, Associations between nutrition and behavior in 5-year-old children, *Nutrition Reviews* (supplement), May 1986, pp. 151–158.
15. E. H. Wender and M. V. Solunto, Effects of sugar on aggressive and inattentive behavior in children with attention deficit disorder with hyperactive and normal children, *Pediatrics* 88 (1991): 960–966.
16. S. Saravis, Aspartame: Effects on learning, behavior, and mood, *Pediatrics* 86 (1990): 75–83.
17. J. Bachorowski and coauthors, Sucrose and delinquency behavioral assessment, *Pediatrics* 86 (1990): 244–253.
18. D. H. Morris, Diet and behavior: Sugar (sucrose) and criminal behavior, *Food and Nutrition News* 58, no. 1 (1986): 5–6.
19. J. L. Rapoport, Diet and hyperactivity, *Nutrition Reviews* (supplement), May 1986, pp. 158–162; D. A. Gans, Sucrose and unusual childhood behavior, *Nutrition Today*, May/June 1991, pp. 8–14.
20. Gum disease largest threat to dental health, *Tallahassee Democrat*, 12 March 1987.
21. A. Sheiham, Why free sugar consumption should be below 15 kg per person per year in industrial countries: the dental evidence, *British Dental Journal* 171 (1991): 63–65.
22. B. G. Bibby and coauthors, Oral food clearance and the pH of plaque and saliva, *Journal of the American Dental Association* 112 (1986): 333–337.
23. Dr. Thomas Truhe as quoted in E. Whitford, Dentists target starch as real cavity friend, *Atlanta Constitution*, 26 March 1991, pp. D1, D10.
24. Sheiham, 1991.
25. National Research Council Committee on Diet and Health, *Diet and Health: Implications for Reducing Chronic Disease Risk* (Washington, D.C., National Academy Press, 1989), p. 279.
26. B. Szepesi, Carbohydrates, *Present Knowledge In Nutrition*, 6th ed. (Washington, D.C.: Nutrition Foundation, 1990), pp. 47–55.
27. WHO study group on Diet, Nutrition and Preventing Noncommunicable Diseases, Diet, nutrition and the prevention of chronic diseases, *Nutrition Reviews* 49 (1991): 291.
28. W. L. Dills, Sugar alcohols as bulk sweeteners, *Annual Review of Nutrition* (1989): 161–186.
29. E. K. Salminen and coauthors, Xylitol vs glucose: effect on the rate of gastric emptying and motilin, insulin, and gastric inhibitory polypeptide release, *American Journal of Clinical Nutrition* 49 (1989): 1228–1232.
30. S. Cohen and coauthors, Saccharin and urothelial proliferation: A threshold phenomenon, *FASEB Journal* 6 (1992): A1594.
31. Quantitative Regulation (180.37), D. Plumb, FDA Center for Food and Nutrition Safety, Personal communication, 6 July 1992.
32. National Research Council, *Evaluation of cyclamate for carcinogenicity* (Washington, D.C.: National Academy Press, 1985), pp. 2–8.
33. A bibliography of 167 research articles on aspartame can be found in J. Van de Kamp, Adverse effects of aspartame, *Current Bibliographies in Medicine* (Washington, D.C.: Government Printing Office, 1991).
34. Aspartame, *FDA Consumer*, October 1991, p. 35.
35. L. Tollefson and R. J. Barnard, An analysis of FDA passive surveillance reports of seizures associated with consumption of aspartame, *Journal of the American Dietetic Association* 92 (1992): 598–601.
36. Health and Welfare Canada, *Nutrition Recommendations*, (Ottawa: Canadian Government Printing Centre, 1990): p. 190.
37. J. P. Heybach and J. L. Smith, Intake of aspartame in 19–50 year old women from the USDA continuing survey of food intakes by individuals (CSFII 85) *FASEB Journal* 2 (1988): A1615; H. H. Butchko and F. N. Kotsonis, Acceptable daily intake vs actual intake: The aspartame example, *Journal of the American College of Nutrition* 10 (1991): 258–266.

38. L. A. Chen and E. S. Parkam, College student's use of high-intensity sweeteners is not consistently associated with sugar consumption, *Journal of the American Dietician Association* 91 (1991): 686–690.
39. M. G. Tordoff and M. I. Friedman, Drinking saccharin increases food intake and preference—I. Comparison with other drinks, *Appetite* 12 (1989): 1–10; M. G. Tordoff and M. I. Friedman, Drinking saccharin increases food intake and preference—II. Hydrational factors, *Appetite* 12 (1989): 11–21; M. G. Tordoff and M. I. Friedman, Drinking saccharin increases food intake and preference—III. Sensory and associative factors, *Appetite* 12 (1989): 23–36; M. G. Tordoff and M. I. Friedman, Drinking saccharin increases food intake and preference—IV. Cephalic phase and metabolic factors, *Appetite* 12 (1989): 37–56.
40. J. E. Blundell and A. J. Hill, Paradoxical effects of an intense sweetener (aspartame) on appetite, *Lancet* 1 (1986): 1092–1093.
41. Saccharin consumption increases food consumption in rats, *Nutrition Reviews* 48 (1990): 163–165.
42. B. J. Rolls, Effects of intense sweeteners on hunger, food intake, and body weight: A review, *American Journal of Clinical Nutrition* 53 (1991): 872–878.
43. P. J. Rogers and coauthors, Uncoupling sweet taste and calories: Comparison to the effects of glucose and three intense sweeteners on hunger and food intake, *Physiology and Behavior* 43 (1988): 547-552.
44. V. M. Sardesai and T. H. Waldshan, Natural and synthetic intense sweeteners, *Journal of Nutritional Biochemistry* 2 (1991): 236–244.
45. P. J. Rogers and J. E. Blundell, Separating the actions of sweetness and calories: Effects of saccharin and carbohydrates on hunger and food intake in human subjects, *Physiology and Behavior* 45 (1989): 1093–1099.
46. Rolls, 1991.
47. P. J. Rogers, H. C. Pleming, and J. E. Blundell, Aspartame ingested without tasting inhibits hunger and food intake, *Physiology and Behavior* 47 (1990): 1239–1243; P. J. Rogers, P. Keedwell, and J. E. Blundell, Further analysis of the short-term inhibition of food intake in humans by the dipeptide L-aspartyl-L-phenylalanine methylester (aspartame), *Physiology and Behavior* 49 (1991): 739–743.
48. B. J. Rolls, L. J. Laster, and A. Summerfelt, Hunger and food intake following consumption of low-calorie foods, *Appetite* 13 (1989): 115–127.
49. D. J. Cantry and M. M. Chan, Effects of consumption of caloric vs noncaloric sweet drinks on indices of hunger and food consumption in normal adults, *American Journal of Clinical Nutrition* 53 (1991): 1159–1164.
50. Position of the American Dietetic Association: Use of nutritive and nonnutritive sweeteners, *Journal of the American Dietetic Association* 93 (1993): 816–821.

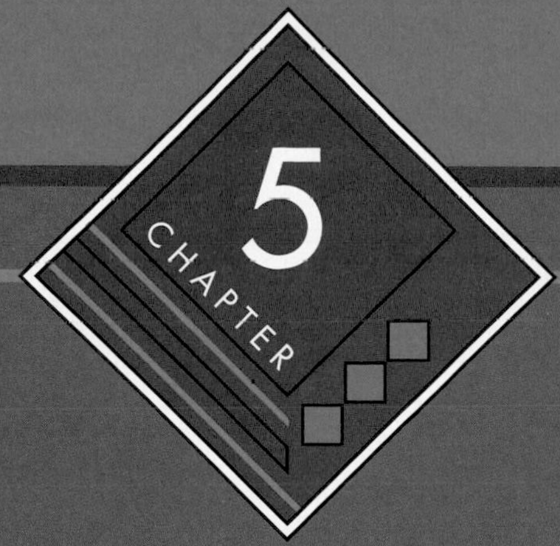

The Lipids: Fats, Oils, Phospholipids, and Sterols

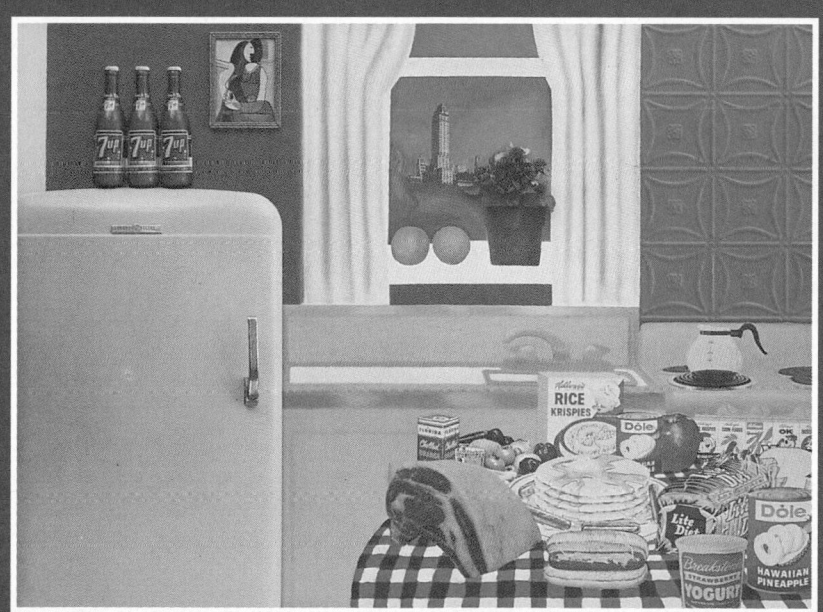

Contents

Still life painting, 30, 1963, by Tom Wesselmann. Assemblage, oil, enamel and synthetic polymer paint on composition with collage of printed advertisements, plastic artificial flowers, etc., 48 1/2 × 66 × 4". Collection, The Museum of Modern Art, New York. Gift of Philip Johnson.

Your bill from a medical laboratory reads, "Blood **lipid** profile—$125." A health care provider reports, "Your blood **cholesterol** is high." Your physician advises, "You must cut down on the **fats** and **oils** in your diet." Blood lipids, cholesterol, fats, and oils—all both contribute to health and detract from it.

lipid (LIP-id) a family of compounds soluble in organic solvents but not in water. Lipids include triglycerides (fats and oils), phospholipids, and sterols.

cholesterol (koh-LESS-ter-all) a member of the group of lipids known as sterols; a soft waxy substance manufactured in the body for a variety of purposes and also found in animal-derived foods.

fats lipids that are solid at room temperature (70°F or 25°C).

oils lipids that are liquid at room temperature (70°F or 25°C).

triglycerides (try-GLISS-er-ides) one of the three main classes of dietary lipids and the chief form of fat in foods. A triglyceride is made up of three units known as fatty acids and one unit called glycerol. (Fatty acids and glycerol are defined later.)

phospholipids (FOSS-foh-LIP-ids) one of the three main classes of lipids. These lipids are similar to triglycerides but each has a phosphorus-containing acid in place of one of the fatty acids. Phospholipids are present in all cell membranes.

lecithin (LESS-ih-thin) a phospholipid, a major constituent of cell membranes, manufactured by the liver and also found in many foods.

sterols (STEER-alls) one of the three main classes of lipids; lipids with a structure similar to that of cholesterol.

◆ Introduction to Fats

The lipids in foods and in the human body fall into three classes. About 95 percent are **triglycerides.** Other classes of the lipid family are the **phospholipids** (of which **lecithin** is one) and the **sterols** (cholesterol, just mentioned, is the best known of these).

No doubt you have been expecting to hear that these fat-related compounds have the potential to harm your health. It may come as a surprise to hear that lipids are also valuable. In fact, lipids are absolutely necessary, and some lipids must be present in your foods if you are to maintain good health. Luckily traces of fats and oils are present in almost all foods, so you needn't make it a point to eat any extra.

Usefulness of Fats

When people speak of fat, they are usually speaking of triglycerides. The term *fat* is more familiar, though, and we will use it here. Fat is the body's chief storage form for the energy from food eaten in excess of need. The storage of fat is a valuable survival mechanism for people who must live a feast-or-famine existence: stored during times of plenty, it enables them to remain alive during times of famine. In addition, fats provide most of the energy needed to perform much of the body's work, especially muscular work.

Most body cells can store only limited fat, but some cells are specialized for storing fat. These, the fat cells, seem able to expand almost indefinitely. The more fat they store the larger they grow. An obese person's fat cells may be many times the size of a thin person's. A fat cell is shown in Figure 5-1.

You may be wondering why the carbohydrate glucose is not the body's major form of stored energy. As mentioned in Chapter 4, the stored form of glucose is glycogen. One characteristic of glycogen is that it holds a great deal of water, and as a result, it is quite bulky and heavy. The body cannot store enough glycogen to provide energy for very long. Fats, however, pack tightly together without water and can store much more energy in a small space.[1] The body fat found on a normal-weight, healthy person contains sufficient energy to fuel a marathon run to the finish or to give to a sick person who cannot eat the energy to battle disease with minimum assistance from food.

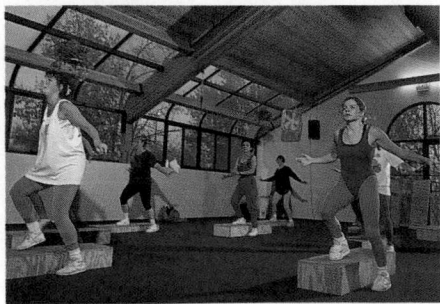

Body fat supplies much of the fuel these muscles need to do their work.

By the same token, foods rich in fat are valuable in many situations. A gram of fat or oil delivers over twice as many calories as a gram of carbohydrate. A hunter or hiker needs to consume a large amount of food energy to travel long distances or to survive in intensely cold weather. As Figure 5-2 shows, such a person can carry more energy in fat-rich foods than in carbohydrate-rich foods. On the other hand, high-fat foods may deliver many *unneeded* calories in only a few bites to the person who is not expending much energy in physical work.

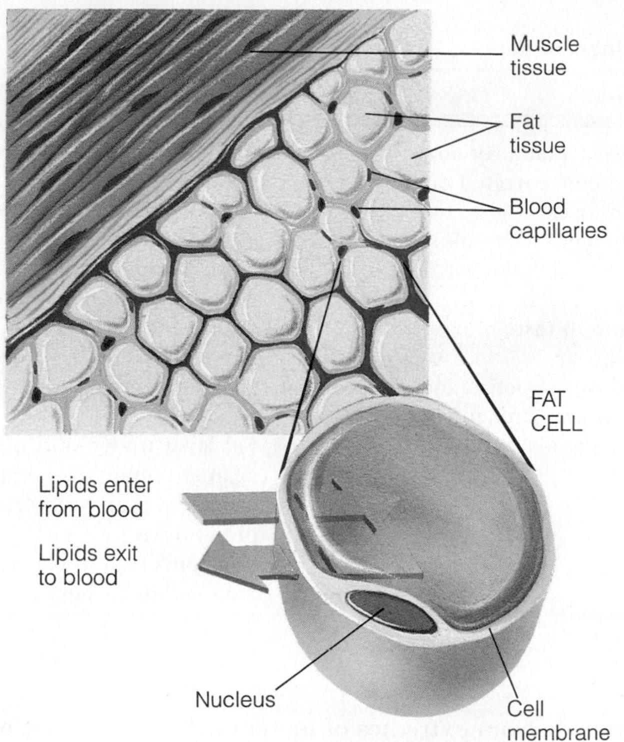

Figure 5-1

A FAT CELL
Within the fat cell, lipid is stored in a droplet. This droplet can greatly enlarge, and the fat cell membrane will grow to accommodate its swollen contents. More about fat cells and obesity—Chapter 9.

People like high-fat foods. Fat carries with it many dissolved compounds that give foods enticing aromas and flavors, such as the aroma of frying bacon or french fries. In fact, when a person's appetite is poor, foods flavored with some fat may tempt that person to eat again. Some fat in food also slows digestion, lending **satiety** to a meal. People feel fuller longer after eating meals that include fat. Fats also help make foods tender.

In the body, fat serves many purposes. Pads of fat surround the vital organs. They serve as shock absorbers; thanks to the fat pads cushioning your internal organs, you can ride a horse or a motorcycle for many hours with no serious internal injuries. The fat blanket under the skin also

satiety (sat-EYE-uh-tee) the feeling of fullness or satisfaction that people feel after meals. Fat provides more satiety than carbohydrate or protein because it slows the stomach's motility.

1 g carbohydrate = 4 calories
1 g fat = 9 calories (but see this chapter's Controversy)
1 g protein = 4 calories

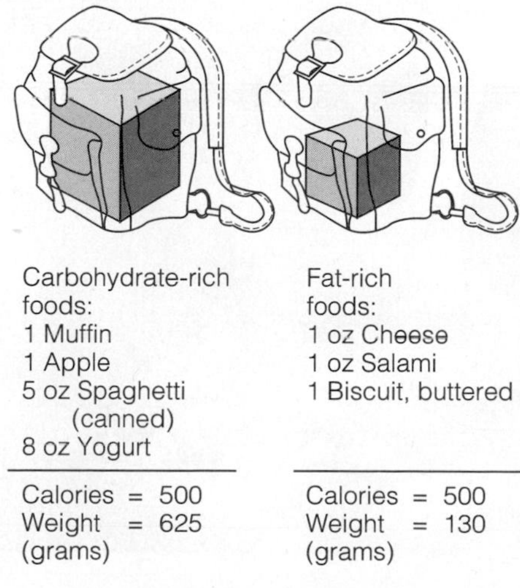

Carbohydrate-rich foods:	Fat-rich foods:
1 Muffin	1 oz Cheese
1 Apple	1 oz Salami
5 oz Spaghetti (canned)	1 Biscuit, buttered
8 oz Yogurt	
Calories = 500	Calories = 500
Weight (grams) = 625	Weight (grams) = 130

Figure 5-2

TWO LUNCHES
Both lunches contain the same number of calories, but the fat-rich lunch takes up less space and weighs less.

essential fatty acids fatty acids needed by the body but not made by the body in amounts sufficient to meet physiological need.

Table 5-1
The Usefulness of Fats

Fats in Food	Fats in the Body
■ Provide essential fatty acids. ■ Provide a concentrated energy source in foods. ■ Carry fat-soluble vitamins. ■ Provide raw material for making needed products. ■ Contribute to taste and smell of foods. ■ Stimulate the appetite and provide satiety after meals. ■ Help make foods tender.	■ Are the body's chief form of stored energy. ■ Provide most of the energy to fuel muscular work. ■ Serve as an emergency fuel supply in times of illness and diminished food intake. ■ Fat pads inside body cavity protect internal organs from shock. ■ Fat layer under skin insulates against temperature extremes. ■ Form the major material of cell membranes. ■ Are converted to other compounds as needed.

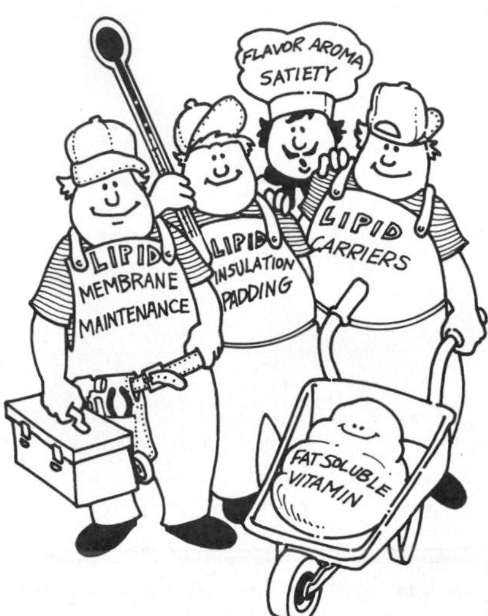

Lipids are useful in foods and are necessary in the body (see Table 5-1).

insulates the body from extremes of temperature, thus assisting with internal climate control.

Some essential nutrients are soluble in fat and therefore are found mainly in foods that contain fat. These nutrients are the **essential fatty acids** and the fat-soluble vitamins: A, D, E, and K. A later section shows that the essential fatty acids serve as raw materials from which the body makes molecules it needs. Lipids are also important to all the body's cells as part of their surrounding envelopes, the cell membranes. Table 5-1 sums up the ways fat is useful, both in foods and in the body.

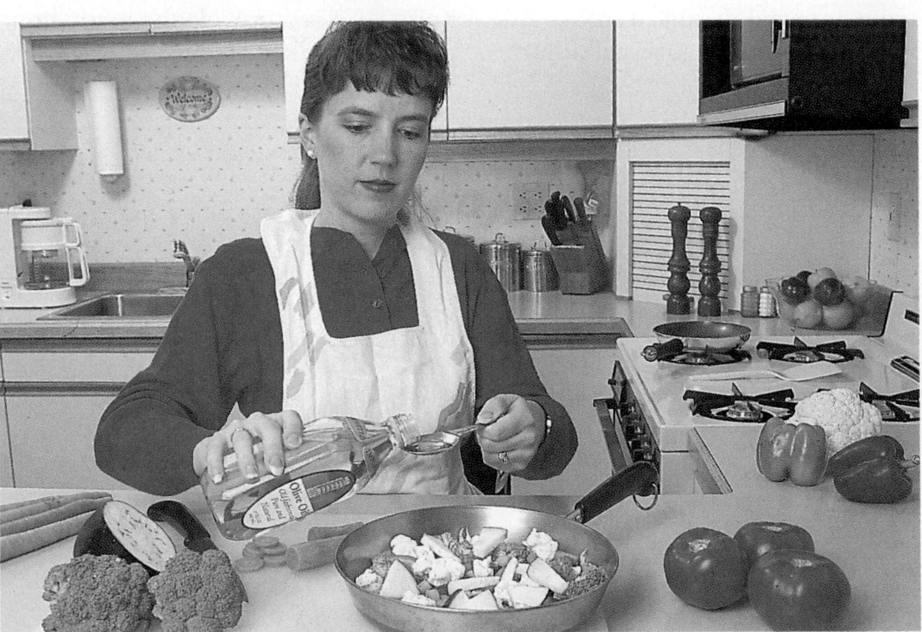

Small amounts of fat offer eaters both pleasure and needed nutrients.

KEY POINT Lipids not only provide energy reserves but also lend satiety to meals, enhance food's aroma and flavor, cushion the vital organs, protect the body from temperature extremes, carry the fat-soluble nutrients, serve as raw materials, and provide the major material of which cell membranes are made.

Harmful Potential of Fats

High dietary fat intakes are associated with serious diseases. A person who chooses a diet too high in certain fats may be inviting the risk of heart and artery disease, or **cardiovascular disease (CVD).**[2] Heart disease is this nation's number-one killer of adults. The person who eats a high-fat diet also incurs a greater-than-average risk of developing some forms of cancer, another leading killer disease.[3] Much research has focused on connections between diet and disease and it takes a whole chapter to show the connections (Chapter 11). Here, a few points about fats and heart health are presented because they underlie dietary recommendations concerning fats (Table 5-2), and a later section of this chapter provides a few more details.

Of great importance in regard to fat and disease is a medical test, the blood lipid profile, which reveals the amounts of various lipids, especially

cardiovascular disease (CVD) disease of the heart and blood vessels. The two most common forms of CVD are *atherosclerosis* and *hypertension* (Chapter 11).

Table 5-2
Recommendations Concerning Intakes of Fats

1. Total Fat[a]

   Dietary Guidelines
   - Choose a diet low in fat.

   World Health Organization
   - Lower limit for total fat intake: 15 percent of total calories from fat.
   - Upper limit for total fat intake: 30 percent of total calories from fat.

2. Saturated Fat

   Dietary Guidelines
   - Choose a diet low in saturated fat.

   World Health Organization
   - Lower limit for saturated fat intake: 0 percent of total calories from saturated fat.
   - Upper limit for saturated fat intake: 10 percent of total calories from saturated fat.

3. Polyunsaturated Fatty Acids

   World Health Organization
   - Lower limit for polyunsaturated fat intake: 3 percent of total calories from polyunsaturated fatty acids.
   - Upper limit for polyunsaturated fat intake: 7 percent of total calories from polyunsaturated fatty acids.

4. Cholesterol

   Dietary Guidelines
   - Choose a diet low in cholesterol.

   World Health Organization
   - Lower limit for cholesterol intake: 0 milligrams cholesterol per day.
   - Upper limit for cholesterol intake: 300 milligrams cholesterol per day.

[a]Includes monounsaturated fatty acids.

Rule of thumb: to estimate the number of fat grams allowed in a day to limit fat calories to 30 percent of total, use this method.

General equation:

$$\frac{\text{total energy need (in calories) drop last digit}}{3} = \text{g fat/day}$$

Examples:

$$\frac{200\cancel{0}}{3} = 67 \text{ g fat/day}$$

$$\frac{250\cancel{0}}{3} = 83 \text{ g fat/day}$$

Source: K. McNutt, Fat traps, tips, and tricks, *Nutrition Today*, May/June 1992, pp. 47–49.

triglycerides and cholesterol, found in the blood. It also identifies the protein carriers with which these lipids are traveling. The results of this test tell much about a person's risk of CVD. The blood cholesterol level is especially telling, and it bears on the question of whether people should avoid foods containing fat, foods containing cholesterol, or both.

Most important in regard to CVD is *blood* cholesterol.* A person's blood cholesterol concentration is considered to be a predictor of that person's likelihood of suffering a fatal heart attack or stroke and the higher the cholesterol, the earlier the episode is expected to be. Blood cholesterol is one of the three major risk factors for CVD (the other two are smoking and high blood pressure, or hypertension). The importance of blood cholesterol cannot be overemphasized.

Now, what does *food* cholesterol have to do with *blood* cholesterol? The answer is that ordinary food *fats* (triglycerides) raise blood cholesterol more than food *cholesterol* does. People often fail to understand this point. When told that cholesterol doesn't matter as much as fat, people often jump to the wrong conclusion—that blood cholesterol doesn't matter. It does matter. High *blood* cholesterol is an indicator of risk for CVD. The main dietary factor associated with elevated blood cholesterol is a high *food fat* intake. In comparison, dietary cholesterol alone makes only a minor contribution.[4]

Heredity modifies everyone's ability to handle food cholesterol somewhat, but a few individuals have inherited a total inability to clear from their blood the cholesterol they have eaten and absorbed. This condition is rare but well known because the study of it led to the discovery of how cholesterol is transported in the body. People with a genetic tendency toward high blood cholesterol must strictly limit fats and refrain from eating cholesterol in foods; perhaps this is where the general public's fear of food cholesterol has come from. The majority of people can eat eggs, liver, and other cholesterol-containing foods in moderation without fear of incurring high blood cholesterol.

An effective dietary weapon against high blood cholesterol is to trim the fat from foods. The photos of Figure 5-3 show that food trimmed of fat is also trimmed of much of its energy. A pork chop trimmed of its border of fat loses almost 100 calories. A plain baked potato has half the calories of one with butter and sour cream. Choosing nonfat milk over whole milk provides a large saving of fat and calories; and so forth. The single most effective step you can take to reduce a food's potential for elevating blood cholesterol is to eat it without the fat.

One more distinction must be made about food fats as they relate to CVD. Triglycerides come in two varieties, saturated and unsaturated, and the saturated type is implicated in raising blood cholesterol. The next section of this chapter describes the differences between saturated and unsaturated fats.

KEY POINT An important distinction: it is not the cholesterol in foods but total fat intake, and especially saturated fat intake, that is the major dietary factor that raises blood cholesterol. Elevated blood cholesterol is a risk factor for cardiovascular disease.

***Blood*, *plasma*, and *serum* cholesterol all refer to about the same thing; this book uses the term *blood* cholesterol. Plasma is blood with the cells removed; in serum the clotting factors are also removed. The concentration of cholesterol is not much altered by these treatments.

Figure 5-3

FOOD FAT AND CALORIES

Fat hides calories in food. When you trim fat, you trim calories.

Pork chop with ½ inch of fat (353 calories; 225 calories from fat).

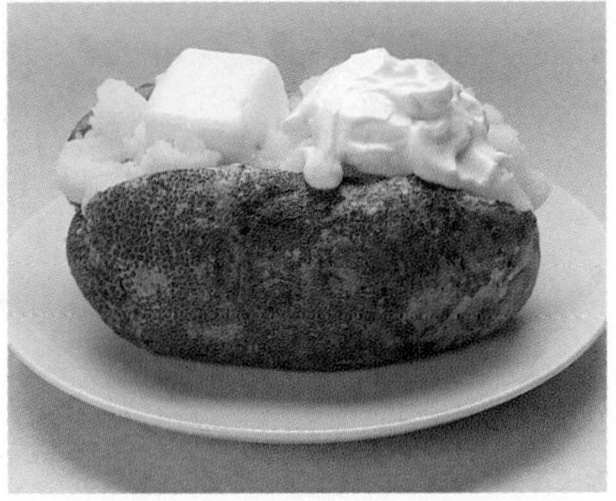

Potato with 1 tablespoon butter and 1 tablespoon sour cream (350 calories; 126 calories from fat).

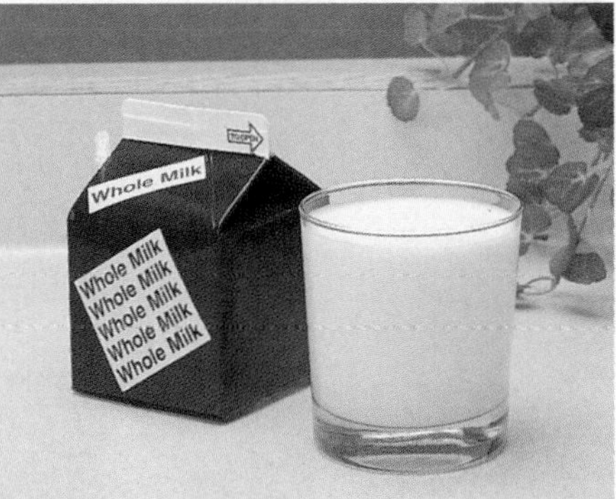

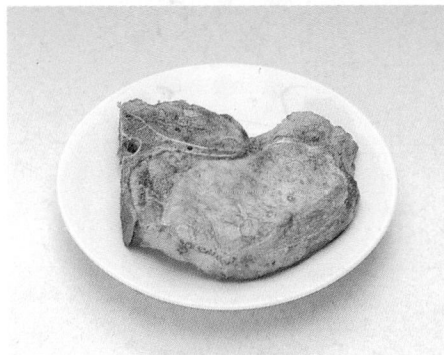

Whole milk, 1 cup (150 calories; 72 calories from fat).

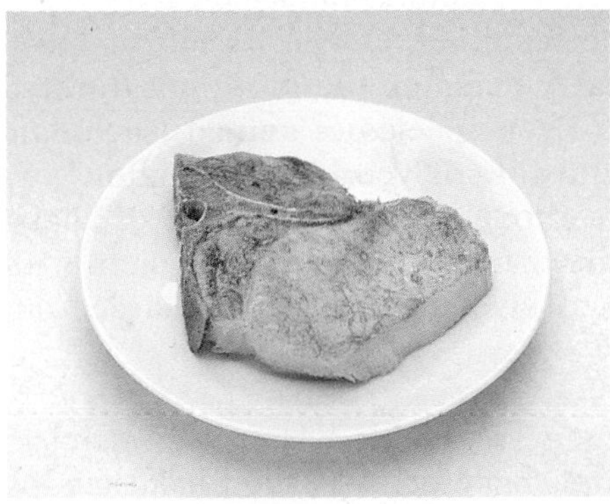

Pork chop with fat trimmed off (265 calories; 117 calories from fat).

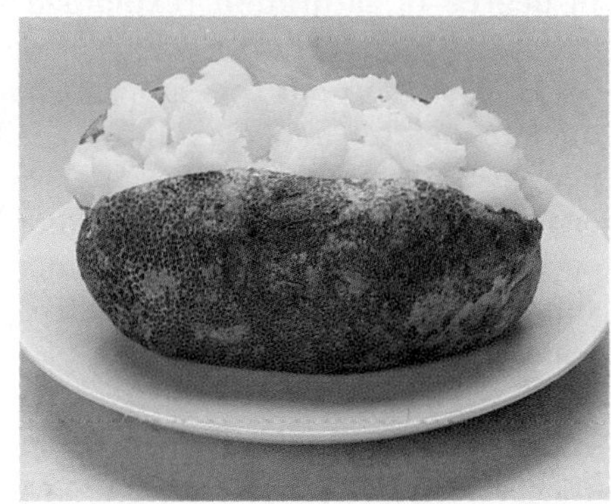

Plain potato (220 calories; fewer than 9 calories from fat).

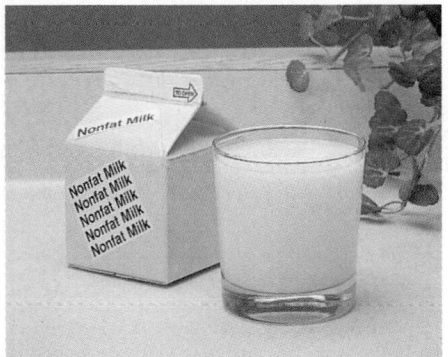

Nonfat milk, 1 cup (90 calories; fewer than 9 calories from fat).

◆ A Close Look at Fats

As mentioned, the term *fat* refers to triglycerides, the major form of lipid found in foods. Triglycerides, in turn, are made of building blocks, fatty acids and glycerol.

Triglycerides: Fatty Acids and Glycerol

Very few **fatty acids** are found free in the body or in foods. Usually the fatty acids are incorporated into large, complex compounds: triglycerides. The name almost explains itself: three fatty acids *(tri)* are attached to a molecule of **glycerol.** Figure 5-4 shows how glycerol and three fatty acids combine to make a triglyceride molecule. Tissues all over the body can easily assemble triglycerides or disassemble them whenever the need strikes. Many triglycerides, especially those eaten in fatty foods, are transported to the fat depots—muscles, breasts, the insulating fat layer under the skin, and others—where they are stored.

fatty acids organic acids composed of carbon chains of various lengths. Each fatty acid has an acid end and hydrogens attached to all of the carbon atoms of the chain.

glycerol (GLISS-er-all) an organic compound, three carbons long, of interest here because it serves as the backbone for triglycerides.

Figure 5-4

TRIGLYCERIDE FORMATION
Glycerol, a small, water-soluble carbohydrate derivative, plus three fatty acids, equals a triglyceride.

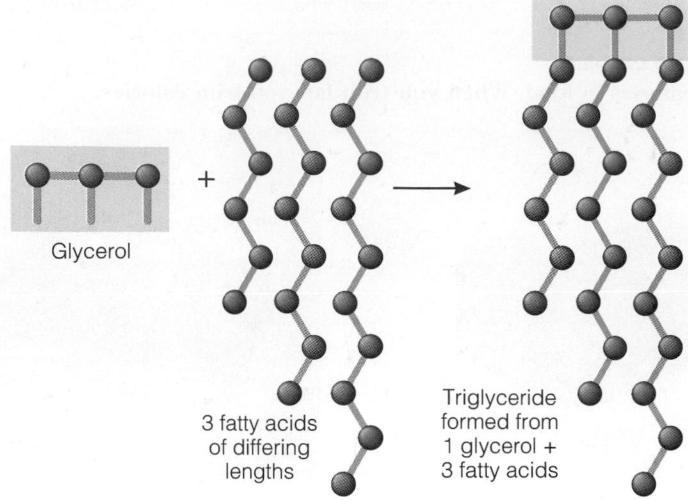

saturated fatty acid a fatty acid carrying the maximum possible number of hydrogen atoms (having no points of unsaturation). A saturated fat is a triglyceride that contains three saturated fatty acids.

point of unsaturation a site in a molecule where the bonding is such that additional hydrogen atoms can easily be added.

unsaturated fatty acid a fatty acid that lacks some hydrogen atoms and has one or more points of unsaturation. An unsaturated fat is a triglyceride that contains one or more unsaturated fatty acids.

monounsaturated fatty acid a fatty acid containing one point of unsaturation.

oleic (oh-LAY-ic) **acid** a monounsaturated fatty acid found in animal and vegetable oils.

polyunsaturated fatty acid (PUFA) a fatty acid in which two or more points of unsaturation occur.

Fatty acids may differ from one another in two ways: in chain length and in degree of saturation (explained next). Depending on which fatty acids are incorporated into a triglyceride, the resulting fat will be soft or hard. Those that contain the shorter-chain fatty acids or the more unsaturated ones are softer and melt more readily. Each species of animal (including people) makes its own characteristic kinds of triglycerides, a function governed by genetics. Fats in the diet can, though, affect the types of triglycerides made. For example, animals raised for food can be fed diets with softer or harder triglycerides in them to give them softer or harder fat, whichever consumers demand.

KEY POINT The body combines three fatty acids with one glycerol to make a triglyceride, its storage form of fat. Fatty acids in food influence the composition of fats in the body.

Saturated versus Unsaturated Fatty Acids

Saturation, the term that identifies fats that raise risks of CVD, refers to a fatty acid's chemical structure—specifically to the number of hydrogens the fatty-acid chain is holding. If every available bond from the carbons is holding a hydrogen, the chain forms a **saturated fatty acid;** it is filled to capacity with hydrogen. The zigzag structure on the left in Figure 5-5 represents a saturated fatty acid.

Sometimes, especially in the fatty acids of plants and fish, there is a place in the chain where hydrogens are missing, an "empty spot," or **point of unsaturation.** A fatty acid carbon chain that possesses one or more points of unsaturation is an **unsaturated fatty acid.** If there is one point of unsaturation, then it is a **monounsaturated fatty acid: oleic acid** is an example (see the second structure in Figure 5-5). If there are two or more points of unsaturation, then it is a **polyunsaturated fatty acid** (examples follow in the next section; and see the third structure in Figure 5-5). You sometimes see polyunsaturated fatty acids abbreviated as **PUFA.**

The degree of saturation of fatty acids in a fat affects the temperature at which the fat melts. Generally, the more unsaturated the fatty acids of a fat the more liquid the fat is at room temperature. In contrast, the more

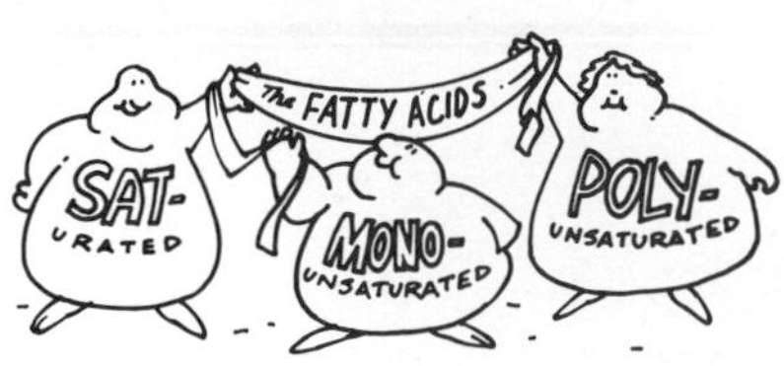

A trio of fatty acids—saturated, monounsaturated, and polyunsaturated.

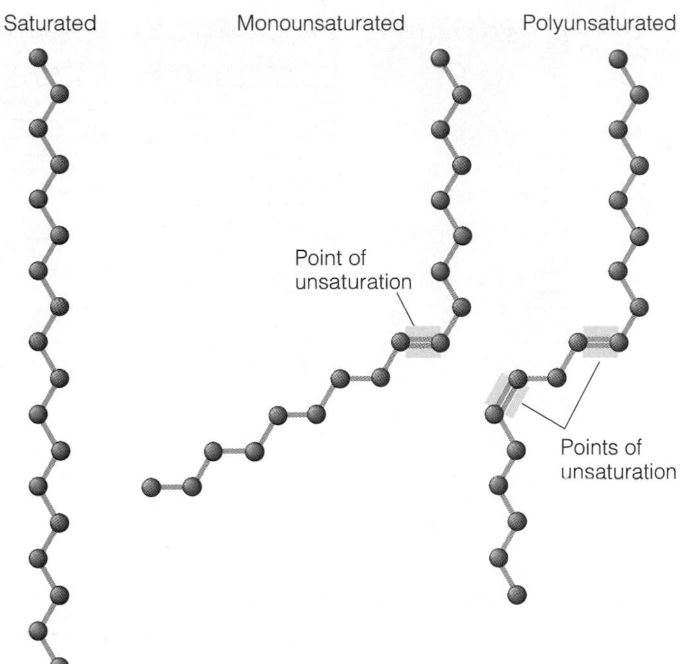

Figure 5-5

THREE FATTY ACIDS
The more carbon atoms in a fatty acid, the longer its length. The more hydrogen atoms attached to those carbons, the more saturated the fatty acid.

saturated a fat the firmer it is. Thus of three fats—lard (which comes from pork), chicken fat, and safflower oil—lard is the most saturated and the hardest; chicken fat is less saturated and somewhat soft; and safflower oil, which is the most unsaturated, is a liquid at room temperature. Chicken is recommended over pork for people avoiding saturated fats. Thus if a health care provider recommends limiting **saturated fats** and using **monounsaturated fats** or **polyunsaturated fats,** you can judge by the hardness of the fats which ones to choose. To determine whether an oil you use contains saturated fats, place the oil in a clear container in the refrigerator and watch for cloudiness. The least saturated oils remain clearest.

saturated fats triglycerides in which all the fatty acids are saturated.

monounsaturated fats triglycerides in which one or more of the fatty acids has one point of unsaturation (monounsaturated).

polyunsaturated fats triglycerides in which one or more of the fatty acids has more than one point of unsaturation (polyunsaturated).

Generally speaking, vegetable and fish oils are rich in polyunsaturates. Some vegetable oils, especially olive oil, are also rich in monounsaturates, and animal fats are generally the most saturated. But you have to know your oils. To obtain polyunsaturated oils, it is not enough to choose foods with labels claiming plant oils over those containing animal fats. Some nondairy whipped dessert toppings use coconut oil, one of the so-called tropical oils, in place of cream (butterfat). Coconut oil does come from a plant, but it disobeys the rule that plant oils are more liquid than animal fats; coconut oil is actually more saturated than cream and seems to add to heart disease risk. Palm oil, used frequently in food processing, is also highly saturated and seems to affect blood lipids in ways not yet fully understood, but has not been proved to add to heart disease risk.[5]

A benefit to health is seen when monounsaturated fat is used in place of saturated fat in the diet.[6] Olive oil probably does not harm the health of the heart, and may even benefit it. The people of Mediterranean regions consume large quantities of olive oil and enjoy low rates of cardiovascular disease. Lately canola oil, another rich source of monounsaturated fatty acids, has appeared on grocers' shelves. Figure 5-6 compares fats and oils in terms of their percentages of saturated, monounsaturated, and polyunsaturated fatty acids.

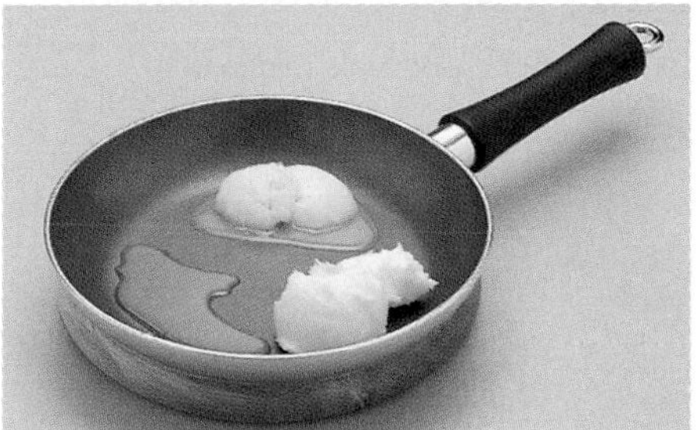

The more unsaturated a fat, the more liquid it is at room temperature. The more saturated a fat, the higher the temperature at which it melts.

Figure 5-6

FATTY ACID COMPOSITION OF COMMON FOOD FATS

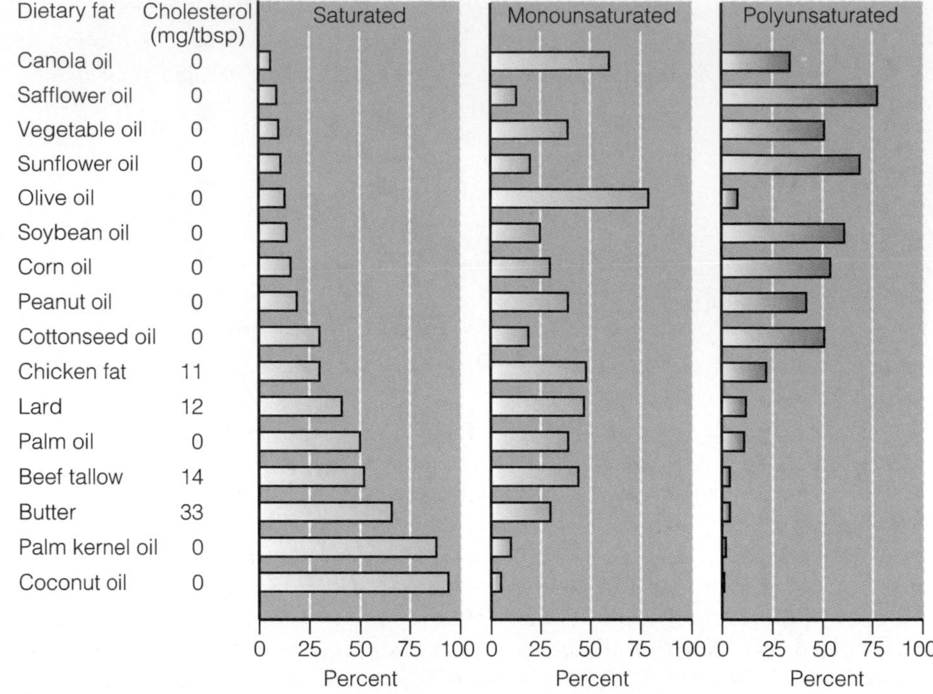

linoleic (lin-oh-LAY-ic) **acid** and **linolenic** (lin-oh-LEN-ic) **acid** polyunsaturated fatty acids, essential nutrients for human beings.

KEY POINT Fatty acids are energy-rich carbon chains that can be saturated (filled with hydrogens) or monounsaturated (with one point of unsaturation) or polyunsaturated (with more than one point of unsaturation). The degree of saturation of the fatty acids in a fat determines the fat's softness or hardness.

Essential Polyunsaturated Fatty Acids

The human body can use carbohydrate, fat, or protein to synthesize nearly all the fatty acids it needs. Two are well-known exceptions: **linoleic acid** and **linolenic acid.** These two polyunsaturated fatty acids, which the body needs for its basic functions, cannot be made from other substances in the body or from each other. They must be supplied by the diet; they are therefore essential nutrients. These essential fatty acids are found in small amounts in the oils of plants and cold-water fish and are readily stored in the adult body. Both serve as raw materials from which the body makes hormonelike substances that regulate a wide range of body functions: blood pressure, blood clot formation, blood lipid regulation, the immune response, the inflammation response to injury and infection, and many others.[7]* They also serve as structural parts of cell membranes.

To read about a possible relationship between polyunsaturated fatty acids and cancer, see Chapter 11.

A deficiency of an essential fatty acid in the diet leads to observable changes in cells, some more subtle than others. When the diet is deficient in *all* of the polyunsaturated fatty acids, symptoms of growth retardation, reproductive failure, skin abnormalities, and kidney and liver disorders appear. Luckily these deficiency disorders are seldom seen except when intentionally induced in research. They sometimes do arise, however, when inadequate diets are provided by mistake. One such mistake is to feed hos-

*The hormonelike derivatives referred to here are short-lived *eicosanoid* (eye-COSS-a-noid) compounds, such as prostaglandins and thromboxanes.

pital clients a formula through a vein that provides no polyunsaturated fatty acids for long periods. Another is to feed infants exclusively on a formula that lacks polyunsaturated fatty acids. Normal food, and especially a balanced diet that includes grains, seeds, nuts, leafy vegetables, and fish, supplies all the needed forms of fatty acids in abundance and prevents deficiencies.

Linoleic acid is the primary member of a group of fatty acids named by their chemical structure as the **omega-6 fatty acid** family. The body can convert linoleic acid to the other members of its omega-6 family that play active parts in body functioning. One of these plays a critical role in the cell membranes that define and protect each cell of the body. Any diet that contains vegetable oils, seeds, nuts, and whole-grain products supplies enough linoleic acid to meet the body's needs. Almost everyone eats enough (see the right-hand side of Figure 5-7 on the next page).

Linolenic acid is the primary member of the **omega-3** family of fatty acids. This family has only recently been appreciated for its role in health. Someone thought to ask the question why the native people of Greenland and Alaska, who eat a diet very high in fat, have such a low death rate from heart disease.[8] The trail led to the abundance of fish they eat, then to the oils in those fish, and finally to two omega-3 fatty acids **EPA** and **DHA** in the oils. These fatty acids can be made in the body from linolenic acid, to some extent, or can be derived from some foods, especially fatty fish.

Now researchers recognize distinct roles for EPA and DHA. Their presence is evident in many tissues. They make up a large proportion of the communicating membranes of the brain, and they are needed for normal brain development.[9] EPA and DHA are also especially active in the rods and cones of the retina of the eye.[10] In rats the concentration of products of linolenic acid diminishes with age, leading researchers to wonder if age-related vision changes might be partly due to failure to maintain omega-3 fatty acids in the retina.[11] Omega-3 fatty acids also play roles in male reproductive tissue, in skin integrity, and in the body's inflammatory response.

Human fat tissue can store EPA and DHA, but does so only when dietary intakes exceed the body's immediate needs for the compounds.[12] Many North Americans do not eat much fish and so do not obtain any extra EPA and DHA to store. They do, however, receive plenty of the omega-6 fatty acids, perhaps undesirably high amounts. A comparison with the fish-eating people of Greenland is illuminating. Greenlanders eat more calories, and more of those calories come from omega-3 acids. We eat fewer calories, and more of ours come from omega-6 acids. Indeed, North Americans eat about twice as many omega-6 and half as many omega-3 acids as Greenlanders do. Researchers have speculated that this may be why the heart attack rate here is so much higher than in Greenland.

Human beings can convert some linolenic acid to its active derivatives, but the process in the human body is not as efficient as in fish or some other animals. For this reason, the linolenic acid found in vegetable oils and a few leafy vegetables may not entirely meet the need for omega-3 fatty acids. It may be necessary to eat seafood to obtain these fatty acids (see the left-hand side of Figure 5-7). One investigator in the field made this clear:

> *Because seafood, especially fatty fish, is virtually the only source of the preformed long-chain ω-3 fatty acids EPA and DHA, I'd suggest everyone eat fish regularly, twice a week, if possible. . . . Plant sources [such as canola and soybean oils],*

omega the last letter of the Greek alphabet (ω) used by chemists to refer to the position of the endmost double bond in a fatty acid. Printers and publishers often use the English letter *n* to replace the Greek ω, as in many of this chapter's references.

omega-6 fatty acid long recognized as important in nutrition, a polyunsaturated fatty acid with its endmost double bond six carbons from the end of the carbon chain. Linoleic acid is an example.

omega-3 fatty acid relatively newly recognized as important in nutrition, a polyunsaturated fatty acid with its endmost double bond three carbons from the end of its carbon chain. Linolenic acid is an example.

EPA, DHA omega-3 fatty acids made from linolenic acid in the tissues of fish.

Figure 5-7

ESSENTIAL FATTY ACIDS IN THE FOOD CHAIN

Source: Adapted from ideas in W. E. Connor, M. Neuringer, and S. Reisbick, Essential fatty acids: The importance of n-3 fatty acids in the retina and brain, *Nutrition Reviews* 50 (1992): II21–II29.

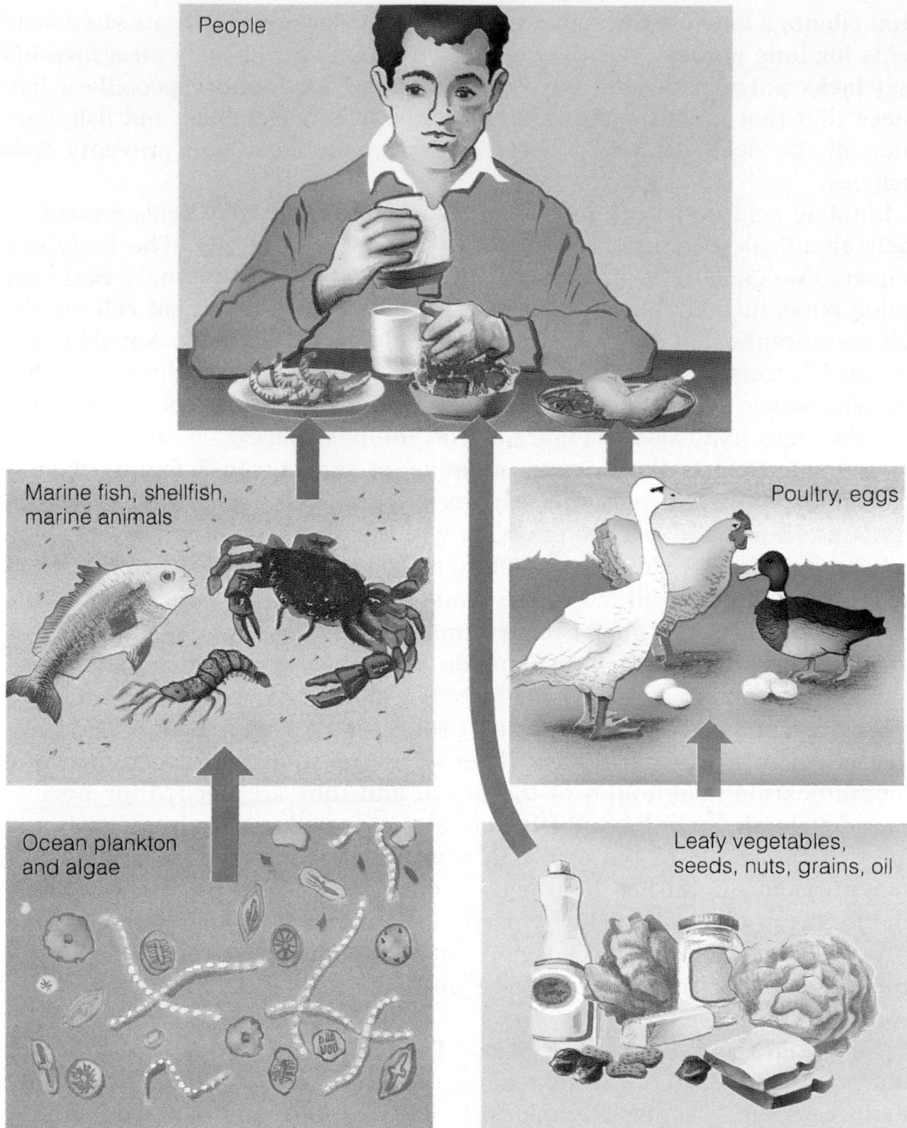

Seafood is a rich source of omega-3 fatty acids. Microscopic marine plants make linolenic acid. Marine animals eat the plants and convert the linoleic acid to related omega-3 acids.

Some land plants and animals are fair sources of omega-3 fatty acids; many are good sources of omega-6 fatty acids.

These fish provide at least 1 gram omega-3 fatty acids, including EPA and DHA, in 100 grams of fish (about 3.5 ounces):*

- Anchovy, European
- Bluefish
- Capelin conch
- Herring, Atlantic, Pacific
- Mackerel, Atlantic, Chub, Japanese horse, or king
- Mullet
- Sablefish
- Salmon, all varieties**
- Saury
- Scad, Muroaji
- Sprat
- Sturgeon, Atlantic or common
- Trout, lake
- Tuna, white albacore or bluefin (not canned light tuna)
- Whitefish, lake

*Fish oil content of fish species varies with season and site of harvest.
**Canned varieties may be high in sodium.

although useful, may not be an adequate substitute for the preformed long-chain fatty acids found in seafood.

JOYCE A. NETTLETON *The Journal Talks with . . .* Journal of the American Dietetic Association *91 (1991): 333.*

This doesn't mean that linolenic and linoleic acids are not important. It does mean that the body may need sources of preformed EPA and DHA in addition to linoleic and linolenic acids. In the future, EPA and DHA may be classed among the essential fatty acids.[13]

No Recommended Dietary Allowances (RDA) for omega-6 and omega-3 fatty acids now exist, but scientists may agree to include them in the future. Meanwhile the advice of the expert quoted above is echoed by many: eat meals of fish two or three times a week, as well as small amounts of vegetable oils, to obtain the right balance between omega-3 and omega-6 intakes. The ratio of intakes of omega-3 to omega-6 fatty acids should be about 1 to 4. This ratio may even turn out to be the key to human requirements: more omega-3 acids may not necessarily be better, but the balance may turn out to be crucial.[14] Purchasing and taking fish oil supplements is not recommended, as this Chapter's Consumer Caution points out.

emulsifier a substance that mixes with both fat and water and that permanently disperses the fat in the water, forming an *emulsion.*

bile an emulsifier made by the liver from cholesterol and stored in the gallbladder. Bile does not digest fat as enzymes do but emulsifies it so that enzymes in the watery fluids may contact it and split the fatty acids from their glycerols for absorption.

KEY POINT Two polyunsaturated fatty acids, linoleic acid (an omega-6 acid) and linolenic acid (an omega-3 acid), are essential nutrients used to make hormonelike substances, to form membranes of the brain, and to support the functioning of the retina of the eye. The omega-6 family includes linoleic acid; seed oils are rich sources. The omega-3 family includes linolenic acid, EPA and DHA. Fish oils are rich sources of EPA and DHA.

Other Members of the Lipid Family

The foregoing sections, half of this chapter, have dealt with just one of the three classes of lipids—the triglycerides and their component fatty acids. These lipids represent 95 percent of all the lipids in the diet and in the body. The word *fat,* used properly, refers to the triglycerides.

The other two classes—phospholipids and sterols—merit a moment's attention, though, because they play important roles in the body. A phospholipid, like a triglyceride, consists of a molecule of glycerol with fatty acids attached, but it contains two, rather than three, fatty acids. In place of the third is a molecule containing phosphorus, which makes the phospholipid soluble in water while its fatty acids make it soluble in fat. This versatility permits any phospholipid to play a role in keeping fats dispersed in water; it can serve as an **emulsifier.**

Lecithins and other phospholipids also play key roles in the structure of cell membranes. Because they are emulsifiers, they have both water-loving and fat-loving characteristics, which enable them to help fats travel back and forth across the lipid-containing membranes of cells into the watery fluids on both sides. Almost magical health-promoting properties, such as the ability to lower blood cholesterol, are sometimes attributed to the group of lipids called lecithin, but the people making the claims are those who stand to gain from selling supplements. Although it is an important lipid to the body, lecithin has no special ability to promote health. A molecule of lecithin is shown in Figure 5-8.

Sterols such as cholesterol are large, complicated molecules consisting of interconnected *rings* of carbon atoms with side chains of carbon, hydrogen, and oxygen attached. Cholesterol serves as the raw material for making another important emulsifier, **bile.** Other sterols are vitamin D, which is made from cholesterol, and several important hormones, the so-called *steroid* hormones, including the sex hormones.

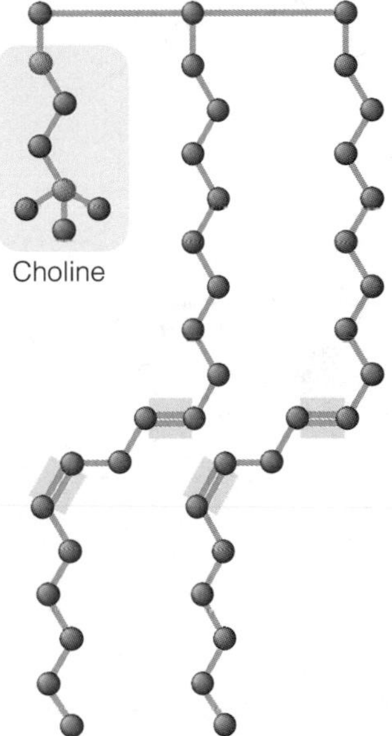

Figure 5-8

A MOLECULE OF LECITHIN

A molecule of lecithin is like a triglyceride but contains only two (polyunsaturated) fatty acids. The third position is occupied by choline (a compound related to the B vitamins). The identity of the two fatty acids can vary, and all of the possible combinations are lecithins.

Fish Oil Supplements

CONSUMER CAUTION Fish oil has received top billing in the news. Readers often see promises such as these: it cures arthritis, it prevents cancer, it reverses heart disease, or it boosts the immune system. While all these claims are based on some research, proof that fish oil can do these things for individuals or populations is lacking. Most research that suggests beneficial effects of fish oil on cancer consists of studies on rats that cannot be directly applied to human beings. The research on heart disease is more convincing than that on cancer, but it does not indicate that people can reverse the effects of other lifestyle habits, such as smoking or being overweight, simply by taking capsules of fish oil. The Food and Drug Administration (FDA) disallows advertisements and labels from claiming that fish oil supplements are effective in disease prevention or treatment because these effects are unproved.[15] However, food choices do seem to make a difference. The choice to replace two or three meals of meat each week with fish can support heart health, especially when the person takes other steps, such as increasing physical activity.[16] Even one fish dish per week may be enough to support the health of the heart.[17]

The idea that fish oil is beneficial and safe in any amount is erroneous. Some evidence indicates that too much fish oil can cause or aggravate illnesses. Concentrated supplements make it easy to overdose, and overdoses can affect hormone levels in ways that may alter blood lipids and blood clotting and may worsen Type II diabetes.[18] Overdoses also may impair immune function, too.[19] Even with low-dose supplements one undesirable effect, elevated LDL cholesterol, occurs. Daily large (7 ounces) servings of fatty fish have also been observed to elevate LDL cholesterol for that matter.[20] A third drawback is that fish oil supplements are made from fish skins and livers, which may have accumulated toxic concentrations of pesticides, heavy metals, and other ocean contaminants that may in turn be concentrated in the pills. Moreover, even without contamination, fish oil naturally contains high levels of the two most potentially toxic vitamins, A and D. When taken over long periods fish oil itself may have unknown long-term toxic effects. Lastly, supplements of fish oil are expensive.

Cholesterol is an important sterol in the structure of brain and nerve cells. In fact, cholesterol is a part of every cell. Like lecithin, cholesterol can be made by the body, so it is not an essential nutrient. But while it is widespread in the body and necessary to its function, it is also the major part of the plaques that narrow the arteries in atherosclerosis, the underlying cause of heart attacks and strokes.

KEY POINT Phospholipids, including lecithin, play key roles in cell membranes; sterols play roles as part of bile, vitamin D, the sex hormones, and other important compounds.

Fish Oil Supplements *continued*

Another potential for harm from taking in too much fish oil may lie in the reactive nature of omega-3 fatty acids in the presence of a reactive form of oxygen. Omega-3 acids are highly unsaturated and so are open to attack by reactive oxygen. This unstable chemical form, known as a **free radical,** is attracted to points of unsaturation. A reaction between the free radical and a fatty acid is dangerous to cells because it starts a chain reaction that destroys neighboring molecules. The delicate fatty-acid-rich membranes of cells are easily damaged by this action. Such reactions can also attack a cell's DNA, an action that may lead to some forms of cancer.[21] Free radical attacks are believed to be important triggers of damage that leads to heart disease. In fact, tissue damage from free radicals has been implicated in over 100 human diseases.[22]

The destructive events just described may be made likely by omega-3 supplements. When research subjects were given fish oil capsules, oxidative cell damage in their bodies increased by 122 percent.[23] Vitamin E in high doses prevented the increase, but most supplements do not contain enough vitamin E to protect cells. Additionally, supplements of fish oil may cause significant losses of body stores of vitamin E and other nutrients that act as **antioxidants.**[24] Antioxidants protect cell lipids against oxidation by offering themselves for destruction instead. With elevated omega-3 fatty acids and diminished antioxidant vitamins, tissues may be more vulnerable to damaging oxidation.

So little is known about the long-term effects of fish oil supplements that taking them is chancy. Besides, eating fish brings other benefits; they are leaner than most other animal protein choices and they are richer in minerals (with the exception of iron). Any benefits from fish oil supplements remain to be proved and may be outweighed by dangers. Go to the source for fish oil—eat fish.

free radical a highly reactive chemical form that can cause destructive changes in nearby chemicals, sometimes setting up a chain reaction.

antioxidant (anti-OX-ih-dant) a compound that protects other compounds from oxygen by itself reacting with oxygen (*anti* means "against"; *oxy* means "oxygen").

hydrogenation(high-droh-gen-AY-shun) the process of adding hydrogen to unsaturated fatty acids to make fat more solid and resistant to the chemical change of oxidation.

emulsification the process of mixing lipid with water, usually through addition of an emulsifier, a compound that attracts both water and fat and prevents the mixture from separating.

Chapter 14 comes back to the topic of seafood safety.

More about vitamin E and other antioxidant vitamins in Chapter 7.

◆ Hydrogenation and Emulsification of Fats

When manufacturers process foods, they often alter the fatty acids in the fat (triglycerides) the foods contain. One major process is **hydrogenation;** another is **emulsification.**

As mentioned, points of unsaturation in fatty acids are like weak spots that are vulnerable to attack by oxygen. Oxidative damage is not confined to fats within body tissues but occurs anywhere oxygen mixes with fats. When the unsaturated points in the oils of food are oxidized, the oils become rancid. This is why cooking oils should be stored in tightly covered

Points of unsaturation are places on fatty acid chains where hydrogen is missing. The bonds that would normally be occupied by hydrogen in a saturated fatty acid are shared, reluctantly, as a double bond between two carbons that both carry a slightly negative charge.

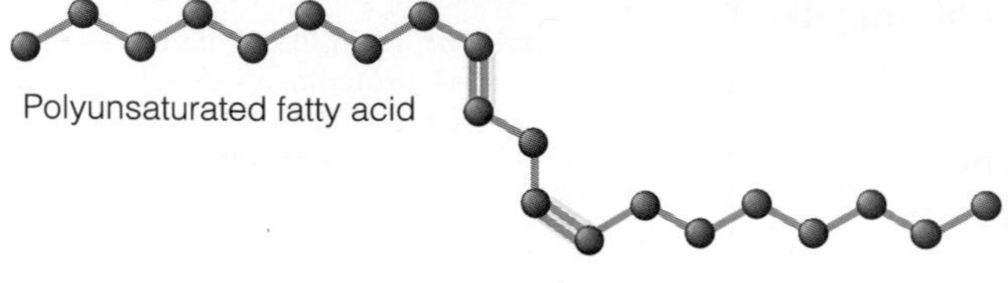

When positively charged hydrogen is made available to one of those bonds, it readily accepts the hydrogen molecules, and in the process, becomes saturated. It no longer has a point of unsaturation.

H+ H+
H+ H+ H+
H+

Hydrogenated fatty acid

Sometimes hydrogenation leaves a fatty acid unsaturated and causes it to change its shape.

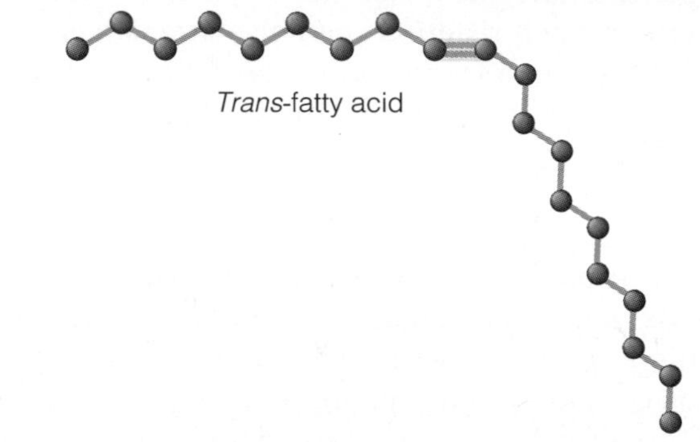

Figure 5-9

HOW HYDROGENATION MAKES FATS MORE SATURATED

containers that exclude air. If stored for long periods, they need refrigeration to retard oxidation.

One way to prevent spoilage of unsaturated fats and also to make them harder is to change their fatty acids chemically by hydrogenation, as shown in Figure 5-9. When food producers want to use a polyunsaturated oil such as corn oil to make a spreadable margarine, for example, they hydrogenate it. They force hydrogen into the oil, some of the unsaturated fatty acids accept the hydrogen, and the oil becomes harder. The product that results is more saturated and more spreadable than the original oil. It is also more resistant to damage from oxidation.

Once hydrogenated, oils lose their unsaturated character and the health benefits that go with it. An alternative to hydrogenation is to add a chemical preservative that will compete for the oxygen and thus protect the oil. The additives are antioxidants, and they work just as vitamin E does, as described earlier. Examples are the well-known additives BHA and BHT listed on snack food labels. Another alternative, already mentioned, is to keep the product refrigerated.

> **smoking point** the temperature at which fat gives off an acrid blue gas.

If you, the consumer, are looking for polyunsaturated oils to include in your diet, hydrogenated oils will not meet your need. Hydrogenated oils are easy to handle and store well. They also have a high **smoking point,** so they are suitable for purposes such as frying. However, hydrogenated oils are more saturated than the oils from which they are made. In contrast, margarines that list liquid oil as the first ingredient are usually the most polyunsaturated. Margarines that are sold in tubs and labeled "soft" are sometimes less saturated than the stick varieties.

Another concern about hydrogenation of fat centers around a change in chemical structure that occurs when polyunsaturated oils are hardened by hydrogenation processing. Some of the unsaturated fatty acids, instead of becoming saturated, end up changing their shapes. This creates unusual products that are not made by the body and that occur naturally in foods to only a limited extent. These changed fatty acids, or ***trans*-fatty acids,** can be taken up into cell membranes, where they may alter membrane functions.

> ***trans*-fatty acids** fatty acids with unusual shapes that can arise when polyunsaturated oils are hydrogenated.

Trans-fatty acids have implications for the body's health. Total fat consumption is associated with cancer susceptibility, and *trans*-fatty acids may act as a part of total fat in this effect. No evidence suggests that *trans*-fatty acids by *themselves* play any specific role in promoting or causing cancer.[25] In terms of the health of the heart and arteries, *trans*-fatty acids are similar to saturated fats in their effects.[26] In fact, some evidence suggests that *trans*-fatty acids may elevate the risk of heart disease to an even greater degree than does regular saturated fat.

When news of *trans*-fatty acids' effects on heart health was first emerging, some people hastily switched from using margarine back to butter, believing oversimplified reports that margarine provided no heart health advantage over butter. It is true that some margarines and shortenings are made from mostly hydrogenated fats and therefore are saturated and contain *trans*-fatty acids. However, some margarines, especially the soft or liquid varieties, are made from unhydrogenated oils. These have long been proved to be less likely to elevate serum cholesterol than the saturated fats of butter. The popular press overstated margarine's villainy as a source of *trans*-fatty acids in the diet. Other foods contribute far more *trans*-fatty acids to the diet than does margarine—and more total fat, too.[27] Fast foods, chips, baked goods, and other commercially prepared foods are high in fats containing up to 50 percent *trans*-fatty acids. Margarines range from zero percent for unhydrogenated varieties to 40 percent for some hydrogenated types.

As for emulsification of fats, this process is commonly used by food processors to blend fat with watery ingredients. No doubt you have encountered salad dressings that separate to form two layers—vinegar on the bottom, oil on top. You have to shake the layers to blend them before pouring the dressing on your salad. Other dressings, also made from vinegar and oil, never separate, for example, mayonnaise. The difference lies in a special ingredient of mayonnaise, the emulsifier lecithin in egg yolks. Lecithin, a phospholipid described earlier, blends the vinegar and oil in a permanent emulsion.

Later sections come back to the topic of fats in food. Now we turn to the body's systems that are designed especially to handle both the fats we eat and those the body makes.

KEY POINT Food fats may be processed by hydrogenation or emulsification. Vegetable margarines are partially hydrogenated oils that are more saturated than the oils they are made from and they contain *trans*-fatty acids. Emulsified fats are those that have been dispersed in water by an emulsifier.

Lipids in the Body

In handling lipids, the body must solve the problem of how to thoroughly mix them with its own watery fluids. The body solves this problem with the use of the emulsifier bile. To digest fats, the digestive system first mixes the fats with its bile-containing digestive juices to permit the fat-digesting enzymes to break the fats down. The role of bile is to emulsify the fat in

Chapter 3 first described the action of bile and gave details of the digestive system.

food in the watery digestive fluids. After fats have been digested, they face another watery barrier, the watery mucus layer that coats the absorptive lining of the digestive tract. Fats must traverse this layer before they may enter the cells of the digestive tract lining. Then the cells face another challenge: to package lipids so that they may travel in the watery fluids of the circulatory system. The next two sections describe the body's superb adaptations to meet all these needs for lipid digestion and transport.

Digestion of Fats

When you partake of animal products such as meat, fish, poultry, or eggs, you are eating fat and protein. When you eat oil-containing plant foods, such as nuts, coconut, or olives, you are eating fat and carbohydrate along with some protein. Of the fats and oils in foods, 95 percent are triglycerides that have been made in living animal or plant tissues, mostly from carbohydrate, the same way the human body makes them.

Food fat can end up in fat stores in the body, but first it has to be digested, absorbed, and transported to its cell destinations. A bite of food in the mouth first encounters the enzymes of saliva. One enzyme, produced by the tongue, acts on long-chain fatty acids, such as those of milk, but the enzyme is thought to play a minor role in fat digestion in adults.[28] In infants, the enzyme plays a major role, because it efficiently digests the fats in milk. Once the food has been chewed and swallowed, it travels to the stomach, where the fat separates from other components and floats as a layer on the top. Since fat does not mix with the stomach fluids, little fat digestion takes place.

By the time fat enters the small intestine, the gallbladder, which stores the liver's output of bile, has contracted and squirted its bile into the intestine. Bile emulsifies fat particles (Figure 5-10), suspending them in the fluid until the fat-digesting enzymes contributed by the pancreas can split

Figure 5-10

THE ACTION OF BILE IN FAT DIGESTION

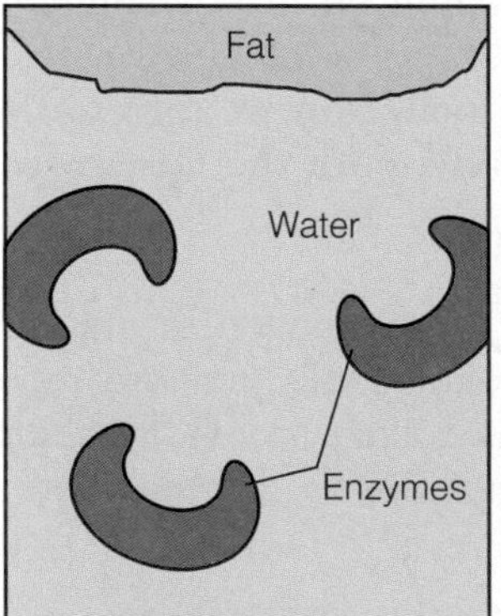

Fat and water tend to separate. Enzymes are in the water and can't get at the fat.

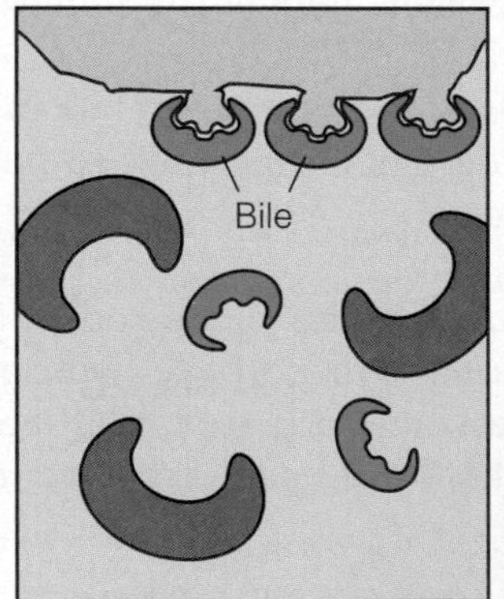

Bile (an emulsifier) arrives. Bile has an affinity for both fat and water and can therefore bring the fat into the water.

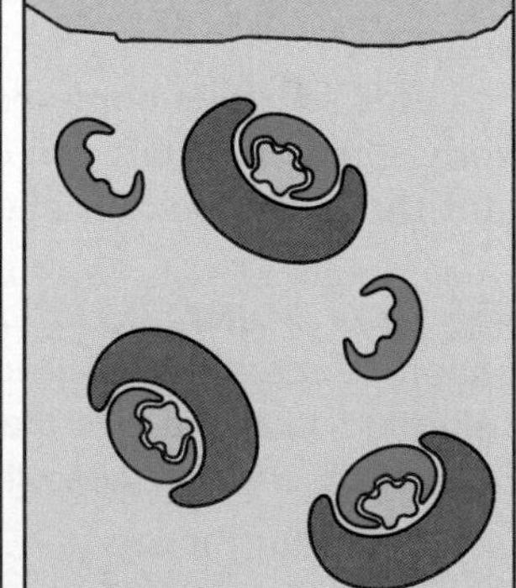

After emulsification, the fat is mixed in the water solution, so fat-digesting enzymes have access to it.

Detergents are emulsifiers and work the same way, which is why they are effective in removing grease spots from clothes. Molecule by molecule, the grease is dissolved out of the spot and suspended in the water, where it can be rinsed away.

them for absorption. A bile molecule works because one of its ends attracts and holds fat, while the other end is attracted to and held by water.

People sometimes wonder how a person without a gallbladder can digest food. The gallbladder is just a storage organ. Without it, the liver still produces bile, but delivers it continuously into the small intestine. People who have had their gallbladders removed must reduce their fat intakes because they can no longer store bile and release it at mealtimes. As a result, their systems can handle only a little fat at a time.

Once the intestine's contents are emulsified, fat-splitting enzymes act on triglycerides to split fatty acids from their glycerol backbones. Free fatty acids, glycerol, and **monoglycerides** cling together in balls surrounded by bile and are shuttled across the watery layer of mucus to the waiting absorptive cells of the intestinal villi.[29] The bile may be absorbed and reused by the body, or it may exit with the feces as was shown in Figure 4-4 of the previous chapter.

The small products of lipid digestion, glycerol and shorter chain fatty acids, can pass directly through the cells of the digestive tract lining into the bloodstream. From there they can travel without help to the tissues that need them.

The larger products of lipid digestion, monoglycerides and long-chain fatty acids, need some help to get to their destinations. Once inside the intestinal cells, they are incorporated into **chylomicrons,** clusters of proteins with the digested lipids. Chylomicrons are a class of **lipoproteins,** described next.

The digestive tract absorbs triglycerides from a meal with up to 98 percent efficiency. In other words, little fat is excreted in feces by a healthy system.[30] The process of fat digestion takes time, though, so the more fat taken in at a meal, the slower the digestive system action becomes. The efficient series of events just described is depicted in Figure 5-11 on the next page.

KEY POINT In the stomach, fats separate from other food components. In the small intestine, bile emulsifies them, enzymes digest them, and the intestinal cells absorb them. Small lipids can travel alone in the blood after absorption, but large lipids must be incorporated into chylomicrons for transport.

monoglycerides (mon-oh-GLISS-er-ides) a product of the digestion of lipids; glycerol molecules with one fatty acid attached (*mono* means "one"; *glyceride* means "a compound of glycerol").

chylomicrons(KYE-low-MY-krons) clusters formed when lipids from a meal are combined with carrier proteins in the intestinal lining. Chylomicrons provide transportation for food fats through the watery body fluids to the liver and other tissues.

lipoproteins (LIP-oh-PRO-teens) clusters of lipids associated with protein, which serve as transport vehicles for lipids in blood and lymph.

LDL (low-density lipoproteins) lipoproteins, containing a large proportion of cholesterol, that transport lipids from the liver to other tissues such as muscle and fat.

Lipid Transport in the Body Fluids

Within the body, many fats travel from place to place as passengers in lipoproteins. For example, the monoglycerides and long-chain fatty acids liberated from digested food fat are too large to be released directly into the bloodstream. Without some mechanism to keep them dispersed, these lipids would separate out and float in globules, disrupting the blood's normal functions. Instead, the intestinal cells allow them to cluster together, and before release, they rejoin them as triglycerides and combine them with protein to form chylomicrons mentioned earlier. The protein and phospholipid in the cluster act as emulsifiers: they attract both water and fat. Their association with both substances enables them to transport lipids in the watery body fluids. The tissues of the body can extract whatever fat they need from these clusters. What is left, the remnants, are picked up by the liver, which dismantles them and reuses their parts. Figure 5-12 on page 163 depicts a lipoprotein.

The chylomicrons are one of three major classes of lipoproteins that the body uses to carry fats from place to place. Other lipoproteins are the **low-density lipoproteins (LDL),** which carry fats made in the liver, and the

Figure 5-11

THE PROCESS OF LIPID DIGESTION AND ABSORPTION

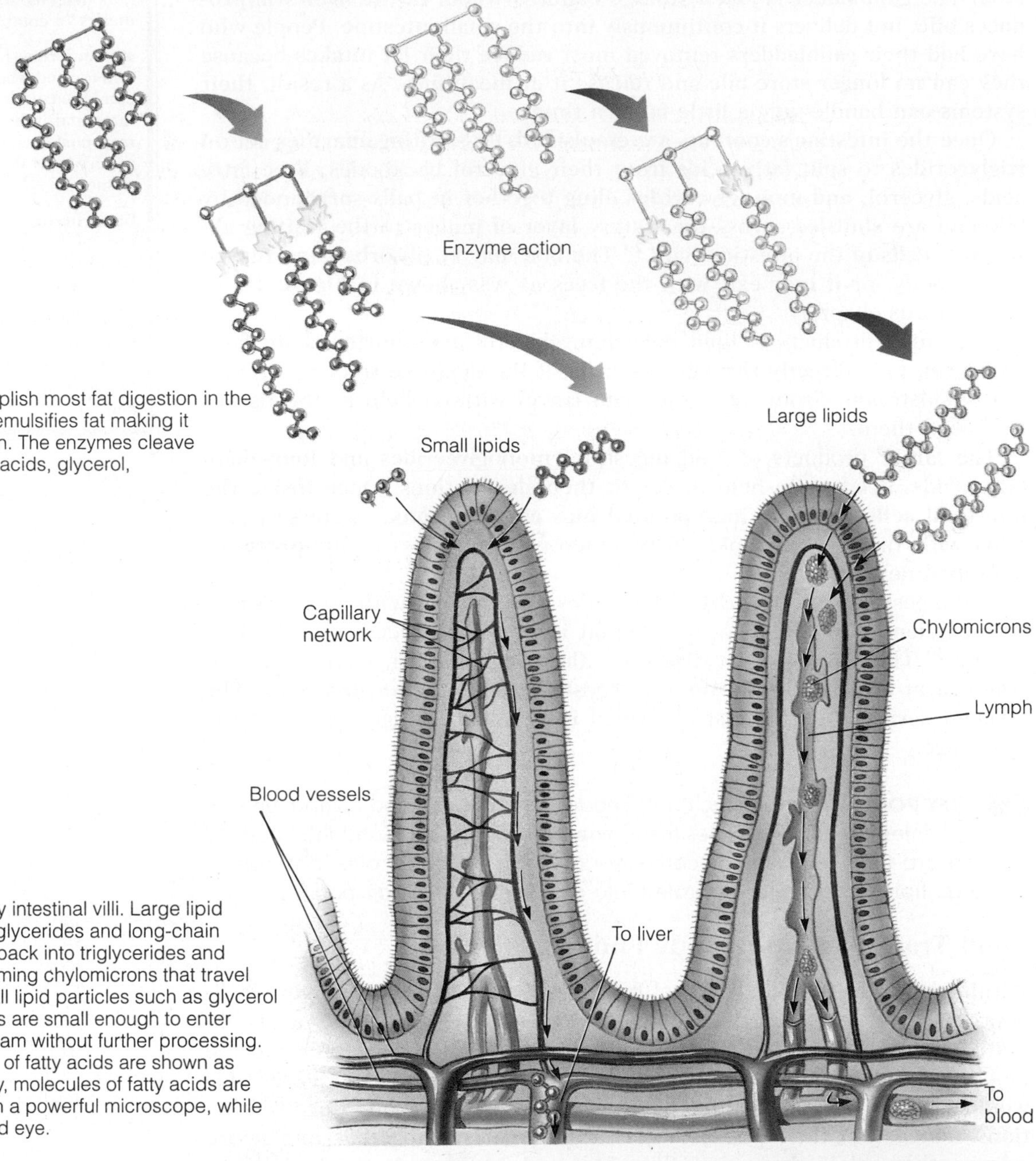

Inside the digestive tract:

Digestive enzymes accomplish most fat digestion in the small intestine where bile emulsifies fat making it available for enzyme action. The enzymes cleave triglycerides into free fatty acids, glycerol, and monoglycerides.

At the intestinal lining:

The parts are absorbed by intestinal villi. Large lipid fragments, such as monoglycerides and long-chain fatty acids are converted back into triglycerides and combined with protein forming chylomicrons that travel in the lymph vessels. Small lipid particles such as glycerol and short-chain fatty acids are small enough to enter directly into the blood stream without further processing. In this diagram,molecules of fatty acids are shown as large objects, but in reality, molecules of fatty acids are too small to see, even with a powerful microscope, while villi are visible to the naked eye.

HDL (high-density lipoproteins) lipoproteins, containing a large proportion of protein, that return cholesterol from storage places to the liver for dismantling and disposal.

high-density lipoproteins (HDL), which carry fats from body cells to the liver.* The carrier proteins for both are made in the liver and both carry large quantities of cholesterol; the HDL also carry many phospholipids.

Lipoproteins are very much on the minds of health care providers who measure people's blood lipid profiles. They are interested not only in the

*Another class of lipoproteins is the very-low-density lipoproteins (VLDL), an early version of the LDL. VLDL become LDL as they lose triglycerides and gain cholesterol.

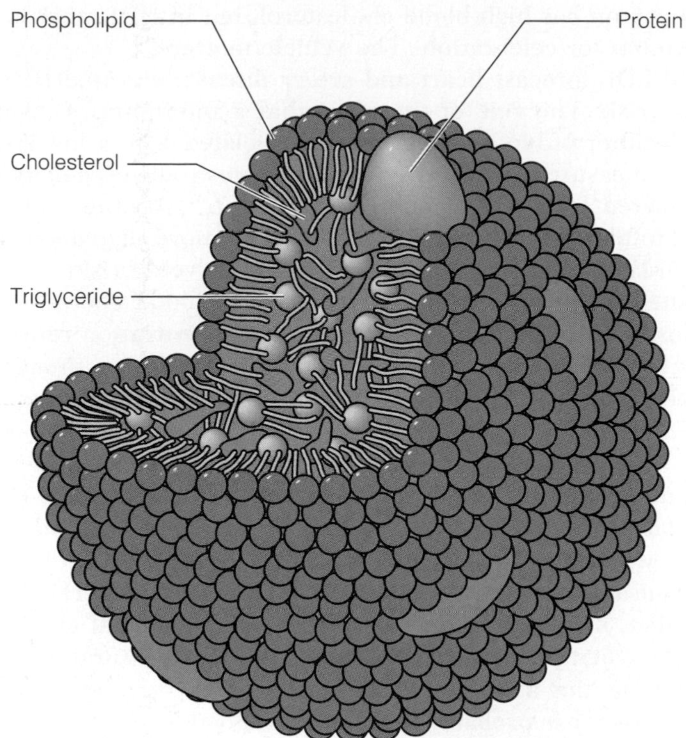

Figure 5-12

A LIPOPROTEIN

An LDL has a high ratio of lipid to protein; an HDL has the reverse—more protein relative to its lipid content.

types of fats in the blood (triglycerides and cholesterol) but also in the lipoproteins that carry them. One distinction among types of lipoproteins is of great importance because it has implications for the health of the heart and blood vessels. That is the distinction between LDL and HDL. The more lipid in the lipoprotein molecule, the lower the density; the more protein, the higher the density. Both LDL and HDL carry lipids around in the blood, but LDL are larger, lighter, and more lipid filled; HDL are smaller, denser, and packaged with more protein. LDL deliver triglycerides and cholesterol from the liver to the tissues; HDL scavenge excess cholesterol and phospholipids from the tissues and return them to the liver for disposal. Elevated LDL concentrations in the blood are a sign of high heart-attack risk, whereas elevated HDL concentrations are associated with a low risk.[31] The next section clarifies this relationship.

KEY POINT Blood and other body fluids are watery, so fats need special transport vehicles to carry them around the body, the lipoproteins. The chief lipoproteins are chylomicrons, LDL, and HDL.

Significance of LDL and HDL

As discussed earlier, cholesterol in foods contributes somewhat to cholesterol in the blood, and excesses of food cholesterol should be avoided. However, dietary cholesterol is not as influential in raising blood cholesterol as is total dietary fat and especially saturated fat, which the body uses to make cholesterol. Now the link to the LDL can be explained. When a person's high blood cholesterol signifies a risk of heart disease, it is because the cholesterol is carried in LDL and is traveling to body tissues to be deposited

there. If a person has high blood cholesterol, but in HDL, that is cause not for concern but for celebration. The vehicle matters.

Elevated LDL forecast heart and artery disease; elevated HDL signify a low disease risk. The rule of thumb is that a minimum of 35 milligrams HDL per deciliter of blood or plasma is associated with a low risk of heart attack. This measurement of HDL amount seems to be especially predictive when compared to the total cholesterol count.[32] Another rule of thumb states that total blood cholesterol should be no more than about four times higher than HDL cholesterol for an acceptable level of risk.

Fortunately, the changes in diet that reduce blood cholesterol concentration mostly do so by reducing LDL. HDL concentration remains for the most part unaffected. The most influential dietary factor thought to *raise* blood cholesterol is a high saturated fat intake.[33] Reducing total fat intake has little effect on blood cholesterol unless the reduction comes from saturated fat.[34] Among fats that *lower* LDL, monounsaturated fats, including olive oil and canola oil, stand out, especially when they take the place of saturated fat in the diet.[35] Other vegetable oils contain mostly polyunsaturated oils, which seem to be only neutral in their effects on blood lipids.[36] When polyunsaturated fat replaces some of the cholesterol-raising saturated fat in the diet, blood cholesterol levels fall. No beneficial change in blood lipids is seen when polyunsaturated fat is added to a saturated-fat rich diet. The heart-protecting action of omega-3 fatty acids from fish mentioned earlier in this chapter is probably unrelated to blood cholesterol.

Some health authorities say all adults should take steps to reduce their blood cholesterol; others say that only those medically identified as at risk for heart disease should do so. In any case, it seems desirable for most people's health's sake to limit saturated fat intake.

What about cholesterol intake? People respond differently. Dietary cholesterol has only a minimal effect on the blood cholesterol of about two-thirds of people. The other third must limit intakes to keep blood cholesterol from rising too high. Eggs, shellfish, liver, and other cholesterol-containing foods are nutritious, however. Cholesterol is unlike salt and sugar in this respect: it cannot be omitted from the diet without omitting nutritious foods. To raise HDL, people should exercise more, lose weight, and, for smokers, quit smoking.

KEY POINT Dietary measures to reduce LDL in the blood are to reduce saturated fat and substitute monounsaturated and polyunsaturated fats for saturated fat. A few people must also reduce cholesterol intake. Cholesterol-containing foods are nutritious and are best used in moderation.

Use of Stored Fat for Energy

When a person's body starts to run out of fuel available from food, it begins to use its stored fat for energy, and also its glycogen, as the last chapter showed. Fat cells respond to the call for energy by dismantling stored fat molecules and releasing their components into the blood. When energy-hungry cells receive these components, they break them down further into small fragments. Finally, each fat fragment is combined with a fragment derived from glucose, and the energy-releasing reaction continues, liberating energy, carbon dioxide, and water.

Thus whenever body fat is broken down to provide energy, carbohydrate must be available as well. Without carbohydrate, ketosis will occur, as de-

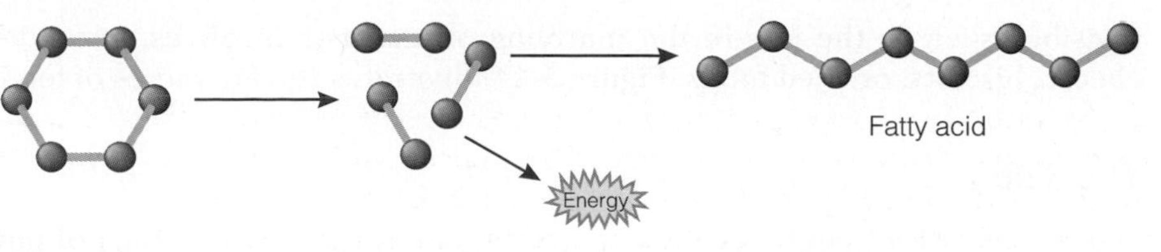
Fatty acid
Energy
Glucose is broken down into fragments.
The fragments can provide immediate energy for the tissues.
If the tissues need no more energy, the fragments can be reassembled, not back to glucose but into fatty acid chains.

Figure 5-13

GLUCOSE TO FAT
Glucose can be used for energy or can be changed into fat and stored.

scribed in the last chapter, and products of incomplete fat breakdown (ketones) will appear in the blood and urine. Because this process and its consequences are so important in weight control, Chapter 9 describes them in greater detail.

The body can also store excess glucose as fat, but this conversion is not energy efficient. Figure 5-13 illustrates a simplified series of steps from carbohydrate to fat. It shows that before excess glucose can be stored as fat, it must first be broken into tiny fragments and then reassembled into fatty acids, steps that require energy to perform. Fat, on the other hand, goes through fewer chemical steps before storage. Thus, given the same number of calories from excess dietary fat or carbohydrate, the body stores more calories from the fat than from the carbohydrate. In short, you may get fatter on fat calories than on the same number of carbohydrate calories. The Controversy that follows this chapter revisits this emerging theory and tells what, if any, significance it holds for meal planners who wish to control the amounts of energy contributed by fats in the diet.

Fat in the Diet

The remainder of this chapter shows you how to choose the right kinds of fat, and in the right amounts, to provide optimal health and pleasure in eating. To start, you must know where the fats are in the food groups.

Three food groups—fats and oils; meat, poultry, and fish; and dairy products—have traditionally accounted for about nine tenths of the fat in the North American diet. Recently people have shifted away from using mostly animal fats toward using fats of vegetable origin. The increasing consumption of vegetable oils has come about because of three factors: (1) their increased use by fast-food chains serving fried foods such as french fries and chicken, (2) a shift away from the use of lard (pork fat), and (3) a shift from butter to margarine. It is a healthy trend that people are choosing unsaturated over saturated fats in their diets. This is countered, however, by a high overall fat intake. Diets high in total fat, while not likely to elevate blood cholesterol, may be associated with high rates of some forms of cancer. Such diets also make obesity likely.

The exchange lists show exactly where the fats are in foods. Two groups always contain fat (the fats and the meats), and two sometimes contain fat (the milk and milk products and the breads). Vegetables and fruits are, if unprocessed, fat free. In their natural states, grains are like fruits and vegetables in that they contain little or no fat. Keep in mind that fats may be visible on foods, such as the fat trimmed from a steak, or they may be

Figure 5-14

FAT IN FOODS

3 g in 1 oz lean meat

8 g in 1 c whole milk

5 g in 1 pat butter or margarine

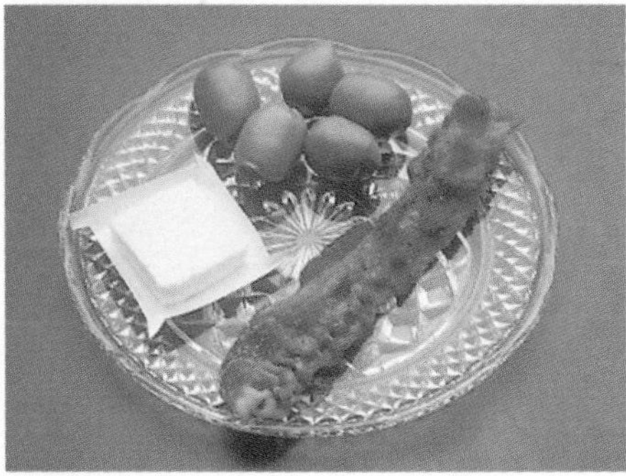

Fat exchanges. Each contributes 5 g fat.

One Exchange	Fat (g)
Milk (1 c)	
Nonfat	Trace
2%	5[a]
Whole	8
Meat (1 oz)	
Lean	3
Medium fat	5½[b]
High fat	8
Peanut butter (1 tbsp)	8[c]
Fat (1 tsp): butter, margarine, or oil	5
Vegetables	0
Fruits	0
Breads, starchy vegetables	0
Sugar	0

[a]5 grams of fat is equal to one teaspoon.
[b]This is often rounded off to 5 g for purposes of diet planning.
[c]The fat in milk and meat is saturated, but the fat in peanut butter is unsaturated.

invisible, such as the fats in the marbling of meat, or in olives, avocados, cheese, biscuits, or fried foods. Figure 5-14 illustrates the fat values of foods.

The Fats

One portion of fat contains about 5 grams (about one teaspoonful) of pure fat, donating 45 calories and negligible protein and carbohydrate. Examples are:

- A teaspoon of butter, margarine, or mayonnaise.
- One eighth of an avocado or five small olives.
- Two large, whole pecans or 1 tablespoon of French dressing.
- Two tablespoons of sour cream or 1 tablespoon of heavy cream.
- Ten large peanuts.
- A strip of crisp bacon.

Many are surprised to find crisp bacon listed as a fat. They know bacon fat is a fat, of course, but think of bacon as meat. Bacon is classified as a fat, however, because its protein content is negligible, even if it is fried crisp and the melted fat is drained away.

KEY POINT One portion of fat contributes 5 grams pure fat and 45 calories. Fats occur naturally in milk products and meats. Fat may be visible in foods or invisible.

The Meats

Meats conceal much of the fat, mostly saturated fat, that people unwittingly consume. Many people, when choosing a serving of meat, don't realize that they are electing to eat a large amount of fat. To help people "see" the fat in meats, the exchange lists present the meats in three categories according to their fat contents: lean, medium-fat, and high-fat meats. Meats in all three categories contain about equal amounts of protein, but because they differ in amounts of fat, their calorie amounts vary significantly. Figure 5-15 lists some examples of lean, medium-fat, and high-fat meats. The complete meat lists are in Appendix D.

A unit of meat on the exchange lists is only 1 ounce of meat. This is a very small amount of meat and is not a serving size; 3 or 4 ounces of meat is thought of as a normal serving size for meal planning. A small, fast-food hamburger, for example, weighs about 3 ounces (three exchanges). Of course, your judgment of what is normal differs from other people's, and you might have to weigh a serving or two of meat to see how much you are eating.

People think of meat as protein food, but calculation of its nutrient content shows a surprising fact. A big (4-ounce), fast-food hamburger contains 26 grams of protein and 35 grams of fat. Because protein offers 4 calories per gram and fat offers 9, the hamburger provides 104 calories from protein and 315 calories from fat. The sandwich calorie total is over 600 calories, with over 50 percent of them from fat. Hotdogs, fried chicken sandwiches, and fried fish sandwiches are also high-fat choices. Because so much of the energy in a meat eater's diet is hidden from view, people can easily overeat on high-fat fast-food choices, and as a consequence may find weight control difficult.

Figure 5-15

SOME EXAMPLES OF LEAN, MEDIUM-FAT, AND HIGH-FAT MEATS

Lean Meat	Medium-fat Meat	High-fat Meat
Beef tenderloin, round steak, chipped beef Chicken or turkey without skin Pork tenderloin, lean ham, Canadian bacon Fish Dry cottage cheese	Chuck roast, cubed steak, meat loaf Pork roast, chops Ground turkey Lamb chops, leg of lamb Liver Canned salmon, tuna in oil Eggs, ricotta cheese, mozzarella cheese	Hamburger, club or rib steaks, corned beef Pork spareribs, sausages Lunch meats Fried chicken or fish Most cheeses, American, Swiss, cheddar
1 lean meat exchange = 1 oz lean meat (3 g fat).	1 medium-fat meat exchange = 1 oz medium-fat meat (5 g fat).	1 high-fat meat exchange = 1 oz high fat meat (8 g fat).

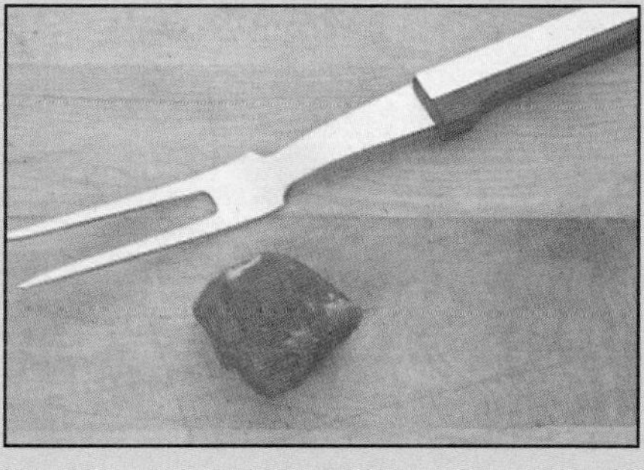

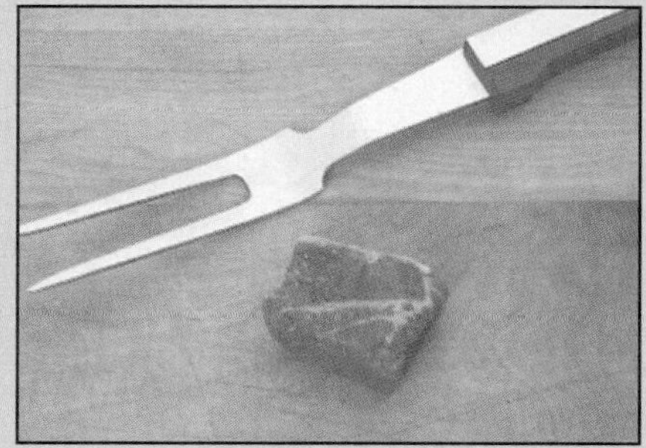

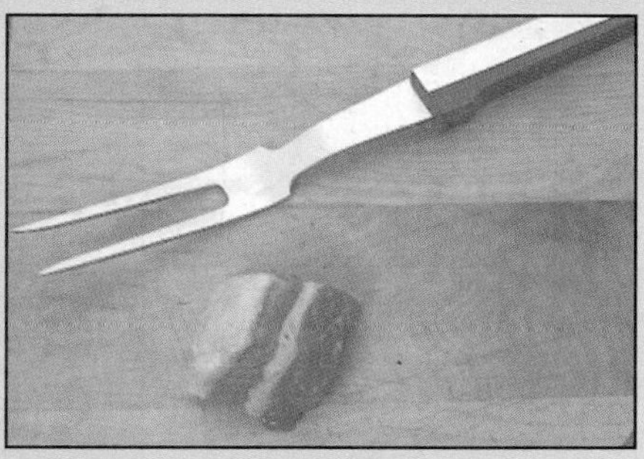

Figure 5-16 on the next page shows that while some fast-food choices can be remarkably high in fat and calories, other choices can be reasonable. Because fast foods are short on variety, let them be part of a lifestyle in which they complement the other parts. Eat differently, often, elsewhere.

Recently some animal breeders have begun producing beef and pork that are lower in fat. This is a help to those shoppers who choose lean cuts: they get less fat in the same quantity of meat. When choosing beef or pork, look for lean cuts named *loin* or *round* from which the fat can be trimmed. Eat small portions, too.

Chicken and turkey meat can also be lean, but processing and frying add fats, especially in "patties," "nuggets," "fingers," or "wings." Chicken wings are mostly skin, and a chicken stores most of its fat just under its skin. The tastiest wing snacks have also been fried in cooking fat (often a saturated type) and then smothered with a buttery, spicy sauce, making wings an extraordinarily high-fat snack. In the same way, watch out for ground turkey or chicken products. Many of these have the skin ground in, and they can be much higher in fat than even lean beef, as Figure 5-17 shows. Their labels may state "lower in fat," but ask yourself, "lower than what?" The box of terms that appeared on Chapter 2's page 53 provided some definitions concerning the fat contents of meats.

KEY POINT Many meats contain large quantities of fat. This is especially true of those that are marbled or have the fat ground in. Ground meats, and even ground turkey, are usually higher in fat than lean meat cuts from which the fat or skin can be trimmed.

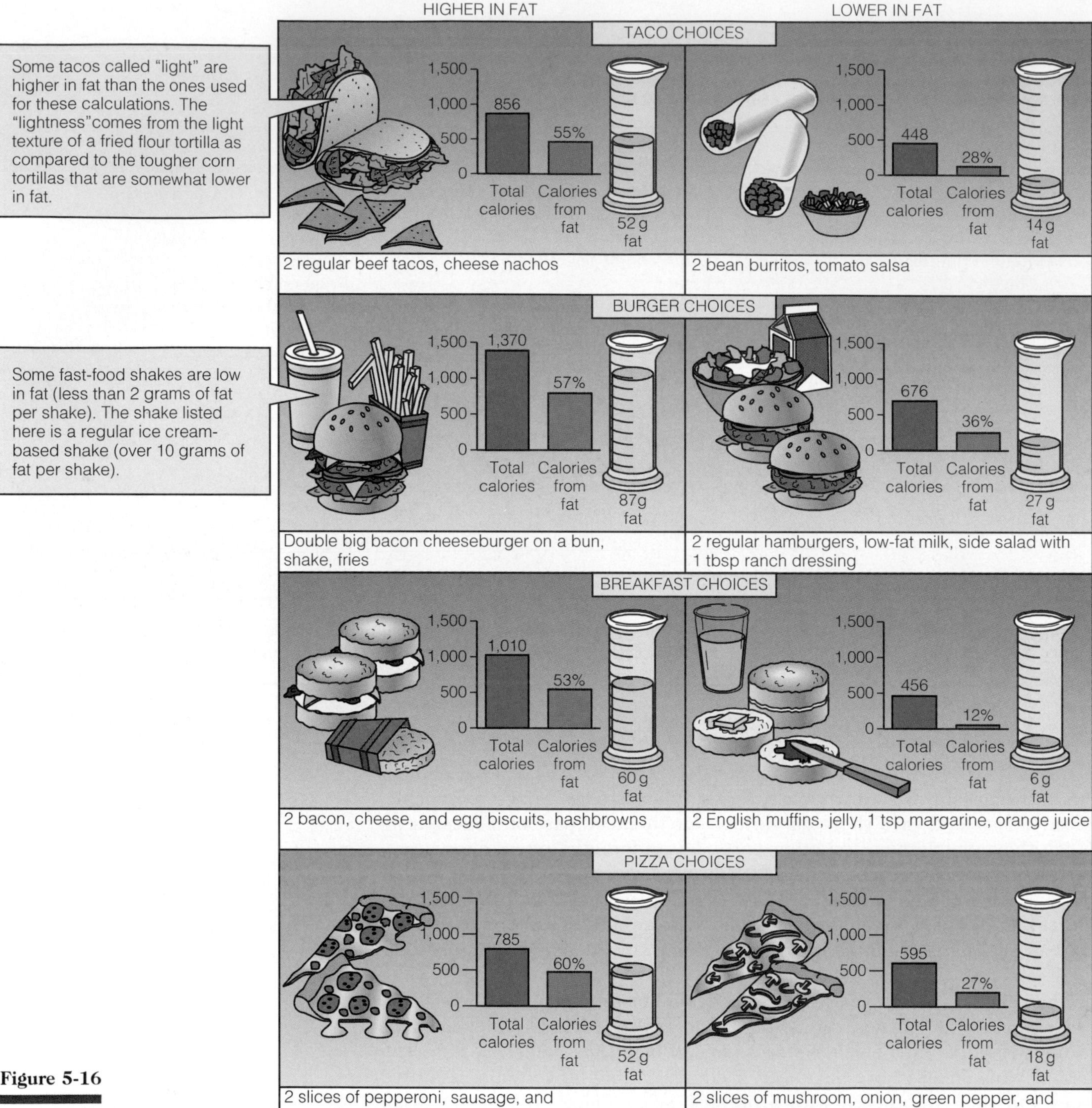

Figure 5-16

FAST-FOOD CHOICES

Other Foods

Figure 5-14 showed earlier that some milk products contain fat. The exchange system views nonfat milk (skim milk) as milk and whole milk as milk with "added" fat. This is because in homogenizing whole milk, milk processors blend in the cream, which otherwise would float and could be removed by skimming. The portion size is 1 cup. A cup of whole milk, then,

Figure 5-17

FAT IN GROUND MEATS

Note that only the ground round, at 7% fat by weight, qualifies to bear the "lean" label. To be called "lean," products must contain fewer than 10 g fat, 4 g saturated fat, and 95 mg cholesterol per 100 grams of food. The numbers that qualify products to be called "extra lean" are, respectively, 5, 2, and 95. The red labels on these packages list rules for safe meat handling, explained in Chapter 14.

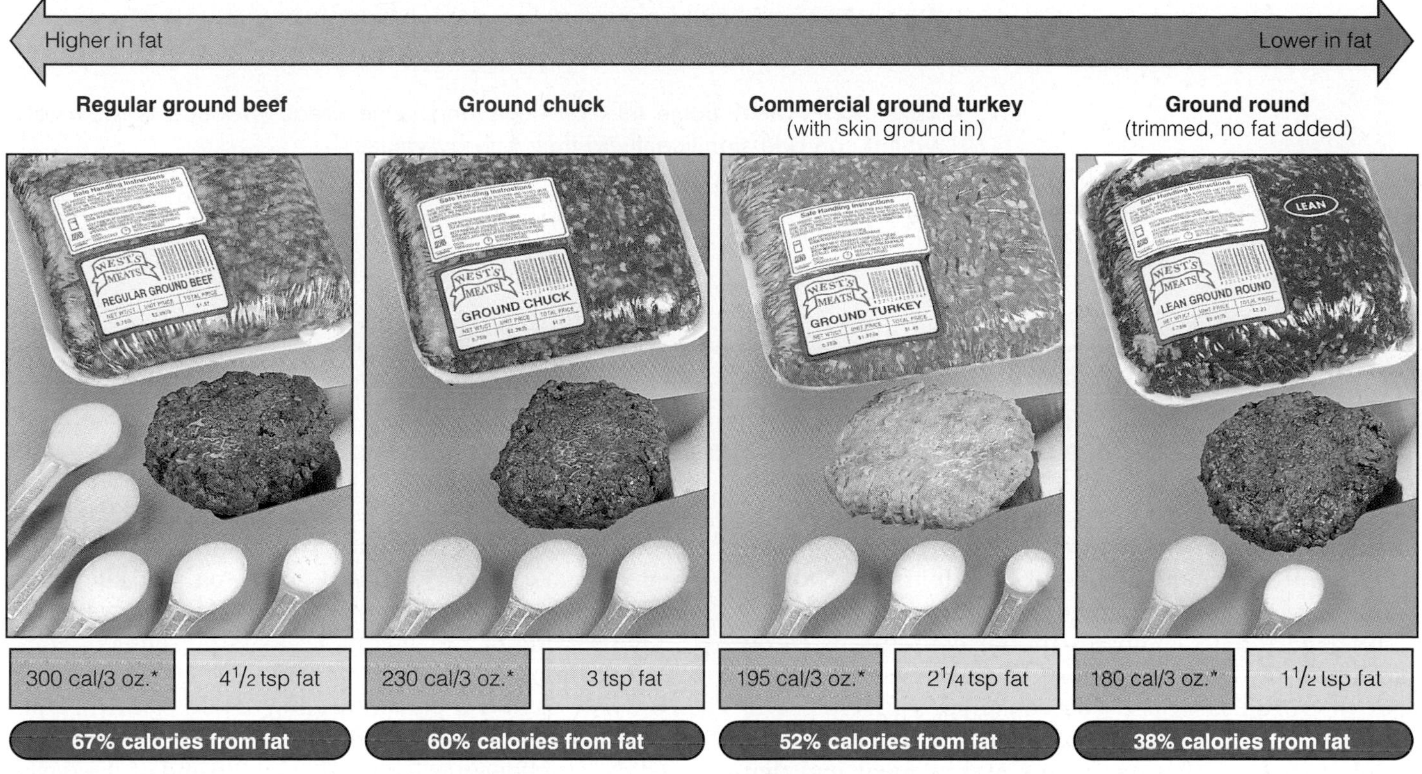
Higher in fat
Lower in fat
Regular ground beef
Ground chuck
Commercial ground turkey
(with skin ground in)
Ground round
(trimmed, no fat added)
WEST'S MEATS
REGULAR GROUND BEEF
GROUND CHUCK
GROUND TURKEY
LEAN GROUND ROUND
LEAN
300 cal/3 oz.*
4 1/2 tsp fat
67% calories from fat
230 cal/3 oz.*
3 tsp fat
60% calories from fat
195 cal/3 oz.*
2 1/4 tsp fat
52% calories from fat
180 cal/3 oz.*
1 1/2 tsp fat
38% calories from fat

*The three-ounce serving used here may seem small to some but it is the largest allowable meat serving according to the Daily Food Guide. Larger servings will, of course, provide more fat and calories than the values listed here.

contains the protein and carbohydrate of skim milk, but in addition contains about 60 added calories of fat. A cup of low-fat (2 percent) milk is halfway between whole and nonfat, with 30 calories of fat. The fat occupies only a teaspoon or two of the volume but nearly doubles the calories in the milk.

Milk and yogurt appear on the milk list, but cream and butter do not. Milk and yogurt are rich in calcium and protein, but cream and butter are not. Cream and butter are on the fat list, which also includes whipped cream, sour cream, and cream cheese. That is why the food group that includes milk is carefully called the "milk, cheese, and yogurt group," and not the "dairy group."

Bread products also sometimes contain fat. Notable are granola and other ready-to-eat cereals, croissants, biscuits, corn bread, dinner rolls, quick breads, French-fried potatoes, potato chips, snack and party crackers, muffins, pancakes, and waffles. Breakfast bars resemble candy bars in their fat and sugar contents.

It may be useful to look back at the set of meals displayed in Figure 2-9 of Chapter 2 to see how their fat contents match with recommended intakes. Chapter 4 praised Monday's meals for their abundant carbohydrate and fiber. The figure used exchange system estimates to determine amounts of fat in the meals and served as an example of how to do so. Vegetables, fruits, and starchy vegetables can be assumed to contain no fat, so the only foods to inspect are the meats, milk, grains, and fats.

Another useful feature of the exchange lists is that they separate the polyunsaturated fat items from the saturated fat items. Of course, which of these you eat makes no difference in the total calories coming from fat. It may, though, make a difference in the unseen condition of your arteries. Processed foods must now state on their labels their contents of total fat and saturated fat in grams, as the following special feature shows.

KEY POINT Some milk products and some bread products contain fat, which can add significantly to their energy values.

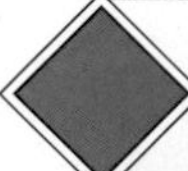

CHECKING OUT FOOD LABELS

How to Read Fat Information on a Food Label

Labels present a great deal of information about fats in foods to those who know where to look. Labels list total fat, saturated fat, and cholesterol contents of foods, in addition to total calories and fat calories in a serving. Here, Figure 5-18 compares the fat contents listed on the labels of three single-portion, microwavable packages of frozen lasagnas. The consumer's first piece of information comes from the names of the products, which announce that one type contains meat and that the other two contain vegetables but no meat. Notice that each package provides a single serving despite slight weight differences. This convenience allows consumers to compare the nutrients in similar single-serving products without taking the products' weights into account.

COMPARING CALORIES AND FAT CALORIES

The calories in the three lasagnas are the first numbers to compare. Lasagna A offers 472 calories per serving, with 252 of them from fat. Lasagna B offers 100 fewer calories in the same size serving, that is, 361 calories with 117 calories from fat. Lasagna C offers just 217 calories, with 9 of them from fat, also in a single serving, this time 11 ounces.

COMPARING TOTAL FAT

Knowing that fat contributes more than twice the calories of either carbohydrate or protein, gram for gram, you might make a guess right away as to which lasagna might offer the most and least fat. A glance at the total grams of fat in each will confirm your guess. You can make a final judgment when you read the label and compare each product to the day's fat allowance.

One serving of Lasagna A, a vegetarian choice, contributes almost half (43 percent) of all the fat allowed in a whole day for a person needing 2,000 calories. The person who chose this food for lunch could easily exceed the fat allowance for the day by the end of the day's meals. Surprisingly, Lasagna B, a meat-containing lasagna, provides only a fifth (20 percent) of the day's fat allowance. This choice leaves room in the day for some other servings of fat-containing foods. Lasagna C, another vegetarian choice, has been specially formulated to provide very little fat indeed—2 percent of calories from fat. With this choice, the eater need not worry about the fat it contributes to the day's total.

COMPARING SATURATED FAT AND CHOLESTEROL

For anyone wishing to avoid heart disease, the amount of saturated fat in a food is also of concern. One way to judge saturated fat in a food is to compare the grams of saturated fat in a serving, listed just below total fat, with the Daily Value for saturated fat. Conveniently, the label provides the percentage of the total allowable saturated fat for a 2,000 calorie diet in its "% Daily Value" column. Cholesterol is also expressed in terms of Percent Daily Value for a person consuming 2,000 calories. Clearly, these three foods vary widely in

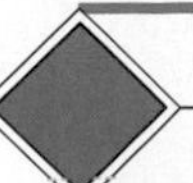

CHECKING OUT FOOD LABELS

How to Read Fat Information on a Food Label *continued*

Figure 5-18

COMPARISON OF THREE DIFFERENT LASAGNAS

A

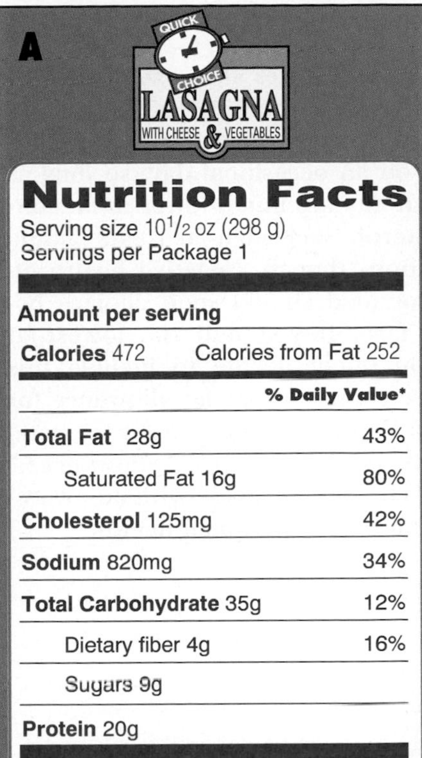

Nutrition Facts

Serving size 10 1/2 oz (298 g)
Servings per Package 1

Amount per serving	
Calories 472	Calories from Fat 252
	% Daily Value*
Total Fat 28g	43%
Saturated Fat 16g	80%
Cholesterol 125mg	42%
Sodium 820mg	34%
Total Carbohydrate 35g	12%
Dietary fiber 4g	16%
Sugars 9g	
Protein 20g	

Vitamin A 25% • Vitamin C <2%
Calcium 50% • Iron 10%

*Percent Daily Values are based on a 2,000 calorie diet. Your daily values may be higher or lower depending on your calorie needs.

	Calories	2,000	2,500
Total Fat	Less than	65g	80g
Sat Fat	Less than	20g	25g
Cholesterol	Less than	300mg	300mg
Sodium	Less than	2,400mg	2,400mg
Total Carbohydrate		300g	375g
Dietary Fiber		25g	30g

Calories per gram
Fat 9 • Carbohydrate 4 • Protein 4

INGREDIENTS, Skim Milk, Ricotta Cheese (Whole milk,Cream, Skim Milk, Vinegar and Salt), Cooked Macaroni, Spinach, Parmesan Cheese, Carrots, Onions, Butter, Soybean Oil, Modified Cornstarch, Bread Crumbs (Enriched Bleached Wheat Flour, Sugar, Corn Syrup, Partially Hydrogenated Soybean Oil, Salt, Yeast, Calcium Propionate, Spice Extractives and BHT),Corn Syrup, Long Grain Rice Meal, Potato Flakes, Malt, Yeast, Vegetable Shortening (Partially Hydrogenated Soybean Oil), Salt, Calcium Propionate, Nonfat Dry Milk Solids, Salt, Romano Cheese (made From Cow's Milk), Mushrooms, Sugar, Salt, Mono- and Diglycerides, Xanthan gum, Spices, Garlic Salt.

B

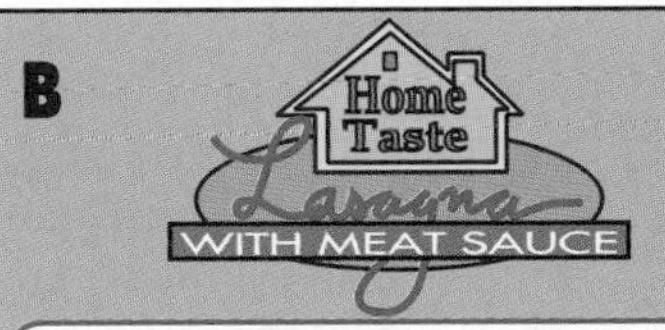

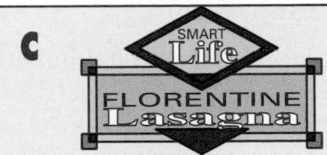

Nutrition Facts

Serving size 10 1/2 oz (298 g)
Servings per Package 1

Amount per serving	
Calories 361	Calories from Fat 117
	% Daily Value*
Total Fat 13g	20%
Saturated Fat 8g	40%
Cholesterol 87mg	29%
Sodium 860mg	36%
Total Carbohydrate 37g	12%
Dietary fiber 0g	
Sugars 8g	
Protein 26g	

Vitamin A 15% • Vitamin C 10%
Calcium 25 % • Iron 10%

*Percent Daily Values are based on a 2,000 calorie diet. Your daily values may be higher or lower depending on your calorie needs.

	Calories	2,000	2,500
Total Fat	Less than	65g	80g
Sat Fat	Less than	20g	25g
Cholesterol	Less than	300mg	300mg
Sodium	Less than	2,400mg	2,400mg
Total Carbohydrate		300g	375g
Dietary Fiber		25g	30g

Calories per gram
Fat 9 • Carbohydrate 4 • Protein 4

INGREDIENTS, Tomatoes, Cooked Macaroni Product, Dry Curd Cottage Cheese, Beef, Low-Moisture Part-Skim Mozzarella Cheese, Dehydrated Onions, Modified Cornstarch, Salt, Parmesan Cheese, Enriched Wheat Flour, Sugar, Spices, Tomato Flavor (Salt, Tomato Paste and Flavorings), Dehydrated Garlic.

C

Nutrition Facts

Serving size 11 oz (312g)
Servings per Package 1

Amount per serving	
Calories 217	Calories from Fat 9
	% Daily Value*
Total Fat 1g	2%
Saturated Fat 0g	0%
Cholesterol 10mg	3%
Sodium 500mg	21%
Total Carbohydrate 34g	11%
Dietary fiber 5g	20%
Sugars 10g	
Protein 18g	

Vitamin A 25% • Vitamin C 25%
Calcium 40 % • Iron 10%

*Percent daily values are based on a 2,000 calorie diet. Your daily values may be higher or lower depending on your calorie needs.

	Calories	2,000	2,500
Total Fat	Less than	65g	80g
Sat Fat	Less than	20g	25g
Cholesterol	Less than	300mg	300mg
Sodium	Less than	2,400mg	2,400mg
Total Carbohydrate		300g	375g
Dietary Fiber		25g	30g

Calories per gram
Fat 9 • Carbohydrate 4 • Protein 4

INGREDIENTS, Tomato Puree, Cooked Enriched Macaroni Product (Durum Semolina,[Niacin, Ferrous Sulfate, Thiamin Mononitrate, Riboflavin], Water, Egg White Solids, Disodium Phopshate, Powdered Cellulose, Soy Protein Isolate, Soy Protein, Vital Wheat Gluten, Guar Gum), Ricotta Cheese (Pasteurized Whey, Pasteurized Milk, Vinegar, Xanthum Gum) Tomatoes, Zucchini, Cheese (Pasteurized Skim-Milk, Water, Natural Flavors, Enzyme, Calcium Chloride, Salt and Vitamin A & D), Carrots, Spinach, Onions, Water, Mushrooms, Concentrated Dealcoholized Burgundy Wine, Sugar, Modified Food Starch, Salt, Spices, Microcrystalline Cellulose, Methylcellulose, Maltodextrin, Hydrolyzed Corn Protein, Xanthum Gum, Guar Gum, Autolyzed Yeast, Calcium Chloride, Citric Acid, Garlic Extractives, Dextrin.

CHECKING OUT FOOD LABELS

How to Read Fat Information on a Food Label *continued*

their saturated fat contents, providing from zero to 80 percent of the Daily Value.

INGREDIENT LIST

Cheeses, meats, butter, oils, and other fats appear on the ingredient lists of products in descending order of predominance by weight. Take a moment to find the fat contributors among the ingredients of each of the products shown in Figure 5-18.

ANALYSIS

To choose wisely among these lasagnas, a consumer must first identify some personal needs with regard to fat, saturated fat, and cholesterol. For example, if the chooser is an athlete with very high energy needs, has normal blood lipid values, has no family history of heart disease, and has trouble gaining enough weight, one of the higher-fat, higher-calorie choices is probably allowable within the context of a balanced diet. Should the person be concerned about high blood cholesterol or have a family history of heart disease, the best choice might be the lasagna lowest in fat, saturated fat, and cholesterol. This same choice might also be most appropriate for the person concerned about body fatness (see the Controversy that follows).

For most people, personal tastes also play a deciding role. If you relish the flavor of the high-fat choice, you probably will not sustain irreparable harm to health should you include it on an occasional day, so long as your other choices that day are much lower in fat, saturated fat, and cholesterol. Such high-fat treats should be used with moderation, though. Negative health effects would be compounded should such choices become standard daily fare. If you find the lowest-fat choice acceptable, you might decide to include this choice at lunch to save room in your fat allowance for a milkshake at dinner. You decide where best to spend your fat, saturated fat, and cholesterol "allowances." Just be sure that your choices are made with an awareness of their impacts on your nutritional health.

Fat Replacers

Fat replacers offer hope for the prevention and treatment of both heart disease and obesity. That hope is based on the assumption that a person using fat substitutes would use them *instead* of fats, not in *addition* to them. People may, though, use fat replacers the way they use artificial sweeteners, and may not reduce their total fat intakes. Or they may reduce their fat intakes but compensate with added calories from carbohydrate. Any reduction in fat may help to shift the body composition to the lean, even if calorie intakes remain steady.[37]

Food chemists have been working for decades on ways to reduce the fat in foods. Today, a thousand new reduced-fat products are among the grocery store choices. Innovations using traditional ingredients such as sugar starch, skim milk, soluble fiber, or egg whites in place of fat have been partly successful.[38] Fat-free bakery goods, cheeses, frozen desserts, and many other products are available that taste rich but offer less than half a gram (less than 5 calories) of fat in a serving. In comparison, a serving of a regular Danish pastry contains 12 grams of fat.

Fat-free products made with traditional ingredients may be tasty, but some people who have tried them say that something is different about them. That "something" is probably a feeling in the mouth that fat provides and that people have come to expect. The familiar flavored granules that mimic the tastes of butter, cheese, or sour cream do not provide the sensation of richness provided by the fatty ingredients they replace. Today, new artificial fats solve this problem by imitating the experience of eating fat—the creaminess as well as the taste—without the calories.[39] They also add tenderness.

Many laboratories are working to develop artificial fats, and a recent review named almost 20 currently under testing. One product the FDA has had under consideration for approval is a calorie-free fat replacement formerly known as sucrose polyester (SPE), now known by its generic name **olestra** (with a lower-case "o"). Olestra is a synthetic combination of sucrose and fatty acids, but unlike either, it is indigestible. Because the body cannot digest it, olestra passes through the digestive tract unabsorbed. Its presence in the digestive tract reduces blood cholesterol concentrations by interfering with fat and cholesterol absorption.

olestra a noncaloric artificial fat made from sucrose and fatty acids; formerly called *sucrose polyester.*

Simplesse the trade name for a protein-based, low-calorie artificial fat, approved by the FDA for use in foods.

Olestra looks, feels, and tastes like dietary fat and can substitute for fats and oils without diminishing the flavor of food, adding calories to the food, or raising blood lipid concentrations. It has the same cooking properties as fats and oils and can be used in products such as shortenings, oils, margarines, snacks, ice creams, and other desserts.

Scientific research on animals and human beings seems to support the safety of olestra as a partial replacement for dietary fats and oils.[40] An undesirable side effect of olestra is its interference with vitamin E absorption, so olestra products may be developed with extra vitamin E added.

Another fat substitute, this one made from protein, goes by the trade name **Simplesse** (with an upper-case "S"). It has been approved by the FDA for use in certain products, such as frozen desserts, mayonnaise, and salad dressings. Simplesse is fabricated by heating and blending proteins from egg whites or milk into tiny round particles. The particles create the *perception* of fat; the tongue perceives them as creamy.

Olestra and Simplesse differ in that olestra is a sucrose polyester, while Simplesse is made of protein. Both the body and the chef use the products differently, too. In the body, Simplesse is digested and absorbed, contributing to energy intake, but olestra passes through essentially unchanged. Simplesse provides 1⅓ calories per gram, a substantial reduction from fat's 9 calories per gram but more than olestra's zero calories. In the kitchen, Simplesse is unsuitable for frying or baking because it gels when heated. Olestra is heat stable and can be used in cooking.

The ideal fat replacement would look, taste, and cook like fat but would not add fat's calories. This is a tall order, but food chemists may be close to filling it.*[41]

*Three of the 20 or so other artificial fats under development are Stellar, made from cornstarch; Oatrim, an extract of oats; and Avicel, made from cellulose derived from wood pulp.

FOOD FEATURE

Defensive Dining

To meet the most important recommendation of almost every nutrition authority—to reduce dietary fats—most people would have to make changes according to the following five principles. The changes would also lower intakes of saturated fat.

1. Eliminate fat as a seasoning and in cooking.
2. Cut down on intake of red meat.
3. Remove the fat from high-fat foods.
4. Replace high-fat foods with specially manufactured lower-fat versions of those foods.
5. Replace high-fat foods with naturally-occurring low-fat alternatives.[42]

With these principles in mind, you can begin to make choices about foods in your diet.

The first arena of choice that you as a consumer face is the grocery store. The right choices here can save many grams of fat at the dinner table. Food labels can reveal much about a processed food's fat content. Once you figure out whether or not a food is high in fat, the choice of whether to consume it depends on how you intend to use it in your diet: as a staple item, or as an occasional treat.

Once at home, one of the most effective steps for reducing fats is to limit fats used as seasonings.[43] This means to omit butter, bacon, or margarine from cooked vegetables, to omit high-fat gravies and sauces, and to omit other last-minute fat additions. Butter and regular margarine contain the same number of calories (45 per teaspoon); diet margarine contains fewer calories because water and fillers have been added. Imitation butter flavoring contains no fat and few calories.

For snacks, use an air popper for popcorn, and then add butter flavoring to the popcorn, if you like it. Keep that flavoring on hand together with other low-fat cooking substitutes such as diet margarine, low-fat salad dressings, nonfat sauce mixes or recipes, and nonstick spray for frying. To replace high-fat ingredients in recipes, check Table 5-3 for hints. These replacements will not change the finished product too much, except for dramatically lowering its contents of fat and saturated fat.

Table 5-3
Substitutes for High-Fat Ingredients

Use	Instead of
Nonfat milk products	Whole milk products
Evaporated nonfat ("skim") milk (canned)	Cream
Yogurt[a] or fat-free sour cream replacer	Sour cream
Reduced-calorie margarine; butter replacers	Butter
Wine, lemon juice, or broth	Butter
Fruit butters	Butter
Part-skim or fat-free ricotta; low-fat or fat-free cottage cheese	Whole-milk ricotta
Part-skim, low-fat, or fat-free cheeses	Regular cheeses
1 tbsp cornstarch (for thickening sauces)	1 egg yolk
Low-fat or fat-free mayonnaise	Regular mayonnaise
Low-fat or fat-free salad dressing (for salads and marinades)	Regular salad dressing
Water-packed canned fish and meats	Oil-packed fish and meats
Lean ground meat and grain mixture	Ground beef
Low-fat frozen yogurt or sherbet	Ice cream
Herbs, lemons, spices, fruits, liquid smoke flavoring, or oil-free dressings	Butter, bacon fat

[a]If the recipe is to be boiled, the yogurt or cottage cheese must be stabilized with a small amount of cornstarch or flour.

If you must add fats, be sure that they are detectable in the food and that you enjoy them. For example, if you use strongly flavored fat, a little goes a long way. Sesame oil, peanut butter, and the fats of strong cheeses are equal in calories to others, but they are so strongly flavored that you can use much less. Try small amounts of grated sapsago, romano, or other hard cheeses to replace larger amounts of less flavorful cheeses.

If you do use oils, trade off among types to obtain the benefits different oils offer. Peanut and safflower oils are especially rich in vitamin E. Olive and canola oil present the heart health benefits associated with monounsaturates, mentioned earlier. Canola also contains omega-3 fatty acids. High temperatures, such as those used in frying, destroy omega-3 acids.

Here are some other tips to update old, high-fat recipes:

- Grill, roast, broil, boil, bake, stir fry, microwave, or poach foods. Don't fry.
- Add a little water or nonfat yogurt to thick, bottled salad dressings. They'll go farther this way and you'll use less oil.
- Cut recipe amounts of meat in half; use only lean meats. Fill in the lost bulk with shredded vegetables, legumes, pasta, grains, or other low-fat items.
- Trim all visible fat and skin from meat and poultry.
- Refrigerate meat pan drippings and broth, and lift off the fat when it solidifies. Then add the defatted broth to a recipe.

All of these suggestions work well when a person carefully plans, selects, purchases, and prepares each meal with the loving attention it deserves. But in the real world, people sometimes fall behind schedule and don't have time to cook, so they eat fast food. Fast foods can be extraordinarily high in fat because so many items are high in meat, are fried, or are made with whole milk. To maintain control of the fat in fast-food meals, review the choices presented earlier in Figure 5-16 and keep these facts in mind:

- Salads are a good choice. Use only about a quarter of the dressing provided or bring your own lowfat dressing.
- If you are really hungry, choose a small hamburger on the side. Hold the mayonnaise: use mustard or ketchup instead.
- Fried fish or chicken sandwiches are at least as high in fat as hamburgers. Broiled sandwiches are far less fatty if you order them made without spreads, dressings, cheese, bacon, or mayonnaise.

By this time you may be wondering if you can realistically make all the changes recommended for your diet and keep high-fat foods completely under control. Be assured that most of the needed changes can easily become habits after a few repetitions. You need not give up all high-fat foods; you need only learn to exercise moderation. The famous French chef Julia Child makes this point about moderation:

> *An imaginary shelf labeled INDULGENCES is a good idea. It contains the best butter, jumbo-size eggs, heavy cream, marbled steaks, sausages and pates, hollandaise and butter sauces, French butter-cream fillings, gooey chocolate cakes, and all those lovely items that demand disciplined rationing. Thus, with these items high up and almost out of reach, we are ever conscious that they are not everyday foods. They are for special occasions, and when that occasion comes we can enjoy every mouthful.*
>
> JULIA CHILD, The Way to Cook, 1989.

You decide what the treats should be and then choose them judiciously, just for pure pleasure. Meanwhile, make sure that your everyday, ordinary choices are those whole, nutrient-dense foods suggested throughout this book. Use the fat-reducing principles presented here to achieve a *diet* with an ideal percentage of fat, and room left over for favorite foods. That way you'll meet all your body's needs for nutrients and never feel deprived.

Notes

1. R. L. Leibel, Fat as fuel and metabolic signal, *Nutrition Reviews* 50 (1992): II12–II16.
2. All major nutrition, health, and governmental agencies concur on this point. For a dissenting view see T. L. V. Ulbright and D. A. T. Southgate, Coronary heart disease: Seven dietary factors, *Lancet* 338 (1991): 985–992.
3. K. K. Carroll, Dietary fats and cancer, *American Journal of Clinical Nutrition* 53 (1991): 1064S–1067S; D. F. Birt, The influence of dietary fat on carcinogenesis: Lessons from experimental models, *Nutrition Reviews* 48 (1990): 1–5; K. L. Erickson and N. E. Hubbard, Dietary fat and tumor metastasis, *Nutrition Reviews* 48 (1990): 6–14.
4. D. M. Hegsted, Dietary fatty acids, serum cholesterol and coronary heart disease in G. J. Nelson, ed., *Health Effects of Fatty Acids* (Champaign, Ill: American Oil Chemists Society, 1991): 50–68.
5. D. Kritchevsky, Preface to the PORIM International Palm Oil Development Conference, *American Journal of Clinical Nutrition* 53 (1991): V.
6. F. H. Mattson, A changing role for dietary monounsaturated fatty acids, *Journal of the American Dietetic Association* 89 (1989): 387–391.
7. C. A. Drevon, Marine oils and their effects, *Nutrition Reviews* 50 (1992): 38–45; A. P. Simopoulos, Omega-3 fatty acids in health and disease and in growth and development, *American Journal of Clinical Nutrition* 54 (1991): 438–463.
8. J. Dyerberg, Linolenate-derived polyunsaturated fatty acids and prevention of atherosclerosis, *Nutrition Reviews* 44 (1986): 125–134; J. P. Middaugh, Cardiovascular deaths among Alaskan Natives, 1980–1986, *American Journal of Public Health* 80 (1990): 282–285.
9. M. A. Crawford, The role of essential fatty acids in neural development: Implications for perinatal nutrition, *American Journal of Clinical Nutrition* 57 (1993): 703S–710S.
10. W. E. Connor, M. Neuringer, and S. Reisbick, Essential fatty acids: The importance of n–3 fatty acids in the retina and brain, *Nutrition Reviews* 50 (1992): II21–II29.
11. Age decreases the omega-3 polyunsaturated fatty acids of the retina, *Nutrition Reviews* 47 (1989): 87–89.
12. D. S. Lin and W. E. Connor, Are the n-3 fatty acids from dietary fish oil deposited in the triglyceride stores of adipose tissue? *American Journal of Clinical Nutrition* 51 (1990): 535–539.
13. A. P. Simopoulos, Summary of the NATO Advanced Research Workshop on Dietary ω-3 and ω-6 Fatty Acids: Biological effects and nutritional essentiality, *Journal of Nutrition* 119 (1989): 521–528.
14. M. D. Boudreau and coauthors, Lack of dose response by dietary n-3 fatty acids at a constant ratio of n-3 to n-6 fatty acids in suppressing eicosanoid biosynthesis from arachidonic acid, *American Journal of Clinical Nutrition* 54 (1991): 111–117.
15. Fish oil supplements, *FDA Consumer*, October 1990, p. 32.
16. K. N. Seidelin, B. Myrup, and B. Fischer-Hansen, n-3 fatty acids in adipose tissue and coronary artery disease are inversely related, *American Journal of Clinical Nutrition* 55 (1992): 1117–1119.
17. K. H. Bønaa, K. S. Bjerve, and A. Nordøy, Habitual fish consumption, plasma phospholipid fatty acids, and serum lipids: The Tromsø Study, *American Journal of Clinical Nutrition* 55 (1992): 1126–1134.
18. S. J. Bhathena and coauthors, Effects of ω-3 fatty acids and vitamin E on hormones involved in carbohydrate and lipid metabolism in men, *American Journal of Clinical Nutrition* 54 (1991): 684–688.

19. K. L. Fritsche, S-C. Huang, and M. Misfeldt, Fish oil and immune function, letter, *Nutrition Reviews* 51 (1993): 24.
20. G. T. Gerhard and coauthors, Comparison of three species of dietary fish: Effects on serum concentrations of low-density-lipoprotein cholesterol and apolipoprotein in normotriglyceridemic subjects, *American Journal of Clinical Nutrition* 54 (1991): 334–339; K. L. Radack, C. C. Deck, and G. A. Huster, n-3 fatty acid effects on lipids, lipoproteins, and apolipoproteins at very low doses: Results of a randomized controlled trial in hypertriglyceridemic subjects, *American Journal of Clinical Nutrition* 51 (1990): 599–605.
21. H. Esterbauer, Cytotoxicity and genotoxicity of lipid oxidation products, *American Journal of Clinical Nutrition* 57 (1993): 779S–786S.
22. B. Halliwell and S. Chirico, Lipid peroxidation: Its mechanism, measurement, and significance, *American Journal of Clinical Nutrition* 57 (1993): 715S–725S; B. Halliwell, J. M. C. Gutteridge, and C. E. Cross, Free radicals, antioxidants, and human disease: Where are we now? *Journal of Laboratory and Clinical Medicine* 119 (1992): 598–620.
23. O. Haglund and coauthors, The effects of fish oil on triglycerides, cholesterol, fibrinogen, and malondialdehyde in humans supplemented with vitamin E, *Journal of Nutrition* 121 (1991): 165–169.
24. M. L. Bierenbaum and coauthors, Effects of canola oil on serum lipids in humans, *Journal of the American College of Nutrition* 10 (1991): 228–233.
25. M. B. Katan and R. P. Mensink, Isomeric fatty acids and serum lipoproteins, *Nutrition Reviews* 50 (1992): 46–48.
26. R. P. Mensink and M. B. Katan, Effect of dietary *trans*-fatty acids on high-density and low-density lipoprotein cholesterol levels in healthy subjects, *New England Journal of Medicine* 323 (1990): 439–445.
27. M. G. Enig and coauthors, Isomeric *trans* fatty acids in the U.S. diet, *Journal of the American College of Nutrition* 9 (1990): 471–486.
28. M. Hamosh, *Lingual and Gastric Lipases: Their Role in Fat Digestion* (Boston: CRC Press, 1990).
29. A. B. R. Thompson, Intestinal aspects of lipid absorption, *Nutrition Today*, July/August 1989, pp. 16–20.
30. D. R. Saunders and J. K. Sillery, Absorption of triglyceride by human small intestine: Dose-response relationship, *American Journal of Clinical Nutrition* 48 (1988): 988–991.
31. NIH Consensus Conference, Triglyceride, high-density lipoprotein, and coronary heart disease, *Journal of the American Medical Association* 269 (1993): 505–510.
32. NIH Consensus Development Panel, Triglyceride, high-density lipoprotein, and coronary heart disease, *Journal of the American Medical Society* 269 (1993): 505–510.
33. D. M. Hegsted, Dietary fatty acids, serum cholesterol, and coronary heart disease, in *Health Effects of Dietary Fatty Acids* (Champaign, Ill.: American Oil Chemists Society, 1991) pp. 50–68; T. L. V. Ulbright and D. A. T. Southgate, Coronary heart disease: Seven dietary factors, *Lancet* 338 (1991): 985–992.
34. D. J. McNamara, Cardiovascular disease, in M. E. Shils, J. A. Olson, and M. Shike eds., *Modern Nutrition in Health and Disease* (Philadelphia: Lea & Febiger, 1994): 1533–1544.
35. Hegsted, 1991; K. R. Norum, Dietary fat and blood lipids, *Nutrition Reviews* 50 (1992): 30–37.
36. Norum, 1992; H. N. Ginsberg and coauthors, Reduction of plasma cholesterol levels in normal men on an American Heart Association step 1 diet or a step 1 diet with added monounsaturated fat, *New England Journal of Medicine* 322 (1990): 574–579; A. Bonanome and coauthors, Carbohydrate and lipid metabolism in patients with non-insulin-dependent diabetes mellitus: Effects of a low-fat, high-carbohydrate diet vs a diet high in monounsaturated fatty acids, *American Journal of Clinical Nutrition* 54 (1991): 586–590.
37. R. W. Foltin and coauthors, Caloric compensation for lunches varying in fat and carbohydrate content by humans in a residential laboratory, *American Journal of Clinical Nutrition* 52 (1990): 969–980.
38. Position of the American Dietetic Association: Fat replacements, *Journal of the American Dietetic Association* 91 (1991): 1285–1288.
39. A. Drewnowski, Sensory properties of fats and fat replacements, *Nutrition Reviews* 50 (1992): II17–II20.
40. K. L. Skare, J. A. Skare, and E. O. Thompson, Evaluation of olestra in short-term genotoxic assays, *Food and Chemical Toxicology* 28 (1990): 69–73; M. Kroger, Can we have our cake and eat it too? *Priorities*, Winter 1989, pp. 37–39.
41. No regulatory clearance needed for NutriFat (abstract), *Journal of the American Dietetic Association* 89 (1989): 426.
42. A. R. Kristal, A. L. Shattuck, and H. J. Henry, Patterns of dietary behavior associated with selecting diets low in fat: Reliability and validity of a behavioral approach to dietary assessment, *Journal of the American Dietetic Association* 90 (1990): 214–220 presents a validated food questionnaire that correlates well with fat intakes; similar principles for reduction of fat by way of meat and milk intakes are found in L. M. Smith-Schneider, M. J. Sigman-Grant, and P. M. Kris-Etherton, Dietary fat reduction strategies, *Journal of the American Dietetic Association* 92 (1992): 34–38.
43. A. R. Kristal and coauthors, Long-term maintenance of a low-fat diet: Durability of fat-related dietary habits in the Women's Health Trial, *Journal of the American Dietetic Association* 92 (1992): 553–559.

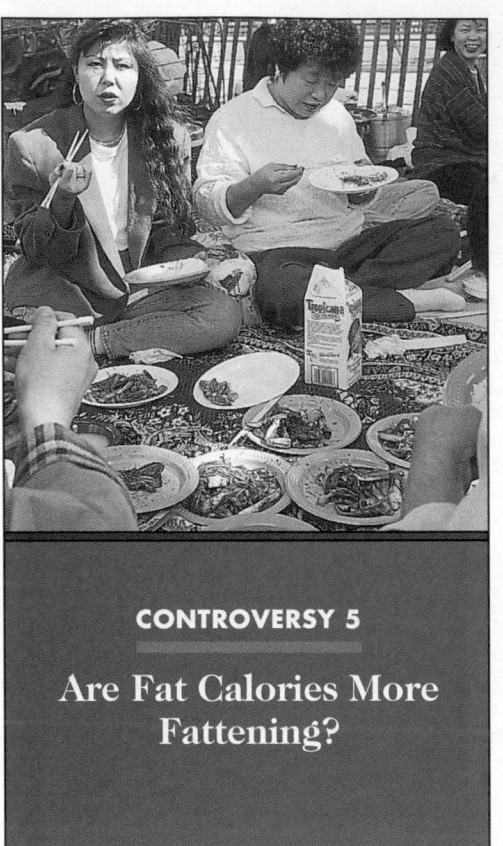

CONTROVERSY 5

Are Fat Calories More Fattening?

For years, nutritionists have taught that the body receives 9 calories from each gram of fat eaten and 4 calories from each gram of protein or carbohydrate. These are the amounts of energy that the nutrients in foods yield when a laboratory scientist burns the foods and measures the heat given off. Logic says that the body should derive the same amounts of energy from foods. After all, a calorie is a calorie, regardless of its source, right? But these tidy numbers pose problems for real people whose bodies do not act according to logic.

Scientists know, too, that each pound of body fat represents 3,500 calories of stored energy. It stands to reason that a person who eats 3,500 extra calories from any nutrient source should gain a pound, and that a person who cuts 3,500 calories from any source should lose a pound. This does not happen. People seem to gain more body fat when they eat extra fat calories than when they eat extra carbohydrate calories, and to lose body fat most efficiently when they limit calories specifically from fat. In short, it may make a great difference to your body fatness whether you choose extra potatoes or extra butter.

Researchers have been investigating the question whether the fat in the diet may influence body fatness more than the diet's total calorie count.[1] This Controversy explores this research.

HIGH-FAT DIETS AND OBESITY As often happens in science, researchers were testing an unrelated theory when they stumbled onto some interesting clues. A study designed to determine whether a fat-rich diet could lead rats to overeat proceeded normally.[2] Rats fed a high-fat diet (42 percent of the calories from fat) voluntarily ate a smaller quantity of food than rats given a lower-fat control diet; thus they consumed the same number of calories as the controls. It was as if the rats had internal calorie counters that determined just how much food they needed to eat to match the energy they expended. This was the expected result.

Then came a surprise. Even though both groups ate the same number of calories of food energy, the rats eating the fat-rich diet became severely obese. The fat-fed rats' body composition changed to over 50 percent body fat, whereas the control rats remained at 30 percent body fat. Thus, it appeared to the researchers that a high-fat diet would induce obesity even when food energy intakes were moderate—in rats, anyway. In rats, total calories eaten cannot explain body fat content; the fat content of the diet seems to play a role too.

This landmark study opened an enormous field of research on human beings. Scientists wanted to see whether people, too, control their calorie intakes with "internal calorie counters" and whether they store more body fat from fat-rich, than from carbohydrate-rich, diets when the calories from both diets are equal.

In one study women ate freely from three different diet plans: a low-fat diet (about 20 percent of calories from fat), a medium-fat diet (about 35 percent), and a high-fat diet (about 50 percent).[3] The foods in each diet plan were similar in taste and appearance; they differed only in the percentages of calories contributed by fat. The women turned out to be unlike rats in that they ate more total calories from the high-fat diet than from the lower-fat diets. The percentage of calories from fat in the diet influenced total calorie intakes strongly—the more fat in the food, the more calories of food energy the women consumed. The women did compensate a little; they did eat a little less total bulk of food when the diet presented more fat.

The reason why the women failed to compensate fully is that fat occupies so little bulk. For example, only 2 teaspoons of fat in an 8-ounce glass of milk nearly doubles the calories from 90 (in nonfat milk) to 150 (in whole milk). Therefore, to successfully keep calories constant while using whole milk in place of nonfat milk, one would have to reduce one's milk portion by more than half. The women did not cut down enough on total food, when the fat content was high, to keep calories constant. Their internal calorie counters were working, but not sensitively enough to prevent them from overconsuming calories, given high-fat foods.

As expected, the women's body weights changed as their fat and calorie intakes changed. Women eating low-fat diets lost weight, while women on high-fat diets gained. Whether the total calories, the total fat, or both were responsible for the weight changes was unclear. Not knowing that this question would arise, the researchers had not designed the experiment to answer it.

Other experiments on people, designed the same way, have produced similar findings. People do tend to overconsume calories when given high-fat diets.[4] This may help to account for the obesity seen in Americans, because the typical diet is high in fat.

WHAT CAUSES WEIGHT GAIN: FAT, CALORIES, OR BOTH? In the rat study described first, it was easy to see that calories of dietary fat contributed more to obesity than the same number of calories from carbohydrate. In human beings, it has been harder to tell what accounts for body fat accumulation. Scientists can control perfectly what rats eat, but often they can only observe and guess what human beings are doing. Because dietary fat contributes to energy intake so dramatically, researchers have difficulty distinguishing which has the greater influence on obesity development.

One group of scientists studied 155 obese men who were eating a "typical American diet"—about 15 percent of total calories from protein, 38 percent from carbohydrate, 41 percent from fat, and 6 percent from alcohol.[5] Their total average food-energy intakes (2,570 calories per day) fell short of current recommendations (2,900 calories per day).[6] Researchers found no correlation between total food-energy intakes and the men's body fat measurements. They did, however, find that the more *fat* a man ate, the fatter was his body and, conversely, that the more carbohydrate a man took in, the lower his body fat. These findings have been repeated over and over, and the consensus seems to be that when people eat diets high in fat, they tend to store body fat efficiently.[7]

Other studies have shown the same relationship holds true in women: those who eat higher-fat diets have higher body-fat contents than total energy intake alone would predict.[8] Once again the data suggest that dietary fat intakes influence body fatness independently of total energy intakes.

In still another study, researchers compared the body composition of 244 adults with the composition of their diets. Those people who ate the highest-fat foods had the highest percentages of body fat.[9] The researchers put these findings to work right away in an experiment on weight gain. They provided either high-fat or moderate-fat diets to men who were attempting to gain weight. To achieve the same amount of weight gain, the men eating high-fat diets required less time and fewer calories than those eating the moderate-fat diets.

UNDERLYING CAUSES OF BODY FAT ACCUMULATION
Research has begun to focus on the biochemical reasons for body fat buildup. What does the body do with the fat and carbohydrate from a meal? Researchers gave men mixed meals of moderate energy value, and found that their bodies used much of the carbohydrate for energy and converted much of the fat into body fat.[10] The underlying mechanism of the body's preference for storing fat over the other energy-yielding nutrients remains to be discovered.

A probable reason why the body stores fat so easily relates to the chemical similarities between food fat and body fat. To convert a molecule of food fat to body fat, the body need only disassemble triglycerides to fatty acids and glycerol, absorb the parts, and put them back together again. To convert a molecule of sucrose to fat, however, the body has to split the glucose from fructose, absorb both monosaccharides, dismantle them into small fragments, then assemble the fragments into fatty acid chains, and finally attach them to a glycerol backbone to make a triglyceride. This work demands many calories of energy. Thus the energy costs of converting dietary fat to body fat are far less than those of converting dietary carbohydrate to body fat. In general, converting dietary fat to body fat requires only 3 percent of the ingested calories; but the conversion of dietary carbohydrate to body fat requires 23 percent of ingested energy.[11] The body wisely chooses to store dietary fat rather than carbohydrate, for it is designed to conserve all possible energy at all opportunities.

Some energy escapes as heat when the body is chemically processing nutrients; the energy lost as heat is called the *thermic effect of food (TEF)*. Only the energy that remains after TEF is spent is available to the body to use immediately or to store as fat.

On average, a person spends about 10 percent of a meal's total energy on TEF, but this varies considerably, depending on the composition of the meal. As dietary carbohydrate increases, the TEF of the meal increases.[12] In contrast, as the percentage of fat in the diet increases, TEF heat production declines.[13] The body literally gives off more heat when a person eats excess carbohydrate than when the person eats the same number of excess calories from fat. Thus while the amount of energy available from foods (as measured in calories) may seem to be the same in diets of different composition, the *efficiency* with which the body uses or stores that energy may vary considerably, depending on the diet's composition.

Some researchers believe the composition of the diet to be as important a factor in the body's fat storage as total energy intake or exercise.[14] One researcher puts it this way, "The single most important thing you can do [to lose weight] is to get the fat out of the diet."[15]

CALORIE VALUES OF NUTRIENTS REVISITED On learning of the research results reported here, people wonder whether the numbers of calories they have learned to assign to grams of fat or carbohydrate are wrong. The numbers are correct for the number of calories of energy present in foods. They may not, however, accurately represent the numbers of calories the body actually derives from foods.

In attempting to determine more accurate numbers, researchers again studied rats. They compared the efficiency of carbohydrate, protein, and fat in providing the body with energy. When compared with carbohydrate (whose energy factor was assumed, as usual, to be 4 calories per gram), fat was so much more efficient that it appeared to provide the equivalent of 11 calories per gram. Of course, fat cannot provide more calories to the body than it contains, so researchers now are questioning the assumption that they started with—that is, the assumption that carbohydrate yields 4 calories per gram. Perhaps the factor for carbohydrate should be only 3 calories per gram. Although carbohydrate in food contains 4 calories per gram, the body may be able to derive only 3 calories per gram from it.

Clearly, from all of the experiments reported here, a diet's total calories are not the only variable that predicts whether fat will be stored or not. The total fat, the total carbohydrate, and the fat-to-carbohydrate ratio of the diet also matter.

A full discussion of why people gain and lose weight is presented later in this book. This Controversy has focused narrowly on the body's efficiency in handling various fuels from the diet. Besides diet composition and the extent to which the body is conditioned, other factors such as genetics, age, smoking, and alcohol intake also influence the body's metabolic efficiency. From what we now know about food fat, though, it is clearly wise for people concerned with weight control to habitually select low-fat, high-carbohydrate foods. This is the recommendation of every leading nutrition authority. It is one of the best ways to lower risks from diseases and to meet the body's needs for nutrients. Now we can add that it is probably also the way a person can control body fatness most easily.

Notes

1. K. R. Westerterp, Food quotient, respiratory quotient, and energy balance, *American Journal of Clinical Nutrition* 57 (1993): 759S–765S.
2. Some of the earliest reports of this effect were from E. B. Forbes and coauthors (1946); the study described here is L. B. Oscai, M. M. Brown, and W. C. Miller, Effect of dietary fat on food intake, growth and body composition in rats, *Growth* 48 (1984): 415–424.
3. L. Lissner, Dietary fat and the regulation of energy intake in human subjects, *American Journal of Clinical Nutrition* 46 (1987): 886–892.
4. A. Tremblay and coauthors, Impact of dietary fat content and fat oxidation on energy intake in humans, *American Journal of Clinical Nutrition* 49 (1989): 799–805.
5. D. M. Dreon and coauthors, Dietary fat:carbohydrate ratio and obesity in middle-aged men, *American Journal of Clinical Nutrition* 47 (1988): 995–1000.
6. Food and Nutrition Board, *Recommended Dietary Allowances*, 10th ed. (Washington, D.C.: National Academy Press, 1989), p. 33.
7. C. Bennet and coauthors, Short-term effects of dietary-fat ingestion on energy expenditure and nutrient balance, *American Journal of Clinical Nutrition* 55 (1992): 1071–1077.
8. T. E. Prewitt and coauthors, Changes in body weight, body composition, and energy intakes in women fed high- and low-fat diets, *American Journal of Clinical Nutrition* 54 (1991): 304–310; I. Romieu, Energy intake and other determinants of relative weight, *American Journal of Clinical Nutrition* 47 (1988): 406–412.
9. Tremblay and coauthors, 1989.
10. O. E. Owen and coauthors, Oxidative and nonoxidative macronutrient disposal in lean and obese men after mixed meals, *American Journal of Clinical Nutrition* 55 (1992): 630–636.
11. G. A. Leveille and P. F. Cloutier, Isocaloric diets: Effects of dietary changes, *American Journal of Clinical Nutrition* 45 (1987): 158–163.
12. R. S. Schwartz and coauthors, The thermic effect of carbohydrate versus fat feeding in man, *Metabolism* 34 (1985): 285–293.
13. Leveille and Cloutier, 1987.
14. W. C. Miller and coauthors, Diet composition, energy intake, and exercise in relation to body fat in men and women, *American Journal of Clinical Nutrition* 52 (1990): 426–430.
15. R. L. Atkinson, Role of diet in obesity treatment, an address presented at the North American Association for the Study of Obesity and Emory University School of Medicine conference Obesity Update: Pathophysiology, Clinical Consequences, and Therapeutic Options, Atlanta, Georgia, August 31–September 2, 1992.

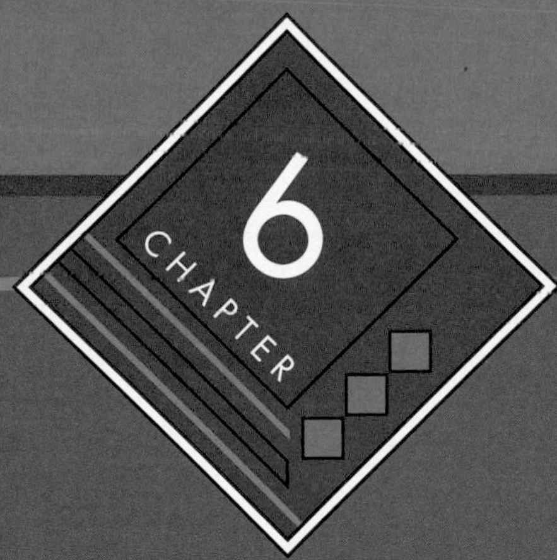

The Proteins and Amino Acids

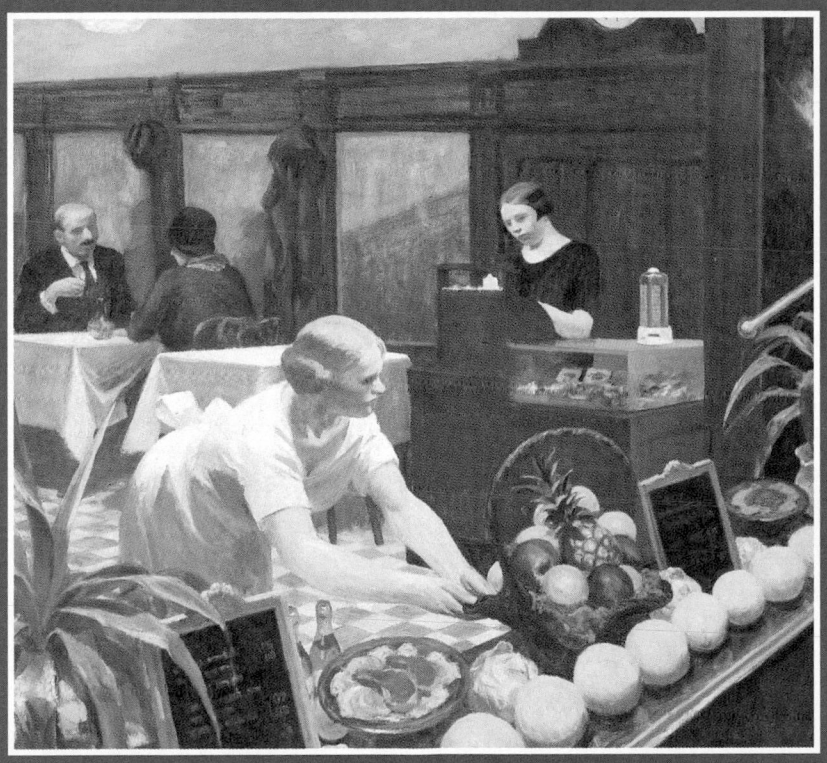

Contents

Edward Hopper, Tables for Ladies; The Metropolitan Museum of Art, George A. Hearn Fund, 1931 (31.62).

proteins compounds composed of carbon, hydrogen, oxygen, *and nitrogen* and arranged as strands of amino acids. Some amino acids also contain the element sulfur.

amino (a-MEEN-o) **acids** building blocks of protein: each has an amine group at one end, an acid group at the other, and a distinctive side chain.

6

The **proteins** are amazing, versatile, and vital cellular working molecules. Without them, life would not exist. First named 150 years ago after the Greek word *proteios* ("of prime importance"), proteins have revealed countless secrets of the ways life processes take place, and they account for many nutrition concerns. Why do we need to eat certain chemical substances (nutrients) and not others? How do we grow? How do our bodies replace the materials they lose? How does blood clot? What gives us immunity? Understanding the nature of the proteins gives us many of the answers to these questions.

Some proteins are working proteins; others form structures. Working proteins include the body's enzymes, antibodies, transport vehicles, hormones, cellular "pumps," and oxygen carriers. Structural proteins include tendons and ligaments, scars, the cores of bones and teeth, the filaments of hair, the materials of nails, and more. All protein molecules have much in common.

The Structure of Proteins

The structure of proteins enables them to perform many vital functions. One key difference from carbohydrates and fats, which contain only carbon, hydrogen, and oxygen atoms, is that proteins contain nitrogen atoms. These nitrogen atoms give the name *amino* (nitrogen containing) to the **amino acids** of which protein is made. Another key difference is that in contrast to the carbohydrates, whose repeating units, glucose molecules, are identical, the amino acids in a strand of protein are different from one another. A strand of amino acids that makes up a protein may contain amino acids of 20 *different* kinds.

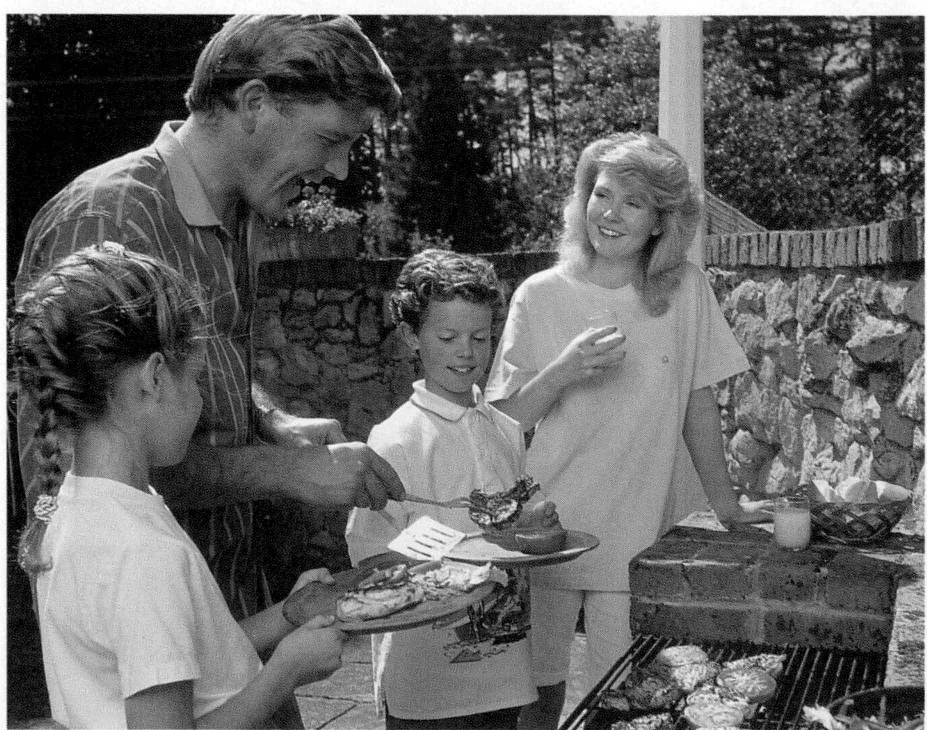

Hair, skin, eyesight, and the health of the whole body depend on protein from food.

Amino Acids

All amino acids have a simple chemical backbone consisting of a single carbon atom with both an **amine group** (the nitrogen-containing part) and an acid group attached to it. This backbone is the same for all amino acids. The differences among amino acids depend on a distinctive structure, the chemical **side chain,** that is also attached to the center carbon of the backbone (Figure 6-1). It is the side chain that gives identity and chemical nature to each amino acid. About 20 amino acids with 20 different side chains make up most of the proteins of living tissue. Other rare amino acids appear in a few proteins.

amine (a-MEEN) **group** the nitrogen-containing portion of an amino acid.

side chain the unique chemical structure attached to the backbone of each amino acid, that differentiates one amino acid from another.

essential amino acids amino acids that cannot be synthesized at all by the body or that cannot be synthesized in amounts sufficient to meet physiological need. Also called *indispensable amino acids.*

The side chains make the amino acids differ in size, shape, and electrical charge. Some are negative, some are positive, and some have no charge (they are neutral). The first part of Figure 6-2 is a diagram of three amino acids, each with a different side chain attached to its backbone. The rest of Figure 6-2 shows how amino acids link to form protein strands. Long strands of amino acids form large protein molecules, and the side chains of the amino acids ultimately help to determine their shapes and behaviors.

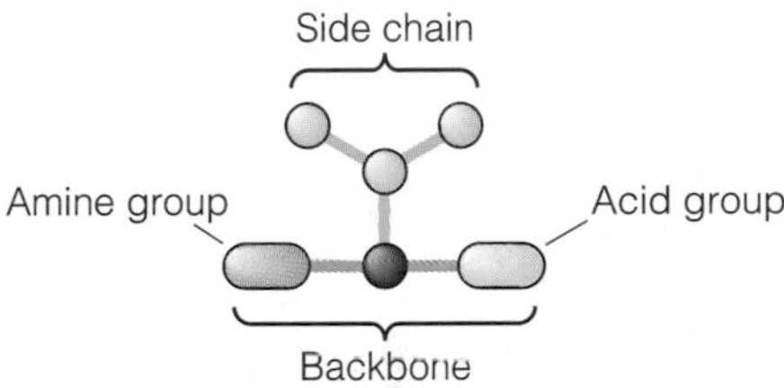

Figure 6-1

AN AMINO ACID

The "backbone" is the same for all amino acids. The side chain differs from one amino acid to the next. The nitrogen is in the amine group.

The body can make about half of the 20 amino acids for itself, given the needed parts: fragments derived from carbohydrate or fat to form the backbones and nitrogen to form the amine groups. Some other amino acids the healthy adult body makes too slowly to meet its need, or cannot make at all. These are the **essential amino acids.** Without these essential nutrients, the body cannot make the proteins it needs to do its work. The indispensability of the essential amino acids makes it necessary to eat often the foods that provide them.

The body not only makes some amino acids, but also breaks protein molecules apart and reuses their amino acids. Both food proteins, after digestion, and body proteins, when they have finished their cellular work, are dismantled to liberate their component amino acids. Pools of such

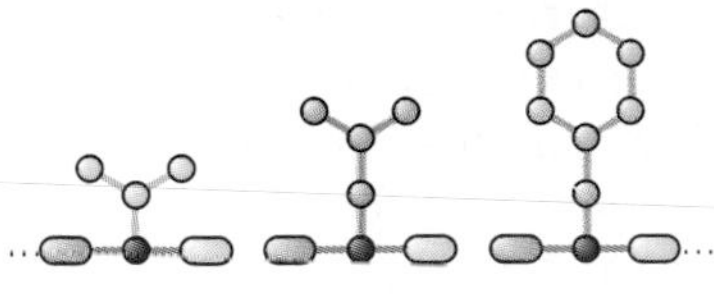

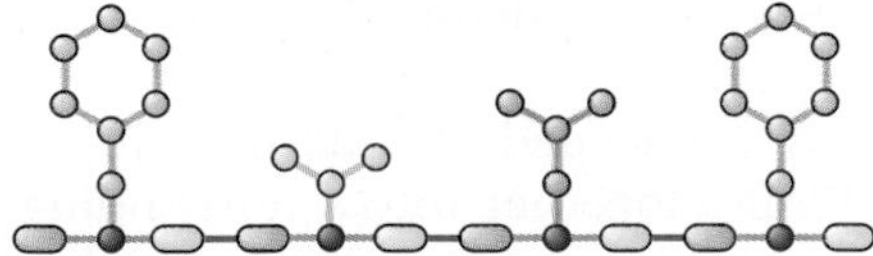

Figure 6-2

DIFFERENT AMINO ACIDS JOIN TOGETHER

This is the basic process by which proteins are assembled.

peptide bond a bond that connects one amino acid with another, making a link in a protein chain.

The essential amino acids:

- Histidine
- Isoleucine
- Leucine
- Lysine
- Methionine
- Phenylalanine
- Threonine
- Tryptophan
- Valine

Other amino acids important in nutrition:

- Alanine
- Arginine
- Asparagine
- Aspartic acid
- Cysteine
- Glutamic acid
- Glutamine
- Glycine
- Proline
- Serine
- Tyrosine

amino acids provide the cells with raw materials from which they can build protein molecules they need. Cells can also use the amino acids for energy and discard the nitrogen atoms as wastes. By reusing amino acids to build proteins, however, the body recycles and conserves a valuable commodity while easing its waste disposal burden.[1]

This recycling system also provides a sort of emergency fund of amino acids that tissues can draw on in times of fuel or protein deprivation. At such times, tissues break down their own proteins, sacrificing working molecules before the ends of their normal lifetimes, to supply energy and protein to body tissues. The body employs a priority system in selecting the tissue proteins to dismantle—it uses the most dispensable ones first.

Not only do amino acids serve as building blocks for proteins, they also perform tasks as amino acids. For example, the amino acid tyrosine forms part of the chemical messengers epinephrine and norepinephrine, which relay nervous system messages throughout the body. Tyrosine also forms the brown pigment melanin responsible for skin, hair, and eye color. It also forms the hormone thyroxine, which helps to regulate the body's metabolic rate. The amino acid tryptophan serves as starting material for the neurotransmitter serotonin and the vitamin niacin.

KEY POINT Proteins are unique among the energy nutrients because they possess nitrogen-containing amine groups and are composed of 20 different amino acid units. Some amino acids are essential, and some are essential only in special circumstances.

Proteins: Strands of Amino Acids

In the first step of making a protein, each amino acid is hooked to the next (this was shown in Figure 6-2). A bond, called a **peptide bond,** is formed between the amino end of one and the acid end of the next. The side chains bristle out from the backbone of the structure, and these give the protein molecule its unique character.

The strand of protein does not remain a straight chain. Figure 6-2 showed only a first step in making proteins, the linking of from several dozen to as many as 300 amino acid units with peptide bonds. The amino acids at different places along the strand are attracted to each other, and this attraction causes some segments of the strand to coil, somewhat like a metal spring. Also, each spot along the coiled strand is attracted to, or repelled from, other spots along its length. This causes the entire coil to fold this way and that, forming a globular structure, as shown in Figure 6-3. Other protein strands form fibrous structures.

The amino acids whose side chains are electrically charged are attracted to water. In the body's watery fluids they therefore orient themselves on the outside of the protein structure. The amino acids whose side chains are neutral are repelled by water and are attracted to one another; these tuck themselves into the center, away from the body fluids. All these interactions among the amino acids and the surrounding fluids result in the unique architecture of each protein.

One final detail may be needed for the protein to become functional. Several strands may clump together into a functioning unit; or a metal ion (mineral) or a vitamin may join to the unit and activate it.

The dramatically different shapes of proteins enable them to perform different tasks in the body. Those of globular shape, such as some proteins

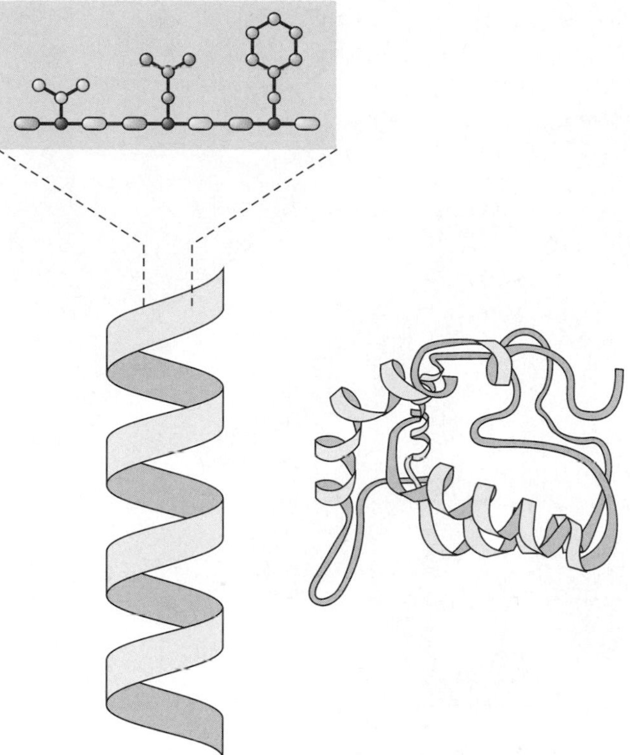

Coiling the strand. The strand of amino acids takes on a spring-like shape as their side chains variously attract and repel each other.

Folding the coil. Once coiled and folded, the protein may be functional as is, or it may need to join with other proteins or add a vitamin or mineral to become active.

Figure 6-3

THE COILING AND FOLDING OF A PROTEIN MOLECULE

of blood, are water soluble. Some are hollow balls, which can carry and store materials in their interiors. In some proteins, several springs of amino acids coil together and form ropelike fibers that can give strength and elasticity to body parts. Some, such as those that form tendons, are more than ten times as long as they are wide, forming stiff, rodlike structures that are somewhat insoluble in water and very strong. Still others act like glue. Among the most fascinating are the **enzymes,** which act on other substances to change them chemically. The variety of proteins is endless. A model of a single, large, globular protein molecule, the **hemoglobin** that carries oxygen in the red blood cells, is shown in Figure 6-4.

enzymes (EN-zimes) protein catalysts (also in Chapter 3). A catalyst is a compound that facilitates a chemical reaction without itself being altered in the process.

hemoglobin the globular protein of red blood cells whose iron atoms carry oxygen around the body.

The great variety of proteins in the world is due to the infinite number of sequences of amino acids that is possible. If you consider the size of the dictionary, in which all of the words are constructed from just 26 letters, you can visualize the variety of proteins that are designed from 20 or so amino acids. The letters in a word must alternate between consonant and vowel sounds, but the amino acids in a protein need follow no such rules. Also, there is no restriction on the length of the chain of amino acids. Thus there are many more possible proteins than possible English words. There may be as many as 10,000 different proteins in a single human cell, each one present in thousands of copies.

The sequences of amino acids that make up a protein molecule are specified by heredity. For each protein there is only one proper amino acid

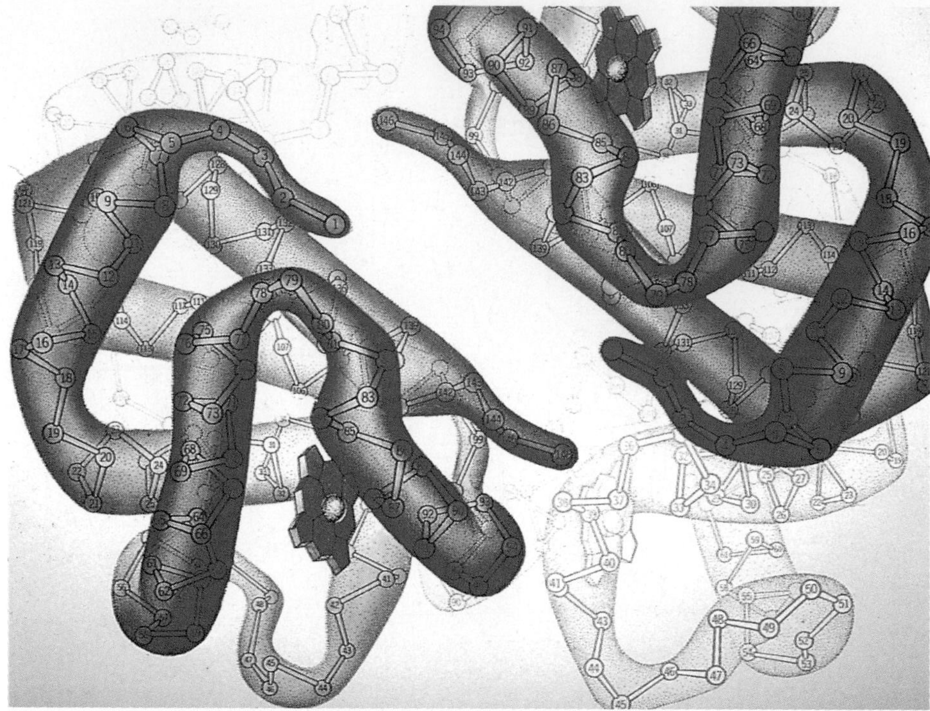

Figure 6-4

THE PROTEIN HEMOGLOBIN
The coiled and looped red structures are the globular proteins; the flat, jagged-edge objects are heme structures; the red center balls are iron atoms. This model represents a molecule of hemoglobin magnified 27 million times.

denaturation the change in shape of a protein brought about by heat, acid, base, alcohol, heavy metals, or other agents.

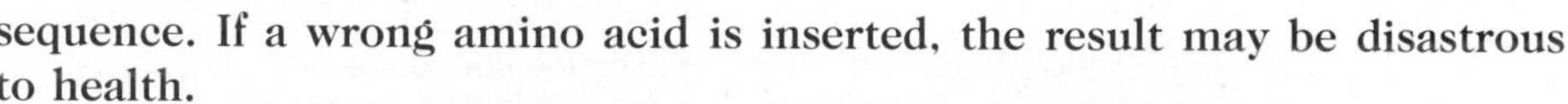

sequence. If a wrong amino acid is inserted, the result may be disastrous to health.

Sickle-cell disease, in which hemoglobin, the oxygen-carrying protein of the red blood cells, is abnormal, is an example of an inherited mistake in the amino acid sequence. Normal hemoglobin contains two kinds of chains. One of the chains in sickle-cell hemoglobin is an exact copy of that in normal hemoglobin. But in the other chain, the sixth amino acid, which should be glutamine, is replaced by valine. The protein is so altered that it is unable to carry and to release oxygen. The red blood cells collapse into crescent shapes instead of remaining disk shaped, as they normally do (Figure 6-5). If too many abnormal, crescent-shaped cells appear in the blood, the result is illness and death. One way to detect the disease is to observe the altered red blood cells under the microscope.

Each person is different from any other human being. What makes you unique are minute differences in your body proteins. These differences are determined by the amino acid sequences of your proteins, which are written into the genetic code you inherited from your parents and they from theirs. At conception each person receives a unique combination of genes. The genes, passed down to a cell from its parent cell, direct the making of all the body's proteins, as shown in Figure 6-6. Notice that genes determine the sequences of the amino acids in the finished protein. Figure 6-7 on page 186 shows genes being copied in preparation for protein synthesis.

KEY POINT Amino acids link into long strands that coil and fold to make a wide variety of different proteins. Each type of protein has a distinctive sequence of amino acids and so has great specificity.

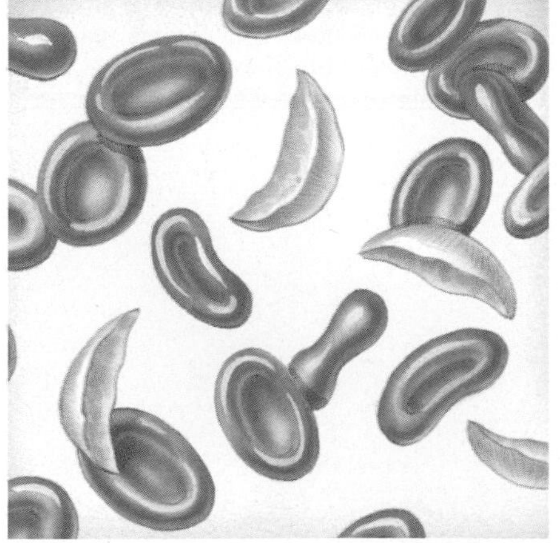

Figure 6-5

NORMAL RED BLOOD CELLS AND SICKLE CELLS

Denaturation of Proteins

Proteins can undergo **denaturation** (distortion of shape) by heat, alcohol, acids, bases, or the salts of heavy metals. The denaturation of a protein is

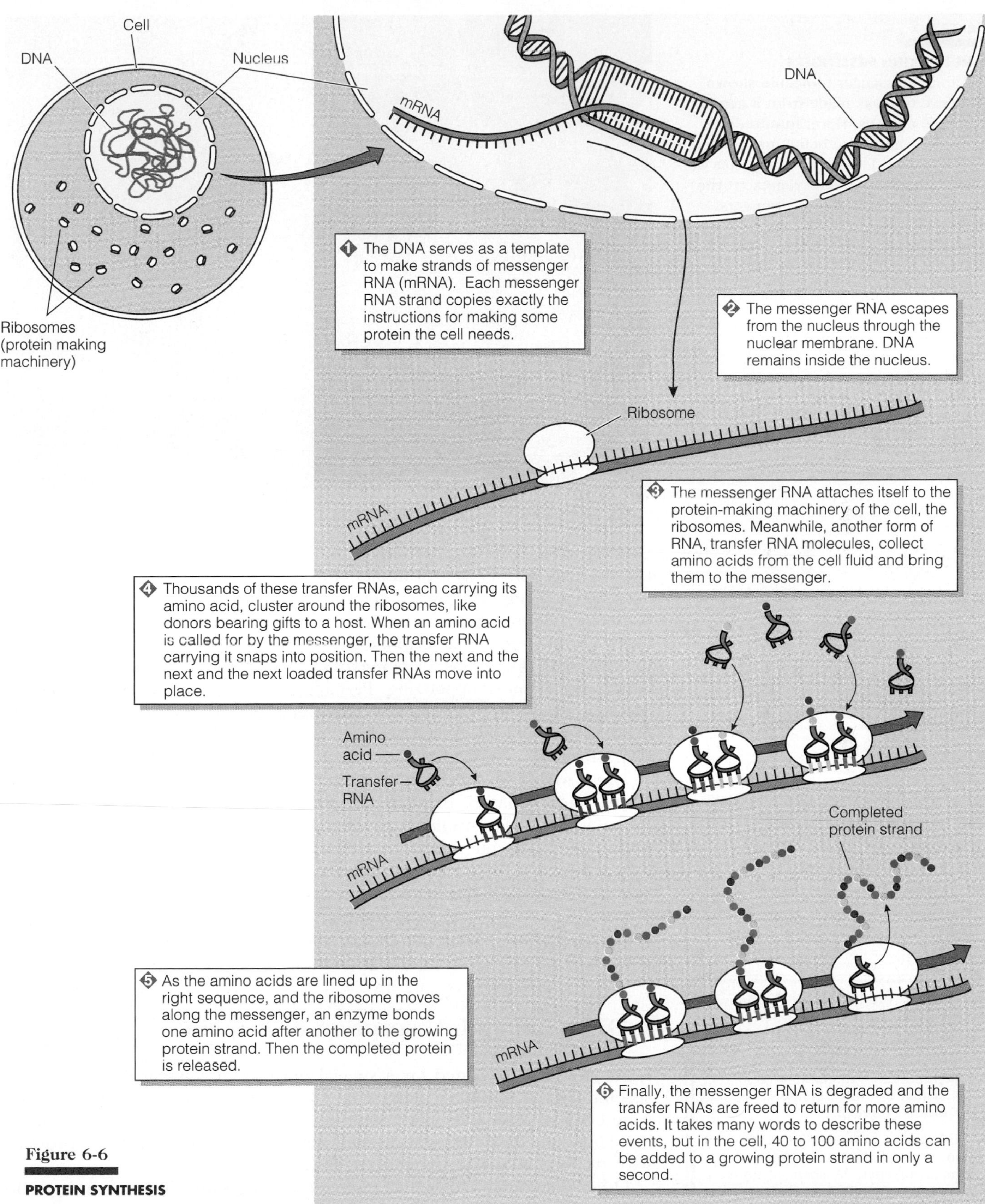

Cell
DNA
Nucleus
Ribosomes (protein making machinery)
mRNA
DNA
1 The DNA serves as a template to make strands of messenger RNA (mRNA). Each messenger RNA strand copies exactly the instructions for making some protein the cell needs.
2 The messenger RNA escapes from the nucleus through the nuclear membrane. DNA remains inside the nucleus.
Ribosome
mRNA
3 The messenger RNA attaches itself to the protein-making machinery of the cell, the ribosomes. Meanwhile, another form of RNA, transfer RNA molecules, collect amino acids from the cell fluid and bring them to the messenger.
4 Thousands of these transfer RNAs, each carrying its amino acid, cluster around the ribosomes, like donors bearing gifts to a host. When an amino acid is called for by the messenger, the transfer RNA carrying it snaps into position. Then the next and the next and the next loaded transfer RNAs move into place.
Amino acid
Transfer RNA
mRNA
Completed protein strand
5 As the amino acids are lined up in the right sequence, and the ribosome moves along the messenger, an enzyme bonds one amino acid after another to the growing protein strand. Then the completed protein is released.
mRNA
6 Finally, the messenger RNA is degraded and the transfer RNAs are freed to return for more amino acids. It takes many words to describe these events, but in the cell, 40 to 100 amino acids can be added to a growing protein strand in only a second.

Figure 6-6

PROTEIN SYNTHESIS

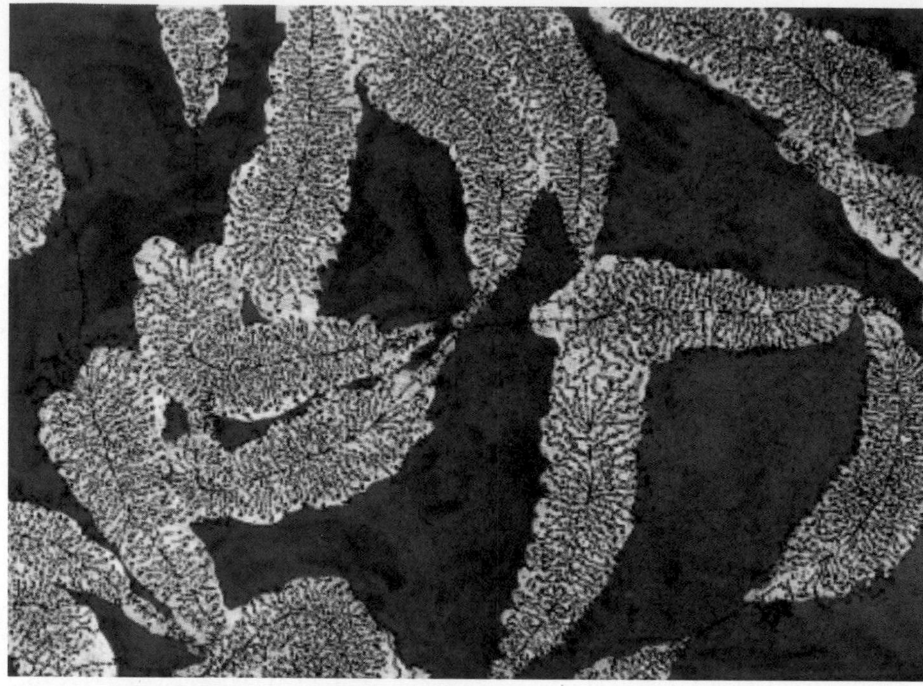

Figure 6-7

GENES MAKING MESSENGERS

The long messenger molecule shown in Figure 6-6 was made from a gene in the cell's nucleus. Here, hundreds of such messengers are being made from several genes. The longest branches on these "Christmas trees" represent the most nearly completed messengers.

the first step in its destruction; thus these agents are dangerous because they damage the body's proteins. However, in digestion, denaturation is useful to the body. During the digestion of a food protein, the stomach acid opens up the protein's structure, permitting digestive enzymes to make contact with the peptide bonds and cleave them. Denaturation also occurs during the cooking of foods. Cooking an egg denatures the proteins of the egg and makes it more appetizing. Perhaps more importantly, cooking denatures two raw-egg proteins: one that binds the B vitamin biotin and the mineral iron and another that slows protein digestion. Thus cooking eggs liberates biotin and iron and aids digestion.

Many well-known poisons are salts of heavy metals like mercury and silver; these denature proteins wherever they touch them. The common first-aid remedy for swallowing a heavy-metal poison is to drink milk. The poison then acts on the protein of the milk rather than on the protein tissues of the mouth, esophagus, and stomach. Later, vomiting is induced to expel the poison that has combined with the milk.

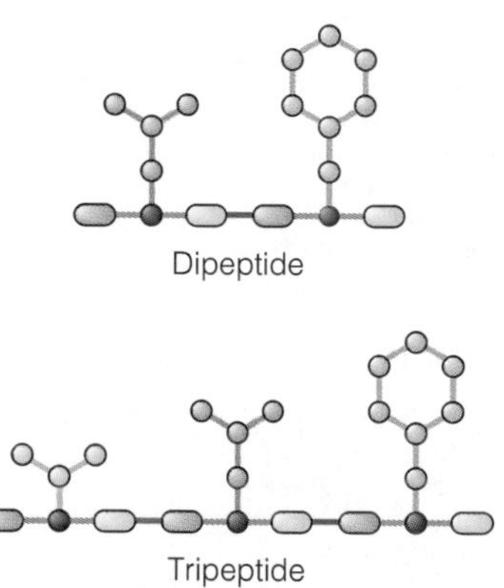

Figure 6-8

A DIPEPTIDE AND TRIPEPTIDE

KEY POINT Proteins can be denatured by heat, acid, bases, alcohol, or the salts of heavy metals. Denaturation may destroy body proteins.

dipeptides (dye-PEP-tides) protein fragments that are two amino acids long. A *peptide* is a strand of amino acids (*di* means "two").

tripeptides (try-PEP-tides) protein fragments that are three amino acids long (*tri* means "three").

polypeptides protein fragments of many (more than ten) amino acids bonded together. (A chain of between four and ten is called an *oligopeptide.*)

Digestion and Absorption of Protein

Each protein is designed for a special purpose in a particular tissue of a specific kind of animal or plant. When a person eats food proteins, whether from cereals, vegetables, beef, fish, or cheese, the body must alter them by breaking them down into amino acids before rearranging them into proteins with its own unique amino acid sequences.

Other than being crushed and moistened with saliva in the mouth, nothing happens to protein until it reaches the very strong acid of the stomach.

There the acid helps to uncoil the protein's tangled strands so that molecules of the stomach's protein-digesting enzyme can attack the peptide bonds. You might expect that the stomach's enzyme itself, being a protein, would be denatured by the stomach's acid. Unlike most enzymes, though, the stomach's enzyme functions best in an acid environment. Its job is to break apart other protein strands into smaller pieces. The stomach lining, which is also made partly of protein, is protected against attack by acid and enzymes by a coat of mucus, secreted by its cells.

Digestion

The whole process of digestion is an ingenious solution to a complex problem. Proteins (enzymes), activated by acid, digest proteins from food, denatured by acid. The mucous coating of the stomach wall protects *its* proteins from being affected by either acid or enzymes. The acid in the stomach is so strong (pH 1.5) that no food is acid enough to make it stronger; the pH of pure vinegar is about 3. It is obvious from this that the stomach is supposed to be acid to do its job.

By the time most proteins slip from the stomach into the small intestine, they are already broken into smaller pieces. Some are single amino acids, some are strands of two or three amino acids (**dipeptides** and **tripeptides**). The majority are longer chains **(polypeptides),** and a few are whole proteins. In the small intestine, alkaline juice from the pancreas neutralizes the acid delivered by the stomach. The pH rises to about 7 (neutral), enabling the next enzyme team to accomplish the final breakdown of the strands. Protein-digesting enzymes from the pancreas and intestine continue working until almost all pieces of protein are broken into small fragments and more single amino acids. Figure 6-8 shows a dipeptide and a tripeptide, and the whole process is summarized in Figure 6-9.

Absorption

The cells all along the small intestine absorb single amino acids. As for dipeptides and tripeptides, the cells that line the small intestine have enzymes on their surfaces that split most of them into single amino acids, and the cells absorb them, too. Then the cells release all the single amino acids into the bloodstream. A few dipeptides, tripeptides, and even larger molecules can escape the digestion process altogether and cross the digestive tract wall to enter the bloodstream. It is thought that these large particles may act as hormones to regulate body functions and provide the body with information about the environment. The larger molecules also may play a role in food allergy via the immune response.[2]

The cells of the small intestine possess different sites for the absorption of different classes of amino acids. Amino acids of the same class compete for the same absorption sites. This means that when a person ingests a large dose of any single amino acid, that one may limit absorption of others in its class. The Consumer Caution entitled "Protein and Amino Acid Supplements" cautions against using single amino acids, partly for this reason.

Once they are circulating in the bloodstream, amino acids are available to be taken up by any cell of the body. The body cells then make proteins,

Mouth

The mouth moistens and crushes protein structures in food.

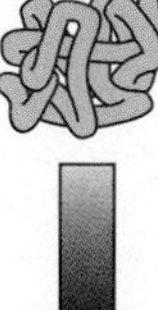

Stomach

Acid denatures protein strands and an enzyme cleaves amino acid strands into dipeptides, tripeptides, and polypeptides.

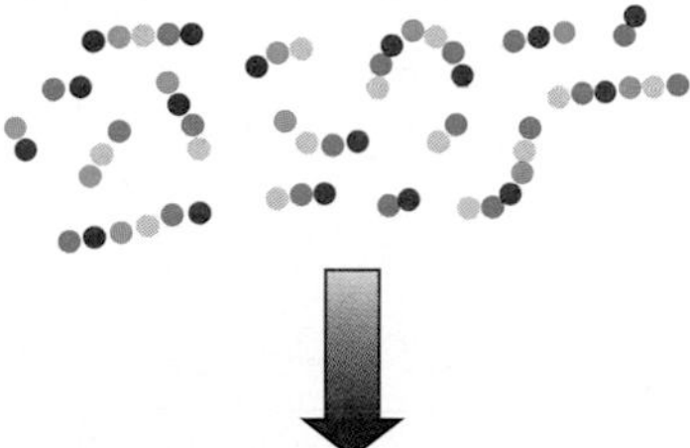

Small intestine

Enzymes from the pancreas and the intestine split peptide chains into tripeptides, dipeptides, and amino acids.

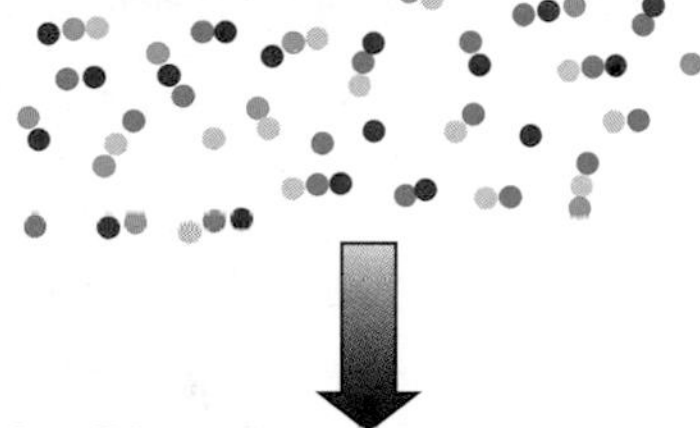

Small intestine

Enzymes on the surface of the small intestine's lining (absorptive cells) split tripeptides and dipeptides. The cells absorb amino acids.

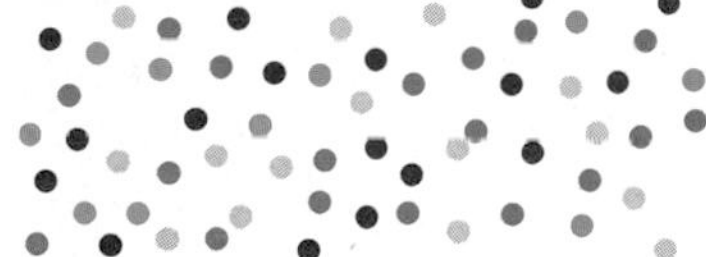

Figure 6-9

HOW PROTEIN IN FOOD BECOMES AMINO ACIDS IN THE BODY

either for their own use or for secretion into lymph or blood for other uses. Alternatively the body cells can use amino acids for energy.

KEY POINT Digestion of protein involves denaturation by stomach acid, then enzymatic digestion in the stomach and small intestine to amino acids, dipeptides, and tripeptides. The cells of the small intestine complete digestion, absorb amino acids and some larger peptides, and release them into the bloodstream.

Muscle work builds muscle; protein supplements do not, and athletes do not need them. Chapter 10 describes how muscles are built and the diet that best supports them.

Protein and Amino Acid Supplements

CONSUMER CAUTION Why do people take protein or amino acid supplements? Athletes take them to build muscle. Dieters take them to spare their bodies' protein while losing weight. People also take individual amino acids, mixtures of two or more amino acids, or products that combine amino acids with other nutrients. Some takers believe the products will cure herpes, induce restful sleep, or relieve pain or depression. Do protein and amino acid supplements really do any of these things? Almost never. Are they safe? No.

Protein supplements are less well digested than protein-rich food and they cost more than food, too. When used as a replacement for such food, they are often downright dangerous. The "liquid protein" diet, advocated some years ago for weight loss, caused deaths in many users. Even the physician-supervised, protein-sparing, modified fast, also based on liquid protein, can cause abnormal heart rhythms.

Amino acid supplements are also unnecessary. The body is designed to handle whole proteins best. It breaks them into manageable pieces (dipeptides and tripeptides), then splits these a few at a time, simultaneously absorbing them into the blood. This bit-by-bit absorption is ideal, because groups of chemically similar amino acids compete for the carriers that absorb them into the blood. An excess of one amino acid can tie up a carrier, and temporarily prevent the absorption of another similar amino acid. When carriers are tied up dealing with an overdose of some on or a few amino acids, some other needed amino acids may pass through the body unabsorbed. The result is a deficiency. The human body evolved without encountering highly concentrated amino acids in the unbalanced arrays found in supplements, and therefore lacks equipment with which to handle them.[3]

Recently, the Food and Drug Administration (FDA) asked a panel of scientists from a well-known scientific research group to review the safety of amino acid supplements.[4] When the scientists began to search the literature for well-controlled studies on the supplements, they found next to none. The panel did find evidence of adverse health effects from amino acids, however, and they therefore concluded that, without appropriate scientific research, no level of intake of these supplements could be considered safe. They also warned that any use of amino acids as dietary supplements is inappropriate, for two reasons. First, some (serine and proline) present a high risk of toxicity. Second, no amino acid supplement performs any nutrient function in the human body.

Protein and Amino Acid Supplements *continued*

The panel also singled out some groups of people they consider to be at especially high risk of harm from amino acid supplements:

- All women of childbearing age.
- Pregnant or lactating women.
- Infants, children, and adolescents.
- Elderly people.
- People with inborn errors of metabolism that affect their bodies' handling of amino acids.
- Smokers.
- People on low-protein diets.
- People with chronic or acute mental or physical illnesses who take amino acids without medical supervision.

Anyone considering taking amino acid supplements should check with a physician first.

Enthusiastic popular reports about two amino acids have led to widespread public use. One is lysine, popularly recommended to prevent or relieve the infections that cause herpes sores on the mouth or genital organs. The other is tryptophan, popularly recommended to relieve pain, depression, and insomnia. Lysine does not relieve or cure herpes infections, and if long-term use helps prevent outbreaks, it does so only in some individuals and with unknown associated risks. Tryptophan has some interesting effects with respect to pain and sleep in responsive individuals, as Controversy 13 explains later.

Some people who elected to take tryptophan developed a blood disorder (EMS, short for *eosinophilia-myalgia syndrome*).* EMS is characterized by severe muscle and joint pain, limb swelling, an elevated white blood cell count, extremely high fever, and, in at least 15 cases, death. Some evidence suggests that changes in procedures at a major Japanese tryptophan processing plant may have introduced contaminants that contributed to the as-yet-incurable disease.[5] FDA has requested a recall of tryptophan supplements made by the company and of all formulas to which they were added.[6] If you own a bottle of tryptophan or a formula containing it, throw it out. It is safer to derive your amino acids from protein-rich foods taken with a little carbohydrate to facilitate their use. A glass of milk or a turkey sandwich is a good choice.

Many of the chapters of this book present evidence on purified nutrients added to foods or taken singly. The Consumer Caution of Chapter 4 showed that the enrichment of a nutritionally inferior food (refined bread) with four added nutrients left it still deficient in many others. The Chapter 5 Consumer Caution showed that fish oil supplements cause side effects. The same is true of amino acids. Even with all that we know about science, it is hard to improve on nature.

---

*An EMS hotline has been established: 1-800-EMS-2829.

hormones as defined in Chapter 3, chemical messengers secreted by a number of body organs in response to conditions that require regulation. Each hormone affects a specific organ or tissue and elicits a specific response.

antibodies (AN-tee-bod-ees; introduced in Chapter 3) large proteins of the blood, produced by the immune system in response to invasion of the body by foreign substances (antigens); they combine with and inactivate them.

immunity (introduced in Chapter 3) specific disease resistance, derived from the immune system's memory of prior exposure to specific disease agents and its ability to mount a swift defense against them.

fluid and electrolyte balance distribution of fluid and dissolved particles among body compartments (see also Chapter 8).

edema (eh-DEEM-uh) the swelling of body tissue caused by leakage of fluid from the blood vessels, seen in (among other conditions) protein deficiency.

The Roles of Proteins in the Body

Only a sampling of the many roles proteins play can be described here, but these should serve to illustrate their versatility, uniqueness, and importance. No wonder their discoverers called them the primary material of life.

Supporting Growth and Maintenance

Amino acids must be continuously available to build the proteins of new tissue. The new tissue may be in an embryo; in a growing child; in new blood needed to replace blood lost in burns, hemorrhage, or surgery; in the scar tissue that heals wounds; or in new hair and nails.

Less obvious is the protein that helps to replace worn-out cells in everyone's body all the time. Each of the millions of red cells of the blood lives for only three or four months. Then each must be replaced by a new cell, produced and released by the bone marrow. The millions of cells that line the intestinal tract live for only three days; they are constantly being shed and need to be replaced. The cells of the skin die and rub off and new ones grow from underneath. Nearly all cells arise, live, and die this way, and while they are living, they constantly make and break down their proteins. Amino acids from food support all the new growth and maintenance of cells and the making of the working parts within them.

Building Enzymes and Hormones

Enzymes are among the most important of the proteins formed in living cells. Thousands of enzymes reside inside a single cell, each one a catalyst that facilitates a specific chemical reaction. Figure 6-10 shows how an enzyme might work.

The body's many **hormones** are messenger molecules, and some are made from amino acids. Various body glands release hormones in response to changes in the internal environment. The hormones then elicit the responses necessary to restore normal conditions. Among hormones made of amino acids is the thyroid hormone, which regulates the metabolic rate of the body. An opposing pair of hormones, insulin and glucagon, maintain blood glucose levels, as was described in Chapter 4. Many other hormones are at work in the body regulating equally critical body functions. Figure 6-11 shows the amino acid sequence of human insulin.

Building Antibodies

Of all the great variety of proteins in living organisms, the **antibodies** demonstrate best that proteins are specific for one organism. Antibodies are formed in response to the presence of foreign particles (usually proteins) that invade the body. The foreign protein may be part of a bacterium, a virus, or a toxin, or it may be present in a food that causes allergy. The body, after recognizing that it has been invaded, manufactures antibodies specially designed to inactivate the foreign protein.

Each antibody is designed specifically to destroy just one invader. An antibody active against one strain of influenza would be of no help to a person ill with another strain. Once the body has learned to make a particular antibody, it remembers. The next time it encounters that same invader, it destroys it even more rapidly. In other words, it develops an **immunity.**

Figure 6-10

ENZYME ACTION

Enzymes are catalysts: they speed up reactions that would happen anyway, but much more slowly. This enzyme works by positioning two compounds, A and B, so that the reaction between them will be especially likely to take place.

Compounds A and B are attracted to the enzyme's active site and park there for a moment in the exact position that makes the reaction between them most likely to occur. They react by bonding together and leave the enzyme as the new compound, AB.

A single enzyme can facilitate several hundred such synthetic reactions in a second. Other enzymes break apart compounds into two or more products or rearrange the atoms in one compound to make another one.

The hormonal system was described in Chapter 3.

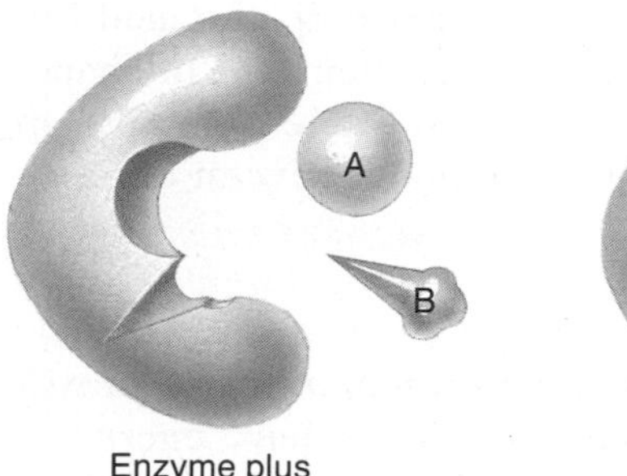

Enzyme plus two compounds, A and B

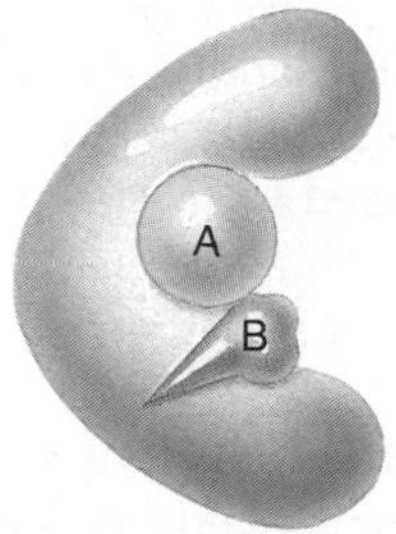

Enzyme complexed with A and B

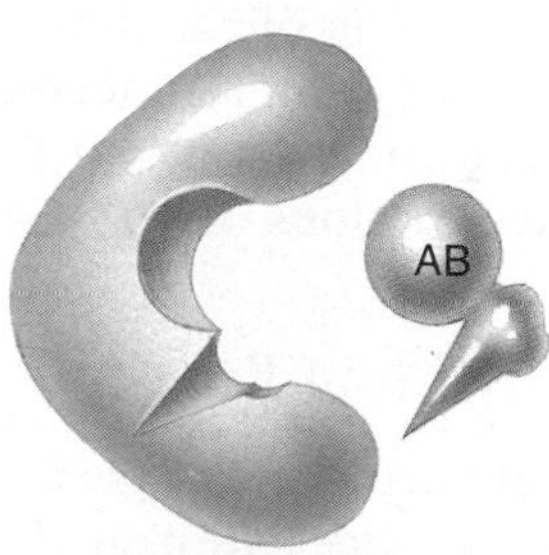

Enzyme plus new compound AB

This molecular memory underlies the principle of immunizations, injections of drugs made from destroyed and inactivated microbes or their products that activate the body's immune defenses. Some immunities are lifelong; others, such as that to tetanus, must be renewed.

Maintaining Fluid and Electrolyte Balance

Proteins help to regulate the quantity of fluids in the compartments of the body to maintain the **fluid and electrolyte balance.** To remain alive, cells must contain a constant amount of fluid. Too much might cause them to rupture; too little would make them unable to function. Although water can diffuse freely into and out of cells, proteins cannot; and proteins attract water. By maintaining stores of internal proteins and also of some minerals, cells retain the fluid they need. Conversely, the cells secrete proteins (and minerals) into the spaces between them to keep the fluid volume constant in those spaces. Thus proper balance is maintained. Should this system begin to fail, too much fluid would collect outside of cells, causing **edema.**

Not only the quantity but also the composition of the body fluids is vital to life. Transport proteins in the membranes of cells correct this composition continuously by transferring substances into and out of cells. For example, sodium is concentrated outside the cells, and potassium is concentrated inside (see Figure 6-12, page 193). A disturbance of this balance can impair the action of the heart, lungs, and brain, triggering a major medical emergency. Cell proteins work daily to avert such a disaster by holding fluids and electrolytes in their proper chambers.

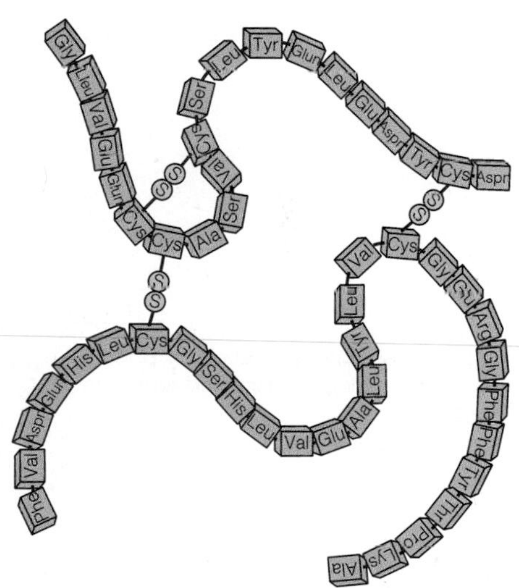

Figure 6-11

AMINO ACID SEQUENCE OF HUMAN INSULIN

This picture shows a refinement of protein structure not mentioned in the text. The amino acid cysteine (cys) has a sulfur-containing side group in it. The sulfur groups on two cysteine molecules can bond together, creating a bridge between two protein strands or two parts of the same strand. Insulin contains three such bridges.

acids compounds that release hydrogens in a watery solution.

bases compounds that accept hydrogens from solutions.

acid-base balance equilibrium between acid and base concentrations in the body fluids.

buffers compounds that help keep a solution's acidity or alkalinity constant.

acidosis (acid-DOSE-iss) blood acidity above normal, indicating excess acid (*osis* means "too much in the blood").

alkalosis (al-kah-LOH-sis) blood alkalinity above normal (*alka* means "base"; *osis* means "too much in the blood").

urea (yoo-REE-uh) the principal nitrogen-excretion product of metabolism, generated mostly by removal of amine groups from unneeded amino acids or from amino acids being sacrificed to a need for energy.

Maintaining Acid-Base Balance

Normal processes of the body continually produce **acids** and their opposite, **bases,** which must be carried by the blood to the organs of excretion. The blood must do this without allowing its own **acid-base balance** to be affected. This feat is another trick of the blood proteins, which act as **buffers** to maintain the blood's normal pH. They pick up hydrogens (acid) when there are too many and release them again when there are too few. The secret is that negatively charged side chains of amino acids can accommodate additional hydrogens, which are positively charged, when necessary.

Blood pH is one of the most rigidly controlled conditions in the body. If it changes too much, the dangerous condition **acidosis** or the opposite, basic condition **alkalosis** can cause coma or death. The hazard of these conditions is due to their effect on proteins. When the proteins' buffering capacity is filled, that is, when they have taken on board all the acid hydrogens they can accommodate—additional acid pulls them out of shape, denaturing them and disrupting many body processes. Table 6-1 sums up the functions of protein discussed in this section and adds several others.

Providing Energy

Only protein can perform all the functions just described, but protein will be sacrificed to provide energy if need be. The body must have energy to live from moment to moment. Obtaining that energy is a high priority for the body.

When amino acids are degraded for energy, their amine groups are stripped off and used elsewhere or are incorporated by the liver into **urea** and sent to the kidney for excretion in the urine. The fragments that remain

The control of water's location by particles is called osmosis and is discussed further in Chapter 8.

Table 6-1
Summary of Functions of Proteins

Growth and Maintenance. Proteins serve as building materials for growth and repair of body tissues.

Enzymes. Proteins facilitate needed chemical reactions.

Hormones. Proteins regulate body processes. Some, but not all, hormones are made of protein.

Antibodies. Proteins form the immune system molecules that fight diseases.

Fluid and Electrolyte Balance. Proteins help to maintain the fluid and mineral composition of various body fluids.

Acid-base balance. Proteins help maintain the acid-base balance of various body fluids by acting as buffers.

Energy. Proteins provide some fuel for the body's energy needs.

Transportation. Proteins help transport needed substances, such as lipids, minerals, and oxygen, around the body.

Blood clotting. Proteins provide the netting on which blood clots are built.

Structural components. Proteins form integral parts of most body structures such as skin, tendons, ligaments, membranes, muscles, organs, and bones.

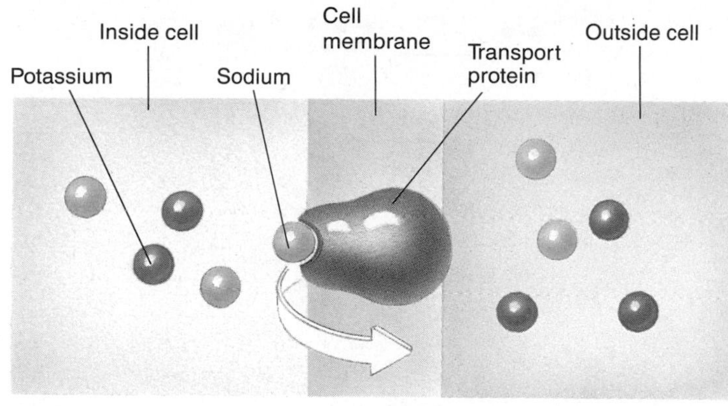

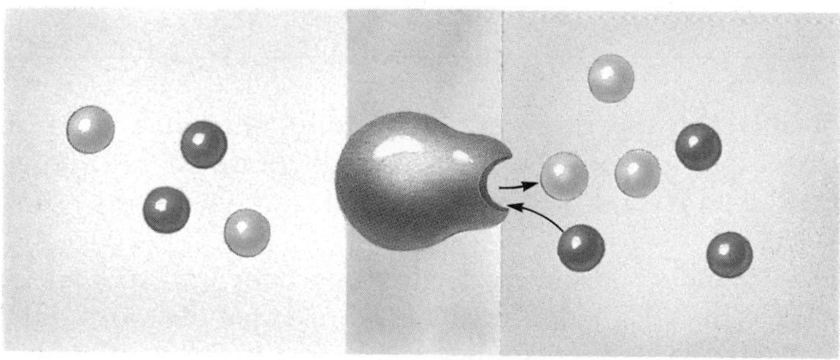

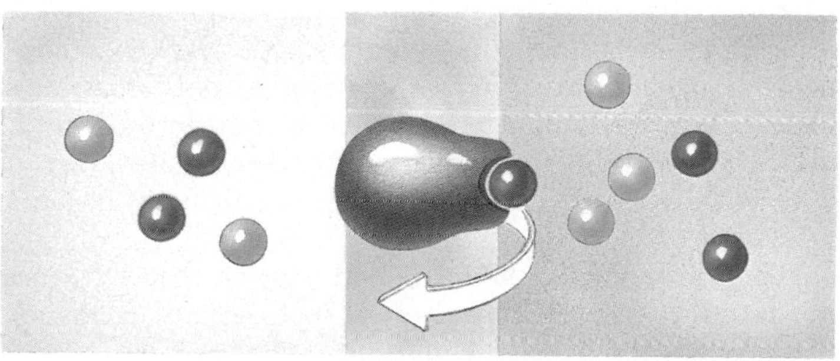

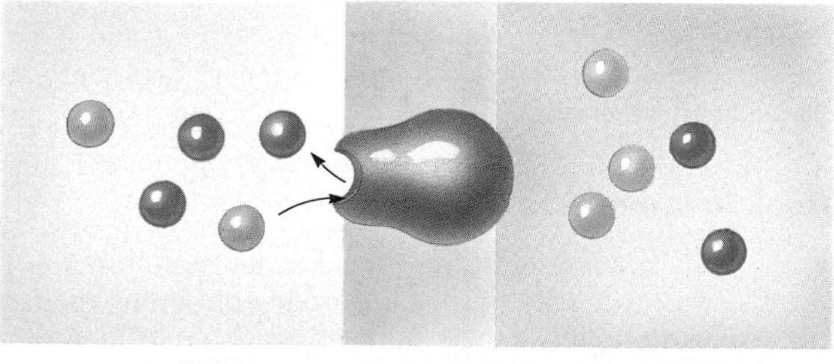

Figure 6-12

PROTEINS TRANSPORT SUBSTANCES INTO AND OUT OF CELLS

A transport protein within a cell membrane acts as a sort of revolving door—it picks up substances on one side of the membrane and flips them to the other side without leaving the membrane itself. The substances being transported here are sodium and potassium. The significance of sodium in fluid and electrolyte balance is discussed in Chapter 8.

are composed of carbon, hydrogen, and oxygen, as are carbohydrate and fat, and can be used to build those substances or can be metabolized like them.

Not only can amino acids supply energy, but many of them can be converted to glucose, as fatty acids can never be. Thus if need be, protein can help to maintain a steady blood-glucose level and so serve the energy needs of the brain.

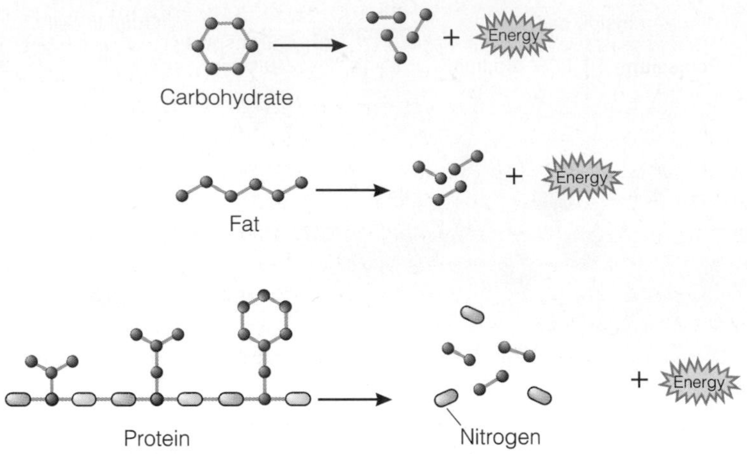

Figure 6-13

THREE DIFFERENT ENERGY SOURCES
Carbohydrate offers energy; fat offers concentrated energy; and protein, if necessary, can offer energy plus nitrogen. The symbols at right are 2-carbon fragments derived from the compounds at left. These fragments "burn" quickly in the presence of oxygen to yield carbon dioxide, water, and energy.

A perspective on the three energy-yielding nutrients, their similarities and differences, should now be clear. Carbohydrate offers energy; fat offers concentrated energy; and protein, if needed, can offer energy plus nitrogen (Figure 6-13).

Only if the protein-sparing energy from carbohydrate and fat is sufficient to power the cells will the amino acids be used for the work only they can perform—making proteins. The body does not make a specialized storage form for protein as it does for carbohydrate and fat. Glucose is stored as glycogen, fat as triglycerides, but body protein is available only as the working molecular and structural components of the tissues. When the need arises, the body dismantles its tissue proteins to obtain amino acids and uses them for energy.[7] Each protein is taken in its own time: first, from the blood and liver; then, from the muscles and other organs. Thus energy deficiency (starvation) always incurs wasting of lean body tissue as well as fat loss.

Athletes and exercisers take note: you cannot build extra muscle tissue by eating extra protein because protein excesses are burned as fuel, converted to glucose, or stored as fat. Chapter 10 gives more details about protein needs of exercisers.

If amino acids are oversupplied, the body has no place to store them. It has no choice but to remove and excrete their amine groups and then to convert the residues to glycogen or fat for energy storage.

KEY POINT When insufficient carbohydrate and fat are consumed to meet the body's energy need, food protein and body protein are sacrificed to supply energy. The nitrogen part is removed from each amino acid, and the resulting fragment is oxidized for energy.

The Fate of an Amino Acid

To review the body's handling of amino acids, let us follow the fate of an amino acid that was originally part of a protein-containing food. When the amino acid arrives in a cell, it may be used in several different ways, depending on the needs of the cell at the time.

The amino acid may be used as is and so become part of a growing protein. It may be altered somewhat to make another needed compound. Alternatively, the cell may dismantle it and use its amine group to build a different amino acid. The remainder may be used for fuel or, if not needed, converted to glucose or fat.

Nearly the same fate awaits the amino acid present in a cell that is starved for energy but has no glucose or fatty acids. This amino acid may be needed to build a vital protein, but without energy, the cell would die. Therefore the amino acid is stripped of its amine group (the nitrogen part), and the remainder of its structure is used for energy. The amine group is excreted from the cell and, finally, from the body in the urine.

Another case in which amino acids are used for energy is when there is a surplus of amino acids and energy-yielding nutrients. In this case the body does not waste this resource. It takes the amino acid apart, excretes the amine group, converts the rest to fat, and then stores the fat in the fat cells.

In summary, then, amino acids in the cell can be used to build proteins; can be converted to other small nitrogen-containing compounds such as the vitamin niacin; or can be converted to some other amino acids. Stripped of their nitrogen, they can be converted to glucose, burned as fuel, or stored as fat.

When not used to build protein or make other nitrogen-containing compounds, amino acids are "wasted," in a sense. This wasting occurs under any of four conditions: (1) when there is not enough energy from other sources; (2) when there is too much protein, so that not all is needed; (3) when there is too much of any amino acid from a supplement; or (4) when the diet's protein is of too-low quality, with too few essential amino acids, as described in the next section.

To prevent the wasting of dietary protein, and permit the synthesis of needed body protein, three conditions must be met. First, the dietary protein must be adequate in quantity. Second, it must supply all essential amino acids in the proper amounts. Third, enough energy-yielding carbohydrate and fat must be present, to permit the dietary protein to be used as such.

KEY POINT Amino acids can be metabolized to protein, nitrogen plus energy, glucose, or fat. They will be metabolized to protein only if sufficient energy is present from other sources. The diet should supply all essential amino acids and a full measure of protein according to guidelines.

legumes (leg-GYOOMS, LEG-yooms) plants of the bean and pea family having roots with nodules that contain special bacteria. These bacteria can trap nitrogen from the air in the soil and make it into compounds that become part of the seed. The seeds are rich in high-quality protein compared with those of most other plant foods.

Amino acids are wasted when:

- Energy is lacking.
- Protein is overabundant.
- An amino acid is oversupplied in supplement form.
- The diet's protein is of too-low quality (too few essential amino acids).

Food Proteins: Quality, Use, and Need

The body responds to different proteins in different ways, depending on many factors: the body's state of health, the food source of the protein, its digestibility, the other nutrients taken with it, and its amino acid assortment. To know whether, say, 30 grams of a particular protein is enough to meet a person's daily needs, it is necessary to account for the effects of these other factors on the body's use of the protein.

Regarding a person's state of health, malnutrition or infection may greatly increase the need for protein while making it hard to eat even normal amounts of food. In malnutrition, digestive enzyme secretion slows, impairing protein digestion. The absorptive surfaces of the digestive tract degenerate, impairing absorption. Diarrhea may result, causing further protein losses. When infection is present, protein is needed for enhanced immune functions as well as for normal functions. This increases the need.

Digestibility affects protein quality profoundly, and it varies from food to food. The protein of oats, for example, is less digestible than that of eggs. Generally, amino acids from animal proteins are best digested and absorbed (over 90 percent). Those from **legumes** follow (about 80 percent). Those from grains and other plant foods vary (from 60 to 90 percent). Cooking

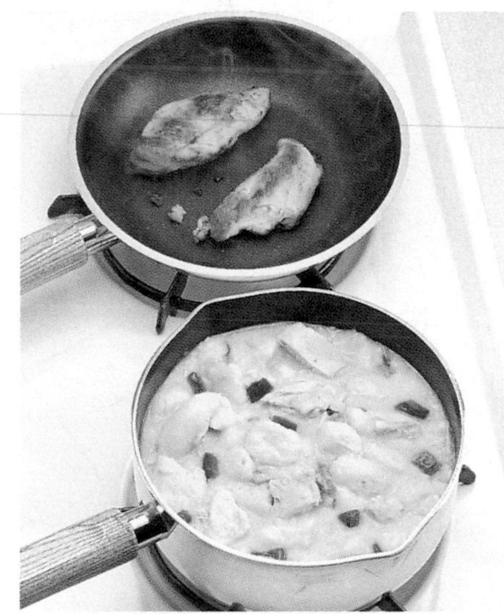

Cooking with moist heat improves protein digestibility in chicken and dumplings, whereas frying makes protein harder to digest.

limiting amino acid a term given to an essential amino acid present in dietary protein in an insufficient amount, so that it limits the body's ability to build protein.

complete proteins proteins containing all the essential amino acids in the right balance.

incomplete proteins proteins lacking, or low in, one or more of the essential amino acids.

mutual supplementation the strategy of combining two incomplete protein sources so that the amino acids in each food make up for those lacking in the other food. Such protein combinations are sometimes called *complementary proteins.*

complementary proteins two or more proteins whose amino acid assortments complement each other in such a way that the essential amino acids missing from each are supplied by the other.

with moist heat generally improves protein digestibility, whereas dry heat methods may impair it.

As for the other nutrients taken with protein, the need for carbohydrate and fat has already been emphasized. To be used efficiently, protein also must be accompanied by the full array of vitamins and minerals.

The quality of a food protein depends partly on its amino acid content. The cells, in making their own proteins, need a full array of amino acids from food, from their own amino acid pools, or from both. If a *nonessential* amino acid (that is, one the cell *can* make) is unavailable from food, the cell will synthesize it and continue attaching amino acids to protein strands being manufactured. If an *essential* amino acid (one the cell *cannot* make) is missing from food, the cells begin to adjust their activities almost immediately.[8] Within a single day of restricted essential amino acid intake, cells begin to conserve by restricting the breakdown of their working proteins and by reducing their use of amino acids for fuel.

These measures help cells to channel the available **limiting amino acid** to its wisest use: making new proteins. Even so, the normally fast rate of protein synthesis slows to a crawl, and cells must make do with the proteins on hand. When the limiting amino acid once again becomes available in abundance, the cells resume normal protein-related activities. If the shortage becomes chronic, however, cells begin to break down their protein-making machinery. This means that even when protein intakes become adequate, protein synthesis lags behind until cells can rebuild the needed machinery. Meanwhile, cells function less and less effectively as their proteins wear out and are only partially replaced.

A diet that is short in any of the essential amino acids thus limits protein synthesis. An earlier analogy likened amino acids to letters of the alphabet. To be meaningful, words must contain all the right letters. For example, a print shop that had no letter "n" in the shop could make no personalized stationery for Jana Johnson. No matter how many J's, a's, o's and s's in the printer's possession, they cannot replace the missing "n"s. Likewise in building a protein molecule, no amino acid can fill the spot of any other.

Partially completed proteins are not held for completion at a later time when the diet may improve. Rather, the partial structures are dismantled, and the component amino acids are returned to the circulation to be made available to other cells. If they are not soon inserted into protein, their amine groups are removed and excreted, and the residues are used for other purposes. The need that prompted the calling for that particular protein will not be met, and since the amine groups are excreted, the body cannot resynthesize the amino acids later.

It follows that all the essential amino acids must be consumed in a balanced diet before the body pools of the essential amino acids dwindle to the point at which body organs are compromised. This presents no problem to people who regularly eat **complete proteins,** such as those of meat, fish, poultry, cheese, eggs, milk, and, new to this list, many soybean products.[9] The proteins of these foods contain ample amounts of all the essential amino acids. An equally sound choice is to eat two **incomplete protein** foods from plants, each of which supplies the amino acids missing in the other. In this strategy, called **mutual supplementation,** the two protein-rich foods are combined to yield **complementary proteins,** that is, proteins containing all the essential amino acids in amounts sufficient to support health. This concept is illustrated in Figure 6-14 on page 198. The two proteins need not even be eaten together, so long as the day's meals supply them both.

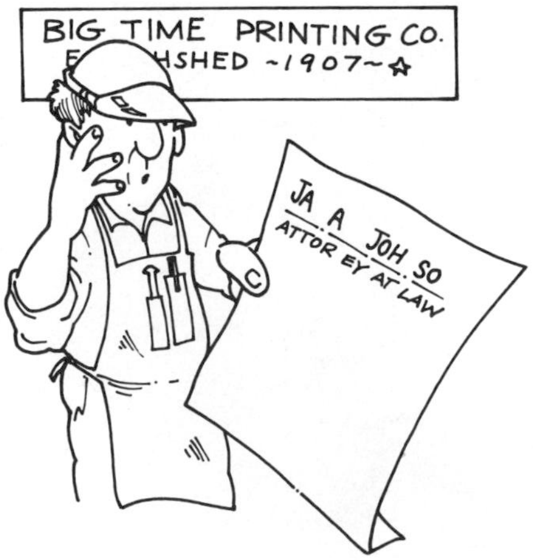

BIG TIME PRINTING CO.
ESTABLISHED ~1907~
JA A JOH SO
ATTOR EY AT LAW

Just as each letter of the alphabet is important in forming whole words, each amino acid must be available to build finished proteins.

Concern about the quality of individual food proteins is of only theoretical interest in settings where food is abundant. Most people in the United States and Canada eat a variety of nutritious foods to meet their energy needs—not just, say, cookies, potato chips, or alcoholic beverages. They would find it next to impossible *not* to meet their protein requirements, even if they were to eat no meat, fish, poultry, eggs, cheese, or soy products. However, while *protein* is usually sufficient in North American diets, future chapters point out that there are *other* nutrients to which people must attend.

Protein quality can make the difference between health and disease when food energy intake is limited (where malnutrition is widespread) or when the selection of foods available is severely limited (where a single food such as potatoes or rice provides 90 percent of the calories). Even then, protein intake may be adequate. To be sure, in these cases, the primary food source of protein must be checked, since its quality is crucial.

protein digestibility-corrected amino acid score (PDCAAS) a measuring tool used to determine protein quality. PDCAAS reflects a protein's digestibility as well as the proportions of amino acids that it provides.

protein efficiency ratio (PER) a measure of protein quality assessed by determining how well a given protein supports weight gain in growing rats. Used to judge the quality of protein in infant formulas and baby foods.

KEY POINT The body's use of a protein depends on the user's health, the protein's digestibility, the nutrients eaten with it, and its amino acid assortment.

Measuring Protein Quality

Researchers have developed many different methods of evaluating the quality of food protein. The most important one for consumers is the **protein digestibility-corrected amino acid score,** or **PDCAAS.** The PDCAAS is the main measure used by those establishing the protein values listed on food labels. One other measure of protein quality, the **protein efficiency ratio (PER),** is also used for measuring the protein quality of infant and baby foods. A difference between the two methods is that the PDCAAS is geared toward protein needed to support the maintenance of body tissue of adults, while the PER is more suitable to identify the best protein sources to support the rapid growth of infants and young children.

All other things being equal, a protein that supplies all the essential amino acids in exactly the right proportions will be most completely used. Chances are that if a diet provides enough of the essential amino acids, then it will meet all the protein needs of the body.[10] A protein that is low in an essential amino acid does not, by itself, support protein synthesis.

Digestibility is also a critical element in evaluating protein sources for human consumption. Simple measures of the total protein contained in a food are not useful by themselves, since, according to those alone, even animal hair or hooves would receive a top score. As the words of its name suggest, the PDCAAS takes into account the digestibility of a protein as well as its amino acid balance. To obtain the PDCAAS, the food is first given a score based on its amino acid balance. Then the score is adjusted to account for the food's digestibility. Some scores are listed in Table 6-2 in the margin. A person trying to choose between peanut butter and chili in the grocery store need never attempt such a calculation, but scientists who must establish adequacy of protein sources for human health worldwide rely on it heavily.[11]

Protein scores are of great importance in dealing with widespread malnutrition, where protein is scarce. For the average well-fed North American, however, eating the highest-quality protein is not necessary. Animal proteins do tend to have slightly higher scores than most plant proteins, but the two can be used in harmony within a diet. The best guarantee of amino acid adequacy is to eat mixtures of foods containing protein in the presence of adequate amounts of energy, vitamins, and minerals.

Table 6-2
PDCAAS of Selected Foods

Food	PDCAAS %
egg white	100
ground beef	100
chicken hot dogs	100
milk protein (casein)	100
nonfat milk powder	100
beef salami	100
tuna	100
soybean protein	94
whole wheat-pea flour	82[a]
chick peas (garbanzos)	69
kidney beans	68
peas	67
sausage, pork	63
pinto beans	61
rolled oats	57
black beans	53
lentils	52
peanut meal	52
whole wheat	40
wheat protein (gluten)	25

[a]An example of mutual supplementation. Combining whole wheat and pea flours yields a protein with a higher PDCAAS than that of either product alone.

Sources: G. Sarwar and F. E. McDonough, Evaluation of protein digestibility-corrected amino acid score method for assessing protein quality of foods, *Journal of the Association of Official Analytical Chemists* 73 (1990): 347–356; G. Sarwar, Digestibility of protein and bioavailability of amino acids in foods, *World Review of Nutrition and Dietetics* 54 (1987): 26–70.

This figure compares the essential amino acids contributed from two incomplete proteins — protein A, which is missing amino acid #2, and protein B, which is missing amino acids #4 and #7.

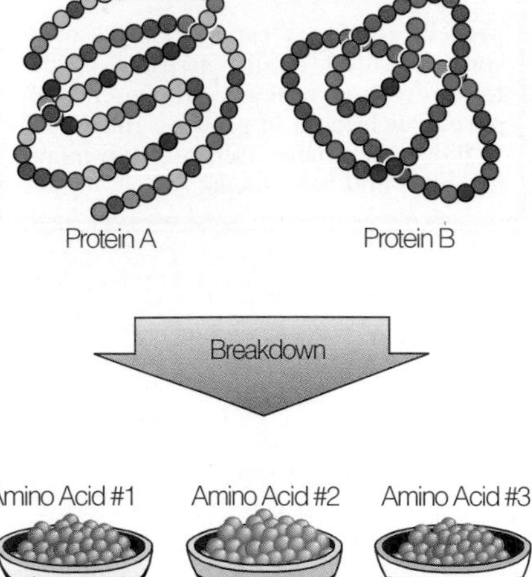

The bowls numbered "1" through "9" represent the nine essential amino acids. Amino acids 1, 3, 5, 6, 8, and 9 are well supplied by either protein A or B. Together, proteins A and B supply sufficient amounts of all the essential amino acids.

Figure 6-14

MUTUAL SUPPLEMENTATION

nitrogen balance the amount of nitrogen consumed compared with the amount excreted in a given time period.

Table 6-3
Recommendations Concerning Intakes of Protein

Recommended Dietary Allowance (RDA)
Adults:[a]

- 0.8 grams protein per kilogram body weight per day.

Dietary Guidelines

- Every day eat 2 to 3 servings to total four to nine ounces daily of cooked dry beans and peas, lean beef or other lean meats, poultry without the skin, fish and shell fish, and occasionally eggs and organ meats.
- Every day choose 2 to 3 servings of lowfat or nonfat milk, yogurt, or cheese.
- Eat a variety of foods to provide small amounts of protein from other sources.

World Health Organization

- Lower limit: 10 percent of total calories from protein.
- Upper limit: 15 percent of total calories from protein.

[a]Recommendations for other population groups are listed on the inside front cover.

KEY POINT The quality of a protein is measured by how much of its nitrogen is retained by the body (digestibility) or by how well the protein supports growth.

The Protein RDA

Menu planners build their meals around the RDA for protein. The RDA is designed to cover the need to replace protein-containing tissue that people lose and wear out every day. Therefore it depends on body size: larger people have a higher protein RDA. The protein RDA also is adjusted to cover additional needs for building new tissue and so is higher for growing children and pregnant and lactating women. The Canadian recommendation for protein is similar and is based on similar assumptions. Table 6-3 above reviews the recommendations concerning dietary protein, first presented in Chapter 2. These ensure that the body is well supplied with the protein it needs.

Underlying the protein RDA are **nitrogen balance** studies, which measure nitrogen lost by excretion compared with nitrogen eaten in food. In healthy adults nitrogen-in (consumed) must equal nitrogen-out (excreted). The laboratory scientist measures the body's daily nitrogen losses in urine, feces, sweat, and skin under controlled conditions and can then estimate the amount of protein needed to replace these losses.*

Under normal circumstances healthy adults are in nitrogen equilibrium, or zero balance, that is, they have at all times the same amount of total protein in their bodies. When nitrogen-in exceeds nitrogen-out, they are said to be in positive nitrogen balance; this means that somewhere in their bodies more proteins are being built than are being broken down and lost. When nitrogen-in is less than nitrogen-out, they are said to be in negative nitrogen balance; they are losing protein. Figure 6-15 illustrates these different states.

*The average protein is 16% nitrogen by weight; that is, each 100 g protein contains 16 g nitrogen. As a rule of thumb, the scientist multiplies the nitrogen's weight by 6.25 to estimate the protein's weight.

Figure 6-15

NITROGEN BALANCE

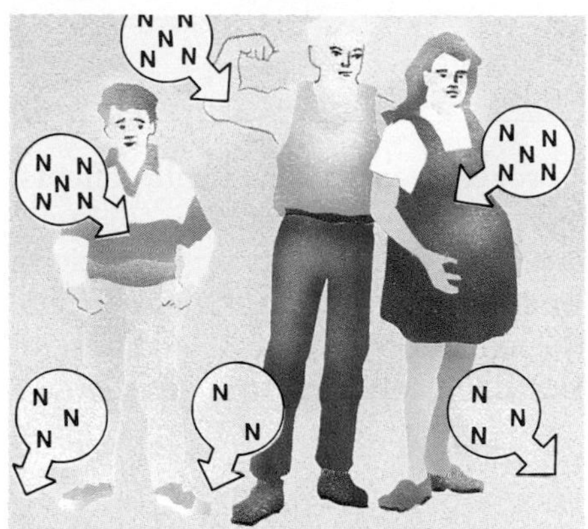

Positive Nitrogen Balance
These people, a growing child, a person building muscle, and a pregnant woman, are all retaining more nitrogen than they are excreting.

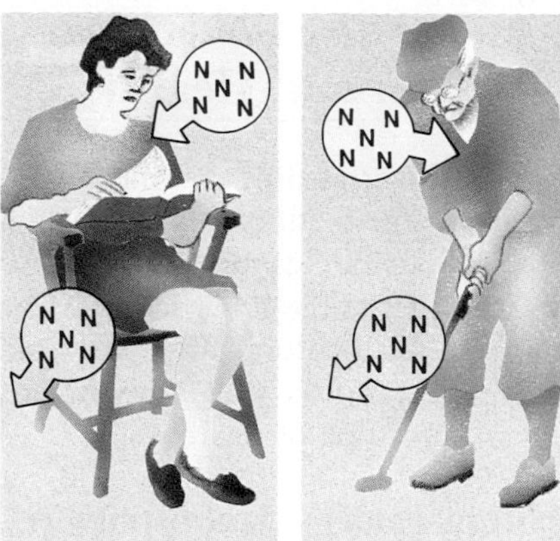

Nitrogen Equilibrium
These people, a healthy college student and a young retiree, are in nitrogen equilibrium.

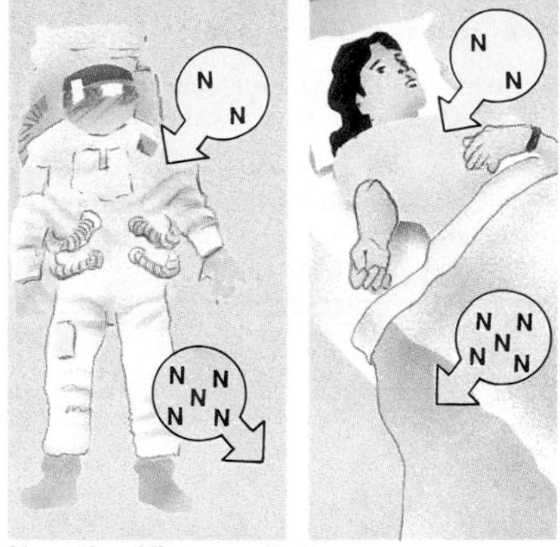

Negative Nitrogen Balance
These people, an astronaut and a surgery patient, are losing more nitrogen than they are taking in.

Growing children add to their bodies new blood, bone, and muscle cells every day. These cells contain protein, so children must have in their bodies more protein, and therefore more nitrogen, at the end of each day than they had at the beginning. A growing child is therefore in positive nitrogen balance. Similarly, when a woman is pregnant she is, in essence, growing a new person; she too must be in positive nitrogen balance until after the birth when she once again reaches equilibrium.

Negative nitrogen balance occurs when muscle or other protein tissue is broken down and lost. Consider the situation when people have to rest in bed for a long time. Their muscles degenerate, and they suffer a net loss of protein. One of several problems faced by the nutritionists responsible for the welfare of astronauts involves the negative nitrogen balance that occurs if astronauts spend many days without gravity in the space capsule. Without the exercise of supporting their bodies' weight, their muscles may waste and weaken. To maintain the muscles, they must do special exercises. The same is true for the bones and calcium, as discussed in Controversy 8.

For healthy adults the RDA for protein has been set at 0.8 grams for each kilogram (or 2.2 pounds) of body weight. Athletes need slightly more, but the increased need is well covered by a regular diet (more in Chapter 10). For infants and children who are growing, the protein RDA, like all nutrient RDA, is higher per unit of body weight.

Protein RDA (adult) = 0.8 g/kg.

To figure your protein RDA:

1. Find your body weight.
2. Convert pounds to kilograms (pounds divided by 2.2 lb/kg equals kilograms).
3. Multiply by 0.8 g/kg to get your RDA in grams per day.

For example:

1. Weight = 110 lb.
2. 110 lb ÷ 2.2 lb/kg = 50 kg.
3. 50 kg × 0.8 g/kg = 40 g.

In making its recommendations for protein intakes, the members of the Committee on RDA took into consideration that the protein in a normal diet would be mixed, that is, a combination of animal and plant protein. They also recognized that not all proteins are used with 100 percent efficiency and that individuals use protein with different efficiencies. Accordingly, the committee made the RDA quite generous. Many normal people can consume less than the RDA for protein and still meet their bodies' needs. What this means in terms of food selections is presented in this chapter's Food Feature.

protein-energy malnutrition (PEM), also called **protein-calorie malnutrition (PCM)** the world's most widespread malnutrition problem, including both kwashiorkor and marasmus and states in which they overlap.

marasmus (ma-RAZ-mus) the calorie-deficiency disease; starvation.

kwashiorkor (kwash-ee-OR-core, kwash-ee-or-CORE) a disease related to malnutrition, with a set of recognizable symptoms, such as edema.

 **KEY POINT** Nitrogen balance compares nitrogen excreted from the body with nitrogen ingested in food. The amount of protein needed daily depends on size and stage of growth. The RDA for adults is 0.8 g of protein per kg of body weight.

◆ Protein and Health

With all the attention that has been paid in recent years to the health effects of starch, sugars, fibers, fats, oils, and cholesterol, protein has been slighted. Protein deficiencies are well known because, together with energy deficiencies, they are the world's leading form of malnutrition. But the health effects of too much protein, and particularly the effects of proteins of different kinds, are far less well known. Let us consider each in turn: deficiency, excess, and type of protein.

Protein-Energy Malnutrition

Protein deficiency and energy deficiency go hand in hand. This combination—**protein-energy malnutrition (PEM)**—is the most widespread form of malnutrition in the world today, affecting over 500 million children. Most often, PEM strikes early in childhood, but it endangers many adults as well. Inadequate food intake leads to poor growth in children and to weight loss and wasting in adults. Stunted growth due to PEM is easy to overlook, because a small child can look perfectly normal. The small stature of children in impoverished nations was once thought to be a "normal" adaptation to the limited availability of food; now it is known to be an avoidable failure of growth due to a lack of food during the growing years.[12]

PEM is prevalent in Africa, Central America, South America, the Near East, and the Far East, but developed countries are not immune. Impoverished people living on U.S. Indian reservations, in inner cities, and in rural areas of the United States, as well as ill people in hospitals, have been diagnosed with PEM. Also, among those who suffer from the eating disorder anorexia nervosa, PEM is almost invariably present.

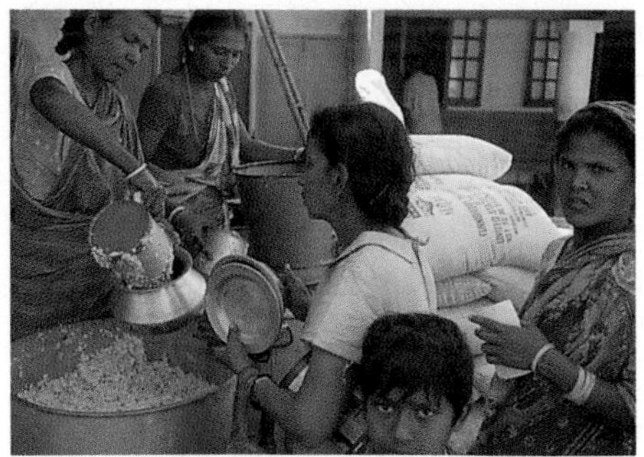

Scant supplies of donated food save some from starvation, but many others go hungry.

PEM seems to take two different forms. In one, the person is shriveled and lean all over; in the other a swollen belly and skin rash are present. These apparent forms of PEM have two different disease names: **marasmus** and **kwashiorkor,** respectively. Marasmus was thought to be caused by energy deficiency and kwashiorkor by protein deficiency. In reality, though, marasmus reflects inadequate food intake and therefore inadequate energy, protein, vitamins, and minerals as well. In addition, diets are rarely deficient in protein when they are adequate in energy. Researchers are currently questioning the validity of classic definitions of the conditions, and may soon change them.[13]* For now, we refer to general starvation as marasmus, and to the special configuration of symptoms in starving children that includes the swollen belly and skin rash as kwashiorkor.

Marasmus occurs most commonly in children from 6 to 18 months of age in overpopulated city slums. Children in impoverished nations subsist on a weak cereal drink with scant energy and protein of low quality; such food can barely sustain life, much less support growth. A starving child often looks like a wizened little old person—just skin and bones.

*A term gaining acceptance for use in place of *kwashiorkor* is *hypoalbuminemic-type* PEM.

Without adequate nutrition, muscles, including the heart muscles, waste and weaken. Brain development is stunted and learning is impaired. Metabolism is so slow that body temperature is subnormal. There is little or no fat under the skin to insulate against cold. Hospital workers find that children with marasmus need to be wrapped up and kept warm. They also need love because they have often been deprived of parental attention as well as food.

dysentery (DISS-en-terry) an infection of the digestive tract that causes diarrhea.

The starving child faces this threat to life by engaging in as little activity as possible—not even crying for food. The body collects all its forces to meet the crisis and so cuts down on any expenditure of protein not needed for the heart, lungs, and brain to function. Growth ceases; the child is no larger at age four than at age two. The skin loses its elasticity and moisture, so it tends to crack; when sores develop, they fail to heal.[14] Digestive enzymes are in short supply, the digestive tract lining deteriorates, and absorption fails. The child can't assimilate what little food is eaten.

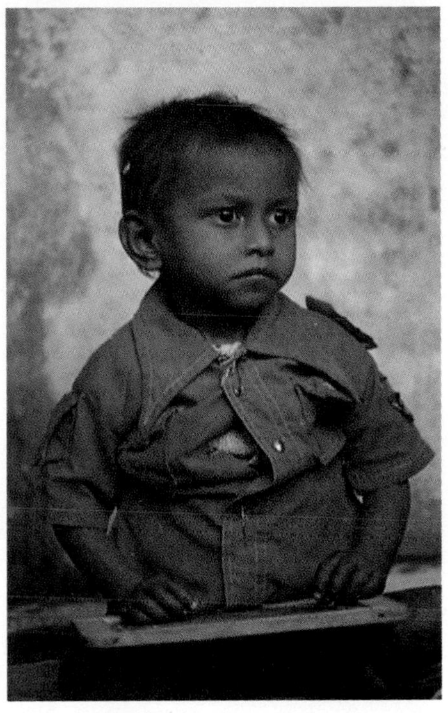

Protein malnutrition impairs learning.

Blood proteins, including hemoglobin, are no longer produced, so the child becomes anemic and weak. The protein and energy needed for immune functions are lacking, which explains the high prevalence of infections in malnourished children. Antibodies to fight off invading bacteria are degraded to provide amino acids for other uses, leaving the child an easy target for infection.[15] Then **dysentery,** an infection of the digestive tract, causes diarrhea, further depleting the body of nutrients, especially minerals. Measles, which might make a healthy child sick for a week or two, kills a child with PEM within two or three days. In fact, infections that occur with malnutrition are responsible for two-thirds of the deaths in young children in developing countries.[16]

If caught in time, the starvation of a child may be reversed by careful nutrition therapy. The fluid balances are most critical. Diarrhea will have depleted the body's potassium and upset other electrolyte balances. The combination of electrolyte imbalances, anemia, fever, and infections often leads to heart failure and sudden death. Careful correction of fluid and electrolyte balances usually raises the blood pressure and strengthens the heartbeat within a few days. Later, nonfat milk, providing protein and carbohydrate, can safely be given; fat is introduced still later, when body protein is sufficient to provide carriers.

The term *electrolyte balance* refers to the proper concentrations of salts within the body fluids (see Chapter 8 for details).

Kwashiorkor is the Ghanaian name for "the evil spirit that infects the first child when the second child is born." In countries where kwashiorkor is prevalent, a young child is weaned from breast milk, which contains high-quality protein designed perfectly to support growth, to a watery cereal with scant protein of low quality. Small wonder the just-weaned child sickens when the new baby arrives.

Some kwashiorkor symptoms very much resemble those of marasmus, but often without severe wasting of body fat. Proteins and hormones that previously maintained fluid balance now are diminished, so that fluid leaks out of the blood and accumulates in the belly and legs, causing edema. The kwashiorkor victim often develops a fatty liver, caused by lack of the protein carriers that transport fat out of the liver.[17] The fatty liver loses some of its ability to clear poisons from the body, prolonging their toxic effects.

PEM is common among the poor, including the hungry and homeless in the United States.[18] Today, millions of people who work to support their children earn so little that they cannot afford nutritious food—one child in eight under the age of 12 is hungry. This situation offers a challenge to nutritionists.[19] Hunger, especially in children, threatens everyone's future. Hungry children do not learn as well as fed children, nor are they competitive. They are ill more often, they have higher absentee rates from school, and when they attend, they cannot concentrate for long. The forces driving poverty and hunger will require many great minds working together to find solutions. Chapter 15 comes back to the topics of hunger, food, and poverty.

KEY POINT Protein deficiency symptoms are always observed when either protein or energy is deficient. Extreme energy deficiency is marasmus; extreme protein deficiency with ample energy is kwashiorkor. The two diseases overlap most of the time and together are called PEM.

Protein Excess

While many of the world's people struggle to obtain enough food and enough protein to keep themselves alive, people in developed countries must consciously limit their protein intakes to avoid excesses. Overconsumption of protein offers no benefits, and may pose health risks. For one thing, as mentioned before, protein-rich foods are often high-fat foods that contribute to obesity with its accompanying health risks. Independently of the effects of fat, high animal protein may raise blood cholesterol, thus contributing to atherosclerosis and heart disease. Infants and children do not adjust well to diets containing large amounts of protein; their body composition is altered. Animals fed experimentally on high-protein diets develop enlarged kidneys and sometimes livers.[20] In human beings, high-protein diets eaten over a lifetime are known to worsen existing kidney problems.[21]

Animals experimentally fed high-protein diets similar to those that Americans typically eat also experience losses of the essential mineral zinc from their tissues as they age.[22] Pregnant women and infants on protein supplements also excrete zinc. Such supplements taken during pregnancy may do more harm than good, even to undernourished women.

Diets high in protein may also accelerate calcium excretion, depleting the bones of their chief mineral.[23] Some experts argue that *food* sources of excess protein do not promote calcium excretion but that protein or amino acid supplements do.[24] In keeping with the first possibility, the Committee on RDA has suggested an upper limit for protein intake of no more than twice the RDA amount, and the World Health Organization (WHO) suggests an even more stringent upper limit of 15 percent of total calories. In a world in which protein deficiency is such a threat to so many, it is ironic that some people in developed countries should be overconsuming protein.

KEY POINT Health risks follow the overconsumption of protein-rich foods.

FOOD FEATURE

Enough, But Not Too Much, Protein

It is clear by now that people in developed nations usually eat more than ample protein. The protein RDA is generous: it more than adequately covers the estimated needs of most people, even those with unusually high requirements.

The meat list and the milk list are the two lists of foods in the exchange system that contribute an abundance of high-quality protein. Two others, the vegetable and grain lists, contribute smaller amounts of proteins, but they can add up to significant quantities. While labels specify the number of protein grams in processed foods, the exchange lists permit you to estimate the protein content of any food (see Figure 6-16).

To illustrate how easy it is to overconsume protein, assume that *your* protein RDA is 50 grams per day. This would divide easily into three meals: 10 grams at breakfast, 20 grams at lunch, and 20 grams at dinner. An egg, a slice of toast, and a glass of milk at breakfast would add up to 18 grams, almost double the allowance for that meal. At lunch a chef's salad with an egg, an ounce of ham, and an ounce of cheese accompanied by a roll would deliver 24 grams; and the greens would be additional. For supper, a 4-ounce piece of chicken, a potato, and vegetable would contribute 33 more. By the time you added more vegetables, the second milk serving, and two more bread/cereal servings, suggested by the Daily Food Guide, you would have added about 20 grams more, exceeding your protein needs for the day by far. Finally, a cup of legumes adds over 10 grams more protein to your day's meals, for a total of more than 100 grams. No wonder most people get more than twice the protein they need.

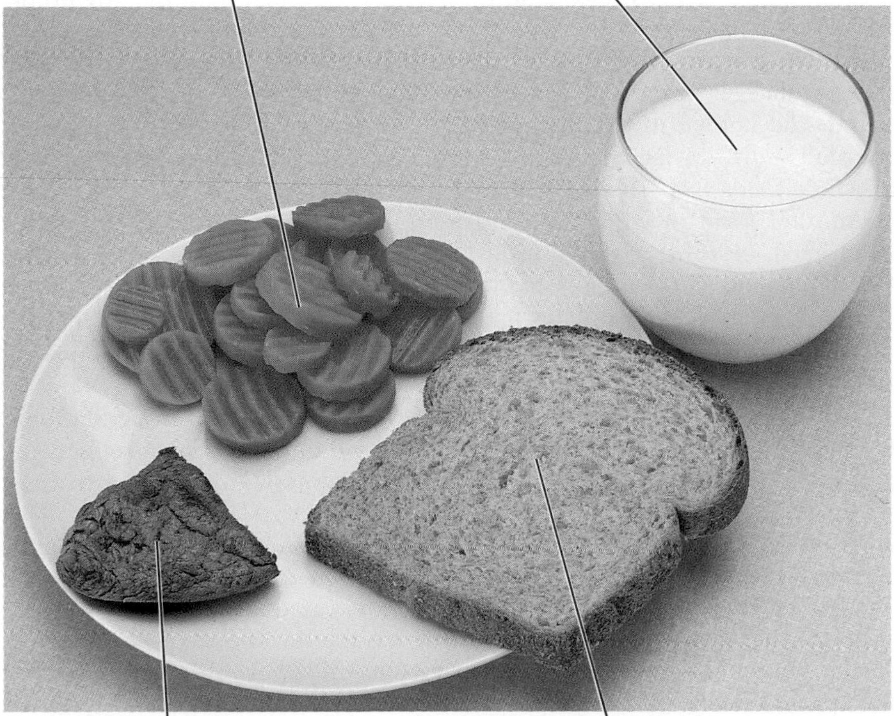

Figure 6-16

PROTEIN IN FOODS

One Exchange	Proteins (g)
Milk (1 c)	8
Vegetable (½ c)	2
Fruit (1 portion)	0
Bread and starchy vegetable (1 slice or ½ c)	3
Meat (1 oz)	7
Fat	0

textured vegetable protein processed soybean protein used in products formulated to look and to taste like meat, fish, or poultry.

tofu (TOE-foo) a curd made from soybeans, rich in protein and often rich in calcium, used in many Asian and vegetarian dishes in place of meat.

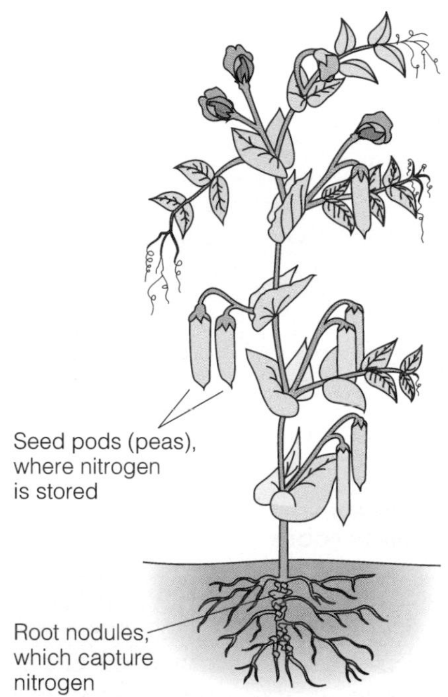

Figure 6-17

A LEGUME

The legumes are such plants as the kidney bean, soybean, garden pea, lentil, black-eyed pea, and lima bean. Bacteria in the root nodules can "fix" nitrogen from the air, contributing it to the beans. Ultimately, thanks to these bacteria, the plant leaves in the soil more nitrogen than it takes out. So efficient at trapping nitrogen are the legumes that farmers often grow them in rotation with other crops to fertilize fields. Legumes are shown among the meat alternatives in Figure 2-4 of Chapter 2.

Protein is critical in nutrition, but too many protein-rich foods in the diet can displace other important foods. Protein-rich foods carry with them a characteristic array of vitamins and minerals, including vitamin B_{12} and iron, but they are notoriously lacking in others—vitamin C and folate, for example. In addition, many protein-rich foods such as meat are high in calories, and to overconsume them is to invite obesity. To keep from vastly overconsuming protein and calories, the person must restrict something. The obvious "something" to restrict is meat.

With the confidence that one's protein intake is ample, one can plan meatless or reduced-meat meals with pleasure. Many interesting, protein-rich meat alternates are available. One of these has already been mentioned: the legumes.

The protein of legumes is of a quality almost comparable to that of meat. Figure 6-17 shows a legume plant's special root system that enables them to make abundant protein. Legumes are also excellent sources of fiber, many B vitamins, iron, calcium, and other minerals. A cup of cooked legumes contains 31 percent of the protein and 42 percent of the iron recommended daily for an adult male. Like meats, though, legumes do not offer every nutrient, and they do not make a complete meal by themselves. They contain no vitamin A, vitamin C, or vitamin B_{12}, and their balance of amino acids can be much improved by using grains and other vegetables with them.

Soybeans are versatile legumes, and people make many products from them. However, the heavy use of soy products in place of meat inhibits iron absorption. The effect can be alleviated by using small amounts of meat and/or foods rich in vitamin C in the same meal with the soy products. Vegetarians sometimes use convenience foods made from **textured vegetable protein** (soy protein) that are formulated to look and to taste like hamburgers or breakfast sausages. Many of these are intended to match the known nutrient contents of animal-protein foods, but often they fall short. A wise vegetarian would instead learn to use combinations of whole foods (see Table 6-4).

Another form in which the nutrients of soybeans are available is as bean curd, or **tofu,** a staple used in many Asian dishes. Thanks to the use of calcium salts when some tofu is made, it can be high in calcium. This information may not be listed on the label of a particular brand, though, and an interested consumer may have to write to the company to find out whether calcium sulfate was used in processing.

The Food Features presented so far show that the recommendations for the three energy-yielding nutrients go hand in hand. If you reduce fat and increase carbohydrate, protein totals automatically come into line with the requirements.

To estimate the amounts of protein in meals such as the Monday and Tuesday meals of Chapter 2, assign each food to the appropriate exchange list, and note its protein value. This was done in Figure 2-9 on pages 56–57. The fruits and fats can be assumed to contain no protein, so the only foods to inspect are the meats, milks, grains, starchy vegetables and breads, and vegetables. This method underestimates the pro-

Table 6-4
Complementary Protein Combinations
Combine foods from two or more of these columns to obtain complete protein.

Grains	Legumes	Seeds and Nuts	Vegetables
Barley	Dried beans	Sesame seeds	Leafy greens
Bulgur	Dried lentils	Sunflower seeds	Broccoli
Cornmeal	Dried peas	Walnuts	Others (see exchange lists)
Oats	Peanuts	Cashews	
Rice	Soy products	Other nuts	
Whole-grain breads		Nut butters	
Pasta			

tein in foods such as sunflower seeds (listed with fats and assigned no protein value) and peas and beans (listed with the breads for their high carbohydrate contents). Still, if you looked up every food in Appendix A and computed the actual protein grams, the total would come to 89 grams, a number very close to the 93 grams obtained much more quickly with the exchange system. For macronutrients such as protein, a difference of just a few grams in the day's total is not significant.

CHECKING OUT FOOD LABELS
How to Read Protein Information on a Food Label

Chapter 6 pointed out that people in this society easily meet, and usually exceed, their needs for protein. Still, the choice of protein-containing foods can make a difference to a person's health. Figure 6-18 on the next page displays labels from two cans of chili, a vegetarian chili and a chili with meat. The protein contributed by each, along with some other nutrients these foods contribute, are of interest to the reader of labels.

PROTEIN VALUES

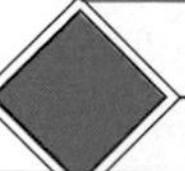

Both labels list protein in grams, as required. The numbers here reflect only protein quantity, not quality. These chilis are almost alike with regard to amount of protein present, and as it turns out, their quality is almost equal. Table 6-2 listed soy protein among the foods highest in protein quality. The soy protein added to the vegetarian chili rates almost as high in quality as the meat added to the other type, making the two products equally supportive with regard to protein needs of adults. This discovery might surprise a consumer who undervalues vegetable protein and believes that only meat supplies protein of value.

Listing the "% Daily Value" for protein on a label is optional, but for manufacturers who choose to do so, the law requires that they use the PDCAAS method to account for the protein's digestibility. Some consumers would like to know how much protein a food contributes toward the day's total. A few manufacturers spend the extra effort to determine this value, but most people need not track protein through the day. Few people who eat normal diets ever become protein deficient.

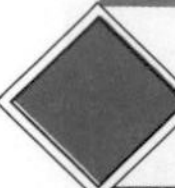

CHECKING OUT FOOD LABELS

How to Read Protein Information on a Food Label *continued*

Figure 6-18

TWO CHILIS

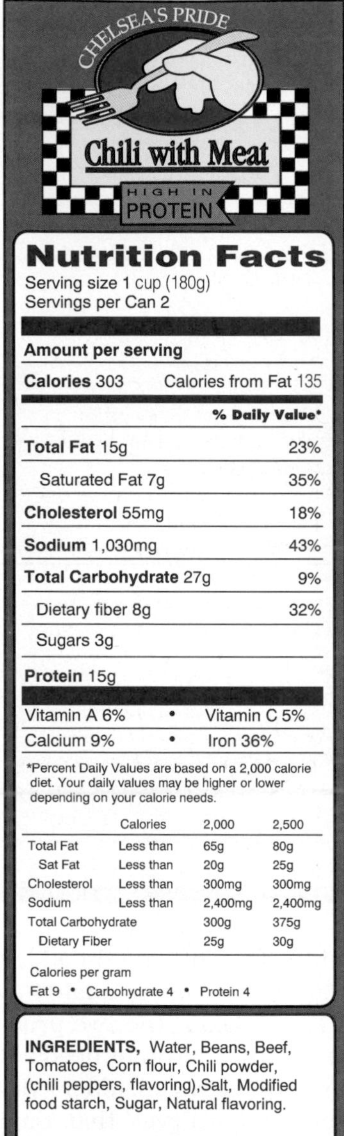

CHELSEA'S PRIDE
Chili with Meat
HIGH IN PROTEIN

Nutrition Facts
Serving size 1 cup (180g)
Servings per Can 2

Amount per serving

Calories 303	Calories from Fat 135
	% Daily Value*
Total Fat 15g	23%
Saturated Fat 7g	35%
Cholesterol 55mg	18%
Sodium 1,030mg	43%
Total Carbohydrate 27g	9%
Dietary fiber 8g	32%
Sugars 3g	
Protein 15g	

Vitamin A 6% • Vitamin C 5%
Calcium 9% • Iron 36%

*Percent Daily Values are based on a 2,000 calorie diet. Your daily values may be higher or lower depending on your calorie needs.

	Calories	2,000	2,500
Total Fat	Less than	65g	80g
Sat Fat	Less than	20g	25g
Cholesterol	Less than	300mg	300mg
Sodium	Less than	2,400mg	2,400mg
Total Carbohydrate		300g	375g
Dietary Fiber		25g	30g

Calories per gram
Fat 9 • Carbohydrate 4 • Protein 4

INGREDIENTS, Water, Beans, Beef, Tomatoes, Corn flour, Chili powder, (chili peppers, flavoring),Salt, Modified food starch, Sugar, Natural flavoring.

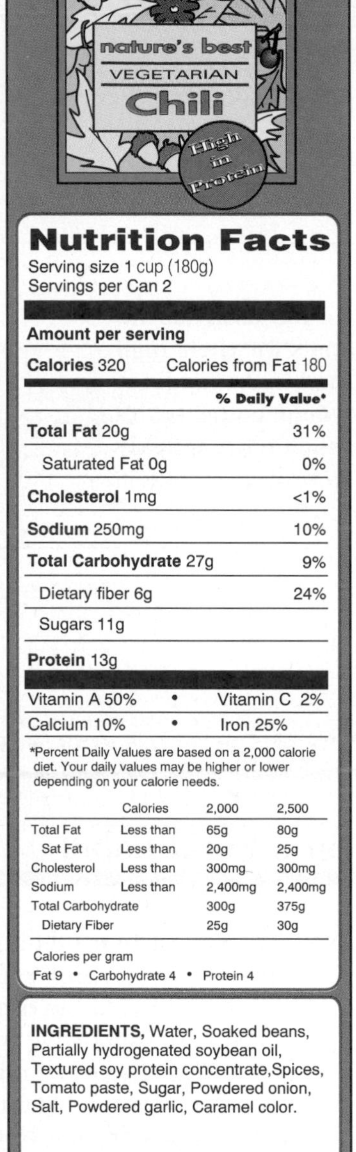

Nutrition Facts
Serving size 1 cup (180g)
Servings per Can 2

Amount per serving

Calories 320	Calories from Fat 180
	% Daily Value*
Total Fat 20g	31%
Saturated Fat 0g	0%
Cholesterol 1mg	<1%
Sodium 250mg	10%
Total Carbohydrate 27g	9%
Dietary fiber 6g	24%
Sugars 11g	
Protein 13g	

Vitamin A 50% • Vitamin C 2%
Calcium 10% • Iron 25%

*Percent Daily Values are based on a 2,000 calorie diet. Your daily values may be higher or lower depending on your calorie needs.

	Calories	2,000	2,500
Total Fat	Less than	65g	80g
Sat Fat	Less than	20g	25g
Cholesterol	Less than	300mg	300mg
Sodium	Less than	2,400mg	2,400mg
Total Carbohydrate		300g	375g
Dietary Fiber		25g	30g

Calories per gram
Fat 9 • Carbohydrate 4 • Protein 4

INGREDIENTS, Water, Soaked beans, Partially hydrogenated soybean oil, Textured soy protein concentrate,Spices, Tomato paste, Sugar, Powdered onion, Salt, Powdered garlic, Caramel color.

DESCRIPTORS AND HEALTH CLAIMS

◆ Of greater concern than grams of protein in a food is what food is delivering the protein. What *other* nutrients does the food offer? For example, beans provide fiber to the diet along with their protein. Foods that provide no significant fiber need not list fiber separately. Both chili types here are based on beans, and both qualify for a "high in fiber" claim. Neither chili type, however, may boast that its high fiber content might help to reduce the likelihood of cardiovascular disease. This is because both of these chilis are so extraordinarily high in fat that they might *contribute* to diseases despite their favorable fiber contents.

Foods that contain any nutrient in amounts that may incur disease risks may not bear any health claims. This is true even for a food that is high in one or more beneficial constituents. Conversely, any food that *does* bear a health claim will reliably contain, in a serving, 20 percent or less of the Daily Values for fat, saturated fat, cholesterol, and sodium. Translated into grams, that means that a food bearing a health claim will contain, per serving, less than 13 grams fat, less than 4 grams saturated fat, less than 60 milligrams cholesterol, and less than 480 milligrams sodium. Can you see how the FDA and USDA officials who wrote the laws governing food labels have worked to ensure that the health claims are meaningful? They are intended to be so well regulated that consumers can easily pick out healthy packaged foods.

FAT IN PROTEIN-RICH FOODS

◆ As mentioned, beans provide an excellent source of fat-free protein in both chili products. How is it, then, that both these products are so perilously high in fat? The sources of fat are clearly indicated on the labels, too, for those who read the ingredients. The meat-containing chili derives its fat from ground beef, its first and therefore predominant ingredient. The vegetarian chili gets its fat from soybean oil, its second most predominant ingredient.

The fat in these two chili selections makes a point about processed foods. Consumers who rely heavily on processed foods turn over the responsibility for food preparation to manufacturers. In doing so, consumers must then accept into their diets whatever ingredients manufacturers decided to use. How much better off nutritionally is the person who makes chili at home from beans, a little lean meat or macaroni, tomatoes, and seasonings with no added fat? If this product bore a label, it could easily qualify to carry many of the health claims allowed on labels of processed foods. No one waves banners for the health-promoting qualities of home-made foods, but those educated in nutrition science advocate home cooking because it returns control to the hands of the consumer.

 Notes

1. V. R. Young and J. S. Marchini, Mechanisms and nutritional significance of metabolic responses to altered intakes of protein and amino acids with reference to nutritional adaptation in humans, *American Journal of Clinical Nutrition* 51 (1990): 270–289.
2. M. L. G. Gardner, Gastrointestinal absorption of intact proteins, *Annual Reviews of Nutrition* 8 (1988): 329–350.
3. H. N. Christensen, Amino acid nutrition: A two-step absorptive process, *Nutrition Reviews* 51 (1993): 95–100.
4. S. A. Anderson and D. J. Raiten, eds., *Safety of Amino Acids Used as Supplements* (Bethesda: Federation of American Societies for Experimental Biology, 1992).
5. D. J. Clauw and P. Katz, Treatment of the eosinophilia-myalgia syndrome, *New England Journal of Medicine* 323 (1990): 417–418; E. A. Belongia, A. N. Mayeno and M. T. Osterholm, The eosinophilia-myalgia syndrome and tryptophan, *Annual Review of Nutrition* 12 (1992): 235–256.
6. L-Tryptophan recall expanded, *FDA Consumer*, June 1991, pp. 38–39.
7. Young and Marchini, 1990.
8. Young and Marchini, 1990.
9. V. R. Young, Soy protein in relation to human protein and amino acid nutrition, *Journal of the American Dietetic Association* 91 (1991): 828–835.
10. Dr. G. P. Webb, Faculty of Science, University of East London, personal communication, 1992.
11. *Protein Quality Evaluation: Report of a Joint FAO/WHO Expert Consultation*, Food and Nutrition paper no. 51 (Rome, Italy: FAO and WHO, 1990).
12. B. Torún and F. Chew, Protein-energy malnutrition in M. E. Shils, J. A. Olson, and M. Shike, eds., *Modern Nutrition in Health and Disease* (Philadelphia: Lea & Febiger, 1994), pp. 950–976 presents a full discussion of PEM.
13. C. Gopalan, The contribution of nutrition research to the control of undernutrition: The Indian experience, *Annual Review of Nutrition* 12 (1992): 1–17; D. B. Jelliffe and E. F. P. Jelliffe, Causations of kwashiorkor: Toward a multifactorial consensus, *Pediatrics* 90 (1992): 110–112.
14. A. P. Delahoussaye and J. L. Jorizzo, Cutaneous manifestations of nutritional disorders, *Dermatologic Clinics* 7 (1989): 559–570.
15. B. D. Woodward and R. G. Miller, Depression of thymus-dependent immunity in wasting protein-energy malnutrition does not depend on an altered ratio of helper ($CD4^+$) to suppressor ($CD8^+$) cells or on a disproportionately large atrophy of the T-cell relative to the B-cell pool, *American Journal of Clinical Nutrition* 53 (1991): 1329–1335; H. P. Redmond and coauthors, Impaired macrophage function in severe protein-energy malnutrition, *Journal of the American Dietetic Association* 91 (1991): 192–195.
16. R. K. Chandra, 1990 McCollum Award Lecture: Nutrition and immunity: Lessons from the past and new insights into the future, *American Journal of Clinical Nutrition* 53 (1991): 1087–1101.
17. M. A. Dhansay, A. J. Benade, and P. R. Donald, Plasma lecithin-cholesterol acyltransferase activity and plasma lipoprotein composition and concentrations in kwashiorkor, *American Journal of Clinical Nutrition* 53 (1991): 512–519.
18. J. C. Wolgemuth and coauthors, Wasting malnutrition and inadequate nutrient intakes identified in a multiethnic homeless population, *Journal of the American Dietetic Association* 92 (1992): 834–839; M. Nestle and S. Guttmacher, Hunger in the United States: Rationale, methods, and policy implications of state hunger surveys, *Journal of Nutrition Education* 24 (1992): 18S–22S.
19. J. M. Dodds, S. L. Parker, and P. S. Haines, Hunger in the 80's and 90's: A challenge for nutrition educators, *Journal of Nutrition Education* 24 (1992): 2S.
20. N. Bouby and coauthors, Role of the urinary concentrating process in the renal effects of high protein intake, *Kidney International* 34 (1988): 4–12.
21. F. E. Ahmed, Effect of diet on progression of chronic renal disease, *Journal of the American Dietetic Association* 91 (1991): 1266–1270.
22. A. R. Sherman, L. Helyar, and I. Wolinsky, Effects of dietary protein concentration on trace minerals in rat tissues at different ages, *Journal of Nutrition* 115 (1985): 607–614.
23. M. G. Holl and L. H. Allen, Comparative effects of meals high in protein, sucrose, or starch on human mineral metabolism and insulin secretion, *American Journal of Clinical Nutrition* 48 (1988): 1219–1225; M. B. Zemel, Calcium utilization: Effect of varying level and source of dietary protein, *American Journal of Clinical Nutrition* 48 (1988): 880–883; R. P. Blank and coauthors, Calcium metabolism and osteoporotic ridge resorption: A protein connection, *Journal of Prosthetic Dentistry* 58 (1987): 590–595; E. Fernandez-Repollet, P. Van Loon, and M. Martinez-Maldonado, Renal and systemic effects of short-term high protein feeding in normal rats, *American Journal of the Medical Sciences* 297 (1989): 348–354; J. C. Howe, Postprandial response of calcium metabolism in postmenopausal women to meals varying in protein level and source, *Metabolism: Clinical and Experimental* 39 (1990): 1246–1252; an article showing no difference in bone mineral content between omnivores and vegetarians is I. F. Hunt and coauthors, Bone mineral content in postmenopausal women: comparison of omnivores and vegetarians, *American Journal of Clinical Nutrition* 50 (1989): 517–523.
24. H. Spencer, L. Kramer, and D. Osis, Do protein and phosphorous cause calcium loss? *Journal of Nutrition* 118 (1988): 657–660.

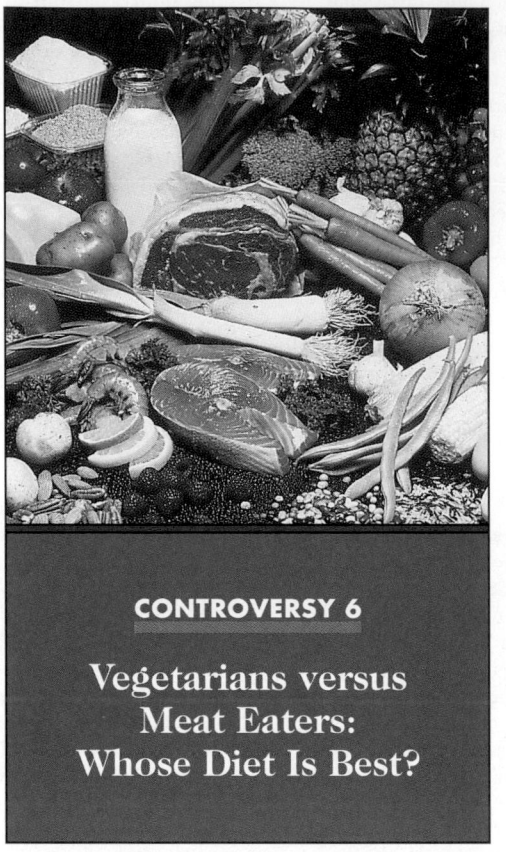

CONTROVERSY 6

Vegetarians versus Meat Eaters: Whose Diet Is Best?

One young professional person rejects all animal products, shuns grains, and seeks out vegetables, fruits, and herbs. Another young professional relishes meat at every meal and usually orders "steak and potatoes; hold the rabbit food." These two have a lot more in common than either would probably believe. Both are extremists in their choices of foods. Both may be jeopardizing their health by way of their rigid, unbalanced daily food intakes. But both vegetarian diets and meat-containing diets have elements in their favor, provided that they are not taken to extremes. This Controversy looks first at the positive health aspects of vegetarian diets, then at the positive aspects of meat-eaters' diets. It concludes by showing how both can maximize the benefits and minimize the risks of their diets.

POSITIVE HEALTH ASPECTS OF VEGETARIAN DIETS Researchers often study vegetarians in an attempt to establish relationships between diet and health. Such research would be easy if the only difference between vegetarians and others was their consumption of meat. However, many vegetarians have adopted lifestyles that differ from those of meat eaters in other ways besides diet. There are exceptions, but typically, vegetarians use no tobacco, use alcohol in moderation if at all, and are more physically active than others. Researchers must account for the effects of lifestyle differences other than diet before they can see how health correlates with diet. Even then, *correlations* are not *causes.* Without more evidence, conclusions must be tentative.

Still, with all these qualifications, research findings are intriguing. They seem to indicate that the vegetarian diet may offer some protection against five conditions: obesity, high blood pressure, heart disease, digestive disorders, and cancer. What is known about these relationships follows.

Obesity Vegetarians tend to maintain healthier body weights than nonvegetarians. Perhaps they consciously control their food intakes and exercise habits. Perhaps their diet, which tends to be low in fat and high in fiber-rich bulky foods, is lower in calories than the average diet based on meat. The especially fattening power of fat, described in Controversy 5, may also be a factor: vegetarians tend to have low fat intakes. In any case, a healthy body weight, combined with high intakes of complex carbohydrates and fiber and a low intake of fat, reduces the risks of several obesity-related diseases.

Blood Pressure In some studies, vegetarians have lower blood pressure than nonvegetarians; in others, there is no difference. Various combinations of lifestyle factors and diet seem to influence blood pressure. Among lifestyle factors, smoking and alcohol intake raise blood pressure, and exercise lowers it. Diet alone may be responsible, however. The effect of a vegetarian diet on blood pressure remains apparent even when all the people being compared are nonsmokers. In one group of volunteers, blood pressure declined during the period when they ate a vegetarian diet and rose again when they resumed eating meat.[1]

Heart Disease Fewer vegetarians suffer from diseases of the heart and arteries than meat eaters, even when the people being compared are all nonsmokers. The dietary factor most directly related to coronary artery disease is fat intake, especially of saturated fat. When vegetarians are fed meat, which contains saturated fat, their lipid profiles change for the worse; when meat eaters are fed a low-fat vegetarian diet, their lipid profiles improve. One study compared two low-fat diets, one vegetarian and another containing lean meats. Both diets lowered blood cholesterol, but the vegetarian diet's effects were greater.[2] People can achieve low blood cholesterol and still eat meat: researchers found lowered blood cholesterol in subjects who ate meat but who also kept intakes of saturated fat to a minimum.[3] In general, the typical vegetarian diet is also higher in dietary fiber than the typical nonvegetarian diet, another factor believed to help control blood lipids.

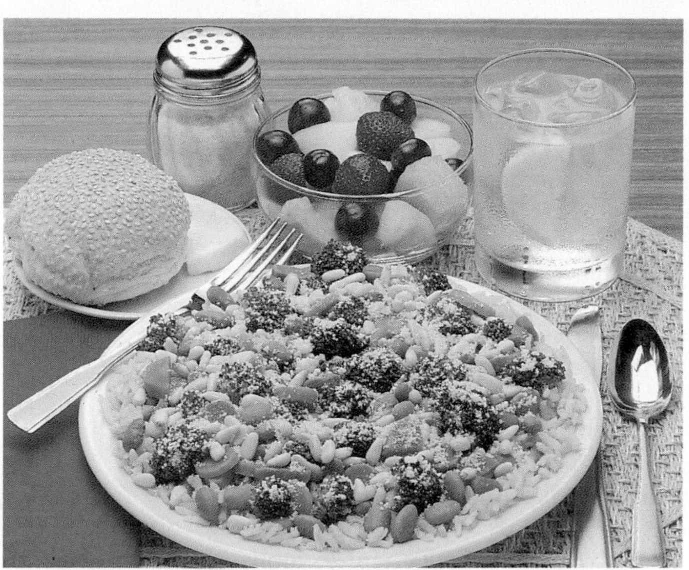

A balanced meal need not include meat to be nutritious.

Protein seems to affect blood cholesterol, too. Diets containing purified proteins from animal sources (milk, fish, and egg) may raise blood cholesterol higher than do similar diets containing purified soybean protein, at least in some animals. When rabbits were fed diets containing 50 percent of calories from purified animal protein along with high cholesterol, the animals suffered rapid advancement of atherosclerosis.[4] Rabbits are naturally vegetarians, though, so this may not be a fair test of what happens in human beings.

In any case, it is suggested that people with high blood cholesterol can lower it by altering the ratio of the animal to vegetable protein in their diets. The typical ratio is 2 to 1; the suggested ratio 1 to 1. In animals, the 1-to-1 ratio maintains blood cholesterol as low as a diet containing vegetable protein alone. For people with blood cholesterol in the lower ranges, though, no effect is seen. Some investigators believe that for these lucky people the type of dietary protein is of little significance.

People eat foods, not purified proteins, so the question of whether animal or vegetable proteins, by themselves, raise or lower blood cholesterol is academic. The purified proteins found in experiments to raise blood cholesterol are milk protein (casein) and the protein of fish. If the whole foods are used instead of the isolated proteins, the contrast between animal and vegetable proteins is not seen. Milk *lowers* blood cholesterol just as soy does, and meals of fish provide benefits to heart health, as Chapter 5 made clear. In conclusion, then, lipids are of significance in the vegetarian heart connection and proteins may not be.

Digestive Disorders Constipation and diverticular disease are less common in people who consume a high-fiber vegetarian or semivegetarian diet than in people who consume a typical meat-based diet. Chapter 4 presented possible ways fiber might influence the health of the digestive tract.

Cancer Seventh-Day Adventists, an often-studied vegetarian group, enjoy a cancer rate of about one half to two thirds that of the rest of the population, even when cancers linked to smoking and alcohol are taken out of the picture. Their low cancer mortality may possibly be due to their low meat intakes, to their high intakes of vegetables and cereal grains, to both—or to other lifestyle factors. In general, low cancer rates correlate with low meat and high fruit, vegetable, and grain intakes.

Some scientific findings support the idea that vegetarian diets may reduce the risks of colon cancer.[5] People with colon cancer seem to eat more meat, less fiber, and more saturated fat than others without colon cancer.[6] Something about high-fat, high-protein, low-fiber diets creates an environment in the human colon that may promote the development of colon cancer.[7]

In general, then, many vegetarians have less risk of developing obesity, high blood pressure, heart disease, digestive disorders, cancer, than do meat eaters.[8] Two million people in the United States follow vegetarian diets. If they plan their diets correctly, they obtain all the nutrients they need to support good health.

POSITIVE HEALTH ASPECTS OF THE MEAT EATER'S DIET The meat-loving character presented at the start of this chapter was exaggerated to make a point. In reality, few people shun all vegetables. Those who really eat like that place themselves in peril of malnutrition. To be healthy, people must either eat foods from all five food groups presented in Chapter 2, or, if they omit foods from one group, they must make careful substitutions to compensate. No substitutes can take the place of fruits and vegetables. This section considers a balanced diet of which meat is a part.

Growth Meat, eggs, and other foods from animal sources support growth well. Without them, children's growth often shows deficits. Populations existing on monotonous cereal diets, either for reasons of meat taboos or of economic necessity, are often found to be malnourished, as revealed by their short stature, low resistance to diseases, short life spans, and high infant mortality. Even in populations with more varied diets, the children who eat the most animal-derived products have been observed to grow the best.[9] Children who eat equal protein amounts, but from plant sources, may not grow as well. These observations and laboratory work have led to a common belief: that animal and dairy products are superior to plants as protein-rich foods. Present-day clinical tests have shown, however, that this impression is erroneous, at least with regard to nutrition of adults.

It is true that animal and dairy foods contain complete, more digestible proteins. It seems to be true that children of milk- and meat-eating populations are generally larger, fatter, and more resistant to infections than are those of grain-eating populations. But it is also true that some children grow normally on a diet of vegetables, legumes, fruits, and grains. It must be carefully planned with knowledge and delivered consistently, however.

Support during Critical Times Meat eaters can generally rely on their diets during critical times of life. For example, a vegetarian woman may enter pregnancy too thin; be too low in iron, zinc, and vitamin B_{12}; and fail to gain enough weight during pregnancy to support the normal growth and development of her fetus. Meat eaters are much less likely to face these problems.

Meat, which contains abundant protein, iron, and food energy in less bulk, can support the growth of children more efficiently. Unlike strict vegetarians, eaters of meats and dairy products can be sure of receiving enough vitamin B_{12}, vitamin D, calcium, iron, and zinc as well as protein, without supplements or fortified foods.

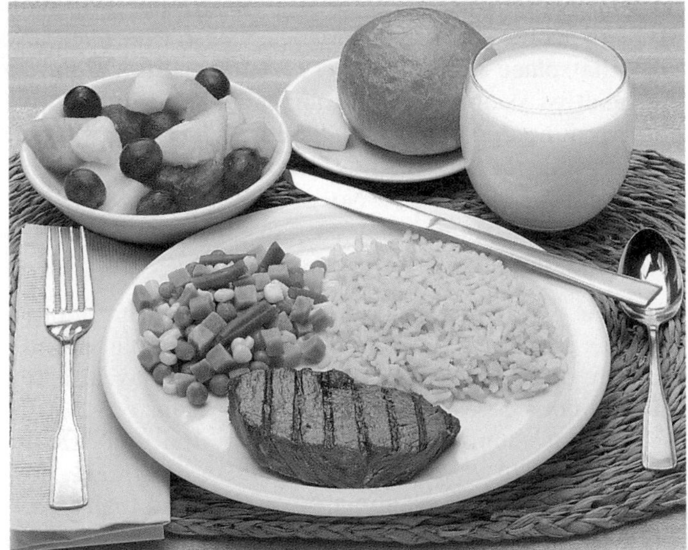

Two meat servings of the size depicted here present the maximum daily meat intake suggested by the Daily Food Guide as health-promoting.

Fertility Some studies raise the question whether vegetarian women have a diminished capacity to conceive. They report that vegetarian women have less of the hormone estrogen in their blood than meat-eating women, and that they more often have irregular menstrual periods.[10] Meat eaters' blood estrogen is considered to be normal, and they have fewer problems with infertility.

Nutrient Adequacy For the vegan who excludes all animal products, achieving adequate energy and nutrient intakes may be difficult, particularly for growing children. Foods of plant origin generally offer much less energy for their bulk than do foods of animal origin. A child's small stomach can hold only so much food, and a vegetarian child may feel full before having eaten enough food to meet nutrient needs. If the food carries little energy per unit of bulk, it may not deliver sufficient energy to support growth.[11] For obesity-prone adults, a bulky diet can be advantageous, but a child fed without meat, milk, or eggs may face stunted growth. Children who consume animal products tend to be taller in height and heavier in weight than vegan children.[12] They are also protected from the vitamin D-deficiency disease rickets, which is especially likely to strike vegans in cold climates.[13]

The only foods that come close to matching the nutrients of meat are legumes, nuts, and the highest-protein cereal grains. Furthermore, even if a child obtains the full RDA of protein from these sources, fiber and other factors in plant foods may make them less available to the body.

Many of the nutrients of meat are also found in milk products and eggs, so vegetarians who consume these foods have few nutrient deficiency concerns.[14] Such foods can adequately support the growth of children.[15]

CONCLUSIONS Both the vegetarian's and the meat eater's diets have the potential to benefit health. Many of the benefits attributed to the vegetarian diet may be due to its low fat content, but a meat eater who keeps fat intakes low gains the same advantages. Diets including the recommended 2- to 3-ounce portions of such meats as turkey breast and fish, as well as providing the needed low-fat grains, fruits, and vegetables, probably support health as well as vegetarian diets. The vegetarian diet's other chief advantage, that it is high in fiber, can also be true of the moderate meat eater's diet.

Conversely, both diets can be high in fat. A vegetarian who dines on cheddar cheese, butter sauces, sour cream, and deep-fried vegetables invites the same health hazards as the overeater of high-fat meats. And both diets can, if not properly balanced, lack nutrients. The vegetarian's diet may lack vitamin B_{12}, vitamin D, calcium, iron, and zinc; the meat eater's diet may lack vitamins A, folate, and C, among others.

For both eaters, then, planning is the key to obtaining adequate nutrients. Those who eliminate meats can follow the Daily Food Guide presented in Chapter 2 (pages 40 and 41). If they permit themselves the use of animal products, they can use milk, cheese, and eggs for protein; if not, they can use legumes and products made from them, such as peanut butter and tofu, to the same extent that meat eaters use meat.

Plant foods, including vegetables, can donate a surprising amount of protein to the diet. When researchers first studied human protein needs, they concluded that vegans could easily become protein deficient unless they balanced their amino acids gram for gram at every meal. Later research showed this investment of effort to be unnecessary. Still, the original impression stuck with the public for years. Researchers still agree that health depends on obtaining adequate amounts of all the amino acids, but they now think the timing is less critical. Amino acid intakes must be balanced over days, not hours. Evidence shows that the liver monitors the amino acid composition of proteins eaten at a meal. If the meal is low in an essential amino acid, the liver breaks down its own proteins to supply it. Later, at the next meal or so when the amino acid is once again abundant, the liver replenishes its protein to be ready for the next occasion. Thus if a protein source such as corn (low in tryptophan, but not in other amino acids) is eaten alone on occasion, the liver cells donate needed tryptophan, thus allowing some protein synthesis to continue temporarily. In a well-nourished person, incomplete proteins occasionally eaten alone cause no harm.

In practice, the possibility of a vegetarian's suffering a protein deficiency due to unbalanced amino acid consumption from plant foods is remote. Only when fruits and certain vegetables define the core of the diet, severely limiting both the *quantity and quality* of its protein, might protein deficiency result. Steady diets based on cassava or fruits are examples. They would soon deplete the body's essential amino acid pool and protein deficiency would ensue. The root vegetable cassava that people of many developing countries use daily contains adequate energy but inadequate protein. Fruits provide adequate energy, but most are low in protein. Advocates of fruitarian (only fruit) diets should include nuts and seeds regularly.

For calcium, if vegetarians don't use milk, they can use soy milk. In addition, the nutrients iron, zinc, and vitamin B_{12} require special attention from strict vegetarians. Meat provides much of the iron and zinc in the meat eater's diet, and vitamin B_{12} is found reliably only in animal-derived foods. Vegetarians can obtain iron from plant foods such as legumes, dark green leafy vegetables, iron-fortified cereals, and whole-grain breads and cereals. Eggs, for those who eat them, can meet vitamin B_{12} needs; vegans must rely on vitamin B_{12}-fortified sources or on supplements.[16] Fermented plant products such as tempeh, made from soy beans, may contain some vitamin B_{12} contributed by the bacteria that did the fermenting, but unfortunately, much of the vitamin B_{12} found in these products may be in an inactive form.[17]

Meat eaters, too, can most easily obtain the nutrients they need by following the Daily Food Guide. If they obtain the recommended servings of fruits, vegetables, and grains, and keep their meat portions moderate, they will fare well nutritionally. For the most part it seems that nonmeat and low-meat diets can both support good health.

This comparison has shown that there is nothing mysterious about either the meat eater's or the vegetarian's diet. Both can be analyzed scientifically. In particular, vegetarianism is not a religion like Buddhism or Hinduism; it is merely an eating plan that selects plant foods to deliver needed nutrients. Some people make much of the distinctions between types of vegetarians first described in Chapter 1—lacto-vegetarians, lacto-ovo vegetarians, and vegans. These distinctions are useful academically, but do not represent uncrossable lines. Many combinations of these categories exist. Some people eat no read meat, but do eat chicken and fish. Some people eat meat only once a week, and use plant protein foods the rest of the time. Many people rely mostly on milk products to meet their protein needs, but eat fish occasionally, and so forth. To force people into the categories of "vegetarians" and "meat eaters" leaves out all these in-between styles of eating that represent large numbers of people and have much to recommend them.

To the person just beginning to study nutrition, consider adopting the attitude that the choice to make is not whether to be a meat eater or a vegetarian, but where along the spectrum to locate yourself. Your preferences, whatever they are, should be honored and the only caveat is that you make your diet adequate, balanced, and varied, and use moderation when choosing high-calorie foods.

Notes

1. L. J. Beilin and coauthors, Vegetarian diet and blood pressure levels: Incidental or causal association? *American Journal of Clinical Nutrition* 48 (1988): 806–810.
2. M. Kestin and coauthors, Cardiovascular disease risk factors in free-living men: Comparison of two prudent diets, one based on lactoovovegetarianism and the other allowing meat, *American Journal of Clinical Nutrition* 50 (1989): 280–287.
3. S. A. Morgan, A. J. Sinclair, and K. O'Dea, Effect on serum lipids of addition of safflower oil or olive oil to very-low-fat diets rich in lean beef, *Journal of the American Dietetic Association* 93 (1993): 644–648.
4. K. K. Carroll, Review of clinical studies on cholesterol-lowering response to soy protein, *Journal of the American Dietetic Association* 91 (1991): 820–827.
5. U. G. Allinger and coauthors, Shift from a mixed to a lactovegetarian diet: Influence on acidic lipids in fecal water—A potential risk factor for colon cancer, *American Journal of Clinical Nutrition* 50 (1989): 992–996.
6. M. B. Grosvenor, Diet and colon cancer, *Nutrition and the M.D.*, April 1989; S. A. Bingham, Meat, starch, and nonstarch polysaccharides and large bowel cancer, *American Journal of Clinical Nutrition* 48 (1988): 762–776.
7. M. I. McBurney, P. J. Van Soest, and J. L. Jeraci, Colonic carcinogenesis: The microbial feast or famine mechanism, *Nutrition and Cancer* 10 (1987): 23–38.
8. J. T. Dwyer, Health aspects of vegetarian diets, *American Journal of Clinical Nutrition* 48 (1988): 712–738; Position of the American Dietetic Association: Vegetarian diets, *Journal of the American Dietetic Association* 88 (1988): 351–355.
9. L. H. Allen and coauthors, Interactive effects of dietary quality on the growth and attained size of young Mexican children, *American Journal of Clinical Nutrition* 56 (1992): 329–333.
10. A. B. Pederson and coauthors, Menstrual differences due to vegetarian and nonvegetarian diets, *American Journal of Clinical Nutrition* 53 (1991): 879–885.
11. C. Jacobs and J. T. Dwyer, Vegetarian children: Appropriate and inappropriate diets, *American Journal of Clinical Nutrition* 48 (1988): 822–825.
12. T. A. B. Sanders, Growth and development of British vegan children, *American Journal of Clinical Nutrition* 48 (1988): 822–825.
13. P. C. Dagnelie, High prevalence of rickets in infants on macrobiotic diets, *American Journal of Clinical Nutrition* 51 (1990): 202–208.
14. Position of The American Dietetic Association, 1988.
15. J. M. O'Connell, Growth of vegetarian children: The Farm Study, *Pediatrics* 84 (1989): 475–481; M. Tayter and K. L. Stanek, Anthropometric and dietary assessment of omnivore and lacto-ovo-vegetarian children, *Journal of the American Dietetic Association* 89 (1989): 1661–1663.
16. D. R. Miller and coauthors, Vitamin B-12 status in a macrobiotic community, *American Journal of Clinical Nutrition* 53 (1991): 524–529.
17. V. Herbert, Vitamin B-12: Plant sources, requirements, and assay, *American Journal of Clinical Nutrition* 48 (1988): 852–858.

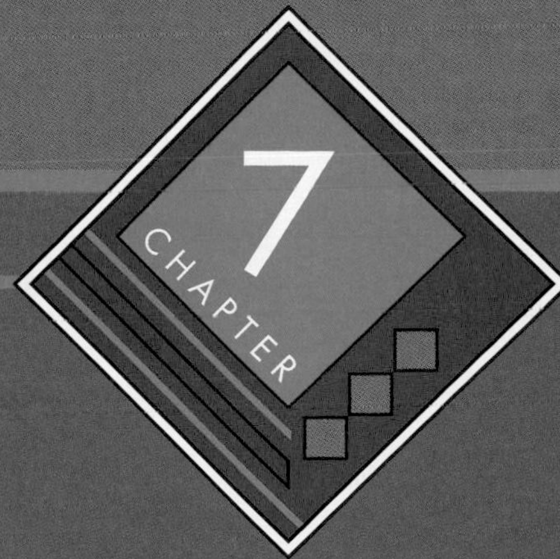

The Vitamins

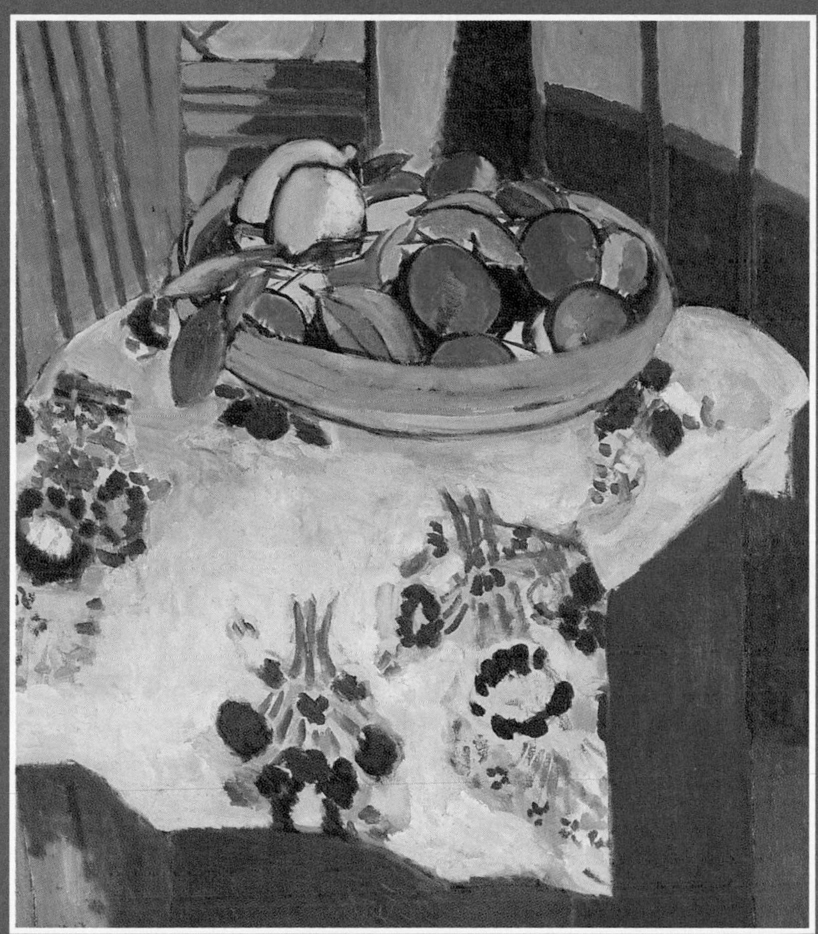

Contents

Henri Matisse, Still Life with Oranges, Musée du Louvre, Photo R.M.N.; © 1992 Les Hertiers Matisse, Paris/ARS, N.Y.

vitamins organic compounds, vital to life, indispensable to body function, needed in minute amounts; noncaloric essential nutrients.

precursors compounds that can be converted into active vitamins; also known as **provitamins.**

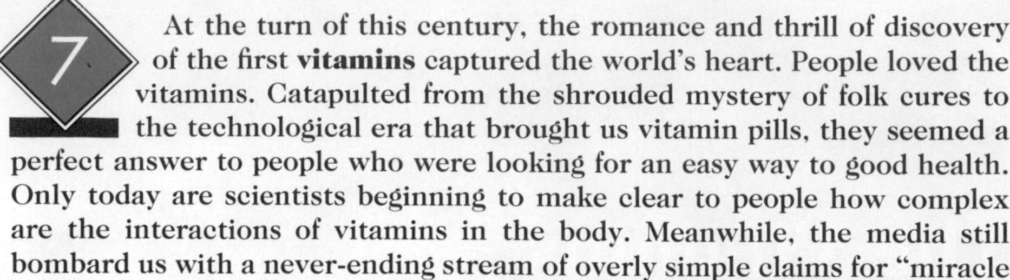

At the turn of this century, the romance and thrill of discovery of the first **vitamins** captured the world's heart. People loved the vitamins. Catapulted from the shrouded mystery of folk cures to the technological era that brought us vitamin pills, they seemed a perfect answer to people who were looking for an easy way to good health. Only today are scientists beginning to make clear to people how complex are the interactions of vitamins in the body. Meanwhile, the media still bombard us with a never-ending stream of overly simple claims for "miracle vitamins," and the supplement business is a multi*billion* dollar industry.

From a review of the history of vitamin discoveries, it is easy to see why people are so impressed. The story line has been repeated over and over with the discovery of each new vitamin. For example, whole groups of people are unable to walk (or are going blind or bleeding profusely) until an alert scientist stumbles onto the substance missing from their diets. According to the plot, the scientist usually confirms the discovery by feeding vitamin-deficient feed to laboratory animals. The animals respond by becoming unable to walk (or going blind or bleeding profusely). Then, miraculously, they recover when the one missing ingredient is restored to their diet. Miraculous cures of people follow as they, too, receive the missing vitamin. On reading dramatic stories like these, people come to believe that vitamins will cure a host of ailments. But the truth is that the only disease a vitamin will cure is the one caused by a deficiency of that vitamin.

The only disease a vitamin can cure is the one caused by a deficiency of that vitamin.

It took a sophisticated knowledge of chemistry and biology to isolate the vitamins and to learn their chemical structures. Today, chemists can synthesize vitamins in the laboratory, and people can therefore take them in supplement form. This development may present some advantages, but it also results in risks, for even if used to cure deficiency, vitamin doses can be too high, and can do harm.

As they were discovered, the vitamins were named, and many were also given letters and numbers. This led to the confusion that still exists today. This chapter uses the names shown in Table 7-1; alternative names are given in Tables 7-3 and 7-4 on pages 249–254.

Previous chapters included Consumer Caution sections on supplements. People take supplements for so many different reasons that this chapter's entire Controversy is devoted to the question whether you may need vitamin (and mineral) supplements and if so, which ones to take. The Consumer Caution section focuses on some emerging knowledge that proposes a special function for certain vitamins and a mineral, the antioxidant nutrients, with regard to cancer and heart disease prevention.

Table 7-1
Vitamin Names

Fat-soluble vitamins
Vitamin A
Vitamin D
Vitamin E
Vitamin K
Water-soluble vitamins
B vitamins
Thiamin
Riboflavin
Niacin
Vitamin B_6
Folate
Vitamin B_{12}
Pantothenic acid
Biotin
Vitamin C

Vitamin names established by the International Union of Nutritional Sciences Committee on Nomenclature, in Nomenclature policy: Generic descriptors and trivial names for vitamins and related compounds, *Journal of Nutrition* 117 (1987): 7–15.

Definition and Classification of Vitamins

A child once defined a vitamin as "what, if you don't eat, you get sick." Although the grammar left something to be desired, the definition was accurate. Less imaginatively, a vitamin is defined as an essential, noncaloric, organic nutrient needed in tiny amounts in the diet. The role of many vitamins is to help make possible the processes by which other nutrients are digested, absorbed, and metabolized, or built into body structures. Although small in size and quantity, the vitamins accomplish mighty tasks, some of which are still being discovered.

Some of the vitamins occur in foods in a form known as **precursors,** or **provitamins.** Once inside the body, these are changed chemically to one or more active vitamin forms. Thus in measuring the amount of a vitamin found in food, it is often most accurate to count not only the amount of the true vitamin but also the vitamin activity potentially available from its precursors. Tables 7-3 and 7-4 on pages 249–254 show which vitamins have precursors.

The vitamins fall naturally into two classes: fat soluble and water soluble. Solubility imparts to vitamins many of their characteristic behaviors and determines how they are absorbed into and transported around the bloodstream, whether they can be stored in the body, and how easily they are lost from the body. In general, fat-soluble vitamins are absorbed, like other fats, into the lymph. They travel in the blood associated with protein carriers. Fat-soluble vitamins can be stored with other lipids in fatty tissues, and because they are stored, they can build up to toxic concentrations. The water-soluble vitamins, on the other hand, are generally absorbed directly into the bloodstream, where they travel freely. They are not stored in tissues to any great extent; rather, excesses are excreted in the urine. Thus the risks of immediate toxicities are not as great as for fat-soluble vitamins, except in cases of extremely high doses. This chapter addresses first the fat-soluble vitamins and then the water-soluble ones. Some of the most important facts will be discussed separately for each vitamin, and the tables at the end of the chapter sum up the basic facts about all of them.

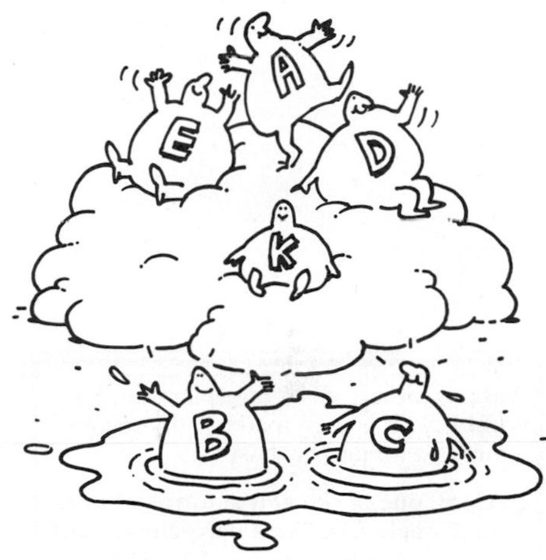

Vitamins fall into two classes—fat soluble and water soluble.

KEY POINT Vitamins are essential, noncaloric nutrients, needed in tiny amounts in the diet, that serve as helpers in cell functions. The fat-soluble vitamins are vitamins A, D, E, and K; the water-soluble vitamins are the B vitamins and vitamin C.

The Fat-Soluble Vitamins

The fat-soluble vitamins—A, D, E, and K—generally occur together in the fats and oils of foods. Like the lipids, these vitamins require bile for absorption. Once absorbed, they are stored in the liver and fatty tissues until the body needs them. For this reason the body can easily survive weeks of consuming foods that lack them, as long as the diet as a whole provides *average* amounts that approximate the Recommended Dietary Allowances (RDA).[1] The capacity to be stored also sets the stage for toxic buildup, should an excess be taken in, especially in the form of supplements. Excesses of vitamins A, D, and K can especially easily reach toxic levels.

Deficiencies of the fat-soluble vitamins are likely when the diet is consistently low in them or when they are inadvertently lost from the digestive tract dissolved in undigested fat. Any disease that produces fat malabsorption (such as liver disease that prevents bile production) can bring about deficiencies of the fat-soluble vitamins. Deficiencies are also likely when people eat diets that are extremely low in fat; such diets interfere with the absorption of these vitamins. A person who uses mineral oil (which the body can't absorb) as a laxative risks losing the fat-soluble vitamins by excretion.

The roles that the fat-soluble vitamins play in the body are diverse. Vitamin A is, among many other things, a visual pigment. Vitamins A and D can act somewhat like hormones, directing cells to convert one substance to another, to store this, or to release that. Vitamin E flows all over the body, preventing oxidative destruction of tissues. Vitamin K is necessary for blood to clot. Each is worth a book in itself.

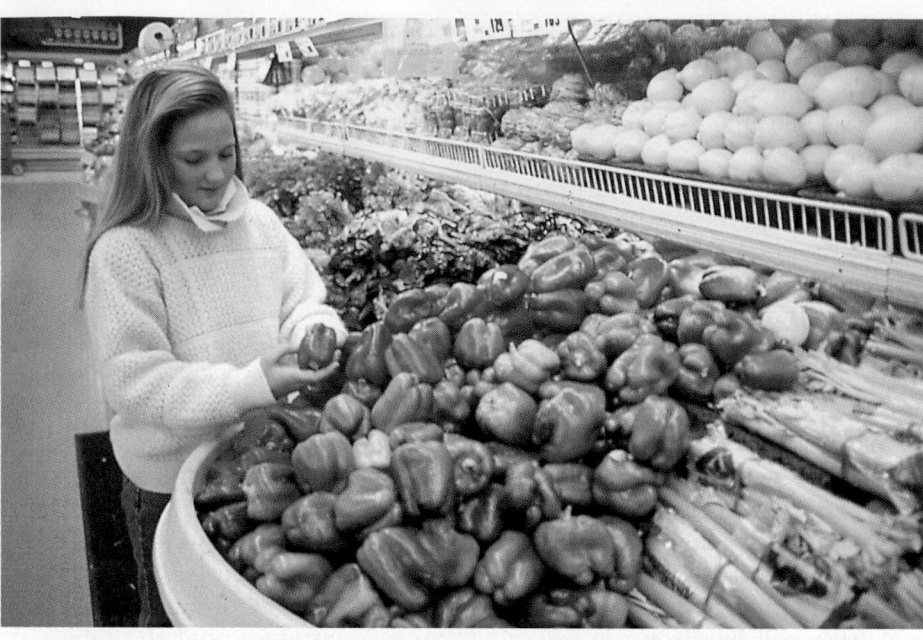

Colorful foods often are rich in vitamins.

beta carotene an orange pigment; a vitamin A precursor made by plants and stored in human fat tissue.

retinol one of the active forms of vitamin A made from beta carotene in animal and human bodies. Other active forms are **retinal** and **retinoic acid.**

retina (RET-in-uh) the layer of light-sensitive nerve cells lining the back of the inside of the eye.

cornea (KOR-nee-uh) the hard, transparent membrane covering the outside of the eye.

rhodopsin the light-sensitive pigment of the cells in the retina; it contains vitamin A (*rhod* refers to the rod-shaped cells; *opsin* means "visual protein").

night blindness slow recovery of vision after exposure to flashes of bright light at night; an early symptom of vitamin A deficiency.

Vitamin A and Beta Carotene

Vitamin A has the distinction of being the first fat-soluble vitamin to be recognized. Today, after more than 75 years of research and revelations, vitamin A and its plant-derived precursor, **beta carotene,** are the focus of attention and intrigue for researchers around the world. Much of this intensive research effort is based on accumulating evidence that both active vitamin A and beta carotene may protect against certain types of cancer.

Vitamin A Vitamin A is certainly one of the most versatile vitamins, with roles in such diverse functions as vision, immune defenses, maintenance of body linings and skin, bone and body growth, normal cell development, and reproduction. In short, vitamin A is needed everywhere. Three forms of vitamin A are active in the body; one of the active forms, **retinol,** is stored in the liver. The liver makes retinol available to the bloodstream and thereby to the body cells. The cells convert retinol to its other two active forms, **retinal** and **retinoic acid,** as needed.

Perhaps the most familiar function of vitamin A is in eyesight. Vitamin A plays two indispensable roles in the eye: in the events of light perception at the **retina** and in the maintenance of a healthy, crystal-clear outer window, the **cornea.**

When light falls on the eye, it passes through the clear cornea and strikes the cells of the retina, bleaching many molecules of the pigment **rhodopsin** that lie within them. Vitamin A is a part of the rhodopsin molecule. The vitamin is broken off when bleaching occurs, initiating the signal that conveys the sensation of sight to the optic center in the brain. The vitamin then reunites with the pigment, but a little vitamin A is destroyed each time this reaction takes place, and fresh vitamin A arriving in the blood regenerates the supply. If the supply is low, a lag occurs before the eye can see again after a flash of bright light at night (see Figure 7-1). This lag in the recovery of night vision, termed **night blindness,** may indicate a vitamin A deficiency. A bright flash of light can temporarily blind even normal, well-

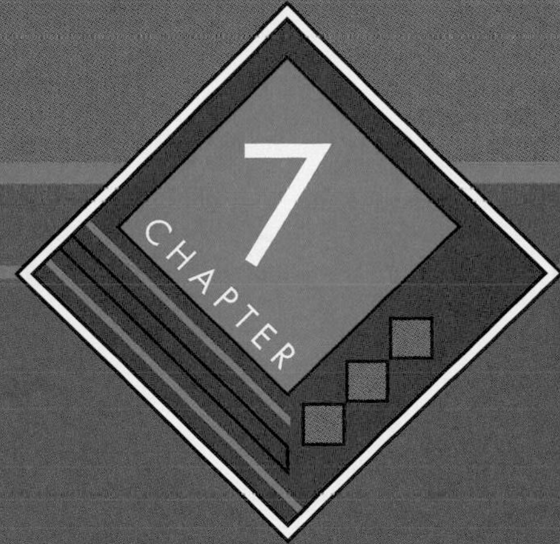

The Vitamins

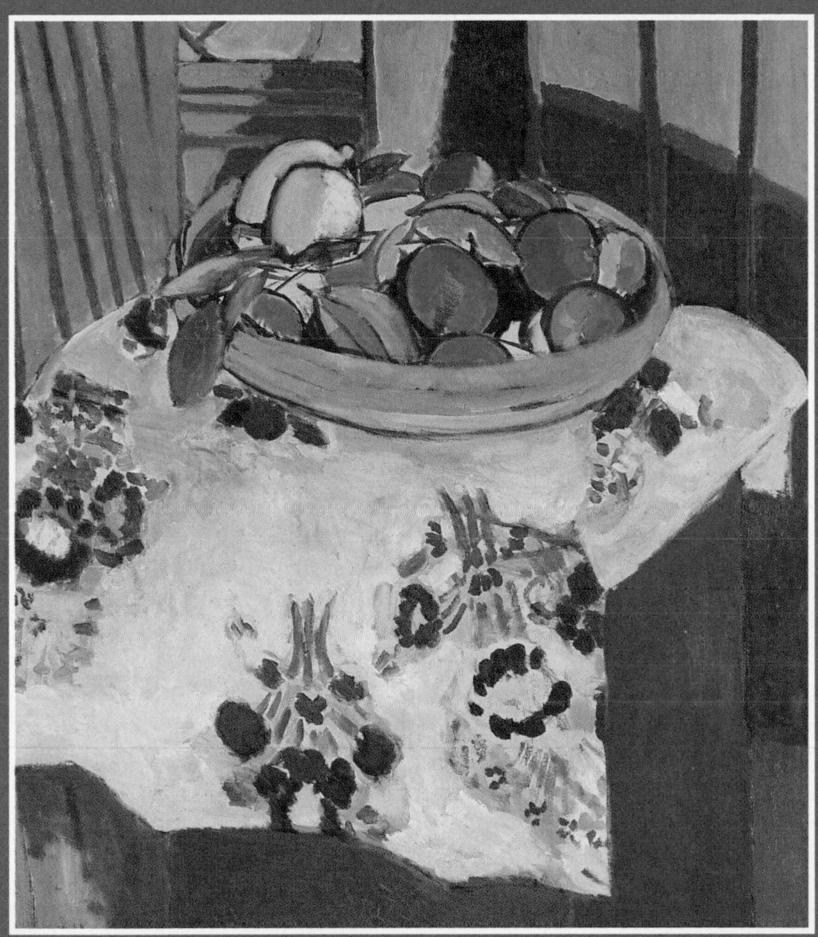

Contents

Henri Matisse, Still Life with Oranges, Musée du Louvre, Photo R.M.N.;

vitamins organic compounds, vital to life, indispensable to body function, needed in minute amounts; noncaloric essential nutrients.

precursors compounds that can be converted into active vitamins; also known as **provitamins.**

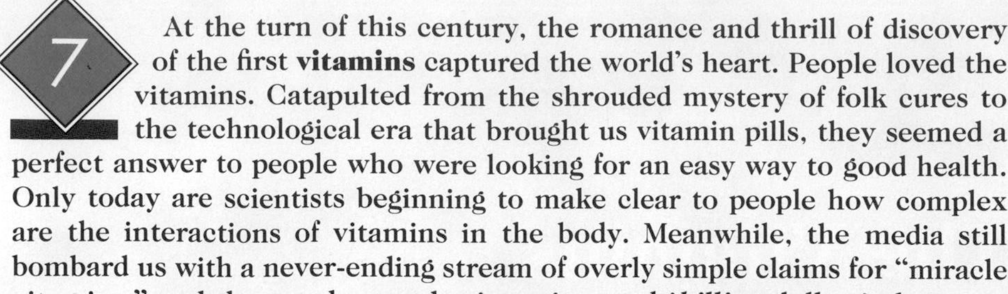

At the turn of this century, the romance and thrill of discovery of the first **vitamins** captured the world's heart. People loved the vitamins. Catapulted from the shrouded mystery of folk cures to the technological era that brought us vitamin pills, they seemed a perfect answer to people who were looking for an easy way to good health. Only today are scientists beginning to make clear to people how complex are the interactions of vitamins in the body. Meanwhile, the media still bombard us with a never-ending stream of overly simple claims for "miracle vitamins," and the supplement business is a multi*billion* dollar industry.

From a review of the history of vitamin discoveries, it is easy to see why people are so impressed. The story line has been repeated over and over with the discovery of each new vitamin. For example, whole groups of people are unable to walk (or are going blind or bleeding profusely) until an alert scientist stumbles onto the substance missing from their diets. According to the plot, the scientist usually confirms the discovery by feeding vitamin-deficient feed to laboratory animals. The animals respond by becoming unable to walk (or going blind or bleeding profusely). Then, miraculously, they recover when the one missing ingredient is restored to their diet. Miraculous cures of people follow as they, too, receive the missing vitamin. On reading dramatic stories like these, people come to believe that vitamins will cure a host of ailments. But the truth is that the only disease a vitamin will cure is the one caused by a deficiency of that vitamin.

The only disease a vitamin can cure is the one caused by a deficiency of that vitamin.

It took a sophisticated knowledge of chemistry and biology to isolate the vitamins and to learn their chemical structures. Today, chemists can synthesize vitamins in the laboratory, and people can therefore take them in supplement form. This development may present some advantages, but it also results in risks, for even if used to cure deficiency, vitamin doses can be too high, and can do harm.

As they were discovered, the vitamins were named, and many were also given letters and numbers. This led to the confusion that still exists today. This chapter uses the names shown in Table 7-1; alternative names are given in Tables 7-3 and 7-4 on pages 249–254.

Table 7-1
Vitamin Names

Fat-soluble vitamins
- Vitamin A
- Vitamin D
- Vitamin E
- Vitamin K

Water-soluble vitamins
- B vitamins
  - Thiamin
  - Riboflavin
  - Niacin
  - Vitamin B_6
  - Folate
  - Vitamin B_{12}
  - Pantothenic acid
  - Biotin
- Vitamin C

Vitamin names established by the International Union of Nutritional Sciences Committee on Nomenclature, in Nomenclature policy: Generic descriptors and trivial names for vitamins and related compounds, *Journal of Nutrition* 117 (1987): 7–15.

Previous chapters included Consumer Caution sections on supplements. People take supplements for so many different reasons that this chapter's entire Controversy is devoted to the question whether you may need vitamin (and mineral) supplements and if so, which ones to take. The Consumer Caution section focuses on some emerging knowledge that proposes a special function for certain vitamins and a mineral, the antioxidant nutrients, with regard to cancer and heart disease prevention.

Definition and Classification of Vitamins

A child once defined a vitamin as "what, if you don't eat, you get sick." Although the grammar left something to be desired, the definition was accurate. Less imaginatively, a vitamin is defined as an essential, noncaloric, organic nutrient needed in tiny amounts in the diet. The role of many vitamins is to help make possible the processes by which other nutrients are digested, absorbed, and metabolized, or built into body structures. Although small in size and quantity, the vitamins accomplish mighty tasks, some of which are still being discovered.

Some of the vitamins occur in foods in a form known as **precursors,** or **provitamins.** Once inside the body, these are changed chemically to one or

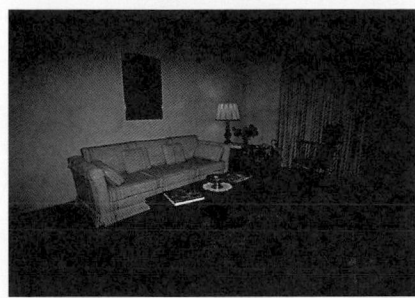

In dim light, you can make out the details in this room.

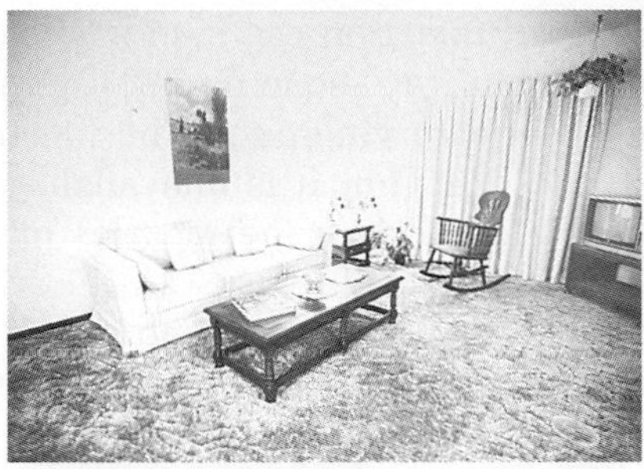

A flash of bright light momentarily blinds you as the pigment in the retina is bleached.

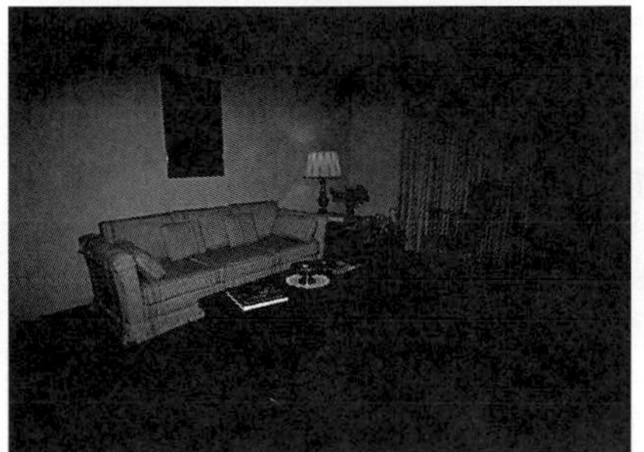

You quickly recover and can see the details again in a few seconds.

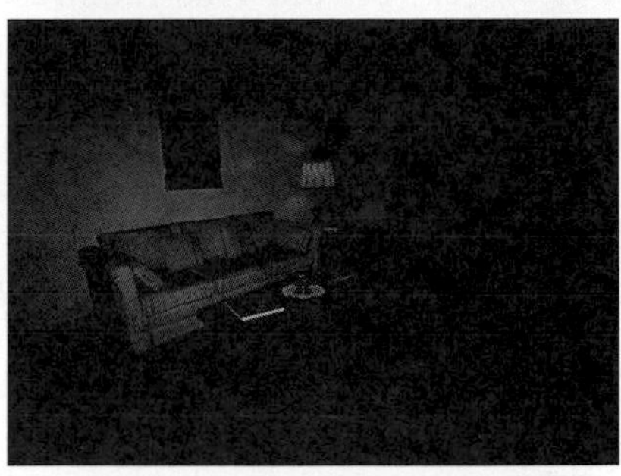

With inadequate vitamin A, you do not recover but remain blind for many seconds; this is night blindness.

Figure 7-1

NIGHT BLINDNESS
This is one of the earliest signs of vitamin A deficiency.

nourished eyes, but if you experience a long recovery period before vision returns, your health care provider may want you to check your vitamin A intake.

A deficiency of vitamin A that has progressed well beyond the night blindness stage may be reflected in an accumulation of a protein, **keratin,** which clouds the eye's outer vitamin A-dependent part, the cornea. The condition is known as **keratinization,** and it can progress to **xerosis** (drying) and then to thickening and permanent blindness, **xerophthalmia.** Tragically, vitamin A-deprived children often become blind from this easily preventable condition. If the deficiency is discovered early, it can be reversed by capsules containing 60,000 RE of vitamin A taken twice each year.[2]

Vitamin A is needed by all **epithelial tissue** (external skin and internal linings), not just by the cornea. The skin and all of the protective linings of the lungs, intestines, vagina, urinary tract, and bladder serve as barriers to infection by bacteria and to damage from other sources. If vitamin A is deficient, some of the cells in these areas are displaced by cells that secrete keratin, the same protein that provides toughness in hair and fingernails. Keratin makes the surfaces dry, hard, cracked, and vulnerable to infection (see Figure 7-2). The cells then fail to function and eventually die. The dead cells accumulate on the surface, and become hosts to bacterial infection. In the cornea, as described, keratinization leads to xerophthalmia; in the lungs, the displacement of mucus-producing cells makes respiratory infections likely; in the vagina, the same process leads to vaginal infections.

The body's other defenses against infections also depend on vitamin A.[3] When the defenses are weak, especially in vitamin A-deficient children, an illness such as measles can become severe. A downward cycle of malnutri-

keratin (KERR-uh-tin) a water-insoluble protein; the normal protein of hair and nails.

keratinization accumulation of keratin in a tissue; a sign of vitamin A deficiency.

xerosis a symptom of vitamin A deficiency in the cornea—drying.

xerophthalmia (ZEER-ahf-THALL-me-uh) hardening of the cornea of the eye in advanced vitamin A deficiency that can lead to blindness (*xero* means "dry"; *ophthalm* means "eye").

epithelial (ep-ih-THEE-lee-ull) **tissue** the layers of the body that serve as selective barriers to the environment. Examples are the cornea, the skin, the respiratory lining, and the lining of the digestive tract.

Retin A, a vitamin A acid cream for acne, is discussed in Chapter 13.

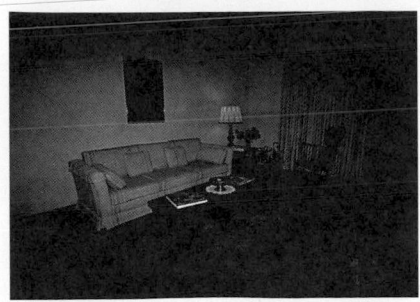

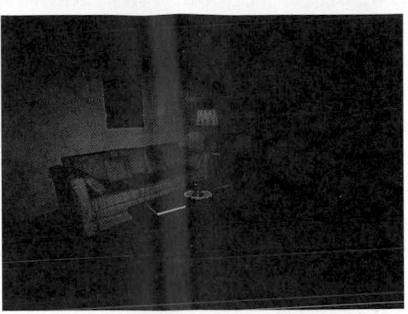

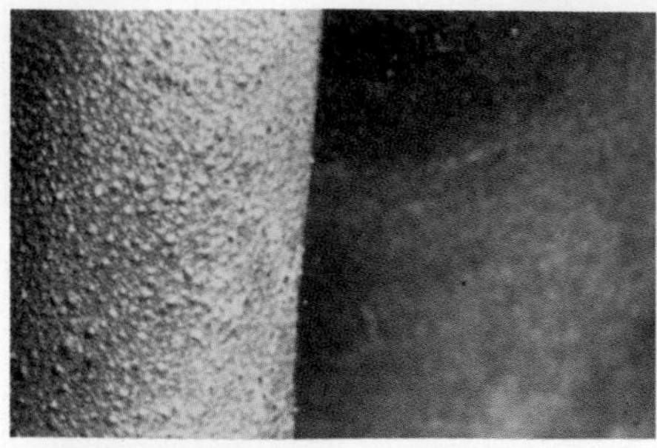

Figure 7-2

THE SKIN IN VITAMIN A DEFICIENCY
The hard lumps reflect accumulations of keratin in the epithelial cells.

tion and infection can set in. The child's body must devote its scanty store of vitamin A to the immune system's fight against measles viruses. But without adequate vitamin A, the infection worsens. More vitamin A is needed for the fight, but it is unavailable, and the infection gains ground. Even if the child survives the measles infection, blindness is likely. The corneas, already damaged by the chronic vitamin A shortage, degenerate rapidly as their meager supply of vitamin A is diverted to the immune system. Vitamin A deficiency-induced blindness often follows bouts of infection.[4] In Asia alone vitamin A deficiency causes blindness in a quarter of a million children each year.[5]

Vitamin A also assists in bone growth. Normal children's bones grow longer, and the children grow taller by remodeling each old bone into a new, bigger version. This requires dismantling the old bone structures and replacing them with new, larger bone parts. Growth cannot take place just by adding on to the small bone; vitamin A is needed in the critical dismantling steps. By helping reshape the jawbone as it grows, vitamin A permits normal tooth spacing. Crooked teeth and poor dental health can result from deficiencies in prenatal or early postnatal life. In children, failure to grow is one of the first signs of poor vitamin A status; when vitamin A is restored in such children, they gain weight and grow taller.[6]

Although relatively rare in developed countries, vitamin A deficiency is a vast problem worldwide, placing a heavy burden on society. More than 5 million of the world's children suffer from signs of vitamin A deficiency—not only blindness but stunted growth, poor appetite, and impaired immunity with resulting infections. In just one country, Indonesia, vitamin A deficiency is responsible for the deaths of 150,000 preschool children each year. In other countries the toll is many times greater.[7] Supplementing such children with vitamin A has reduced their rates of death by as much as half.[8] The World Health Organization (WHO) and UNICEF (the United Nations International Children's Emergency Fund) have declared the elimination of vitamin A deficiency a major goal in their quest to improve child survival throughout the developing world.

The effects of excessive vitamin A intakes during pregnancy are discussed in Chapter 12.

Toxicity presents a danger equal to that of deficiency for people who take excess vitamin A in supplements.[9] Its many symptoms include hair loss, joint pain, stunted growth, bone and muscle soreness, cessation of menstruation, nausea, diarrhea, rashes, and enlargement of the liver and spleen. Children are most likely to be hurt because they need less vitamin A and are more sensitive to overdoses than adults are. Serious toxicity is seen in infants and young children whose overzealous parents have given them more than 10 times the recommended amount for weeks at a time. Children who think vitamin pills are candy may also self-overdose. Early symptoms of overdoses in children are loss of appetite, growth failure, and itching of the skin.

Healthy people can eat vitamin A-rich foods in large amounts without risking toxicity, with the possible exception of liver. One report describes children falling ill after eating liver daily for years, but this is a medical rarity.[10] Inuit people and arctic explorers know that polar bear livers, because the bears eat fish whole (and thus fish livers), contain large amounts of the vitamin and are therefore a dangerous food source.

As far as vitamin A supplements go, the National Research Council (NRC) and other nutrition agencies recommend that people avoid taking supplements in excess of the RDA.[11] A table in Controversy 7 lists a safe dose of vitamin A that will not be toxic even over a long period of time. But the

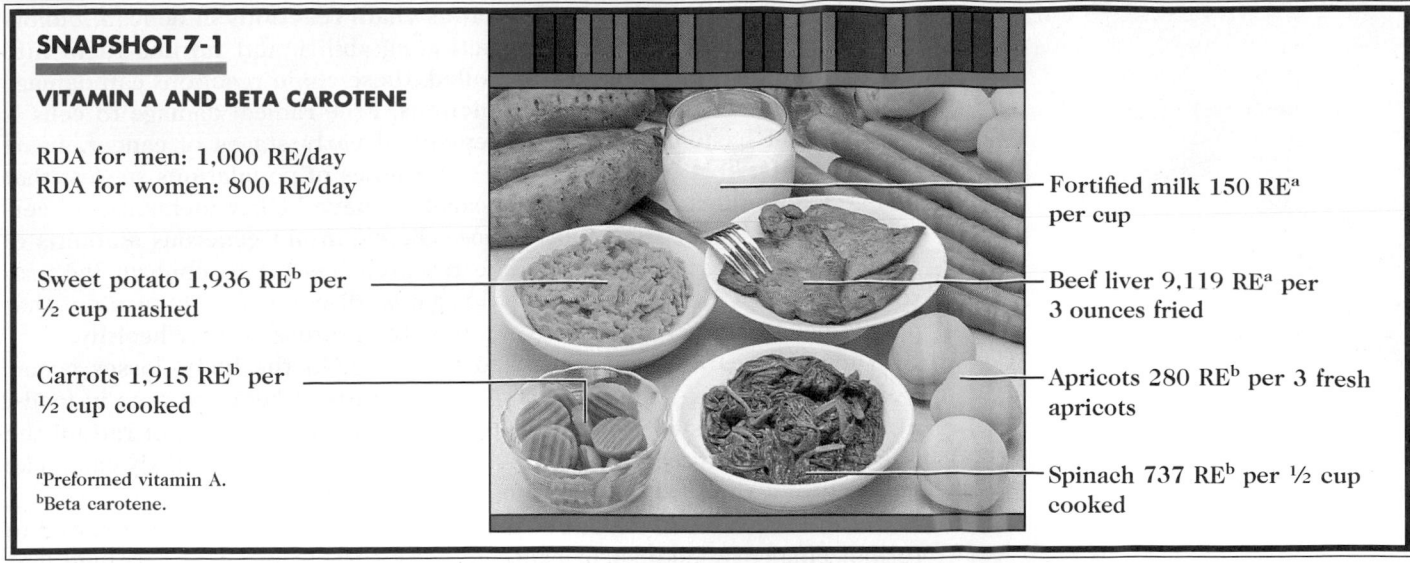

best way to ensure a safe vitamin A intake is to steer clear of supplements and instead to eat foods to obtain it. Snapshot 7-1 shows a sampling of the richest food sources of both preformed vitamin A and beta carotene. This chapter's Food Feature discusses the best ways to obtain sufficient amounts of all of the vitamins.

Studies of typical fast-food meals indicate that in the past, these foods have often been lacking in vitamin A. Recently, however, fast-food restaurants have been offering salads with cheese, carrots, and other vitamin A-rich foods as alternatives to the plain burgers, fries, and cola meals of yesterday. These selections greatly improve the nutritional quality of some fast-food meals.

The amount of vitamin A a person needs is proportional to the person's body weight. Although the RDA for vitamin A is given as a daily amount, the vitamin need not be consumed every day. An average intake that meets the daily RDA over several months is sufficient. According to the RDA, a man needs a daily average of about 1,000 **RE (retinol equivalents);** a woman needs about 800 RE, more during lactation; children need less.

Vitamin A recommendations are expressed in RE, but some food tables still express vitamin A contents using a different unit, the **IU (international unit).** Note that this book's Appendix A uses RE for your convenience, but be careful to notice whether other food tables or supplement labels do. See Appendix C for help in converting the units. People working with the amounts of vitamin A in foods have to remember to make sure that they are all expressed in the same units before making comparisons.

Beta Carotene In plants, vitamin A exists only in its precursor forms. Beta carotene, the most abundant of these precursors, has the highest vitamin A activity. For many years scientists believed beta carotene to be of interest solely as a vitamin A precursor. Eventually researchers began to recognize beta carotene itself as an extremely effective antioxidant in the body. You may recall from Chapter 5 that antioxidants are compounds that protect other compounds (such as DNA in genetic material or the proteins or lipids in cell membranes) from attack by highly reactive molecules known as free

RE (retinol equivalent) a measure of vitamin A activity; the amount of retinol that the body will derive from a food containing vitamin A (preformed retinol) or its precursor carotene.

IU (international unit) a measure of fat-soluble vitamin activity. For methods to convert IU to RE, see Appendix C.

The RDA tables are on the inside front cover.

radicals. Free radicals lead to dangerous chain reactions in delicate biological molecules, disrupting their functioning ability and turning them into free radicals, as well. If left uncontrolled, these chain reactions can damage cell structures and impair tissue functions. Free radical damage to cells is suspected of hastening the advancement of early stages of cancer, heart disease, and a host of other maladies.[12] Studies of populations suggest that people whose diets are low in beta carotene have higher incidences of certain types of cancer than those whose diets contain generous amounts of foods rich in beta carotene.[13] While research has yet to confirm the protective effect of dietary beta carotene against diseases, it may turn out that people need both active vitamin A and beta carotene to stay healthy.

When beta carotene is converted to retinol in the body, losses occur. This is why, rather than expressing the amounts of beta carotene in foods, nutrition scientists use the RE, which expresses the amount of retinol the body actually derives from a plant food after conversion. The body can make one unit of retinol from about three of beta carotene.

Retinol in excess is toxic, but beta carotene is not; it is not converted to retinol efficiently enough to cause toxicity symptoms. Beta carotene has, however, been known to turn people bright yellow if they eat too much. Beta carotene builds up in the fat just beneath the skin and imparts a yellow cast.

Many foods from plants contain beta carotene. Some are such a bright orange color that they decorate the plate. Carrots, sweet potatoes, pumpkins, cantaloupe, and apricots are all rich sources. Another colorful group, *dark* green vegetables such as spinach, other greens, or broccoli, owe their color to chlorophyll and beta carotene. The orange and green pigments together give a deep dark green color to the vegetables. Other colorful vegetables can fool you into thinking they contain beta carotene, such as iceberg lettuce, beets, and sweet corn, but these foods derive their color's from other pigments and are poor sources of beta carotene. As for "white" plant foods such as grains and potatoes, they have none. Recommendations state that a person should eat *deep*-orange or *dark*-green vegetables and fruits at least every other day.

KEY POINT Vitamin A is essential to vision, integrity of epithelial tissue, growth of bone, reproduction, and more. Vitamin A deficiency causes blindness, sickness, and death and is a major problem worldwide. Liver and milk are rich sources of active vitamin A. Overdoses are possible and cause many serious symptoms. The vitamin A precursor in plants, beta carotene, is an effective antioxidant in the body. Brightly colored plant foods are richest in beta carotene.

Vitamin D

Vitamin D is different from all the other nutrients in the body in that the body can synthesize it with the help of sunlight. Therefore, in a sense, vitamin D is not an essential nutrient. Given enough sun, you need consume no vitamin D at all in the foods you eat. Folk wisdom has it that sunshine promotes health and recovery from diseases. People of past generations observed the benefit that sunlight offered those with tuberculosis long before scientists worked out the details.[14] Now vitamin D is appreciated for its role in assisting the tissues of immunity in launching their attacks against infection. However, keep in mind that too much sun is dangerous. It increases many people's risks of skin cancer.

When the sun shines on a cholesterol compound in human skin, the compound is transformed into a vitamin D precursor and is absorbed directly into the blood. Slowly, over the next day and a half or so, the liver and kidneys finish converting the precursor to the active form of vitamin D. Diseases that affect either the liver or the kidneys may impair the conversion of the inactive precursor to the active vitamin and therefore produce symptoms of vitamin D deficiency.

The best-known role of vitamin D is as a member of a large and interacting team of nutrients and hormones that continuously maintain blood calcium levels and thereby bone integrity, especially during growth. Vitamin D ensures that sufficient calcium and phosphorus are available in the blood to support the growing bone structure. Calcium is also indispensable to the proper functioning of all tissues of the body; cells of muscles, nerves, glands, and others all draw calcium from the blood as they need it. The skeleton serves as a vast warehouse of stored calcium, and it is tapped when the blood supply begins to run low. To raise the level of blood calcium, the body can draw from only two other places: from the digestive tract, where food brings calcium in, and from the kidney, which recycles calcium into the body from the blood filtrate destined to become urine. Vitamin D acts, when needed, at all three locations to raise the blood calcium level.

Vitamin D acts like a hormone, a compound manufactured by one organ of the body that acts on other organs or tissues. The bones, intestines, and kidneys all respond to the influence of vitamin D. Scientists are now discovering other vitamin D target organs and cells, including the brain, pancreas, skin, reproductive organs, and some cancer cells.[15] Like vitamin A, vitamin D is also more like a hormone than a vitamin in that it stimulates maturation of cells, including cells of the immune system.[16]

The most obvious sign of vitamin D deficiency is abnormality of the bones. The disease **rickets,** caused in children by vitamin D deficiency, has been recognized for several centuries, and even in the 1700s it was known to be curable by cod-liver oil, which is rich in the vitamin. More than a hundred years later, a Polish physician linked sunlight exposure to prevention and cure of rickets. At the turn of this century, enough was finally known about rickets to reproduce it in laboratory animals. Today the bowed legs, knock knees, and protruding (pigeon) chests of children with rickets are no longer common sights. Tragically, some children still suffer the ravages of rickets largely because of inadequate food due to poverty combined with a lack of sunlight.[17]

Adult rickets, or **osteomalacia,** occurs most often in women with low calcium intakes and little exposure to the sun (therefore little opportunity to make vitamin D) and who have repeated pregnancies and then breastfeed their babies. Under these conditions calcium is withdrawn from the bones but is not picked up efficiently from the intestine or recycled by the kidneys. The bones lose their minerals and protein understructure, becoming porous, soft, and easy to break. The bones of the legs and spine may soften to such an extent that a young woman who is tall and straight at the age of 20 years may, after several pregnancies, become bowlegged and bent by age 30.

Vitamin D is the most potentially toxic of all vitamins. Ingestion of as little as four to five times the recommended daily intake can cause toxicity symptoms including diarrhea, headache, and nausea. If overdoses continue, the vitamin raises the blood mineral level to dangerous extremes, forcing

rickets the vitamin D deficiency disease in children, characterized by abnormal growth of bone, manifested in bowed legs or knock knees, outward-bowed chest, and knobs on the ribs.

osteomalacia (OS-tee-o-mal-AY-shuh) the vitamin D deficiency disease in adults (*osteo* means "bone"; *mal* means "bad"). Symptoms include bending of the spine and bowing of the legs.

Chapter 8 and Controversy 8 present more about bone minerals and their regulation.

Osteoporosis, another bone-weakening disease, is discussed in Controversy 8.

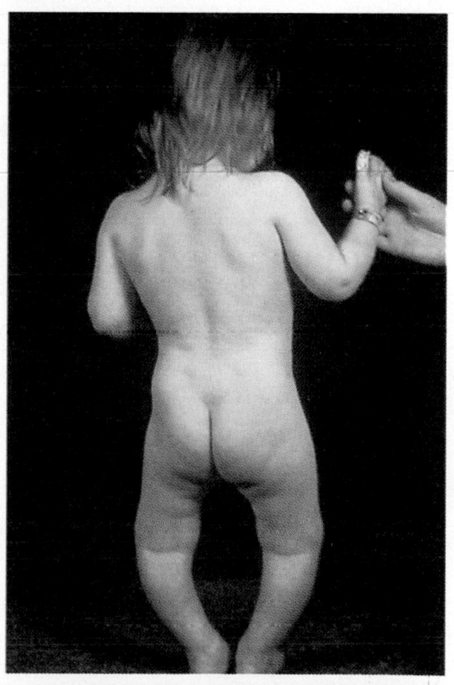

This child has the vitamin D-deficiency disease rickets.

calcium to be deposited in soft tissues such as the heart and kidneys. If calcium deposits form in the arteries of the heart, the consequence of overdosing is death.

The likeliest victims of vitamin D poisoning are infants whose well-intended but misguided parents think that if some is good, more is better. People who take supplements containing vitamin D may also easily overdose, not realizing that their tissues are building up stockpiles of the vitamin. Intakes of only 5 times the RDA have been associated with signs of vitamin D toxicity in young children and adults.[18] The amounts found in foods are safe, but concentrated supplements should be treated with respect and used only on the advice of a physician. Most of the world's population relies on natural exposure to sunlight to maintain adequate vitamin D nutrition.[19]

The sun presents no risk of vitamin D toxicity; the skin breaks down any excess vitamin made there. Even lifeguards on southern beaches are safe from vitamin D toxicity from the sun because the body never makes an overdose. Of course, long sun exposure has *other* undesirable consequences, such as premature wrinkling of the skin and the increased risk of skin cancer mentioned earlier. These dangers may be somewhat reduced by using sunscreens. Unfortunately, sunscreens with sun protection factors (SPF) of 8 and above also prevent vitamin D synthesis. A strategy to solve this dilemma is to apply sunscreen after enough time has elapsed to provide sufficient vitamin D. Production of vitamin D doesn't demand idle hours of sunbathing, though. Just being outdoors, even in lightweight clothing, is sufficient. Dark-skinned people require long exposure to direct sun (up to 3 hours, depending on the climate) for a full day's supply of vitamin D, while light-skinned people need much less time (10 or 15 minutes).[20]

The ultraviolet rays of the sun that promote vitamin D synthesis may be filtered out by clouds, smoke, smog, heavy clothing, window glass, and even window screens. Some types of tanning booths may also stimulate vitamin D synthesis, but the hazards may outweigh any possible benefits. The Food and Drug Administration (FDA) warns that if the lamps are not properly filtered, users of tanning booths risk burns, damage to blood vessels, skin cancer, and damage to the eyes.[21] Daily doses of vitamin D or even sunshine are not necessary because synthesis of vitamin D continues for days *after* exposure to sun and because the body stores in its fat tissue enough vitamin D to last through the dark winter months.

The slower vitamin D production in dark-skinned people may at least partly account for many of today's cases of rickets. In the United States and Canada, almost all cases show up in dark-skinned people who live in smoggy northern cities or who lack exposure to sunlight. Worldwide, rickets is still a major health problem, especially in societies where people traditionally clothe themselves in concealing garments.

As Snapshot 7-2 shows, the few significant food sources of vitamin D are butter, cream, egg yolks, liver, fatty fish such as salmon, and fortified margarine. In the United States and Canada, milk, whether fluid, dried, or evaporated, is usually fortified with vitamin D, so that a daily quart (or liter) will supply the amount of the vitamin recommended for a young adult. That way the young adult who drinks the recommended 2 cups a day receives half the RDA; the other half comes from sun exposure and other food sources. Older adults need half this amount. Children who drink 2 cups or more of milk will have a head start toward meeting their vitamin D needs for growth. Strict vegetarians, and especially their children, may have low

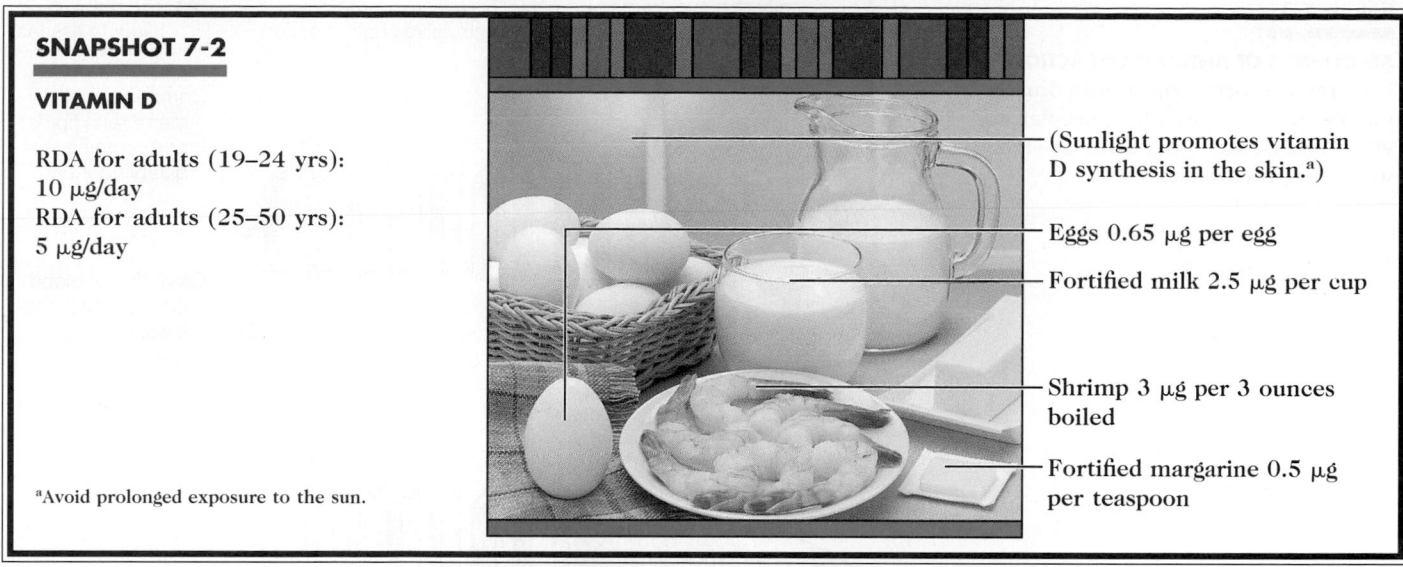

vitamin D intakes because no fortified plant source except margarine exists. In the United States breakfast cereals may be fortified with vitamin D, as their labels indicate.

The RDA for vitamin D is 5 micrograms per day for adults older than 24 years. The RDA is higher during growth or bone formation in pregnancy, lactation, childhood, and adolescence. It remains high in early adult life, while bones continue to gain density. People who are housebound or institutionalized or who work at night may incur (over years) a vitamin D deficiency that leads to deficiency of calcium severe enough to damage their bones. Adults who can tolerate milk receive a source of both vitamin D and calcium; those with sensitivities to milk should seek alternative calcium sources and should make a point of spending time outdoors.

tocopherol (tuh-KOFF-er-all) a kind of alcohol. The active form of vitamin E is *alpha*-tocopherol.

KEY POINT Vitamin D raises blood minerals, notably calcium and phosphorus, permitting bone formation and maintenance. A deficiency in childhood can cause rickets and, in later life, osteomalacia. Vitamin D is the most toxic of all the vitamins, and excesses are dangerous or deadly. People exposed to the sun make vitamin D from cholesterol; fortified milk is an important food source.

Vitamin E

More than 70 years ago, researchers discovered a compound in vegetable oils necessary for reproduction in rats. This compound was named **tocopherol.** *Tokos* is a Greek word meaning "offspring." A few years later, the compound was named vitamin E. Eventually, four different tocopherol compounds were discovered, and each was named by one of the first four letters of the Greek alphabet: alpha, beta, gamma, and delta.

Vitamin E, because it can be oxidized, is like a bodyguard for other substances; it serves as an antioxidant. By being destroyed itself, vitamin E protects the polyunsaturated fats and other fat-soluble substances, such as vitamin A, from oxidation. Vitamin E serves as one of the body's main defenders against oxidative damage by breaking the free radical chain reaction (Figure 7-3).[22]

Figure 7-3

AN EXAMPLE OF ANTIOXIDANT ACTION
Free radical formation occurs during metabolic processes and it accelerates when diseases or other stresses strike, worsening their effects.

1 A chemically reactive oxygen free radical attacks fatty acid, DNA, protein, or cholesterol molecules forming other free radicals.
2 This initiates a rapid, destructive chain reaction.
3 The result is injury to tissues:
Damage to cell-membrane lipids and proteins, disabling them
Precancerous changes in DNA
Oxidation of blood cholesterol initiating steps leading to heart disease
Oxygen free radical
Fatty acids, DNA or cholesterol
Vitamin E
Vitamin E stops the chain reaction by changing the nature of the free radical

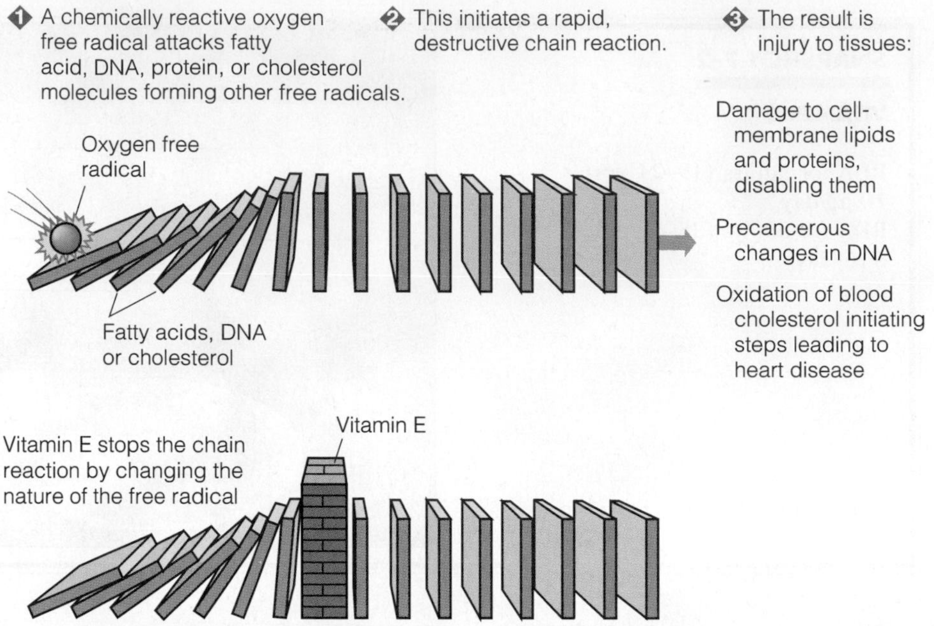

erythrocyte (eh-REETH-ro-sight) **hemolysis** (he-MOLL-ih-sis) rupture of the red blood cells, caused by vitamin E deficiency (*erythro* means "red"; *cyte* means "cell"; hemo means "blood"; *lysis* means "breaking").

Vitamin E exerts an especially important antioxidant effect in the lungs, where the cells are exposed to high oxygen concentrations that can destroy their membranes. As the red blood cells carry oxygen from the lungs to other tissues, vitamin E protects their cell membranes too. Vitamin E also protects the white blood cells that defend the body against disease. Normal nerve development also depends on vitamin E. Vitamin E may also play other roles in normal immunity.[23]

More research is needed to determine whether vitamin E in amounts greater than the RDA can offer protection against disease. Two large epidemiologic studies lend support to this idea. Researchers found that large doses of vitamin E supplements were associated with a significant reduction in the risk of heart disease.[24] So far, the evidence is not strong enough to warrant recommending that healthy people take supplements. More details are presented later on, in the Consumer Caution.

A deficiency of vitamin E produces a wide variety of symptoms in laboratory animals. Most of these symptoms have not been reproduced in human beings, however, despite many attempts. Three reasons have been given for this. First, the vitamin is so widespread in food that it is almost impossible to create a vitamin E-deficient diet. Second, the body stores so much vitamin E in its fatty tissues that a person could not keep on eating a vitamin E-free diet for long enough to deplete these stores and to produce a deficiency. Third, the cells may recycle their working supply of vitamin E, using the same molecules over and over.[25]

The classic vitamin E deficiency symptom in human beings occurs in premature babies. Some of these babies are born before the transfer of the vitamin from the mother to the infant that takes place in the last weeks of pregnancy. Without sufficient vitamin E, the infant's red blood cells rupture **(erythrocyte hemolysis),** and the infant becomes anemic. Researchers have recently recognized a neuromuscular disorder caused by vitamin E deficiency in adults.[26] Common symptoms include loss of muscle coordination and reflexes and impaired vision and speech. Vitamin E treatment corrects these symptoms.

Two other conditions are apparently caused sometimes by vitamin E deficiency in human beings. One is a painful but nonmalignant disease characterized by painful lumps in women's breasts **(fibrocystic breast disease).** This may also be worsened by overuse of caffeine, so it sometimes responds to vitamin E supplements and sometimes to abstinence from caffeine. The other is a leg disorder that involves pain on walking and cramps in the calves at night. The disorder is known as intermittent claudication (*claudicare* means "to limp").

fibrocystic breast disease a harmless condition in which the breasts become lumpy and painful; caused sometimes by vitamin E deficiency and sometimes associated with caffeine toxicity (*fibro* means "fibrous tissue"; *cyst* means "closed sac").

In human beings, vitamin E deficiency is usually associated with diseases, notably those that cause malabsorption of fat. These include disease or injury of the liver (which makes bile, necessary for digestion of fat), the gallbladder (which delivers bile into the intestine), and the pancreas (which makes fat-digesting enzymes), as well as a number of hereditary diseases involving digestion and use of nutrients.

It may be, however, that rare vitamin E deficiencies are seen in people without diseases. People in whom they are most likely are those who for years eat diets extremely low in fat; or who use fat substitutes, such as diet margarines and salad dressings, as their only sources of fat; or who consume diets composed largely of highly processed or "convenience" foods, since vitamin E is destroyed by extensive heating in the processing of these foods.

Although vitamin E deficiency is rare, many horror stories have been told about vitamin E deficiency diseases in human beings. Extravagant claims have been made that it cures all sorts of things because it affects animals' hearts, muscles, and reproductive systems. Vitamin E deficiency does not, however, affect the organs of human beings in the same ways. While research has revealed possible roles for vitamin E, it has also clearly discredited claims that vitamin E improves athletic endurance and skill, enhances sexual performance, or cures sexual dysfunction in males.

The RDA for vitamin E is based on body size: it is 8 milligrams a day for women, 10 for men. Note that the RDA gives values for vitamin E in units known as alpha TE (alpha tocopherol equivalents). One of these units, 1 alpha TE, equals 1 milligram of active vitamin E. The need for vitamin E rises as polyunsaturated oil intake rises, because the oil requires antioxidant protection by the vitamin. Normally, people whose oil intakes are high receive ample vitamin E along with the oil. People who need vitamin E supplements are, as mentioned, people with very low fat intakes as well as people with diseases impairing fat absorption, which cause vitamin E deficiency.

Cases of vitamin E toxicity are rare. The medical literature contains isolated reports of adverse effects on laboratory animals and of nausea, intestinal distress, and other vague complaints in human beings. Large doses may augment the effects of anticoagulant medication used to oppose unwanted blood clotting; people taking such drugs risk uncontrollable bleeding when they also take large doses of vitamin E. However, for most individuals, daily doses below 300 milligrams are probably harmless.

Vitamin E is widespread in foods. About 20 percent of the vitamin E people consume comes from vegetable oils and products made from them, such as margarine, salad dressings, and shortenings (Snapshot 7-3). Another 20 percent comes from fruits and vegetables. Fortified cereals and other grain products contribute about 15 percent of the vitamin E in the diet, and meats, poultry, fish, eggs, nuts, and seeds contribute smaller percent-

SNAPSHOT 7-3

VITAMIN E

RDA for men: 10 mg/day
RDA for women: 8 mg/day

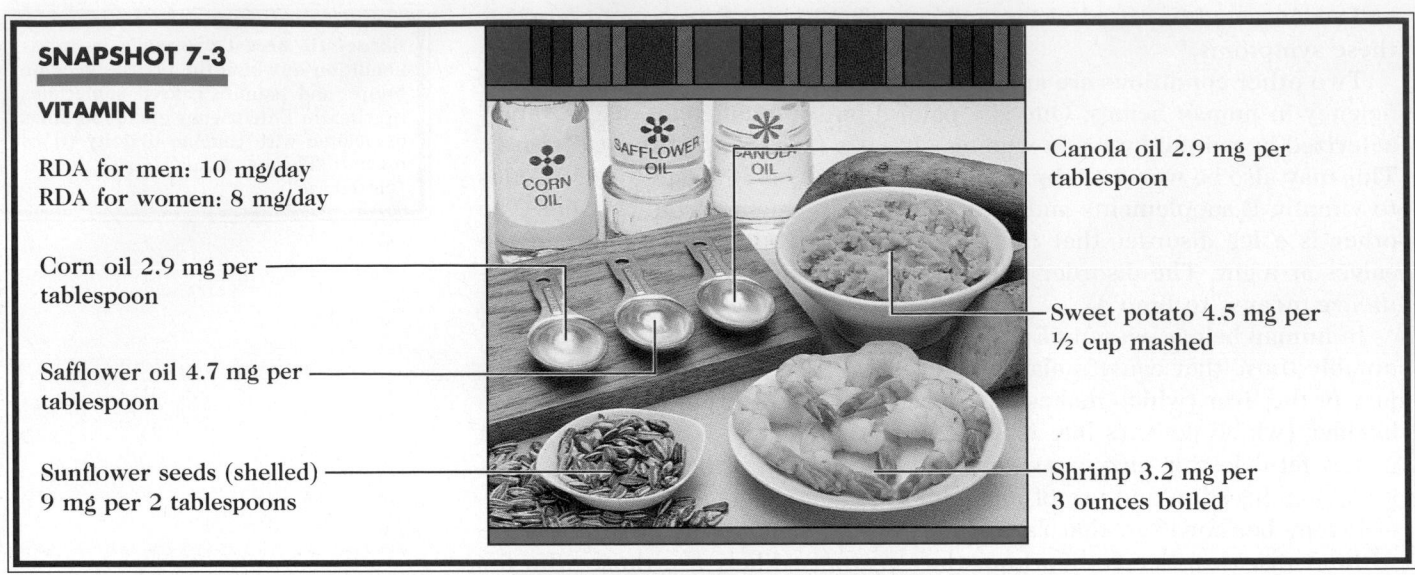

ages.[27] Wheat germ oil and soybean oil are rich in vitamin E. Animal fats, such as milk fat or the fat of meats, have negligible vitamin E. Oil that has been heated to frying temperatures and food fried in oil retain little intact vitamin E. Most processed and convenience foods do not contribute enough vitamin E to ensure adequate intakes.

KEY POINT Vitamin E acts as an antioxidant in cell membranes and is especially important for the integrity of cells that are constantly exposed to high oxygen concentrations, namely the lungs and blood cells, both red and white. Vitamin E deficiency is rare in human beings, but it does occur in newborn premature infants. The vitamin is widely distributed among plant foods; toxicity is rare.

Vitamin K

Vitamin K is the fat-soluble vitamin necessary for the synthesis of at least four proteins involved in blood clotting. If blood cannot clot, then wounds may bleed for a dangerously long time; this is why people's blood is drawn to measure clotting time before they go into surgery. Vitamin K is sometimes administered before operations to reduce bleeding in surgery. Vitamin K may be of value at this time, but only if a vitamin K deficiency exists. Vitamin K does not improve clotting in those with other bleeding disorders, such as the genetic disease hemophilia.

K stands for the Danish word *koagulation* (clotting).

In some heart problems there is a need to *prevent* the formation of clots within the circulatory system. This is popularly referred to as "thinning" the blood. One of the best-known medicines for this purpose is dicumarol, which interferes with the action of vitamin K in promoting clotting. Vitamin K therapy is necessary for people taking dicumarol if uncontrolled bleeding occurs.

Vitamin K is necessary for the synthesis of a key protein in bone formation.[28] Together with the more famous bone vitamin, vitamin D, vitamin

SNAPSHOT 7-4

VITAMIN K[a]

RDA for men:
(19–24 yrs) 70 μg/day
(25–50 years) 80 μg/day
RDA for women:
(19–24 yrs) 60 μg/day
(25–50 yrs) 65 μg/day

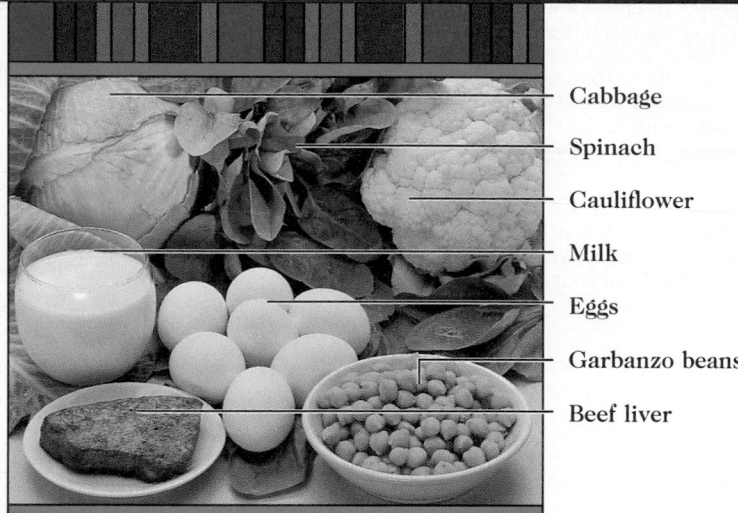

[a]Techniques to analyze vitamin K in foods are changing rapidly. Values based on the newest analytical techniques are not yet available.

K ensures that the bones produce this protein normally so that bones can bind the minerals they need to form normally.

Like vitamin D, vitamin K can be obtained from a nonfood source—in this case, the intestinal bacteria. Billions of bacteria normally reside in the intestines, and some of them synthesize vitamin K. The extent to which the body uses the vitamin K synthesized by these bacteria is not known. People may obtain about half of their daily needs from this source.

It seems unlikely that many U.S. adults experience vitamin K deficiency, even if they seldom eat vitamin K-rich foods.[29] Exceptions are newborn infants whose intestinal tracts are not yet inhabited by bacteria and people who have taken antibiotics that have killed their intestinal bacteria. Supplements of the vitamin are needed in these cases.

Vitamin K is not toxic in the range of amounts commonly consumed from natural sources, but toxicity can result when supplements of a synthetic version of vitamin K are given, especially to infants or to pregnant women. Toxicity induces breakage of the red blood cells and release of their pigment, which colors the skin yellow.* Vitamin K toxicity also causes brain damage. Because the vitamin K contained in supplements can easily reach toxic levels, it is available as a single vitamin only by prescription.

An RDA for vitamin K was published for the first time in 1989 (see the RDA tables on the inside front cover). Snapshot 7-4 shows that vitamin K's richest plant food sources are dark-green leafy vegetables, which provide from 50 to 800 micrograms per 3-ounce serving, and members of the cabbage family. There is also one rich animal food source, liver.[30] Milk, meats, eggs, cereals, and fruits provide smaller, but still significant amounts. Food tables do not include vitamin K contents of foods because they are not known with sufficient precision.

*A toxic dose of a vitamin K compound such as *menadione* causes the liver to release the blood cell pigment *(bilirubin)* into the blood (instead of excreting it into the bile) and leads to *jaundice.* When bilirubin invades the brain of an infant, the condition is often fatal.

coenzyme (co-EN-zime) a small molecule that works with an enzyme to promote the enzyme's activity. Many coenzymes have B vitamins as part of their structure (*co* means "with").

The water-soluble vitamins require special measures in food preparation to avoid losing or destroying them. See the Food Feature of Chapter 14.

Figure 7-4

COENZYME ACTION

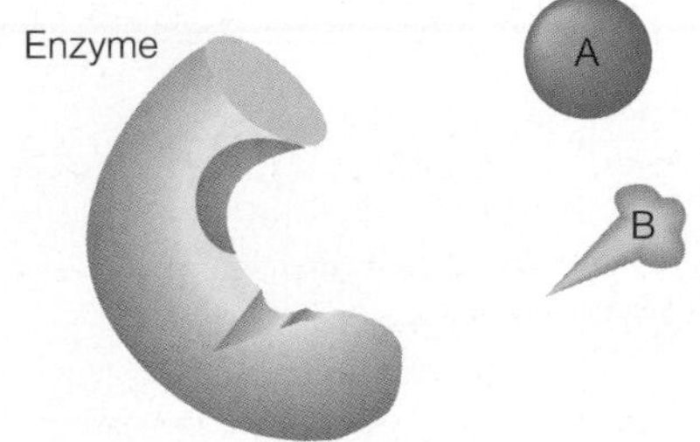

Without the coenzyme, compounds A and B don't respond to the enzyme.

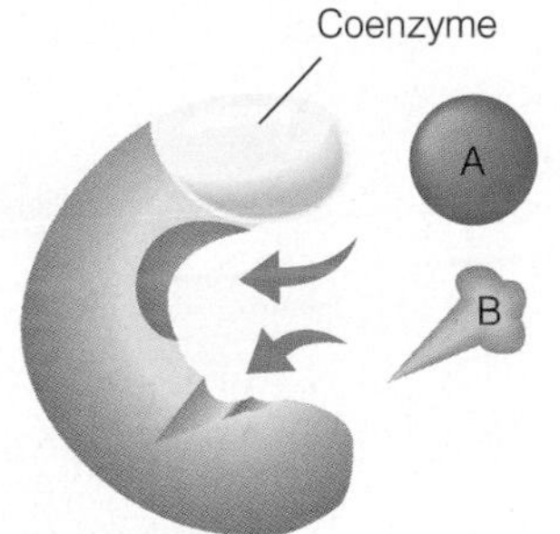

With the coenzyme in place, compounds A and B are attracted to the active site on the enzyme, and they react.

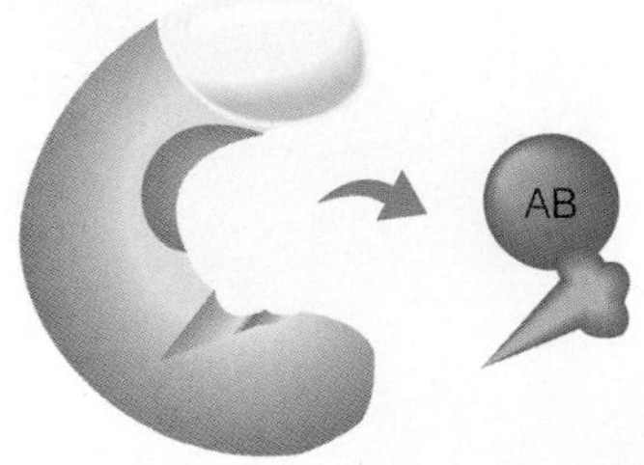

The reaction is completed with the formation of a new product. In this case the product is AB.

KEY POINT Vitamin K is necessary for blood to clot; deficiency causes uncontrolled bleeding. The bacterial inhabitants of the digestive tract produce vitamin K, and most people derive about half their requirement from them and half from food. Excesses are toxic.

The Water-Soluble Vitamins

All of the other vitamins, the B vitamins and vitamin C, are water soluble. Cooking and washing water can leach them out of foods. The body absorbs them easily and just as easily excretes them in the urine. Under ordinary circumstances, you need not be concerned about consuming modest excesses. Some of the water-soluble vitamins can remain in the lean tissues for periods of a month or more, but these tissues are actively exchanging materials with the body fluids at all times. At any time, the vitamins may be picked up by the extracellular fluids, carried away by the blood, and excreted in the urine. Generally, the RDA committee suggests that you make sure your three-day intake average meets the RDA by choosing foods that are rich in water-soluble vitamins.[31]

Foods never deliver toxic doses of the water-soluble vitamins, but the large doses concentrated in vitamin supplements can reach toxic levels. Normally, though, the most likely hazard to the taker is to the wallet. As one person aptly noted, "If you take supplements of the water-soluble vitamins, you may have the most expensive urine in town."

The B Vitamins and Their Relatives

The B vitamins act as part of coenzymes. A **coenzyme** is a small molecule that combines with an enzyme to make it active. (Recall that enzymes are large proteins that do the body's building, dismantling, and other work; see pages 190–191.) Sometimes the vitamin part of the enzyme is the active site, where the chemical reaction takes place. The substance to be worked on is attracted to the active site and snaps into place; the reaction proceeds instantaneously. The shape of each enzyme predestines it to accomplish just one kind of job. Without its coenzyme, however, the enzyme is as useless as a sewing machine without its needle. Figure 7-4 shows how a coenzyme enables an enzyme to do its job.

Each B vitamin has its own special character, and the amount of detail known about each one is overwhelming. To simplify things, this introduction to them describes some of the ways in which the B vitamins work together as a group and emphasizes the consequences of deficiencies. The sections that follow present more details about the vitamins as individuals.

B Vitamin Roles in Metabolism

Figure 7-5 shows some body organs and tissues in which the B vitamins help the body metabolize carbohydrates, lipids, and amino acids. It is not presented to teach details; that is best left to courses in biochemistry. The purpose of the figure is to give an impression of where the B vitamins work together with enzymes in the metabolism of energy nutrients and in the making of new cells. A few details are presented in the figure legend.

Many people mistakenly believe that B vitamins give you energy. They do not, at least not directly. The energy-yielding nutrients, carbohydrate,

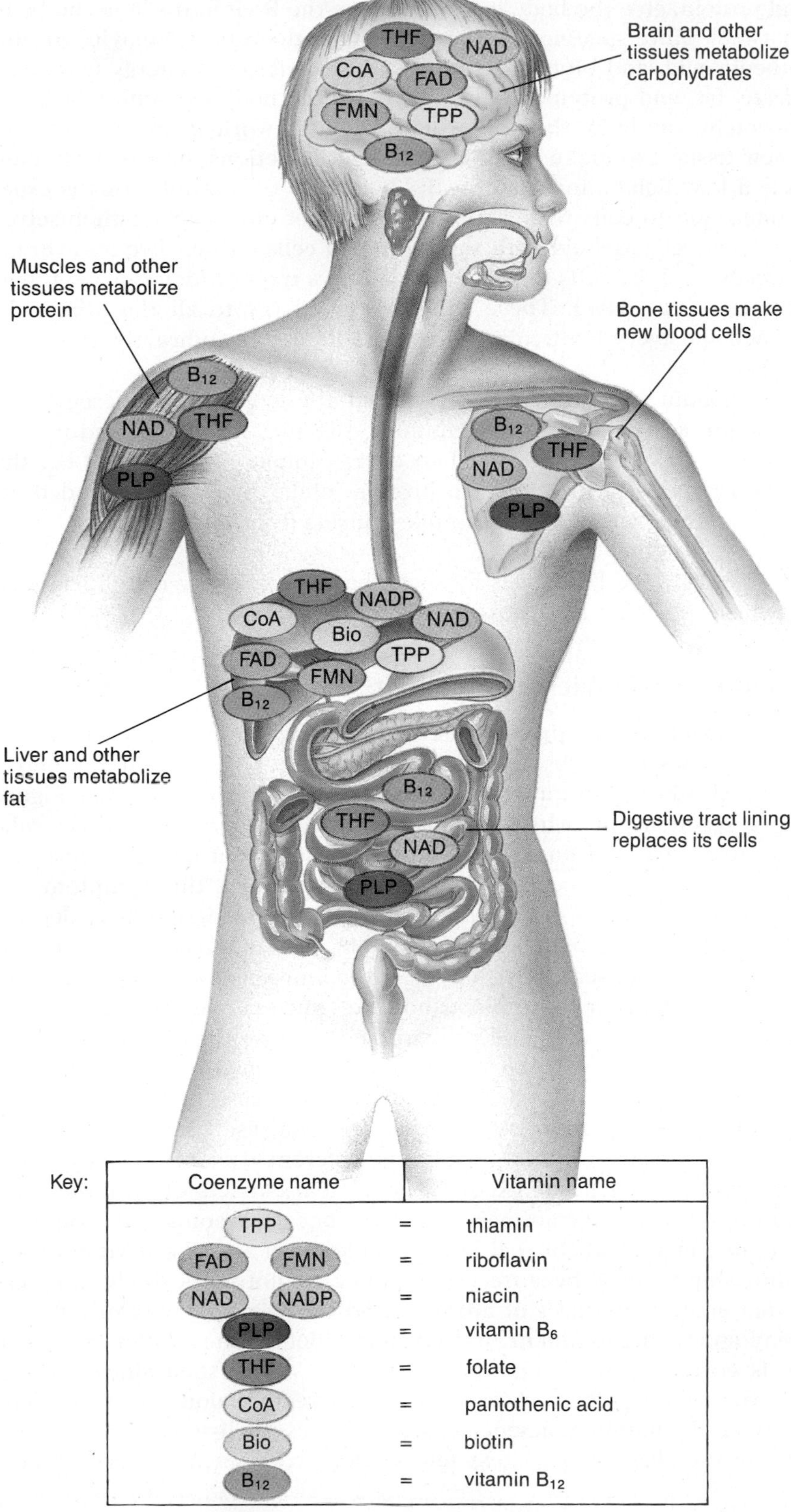

Coenzyme name		Vitamin name
TPP	=	thiamin
FAD FMN	=	riboflavin
NAD NADP	=	niacin
PLP	=	vitamin B_6
THF	=	folate
CoA	=	pantothenic acid
Bio	=	biotin
B_{12}	=	vitamin B_{12}

Figure 7-5

SOME ROLES OF THE B VITAMINS IN METABOLISM: EXAMPLES

This figure does not attempt to teach intricate biochemical pathways or names of B vitamin-containing enzymes. Its sole purpose is to show a few of the many tissue functions that depend on B vitamin-containing enzymes. The B vitamins work in every cell, and this displays less than 1/1000th of what they actually do.

Every B vitamin is part of one or more coenzymes that make possible the body's chemical work. For example, the niacin coenzymes are necessary for most of the energy pathways. The thiamin and riboflavin coenzymes are also important in the energy pathways. The folate and vitamin B_{12} coenzymes are necessary for the making of RNA and DNA and thus new cells. The vitamin B_6 coenzyme is necessary for the processing of amino acids, and therefore, of protein. Many other relationships are also critical to metabolism.

thiamin (THIGH-uh-min) a B vitamin involved in the body's use of fuels.

fat, and protein, give the body fuel for energy; the B vitamins help the body use that fuel. More specifically, the B vitamins thiamin, riboflavin, niacin, pantothenic acid, and biotin participate in the release of energy from carbohydrate, fat, and protein. Vitamin B_6 helps the body use amino acids to make protein; the body then puts the protein to work in many ways—to build new tissues, to make hormones, to fight infections, or as energy fuel, to name a few. Folate and vitamin B_{12} help cells to multiply; this is especially important to cells with short life spans that must replace themselves rapidly. Such cells include both the red blood cells (which live an average of six weeks) and the cells that line the digestive tract (which replace themselves every three days). These cells deliver energy to all the others. In short, each and every B vitamin is involved, directly or indirectly, in energy metabolism.

The B vitamin amounts that people need are determined differently for each vitamin. For three of the B vitamins, thiamin, riboflavin, and niacin, recommendations are proportional to energy intake. For vitamin B_6, the recommendation is proportional to protein intake. The recommended intakes are summarized in the RDA tables (inside front cover).

KEY POINT The B vitamins facilitate the work of every cell. Some help generate energy, others help make protein and new cells.

B Vitamin Deficiencies and Toxicities

As long as B vitamins are present, their presence is not felt. Only when they are missing does their absence manifest itself in a lack of energy and a multitude of other symptoms, as you can imagine after looking at Figure 7-5. The reactions by which B vitamins facilitate energy release take place in every cell, and no cell can do its work without energy. Thus in a B-vitamin deficiency, every cell is affected. Among the symptoms of B-vitamin deficiencies are nausea, severe exhaustion, irritability, depression, forgetfulness, loss of appetite and weight, pain in muscles, impairment of the immune response, loss of control of the limbs, abnormal heart action, severe skin problems, teary or bloodshot eyes, and many more. Because cell renewal depends on energy and protein, and because these depend on the B vitamins, the digestive tract and the blood are invariably damaged. In children, full recovery may be impossible. In the case of a thiamin deficiency, for example, permanent brain damage can result.

In academic discussions of the vitamins, different sets of deficiency symptoms are given for each one. Actually such clear-cut sets of symptoms are found only in laboratory animals that have been fed contrived diets that lack just one ingredient. In real life, a deficiency of any one B vitamin seldom shows up by itself because people don't eat nutrients singly; they eat foods that contain mixtures of nutrients. Still the deficiency of one B vitamin may appear predominant in a cluster of deficiencies. Often, if a deficiency is corrected by giving wholesome food rather than single supplements, the subtler deficiencies will be corrected along with it. The symptoms of B vitamin deficiencies and toxicities are listed in Table 7-4 at the end of the chapter. The next few sections treat each B vitamin separately.

Thiamin and Riboflavin All cells use **thiamin,** which plays a critical role in their energy metabolism. Thiamin also occupies a special site on the nerve cell membrane. Consequently, nerve processes and their responding tissues, the muscles, depend heavily on thiamin.

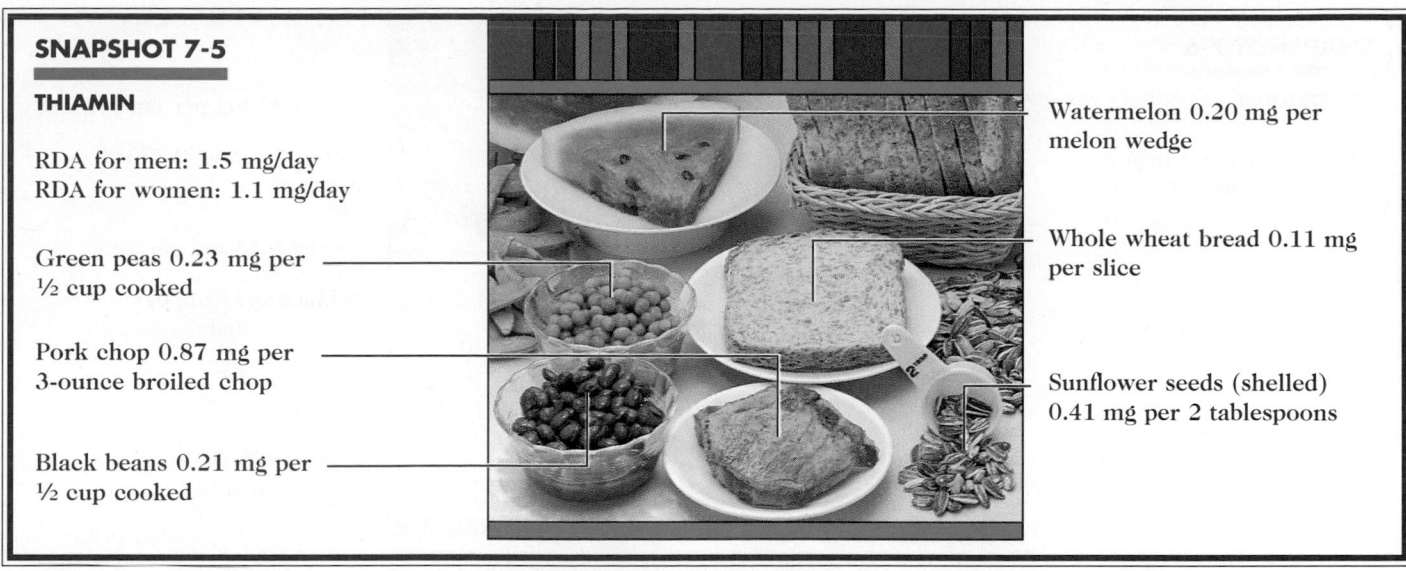

The thiamin deficiency disease **beriberi** was first observed in the Far East, where rice provided 80 to 90 percent of the total calories most people consumed and therefore was their principal source of thiamin. When the custom of polishing rice (removing its brown coat, which contained the thiamin) became widespread, beriberi swept through the population like an epidemic. Scientists wasted years of time and effort hunting for a microbial cause of beriberi before they realized that the cause of beriberi was not something present in the environment but something absent from it.

beriberi the thiamin-deficiency disease, characterized by loss of sensation in the hands and feet, muscular weakness, advancing paralysis, and abnormal heart action.

riboflavin (RIBE-o-flay-vin) a B vitamin.

Just before the year 1900, an observant physician working in a prison in the Far East discovered that beriberi could be cured with proper diet. The physician noticed that the chickens at the prison developed a stiffness and weakness similar to that of the prisoners who had beriberi. The chickens were being fed the rice left on the plates of prisoners. When the rice bran, which had been discarded in the kitchen, was given to the chickens, their paralysis was cured. As might be expected, the doctor met resistance when he tried to feed the rice bran, the "garbage," to the prisoners. Later, extracts of rice bran were used to prevent infantile beriberi; still later, thiamin was synthesized.

Thiamin occurs in small amounts in many nutritious foods. Pork, ham, leafy green vegetables, whole-grain cereals, and legumes are especially rich in thiamin (see Snapshot 7-5 above). People who keep empty-calorie foods to a minimum and include ten or more servings of nutritious foods each day will easily meet their thiamin needs.

People addicted to alcohol, though, may develop thiamin deficiency. Alcohol can contribute energy, but carries almost no nutrients with it and often displaces food. In addition, alcohol causes excretion of thiamin in the urine, doubling the risk of deficiency.

Like thiamin, **riboflavin** plays a role in the energy metabolism of all cells. When thiamin is deficient, riboflavin may be lacking too, but the deficiency symptoms may be unseen because those of thiamin deficiency are more severe. Foods that remedy the thiamin deficiency invariably also contain some riboflavin, so they clear up both deficiencies. People obtain as much as half of their riboflavin from milk and milk products such as cheese. Green

SNAPSHOT 7-6

RIBOFLAVIN

RDA for men: 1.7 mg/day
RDA for women: 1.3 mg/day

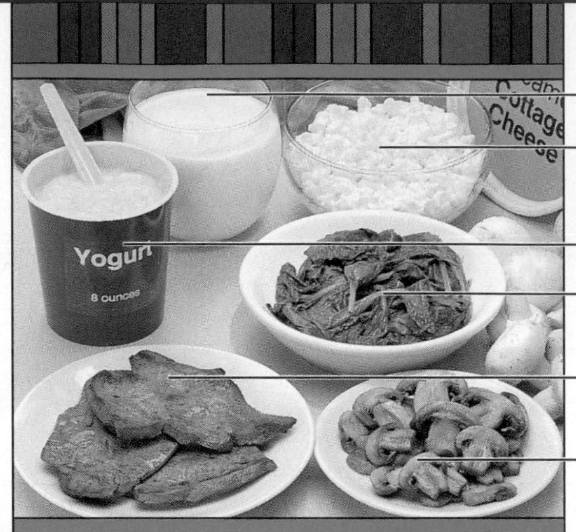

Milk 0.34 mg per cup

Cottage cheese 0.37 mg per cup

Yogurt 0.53 mg per cup

Spinach 0.21 mg per ½ cup cooked

Beef liver 3.5 mg per 3 ounces fried

Mushrooms 0.23 mg per ½ cup cooked

niacin a B vitamin needed in energy metabolism. Niacin can be eaten preformed, or can be made in the body from tryptophan, one of the amino acids. Other forms of niacin are *nicotinic acid, niacinamide, nicotinamide.*

pellagra (pell-AY-gra) the niacin-deficiency disease (*pellis* means "skin"; *agra* means "rough"). Symptoms include the "4 Ds": diarrhea, dermatitis, dementia, and, ultimately, death.

niacin equivalents the amount of niacin present in food, including the niacin that can theoretically be made from its precursor tryptophan, present in the food.

leafy vegetables, whole grain breads and cereals, and some meats contribute the rest of the riboflavin in people's diets (Snapshot 7-6 above).

Niacin The vitamin **niacin,** like thiamin and riboflavin, participates in the energy metabolism of every body cell. The niacin-deficiency disease **pellagra** appeared in Europe in the 1700s when corn from the New World came into wide acceptance as a staple food. At about the turn of this century in the United States, pellagra was devastating people's lives throughout the South and Midwest. Hundreds of thousands of pellagra victims were thought to be suffering from a contagious disease until this dietary deficiency was pinned down. The disease still occurs in poorly nourished people of today's urban slums and particularly in those with alcohol addiction. Pellagra is also still common in parts of Africa and Asia.

Early workers seeking the cause of pellagra observed that well-fed people *never* got it. From there they defined a diet that reliably produced the disease—one of cornmeal, pork fat, and molasses. Corn happens not only to be low in protein, but also to lack tryptophan, the amino acid from which niacin is made. Salt pork contains too little protein to compensate; and molasses is virtually protein free.

Figure 7-6 shows the skin disorder associated with pellagra. For comparison, Figure 7-7 shows a skin disorder associated with vitamin B_6 deficiency, a reminder that any nutrient deficiency affects the skin and all other cells. The skin just happens to be the organ you can see.

The key nutrient that prevents pellagra is niacin, but any protein containing sufficient amounts of the amino acid tryptophan will serve in its place. Tryptophan, which is abundant in almost all proteins (but is unavailable from the protein of corn), is converted to niacin in the body. In fact, it is possible to cure pellagra by administering tryptophan alone. Thus a person eating more than adequate protein (as most people do) will not be deficient in niacin. The amount of niacin in a diet is therefore stated in terms of **niacin equivalents,** a measure that takes available tryptophan into account. Snapshot 7-7 shows some food sources of niacin.

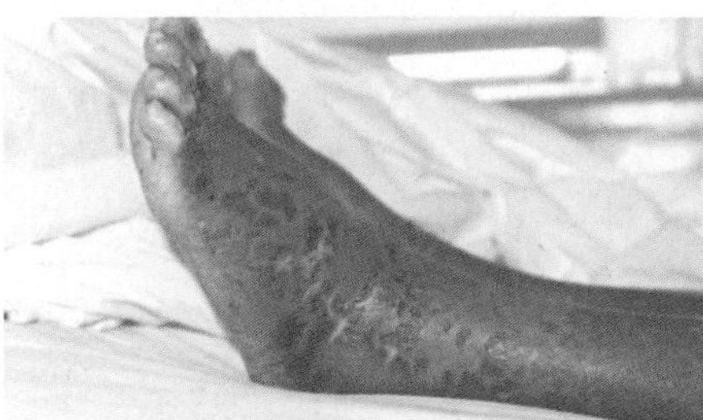

Figure 7-6

PELLAGRA
The typical dermatitis of pellagra develops on skin that is exposed to light.

SNAPSHOT 7-7

NIACIN

RDA for men: 19 mg/day
RDA for women: 15 mg/day

Baked potato 3.3 mg per whole small potato

Mushrooms 7 mg per ½ cup cooked

Tuna (in water) 11.3 mg per 3 ounces

Pork chop 4.4 mg per 3-ounce broiled chop

Chicken breast 11.7 mg per 3 ounces cooked

Certain forms of niacin supplements in amounts 10 times or more the RDA cause "niacin flush," a dilation of the capillaries of the skin with perceptible tingling that, if intense, can be painful. Some physicians administer large niacin doses as part of their arsenal of drugs against atherosclerosis. When used this way, niacin leaves the realm of nutrition to become a pharmacological agent, a drug. As with any drug, self dosing with niacin is ill advised; large doses may injure the liver, cause ulcers, and produce some symptoms of diabetes.[32]

folate (FOH-late) a B vitamin that acts as part of a coenzyme important in the manufacture of new cells. Other names for folate are *folacin*, and *folic acid*.

Folate and Vitamin B_{12} These two vitamins work closely together on many body projects, so they are presented here as a team. The vitamin **folate** is required to make all new cells. Folate helps synthesize the DNA needed for the new cells. Deficiencies may result from an inadequate intake, impaired absorption, increased excretion, or increased metabolic need for the vitamin.

Of all the vitamins, folate seems to be most vulnerable to interactions with medications. Ten major groups of drugs have been shown to interfere with the body's use of folate, including aspirin and its relatives and antacids. Use of these drugs to relieve an occasional headache or upset stomach presents no concern, but frequent users may need to attend to their folate intakes. These include people with chronic pain or ulcers who rely heavily on aspirin or antacids as well as those who smoke or take oral contraceptives or anticonvulsants.[33]

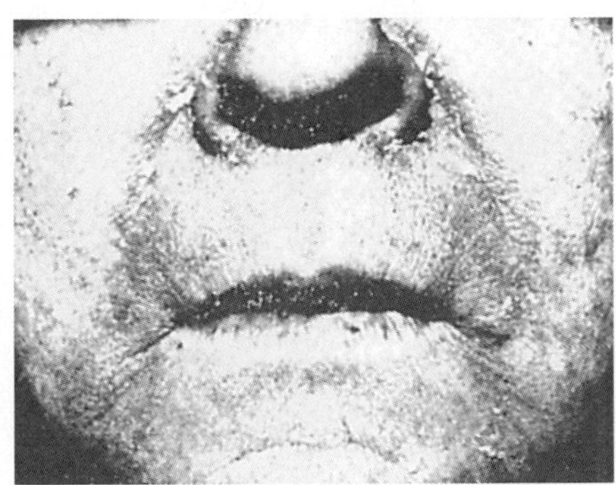

Figure 7-7

VITAMIN B_6 DEFICIENCY

In this dermatitis, the skin is greasy and flaky, unlike the skin affected by the dermatitis of pellagra.

Because the blood cells and digestive tract cells divide most rapidly, they are most vulnerable to deficiency. As a result, deficiencies of folate cause anemia and abnormal digestive function. In the United States a significant number of cases of folate-deficiency anemia occur yearly. Folate deficiency is especially prevalent among pregnant women, whose need is great because of rapid cell multiplication. Folate deficiency during pregnancy has been linked to the birth defects known as neural tube defects, an association discussed in Controversy 7 and Chapter 12.

Folate, as its name, derived from the word *foliage*, implies, is abundant in green, leafy vegetables such as spinach and turnip greens (see Snapshot

SNAPSHOT 7-8

FOLATE

RDA for men: 200 μg/day
RDA for women: 180 μg/day

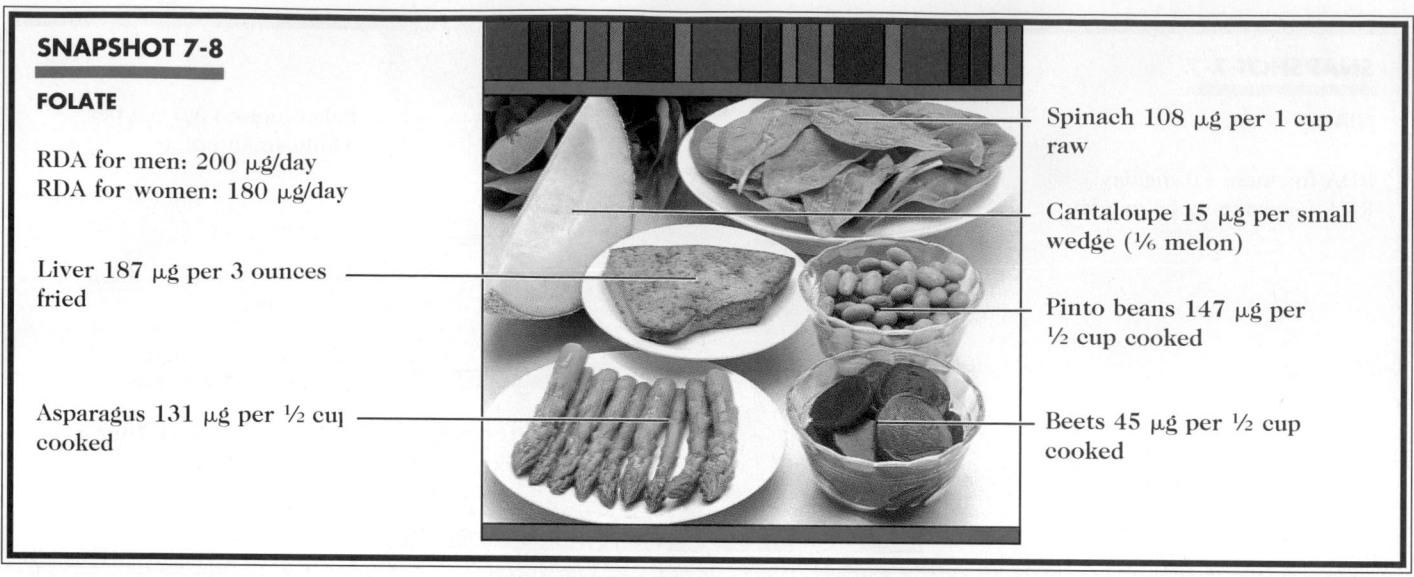

vitamin B_{12} a B vitamin that enables folate to get into cells and also helps maintain the sheath around nerve cells. Vitamin B_{12}'s scientific name, not often used, is *cyanocobalamin.*

intrinsic factor a factor found inside a system. The intrinsic factor necessary to prevent pernicious anemia is now known to be a compound that helps in the absorption of vitamin B_{12}.

pernicious (per-NISH-us) **anemia** vitamin B_{12} deficiency disease, caused by lack of intrinsic factor and characterized by large, immature red blood cells and damage to the nervous system. *Pernicious* means "highly injurious or destructive."

7-8). Fresh, uncooked vegetables and fruits are the best sources of folate, because heat destroys as much as half the folate in foods. Eggs also contain some folate. Orange juice and legumes are rich in folate, although the absorption of folate from these foods may be limited because they contain factors that may interfere with folate absorption.[34] Some research suggests that milk may enhance the absorption of folate, although it is unclear which constituent in milk does so.[35]

Folate, with the help of **vitamin B_{12},** works to make red blood cells. Vitamin B_{12} by itself also serves the body by helping to maintain the sheaths that surround and protect nerve fibers. It also may influence the cells that build bone tissue.[36]

The absorption of vitamin B_{12} requires an **intrinsic factor,** a compound made inside the body. The design for this factor is carried in the genes. The intrinsic factor is synthesized in the stomach, where it attaches to the vitamin; the complex then passes to the small intestine and is absorbed into the bloodstream. A few people have an inherited defect in the gene for intrinsic factor, which makes vitamin B_{12} absorption abnormal, beginning in mid-adulthood. Without normal absorption of vitamin B_{12} from food, they develop deficiency symptoms. In this case or in the case of stomach injury that limits production of intrinsic factor, vitamin B_{12} must be supplied by injection to bypass the defective absorptive system. The vitamin B_{12} deficiency caused by lack of intrinsic factor is known as **pernicious anemia.**

Without sufficient vitamin B_{12}, folate fails to do its blood-building work, so vitamin B_{12} deficiency causes an anemia identical to that caused by folate deficiency. The blood symptoms of deficiencies of either folate or vitamin B_{12} include the presence of large, immature red blood cells. Giving extra folate will clear up this blood condition, but it is a poor choice, because the deficiency of vitamin B_{12} can continue, undetected. Vitamin B_{12}'s other functions then become compromised, and the results can be devastating: damaged nerve sheaths, creeping paralysis, and general malfunctioning of nerves and muscles. A physician may notice cues to the B_{12} problem, but it is hard to diagnose correctly. More likely, the damage will proceed unchecked.[37]

SNAPSHOT 7-9

VITAMIN B_{12}

RDA for adults: 2 μg/day

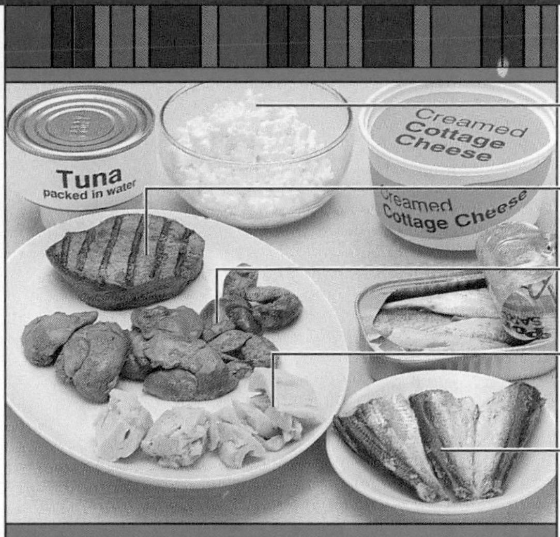

Cottage cheese 1.3 μg per cup

Sirloin steak 2.4 μg per 3 ounce steak cooked

Chicken liver 16.5 μg per 3 ounces cooked

Tuna (in water) 1.8 μg per 3 ounces

Sardines 7.6 μg per 3 ounces

In some cases, even without high folate intakes, vitamin B_{12} deficiency may not produce blood symptoms. Especially in people suffering from psychiatric disorders, nerve damage from vitamin B_{12} deficiency may be difficult to diagnose, and effective treatment can be tragically delayed.[38]

As Snapshot 7-9 shows, vitamin B_{12} is present only in foods of animal origin, not in foods from plants. This places the uninformed, strict vegetarian at special risk. People who give up all foods of animal origin may not show signs of deficiency right away because up to five years' worth of vitamin B_{12} can be stored in the body; but eventually signs develop.[39] Additionally, vegetarians are most likely to be well supplied with folate because, as mentioned earlier, vegetables are rich in folate. A pregnant or lactating woman who is eating such a diet should be aware that her infant can develop a vitamin B_{12} deficiency, even if the mother remains healthy. A deficiency of this vitamin can cause irreversible nervous system damage in the fetus. The birth of an infant with nerve problems can be the mother's first clue to the deficiency. All strict vegetarians, and especially pregnant women, must be sure to use B_{12}-fortified products such as vitamin B_{12}-fortified soy "milk," or to take the appropriate supplements. The Food Feature mentions some vitamin B_{12} sources for the vegetarian.

The way folate masks the anemia of vitamin B_{12} deficiency underlines a point already made several times. It takes a skilled professional to make a correct diagnosis, and the risk you take when you diagnose yourself or listen to would-be experts is clearly serious. A second point should also be underlined here. Since vitamin B_{12} deficiency in the body may be caused either by a lack of the vitamin in the diet or by a lack of intrinsic factor necessary to absorb it, a change in diet alone may not correct it, another reason for seeking professional diagnosis of physical symptoms.

vitamin B_6 a B vitamin. Its three active forms are *pyridoxine*, *pyridoxal*, and *pyridoxamine*.

Vitamin B_6 In the cells, **vitamin B_6** helps to convert one kind of amino acid, of which cells have an abundance, to others that the cells need more of. It also aids in the conversion of tryptophan to niacin and plays important roles in the synthesis of hemoglobin. Vitamin B_6 also assists in releasing stored glucose from glycogen and thus contributes to regulation of blood

SNAPSHOT 7-10

VITAMIN B_6

RDA for men: 2.0 mg/day
RDA for women: 1.6 mg/day

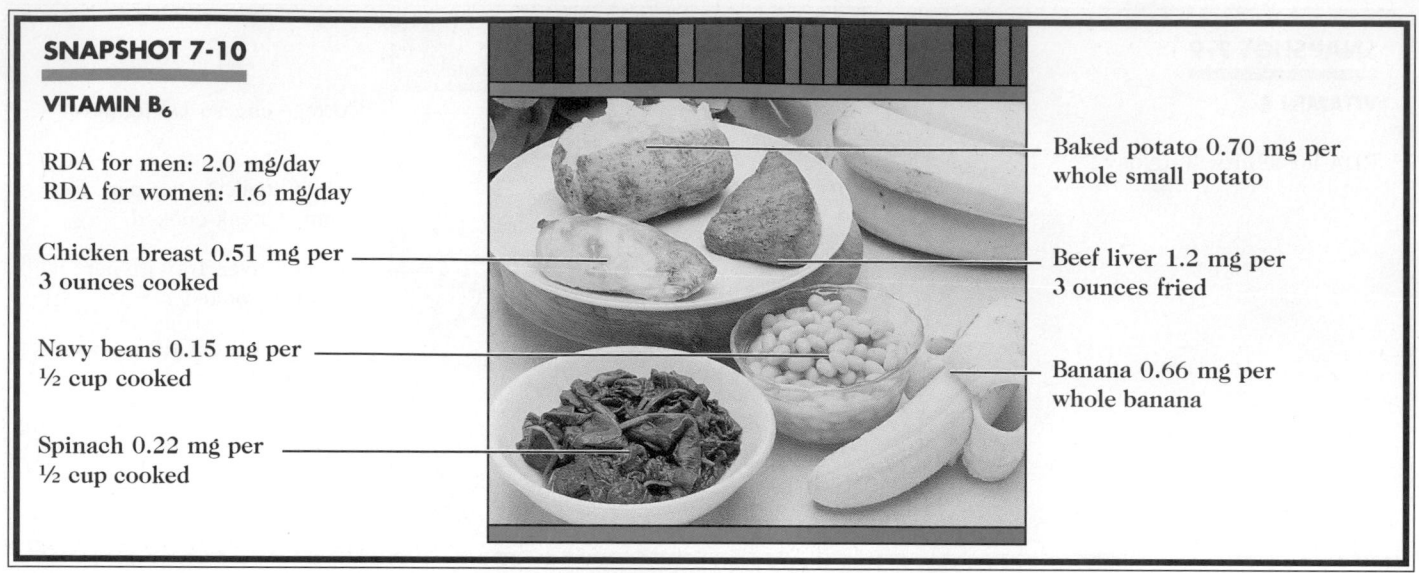

biotin (BY-o-tin) a B vitamin; a coenzyme necessary for fat synthesis and other metabolic reactions.

pantothenic (PAN-to-THEN-ic) **acid** a B vitamin.

The links between PMS and vitamin B_6 are explored in Chapter 13.

glucose. Vitamin B_6 research during the last decade or so has revealed roles for the vitamin in immune function and steroid hormone activity.[40]

Because of these diverse functions, vitamin B_6 deficiency is expressed in general symptoms, such as weakness, irritability, and insomnia. Other symptoms include the greasy dermatitis shown earlier, anemia, and in advanced cases of vitamin B_6 deficiency, convulsions. A shortage of vitamin B_6 also weakens the immune response.[41]

Large doses of vitamin B_6 can be dangerous. The first major report of vitamin B_6 toxicity appeared in 1983. Until that time it was generally believed that, like most of the other water-soluble vitamins, vitamin B_6 could not reach toxic concentrations in the body. The report told of women who took more than 2 grams of vitamin B_6 daily (the RDA for women is less than 2 *milli*grams) for two months or more in an attempt to cure the symptoms of premenstrual syndrome (PMS). The women developed numb feet, then lost sensation in their hands, then became unable to work. Later, in some cases, their mouths became numb. Since the first report of vitamin B_6 toxicity, researchers have seen toxicity symptoms in more than 100 women who took vitamin B_6 supplements for more than 5 years. The women recovered after they stopped taking the supplements. The potential toxicity of vitamin B_6 is yet another reason why people should not self-diagnose and self-prescribe vitamins for their own illnesses. Table 7-4 on pages 251–254 lists common deficiency and toxicity symptoms of vitamin B_6 and other water-soluble vitamins.

Because vitamin B_6 plays many roles in protein metabolism, the RDA for vitamin B_6 is roughly proportional to protein intakes. Meats, fish, and poultry (protein-rich foods), potatoes; leafy, green vegetables; and some fruits are good sources of vitamin B_6 (Snapshot 7-10).

Biotin and Pantothenic Acid Two other B vitamins, **biotin** and **pantothenic acid,** are, like thiamin, riboflavin, and niacin, important in energy metabolism. Biotin is a cofactor for several enzymes active in the metabolism of carbohydrate, fat, and protein. Pantothenic acid was first recognized as a substance that stimulates growth. Pantothenic acid is a component of

SNAPSHOT 7-11

BIOTIN AND PANTOTHENIC ACID[a]

Estimated safe and adequate intake for adults:
Biotin: 30–100 μg/day
Pantothenic acid: 4–7 mg/day

Eggs
Milk
Whole wheat bread
Broccoli, cooked
Chicken breast, cooked
Pinto beans
Beef liver, fried

[a]Information concerning biotin and pantothenic acid in foods is incomplete; deficiencies are rare.

a key coenzyme that makes possible the release of energy from the energy nutrients. It also participates in more than 100 different steps in the synthesis of lipids, neurotransmitters, steroid hormones, and hemoglobin.[42]

Although rare diseases may precipitate deficiencies of biotin and pantothenic acid, both vitamins are widespread in foods (Snapshot 7-11). Healthy people eating ordinary diets are not at risk for deficiencies.

inositol (in-OSS-ih-tall) a nonessential nutrient.

lipoic (lip-OH-ic) **acid** a nonessential nutrient.

choline (KOH-leen) a nonessential nutrient.

KEY POINT Historically famous B vitamin deficiency diseases are beriberi (thiamin), pellagra (niacin), and pernicious anemia (vitamin B_{12}). Pellagra can be prevented by adequate protein because the amino acid tryptophan can be converted to niacin in the body. A high intake of folate can mask the blood symptom of vitamin B_{12} deficiency but will not prevent the associated nerve damage. Vitamin B_6 is important in amino acid metabolism and can be toxic in excess. Biotin and pantothenic acid are important to the body and are abundant in food.

Non-B Vitamins

The section on the B vitamins has left a few compounds unrecognized that are sometimes *called* B vitamins. These are **inositol, lipoic acid,** and **choline.** They might more appropriately be called *nonvitamins* because they are not essential nutrients for human beings. Deficiencies can, however, be induced in laboratory animals for experimental purposes. Like the B vitamins described above, they serve as coenzymes in metabolism. Even if they were essential in human nutrition, supplements would be unnecessary because they are abundant in foods.

In addition to inositol, lipoic acid, and choline, other substances have been mistakenly thought essential in human nutrition because they are needed for growth by bacteria or other life forms. These substances include PABA (para-aminobenzoic acid), bioflavonoids ("vitamin P" or hesperidin), and ubiquinone (coenzyme Q). Other names you may hear are "vitamin B_{15}," or pangamic acid (a hoax); "vitamin B_{17}" (laetrile or amygdalin, not

Links between choline and brain function are discussed in Controversy 13.

scurvy the vitamin C deficiency disease.

ascorbic acid one of the active forms of vitamin C (the other is dehydroascorbic acid).

a cancer cure and not a vitamin by any stretch of the imagination); "vitamin B_T" (carnitine, an important piece of cell machinery but not a vitamin), and more.

KEY POINT Many substances that people claim are B vitamins are not, although some may have nonnutrient effects or may be useful as drugs. Among them are inositol, lipoic acid, and choline.

Vitamin C

Two hundred odd years ago, any man who joined the crew of a seagoing ship knew he had only half a chance of returning alive—not because he might be slain by pirates or die in a storm but because he might contract **scurvy,** a dread disease that might kill as many as two thirds of a ship's men on a long voyage. Only ships that sailed on short voyages, especially around the Mediterranean Sea, were safe from this disease. It was not known at the time that the special hazard of long ocean voyages was that the ship's cook used up his fresh fruits and vegetables early and relied for the duration of the voyage on cereals and live animals.

The first nutrition experiment to be conducted on human beings was devised nearly 250 years ago to find a cure for scurvy. A British physician divided some sailors with scurvy into groups. Each group received a different test substance: vinegar, sulfuric acid, seawater, oranges, or lemons. The ones receiving the citrus fruits were cured within a short time. Sadly, it was 50 years before the British Navy made use of the information and required all its vessels to provide lime juice to every sailor daily. The term ***limey*** was applied to the British sailors in mockery because of this requirement. The name later given to the vitamin, **ascorbic acid,** literally means "no-scurvy acid."

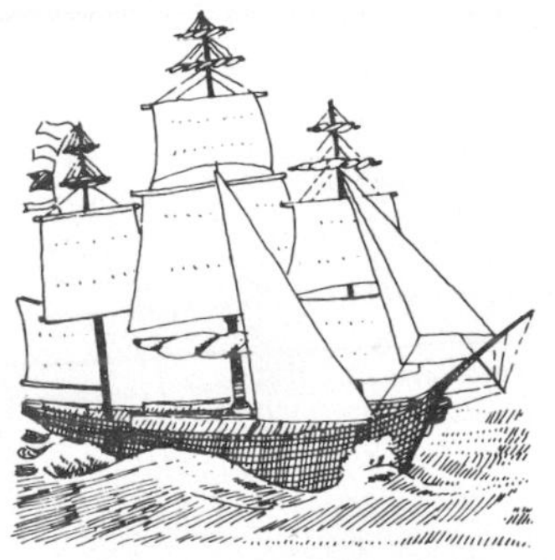

Long voyages without fresh fruits and vegetables spelled death by scurvy for the crew.

Since vitamin C is a water-soluble vitamin like the B vitamins, you might expect its mode of action to be like that of the B vitamins. To some extent, in some situations, vitamin C does help a specific enzyme perform its job just as the B vitamins do. In others, vitamin C acts in a more general way, as an antioxidant. Many substances found in foods and important in the body can be destroyed by oxidation. Remember the roles of beta carotene and vitamin E in protecting fat-soluble substances. Vitamin C works in much the same way with water-soluble substances, protecting them from oxidation by being oxidized itself. In the intestines, vitamin C protects iron from oxidation and so promotes its absorption. The antioxidant roles of vitamin C are the focus of extensive study, especially in relation to disease prevention, as the following Consumer Caution section points out.

Antioxidant Nutrients, Cancer, and Heart Disease

CONSUMER CAUTION In the last decade or so, intensive research efforts have given scientists a new understanding of the role of dietary factors in protecting people against cancer and other diseases. Accumulating evidence gives weight to the importance of the antioxidant functions of beta carotene (provitamin A), vitamin C, and vitamin E in preventing disease-causing damage to cells and tissues.

Antioxidant Nutrients, Cancer, and Heart Disease *continued*

CONSUMER CAUTION Before you race out to buy bottles of antioxidant supplements, though, recall the information in Chapter 1. It stated that only after rigorous, repeated testing can preliminary findings be considered confirmed. Scientists and medical and health experts around the world are working as fast as they can to clarify and confirm the roles of antioxidant nutrients in disease prevention.[43] They are excited about the potential importance of their work. Epidemiological evidence shows a correlation between low intakes of the antioxidant nutrients and a high incidence of disease. Laboratory studies with animals and cells seem to back up the findings. Here is what the research has shown so far.

Normal body processes result in the formation of unstable free radicals, highly reactive molecules often containing oxygen.* Free radicals set up destructive chain reactions that damage proteins, DNA, and unsaturated fatty acids inside cells. Physical stresses such as injury, infection, radiation exposure, or even excessive exercise greatly accelerate the formation of radicals in affected tissues, thus amplifying the total harmful effects. The body maintains many defenses against such damage.[44]

Many studies have shown that beta carotene, apart from its role in forming vitamin A, offers a degree of protection against cancer in animals.[45] However, the protective effects vary depending on the experimental conditions, the types of animals tested, and the cancer types and sites.

Research on human beings also produces diverse results. Researchers have for years been comparing populations that have high cancer rates with populations that have low cancer rates but who are similar in other characteristics—for example, smoking history and age. The researchers have collected diet information and/or blood samples and compared findings. Diet studies show that low intakes of vegetables and fruits, and specifically of those containing beta carotene and its relatives, are consistently linked with an increased incidence of lung cancer.[46] Blood studies show that low concentrations of beta carotene in the blood are consistently associated with the development of lung cancer.[47] The researchers note, however, that other constituents of fruits and vegetables have not been ruled out and may turn out to be responsible for the effect.

The role of vitamin C in the prevention of cancer is still being studied as well. Large-scale studies of populations offer strong support for a protective effect of vitamin C against certain types of cancer (cancer of the mouth, larynx, and esophagus, in particular).[48] In a dozen or so different studies, researchers have identified individuals with and without cancer and have assessed their dietary intakes of vitamin C.[49] They have found that people with high vitamin C intakes had lower

---

*Common biological radicals include $O_2^{\bullet -}$ (superoxide), H_2O_2 (hydrogen peroxide), and $OH^{\bullet}$ (hydroxyl) molecules, referred to as *reactive oxygen species.*

(continued on the next page)

Antioxidant Nutrients, Cancer, and Heart Disease *continued*

Figure 7-8

VITAMIN C RECOMMENDATIONS FROM SEVERAL SOURCES

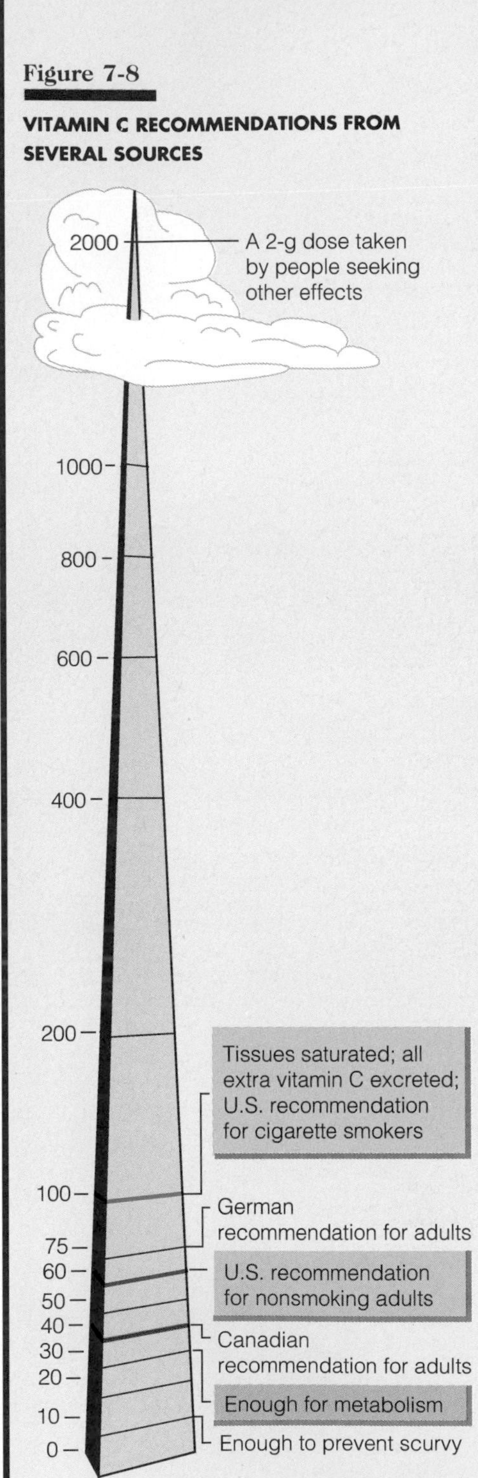

CONSUMER CAUTION risks of cancer than did people with low intakes. Some research suggests that vitamin C protects against stomach cancer by way of its antioxidant function.[50]

Evidence for a protective role of vitamin E against cancer is less consistent than for beta carotene and vitamin C. However, results of a large population study showed that people with low blood concentrations of vitamin E had a greater risk of certain cancers than those with higher concentrations of blood vitamin E.[51]

The correlations of high intakes of the antioxidant nutrients beta carotene, vitamin C, and vitamin E with low cancer risks may reflect some general benefits of eating diets rich in fruits and vegetables and low in fat. The findings thus far do not support the taking of vitamin supplements to prevent cancer. Moreover, no evidence suggests that they may improve the course of cancer once started. Many questions must be answered before supplementation can be recommended, if ever, as a strategy to prevent cancer. For example, which nutrients affect which cancers, and how? What are the optimal doses to reduce risk? What are the potential adverse effects of supplementation?

The findings relating cancer to diet do, however, offer strong support for recommendations to increase consumption of fruits and vegetables, recommendations that are for foods, not for supplements. Foods contain combinations of substances not found in any pill: many vitamins, fiber, the mineral selenium (also an antioxidant), other minerals, along with many nonnutrients. Researchers acknowledge that some of the factors in fruits and vegetables that offer the benefit of protection against cancer remain mysterious. In other words, the cast of characters in the story of the antioxidant nutrients and cancer is still incomplete. Until all the characters have had a chance to audition, don't try to predict who will get the starring role.

In the case of heart disease, the situation is different. At least for one antioxidant nutrient, vitamin E, doses beyond those normally obtained from food are statistically linked with lower risks of heart disease. During the 1980s, a study of almost 90,000 nurses first suggested a connection to vitamin E supplements and reduced heart disease risk. Other studies that followed confirmed that for both men and women, daily vitamin E doses of between 100 and 400 IU are linked with lower risks of heart disease.[52] Daily doses lower than 100 IU demonstrated no connection to reduced risk, while for doses greater than 400 IU the connection did not grow stronger. Experts are not yet ready to make public recommendations concerning vitamin E, but when results of research currently underway become available, such recommendations seem likely.

As for vitamin C, Figure 7-8 demonstrates that intakes vary widely. Notice, however that the official recommendations are all within the same rather narrow range.

Vitamin C is required for the production and maintenance of **collagen,** a protein substance that forms the base for all connective tissues in the body: bones, teeth, skin, and tendons. Collagen forms the scar tissue that heals wounds, the reinforcing structure that mends fractures, and the supporting material of capillaries that prevents bruises.

collagen (COLL-a-jen) the chief protein of most connective tissues, including scars, ligaments, and tendons, and the underlying matrix on which bones and teeth are built.

Vitamin C also enhances the immune response and so protects against infection. The relationship between vitamin C and the common cold is discussed in Chapter 11. The vitamin is also important to the production of thyroxin, the hormone that regulates basal metabolic rate and body temperature.

In times of stress, the body's vitamin C pool dwindles, because it is involved in the release of the stress hormones from the adrenal gland. Vitamin makers have used this fact to sell "stress-formula" supplements that are largely vitamin C with B vitamins added. In truth, the amount of extra vitamin C used up during stress is well within the safety margin of the RDA. If you are under stress (and who isn't?), generous servings of vitamin C-rich fruits and vegetables will still more than cover your needs.

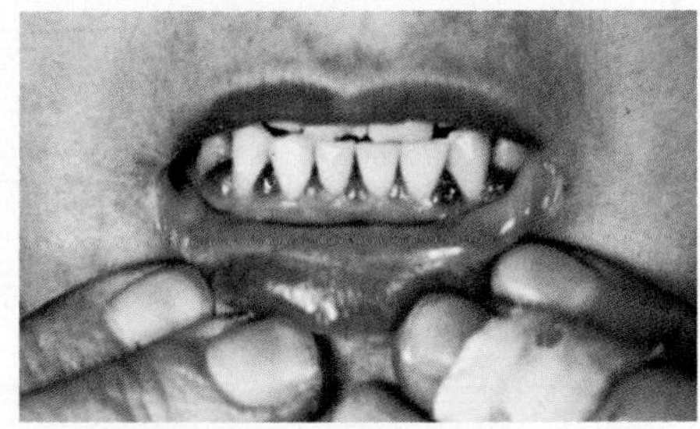

Figure 7-9

SCURVY

Vitamin C deficiency causes breakdown of collagen, which supports the teeth.

Cigarette smoking, among its many harmful effects, interferes with the use of vitamin C. Smokers therefore need to obtain more vitamin C in their diets. Consumption of extra vitamin C can normalize blood levels but cannot protect against the damage caused by smoking.

Most of the symptoms of scurvy can be attributed to the breakdown of collagen in the absence of vitamin C: loss of appetite, growth cessation, tenderness to touch, weakness, bleeding gums (shown here in Figure 7-9), loose teeth, swollen ankles and wrists, and tiny red spots in the skin where blood has leaked out of capillaries. One symptom, anemia, reflects an important role already mentioned, that vitamin C helps the body to absorb and to use iron.

In the United States scurvy is seldom seen today except in infants who are fed only cow's milk, in the elderly, and in people addicted to alcohol. Breast milk and infant formula supply enough vitamin C, but infants who are fed cow's milk and receive no vitamin C in formula, fruit juice, or other outside sources are at risk.[53] Low intakes of fruits and vegetables and a poor appetite for food in general lead to low vitamin C intakes, and are not uncommon among people 65 years of age and older.[54]

The adult RDA for vitamin C of 60 milligrams is midway between two extremes. At one extreme is the requirement, 10 milligrams per day, which is all you need to prevent the symptoms of scurvy from appearing. At the other extreme is the amount at which the body's pool of vitamin C is full to overflowing: about 100 milligrams per day.[55] The RDA for smokers is set at the high end, 100 milligrams, because this amount is needed to maintain blood levels comparable to those of nonsmokers.[56] Other authorities have set different standards. For example, Canada recommends 30 milligrams per day and Germany 75.

The easy availability of vitamin C in pill form and the publication of books recommending vitamin C to prevent and cure colds and cancer have led thousands of people to take large doses of vitamin C. The widespread use of megadoses of vitamin C has enabled researchers to study their toxic effects. Effects that are theoretically possible (but that have not been seen with intakes as high as 3 grams a day) include formation of kidney stones, upset of the acid-base balance, and interference with the action of vitamin E.

SNAPSHOT 7-12

VITAMIN C

RDA for adults: 60 mg/day

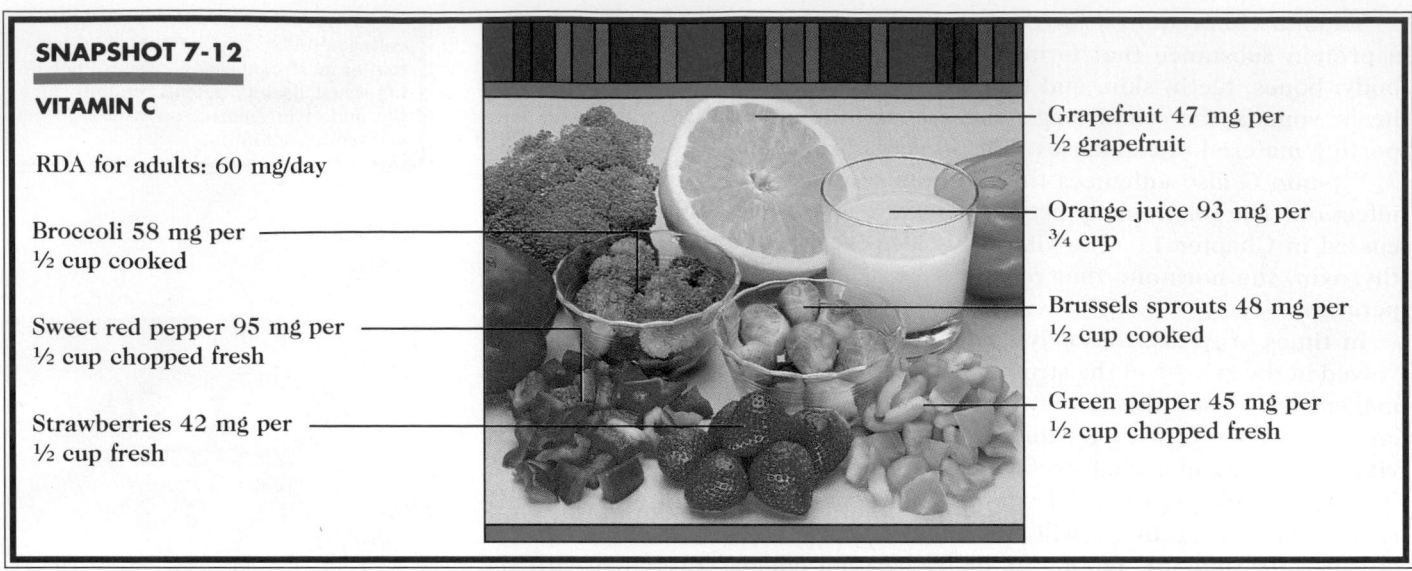

Chapter 11's Consumer Caution comes back to the arguments surrounding vitamin C and diseases.

Other adverse effects, however, have been seen often enough to warrant concern. Nausea, abdominal cramps, and diarrhea are often reported. Several instances of interference with medical regimens are known. Large amounts of vitamin C excreted in the urine can obscure the results of tests used to detect diabetes, giving a false-positive result in some instances and a false-negative result in others. People taking medications to prevent blood clotting may unwittingly abolish their effect if they also take massive doses of vitamin C.[57]

The published research on large doses of vitamin C reveals few instances in which consuming more than 100 to 300 milligrams a day is beneficial. Adults may not be taking major risks if they dose themselves with 1 to 2 grams a day, but doses approaching 10 grams are clearly unsafe. In short, the range of safe vitamin C intakes seems to be broad. Between the absolute minimum of 10 milligrams a day and the reasonable maximum of 2,000 milligrams, nearly everyone should be able to find a suitable intake. People who venture outside these limits do so at their own risk. Vitamin C from food sources such as those shown in Snapshot 7-12 is always safe.

This chapter has addressed all thirteen of the vitamins. It closes with Tables 7-3 and 7-4 on pages 249–254 to sum up the basic facts about each one.

KEY POINT Vitamin C, an antioxidant, is needed for proper maintenance of the connective tissue protein collagen, protects against infection, and helps in iron absorption. The theory that vitamin C prevents or cures colds or cancer is not well supported by research. Vitamin C megadoses may be hazardous. Ample vitamin C can be obtained from foods.

FOOD FEATURE

Choosing Foods Rich in Vitamins

Most people, on learning how important the vitamins are to their health, want to choose foods that are vitamin rich. One way to identify such foods is to look at the vitamins in single servings. This method is shown in Figure 7-10 on pages 244–245. Another useful way to pick foods for vitamin richness is to compare them on a vitamin-per-calorie basis; this method is shown later.

The colors in Figure 7-10 represent the various food groups: white is for the milks and milk products, green for vegetables, purple for fruits, brown for legumes, gold for breads and cereals, and red for meat, fish, and poultry. For the most part, the serving sizes in these figures are those that people might realistically eat. For example, 3 ounces is used for most meats. The vegetable serving size is 1 cup. In terms of the exchange lists, the meat portion is 3 exchanges; the vegetable portion is 2.

Some people, after viewing a figure such as this, are led to believe that to meet their vitamin needs, they must memorize the richest sources of each vitamin and include those foods daily. This is a false notion and can lead people to limit the variety of foods they choose while overemphasizing the components of a few foods. While it is reassuring to know that your carrot-raisin salad at lunch provided more than the entire Daily Value amount for vitamin A, it is a mistake to think that you must then go on to select equally rich sources of all the other vitamins. Such rich sources do not exist for many vitamins. Rather, foods work in harmony to provide the nutrients. For example, a baked potato, while not a star performer among vitamin C providers, contributes substantially to a day's need for this nutrient and contributes some thiamin too. By the end of the day, assuming that your food choices were made with reasonable care, the bits of thiamin, vitamin B_6, and vitamin C from each serving of food have accumulated to make a more than adequate total diet.

With a few exceptions, nutritious foods generally provide small quantities of thiamin, as shown by Figure 7-10. A few meats are exceptionally good thiamin sources; these are members of the pork family. As you can see in the graph, one small pork chop (275 calories) provides over half of the Daily Value for thiamin, but again, this does not suggest that you eat pork every day. Legumes and grains are also good, low-fat sources, and they provide beneficial fiber and nutrients lacking from meats. On the other hand, beans lack the vitamin B_{12} provided by meats. Peanut butter is a good source of thiamin as it is of most B vitamins, but its high fat and calorie contents call for moderation in its use.

The vitamin B_6 data provide another insight to support the argument for variety. From just the few foods listed here, you can see that no one source can provide the whole day's requirement but that a variety of meats, fish, and poultry; potatoes; and a few vegetables and fruits can work together to supply it.

Folate and vitamin C are represented in foods in the last two graphs of Figure 7-10. These nutrients are both richly supplied by fruits and vegetables. The richest source of either may be only a moderate source of the other, but the recommended servings of fruits and vegetables in

Figure 7-10

FOOD SOURCES OF VITAMINS SELECTED TO SHOW A RANGE OF VALUES—COMMONLY EATEN PORTIONS RANKED RICHEST TO POOREST

Food	Serving size (energy)	R.E.
VITAMIN A		
Beef liver	3 oz fried (185 cal)	9,123
Sweet potato	1 whole baked (117 cal)	2,486
Carrot	1 whole fresh (31 cal)	2,024
Spinach	1 c fresh cooked (42 cal)	1,474
Butternut squash	1 c baked (82 cal)	1,435
Winter squash	1 c mashed (96 cal)	872
Cantaloupe	1/2 (93 cal)	860
Tomatoes	1 c cooked (65 cal)	178
Milk, nonfat	1 c (85 cal)	149
Cheddar cheese	1 oz (114 cal)	86
Summer squash	1 c cooked (36 cal)	52
Peach	1 fresh medium (37 cal)	47
Apple	1 fresh medium (81 cal)	7
Sirloin steak	3 oz lean (165 cal)	0
Whole-wheat bread	1 slice (70 cal)	0
Baked potato	1 whole (220 cal)	0

Food	Serving size (energy)	mg
VITAMIN E		
Sunflower seeds	1/4 c dry (205 cal)	18
Sweet potato	1 baked (117 cal)	7
Sunflower seed oil	1 tbs (120 cal)	6.5
Cottonseed oil	1 tbs (120 cal)	5
Safflower oil	1 tbs (120 cal)	4.5
Peanut butter	1/4 c chunky (377 cal)	4
Shrimp	3 oz boiled (84 cal)	3
Corn oil	1 tbs (120 cal)	2.5
Canola oil	1 tbs (120 cal)	2.5
Peanuts	1 oz (167 cal)	2
Salmon, broiled/baked	3 oz (184 cal)	2
Apple	1 fresh medium (81 cal)	1.5
Parsley	1 tbs fresh chopped (1 cal)	1
Cheddar cheese	1 oz (114 cal)	0.5
Whole-wheat bread	1 slice (70 cal)	0

Food	Serving size (energy)	mg
THIAMIN		
Pork chop	3.1 oz broiled (275 cal)	0.87
Sunflower seeds	1/4 c dry (205 cal)	0.82
Black beans	1 c cooked (228 cal)	0.42
Green peas	1 c cooked (124 cal)	0.46
Watermelon	1 slice (154 cal)	0.39
Oatmeal	1 c cooked (145 cal)	0.26
Oysters	1 c raw (169 cal)	0.25
Baked potato	1 whole (220 cal)	0.22
Orange juice	1 c, fresh (111 cal)	0.22
Sirloin steak	3 oz lean (165 cal)	0.15
Whole-wheat bread	1 slice (70 cal)	0.10
Milk, nonfat	1 c (85 cal)	0.09
Summer squash	1 c cooked (36 cal)	0.08
Cabbage	1 c raw shredded (17 cal)	0.03
Apple	1 fresh medium (81 cal)	0.02
Cheddar cheese	1 oz (114 cal)	0.01

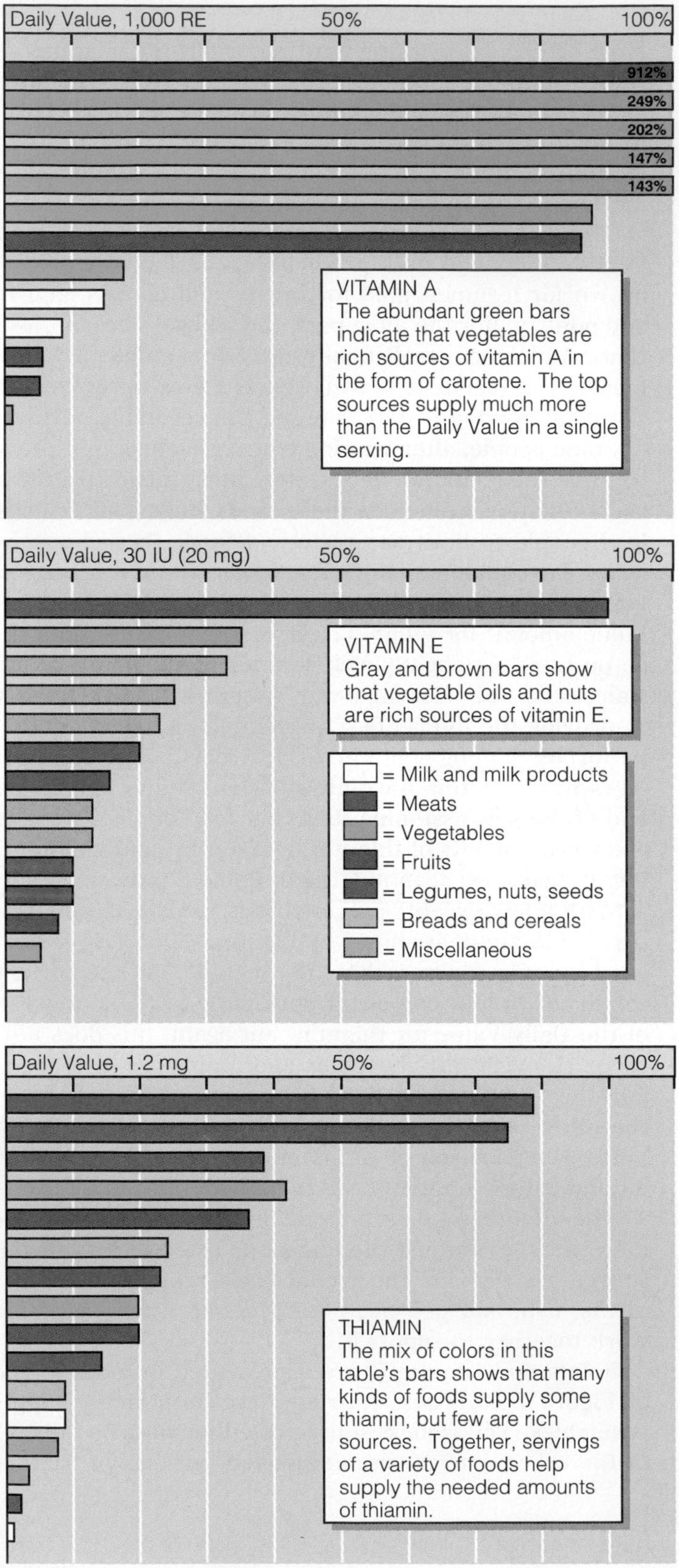

Daily Value, 1,000 RE
50%
100%
912%
249%
202%
147%
143%
VITAMIN A
The abundant green bars indicate that vegetables are rich sources of vitamin A in the form of carotene. The top sources supply much more than the Daily Value in a single serving.
Daily Value, 30 IU (20 mg)
50%
100%
VITAMIN E
Gray and brown bars show that vegetable oils and nuts are rich sources of vitamin E.
= Milk and milk products
= Meats
= Vegetables
= Fruits
= Legumes, nuts, seeds
= Breads and cereals
= Miscellaneous
Daily Value, 1.2 mg
50%
100%
THIAMIN
The mix of colors in this table's bars shows that many kinds of foods supply some thiamin, but few are rich sources. Together, servings of a variety of foods help supply the needed amounts of thiamin.

Figure 7-10

FOOD SOURCES OF VITAMINS SELECTED TO SHOW A RANGE OF VALUES—COMMONLY EATEN PORTIONS RANKED RICHEST TO POOREST (cont.)

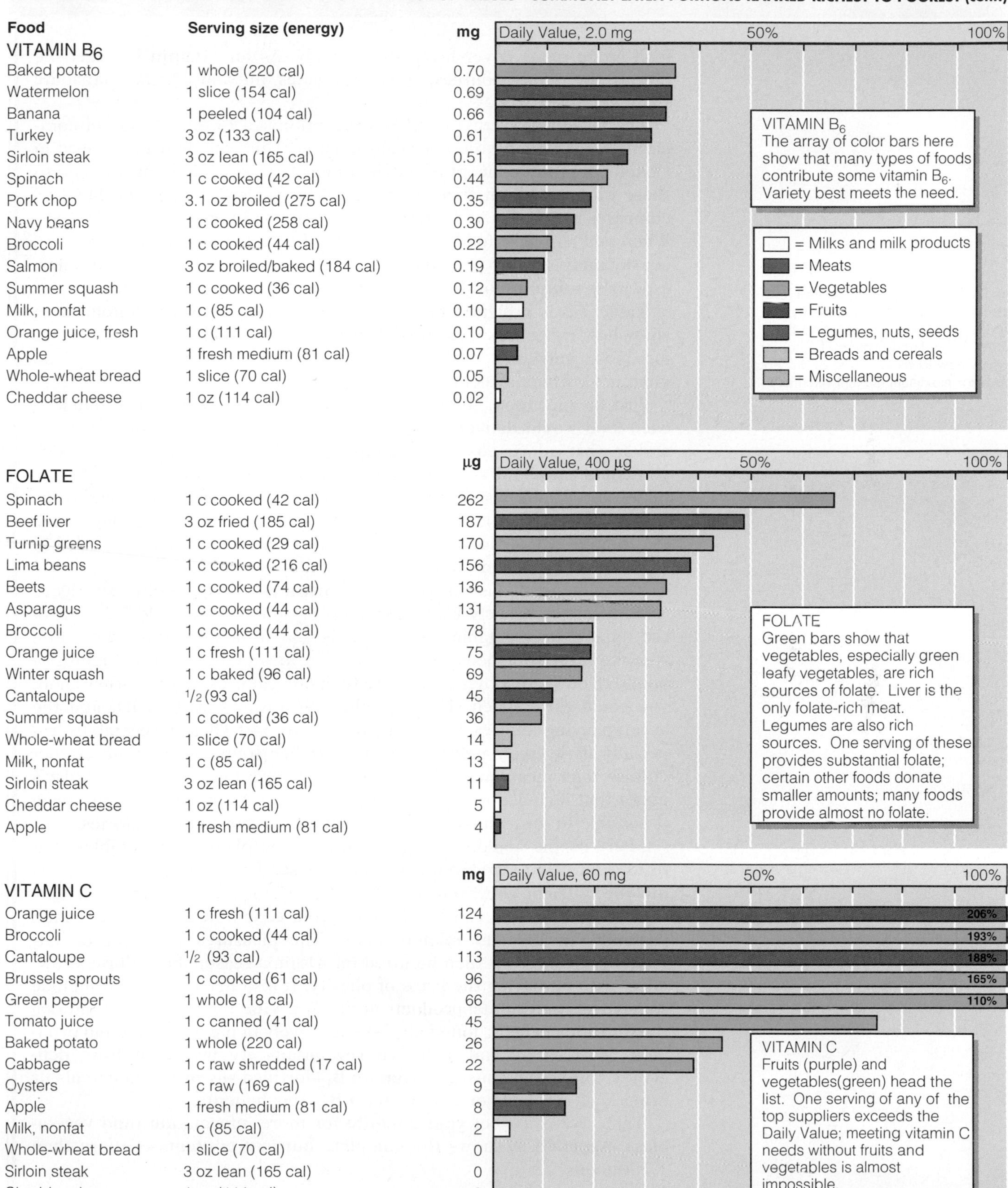
Food
Serving size (energy)
mg
Daily Value, 2.0 mg
50%
100%
VITAMIN B_6
Baked potato 1 whole (220 cal) 0.70
Watermelon 1 slice (154 cal) 0.69
Banana 1 peeled (104 cal) 0.66
Turkey 3 oz (133 cal) 0.61
Sirloin steak 3 oz lean (165 cal) 0.51
Spinach 1 c cooked (42 cal) 0.44
Pork chop 3.1 oz broiled (275 cal) 0.35
Navy beans 1 c cooked (258 cal) 0.30
Broccoli 1 c cooked (44 cal) 0.22
Salmon 3 oz broiled/baked (184 cal) 0.19
Summer squash 1 c cooked (36 cal) 0.12
Milk, nonfat 1 c (85 cal) 0.10
Orange juice, fresh 1 c (111 cal) 0.10
Apple 1 fresh medium (81 cal) 0.07
Whole-wheat bread 1 slice (70 cal) 0.05
Cheddar cheese 1 oz (114 cal) 0.02
VITAMIN B_6
The array of color bars here show that many types of foods contribute some vitamin B_6. Variety best meets the need.
= Milks and milk products
= Meats
= Vegetables
= Fruits
= Legumes, nuts, seeds
= Breads and cereals
= Miscellaneous
µg
Daily Value, 400 µg
50%
100%
FOLATE
Spinach 1 c cooked (42 cal) 262
Beef liver 3 oz fried (185 cal) 187
Turnip greens 1 c cooked (29 cal) 170
Lima beans 1 c cooked (216 cal) 156
Beets 1 c cooked (74 cal) 136
Asparagus 1 c cooked (44 cal) 131
Broccoli 1 c cooked (44 cal) 78
Orange juice 1 c fresh (111 cal) 75
Winter squash 1 c baked (96 cal) 69
Cantaloupe 1/2 (93 cal) 45
Summer squash 1 c cooked (36 cal) 36
Whole-wheat bread 1 slice (70 cal) 14
Milk, nonfat 1 c (85 cal) 13
Sirloin steak 3 oz lean (165 cal) 11
Cheddar cheese 1 oz (114 cal) 5
Apple 1 fresh medium (81 cal) 4
FOLATE
Green bars show that vegetables, especially green leafy vegetables, are rich sources of folate. Liver is the only folate-rich meat. Legumes are also rich sources. One serving of these provides substantial folate; certain other foods donate smaller amounts; many foods provide almost no folate.
mg
Daily Value, 60 mg
50%
100%
VITAMIN C
Orange juice 1 c fresh (111 cal) 124 206%
Broccoli 1 c cooked (44 cal) 116 193%
Cantaloupe 1/2 (93 cal) 113 188%
Brussels sprouts 1 c cooked (61 cal) 96 165%
Green pepper 1 whole (18 cal) 66 110%
Tomato juice 1 c canned (41 cal) 45
Baked potato 1 whole (220 cal) 26
Cabbage 1 c raw shredded (17 cal) 22
Oysters 1 c raw (169 cal) 9
Apple 1 fresh medium (81 cal) 8
Milk, nonfat 1 c (85 cal) 2
Whole-wheat bread 1 slice (70 cal) 0
Sirloin steak 3 oz lean (165 cal) 0
Cheddar cheese 1 oz (114 cal) 0
VITAMIN C
Fruits (purple) and vegetables(green) head the list. One serving of any of the top suppliers exceeds the Daily Value; meeting vitamin C needs without fruits and vegetables is almost impossible.

food group plans cover both needs amply. As for vitamin E, vegetable oils are the richest sources. Some vegetables, nuts, and fruits contribute some vitamin E, too.

The beginning of this Food Feature promised to offer a way of comparing foods on a vitamin-per-calorie basis. This way, first introduced in Chapter 1 as the concept of nutrient density, is especially meaningful to those who must limit their energy intakes. Table 7-2 on pages 247–248 compares how much of a vitamin foods contribute on a per-calorie basis. When you compare foods on this basis, the vegetables suddenly assume considerably greater prominence as rich sources of all of the vitamins, especially useful if you like to consume large quantities of them.

The foods listed in the tables here are assumed to have been prepared and processed in ways that conserve their nutrients. The Food Feature of Chapter 14 reveals how to select, store, and prepare foods for maximum nutrient retention.

Table 7-2 is designed to make several points. It is also intended to show how ridiculous it is to try to use any one food to meet the needs for most nutrients. Notable exceptions are vitamin A, folate, and vitamin C, which are concentrated in a few foods.

Just for fun, then, the right side of each section shows how much of each food would deliver your entire need of the nutrient for the day—and at what calorie cost. For example, to get your vitamin A for the day, you could eat about a cup of almost any kind of dark green, leafy vegetables. You could also eat half a carrot or 1 bite of cooked beef liver. Notice, though, that all the apples in Washington can't meet a day's need for vitamin A. Poor food sources of every vitamin have been included in every table to remind you to keep your diet balanced.

The vitamin B_6 part of the table illustrates another point. In Figure 7-10, meats rank fairly high as vitamin B_6 sources. In Table 7-2, four of the top six are vegetables. The point is that while you *could* eat sirloin steak to meet your need for vitamin B_6, you would have to eat almost a pound to do so, together with more than 600 calories. On the other hand, you could eat spinach (if you could wolf down 3 cups of it), and the accompanying calories would amount to only 140. Clearly vegetables (especially dark green vegetables) are a richer source of vitamin B_6 *per calorie* than meats are—that is, they are more nutrient dense. A day's meals that included generous servings of several vegetables would make it possible to meet nutrient needs without overconsuming calories.

Many people couldn't imagine eating large plates of vegetables, but from a nutrition standpoint, it makes sense. The calorie cost is almost nil; the nutrient contributions are highly significant; and the nutrients that are still needed can be obtained from economical portions of milk products, meats, and related foods. The pleasures of sweet or fat-containing foods can then be fitted in, within a reasonable calorie allowance, without paying the price of obesity. It also makes sense to include some meats and animal products in the diet. Vitamin B_{12} is unique among the nutrients in being found almost exclusively in meats and animal products. Meat eaters and lacto-ovo vegetarians are protected from deficiency, but vegans must use vitamin B_{12}-fortified soy milk and cereals or other such products or take vitamin B_{12} supplements.

Table 7-2 can whet your appetite for more information (and vegetables). Appendix A shows the complete nutrient contents of more than 1,700 foods.

Table 7-2
Serving Sizes and Energy Amounts Required to Meet the Daily Value from Single Sources

If You Wanted 100% of the Daily Value from This Food	You Would Have to Eat This Size Serving
Vitamin A	
Carrot, whole fresh	0.5 carrot (16 cal)
Beef liver, fried	0.3 oz (19 cal)
Dandelion green, cooked	0.8 c (28 cal)
Spinach, cooked	0.7 c (29 cal)
Turnip greens, cooked	1.3 c (38 cal)
Sweet potato, baked	0.4 potato (47 cal)
Butternut squash, baked	0.7 c (58 cal)
Cantaloupe melon	0.6 melon (113 cal)
Broccoli, cooked	4.5 c (207 cal)
Nonfat milk	6.7 c (576 cal)
Oysters, raw	4.5 c (720 cal)
Cheddar cheese	11 oz (1,254 cal)
Apple, fresh medium	too much (too many cal)
Sirloin steak, lean	too much (too many cal)
Sole/flounder, baked	too much (too many cal)
Whole wheat bread	too much (too many cal)
Thiamin	
Mushrooms, raw sliced	20 c (360 cal)
Green peas, cooked	3.2 c (403 cal)
Sunflower seeds, dry	0.5 c (410 cal)
Pork chop	5.3 oz (468 cal)
Broccoli, cooked	11 c (506 cal)
Watermelon	3.8 sl (578 cal)
Turnip greens, cooked	20 c (580 cal)
Oysters, raw	5.3 c (848 cal)
Whole wheat bread	14 sl (980 cal)
Nonfat milk	17 c (1,462 cal)
Sole/flounder, baked	100 oz (3,960 cal)
Sirloin steak, lean	42 oz (2,544 cal)
Apple, fresh medium	100 apples (8,000 cal)
Cheddar cheese	too much (too many cal)
Folate	
Romaine lettuce, chopped	5.3 c (48 cal)
Spinach, cooked	1.5 c (62 cal)
Turnip greens, cooked	2.3 c (67 cal)
Parsley, chopped fresh	3.6 c (72 cal)
Asparagus, cooked	2.3 c (101 cal)
Broccoli, cooked	3.7 c (170 cal)
Mushrooms, raw sliced	25 c (450 cal)
Beef liver, fried	7.9 oz (481 cal)
Lima beans, cooked	2.3 c (598 cal)
Whole wheat bread	25 sl (1,750 cal)
Nonfat milk	25 c (2,150 cal)
Oysters, raw	17 c (2,720 cal)
Apple, fresh medium	100 apples (8,000 cal)
Sirloin steak, lean	10 lb (9,600 cal)
Cheddar cheese	100 oz (11,400 cal)

(table continued on next page)

Table 7-2
Serving Sizes and Energy Amounts Required to Meet the Daily Value from Single Sources (continued)

If You Wanted 100% of the Daily Value from This Food	You Would Have to Eat This Size Serving
Vitamin B_6	
Spinach, cooked	4.5 c (185 cal)
Mustard greens, cooked	11 c (231 cal)
Cauliflower, cooked	8 c (240 cal)
Broccoli, cooked	6.3 c (290 cal)
Banana, peeled	3 banana (315 cal)
Watermelon	2.9 sl (441 cal)
Chicken breast, roasted	4 halves (568 cal)
Navy beans, cooked dry	2.8 c (630 cal)
Tuna, canned	14 oz (635 cal)
Baked potato, whole	2.9 potato (638 cal)
Sunflower seeds, dry	1 c (820 cal)
Sole/flounder, baked	21 oz (840 cal)
Sirloin steak, lean	20.5 oz (1,248 cal)
Nonfat milk	20 c (1,720 cal)
Apple, fresh medium	25 apples (2,000 cal)
Whole wheat bread	33 sl (2,310 cal)
Cheddar cheese	100 oz (11,400 cal)
Vitamin C	
Green peppers, whole	0.6 pepper (11 cal)
Parsley, chopped fresh	1.2 c (24 cal)
Cauliflower, cooked	0.9 c (27 cal)
Broccoli, cooked	0.6 c (28 cal)
Strawberries, fresh	0.7 c (32 cal)
Papaya, whole fresh	0.3 papaya (35 cal)
Brussels sprouts, cooked	0.6 c (36 cal)
Mustard greens, cooked	1.8 c (38 cal)
Cantaloupe melon	¼ melon (47 cal)
Orange, fresh medium	0.9 orange (54 cal)
Grapefruit juice, fresh	0.6 c (58 cal)
Oysters, raw	0.8 c (128 cal)
Apple, fresh medium	7.7 apples (616 cal)
Nonfat milk	33 c (2,838 cal)
Sole/flounder, baked	150 oz (6,000 cal)
Cheddar cheese	too much (too many cal)
Whole wheat bread	too much (too many cal)
Vitamin E	
Sweet potato, baked	2.9 potato (334 cal)
Sunflower seeds, dry	0.28 c (227 cal)
Cottonseed oil	4 tbs (480 cal)
Safflower oil	4.4 tbs (522 cal)
Peanut butter, chunky	1.3 c (1885 cal)
Shrimp, boiled	20 oz (560 cal)
Corn oil	7.7 tbs (923 cal)
Canola oil	7.7 tbs (923 cal)
Peanuts	10 oz (1,670 cal)
Salmon, broiled	30 oz (1,840 cal)
Apple, fresh medium	12.5 apples (1,013 cal)
Parsley, fresh chopped	20 tbs (20 cal)
Cheddar cheese	33.3 oz (3,800 cal)

Table 7-3
The Fat-Soluble Vitamins—Functions, Deficiencies, and Toxicities

Vitamin A

Other Names

Retinol, retinal, retinoic acid; main precursor is beta carotene

Chief Functions in the Body

Vision: health of cornea, epithelial cells, mucous membranes; skin health; bone and tooth growth; reproduction; hormone synthesis and regulation; immunity; cancer protection

Deficiency Disease Name

Hypovitaminosis A

Significant Sources

Retinol: fortified milk, cheese, cream, butter, fortified margarine, eggs, liver

Beta carotene: spinach and other dark, leafy greens; broccoli; deep orange fruits (apricots, cantaloupe) and vegetables (squash, carrots, sweet potatoes, pumpkin)

	Deficiency Symptoms	Toxicity Symptoms
BLOOD/CIRCULATORY SYSTEM	Anemia (small-cell type)[a]	Red blood cell breakage, nosebleeds
BONES/TEETH	Cessation of bone growth, painful joints; impaired enamel formation, cracks in teeth, tendency to decay	Bone pain; growth retardation; increase of pressure inside skull mimicking brain tumor; headaches
DIGESTIVE SYSTEM	Diarrhea, changes in lining	Abdominal cramps and pain, nausea vomiting, diarrhea, weight loss
IMMUNE SYSTEM	Depression; frequent respiratory, digestive, bladder, vaginal, and other infections	Overreactivity
NERVOUS/MUSCULAR SYSTEMS	Night blindness (retinal)	Blurred vision, pain in calves, fatigue, irritability, loss of appetite
SKIN AND CORNEA	Keratinization, corneal degeneration leading to blindness,[b] rashes	Dry skin, rashes, loss of hair
OTHER	Kidney stones, impaired growth	Cessation of menstruation, liver and spleen enlargement

Vitamin D

Other Names

Calciferol, cholecalciferol, dihydroxy vitamin D; precursor is cholesterol

Chief Functions in the Body

Mineralization of bones (raises blood calcium and phosphorus via absorption from digestive tract, and by withdrawing calcium from bones and stimulating retention by kidneys)

Deficiency Disease Name

Rickets, osteomalacia

Significant Sources

Self-synthesis with sunlight; fortified milk or margarine, eggs, liver, small fish (sardines)

	Deficiency Symptoms	Toxicity Symptoms
BLOOD/CIRCULATORY SYSTEM		Raised blood calcium
BONES/TEETH	Abnormal growth, misshapen bones (bowing of legs), soft bones, joint pain, malformed teeth	
NERVOUS SYSTEM	Muscle spasms	Excessive thirst, headaches, irritability, loss of appetite, weakness, nausea
OTHER		Kidney stones, stones in arteries, mental and physical retardation

[a]Small-cell anemia is termed *microcytic anemia;* large-cell type is *macrocytic* or *megaloblastic anemia.*

[b]Corneal degeneration progresses from *keratinization* (hardening) to *xerosis* (drying) to *xerophthalomia* (thickening, opacity, and irreversible blindness).

(continued)

Table 7-3
The Fat-Soluble Vitamins—Functions, Deficiencies, and Toxicities (continued)

Vitamin E		
Other Names	**Deficiency Symptoms**	**Toxicity Symptoms**
Alpha-tocopherol, tocopherol	BLOOD/CIRCULATORY SYSTEM	
Chief Functions in the Body	Red blood cell breakage, anemia	Augments the effects of anticlotting medication
Antioxidant (detoxification of strong oxidants), stabilization of cell membranes, regulation of oxidation reactions, protection of PUFA and vitamin A	DIGESTIVE SYSTEM	
		General discomfort
	NERVOUS/MUSCULAR SYSTEM	
Deficiency Disease Name	Degeneration, weakness, difficulty walking, leg cramps	
(No name)	OTHER	
Significant Sources	Fibrocystic breast disease	
Polyunsaturated plant oils (margarine, salad dressings, shortenings), green and leafy vegetables, wheat germ, whole-grain products, nuts, seeds		

Vitamin K		
Other Names	**Deficiency Symptoms**	**Toxicity Symptoms**
Phylloquinone, naphthoquinone	BLOOD/CIRCULATORY	
Chief Functions in the Body	Hemorrhaging	Interference with anticlotting medication; vitamin K analogues may cause jaundice
Synthesis of blood-clotting proteins and a blood protein that regulates blood calcium		
Deficiency Disease Name		
(No name)		
Significant Sources		
Bacterial synthesis in the digestive tract; liver, green leafy vegetables, cabbage-type vegetables, milk		

Table 7-4
The Water-Soluble Vitamins—Functions, Deficiencies, and Toxicities

Thiamin		
Other Names	**Deficiency Symptoms**	**Toxicity Symptoms**
Vitamin B_1	BLOOD/CIRCULATORY SYSTEM	
Chief Functions in the Body	Edema, enlarged heart, abnormal heart rhythms, heart failure	(No symptoms reported)
Part of a coenzyme used in energy metabolism, supports normal appetite and nervous system function	NERVOUS/MUSCULAR SYSTEMS	
Deficiency Disease Name	Degeneration, wasting, weakness, pain, low morale, difficulty walking, loss of reflexes, mental confusion, paralysis	(No symptoms reported)
Beriberi		
Significant Sources		
Occurs in all nutritious foods in moderate amounts; pork, ham, bacon, liver, whole grains, legumes, nuts		
Riboflavin		
Other Names	**Deficiency Symptoms**	**Toxicity Symptoms**
Vitamin B_2	MOUTH, GUMS, TONGUE	
Chief Functions in the Body	Cracks at corners of mouth[c] magenta tongue	(No symptoms reported)
Part of a coenzyme used in energy metabolism, supports normal vision and skin health	NERVOUS SYSTEM AND EYES	
Deficiency Disease Name	Hypersensitivity to light,[d] reddening of cornea	(No symptoms reported)
Ariboflavinosis	OTHER	
Significant Sources	Skin rash	(No symptoms reported)
Milk, yogurt, cottage cheese, meat, leafy green vegetables, whole-grain or enriched breads and cereals		

[c]Cracks at the corners of the mouth are termed *cheilosis* (kee-lOH-sis).
[d]Hypersensitivity to light is *photophobia*.

(continued)

Table 7-4
The Water-Soluble Vitamins—Functions, Deficiencies, and Toxicities (continued)

Niacin

Other Names	Chief Functions in the Body	Deficiency Disease Name	Significant Sources
Nicotinic acid, nicotinamide, niacinamide, vitamin B_3; precursor is dietary tryptophan	Part of a coenzyme used in energy metabolism; supports health of skin, nervous system, and digestive system	Pellagra	Milk, eggs, meat, poultry, fish, whole grain and enriched breads and cereals, nuts, and all protein-containing foods

	Deficiency Symptoms	Toxicity Symptoms
DIGESTIVE SYSTEM	Diarrhea	Diarrhea, heartburn, nausea, ulcer irritation, vomiting
MOUTH, GUMS, TONGUE	Black, smooth tongue[e]	
NERVOUS SYSTEM	Irritability, loss of appetite, weakness, dizziness, mental confusion progressing to psychosis or delirium	Fainting, dizziness
SKIN	Flaky skin rash on areas exposed to sun	Painful flush and rash ("niacin rush"), sweating
OTHER		Abnormal liver function, low blood pressure

Vitamin B_6

Other Names	Chief Functions in the Body	Deficiency Disease Name	Significant Sources
Pyridoxine, pyridoxal, pyridoxamine	Part of a coenzyme used in amino acid and fatty acid metabolism, helps convert tryptophan to niacin, helps make red blood cells	(No name)	Green and leafy vegetables, meats, fish, poultry, shellfish, legumes, fruits, whole grains

	Deficiency Symptoms	Toxicity Symptoms
BLOOD/CIRCULATORY SYSTEM	Anemia (small-cell type)[a]	Bloating
MOUTH, GUMS, TONGUE	Smooth tongue[e]	
NERVOUS/MUSCULAR SYSTEMS	Abnormal brain wave pattern, irritability, muscle twitching, convulsions	Depression, fatigue, impaired memory, irritability, headaches, numbness, damage to nerves, difficulty walking, loss of reflexes, weakness, restlessness
SKIN	Irritation of sweat glands, rashes, greasy dermatitis	
OTHER	Kidney stones	

[a]Small-cell anemia is termed *microcytic anemia;* large-cell type is *macrocytic* or *megaloblastic anemia.*
[e]Smoothness of the tongue is caused by loss of its surface structures and is termed *glossitis* (gloss-EYE-tis).

(table continued on next page)

Table 7-4
The Water-Soluble Vitamins—Functions, Deficiencies, and Toxicities (continued)

Folate		
Other Names	**Deficiency Symptoms**	**Toxicity Symptoms**
Folic acid, folacin, pteroylglutamic acid	BLOOD/CIRCULATORY SYSTEM	
	Anemia (large-cell type)[a]	
Chief Functions in the Body	DIGESTIVE SYSTEM	
Part of a coenzyme used in new cell synthesis	Heartburn, diarrhea, constipation	
	IMMUNE SYSTEM	
Deficiency Disease (No name)	Suppression, frequent infections	
Significant Sources	MOUTH, GUMS, TONGUE	
	Smooth red tongue[e]	
Leafy green vegetables, legumes, seeds, liver	NERVOUS SYSTEM	
	Depression, mental confusion, fainting	
	OTHER	
	Masks of vitamin B_{12} deficiency	
Vitamin B_{12}		
Other Names	**Deficiency Symptoms**	**Toxicity Symptoms**
Cyanocobalamin	BLOOD/CIRCULATORY SYSTEM	
Chief Functions in the Body	Anemia (large-cell type)[a]	(No toxicity symptoms known)
Part of a coenzyme used in new cell synthesis, helps maintain nerve cells	MOUTH, GUMS, TONGUE	
	Smooth tongue[e]	
	NERVOUS SYSTEM	
Deficiency Disease (No name[f])	Fatigue, degeneration progressing to paralysis	
Significant Sources	SKIN	
Animal products (meat, fish, poultry, milk, cheese, eggs)	Hypersensitivity	
Pantothenic Acid		
Other Names	**Deficiency Symptoms**	**Toxicity Symptoms**
(None)	DIGESTIVE SYSTEM	
Chief Functions in the Body	Vomiting, intestinal distress	
Part of a coenzyme used in energy metabolism	NERVOUS SYSTEM	
	Insomnia, fatigue	
Deficiency Disease (No name)	OTHER	
Significant Sources		Water retention (infrequent)
Widespread in foods		

[f]The name *pernicious anemia* refers to the vitamin B_{12} deficiency caused by lack of intrinsic factor, but not to that caused by inadequate dietary intake.

(continued)

Table 7-4
The Water-Soluble Vitamins—Functions, Deficiencies, and Toxicities (continued)

Biotin		
Other Names	**Deficiency Symptoms**	**Toxicity Symptoms**
(None)	BLOOD/CIRCULATORY SYSTEM	
Chief Functions in the Body	Abnormal heart action	(No toxicity symptoms reported)
Part of a coenzyme used in energy metabolism, fat synthesis, amino acid metabolism, and glycogen synthesis	DIGESTIVE SYSTEM	
	Loss of appetite, nausea	
	NERVOUS/MUSCULAR SYSTEMS	
Deficiency Disease (No name)	Depression, muscle pain, weakness, fatigue	
Significant Sources	SKIN	
Widespread in foods	Drying, rash, loss of hair	
Vitamin C		
Other Names	**Deficiency Symptoms**	**Toxicity Symptoms**
Ascorbic acid	BLOOD/CIRCULATORY SYSTEM	
Chief Functions in the Body	Anemia (small-cell type),[a] atherosclerotic plaques, pinpoint hemorrhages	
Collagen synthesis (strengthens blood vessel walls, forms scar tissue, matrix for bone growth), antioxidant, thyroxine synthesis, amino acid metabolism, strengthens resistance to infection, helps in absorption of iron	DIGESTIVE SYSTEM	
		Nausea, abdominal cramps, diarrhea, excessive urination
	IMMUNE SYSTEM	
	Suppression, frequent infections	
	MOUTH, GUMS, TONGUE	
Deficiency Disease Name	Bleeding gums, loosened teeth	
Scurvy	MUSCULAR/NERVOUS SYSTEMS	
Significant Sources	Muscle degeneration and pain, hysteria, depression	Headache, fatigue, insomnia
Citrus fruits, cabbage-type vegetables, dark green vegetables, cantaloupe, strawberries, peppers, lettuce, tomatoes, potatoes, papayas, mangos	SKELETAL SYSTEM	
	Bone fragility, joint pain	
	SKIN	
	Rough skin, blotchy bruises	Rashes
	OTHER	
	Failure of wounds to heal	Interference with medical tests; aggravation of gout symptoms; deficiency symptoms may appear at first on withdrawal of high doses

[a]Small-cell anemia is termed *microcytic anemia;* large-cell type is *macrocytic* or *megaloblastic anemia.*

Notes

1. Food and Nutrition Board, *Recommended Dietary Allowances*, 10th ed. (Washington, D.C.: National Academy of Sciences, 1989), p. 20.
2. K. P. West, G. R. Howard, and A. Sommer, Vitamin A and infection: Public health implications, *Annual Review of Nutrition* 9 (1989): 63–86.
3. West and coauthors, 1989.
4. West and coauthors, 1989.
5. C. Carlier and coauthors, Prevalence of malnutrition and vitamin A deficiency in the Diourbel, Fatik, and Kolack regions of Senegal: Epidemiological study, *American Journal of Clinical Nutrition* 53 (1991): 70–73.
6. K. P. West and coauthors, Vitamin A supplementation and growth: A randomized community trial, *American Journal of Clinical Nutrition* 48 (1988): 1257–1264; Muhilal and coauthors, Vitamin A-fortified monosodium glutamate and health, growth, and survival of children: A controlled field study, *American Journal of Clinical Nutrition* 48 (1988): 1271–1276.
7. West and coauthors, 1989.
8. Muhilal (no initials) and coauthors, 1988; L. Rahmathullah and coauthors, Reduced mortality among children in southern India receiving a small weekly dose of vitamin A, *New England Journal of Medicine* 323 (1990): 929–935; K. P. West, Jr. and coauthors, Efficacy of vitamin A in reducing preschool child mortality in Nepal, *Lancet* 338 (1991): 67–71; N. M. P. Daulaire and coauthors, Childhood mortality after a high dose of vitamin A in high risk populations, *British Medical Journal* 304 (1992): 207–210.
9. J. N. Hathcock and coauthors, Evaluation of vitamin A toxicity, *American Journal of Clinical Nutrition* 52 (1990): 183–202.
10. T. O. Carpenter and coauthors, Severe hypervitaminosis A in siblings: Evidence of variable tolerance to retinol intake, *Journal of Pediatrics* 111 (1987): 507–512.
11. J. N. Hathcock and coauthors, Evaluation of vitamin A toxicity, *American Journal of Clinical Nutrition* 52 (1990): 183–202.
12. A. T. Diplock, Antioxidant nutrients and disease prevention: An overview, *American Journal of Clinical Nutrition* 53 (1991): 189S–193S; B. Halliwell, J. M. C. Gutteridge, and C. E. Cross, Free radicals, antioxidants, and human disease: Where are we now? *Journal of Laboratory and Clinical Medicine* 119 (1992): 598–620.
13. Diplock, 1991.
14. Study sheds light on TB resistance, *Science News* 133 (1988): 60.
15. A. W. Norman, Intestinal calcium absorption: A vitamin-D-hormone-mediated adaptive response, *American Journal of Clinical Nutrition* 51 (1990): 290–300.
16. H. Reichel, H. P. Koeffler, and A. W. Norman, The role of the vitamin D endocrine system in health and disease, *New England Journal of Medicine* 320 (1989): 980–991; J. W. Pike, Vitamin D_3 receptors: Structure and function in transcription, *Annual Review of Nutrition* 11 (1991): 189–216.
17. Single day therapy for nutritional rickets, *Pediatric Notes* 16 (1992): 66.
18. Food and Nutrition Board, 1989, pp. 94–95.
19. A. R. Webb and M. F. Holick, The role of sunlight in the cutaneous production of vitamin D_3, *Annual Review of Nutrition* 8 (1988): 375–399.
20. Webb and Holick, 1988.
21. D. Farley, Tanning salon sees the light, *FDA Consumer*, December 1986/January 1987, pp. 37–38.
22. L. Packer, Protective role of vitamin E in biological systems, *American Journal of Clinical Nutrition* 53 (1991): 1050S–1055S.
23. S. N. Meydani and coauthors, Vitamin E supplementation enhances cell-mediated immunity in healthy elderly subjects, *American Journal of Clinical Nutrition* 52 (1990): 557–563.
24. M. J. Stampfer and coauthors, Vitamin E consumption and the risk of coronary disease in women, *New England Journal of Medicine* 328 (1993): 1444–1449; E. B. Rimm and coauthors, Vitamin E consumption and the risk of coronary disease in men, *New England Journal of Medicine* 328 (1993): 1450–1456.
25. J. Raloff, Vitamin E fights radicals—again and again, *Science News* 27 (1989): 327.
26. R. J. Sokol, Vitamin E deficiency and neurologic disease, *Annual Review of Nutrition* 8 (1988): 351–373.
27. S. P. Murphy, A. F. Subar, and G. Block, Vitamin E intakes and sources in the United States, *American Journal of Clinical Nutrition* 52 (1990): 361–367.
28. P. A. Price, Role of vitamin-K-dependent proteins in bone metabolism, *Annual Review of Nutrition* 8 (1988): 565–583.
29. Food and Nutrition Board, 1989, pp. 107–114.
30. J. W. Suttie, Vitamin K and human nutrition, *Journal of the American Dietetic Association* 92 (1992): 590.
31. Food and Nutrition Board, 1989, p. 20.
32. Y. Henkin, K. C. Johnson, and J. P. Segrest, Rechallenge with crystalline niacin after drug-induced hepatitis from sustained-release niacin, *Journal of the American Medical Association* 264 (1990): 241–243.
33. L. B. Bailey, The role of folate in human nutrition, *Nutrition Today*, September/October 1990, pp. 12–19.
34. J. F. Gregory, Chemical and nutritional aspects of folate research: Analytical procedures, methods of folate synthesis, stability, and bioavailability of dietary folates, *Advances in Food and Nutrition Research* 33 (1989): 1–101; as cited in L. B. Bailey, Evaluation of a new Recommended Dietary Allowance for folate, *Journal of the American Dietetic Association* 92 (1992): 463–468, 471; How do foods affect folate bioavailability? *Nutrition Reviews* 48 (1990): 326–328.
35. N. Swiatlo and coauthors, Relative folate bioavailability from diets containing human, bovine, and goat milk, *Journal of Nutrition* 120 (1990): 172–177.
36. R. Carmel and coauthors, Cobalamin and osteoblast-specific proteins, *New England Journal of Medicine* 319 (1988): 70–75.
37. J. Lindenbaum and coauthors, Neuropsychiatric disorders caused by cobalamin deficiency in the absence of anemia or macrocytosis, *New England Journal of Medicine* 318 (1988): 1720–1728.
38. Unrecognized cobalamin-responsive neuropsychiatric disorders, *Nutrition Reviews* 47 (1989): 208–210.
39 V. Herbert, Vitamin B_{12}: Plant sources, requirements, and assay, *American Journal of Clinical Nutrition* 48 (1988): 852–858.
40. S. N. Meydani and coauthors, Vitamin B_6 deficiency impairs interleukin 2 production and lymphocyte proliferation in elderly adults, *American Journal of Clinical Nutrition* 53 (1991): 1275–1280; J. E. Leeklem, Vitamin B_6: Of reservoirs, receptors, and requirements, *Nutrition Today*, September/October 1988, pp. 4–10.
41. A. H. Merrill, and F. S. Burnham, Vitamin B-6, in *Present Knowledge in Nutrition*, 6th ed., ed. M. L. Brown (Washington, D.C.: Nutrition Foundation, 1990), pp. 155–162.
42. W. O. Song, Pantothenic acid: How much do we know about this B-complex vitamin? *Nutrition Today*, March/April 1990, pp. 19–25.
43. Diplock, 1991.
44. T. Byers and G. Perry, Dietary carotenes, vitamin C, and

vitamin E as protective antioxidants in human cancers, *Annual Review of Nutrition* 12 (1992): 139–159.
45. N. I. Krinsky, Effects of carotenoids in cellular and animal systems, *American Journal of Clinical Nutrition* 52 (1991): 238S–246S.
46. R. G. Ziegler, Vegetables, fruits, and carotenoids and the risk of cancer, *American Journal of Clinical Nutrition* 53 (1991): 251S–259S.
47. H. B. Stahalein and coauthors, Beta-carotene and cancer prevention: The Basel Study, *American Journal of Clinical Nutrition* 53 (1991): 265S–269S.
48. G. Block, Vitamin C and cancer prevention: The epidemiologic evidence, *American Journal of Clinical Nutrition* 53 (1991): 270S–282S.
49. Block, 1991.
50. S. R. Tannenbaum, J. S. Wishnok, and C. D. Leaf, Inhibition of nitrosamine formation by ascorbic acid, *American Journal of Clinical Nutrition* 53 (1991): 247S–250S.
51. P. Knekt and coauthors, Vitamin E and cancer prevention, *American Journal of Clinical Nutrition* 53 (1991): 283S–286S.
52. Stampfer, 1993; Rimm, 1993.
53. Food and Nutrition Board, 1989, pp. 115–124.
54. B. J. Rolls, Aging and appetite, *Nutrition Reviews* 50 (1992): 422–426; Are older Americans making better food choices to meet diet and health recommendations? *Nutrition Reviews* 51 (1993): 20–22.
55. D. A. Bender, Ascorbic acid, in *Nutritional Biochemistry of the Vitamins* (New York, N.Y.: Cambridge University Press, 1992), pp. 360–389; Food and Nutrition Board,1989, p. 117.
56. Food and Nutrition Board, 1989, p. 119.
57. R. A. Jacob, Vitamin C in M. E. Shils, J. A. Olson, and M. Shike, eds., *Modern Nutrition in Health and Disease* (Philadelphia: Lea & Febiger, 1994) pp. 432–448.

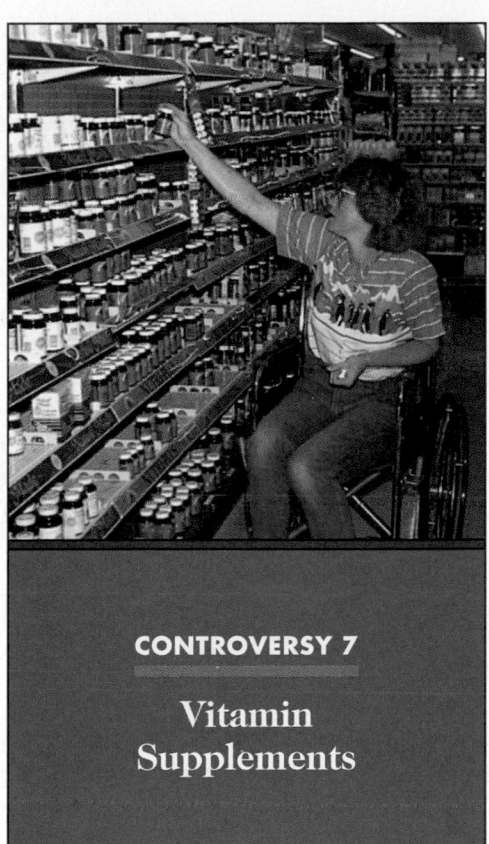

CONTROVERSY 7

Vitamin Supplements

Who should take **supplements?** Almost 40 percent of the population does take them regularly, collectively spending billions of dollars a year on them.[1] But who really needs them? No one? Everyone? Some people? Which people? And which supplements should they take? This Controversy addresses these questions—although, as you will see, the answers are not always clear-cut. The Consumer Caution section of Chapter 7 has already addressed the question whether taking supplements of the antioxidant nutrients is warranted and left the answer up to you, the reader.

MULTIVITAMIN—MINERAL SUPPLEMENTS When people think of supplements, they often think only of vitamins, but vitamins are no more important than minerals, of course. People whose diets lack several vitamins, for whatever reason, probably lack several minerals as well. If there is no way for these people to eat enough nutritious foods to meet their needs, then vitamin-mineral supplements, not just vitamins, may be appropriate. Who, then, might need vitamin-mineral supplements?

According to several experts, several groups of people exist in the U.S. population whose diets put them at risk of developing nutrient deficiencies. This may seem surprising, for the history of nutrition suggests that our health care system and nutrition programs wiped out the nutrient deficiency diseases many decades ago. In fact, the major, overt deficiency diseases such as scurvy, pellagra, and beriberi are very seldom seen today, but deficiencies do still occur. They are called **subclinical,** or **marginal deficiencies:** states of unwellness shy of the classical, full-blown nutrient deficiencies. In contrast to the classical deficiencies, which present a multitude of symptoms and are easy to recognize, subclinical deficiencies are subtle and easy to overlook.

People who may have subclinical deficiencies, or who risk developing them, include the following:

- People such as habitual dieters whose energy intakes are too low to deliver the needed amounts of nutrients.
- People who are elderly.
- People with diseases of the liver, gallbladder, pancreas, or digestive system, whose illnesses impair their absorption of nutrients or who eat little food.
- People who are taking medications that interfere with their bodies' use of specific nutrients.
- Pregnant women and women who are breastfeeding their infants, whose nutrient needs are unusually high.[2]

In all cases, the first remedy for these people should be to attempt to improve their diets so that they obtain the nutrients they need from foods. If that is truly impossible, though, then a multivitamin-mineral supplement that supplies approximately the RDA amount of every nutrient may be appropriate.

NUTRIENT SUPPLEMENTS FOR SPECIAL PROBLEMS Special nutrient supplements may also be appropriate in special cases. Consider the case of the woman who loses a lot of blood and therefore a lot of iron and other blood-building nutrients in menstruation each month. Such a woman may be able to eat in such a way as to make up for all nutrient deficits except that of iron, and for iron, she may need a supplement. The next chapter shows ways for women to try to obtain enough iron in their diets, but also shows that it is hard to do. It also cautions that a competent health care provider's advice is prerequisite to making the decision whether supplementation is appropriate.

bioavailability absorbability, the individual differences in nutrients' ease of absorption.

subclinical deficiency a nutrient deficiency that has no detectable (clinical) symptoms. The term is often used to scare consumers into buying unneeded nutrient supplements. Also called a **marginal deficiency.**

supplements preparations (such as pills, powders, or liquids) containing nutrients; not foods. Breakfast cereals that contain "100 percent of the U.S. RDA" for certain nutrients are defined by law as dietary supplements, not foods.

People who are intolerant to lactose or allergic to milk may have calcium intakes too low to forestall the bone degeneration of old age, osteoporosis.[3] For them, calcium supplements may be appropriate. The Controversy of the next chapter offers perspective on the idea that food choices cannot meet calcium needs.

For people whose medications impair nutritional health by interfering with specific nutrients, specific nutrient supplements may be appropriate. Health care providers watch for these interactions and prescribe appropriate supplements with medication. Drug-nutrient interactions are so numerous, and can have such a devastating impact on nutritional health, that they have become the subject of a specialty area within nutrition. Whole textbooks are written about drug-nutrient interactions, as is Controversy 12 of this book.[4]

Routine health care for pregnancy and lactation may include special supplements of iron, calcium, and folate. Each newborn routinely needs a single dose of vitamin K at birth. Infants may need supplements, depending on whether they are receiving formula or not and on whether their water is low in fluoride or not.

Others for whom health care providers may elect special supplementation may include people being treated for addictions to alcohol or other drugs and people who have undergone the stresses of surgery, injury, or prolonged illness. Also, strict vegetarians may add to their diets supplemental vitamin B_{12}, iron, and zinc.

Later chapters discuss some of these special cases. Iron supplements receive attention in Chapter 8; calcium supplements in Controversy 8; antioxidant nutrient supplements in Chapter 11; supplements for pregnancy and infancy in Chapter 12; and supplements that improve immunity in the elderly in Chapter 13.

THE SPECIAL CASE OF FOLATE In 1992, the United States Public Health Service made an unprecedented recommendation. It advised all women of childbearing age to consume more than double the RDA for folate: 400 micrograms a day.[5] This might lead women to head to the drugstore to buy folate supplements, but the Public Health Service did not say to take supplements. They stated only that women should obtain ample folate in their diets.

The reason is this. Folate deficiency is associated with a group of devastating birth defects known as neural tube defects. These defects affect 1 in every 1,000 births, making them the second most common form of birth defect after Down's syndrome. Neural tube defects range from slight problems in the spine to mental retardation, severely diminished brain size, and death shortly after birth.[6]

Neural tube defects arise in the first days or weeks of pregnancy, long before most women even suspect that they are pregnant. A woman may already have sustained irreversible damage to her developing embryo even before she misses a menstrual period, learns she is pregnant, and receives advice on folate from her health care provider. By recommending that women obtain extra folate *before* pregnancy, the Public Health Service hopes to prevent about half of all neural tube defects (the other half is attributable to causes other than folate deficiency), and to see many more of these infants born normal.[7]

With some forethought and planning, women can obtain the recommended amount of folate from foods. Just three half-cup servings of vegetables richest in folate, for example, can provide about 400 micrograms of folate:

- ½ cup cooked asparagus: 130 micrograms.
- ½ cup chickpeas (garbanzo beans): 140 micrograms.
- ½ cup cooked spinach: 130 micrograms.

Together with the other foods eaten in a day, foods such as these would more than meet the recommended 400 microgram intake. At this writing, a proposal by the Food and Drug Administration (FDA) would list folate among nutrients added to staple grain foods such as bread and rice. The move would bring more women's intakes in line with the 400 microgram target.

High folate doses from supplements are a threat. Until recently, folate was not sold freely over the counter as a single supplement because in its presence a dangerous vitamin B_{12} deficiency can advance unnoticed. One study reported that 800 micrograms, the amount of folate in just two of many types of multivitamin pills, can alter zinc metabolism in men; effects in pregnant women are unknown.[8] Supplements of folate and iron may reduce zinc absorption and so retard fetal growth.[9] Other studies raise other questions about folate safety, and point to the need for more research.[10] Prescription folate supplements contain huge therapeutic doses of about 200 times the RDA. While safety questions remain, such doses have been recommended for women who have already given birth to infants with neural tube defects. The doses seem to be effective in preventing such defects in future infants.[11]

While research on folate supplements continues, the advice we would give to women of childbearing age would be to strive to include folate-containing foods in the diet each day. To those who have a history of neural tube defects in their families, we would recommend obtaining 400 micrograms of folate per day. This amount is safe for most people and may be protective.[12] Then when a woman decides to become pregnant, she should seek medical advice on folate before doing so.

SUPPLEMENT RISKS AND PROBLEMS "So many people seem to need supplements for one thing or another why shouldn't everyone take a multivitamin-mineral supplement to make sure to cover all these needs?" Such logic does lead many people to do exactly that, but supplement-taking is risky, and the risks deserve time equal to the time given to the benefits.

When people self-prescribe supplements, they have to choose doses. "I'll take one of these a day," a person may say, or "I'll take two of these and three of those a day." Whatever the choice, the higher the dose, the greater the risk of harm. High doses of most nutrients are dangerous. People's tolerances for high doses of nutrients vary, just as their risks of deficiencies vary. Amounts that some can tolerate may not be safe for others, and no one knows who falls into which category. Toxic overdoses of vitamins and minerals may be more common than we realize.* Only a few alert health care providers are equipped to recognize the signs of short-term acute toxic doses.

It is impossible to say just how much of a nutrient is too much. Assuming, however, that it is best to err on the conservative side, Table C7-1 presents suggested limits for vitamin and mineral doses in supplements.

Table C7-1
Vitamin and Mineral Doses for Supplements

Substance	Safe Range of Intakes
Vitamins	
Vitamin A	75 to 750 RE[a]
Vitamin D	10 μg[a] (up to age 18) 5 μg[a] (adults)
Vitamin E	6 to 30 mg[a]
Thiamin	1 to 2 mg
Riboflavin	1 to 2 mg
Niacin (as niacinamide)	10 to 20 mg
Vitamin B_6	1.5 to 2.5 mg
Folate	0.1 to 0.4 mg (in multivitamin form)
Vitamin B_{12}	3 to 10 μg
Pantothenic acid	5 to 20 mg (in multivitamin form)
Biotin	Not recommended in supplement form
Vitamin C	50 to 100 mg
Minerals	
Calcium	400 to 800 mg
Phosphorus	No need to supplement
Magnesium	No need to supplement
Iron	10 to 39 mg (women)
Zinc	10 to 25 mg (adults)
Iodine	Not recommended in supplement form

[a]Some supplements are measured in International Units (IU). To convert to RDA-compatible units, see Appendix C.

Source: Parts adapted from the American Medical Association's Council on Scientific Affairs, Vitamin preparations as dietary supplements and as therapeutic agents, *Journal of the American Medical Association* 257 (1987): 1929–1936; Food and Nutrition Board, *Recommended Dietary Allowances,* 10th ed. (Washington, D.C.: National Academy of Sciences, 1989); PHS recommends folic acid for women of childbearing age, *FDA Consumer,* December 1992, p. 3.

Still more worrisome than short-term, acute overdose effects are the effects of chronic, low-level nutrient toxicity in which the effects develop subtly and slowly. No doubt many of these cases go unrecognized. An example is that of a woman who took just 1,000 RE (5,000 IU) of vitamin A a day, an amount typically found in vitamin-mineral supplements—but she took this dose daily for ten years. Then she was diagnosed with liver disease. Only when she discontinued the supplement did the condition clear up.[13] In view of the potential hazards that supplements present, some authorities believe they should be required to bear warning labels, but such labels are not yet planned.

Another problem arises when people who are already ill are led to believe that high doses of vitamins or minerals can be therapeutic or can strengthen the immune system. These claims are exceedingly common, as this report by a watchdog group illustrates:

> *In 1989, volunteers of the Consumer Health Education Council (CHEC) telephoned 41 Houston-area health food stores and asked to speak with the person who provided nutrition advice. The callers explained that they had a brother sick with AIDS. . . . All 41 retailers offered products they said could strengthen the brother's immune system. . . . Thirty said they sold products that would cure AIDS.*[14]

Other such inquiries led to wrong-headed advice from salespeople urging that customers use supplements to treat headaches, dizziness, fatigue, kidney stones, abnormal thirst (a diabetes warning sign), glaucoma (a progressive eye-destroying disease), sudden weight loss (a serious medical symptom), and to prevent contracting the virus that causes AIDS (none of the salespeople mentioned using condoms). Meanwhile, few salespeople recommended that the callers obtain medical advice.

*One report estimates accidental nutrient overdoses in 1990 at more than 1,300. Centers for Disease Control, as cited in *Hype and Hope: The Cost of Vitamins,* 1992 (New York City Department of Consumer Affairs, 42 Broadway, New York, NY 10004), p. 2.

The FDA's hands are tied in protecting consumers against this widespread fraud, because the FDA can only regulate foods and drugs. The current law excludes supplements from the drug category even though they are often sold with *spoken* promises of druglike actions. The law also exempts them from meeting many of the standards applied to foods. As a result, supplements need not pass the tests of safety and effectiveness applied to drugs; they must only prove that the contents of the bottles are pure, as foods must do. FDA cannot currently limit or ensure the potency of most supplements, and it cannot limit the number of nutrients or other ingredients in the preparations.[15] Neither can it require or enforce expiration dates on labels to ensure that products have not disintegrated from age before they are sold. FDA also cannot require warnings concerning overdoses. In fact, government agencies are specifically prohibited from requiring even minor changes on supplement labels until the second half of the 1990s.[16] To remedy this deplorable situation, a 12-person FDA Dietary Supplement Task Force is holding hearings to explore the entire issue of how to regulate dietary supplements in the future.[17]

Another argument against the use of supplements is that no one knows exactly how to formulate the "ideal" supplement. What nutrients should be included? How much of each? And how should an individual choose a supplement, since no one's needs are exactly like anyone else's? Surveys of supplement takers have repeatedly shown that little relationship exists between the nutrients people take in pills and the ones they actually need. Often they take supplements containing just the nutrients they need least—and still miss out on the nutrients they are failing to derive from their diets.

Also, supplements may lull their takers into a false sense of security. A person may eat irresponsibly, thinking, "My supplement will cover my needs." Or, experiencing the warning signs of a disease, a person may postpone seeking a diagnosis, thinking, "I'll just take a nutrient supplement to make this go away." Such self-diagnosis is dangerous at best.

Other invalid reasons why people may take supplements include:

- They feel insecure about the amounts of nutrients in the food supply.
- They falsely believe that supplements can provide energy.
- They have faith that supplements will help them cope with stress.
- They wish to build lean body tissue without physical work, or wrongly believe that supplements will build muscles faster than work alone.
- They want to prevent or cure conditions from the common cold to cancer.

Ironically, one study found that supplement users perceived themselves as less healthy overall than nonusers.[18] Even more ironically, states of unhealthiness today are far more likely to be due to overnutrition and poor lifestyle choices than to nutrient deficiencies. People with risk factors for heart disease, cancer, and the other major diseases of today may wish they could just take vitamin pills to gain health. The truth, that they need to make efforts to change their eating and exercise habits, is harder to swallow.

Another problem is that of **bioavailability.** In general, nutrients are absorbed best from foods, in which they are dispersed among other ingredients that facilitate their absorption. In contrast, some supplement pills fail to dissolve, and so pass through the system unabsorbed. Also, nutrients taken in pure, concentrated form are likely to interfere with each other's absorption or even with the absorption of the nutrients in foods eaten at the same time. Minerals provide examples: zinc hinders copper and calcium absorption, iron hinders zinc absorption, calcium hinders magnesium and iron absorption, and magnesium hinders calcium and iron absorption. Interference among nutrients also takes place when people use *foods* that are fortified with added minerals, another reason to rely on ordinary foods for optimal absorption of nutrients.[19]

Although minerals provide the most familiar and best-documented examples, other types of interference among nutrients are now being seen. The vitamin A precursor beta carotene, long thought to be completely nontoxic, has recently been shown to interfere with vitamin E metabolism when taken over the long term as a dietary supplement.[20]

In view of all the negatives associated with supplement taking, several nutrition societies have indicated that most people should *not* use them.[21] These experts urge that whenever a person's diet is inadequate, the action to take is not to add supplements but to improve food choices and eating patterns.[22]

SELECTION OF A MULTINUTRIENT SUPPLEMENT Now the question is, do *you* need a supplement? From the foregoing, if you choose to take one, you do so at some risk. However, if you fall into one of the categories already noted, and if you cannot meet your nutrient needs from foods, a supplement may be in order.

The next question is, which supplement to choose? A shopper faces a bewildering array of containers on the drugstore counter, each one with clever, and usually deceptive, ads on the labels—"For vitality!" "Infants only!" "For those with active lives!" "Time release!" "Stress formula!" Sometimes pictures of people having fun, looking sexy, and feeling healthy imply that supplements can confer these assets on the taker.

The first step in escaping the clutches of the health hustlers is to imagine that you can simply white out the picture of the sexy people on the beach and the meaningless, glittering generalities like "new and improved." No matter how lovely the container, you are shopping for the contents—a nutrient supplement. (If a pretty container is what you need, you can get one for less in housewares.) After you have whited out the label claims, all you have left is the list of ingredients, what form they are in, and the price. From here you can make a rational decision based on facts.

You have two basic questions to answer. The first question: What form do you want—chewable, liquid, or pills? If you'd rather drink your vitamins and minerals than chew them, fine. Remember, you whited out *infant* on the labels, so now those bottles are just liquid supplements. The second question: Who are you? What vitamins and minerals do *you* need? The RDA table on the inside front cover and the table for Canadians (Appendix B) are the standards appropriate for virtually all reasonably healthy people. If you aren't healthy, see your health care provider.

Generally an appropriate supplement provides all the RDA nutrients in amounts smaller than, equal to, or very close to the RDA.[23] Avoid any preparation that, in a daily dose, provides more than the RDA of vitamin A, D, or any mineral or more than ten times the RDA for *any* nutrient. A warning: Expect to reject about 80 percent of available preparations when you choose according to these criteria; be choosy where your health is concerned. Other warnings follow.

Avoid preparations presenting high doses of iron (more than 10 milligrams per day) except for menstruating women. People who menstruate need more iron, but people who don't, don't. Once in the body, iron is hard to get rid of and an excess of iron can cause problems, just as a deficiency can.

Avoid "organic" or "natural" preparations. They are no better than standard types, but they cost much more. The word *synthetic* may sound like "fake," but to synthesize just means to put together, and such supplements are identical to vitamins synthesized by plants and animals. Also disregard "time-release" claims. These supplements differ little from other types, but fetch a higher price. Your body can't tell the difference, but your wallet can.

Avoid products that make "high-potency" claims. More is not better. The RDA is more than enough. You do eat foods, too, after all, so you get well over RDA amounts of vitamins and minerals.

Avoid therapeutic doses (or higher) unless your physician has prescribed them. Nutrients can build up and cause unexpected problems. For example, a man who takes vitamins and begins to lose his hair may think it means he needs *more* vitamins, when in fact hair loss may be an early sign of vitamin A overdose.

Avoid preparations that contain items not needed in human nutrition, such as choline and inositol. It's not that those particular items will harm you, but that they reveal a marketing strategy that makes the whole mix suspect. The manufacturer may want you to believe that its brand of pills contains the latest "new" nutrient that other brands omit, but in fact, for every valid discovery of this kind there are 999,999 frauds.

Avoid "stress formulas." Although the stress response depends on certain B vitamins and vitamin C, the RDA amount provides all that is needed of these, even during final examinations at school.

Avoid pills containing ground parsley, alfalfa, and other vegetable components. They may deliver a few of the same nutrients as a plate of salad or broccoli, but salad and broccoli are much more nutritious—and much cheaper.

Avoid geriatric "tonics." They are generally poor in vitamins and minerals and yet may be so high in alcohol as to threaten inebriation. The liquids designed for infants are more complete.

Local or store brands are just as good as national brands. If they are less expensive, it is not because they are inferior but because the price does not have to cover the cost of national advertising. (One full-page color ad in a national magazine costs upwards of $95,000.) In fact, both expensive and inexpensive pills may have been made in the same batch, only packaged differently.

Steer clear of high doses. Think of the original Stone-Age person, who had to depend only on foods for life and health. Only if the foods available to Stone-Age people could have supplied the amount of a nutrient being advocated, is it safe for us to ingest that amount.

By this standard, the doses some people take are clearly excessive. To obtain 840 milligrams of vitamin E from its best food source, wheat germ, for example, you would have to eat 15 pounds of wheat germ, yet some people take supplements containing more than 840 milligrams of vitamin E every day. To obtain 5 grams of vitamin C, you would have to eat 19 pounds of oranges, yet some people consume more than that much vitamin C daily from supplements.

Our ancestors survived for centuries without nutrient supplements and arrived successfully at the point of producing us. On this basis alone, it can be argued that we must need no more vitamins or minerals than *we* can obtain from food. That much, but not more, would be reasonable to look for in a supplement.

But, come to think of it, if all the nutrients we need can come from foods, are you sure you cannot get them from foods yourself? Foods have much more to recommend them than do supplements. Nutrients in foods come in an infinite variety of combinations with a multitude of different carriers, absorption facilitators, compounds to prevent oxidation, and other benefits. They come with water, fiber, and a host of beneficial and interesting nonnutrients. Foods stimulate the digestive tract to keep it healthy. They come with calories, but you have to eat some calories each day, so why not ask nutritious foods to deliver them? They offer pleasure, satiety, and opportunities for socializing while eating. In no way can nutrient supplements hold a candle to foods as a means of meeting human health needs.[24]

Notes

1. M. M. Bender and coauthors, Trends in prevalence and magnitude of vitamin and mineral supplement usage and correlation with health status, *Journal of the American Dietetic Association* 92 (1992): 1096–1101.
2. National Research Council, *Diet and Health: Implications for Reducing Chronic Disease Risk* (Washington, D.C.: Government Printing Office, 1991), pp. 511–515; D. Herber, W. Mertz, and R. E. Schucker, Food versus pills versus fortified foods, *Dairy Council Digest*, March-April 1987; A. E. Harper, Nutrition insurance—A skeptical view, *Nutrition Forum*, May 1987, pp. 33–37.
3. National Research Council, 1991; Herber, Mertz, and Schucker, 1987; Harper, 1987.
4. An example of such a book is D. A. Roe, *Drug-Induced Nutritional Deficiencies* (Westport, Conn.: AVI). Look for the latest edition.
5. Centers for Disease Control and Prevention, Recommendations for use of folic acid to reduce number of spina bifida cases and other neural tube defects, *Journal of the American Medical Association* 269 (1993): 1233, 1236, 1238.
6. J. M. Scott, P. N. Kirke, and D. G. Weir, The role of nutrition in neural tube defects, *Annual Review of Nutrition* 10 (1990): 277–295.
7. J. L. Mills and coauthors, Maternal vitamin levels during pregnancies producing infants with neural tube defects, *Journal of Pediatrics* 120 (1992): 863–871; A. E. Czeil and I. Dudás, Prevention of the first occurrence of neural-tube defects by periconceptional vitamin supplementation, *New England Journal of Medicine* 327 (1992): 1832–1835; Scott, Kirke, and Weir, 1990.
8. USDA human nutrition research and education report, *Nutrition Today*, November/December 1991, p. 5.
9. K. Simmer and coauthors, Are iron-folate supplements harmful? *American Journal of Clinical Nutrition* 45 (1987): 122–125 as cited by V. Herbert, Folate and neural tube defects, *Nutrition Today*, November/December 1992, pp. 30–33.
10. C. E. Butterworth and T. Tamura, *American Journal of Clinical Nutrition* 50 (1989): 353–358.
11. D. Rush, Folate supplements and neural tube defects, *Nutrition Reviews* 50 (1992): 25–26.
12. W. C. Willett, Folic acid and neural tube defect: Can't we come to closure? *American Journal of Public Health* 82 (1992): 666–668.
13. R. Oren and Y. Ilan, Reversible hepatic injury induced by long-term vitamin A ingestion, *American Journal of Medicine* 93 (1992): 703–704.
14. Advice from health food stores, *Priorities*, Spring 1992, p. 31.
15. Legislative highlights, *Journal of the American Dietetic Association* 91 (1991): 1221–1222.
16. Congress delays supplement labeling rules, *Journal of the American Dietetic Association* 92 (1992): 1461.
17. S. Barrett, Another vitamin war has begun, *Priorities*, Summer 1992, pp. 28–31.
18. Bender and coauthors, 1992.
19. Herber, Mertz, and Schucker, 1987.
20. M. J. Xu, P. M. Plezia, D. S. Alberts, and coauthors, Reduction in plasma or skin alpha-tocopherol concentration with long-term oral administration of beta-carotene in humans and mice, *Journal of the National Cancer Institute* 84 (1992): 1559–1565.
21. The societies that joined to make this statement were the American Dietetic Association, the American Society for Clinical Nutrition, and the American Institute of Nutrition. The American Medical Association reviewed it and endorsed it. Herber, Mertz, and Schucker, 1987.
22. Herber, Mertz, and Schucker, 1987.
23. L. S. Bell and M. Fairchild, Evaluation of commercial multivitamin supplements, *Journal of the American Dietetic Association* 87 (1987): 341–343.
24. *Hype and Hope: The Cost of Vitamins* is a 57-page report that helps consumers avoid worthless supplements. It is available for $3 from the New York City Department of Consumer Affairs, 42 Broadway, New York, NY 10004.

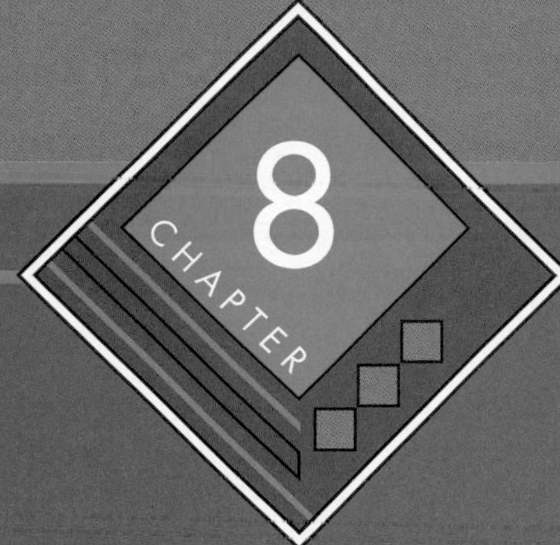

Water and Minerals

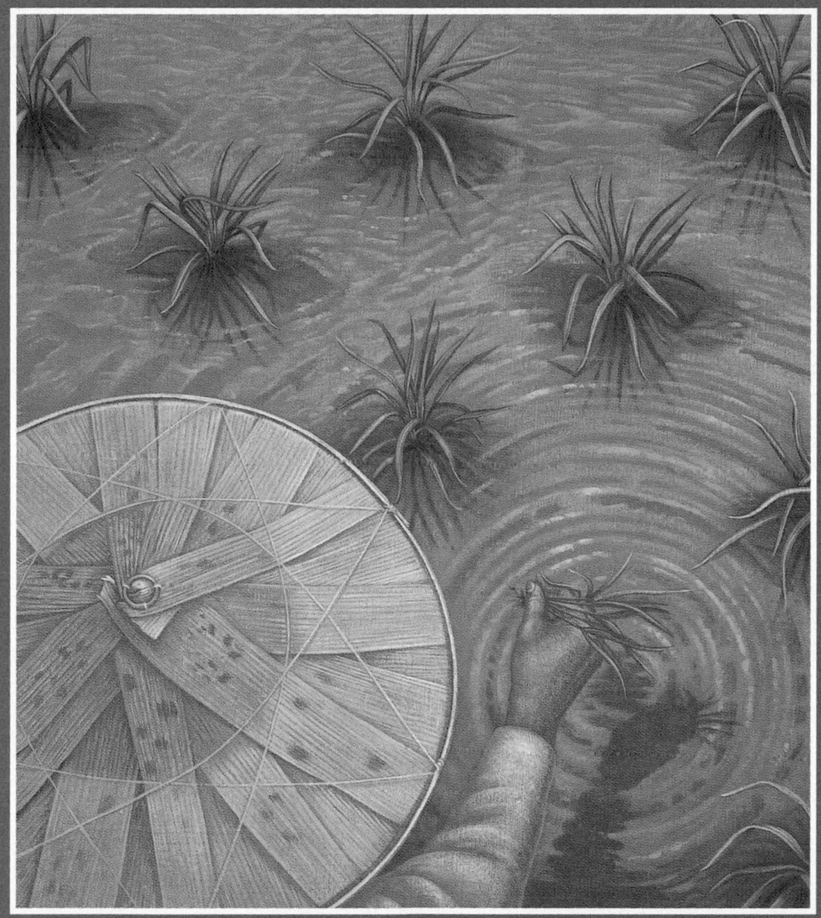

Contents

minerals naturally occurring, inorganic, homogeneous substances; chemical elements.

major minerals essential mineral nutrients found in the human body in amounts larger than 5 grams.

trace minerals essential mineral nutrients found in the human body in amounts less than 5 grams.

8

"Ashes to ashes and dust to dust." This familiar biblical quotation reminds us of our mortality. Perhaps we need this reminder to put our own importance into perspective. It is true that when the life force leaves the body, what is left behind ultimately becomes nothing but a small pile of ashes. Carbohydrates, proteins, fats, vitamins, and water are present at first, but they soon disappear.

The carbon atoms in all the carbohydrates, fats, proteins, and vitamins combine with oxygen to produce carbon dioxide, which vanishes into the air; the hydrogens and oxygens of those compounds unite to form water; and this water, along with the water that was a large part of the body weight, evaporates. The ashes that are left behind are the **minerals,** a small pile that weighs only about 5 pounds. The pile is not impressive in size, but when you consider the tasks these minerals perform, you may realize their great importance in living tissue.

Consider calcium and phosphorus. If you could separate these two minerals from the rest of the pile, you would take away about three fourths of the total. Crystals made of these two minerals, plus a few others, form the structure of the bones and so provide the architecture of the skeleton.

Run a magnet through the one fourth of the pile that remains, and pick up the iron. It would not fill a teaspoon, but it is billions of billions of iron atoms. As part of hemoglobin, these iron atoms have the special property of being able to attach to oxygen and to make it available at the sites where metabolic work is taking place, inside the cells.

If you were able to extract all the other minerals, leaving only copper and iodine in the pile of ashes, you would want to close the windows before you did it. A slight breeze would blow these remaining bits of dust away. Yet the amount of copper remaining in the dust is necessary for iron to hold and to release oxygen, and iodine is the critical mineral in the thyroid hormones. Figure 8-1 shows the amounts of **major minerals** and a few of the **trace minerals** in the human body. Other minerals such as gold and aluminum, while present in the body, are not known to be nutrients.

That a distinction is made between the major and the trace minerals doesn't mean that one group is more important in the body than the other. A daily deficiency of a few micrograms of iodine is just as serious as a deficiency of several hundred milligrams of calcium. Major minerals and trace

Figure 8-1

MINERALS IN A 60-KILOGRAM PERSON
The major minerals are those present in amounts larger than 5 grams (a teaspoon). The essential trace minerals number a dozen or more; only four are shown. A pound is about 454 grams; thus only calcium and phosphorus appear in amounts larger than a pound.

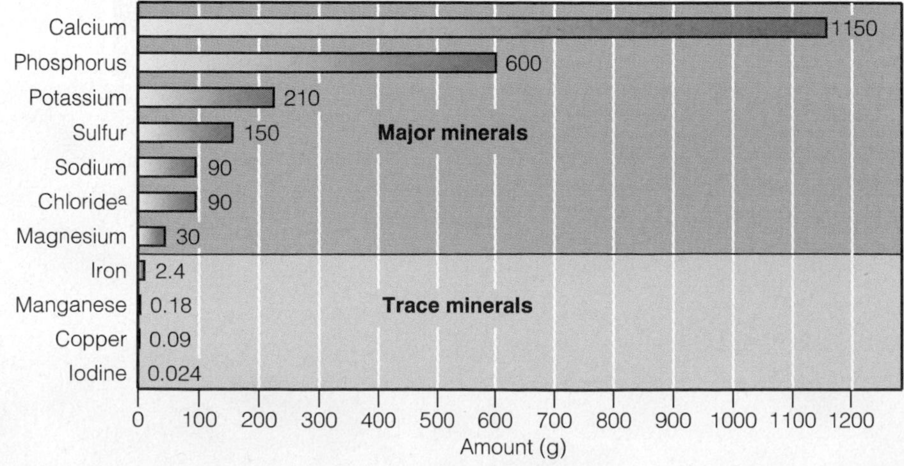

[a] Chlorine appears in the body as the chloride ion.

minerals all play specific roles. However, because the major minerals are present in larger total quantities, they influence the body fluids, thereby affecting the whole body in a general way.

A person can drink pure water, but in the body, that water mingles with minerals to become fluids in which all life processes take place. This chapter begins with a discussion of water—the most indispensable nutrient of all—and the major minerals that characterize the body's fluids and regulate their distribution within the body. Then the chapter discusses the specialized roles of the minerals.

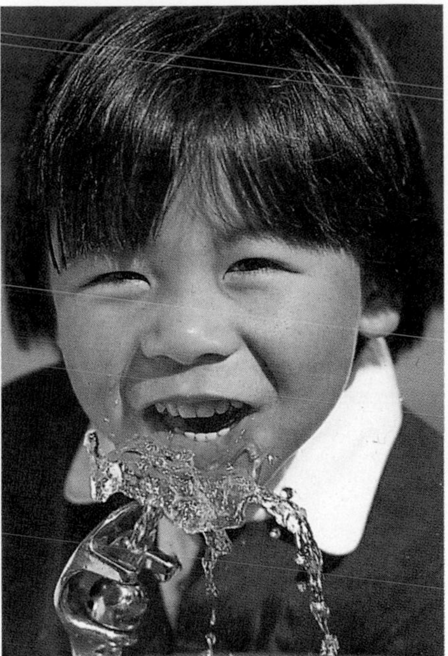

Water is the most indispensable nutrient.

◆ Water

You began as a single cell bathed in a nourishing fluid. As you became a beautifully organized, air-breathing body of billions of cells, each of your cells had to remain next to water to remain alive. Water brings to each cell the exact ingredients the cell requires and carries away the end products of its life-sustaining reactions.

Water in the body is not simply a river coursing through the arteries, capillaries, and veins. Some of the water is part of the chemical structure of compounds that form the cells, tissues, and organs of the body. For example, proteins hold water molecules within them. This water is locked in and is not readily available for any other use. Water also participates actively in many chemical reactions.

As the medium for the body's traffic of nutrients and waste products, water is nearly a universal solvent. Luckily for our physical integrity, this is not quite the case, but water does dissolve amino acids, glucose, minerals, and many other substances needed by the cells. Fatty substances are specially packaged with water-soluble proteins so that they too can travel freely in the blood and lymph. The water of the body fluids is thus the transport vehicle for all the nutrients.

Boasting scientist: I'm working on discovering the universal solvent.

Skeptical farmer: Is that so? Well, when you've got it, what are you going to keep it in?

Another important characteristic of water is its incompressibility. Its molecules resist being crowded together. Thanks to this characteristic, water can act as a lubricant and a cushion for the joints. For the same reason it can protect a sensitive tissue such as the spinal cord from shock. The fluid that fills the eye serves in a similar way to keep optimal pressure on the retina and lens. The unborn infant is cushioned against shock by the bag of amniotic fluid in which it develops. Water also lubricates the digestive tract and all tissues moistened with mucus.

Still another of water's special features is its heat-regulating capacity. This characteristic of water is familiar to coastal dwellers who know that land surrounded by water is protected from wide variations in temperature from day to night. Water itself changes temperature slowly; at night, when the land cools, the water gives up its heat gradually to the air, moderating the coolness of the night. In contrast, the desert varies widely in temperature from day to night because it is dry. Similarly, water helps to maintain body temperature. A great deal of heat is required to change water from a liquid to a gas, so when we sweat, the evaporating water carries off large quantities of body heat. To sum up, water:

- Carries nutrients and waste products throughout the body.
- Actively participates in many chemical reactions.
- Serves as the solvent for minerals, vitamins, amino acids, glucose, and a multitude of other small molecules.

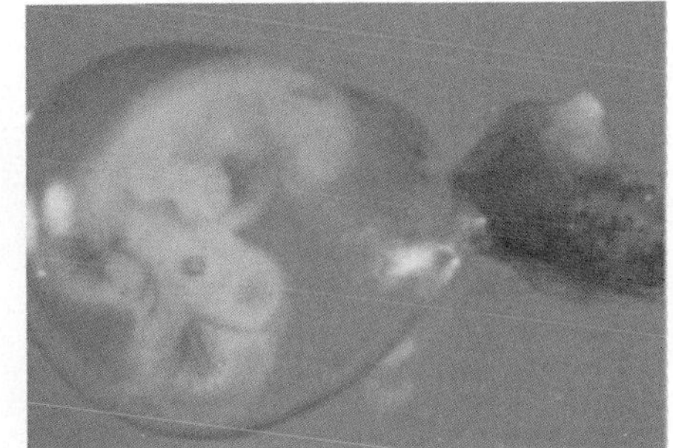

Human life begins in water.

dehydration loss of water. The symptoms progress rapidly from thirst to weakness to exhaustion and delirium, and end in death.

water intoxication the rare condition in which body water content is too high. Symptoms are headache, muscular weakness, lack of concentration, poor memory, and loss of appetite.

water balance the balance between water intake and water excretion, which keeps the body's water content constant.

- Acts as a lubricant and cushion around joints.
- Serves as shock absorber inside the eyes, spinal cord, and amniotic sac surrounding a fetus in the womb.
- Aids in maintaining the body's temperature.

KEY POINT Water provides the medium for transportation, and chemical reactions, acts as a solvent, and provides shock protection, lubrication, and temperature regulation in the human body.

Water Balance

Water makes up about 60 percent of the body's weight. It is such an integral part of us that people seldom are conscious of its importance, unless they are deprived of it. You can survive a deficiency of any of the other nutrients for a long time, in some cases even for months or years, but you can survive only a few days without water. Since the body's self-purification process requires that it excrete at least a pint of water a day, a person must consume that much each day to avoid life-threatening losses.

The total amount of fluid in the body is kept constant by delicate balancing mechanisms. Imbalances can occur, such as **dehydration** and **water intoxication,** but the balances are restored to normal as promptly as the body can manage it. Both intake and excretion are controlled to maintain **water balance.**

Water Intake

Thirst and satiety govern water intake. When the blood is too concentrated (having lost water but not salt and other dissolved substances), the molecules and particles in the blood attract water out of the salivary glands. The mouth becomes dry as a result, and you drink to wet your mouth. The brain center known as the hypothalamus (described in Chapter 3) also monitors the concentration of the blood. When the blood is too concentrated, the hypothalamus initiates impulses that stimulate drinking behavior. The volume of the blood also plays a role: thirsty animals drink until nerves in their hearts, known as stretch receptors, are stimulated enough to turn off the drinking.[1] Thus thirst adjusts to provide a water intake that exactly meets the need.

Thirst lags behind water lack. A water deficiency that develops slowly can switch on drinking behavior in time to prevent serious dehydration, but one that develops fast may not. Also, thirst itself does not remedy a water deficiency; drinking does. You have to notice that you are thirsty, pay attention, and take the time to get a drink. The athlete, the long-distance casual runner, the gardener in hot weather, and the elderly person whose thirst sensation may be blunted can experience serious dehydration. They need to be alert to their thirst signals and to drink promptly in response to them. (Chapter 10 offers more on the fluid needs of active people.)

Water Excretion

Water excretion is governed by the brain and the kidneys. The hypothalamus senses when the blood's sodium concentration is too high or blood volume or blood pressure is too low. Then it calls forth a hormone from the pituitary gland that directs the kidneys to shift water back into the bloodstream from the pool destined for excretion. The kidneys themselves also respond to the sodium concentration in the blood passing through them and secrete regulatory substances of their own. The net result is that the more water the body needs, the less it excretes. Still, there is a minimum amount of water that the body must excrete to carry off waste materials in the urine and feces, to generate sweat, and to evaporate from the lungs, and a minimum must be consumed each day to replace that water. Figure 8-2 shows how intake and excretion naturally balance out.

hard water water with high calcium and magnesium concentrations.

soft water water with a high sodium concentration.

bottled water drinking water sold in bottles.

Water Sources and Recommendations

In addition to water itself and other beverages made of water, nearly all foods contain water. Most fruits and vegetables contain large quantities of water, up to 95 percent; many meats and cheeses contain at least 50 percent. The energy-yielding nutrients in foods give rise to additional water as the body breaks them down.

Water needs vary greatly depending on the foods a person eats, the environmental temperature and humidity, the person's activity level, and other factors. The Committee on Recommended Dietary Allowances (RDA) recommends that under normal dietary and environmental conditions adults should consume between 1 and 1½ milliliters of water for each calorie spent in the day.[2] For the person who expends about 2,000 calories a day, this works out to 2 to 3 liters, or about 6 to 8 cups. Sweating increases water needs.

Water naturally occurs as **hard water** or **soft water,** a distinction that affects health with regard to three minerals. Hard water has high concentrations of calcium and magnesium. Soft water's principal mineral is sodium. In practical terms, soft water makes more bubbles with less soap; hard water leaves a ring on the tub, a jumble of rocklike crystals in the teakettle, and a gray residue in the wash. Soft water may seem the more desirable, and homeowners may even purchase water softeners that remove magnesium and calcium and replace them with sodium. However, soft water appears to contribute to a higher incidence of hypertension and heart disease in areas where it is used. Hard water may oppose these conditions.

Soft water also more easily dissolves certain metals, such as cadmium and lead, from pipes. Cadmium is not an essential nutrient. In fact, it can harm the body, affecting at least some enzymes by displacing zinc from its normal sites of action. Cadmium is also suspected of promoting hypertension. Lead is another toxic metal, and the body seems to absorb it more readily from soft than from hard water, possibly because the calcium in hard water protects against its absorption. Old plumbing may contain cadmium or lead. People who live in old buildings should run the cold water tap a minute before drawing water for use at breakfast to flush out harmful minerals. This will flush out the water that collected metals from the pipes during the night.

Many people turn to **bottled water** as an alternative to tap water. As the Consumer Caution points out, bottled water may or may not contain more health-promoting mineral arrays than ordinary tap water does.

KEY POINT Hard water is high in calcium and magnesium. Soft water is high in sodium, and it dissolves cadmium and lead from pipes.

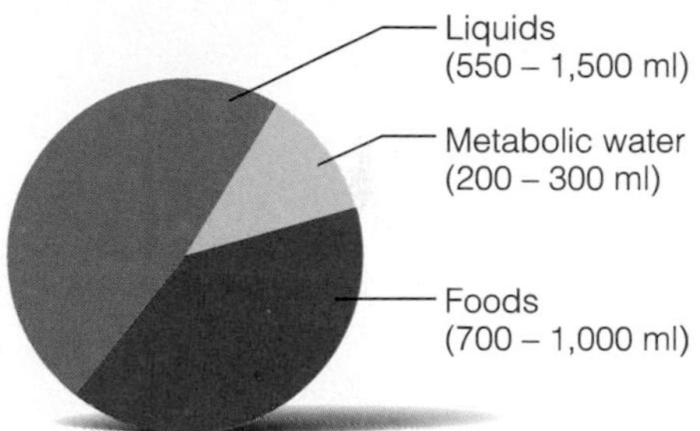

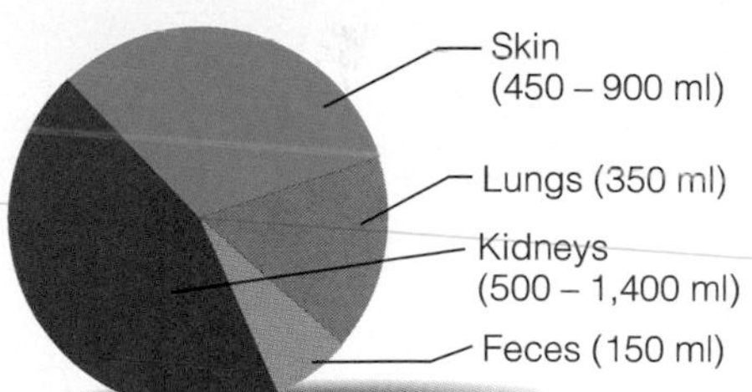

Figure 8-2

WATER BALANCE

Water enters the body through consumption of liquids and foods, and some water is created in the body as a by-product of metabolic processes. Water leaves the body through the evaporation of sweat, in the moisture of exhaled breath, in the urine, and in the feces.

Bottled Water

surface water water that comes from lakes, rivers, and reservoirs.

ground water water that comes from underground aquifers.

aquifers underground rock formations containing water that can be drawn to the surface for use.

CONSUMER CAUTION Many people are concerned about the safety of their water supplies because contaminated water can harm people's health. Households, traffic, industry, and agriculture all add pollutants to environmental water and thereby degrade its quality. Hundreds of contaminants, including disease-causing bacteria and viruses from human wastes, toxic pollutants from highway fuel runoff, spills and heavy metals from industry, and organic chemicals such as pesticides from agriculture, have been detected in public drinking water.

Public water systems have been devised to treat water to at least partly remove these hazards. Treatment includes the addition of a disinfectant (usually chlorine) to kill microorganisms. Private well water is usually not chlorinated or cleansed, so the 40 million Americans who drink water from private wells are especially likely to encounter microorganisms in their water. The Environmental Protection Agency (EPA) is responsible for ensuring that public water systems meet minimum standards for protection of public health. Critics charge that the laws are inadequate to protect drinking water and those in place are not enforced.

Many people feel unsure of the safety of their public drinking water and so seek an alternative water source. As a result, sales of bottled water have boomed. About 1 in 15 households uses bottled water as its main drinking water source, believing it to be safer than tap water and therefore worth its substantial price.

Unfortunately, bottled water is just as vulnerable to contamination as tap water is. After all, whether water comes from the tap or is poured from a bottle, *all* water comes from the same sources, **surface water** and **ground water.** Each of these sources supplies water for about half of the population.

Surface water comes from lakes, rivers, and reservoirs and provides drinking water for most of the nation's major cities. Surface water is easily contaminated by acid rain; runoff from highways; pesticide, fertilizer, and animal waste runoff from agricultural areas; and industrial wastes. These contaminants run directly from pavements, septic tanks, farm lands, and industrial areas into streams that feed surface water bodies.

Surface water moves faster than groundwater and so is somewhat cleansed by aeration and sunlight. It is also filtered by the plants and microorganisms that live in it. These processes can remove some contaminants, but some others may stay in the water.

Ground water comes from **aquifers,** underground rock formations saturated with water. People in rural areas rely mostly on ground water pumped up from private wells. Ground water is susceptible to contamination from hazardous waste sites, dumps, oil and gasoline pipelines, and landfills, as well as downward seepage from surface water bodies. Ground water moves slowly and lacks aeration and exposure to sunlight, so contaminants break down more slowly in ground water than in surface water. Ground water, however, must "percolate," or seep through soil, sand, and rock, to reach the aquifer. Percolation filters out some, but not all, of the contaminants.

Bottled Water *continued*

Bottled water is classed as a food, so it is regulated by the Food and Drug Administration (FDA). The FDA has proposed bottled water standards that impose limits for about 50 chemicals and other contaminants.[3] Still, problems of bottled waters are unlikely to improve from new rules alone. Today's problems of infrequent testing for contaminants and sporadic inspection of processing plants[4] must also be solved before bottled water can be assumed to be as healthful, pure, and sanitary as U.S. tap water.

Overwhelmingly, the people who buy bottled water say that taste is their primary reason for doing so. Some people simply prefer the taste of bottled water over the taste of water from their taps. Most water bottling plants disinfect their products with ozone, a form of oxygen, and, unlike chlorine, ozone leaves no flavor or odor in the water. Another reason is to avoid public water that consistently tests positive for one or more chemical or other contaminants. Test records are available through city or state public health departments and can be fascinating reading to those who wish to discover how pure their tap water is.

As a consumer, what should you look for when buying bottled water? Concerning labeling, no legal definitions yet exist for the names applied to bottled water, such as **distilled water; mineral water; purified water; seltzer, soda,** or **tonic water;** and **spring water,** but such definitions are forthcoming (Table 8-1). Meanwhile, here are a few guidelines.[5]

First, determine if the bottling company is a member of the International Bottled Water Association (IBWA). The IBWA is a trade group that represents about 90 percent of the domestic bottled water market and 35 imported brands. The IBWA supports FDA's proposed regulations.

Also determine the water's source. If the bottled water comes from a public source, what kind of treatment processes have been used to remove contaminants? If the bottled water comes from a spring or stream, where is it located? Is the area agricultural, residential, industrial, or undeveloped? Under the proposed rules, bottled water from municipal sources will be labeled as such unless it has been distilled or purified.

Buy water bottled in glass containers, if possible. Studies have not been conducted to determine the contamination effects of plastic packaging on water.

Also, if your water is dispensed from a water cooler, disinfect the cooler once a month by running half a gallon of white vinegar through it. Remove the vinegar residue by rinsing the cooler with 4 or 5 gallons of tap water. The bacterial content of water coolers has been found to be considerably higher than that recommended by the government. Bacterial and mold growths can cause serious infection and disease in those who ingest water contaminated with them.

Sales of bottled water show little sign of slowing down as more and more people question the safety of their water. Before you spend your money though, be sure that you are getting a quality product in return.

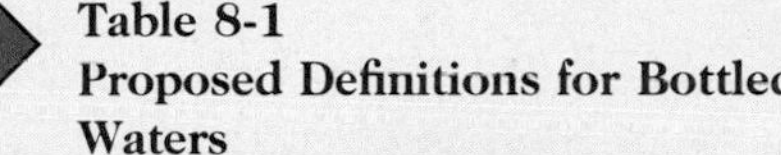

Table 8-1
Proposed Definitions for Bottled Waters

These terms may soon define bottled water

- **distilled water** water that has been processed by vaporization to remove all dissolved minerals.
- **mineral water** water obtained from geologically and physically protected underground sources.
- **purified water** water treated by any of a number of chemical or physical processes that remove dissolved solids, including minerals.
- **seltzer, soda, or tonic waters** legally, soft drinks, not regulated as water. Also called *carbonated water.*
- **spring water** water obtained from an underground source that flows naturally to the surface.

salts compounds composed of charged particles (ions). An example is potassium chloride (K^+Cl^-).

ions (EYE-ons) electrically charged particles, such as sodium (positively charged) or chloride (negatively charged).

electrolytes compounds that partly dissociate in water to form ions, such as the potassium ion (K^+) and the chloride ion (Cl^-).

fluid and electrolyte balance maintenance of the proper amounts and kinds of fluid and minerals in each compartment of the body.

fluid and electrolyte imbalance failure to maintain the proper amount and kind of fluid in every body compartment; a medical emergency.

acid-base balance maintenance of the proper degree of acidity in each of the body's fluids.

Body Fluids and Minerals

About 40 percent of the body's water weight is inside the cells, and about 15 percent bathes the outsides of the cells. The remainder fills the blood vessels. Special provisions are needed to ensure that cells do not collapse when water leaves them or swell up when too much water enters them. The cells cannot pump water across their membranes because water slips in and out freely. They can, however, pump minerals across their membranes. The major minerals form **salts** that dissolve in the body fluids; the cells direct where the salts go; and this determines where the fluids flow, because water follows salt.

When mineral (or other) salts dissolve in water, they separate into single, electrically charged particles known as **ions.** Unlike pure water, which conducts electricity poorly, ions dissolved in water carry electrical current. For this reason, the electrically charged ions are called **electrolytes.** Figure 8-3 shows how the body uses electrolytes to move its fluids around. Figure 6-12 of Chapter 6 showed that proteins form the pumps that move mineral ions across cell membranes. The successful result is **fluid and electrolyte balance,** the proper amount and kind of fluid in every body compartment.

If something happens to overwhelm the fluid balance, severe illness can result quickly, since fluid can shift rapidly from one compartment to another. For example, in vomiting or diarrhea, the loss of water from the intestinal tract pulls fluid from between the cells in every part of the body. Fluid then leaves the inside of the cells to restore balance. Meanwhile the kidneys detect the water loss and attempt to retrieve water from the pool destined for excretion. To do this they raise the sodium concentration outside the cells, and this pulls still more water out of them. When this happens, the very serious condition of **fluid and electrolyte imbalance** occurs. Water and minerals lost in vomiting or diarrhea ultimately come from every body cell. This loss disrupts the functioning of the heart and threatens life. It is a cause of fatality among those with eating disorders.

Controversy 10 describes the problems of eating disorders.

The minerals help manage still another balancing act, the **acid-base balance,** or pH, already mentioned in Chapter 6. Among the major minerals, some, when dissolved in water, give rise to acids, some to bases. A small percentage of water molecules (H_2O) also exist as positive and negative

Figure 8-3

FLUIDS AND ELECTROLYTES
Water flows in the direction of the more highly-concentrated solution.

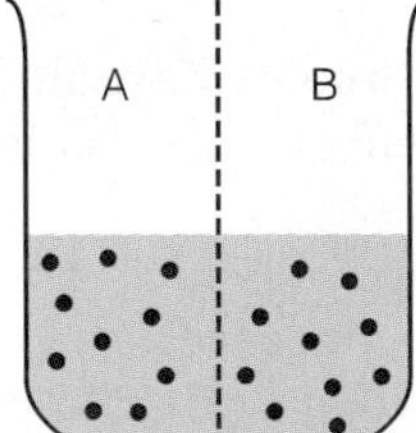

1. With equal numbers of dissolved particles on both sides, water levels remain equal.

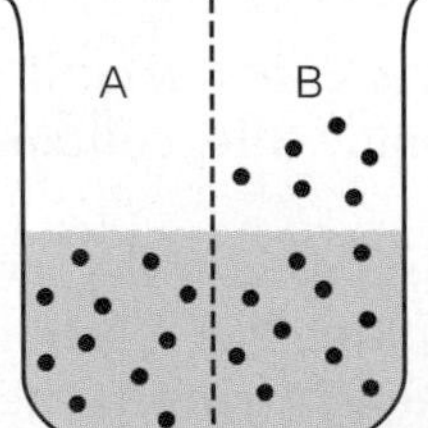

2. Now additional particles are added to increase the concentration on side B. Particles cannot flow across the divider (in the case of a cell, the divider is a membrane).

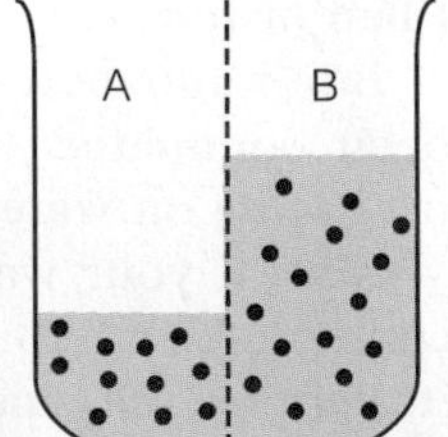

3. Water can flow both ways across the divider, but tends to move from side A to side B, where there is a greater concentration of dissolved particles. The *volume* of water increases on side B, and the *concentrations* on sides A and B become equal.

ions; H (positive) and OH (negative). Excess H ions in a solution make it an acid; they lower the pH; excess OH ions make it a base; they raise pH.

The body's proteins and some of its mineral salts help prevent changes in the acid-base balance of its fluids by serving as **buffers**—molecules that gather up or release H ions as needed to maintain the correct pH. The kidneys help to control the pH balance by excreting more or less acid (H ions). The lungs help also by excreting more or less carbon dioxide. (In solution in the blood, carbon dioxide forms an acid, carbonic acid.) The maintenance of the acid-base balance by means of these tight controls permits all other life processes to take place.

buffers compounds that can help to keep the acidity of a solution from changing by neutralizing acids and bases.

hydroxyapatite the chief crystal of bone, formed from calcium and phosphorus. (See also *fluorapatite*, p. 290)

KEY POINT Water makes up about 60 percent of the body's weight. Water losses from the body necessitate intake of an equal amount of water to maintain balance. Electrolytes help keep fluids in their proper compartments and help buffer these fluids, permitting all life processes to take place.

The Major Minerals

While all the major minerals help to maintain the balances just described, each also plays some special roles of its own. These roles are described in the following sections and are summarized in Table 8-7 on pages 298–300. The order does not imply that the first are the most important.

Calcium

Major minerals:
- Calcium
- Chloride
- Magnesium
- Phosphorus
- Potassium
- Sodium
- Sulfur

As Figure 8-1 showed, calcium is by far the most abundant mineral in the body. Nearly all (99 percent) of the body's calcium is stored in the bones, where it plays two important roles. First, it is an integral part of bone structure. Second, bone calcium serves as a bank that can release calcium to the body fluids if even the slightest drop in blood calcium concentration occurs. Many people have the idea that calcium (and the other minerals of bone), once deposited in bone, stays there forever—that once a bone is built, it is inert, like a rock. Not so. The minerals of bones are in constant flux, with formation and dissolution taking place every minute of the day and night.

Calcium and phosphorus are essential to the formation of bone (Figure 8-4). As bones begin to form, calcium phosphate salts, along with some other minerals, particularly fluoride, lay down crystals on a foundation material composed of the protein collagen. These crystals, called **hydroxyapatite,** invade the collagen and gradually lend more and more rigidity to the maturing bones until they are able to support the weight they will have to carry. Thus the long leg bones of children can support their weight by the time they have learned to walk.

The formation of teeth follows a pattern similar to that of bones. Hydroxyapatite crystals form on a collagen matrix to create the dentin that gives strength to the teeth (see Figure 8-5). Calcification of the "baby" teeth occurs in the gums during the latter half of the infant's time in the womb. The calcification of the permanent teeth takes place during early childhood, up to about the age of three; that of the "wisdom" teeth begins at about the age of ten. The turnover of minerals in teeth is not as rapid as in bone, but some withdrawal and redepositing does take place throughout life. Fluoride hardens and stabilizes the crystals of both bones and teeth, opposing the withdrawal of minerals from them.

Figure 8-4

A BONE

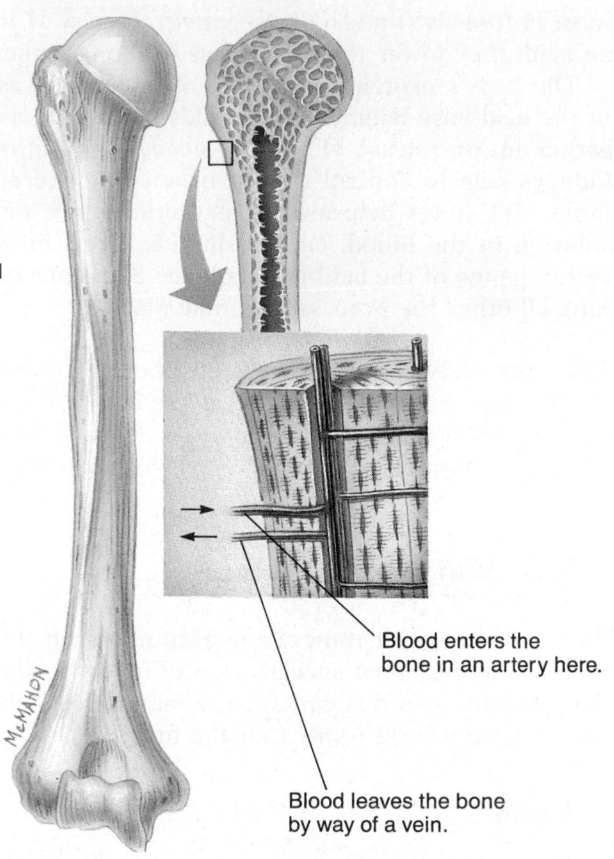
Blood travels in capillaries throughout the bone. It brings nutrients to the cells that maintain the bone's structure, and carries away waste materials from those cells. It picks up and deposits minerals as instructed by hormones.
This bone derives its structural strength from the lacy network of crystals that lie along the bone's lines of stress. If minerals are withdrawn to cover deficits elsewhere in the body, the bone will grow weak, and ultimately will bend or crumble.
Blood enters the bone in an artery here.
Blood leaves the bone by way of a vein.
McMAHON

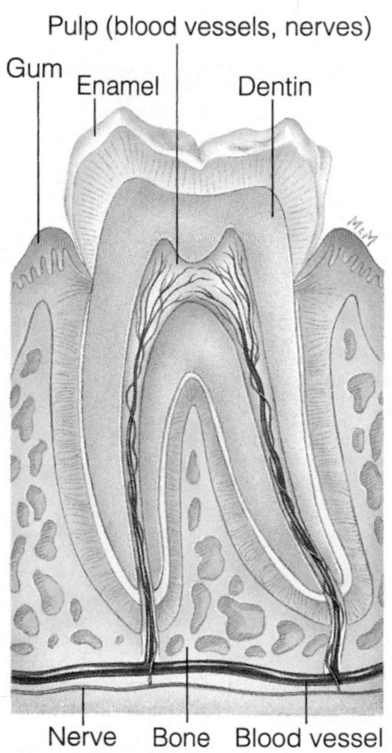
Pulp (blood vessels, nerves)
Gum
Enamel
Dentin
Nerve
Bone
Blood vessel

Figure 8-5

A TOOTH

The inner layer of dentin is bonelike material that forms on a protein (collagen) matrix. The outer layer of enamel is harder than bone. Both dentin and enamel contain hydroxyapatite crystals (made of calcium and phosphorus). The crystals of enamel may become even harder when exposed to the trace mineral fluoride.

Calcium in Body Fluids

Only about 1 percent of the body's calcium is in the fluid that bathes and fills the cells, but this minute amount plays these major roles:

- It regulates the transport of ions across cell membranes and is particularly important in nerve transmission.
- It helps maintain normal blood pressure (see Chapter 11).
- It is essential for muscle contraction and therefore for the heartbeat.
- It is involved in the secretion of hormones, digestive enzymes, and neurotransmitters.
- It plays an essential role in the clotting of blood.

Because of its importance, blood calcium is tightly controlled.

Calcium Balance

Cells need continuous access to calcium, so the body maintains a constant calcium concentration in the blood. The skeleton serves as a bank from which the blood can borrow and return calcium as needed. Withdrawals and deposits of calcium are not at the mercy of the amount taken in food but are regulated by hormones sensitive to blood calcium.* This means that

*Calcitonin, made in the thyroid gland, is secreted whenever the calcium concentration in the blood rises too high. It acts to stop withdrawal from bone and to slow absorption from the intestine. Parathormone, from the parathyroid glands, has the opposite effect.

you could go without adequate dietary calcium for years and not suffer noticeable symptoms. Only later in life would you suddenly discover that your calcium savings account had dwindled to the point at which the integrity of your skeleton could no longer be maintained. This would mean that throughout your adult years you were developing the fragile bones of **osteoporosis,** or **adult bone loss.** Osteoporosis constitutes a major health problem for many older people whose bones suddenly begin to shatter. The problem and its possible causes and prevention are the topics of this chapter's Controversy.

Calcium deficiencies are widespread, due largely to losses in adulthood. To protect against these losses, high calcium intakes are recommended early in life. A too-low calcium intake during the growing years may prevent achievement of maximum **peak bone mass** and density.[6] Too little calcium packed into the skeleton during childhood and young adulthood strongly predicts susceptibility to osteoporosis later in adulthood.[7]

The body is sensitive to an increased need for calcium, although it sends no signals to the conscious brain indicating calcium need. Instead it quietly increases its absorption of the mineral from the intestine and prevents its loss from the kidneys, thus conserving it. For example, more calcium is needed for growth, so infants and children absorb up to 75 percent of ingested calcium; and pregnant women, about 50 percent. Other adults, who are not growing, absorb about 30 percent.[8] The body also absorbs a higher percentage of calcium when less total calcium is provided in the diet. Deprived of calcium for months or years, an adult may double the calcium absorbed; when supplied for years with abundant calcium, the same person may absorb only a third the normal amount. These adjustments take time. A person accustomed to high calcium intakes who suddenly cuts back is likely to lose calcium from bone stores while the body adapts to the new level of intake.

osteoporosis (OSS-tee-oh-pore-OH-sis), also known as **adult bone loss,** a condition of older persons in which the bones become porous and fragile (*osteo* means "bones"; *poros* means "porous").

peak bone mass the highest attainable bone density for an individual, developed during the first three decades of life.

kefir a yogurt-based beverage.

In vitamin D deficiency:

- Rickets causes the bones of children to be soft and malformed.
- Osteomalacia causes the bones of adults to soften and bend.

In osteoporosis:

- Bones of older adults become brittle and fragile.

Read about calcium supplements in Controversy 8.

Meeting the Calcium RDA

Because the human body can adjust its calcium absorption to varying levels of intake, setting recommended allowances is difficult. The U.S. and Canadian recommendations for calcium intake are high, especially for young people up to the age of 24 years. The high intake recommendations are perhaps appropriate because people develop their peak bone mass during this time. After 30 years of age or so, the skeleton no longer adds significantly to bone density. After about 40 years of age, regardless of calcium intake, bones begin to lose density.[9] Thus obtaining enough calcium during the young years of life ensures that the skeleton will start out with enough mass to minimize bone losses through life. This is why the RDA for calcium has been set at 1,200 milligrams daily for young adults up to the age of 24 years. After 24 years, the RDA is lowered to 800 milligrams a day because the opportunity to build strong bones may have passed and the lower amount is sufficient to maintain bone tissue.

Milk and milk products are traditional sources of calcium for people who can tolerate them. Table 8-2 shows the current milk recommendations that help to meet the RDA for various age groups. People who do not use milk because of lactose intolerance, dislike, or allergy must obtain calcium from other sources. Care is needed, though; *wise* substitutions must be made. Most of milk's many sisters are recommended choices: yogurt, **kefir,** buttermilk, cheese (especially the low-fat or nonfat varieties), and, for people

Table 8-2
Recommended Fluid Milk Intakes

Age	Recommended Daily Intake
Children	2 cups
Teenagers	3 cups
Adults	2 cups
Pregnant or lactating women	3 cups
Pregnant or lactating teens	4 cups

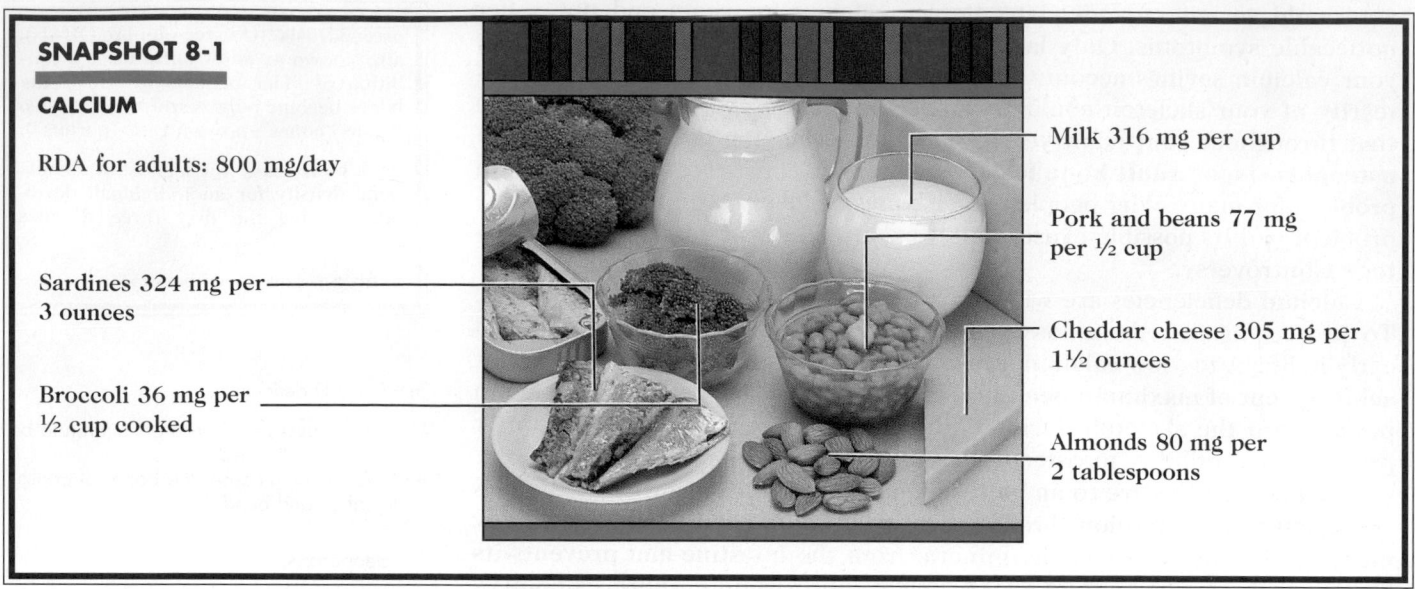

SNAPSHOT 8-1

CALCIUM

RDA for adults: 800 mg/day

nori a type of seaweed popular in Asian, particularly Japanese, cooking.

who can afford the calories, ice milk. Cottage cheese and frozen yogurt desserts contain about half the calcium of milk, with 2 cups being equivalent in calcium to 1 cup of milk. Butter, cream, and cream cheese contain negligible calcium, being almost pure fat. Snapshot 8-1 shows rich calcium sources.

If no milk product is acceptable as is, consider tinkering with it to make it work. Add chocolate to milk; fruit to yogurt; or nonfat milk powder to *any* dish—meatloaf, cookies, hamburgers, gravies, soups, casseroles, puddings, even beverages such as coffee or tea, hot or iced. Only 5 heaping tablespoons offer the equivalent of a cup of fresh milk.

For the many people who cannot use milk and milk products, oysters are a rich source. So are small fish such as canned sardines or other canned fishes prepared with their bones. Another rich source is stocks or extracts made from bones. The Vietnamese people's tradition of making such a stock helps account for their adequate calcium intake without the use of milk. To make a high-calcium extract, soak cracked bones from chicken, turkey, pork, or fish in vinegar; then slowly boil them until the bones become soft. The bones release calcium into the acid medium, and most of the vinegar taste boils off. Use the stock in place of water to cook soup, vegetables, rice, or stew. One *tablespoon* of such stock may contain over 100 milligrams of calcium.

Among vegetables, broccoli, beet greens, and kale are good sources of available calcium. So are collard and mustard greens, watercress and parsley, and probably some seaweeds, such as the **nori** popular in Japanese cookery. Certain other foods, including spinach, swiss chard, and rhubarb, appear equal to milk in calcium contents but actually provide no calcium, or very little, to the body because they contain binders that prevent calcium's absorption. Of course, the presence of calcium binders does not make greens inferior foods. Dark greens are a superb source of riboflavin, virtually indispensable for the vegan or anyone else who does not drink milk. Greens also are rich in iron, beta carotene, and dozens of other essential nutrients.

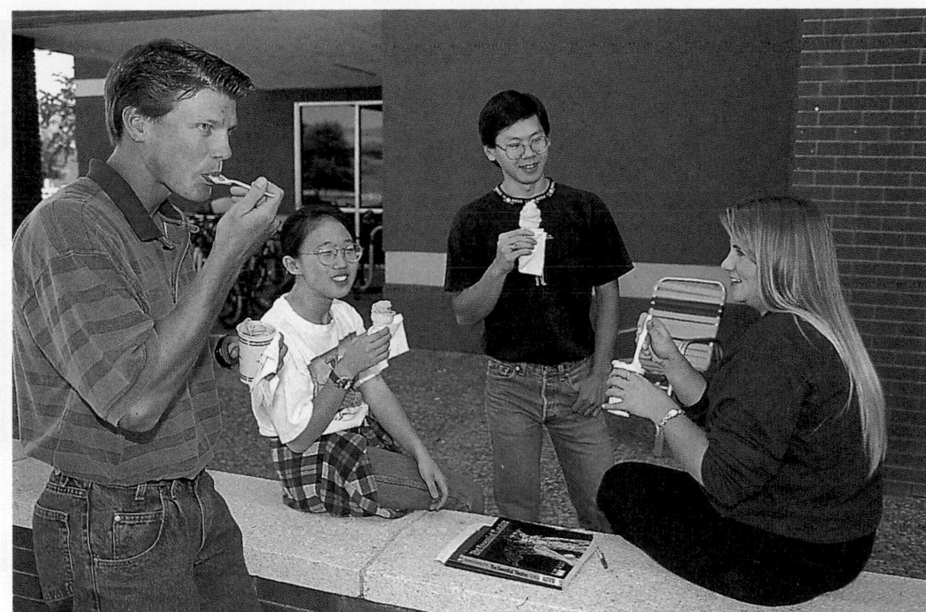

Calcium in a delicious form.

Next in order of preference among nonmilk sources of calcium are foods that contain large amounts of calcium salts by an accident of processing or by intentional fortification. In the processed category are bean curd (**tofu:** calcium salt is often used to coagulate it); canned tomatoes (firming agents donate 63 milligrams per cup of tomatoes); stone-ground or self-rising flour; stone-ground whole or self-rising cornmeal; and blackstrap molasses.

tofu a curd made from soybeans, rich in protein and often high in calcium; used in many Asian and vegetarian dishes in place of meat.

Among food products specially fortified to add calcium to people's diets, the richest in calcium is high-calcium milk itself, that is, milk with extra calcium added, which provides more calcium per cup than any natural milk, 500 milligrams per 8 ounces. Then comes calcium-fortified orange juice, with 300 milligrams per 8 ounces, a good choice because the bioavailability of its calcium compares favorably with that of milk. Calcium-fortified soy milk can also be prepared so that it contains more calcium than whole cow's milk. Soy-based infant formula is fortified with calcium, and no law forbids adults to use it in cooking for themselves.

Finally, there are supplements intended to meet calcium needs without regard to needs for energy or other nutrients. Most people who take calcium supplements do so in hopes of warding off osteoporosis. However, as Controversy 8 points out, supplements are not magic bullets against bone loss.

KEY POINT Calcium makes up bone and tooth structure and plays roles in nerve transmission, muscle contraction, and blood clotting. Calcium absorption increases when there is a dietary deficiency or an increased need such as during growth. Milk and milk products are rich calcium sources, as are fish with bones, certain green vegetables, and calcium-fortified foods.

Phosphorus

Phosphorus is the second most abundant mineral in the body. About 85 percent of it is found combined with calcium in the crystals of the bones and teeth.

SNAPSHOT 8-2

PHOSPHORUS

RDA for adults: 800 mg/day

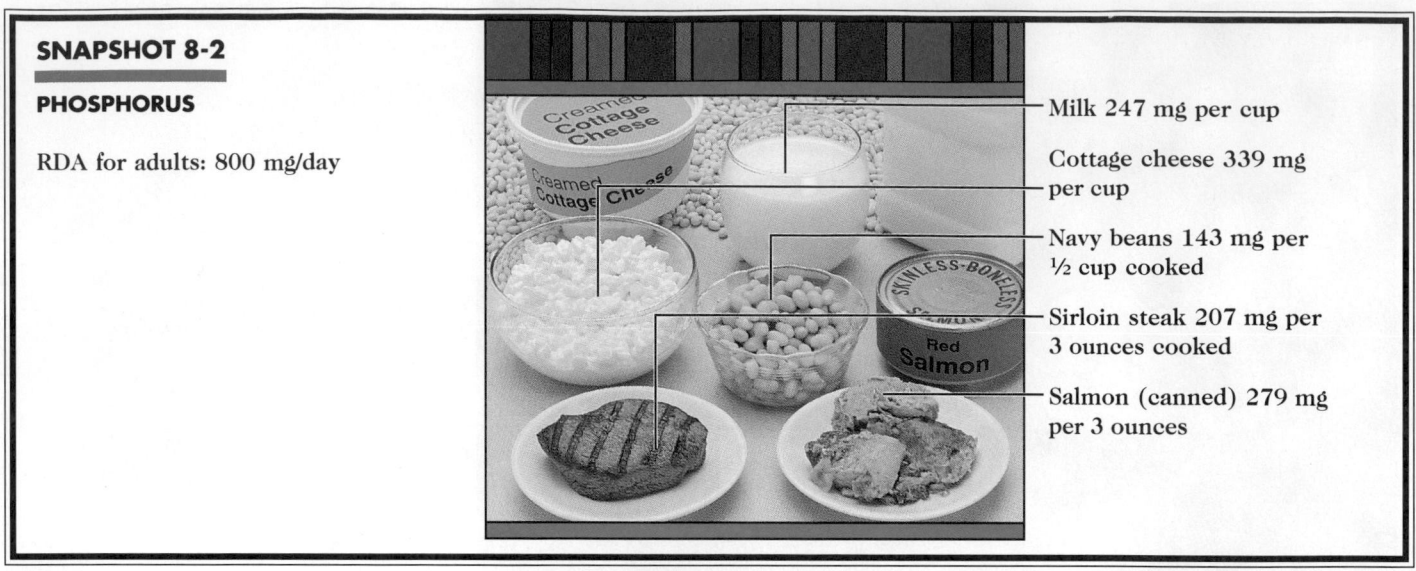

Note: The mineral is *phosphorus*. The adjective form is spelled with an *-ous* (as in *phosphorous salts*).

The concentration of phosphorus in the blood is less than half that of calcium, but its functions are critical to life. Phosphorous salts buffer the acid-base balance of cellular fluids. Each cell also depends on phosphorus as part of its genetic material, thus making phosphorus essential for growth and renewal of tissues. In cells' metabolism of energy nutrients, phosphorous compounds handle energy and work with many enzymes and vitamins to extract the energy from nutrients. Recall from Chapter 5 that phosphorus is part of molecules of certain lipids, phospholipids, that form the membranes surrounding each cell and its parts.

As Snapshot 8-2 shows, animal protein is the best source of phosphorus because phosphorus is so abundant in the cells of animals. Recommended intakes for phosphorus are the same as those for calcium, except during infancy. Luckily, needs for phosphorus are easily met by almost any diet, and deficiencies are unknown.

KEY POINT Most of the phosphorus in the body is in the bones and teeth. Phosphorus in the blood helps maintain acid-base balance, is part of the genetic material in cells, assists in energy metabolism, and is part of cell membranes. Deficiencies of phosphorus are unknown.

Magnesium

Magnesium barely qualifies as a major mineral: only about 1¾ ounces are present in the body of a 130-pound person, over half of it in the bones. Most of the rest is in the muscles, heart, liver, and other soft tissues, with only 1 percent in the body fluids. The supply of magnesium in the bones can be tapped to maintain a constant blood level whenever dietary intake falls too low. The kidney can also act to conserve magnesium.

Magnesium is critical to the operation of hundreds of enzymes, and it directly affects the metabolism of potassium, calcium, and vitamin D. Magnesium acts in the cells of all the soft tissues, where it is part of the protein-making machinery and is necessary for the release of energy. Magnesium

SNAPSHOT 8-3

MAGNESIUM

RDA for men: 350 mg/day
RDA for women: 280 mg/day

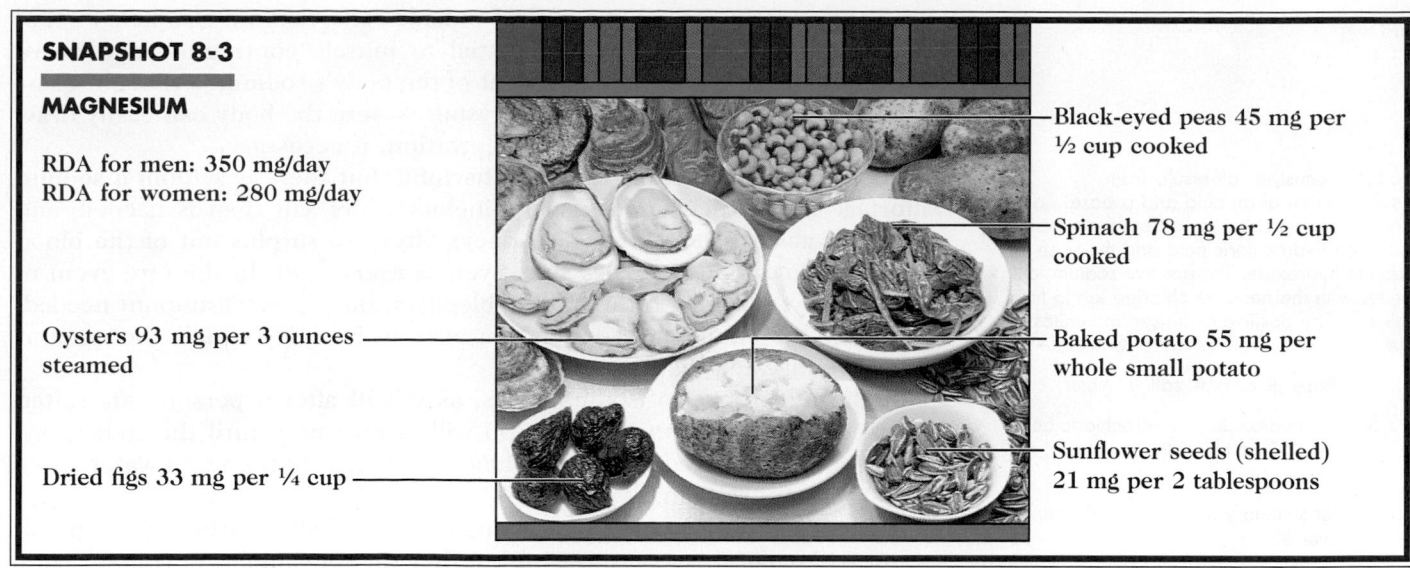

helps muscles relax after contraction and promotes resistance to tooth decay by holding calcium in tooth enamel.

Deficiency of magnesium may occur as a result of inadequate intake, vomiting, diarrhea, alcoholism, or protein malnutrition. It may also occur in hospital clients who have been fed fluids lacking nutrients into a vein for too long; or in persons using diuretics.

People whose drinking water has a high magnesium content experience a lower incidence of sudden death from heart failure than other people. It seems likely that magnesium deficiency makes the heart unable to stop itself from going into spasms once it starts.[10] Magnesium deficiency may also cause larger than normal amounts of cholesterol to be deposited in arteries, promoting heart disease.[11] Such a deficiency also causes hallucinations that can be mistaken for mental illness or drunkenness.

Chapter 10 discusses magnesium in relation to the exercising body.

Dietary intakes of magnesium average about three-quarters of the RDA for both men and women in the United States. Dietary surveys that determined this, however, did not account for the nutrient contribution of water. In various parts of the country, water can contribute significantly to magnesium intakes, so people living in those regions need less from food.

Despite intakes below the RDA, overt deficiency symptoms in normal, healthy people are rare.[12] Snapshot 8-3 above shows magnesium-rich foods. Magnesium is easily washed and peeled away from foods during processing, so slightly processed or unprocessed foods are the best choices.

Sodium

Salt has been known throughout recorded history. The Bible's saying "You are the salt of the earth" means that a person is valuable. If, on the other hand, "you are not worth your salt," you are worthless. Even the word *salary* comes from the word *salt.* Sodium is the positive ion in the compound sodium chloride (table salt) and other salts and contributes 40 percent of its weight. Thus a person who consumes a gram of salt consumes 400 milligrams of sodium. As already mentioned, sodium is the chief ion used to maintain the volume of fluid outside cells. Sodium also helps maintain acid-base balance and is essential to muscle contraction and nerve transmission. About 30 to 40 percent of the body's sodium is thought to be stored on the surface of the bone crystals, where the body can easily draw upon it to replenish the blood concentration, if necessary.

To the chemist, a salt results from neutralization of an acid and a base. Sodium chloride, table salt, results from the reaction between hydrochloric acid and the base sodium hydroxide. The positive sodium ion unites with the negative chloride ion to form the salt. The positive hydrogen ion unites with the negative hydroxide ion to form water.

Base + acid = salt + water.

Sodium hydroxide + hydrochloric acid = sodium chloride + water.

For a brief summary of the kidneys' action, see Chapter 3.

A deficiency of sodium would be harmful, but there is seldom a sodium shortage in the diet. Foods usually include more salt than is needed, and the body absorbs it freely. The kidneys filter the surplus out of the blood into the urine. They can also sensitively conserve salt. In the rare event of a deficiency, they can return to the bloodstream the exact amount needed. Normally the amount of sodium you excrete in a day equals the amount you have ingested that day.

If the blood level of sodium rises, as it will after a person eats salted foods, thirst ensures that the person will drink water until the sodium-to-water ratio is restored. Then the kidneys can excrete the extra water along with the extra sodium.

Dieters sometimes think that eating too much salt or drinking too much water will make them gain weight, but they do not gain fat, of course. They gain water, but they excrete this excess water immediately. Excess salt is excreted as soon as enough water is drunk to carry the salt out of the body. From this perspective, then, the way to keep body salt (and "water weight") under control is to drink more, not less, water.

The connection of salt with high blood pressure in salt-sensitive people is well known. Most people have learned that they should not consume too much sodium. Some question has arisen recently, however, about whether the culprit in relation to high blood pressure is sodium alone, the particular combination of sodium and chloride, or even the chloride ion alone. Chapter 11 describes the effects of these and other factors on blood pressure.

If blood sodium drops, body water is lost, and both water and sodium must be replenished to avert emergency. Overly strict use of low-sodium diets in the treatment of hypertension, kidney disease, or heart disease can deplete the body of needed sodium; so can vomiting, diarrhea, or heavy sweating. Under normal conditions of sweating due to exercise, salt losses may easily be replaced later in the day with ordinary foods.

Diets rarely lack sodium. For this reason no RDA has been set; instead, the RDA committee estimated the *minimum* sodium requirement for adults to be 500 milligrams.[13] The National Research Council (NRC) recommendations emphasize moderation, not adequacy, and thus set a maximum intake of *salt* at 6 grams (2,400 milligrams sodium). The most recent food intake survey in the United States estimates that men consume an average of 3,300 milligrams of sodium a day.[14] Cultures vary in their use of salt. Asian people, whose staple sauces and flavorings are based on soy sauce and monosodium glutamate (MSG or Accent), consume the equivalent of about 30 to 40 grams of salt per day. In China, Japan, and Korea, the prevalence of high blood pressure is equal to or greater than that of the United States.[15]

One of the most important favors you can do yourself, especially if you have heart disease in your family, is to learn to control your salt intake. An obvious step is to control your use of the saltshaker, but this source may account for as little as 15 percent of your total salt intake. A more productive step may be to limit intakes of processed foods, the source of up to 75 percent of the salt in most people's diets.[16] (The other 10 percent occurs naturally in foods.) This chapter's Food Feature shows how to cut down on

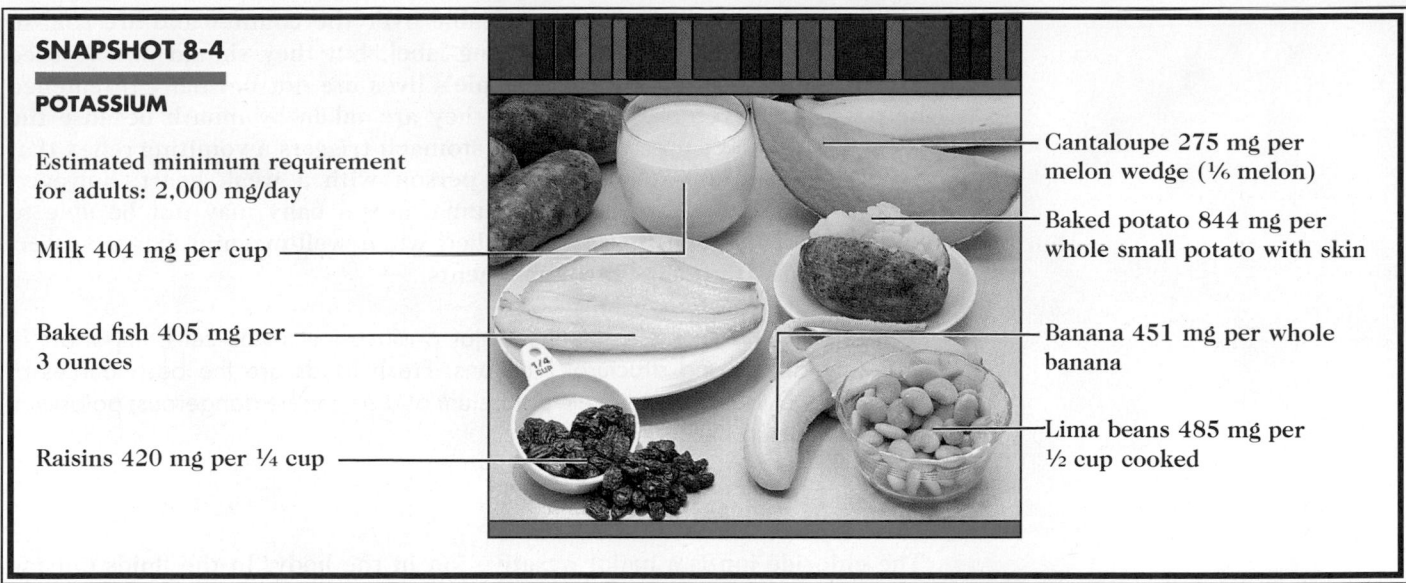

salt. A table in that section shows how processing adds sodium to foods while depleting another mineral of interest, potassium.

> **diuretics** (dye-you-RET-ics) medications causing increased urinary water excretion.

KEY POINT Sodium is the main positively charged ion outside the body's cells. Sodium attracts water. Thus too much sodium (or salt) may aggravate hypertension. Diets rarely lack sodium.

Potassium

Potassium is the principal, positively charged ion inside body cells. It plays a major role in maintaining fluid and electrolyte balance and cell integrity. It is also critical to maintaining the heartbeat. The sudden deaths that occur during fasting or severe diarrhea and in kwashiorkor children are thought to be due to heart failure caused by potassium loss.

Kwashiorkor was described in Chapter 6.

Dehydration leads to potassium loss from inside cells. It is especially dangerous because potassium loss from brain cells makes the victim unaware of the need for water. Because of this adults are warned not to take **diuretics** (water pills) that cause potassium loss except under a physician's supervision. When taking such diuretics, a person should alert all other health care providers to their use. Any physician prescribing such diuretics will tell the client to eat potassium-rich foods to compensate for the losses. Depending on the diuretic, the physician may also advise a lower sodium intake.

A dietary deficiency of potassium is unlikely in healthy people, although low potassium intakes are possible with diets low in fresh fruits and vegetables. Because potassium is found inside all living cells and because cells remain intact unless foods are processed, the richest sources of potassium are *fresh* foods of all kinds. Bananas, despite their fame as a rich potassium source, are just moderate. Bananas, however, are available everywhere, are easy to chew, and have a sweet taste that almost everyone likes. As Snapshot 8-4 above shows, foods of all kinds offer abundant potassium. Most whole vegetables and fruits are outstanding.

Unlike sodium, potassium may exert a positive effect against hypertension and related ills. See Chapter 11 for details.

Potassium chloride pills are available over the counter and are sold in health food stores without a warning label, but they should not be used except on a physician's advice. People's lives are not normally threatened by potassium overdoses as long as they are taken by mouth because the presence of excess potassium in the stomach triggers a vomiting reflex that expels the unwanted substance. A person with a weak heart, however, should not be put through this trauma, and a baby may not be able to withstand it. Several infants have died when well-meaning parents overdosed them with potassium supplements.

KEY POINT Potassium is the major positive ion inside cells, important in many metabolic and structural functions. Fresh foods are the best sources of potassium. Diuretics can deplete potassium and so can be dangerous; potassium excess can also be dangerous.

Other Major Minerals

The chloride ion is a major negative ion in the body. In the fluids outside the cells, it accompanies sodium; inside the cells it occurs primarily in association with potassium. Thus it helps to maintain the crucial fluid balances (acid-base and electrolyte balances) mentioned in the earlier discussion of water. The chloride ion also plays a special role as part of the hydrochloric acid that maintains the strong acidity of the stomach. Its principal food source is salt, both added and naturally occurring in foods. In its elemental form, chlorine forms a deadly green gas; dissolved in fluid, chlorine can be useful as a disinfectant, but it must be handled carefully.

The body does not use sulfur by itself as a nutrient; rather it is present in essential nutrients that the body does use, such as thiamin and all proteins. It plays its most important role in helping strands of protein to assume a particular shape. Skin, hair, and nails contain some of the body's more rigid proteins, which have high sulfur contents.

There is no recommended intake for sulfur, and deficiencies are unknown. The summary table at the end of this chapter presents the main facts on the major minerals.

KEY POINT Chloride is the body's major negative ion inside and outside of cells. It is essential to the acid-base balance and is part of the stomach's hydrochloric acid necessary to digest protein. Sulfur is also considered a major mineral, although it occurs only as part of other compounds such as protein.

Table 8-3
Trace Minerals

RDA Nutrients
Iron Zinc Iodine Selenium
Safe and Adequate Daily Dietary Intakes Established
Copper Manganese Fluoride Chromium Molybdenum
Known Essential for Animals; Human Requirements under Study
Arsenic Nickel Silicon Boron
Known Essential for Some Animals; No Evidence That Intake by Humans is Ever Limiting; No RDA Necessary
Cobalt
The evidence for requirements and essentiality is weak for the trace minerals cadmium, lead, lithium, tin, and vanadium.

The Trace Minerals

Laboratory techniques developed in the last two decades have enabled scientists to detect minerals in smaller and smaller quantities in living cells. Knowledge of the "new" trace elements is evolving from this research. An obstacle to determining their precise roles lies in the difficult task of providing an experimental diet lacking in the one element under study. Thus research in this area is limited mostly to the study of laboratory animals, which can be fed highly refined, purified diets in environments that are free of all contamination. Whole books have been published on the trace minerals alone, and research is still rapidly expanding knowledge about them. As Table 8-3 shows, the Committee on RDA has established recommended dietary allowances for the best known trace elements—iron, zinc, iodine, and selenium. Tentative ranges for safe and adequate daily intakes of others are also published. Still others are recognized as essential nutrients for some animals, but have not been proven to be required for human beings.

goiter (GOY-ter) enlargement of the thyroid gland due to iodine deficiency.

cretinism (CREE-tin-ism) severe mental and physical retardation of an infant caused by the mother's iodine deficiency during her pregnancy.

Iodine

Iodine is needed by the body in an infinitesimally small quantity, but its principal role in human nutrition makes obtaining this amount critical. Iodine is a part of thyroxine, the hormone responsible for regulating the basal metabolic rate. Iodine must be available for thyroxine to be synthesized.

When the iodine concentration of the blood is low, the cells of the thyroid gland enlarge in an attempt to trap as many particles of iodine as possible. Sometimes the gland enlarges until it makes a visible lump in the neck, a **goiter.** People with the condition suffer sluggishness and weight gain. In a pregnant woman, severe iodine deficiency causes the extreme and irreversible mental and physical retardation of the infant known as **cretinism.** Much of the mental retardation can be averted if the pregnant woman's deficiency is detected and treated in time, but if it goes uncorrected, the child may live his or her whole life with an IQ as low as 20 (100 is average). Iodine deficiency is one of the world's most common preventable causes of mental retardation.[17]

The iodine in food varies. Generally it reflects the soil in which plants are grown or on which animals graze. Iodine is plentiful in the ocean, so seafood is a completely dependable source. In the central parts of the United States that were never under the ocean, the soil is poor in iodine. In those areas the use of iodized salt and the consumption of foods shipped in from other, iodine-rich areas have been necessary to wipe out the iodine deficiency that once was widespread. Surprisingly, sea salt delivers little iodine to the eater because iodine becomes a gas and escapes into the air during the salt-drying process.

In iodine-poor regions, the iodization of salt has all but eliminated the widespread misery caused there earlier by goiter and cretinism. However, goiter is still prevalent in developing nations. In the United States, salt box labels state whether salt is iodized; in Canada all table salt is iodized.

A dramatic increase in iodine intakes in the United States concerns some observers. Excessive intakes of iodine can cause an enlargement of the thyroid gland resembling goiter, which in infants can block the airways and cause suffocation.[18] Intakes reached an all-time high of 800 micrograms per person per day in 1974; since then, intakes declined somewhat but are still several times the RDA of 150 micrograms. The toxic level at which detectable harm results is thought to be over 2,000 micrograms per day for an adult, an amount only a few times higher than the amount most people receive daily. Like chlorine and fluorine, iodine is a deadly poison in large amounts.

Much of the excess iodine in U.S. diets today comes from bakery products and from milk. The baking industry uses dough conditioners and most dairies feed cows iodine-containing medications and use iodine to disinfect milking equipment. One cup of milk supplies nearly the RDA of iodine, and so does less than a half teaspoon of iodized salt.[19] Both the dairy and bakery industries have been reducing their use of iodine compounds, but the emergence of this problem points to a need for continued surveillance of the food supply.

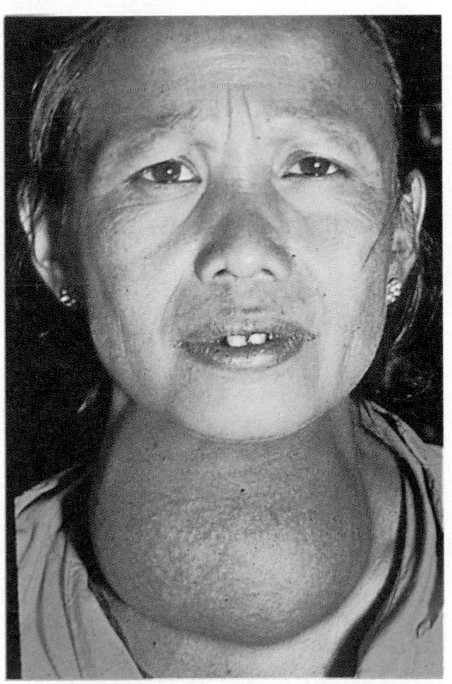

In iodine deficiency, the thyroid gland enlarges—a condition known as simple goiter.

hemoglobin (HEEM-oh-globe-in) the oxygen-carrying protein of the blood; found in the red blood cells (*hemo* means "blood"; *globin* means "spherical protein").

myoglobin (MYE-o-globe-in) the oxygen-holding protein of the muscles (*myo* means "muscle").

iron deficiency the condition of having depleted iron stores which, at the extreme, causes iron-deficiency anemia.

iron-deficiency anemia one of the anemias characterized by red blood cell shrinkage and color loss caused by iron deficiency. Accompanying symptoms are weakness, apathy, headaches, pallor, intolerance to cold, and inability to pay attention. (For other anemias, see index).

KEY POINT Iodine is part of the hormone thyroxine, which influences energy metabolism. The deficiency diseases are goiter and cretinism. Iodine occurs naturally in seafood and in foods grown on land that was once covered by oceans; it is an additive in milk and bakery products. Large amounts are poisonous.

Iron

Every living cell, whether plant or animal, contains iron. Most of the iron in the body is a component of the proteins **hemoglobin** in red blood cells and **myoglobin** in muscle cells. Hemoglobin in the blood carries oxygen from the lungs to tissues throughout the body. Myoglobin carries and stores oxygen for the muscles. Both hemoglobin and myoglobin contain iron, and the iron helps them to carry and hold oxygen and then release it.

All the cells need oxygen because they release carbon and hydrogen atoms as they break down energy nutrients. The oxygen combines with these atoms to form the waste products carbon dioxide and water; thus the body constantly needs fresh oxygen and nutrients to keep the cells going. As cells use up and excrete their oxygen (as carbon dioxide and water), red blood cells shuttle between metabolizing tissues and lungs to bring in fresh oxygen supplies. Besides helping hemoglobin to carry oxygen around and myoglobin to hold it in muscles, iron helps many enzymes in energy pathways to use oxygen. Iron is also needed to make new cells, amino acids, hormones, and neurotransmitters.

Iron is clearly the body's gold, a precious mineral that is hoarded and closely guarded. The liver packs new red blood cells with iron sent from the bone marrow and ships them out to the blood, where they live for about three to four months. When those red blood cells die, the spleen and liver break them down, save their iron, and send it back to the bone marrow to be kept for reuse. Only tiny losses of iron occur in the clipping of nails, the cutting of hair, the shedding of skin cells, and, if bleeding occurs, the loss of blood.

The body also has special provisions for obtaining iron. Normally, only about 10 to 15 percent of dietary iron is absorbed; but if the body's supply is diminished or if the need increases for any reason (such as pregnancy), absorption increases.

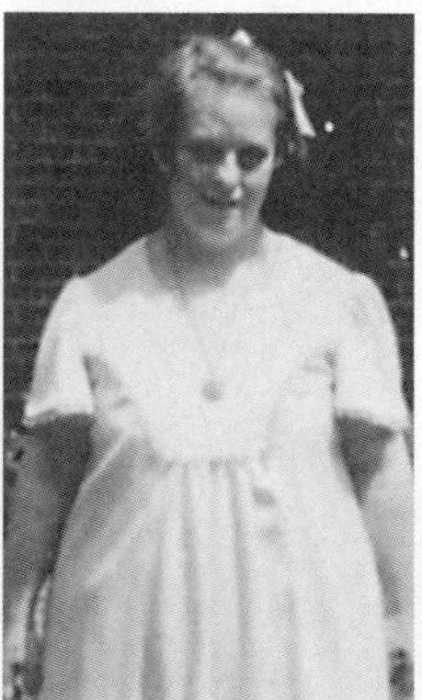
An adult with cretinism—her mother was iodine deficient while pregnant with her.

Iron Deficiency If absorption cannot compensate for losses or low dietary intakes then iron stores are used up and iron deficiency sets in. Iron deficiency and anemia are not one and the same, though they often go hand in hand. The distinction between **iron deficiency** and **iron-deficiency anemia** is an important one. People may be iron deficient without being anemic. The term *iron deficiency* refers to depleted iron stores without regard to the degree of depletion or the presence of anemia. The term *anemia* refers to severe depletion of iron stores resulting in low blood hemoglobin.

Without iron, the body becomes unable to make enough hemoglobin to fill its new blood cells. A sample of iron-deficient blood examined under the microscope shows smaller cells that are a lighter red than normal (see Figure 8-6). The undersized cells contain too little hemoglobin and thus deliver too little oxygen to the tissues. This limits cells' energy metabolism. Some of the symptoms of iron-deficiency anemia, such as tiredness, apathy, and a tendency to feel cold, reflect energy deficiency.

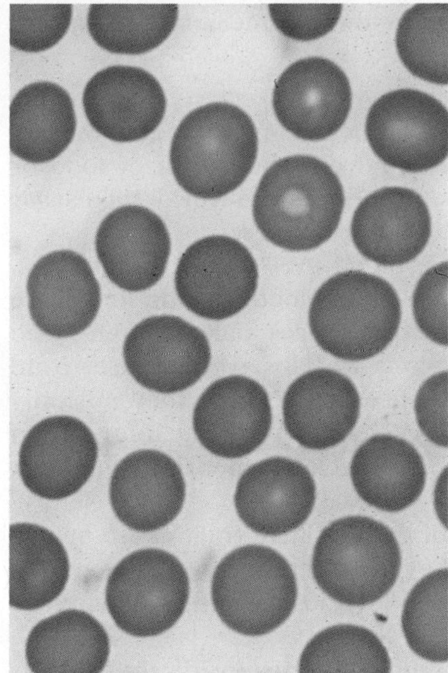

Normal blood cells. Both size and color are normal.

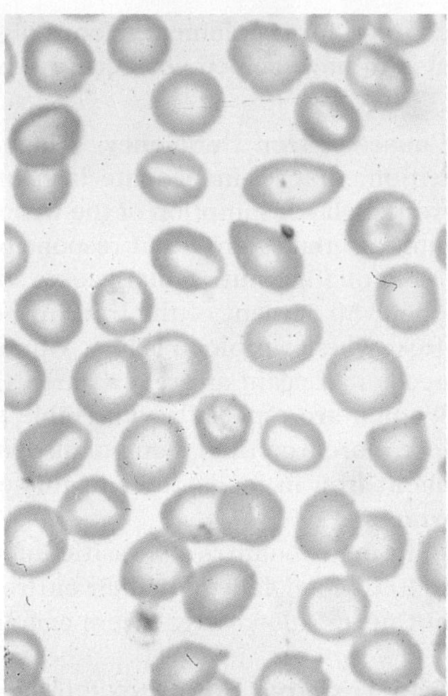

Blood cells in iron-deficiency anemia. These cells are small and pale because they contain less hemoglobin.

Figure 8-6

NORMAL AND ANEMIC BLOOD CELLS

Long before the red blood cells are affected and anemia is diagnosed, though, people exhibit the impact of iron deficiency in their behavior. Even at slightly lowered iron levels, physical work capacity and productivity are impaired. With reduced energy available to work, play, think, or learn, people simply do these things less. Because they work and play less, they become less physically fit. Many of the symptoms associated with iron deficiency are easily mistaken for behavioral or motivational problems. Children deprived of iron become restless, irritable, and unable to pay attention. Such symptoms disappear when iron intake improves.

A curious symptom seen in some people with iron deficiency is an appetite for ice, clay, paste, and other nonnutritious substances. Such people have been known to eat as many as eight trays of ice in a day. This behavior has been observed in poverty-stricken women and children who are deficient in either iron or zinc and has been given the name **pica.** When caused by iron deficiency, pica clears up dramatically within days after iron is given, even if anemia is present and the red blood cells have not yet responded.

pica (PIE-ka) a craving for nonfood substances. Also known as **geophagia** (gee-oh-FAY-gee-uh) when referring to clay eating, **pagophagia** (pag-oh-FAY-gee-uh) when referring to ice craving. (*Geo* means "earth"; *pago* means "frost"; *phagia* means "to eat.")

Feeling fatigued, weak, and apathetic is a sign that something is wrong. It is not a sign that you necessarily need iron or other supplements. Two actions are called for: first, get your diet in order; then, if symptoms persist for more than a week or two, consult a physician for a diagnosis.

Prevalence of Iron Deficiency Worldwide, iron deficiency is the most common nutrient deficiency.[20] Iron-deficiency anemia affects an estimated 15 percent of the world's population, with the highest prevalence in developing countries.[21] Infants (six months old or older), young children, and pregnant women are especially vulnerable. In the United States the iron status of infants and young children has improved in the last decade thanks to more widespread breastfeeding and greater use of iron-fortified infant formula.[22] For children from low-income families, the Special Supplemental Food Program for Women, Infants, and Children (WIC), which provides

iron overload the state of having more iron in the body than it needs or can handle. Too much iron is toxic and can damage the liver.

coupons for supplemental foods high in iron to low-income families, appears also to have helped correct iron deficiency.[23]

Causes of Iron Deficiency The cause of iron deficiency is usually malnutrition, that is, inadequate iron intake, either from sheer lack of food or from high consumption of the wrong foods. In the Western world, high sugar and fat intakes are often responsible for low iron intakes.

Among nonnutritional causes of anemia, blood loss is the primary one. About 80 percent of the iron in the body is in the blood, so iron losses are great whenever blood is lost. Women's menstrual losses make women's iron needs half again as great as men's, but anyone who loses blood loses iron. Women are especially vulnerable to iron deficiency because they not only lose more iron than men but also, on average, eat less food. The information about iron in foods, later in this chapter, is especially important for most women.

In many countries parasitic infections of the digestive tract cause people to lose blood daily. For their entire lives they may feel tired and unenergetic but never know why. Ulcers can also cause blood loss leading to anemia.

Iron Toxicity Iron is toxic in large amounts, and once inside the body, it is difficult to excrete. The body's defense against iron poisoning is a control system: the intestinal cells trap some of the iron and hold it within their boundaries. When they are shed, these cells carry out of the intestinal tract the excess iron that they collected during their brief lives.

Some individuals, however, are poorly defended against iron toxicity. Once considered rare, **iron overload** has emerged as an important iron disorder.[24] Iron overload is caused by a hereditary defect that causes the intestine to helplessly absorb excess iron. Tissue damage occurs, especially in iron-storing organs such as the liver. Infections are likely because bacteria thrive on iron-rich blood. The effects are most severe in alcohol abusers because alcohol damages the intestine, further impairing its defenses against absorbing too much iron.

Iron overload occurs in more men than women. An argument against widespread fortification of foods with iron is that it might put still more men at risk of iron overload. Although the incidence of iron overload seems to have increased over the past few decades, survey data indicate that iron fortification and dietary iron supplements have not contributed to the problem.[25] Most likely, the apparent increase in incidence is due to greater awareness among physicians and enhanced accuracy in diagnosis.[26] Widespread iron fortification of foods makes it difficult for susceptible people to follow a low-iron diet.

Recent research has posed some new questions regarding people's iron stores. Researchers in Finland studied about 2,000 healthy men for three years.[27] The researchers tracked about 20 risk factors for heart attacks, including smoking, blood pressure, cholesterol, and serum ferritin (the protein that carries iron in the blood). At the end of the three years, the risk of heart attack was twice as great for men with high serum ferritin concentrations. The only stronger predictor of heart attack was smoking. In the laboratory, iron acts as a powerful catalyst in oxidation reactions that yield free radicals. Free radical damage is believed to instigate lipid changes that damage the arteries, leading to heart disease. Cells normally stow away their iron atoms securely inside organic molecules such as hemoglobin or ferritin, but the atoms can be released under some conditions. Once free, iron atoms actively promote free radical reactions inside the body.[28] In this way, iron in the body may turn out to have some bearing on the development of heart disease, but much more work is needed to clarify the association.

Table 8-7 on pages 298–300 summarizes the effects of iron toxicity. Be forewarned against unnecessarily taking supplements that contain high doses of iron, and keep such pills safely out of children's reach. Iron supplements are the number one cause of fatal accidental poisonings among U.S. children under three years old.[29]

heme (HEEM) the iron-containing portion of the hemoglobin and myoglobin molecules.

MFP factor a factor (identity unknown) present in **M**eat, **F**ish, and **P**oultry that enhances the absorption of nonheme iron present in the same foods or in other foods eaten at the same time.

phytates compounds present in plant foods (particularly whole grains) that bind iron and prevent its absorption.

Iron Recommendations and Sources

The iron RDA is 10 milligrams a day for men and older women. For women of childbearing age, the RDA is higher, 15 milligrams, to replace menstrual losses. During pregnancy, a woman needs double this amount, 30 milligrams. Adult men experience iron-deficiency anemia rarely. Should a man have a *low* hemoglobin concentration, this alerts his health care provider to examine him for a blood-loss site.

To be sure to meet iron needs, it is best to rely on foods, since the iron from supplements is far less well absorbed than that from food. However, the usual Western mixed diet provides only about 5 to 6 milligrams of iron in each 1,000 calories, not enough for some people. An adult male who eats upwards of 2,500 calories a day has no trouble meeting his RDA of 10 milligrams, but a woman who eats fewer calories and needs *more* iron understandably does have trouble meeting her 15-milligram RDA. To meet it, she must select high-iron, low-calorie foods from each food group.

Dietary factors that increase iron absorption:

- Vitamin C
- MFP factor

Factors that hinder iron absorption:

- Tea
- Coffee
- Calcium and phosphorus
- Phytates and fiber

Iron occurs in two forms in foods: as **heme** iron, bound into the iron-containing part of hemoglobin and myoglobin in meat, poultry, and fish; and as nonheme iron, the kind in foods from plants and the nonheme iron in meats. Its form affects its absorption. Heme iron is much more reliably absorbed than is nonheme iron. Healthy people with adequate iron stores absorb heme iron at a fairly constant rate of about 23 percent over a wide range of meat intakes. People absorb nonheme iron at rates of 2 to 20 percent, depending on dietary factors and iron stores.

Meat, fish, and poultry contain a factor **(MFP factor)** other than heme that promotes the absorption of nonheme iron from other foods eaten with it. Vitamin C proves to be a potent promoter of iron absorption and can triple nonheme iron absorption from foods eaten in the same meal.[30] A system of calculating the amount of iron absorbed from a meal, based on these factors, is presented in Table 8-4.

Some factors impair iron absorption. These include tea, coffee, the calcium and phosphorus in milk, and the **phytates** and fiber in whole-grain cereals. The effect of soy on iron absorption is controversial; some studies have concluded that soy inhibits iron absorption, others indicate no effect. Snapshot 8-5 shows iron amounts in food regarded as rich iron sources.

The amount of iron ultimately absorbed from a meal depends on the interaction between promoters of iron absorption and inhibitors. When you eat meat with legumes (for example, ham and beans or chili with beans and meat), MFP factor enhances iron absorption from both. The vitamin C from a slice of tomato and a leaf of lettuce in a sandwich will enhance iron absorption from the bread. The meat and tomato in spaghetti sauce help the eater to absorb the iron from the spaghetti. A sauce cooked in an iron pan draws iron from this source, too.

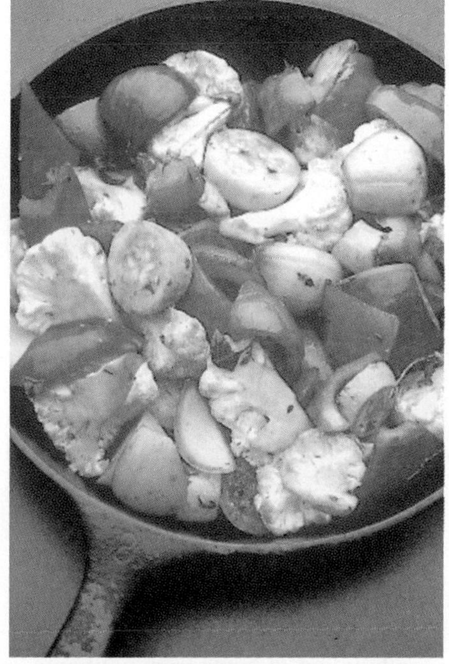

The old-fashioned iron skillet adds supplemental iron to foods.

Table 8-4
Calculation of Iron Absorbed from Meals

Three factors go into the calculation of the amount of iron absorbed from a meal: first, how much of the iron in the meal was heme and how much was nonheme iron; second, how much vitamin C was in the meal; and third, how much total meat, fish, and poultry (MFP) was consumed. (It is assumed your iron stores are moderate; otherwise, you'd have to take this into consideration, too.) Write down the foods you eat at a typical meal, look up their iron content in Appendix A of the text, and then answer these questions:

1. How much iron was from animal tissues (MFP)? _____ mg.
2. 40% of (1), on the average, is heme iron: (1) _____ mg × 0.40 = _____ mg heme iron.
3. How much iron was from other sources? _____ mg.
4. This (3), plus 60% of (1), is nonheme iron: (3) _____ mg + 0.60 × (1) _____ mg = _____ mg nonheme iron.
5. How much vitamin C was in the meal? Less than 25 mg is low; 25 to 75 mg is medium; more than 75 mg is high. _____ mg.
6. How much MFP was in the meal? Less than 1 oz lean MFP is low; 1 to 3 oz is medium; more than 3 oz is high.[a] _____ oz.
7. Now calculate the heme iron absorbed. You absorbed 23% of the heme iron, or (2) _____ mg × 0.23 = _____ mg heme iron absorbed.
8. Now, take your best score from (5) and (6). If either vitamin C or MFP was high or if both were medium, the availability of your nonheme iron was high. If neither was high, but one was medium, the availability of your nonheme iron was medium. If both were low, your nonheme iron had poor availability. You absorbed:
   - High availability: 8% of the nonheme iron.
   - Medium availability: 5% of the nonheme iron.
   - Poor availability: 3% of the nonheme iron.
9. Now calculate the nonheme iron absorbed. You absorbed _____ % of the nonheme iron, or (4) _____ mg × _____ = _____ mg nonheme iron absorbed.
10. Add the heme and nonheme iron from (7) and (9) together:
    - _____ mg heme iron absorbed.
    - _____ mg nonheme iron absorbed.

    Total = _____ mg iron absorbed.

The RDA assumes you will absorb 10% of the iron you ingest. Thus, if you are a man over age 18 or a woman over age 50 (RDA 10 mg), you need to absorb 1 mg per day. If you are a woman 11 to 50 years old (RDA 15 mg), you need to absorb 1.5 mg per day. If you have higher menstrual losses than the average woman, you may need still more.

[a]We have adapted the calculation of Monsen and coauthors, stating it in ounces. Her actual numbers are less than 23 g cooked meat, low; 23 to 46 g, medium: and 69 g or more, high.

Source: E. R. Monsen and coauthors, Estimation of available dietary iron, *American Journal of Clinical Nutrition* 31 (1978): 134–141.

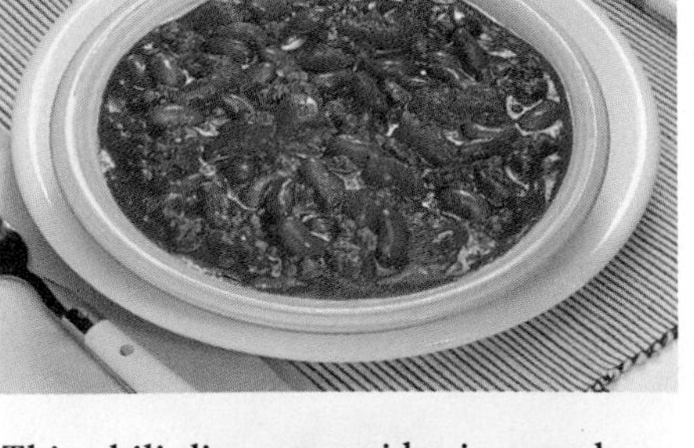

This chili dinner provides iron and MFP from meat, iron from legumes, and vitamin C from tomatoes. The combination of heme iron, nonheme iron, MFP, and vitamin C helps to achieve maximum iron absorption.

Foods cooked in iron pans contain iron salts somewhat like those in supplements. The iron content of 100 grams of spaghetti sauce simmered in a glass dish is 3 milligrams, but it is 87 milligrams when the sauce is cooked in a black iron skillet. Even in the short time it takes to scramble eggs, a cook can triple the eggs' iron content by scrambling them in an iron pan. Similarly, the reason why dried peaches or raisins contain more iron

SNAPSHOT 8-5

IRON

RDA for men: 10 mg/day
RDA for women: 15 mg/day

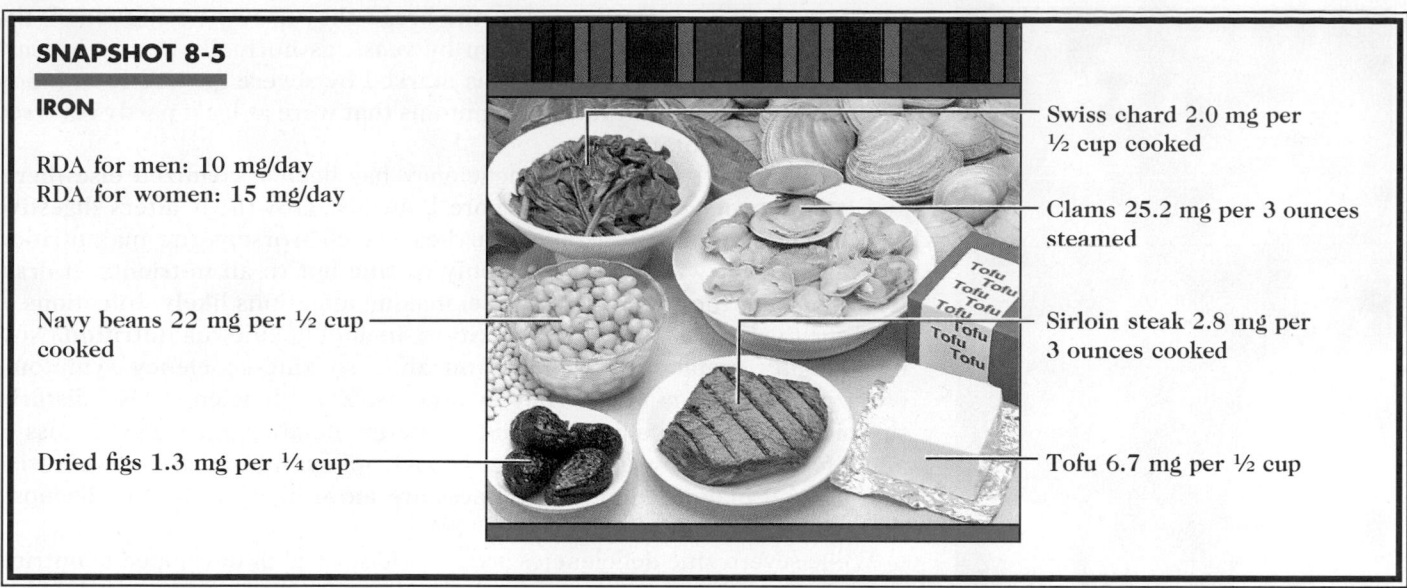

than the fresh fruit is because they are dried in iron pans. This iron is in the ferric form, an inorganic salt that is not as well absorbed as that from meat, but some does get into the body.

KEY POINT Most iron in the body is contained in hemoglobin and myoglobin or occurs as part of enzymes in the energy-yielding pathways. Iron-deficiency anemia is a problem worldwide. Iron is lost through menstruation and other bleeding; the shedding of intestinal cells protects against overload. Too much iron is toxic. For maximum iron absorption, use meat, other iron sources, and vitamin C together.

Zinc

Zinc occurs in a very small quantity in the body, but works with proteins in every organ as a helper for more than 100 enzymes. Zinc works with enzymes that:

- Make parts of cells' genetic material.
- Make heme in hemoglobin.
- Help the pancreas with its digestive functions.
- Help metabolize carbohydrate, protein, and fat.
- Liberate vitamin A from storage in the liver.
- Dispose of damaging free radicals.

Zinc also affects behavior and learning, assists in immune function, and is essential to wound healing, sperm production, taste perception, fetal development, and growth in children. Zinc is needed to produce the active form of vitamin A in visual pigments. When zinc deficiency occurs, it impairs all these and other functions. Even a mild zinc deficiency can result in impaired immunity, abnormal taste, and abnormal vision in the dark.[31]

Zinc deficiency in human beings was first reported in the 1960s from studies with growing children and adolescent boys in the Middle East. The native diets were typically low in animal protein and high in whole grains and beans; consequently they were high in fiber and phytates, which bind

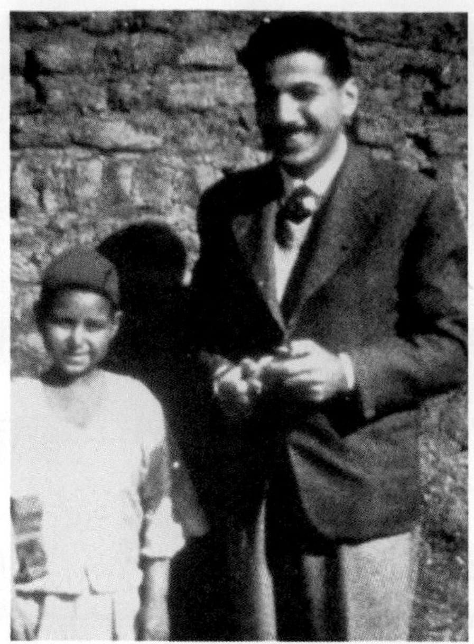

A zinc-deficient teenager and a well-nourished adult man. The Egyptian boy in the picture is 17 years old but is only 4 feet tall, the height of a 7-year-old in the United States. His genitalia are like those of a six-year-old. The retardation is rightly ascribed to zinc deficiency because it is partially reversible when zinc is restored to the diet.

zinc as well as iron. Furthermore, the bread they ate was unleavened; the phytates had not been broken down by yeast, as normally occurs in leavened bread. The zinc deficiency was marked by severe growth retardation and arrested sexual maturation, symptoms that were at least partly reversed by zinc supplementation.

Since the first reports, zinc deficiency has been recognized elsewhere, and it is known to affect much more than just growth. It alters digestive function profoundly and causes diarrhea, which worsens the malnutrition already present, with respect not only to zinc but to all nutrients. It drastically impairs the immune response, making infections likely. Infections of the intestinal tract worsen malnutrition, including zinc malnutrition. Normal vitamin metabolism depends on zinc, so zinc-deficiency symptoms often include vitamin-deficiency symptoms. Zinc deficiency also disturbs thyroid function and slows the body's energy metabolism. It causes loss of appetite and slows wound healing. In fact, its symptoms are so pervasive that general malnutrition and sickness are more likely to be the diagnosis than zinc deficiency alone.

While severe zinc deficiencies are not widespread in developed countries, they occur among some groups, including pregnant women, young children, the elderly, and the poor. Among these people, poor growth, poor appetite, and impaired taste sensitivity may indicate zinc deficiency. When pediatricians or other health workers evaluating children's health note poor growth accompanied by poor appetite, they should think zinc.

Zinc is toxic in large quantities, and zinc supplements can cause serious illness or even death in high enough doses. Doses of zinc only a few milligrams above the RDA, especially when taken regularly over time, lower the body's copper content, an effect that, in animals, leads to degeneration of the heart muscle. In high doses, zinc also alters cholesterol metabolism and appears to accelerate the development of atherosclerosis. High doses of zinc can also inhibit iron absorption from the digestive tract.[32] In the blood, a protein that carries iron from the digestive tract to tissues that need it also carries some zinc. If this protein is burdened with excess zinc, then little or no room is left for iron to be picked up from the intestine. The opposite is also true; too much iron leaves little room for zinc to be picked up, thus impairing zinc absorption. Zinc and iron are often found together in foods, but food sources never cause imbalances like these in the body. Supplements, though, can easily do so.

Unlike excess iron, excess zinc can escape from the body. The pancreas secretes zinc-rich juices into the digestive tract, and some of these are excreted. Still, overdoses from zinc supplements can overwhelm the route of escape and cause toxicity. For zinc, then, supplements should be avoided unless prescribed by a physician. Foods, on the other hand, are safe sources.

Meats, shellfish, and poultry are top providers of zinc (see Snapshot 8-6). Among plant sources, some legumes and whole grains are rich in zinc, but the zinc is not as well absorbed from them as from meat. The RDA of 15 milligrams per day for men and 12 milligrams per day for women is probably not met by most people; the average intake is probably closer to 10 milligrams. Vegetarians are advised to eat varied diets that include whole-grain breads well leavened with yeast, which improves the availability of zinc.

KEY POINT Zinc assists enzymes in all cells. Deficiencies in children cause growth retardation with sexual immaturity. Zinc is toxic in large amounts. Animal foods are the best sources.

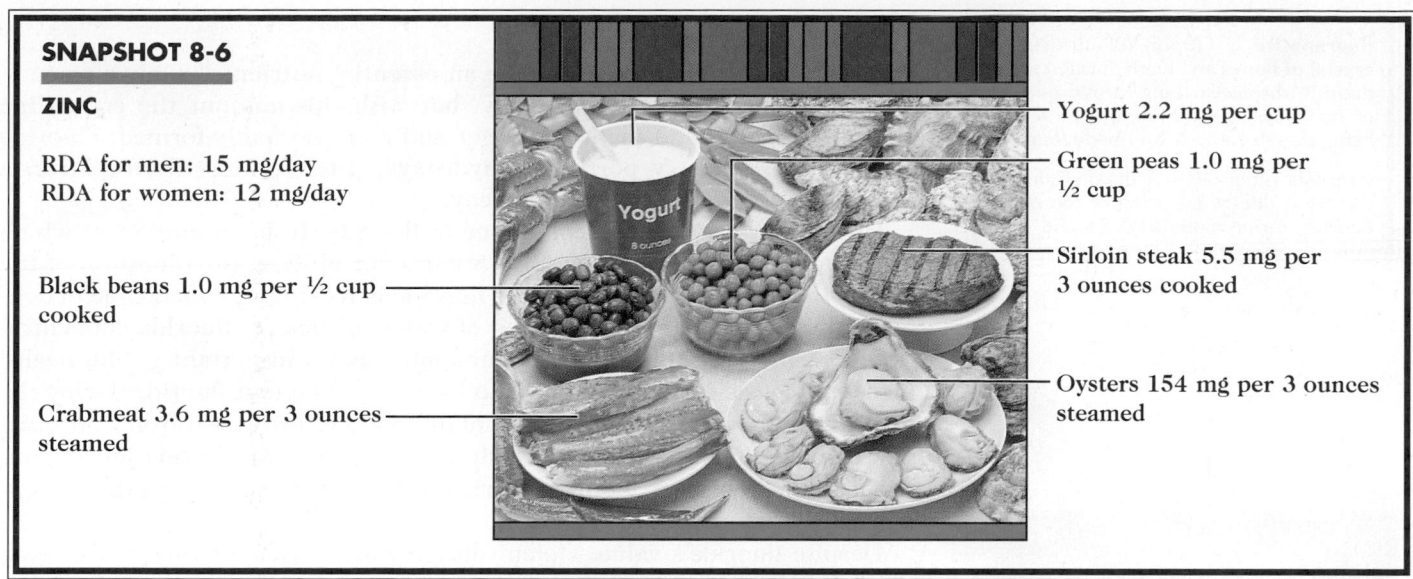

Selenium

Selenium has been attracting attention for its role in assisting vitamin E in protecting vulnerable body chemicals from oxidation. Selenium has a sparing effect on vitamin E because it can take the place of vitamin E in some antioxidant activities. The question of whether selenium protects against the development of cancers is currently under investigation. So far the results are inconclusive. Among the most recent discoveries about selenium is a role for the mineral in the hormone that regulates the body's rate of metabolism, thyroid hormone.[33]

A deficiency of selenium in people can open the way for a specific type of heart disease (unrelated to the heart disease discussed in Chapters 5 and 11). The condition, first identified in China among people from areas with selenium-deficient soils, led researchers to connect selenium deficiency to this disease, thus elevating the mineral to its rightful place among the essential nutrients (see the inside front cover; page B lists selenium's RDA value). The soils in the United States and Canada grow foods that supply plenty of selenium.

In laboratory animals, selenium deficiency is hard to produce. To induce it, selenium-free diets must be fed to two generations of animals. Anyone who eats a normal diet composed of mostly unprocessed foods need not worry about selenium. It is widely distributed in foods such as meats and shellfish and in vegetables and grains grown on selenium-rich soil. From current indications, it is likely that most people in the United States receive well over the RDA amount.[34]

Toxicity is possible, especially when people take selenium supplements over a long period. Selenium toxicity brings on symptoms such as hair loss, diarrhea, and nerve abnormalities. Selenium supplements taken inappropriately as an anticancer agent make selenium toxicity likely.[35]

KEY POINT Selenium works with vitamin E to protect body compounds from oxidation. A deficiency induces a disease of the heart. Deficiencies in developed countries are rare, but toxicities occur from overuse of supplements.

fluorapatite (floor-APP-uh-tight) a crystal of bones and teeth, formed when fluoride displaces the hydroxy portion of hydroxyapatite. Fluorapatite resists being dissolved back into body fluid.

fluorosis (floor-OH-sis) discoloration of the teeth due to ingestion of too much fluoride during tooth development.

Fluoride

Fluoride has not been proven to be an essential nutrient.[36] Only a trace of fluoride occurs in the human body, but with this amount the crystalline deposits in bones and teeth are larger and more perfectly formed. Fluoride replaces the hydroxy portion of hydroxyapatite, forming **fluorapatite,** a crystal that is more resistant to decay.

Drinking water is the usual source of fluoride. In communities in which the water contains too much, 2 to 8 parts per million, discoloration of the teeth, **fluorosis,** may occur. Where fluoride is lacking, the incidence of dental decay is very high. Fluoridation of water to raise its fluoride concentration to 1 part per million is recommended as an important public health measure. Those fortunate enough to have had sufficient fluoride during the tooth-forming years of infancy and childhood are protected from tooth decay throughout life.[37] Figure 8-7 shows the extent of fluoridation nationwide; states that have adopted fluoridation in more than half of their counties are shown in color.

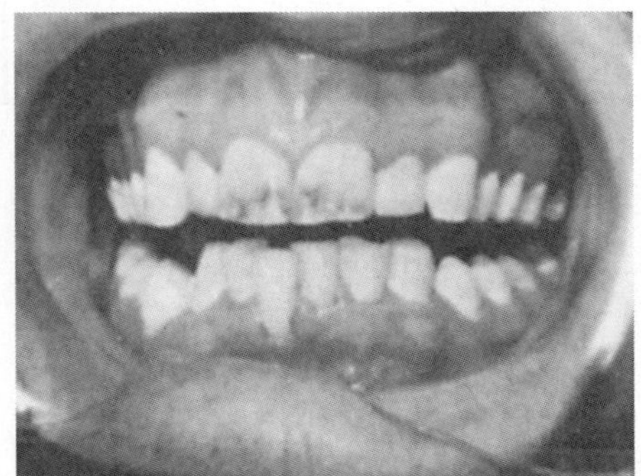

Fluorosis

Despite fluoride's value, violent disagreement often surrounds the decision concerning fluoridation of community water. Proponents argue that fluoridation is an obvious, safe, and cost-effective measure to help prevent dental caries in the young. Opponents argue that altering the community water supply is "unnatural" and deprives its consumers of the freedom to refuse to take fluoride. They fear accidental overdoses, perhaps mistaking the relatively nontoxic salt sodium *fluoride* for the highly volatile gas *fluorine,* which is deadly in excess. They may claim that communities using fluoridated water have an increased cancer rate, but studies on this show no connection.

On the basis of the accumulated evidence of its beneficial effects, fluoridation has been endorsed by the National Institute of Dental Health, the

Figure 8-7

FLUORIDATION IN THE UNITED STATES

Source: Fluoridation Census 1989 Summary, U.S. Department of Health and Human Services, Public Health Service, Centers for Disease Control and Prevention, National Center for Prevention Services, Division of Oral Health, Atlanta, GA, April 1993.

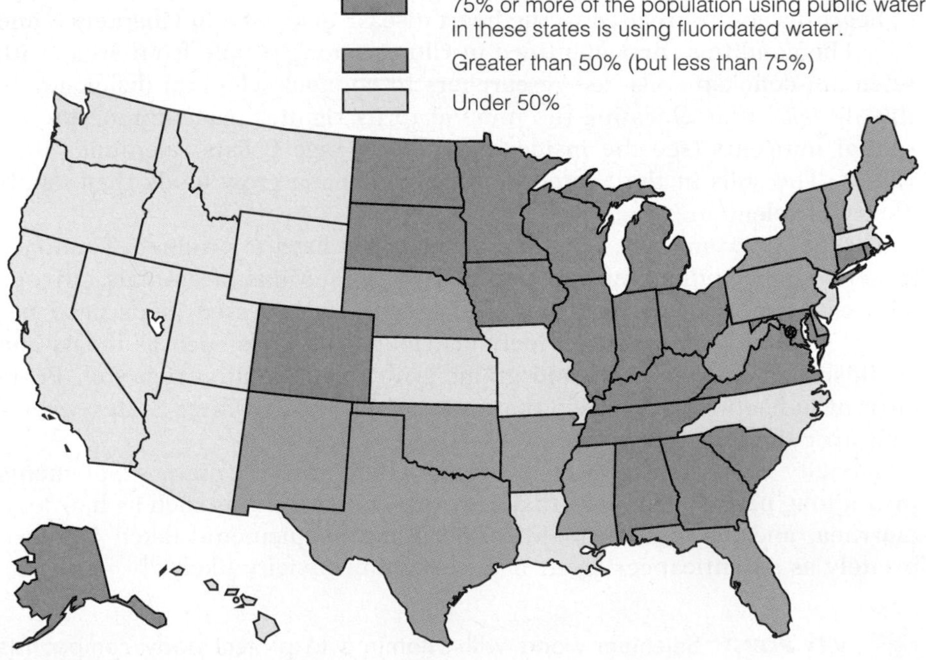

American Medical Association, the National Cancer Institute, and the National Nutrition Consortium. The allegation that it causes cancer has no basis in fact and has been refuted by the National Cancer Institute, the American Cancer Society, and the National Institute of Dental Research.

Now that fluoride has been added to many water supplies, the amounts in foods processed with use of that water are increasing. The total fluoride consumed by certain populations may therefore be greater than expected. No hazard exists at present levels of fluoride consumption, but continued monitoring is important.

KEY POINT Fluoride stabilizes bones and makes teeth resistant to decay. Excess fluoride discolors teeth; large doses are toxic.

Chromium

Chromium works closely with the hormone insulin, facilitating the uptake of glucose into cells and the release of its energy. Chromium occurs in foods in association with several different complexes. Early research identified chromium as part of a small organic compound given the name **glucose tolerance factor (GTF).**[38] Researchers suggest the term "biologically active chromium" to describe the chromium-containing compound because in this form, chromium is easily used by the body. When chromium is lacking, insulin action is impaired, resulting in a diabeteslike condition of high blood glucose.[39] In addition, diets that are high in simple sugars deplete the body's supply of chromium.[40]

Although chromium is present in a variety of foods, it is estimated that 90 percent of U.S. adults consume less than the recommended minimum intake of 50 micrograms a day.[41] Chromium is easily lost during food processing, as are other trace minerals. As people find themselves more pressed for time and depend more heavily on refined foods, chromium deficiencies become more likely. The best chromium food sources are liver, whole grains, nuts, and cheeses.

KEY POINT Chromium works with the hormone insulin to control blood glucose concentration. Many adults in the United States have low dietary intakes of chromium.

glucose tolerance factor (GTF) one name given to a form of chromium thought to be biologically active; a complex of chromium and several small organic molecules.

Copper

Among copper's most vital roles are to help form hemoglobin and collagen. Copper is needed in many enzymes. Copper, like iron, assists in many of the reactions related to the release of energy.

Copper deficiency is rare but not unknown. It has been seen in children with protein deficiency and iron-deficiency anemia, and it can severely disturb growth and metabolism. Excess zinc interferes with copper absorption and can cause deficiency. Copper toxicity from foods is unlikely, but supplements can cause it. The best food sources of copper include organ meats, seafood, nuts, and seeds.

KEY POINT Copper is needed to form hemoglobin and collagen and in many other body processes. Copper deficiency is rare.

Other Trace Minerals

As is true of fluoride, chromium, and copper, estimated safe and adequate daily dietary intakes are established for two other trace minerals, *molybdenum* and *manganese.* Molybdenum functions as part of several metal-containing enzymes, some of which are giant proteins. Manganese works with dozens of different enzymes that facilitate many different body processes.

Several other trace minerals are now recognized as important to health. Research suggests that dietary lack of *boron* may be one factor that enhances susceptibility to osteoporosis by way of its effects on calcium metabolism.[42] The richest food sources of boron are noncitrus fruits, leafy vegetables, nuts, and legumes. *Cobalt* is recognized as the mineral in the large vitamin B_{12} molecule; the alternative name for vitamin B_{12}, cobalamin, reflects its presence. *Nickel* is important for the health of many body tissues; deficiencies harm the liver and other organs. *Silicon* is known to be involved in bone calcification, at least in animals. The future may reveal that many other trace minerals also play key roles: barium, cadmium, lead, lithium, mercury, silver, tin, vanadium. Even arsenic, a known poison and carcinogen, may turn out to be essential in tiny quantities.

As research on the trace minerals continues, many interactions among them are also coming to light. An excess of one may cause a deficiency of another. A slight manganese overload, for example, may aggravate an iron deficiency. A deficiency of one may open the way for another to cause a toxic reaction. Iron deficiency, for example, makes the body much more susceptible to lead poisoning than it normally is. Good food sources of one are poor food sources of another, and factors that cooperate with some trace elements oppose others. Vitamin C, for example, enhances the absorption of iron and depresses that of copper. The continuous outpouring of new information about the trace minerals is a sign that we have much more to learn.

All of the trace minerals are toxic in excess. The hazards of overdoses are among the chief risks faced by people who take multiple nutrient supplements. The way to obtain the trace minerals is from food, which is not hard to do. You need only eat a variety of whole foods in the amounts recommended in the Daily Food Guide. Some claim that organically grown foods contain more trace minerals than those grown on chemical fertilizers. Organic fertilizers do contain more trace minerals than do refined chemical fertilizers, and plants do take up some of the minerals they are given, so this claim may turn out to be valid. Table 8-7 on pages 298–300 sums up what this chapter has said about the minerals and fills in some additional information. The next section provides details about controlling intakes of foods high in sodium chloride for the purpose of controlling hypertension.

KEY POINT Many different trace elements play important roles in the body. All of the trace minerals are toxic in excess.

FOOD FEATURE

Controlling Salt Intake

The role of diet, and specifically of salt, in the *prevention* of hypertension has been debated. The evidence is inconclusive. The value of a low-salt diet in the treatment of *established* hypertension is unquestioned, however. Studies have shown that even mild restriction of salt can produce a modest but definite fall in blood pressure in many people.

One of the problems that plagues people attempting to understand the links between salt and hypertension is the need to distinguish between *sodium* and *sodium chloride*, or *salt*. The chloride ion may be as important as the sodium ion, and salt may be what people need to limit. Most advice is still phrased in terms of sodium, though, so that people are forced to avoid more products than necessary, such as baking soda (sodium bicarbonate) and other sodium salts. Most guidelines to reduce dietary sodium intake also reduce salt intake, so here are some recommendations for those who wish to reduce their salt *and* sodium intakes.

First, remember that salt poured from the salt shaker contributes little to most people's total salt consumption, but processed foods and fast foods contribute greatly. Whole, unprocessed foods contain only small amounts of salt naturally, and these foods plus the water you drink contain enough salt to meet the needs for sodium and chloride. Use many more whole foods and you will have accomplished a tremendous reduction in your salt intake. Notice, too, from Table 8-5, that in each food group the least processed foods are not only lowest in sodium but also highest in potassium, an added benefit. No recommendation has been

Table 8-5
Processing Reduces Potassium, Increases Sodium in Foods

Food	Potassium (mg)	Sodium (mg)	Ratio
Milk Foods			
Milk (whole), 1 c	368	119	3:1
Chocolate pudding, 1 c (home cooked)	424	268	2:1
Chocolate pudding, 1 c (instant)	432	738	1:2
Meats			
Beef roast (cooked), 3 oz	252	54	5:1
Corned beef (canned), 3 oz	116	855	1:7
Chipped beef, 3 oz	377	2949	1:8
Vegetables			
Corn (cooked), 1 c	226	8	28:1
Creamed corn (canned), 1 c	344	730	1:2
Cornflakes, 1 c	20	228	1:11
Fruits			
Peaches (fresh), 1	171	1	171:1
Peaches (canned), 1	150	10	15:1
Peach pie, 1 piece	149	288	1:2
Grains			
Whole-wheat flour, 1 c	486	6	81:1
Whole-wheat bread, 1 slice	34	135	1:4
Wheat crackers, 4	17	69	1:4

made for the potassium-to-sodium ratio of the diet. The RDA tables indicate that a 2-to-1 ratio or higher is acceptable; lower might not be. Figure 8-8 goes on to identify some sources of sodium in the U.S. diet.

In reducing your intakes of processed foods, pay particular attention to those listed in Table 8-6. Also notice that processed foods don't always taste salty. Most people are surprised to learn that a serving of cornflakes contains more sodium than a serving of cocktail peanuts and that a serving of instant chocolate pudding contains still more. In the case of the peanuts, they may *taste* saltier than cornflakes because the salt sits on the surface, allowing faster contact with the salt-sensing taste buds. The sodium of instant pudding originates as sodium-containing thickeners, not from salt itself. The Checking Out Food Labels section identifies the sodium listed on food labels and demonstrates how other minerals and vitamins appear.

If you cook without salt, you may find that just a tiny shake of salt at the table will produce a salty flavor atop your food (remember the peanuts). Then you won't even miss the salt normally added in cooking. Soon you may learn to skip the salt entirely and enjoy the unsalted flavors of foods. Or you may learn to enhance them with salt-free spices such as cinnamon, curry, garlic, ginger, lemon, mustard powder, nutmeg, paprika, parsley, and thyme. Sour flavors, such as lemon juice and vinegar, are especially useful in replacing salt because they enhance what-

Figure 8-8

SOURCES OF SODIUM IN THE U.S. DIET

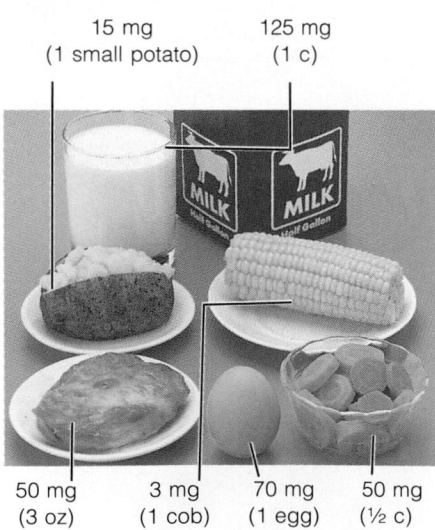

Unprocessed foods that are low in sodium contribute less than 10 percent of the total sodium in the U.S. diet.

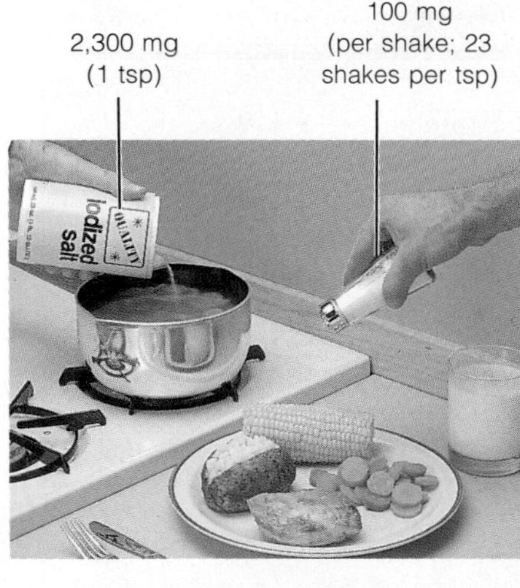

Salt added at home, in cooking or at the table, contributes 15 percent of the total sodium in the U.S. diet.

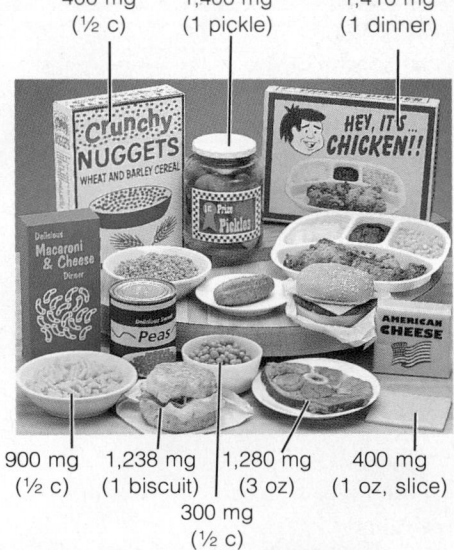

Processed foods such as these contribute 75 percent of the sodium in the U.S. diet.

ever natural salty flavor a food may have. As salt intake gradually decreases, the taste buds adjust, and the taste of food with less salt becomes the preferred taste.

Make substitutions too. In particular, use low-salt canned bouillon and broth and homemade, salt-free stocks. Choose salt-free or low-sodium products whenever they are offered. Many other low-sodium products are available, but in general you can make a low-sodium diet attractive without using these products. Some people, however, like to use them to add variety.

When soft water is used in food products, it may contribute significantly to salt intake. Learn whether your water is hard or soft, and adjust your use of salt accordingly. Be aware that medications, toothpastes, mouthwashes, and other nonfood products may also contain salt.

In salt substitutes the sodium is generally replaced by potassium. Some people don't like the taste of salt substitutes but may find them acceptable if used sparingly. (Don't heat them, though, because they turn bitter.) Often people find foods more acceptable without any salt at all. The use of a potassium-containing salt substitute serves the dual purpose of increasing potassium intake while reducing sodium intake.* Some products contain a combination of regular table salt and salt substitute. Although these products may be more palatable, they also can contribute a significant amount of salt to the diet.

Besides all these considerations, many positive choices are possible. The person who wishes to use diet to prevent or to reduce high blood pressure should limit alcohol intake and should also eat plenty of fresh fruits, vegetables, milk products, legumes, and meats for potassium, calcium, and magnesium. Also it is important to maintain appropriate weight and engage in regular, enjoyable, vigorous physical activity, topics emphasized in the next two chapters.

*People with renal insufficiency should not use salt substitutes containing potassium.

Table 8-6
Foods Especially High in Salt or Sodium

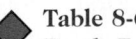

Foods Especially High in Salt or Sodium
Foods prepared in brine, such as pickles, olives, and sauerkraut.
Salty or smoked meat, such as bologna, corned or chipped beef, frankfurters, ham, luncheon meats, salt pork, sausage, and smoked tongue.
Salty or smoked fish, such as anchovies, caviar, salted and dried cod, herring, sardines, and smoked salmon.
Snack items such as potato chips, pretzels, salted popcorn, and salted nuts and crackers.
Bouillon cubes; seasoned salts (including sea salt); MSG; soy sauce, Worcestershire sauce, and barbecue sauce.
Fast foods.
Cheeses, especially processed types.
Canned and instant soups.
Prepared horseradish, catsup, mustard, and salad dressings.

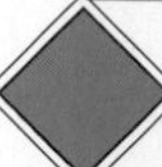

CHECKING OUT FOOD LABELS

How to Read Vitamin and Mineral Information on a Food Label

The FDA and USDA have selected two vitamins and three minerals to be highlighted on labels. These nutrients are well chosen to reflect the health concerns of people today. Vitamins A and C are in short supply in some people's diets. The minerals calcium and iron are included because they, too, are often lacking in the diet. In contrast, sodium is one of the nutrients many people must limit in their diets.

Nutrients such as niacin and potassium, whose listing on labels is optional, are also important in nutrition, of course. But neither deficiencies nor excesses of them are seen in people eating typical diets in the United States. Figure 8-9 presents labels of two cans of food—sweet potatoes and vegetable soup. Search the labels shown there to find each of the five nutrients just named. Not all are in the same place on the label.

NUTRITION FACTS PANEL

Notice that sodium is listed right under fat and cholesterol, rather than appearing in smaller type with vitamin A, vitamin C, calcium, and iron. In our society, consuming too little sodium is almost impossible, while overconsuming it is all too easy. For this reason, sodium takes its place with nutrients for which the *upper* limit is of greatest concern. Of these two foods, the one without added salt is lowest in sodium. Table 2-9 of Chapter 2 defined some sodium terms used on food labels.

PERCENT DAILY VALUE

The Percent Daily Value column compares the sodium in a serving of the food with the recommendation listed in the first column at the bottom of the label. The chart lists the same maximum sodium intake for both calorie levels. That means that a person who eats an extra 500 calories of energy is supposed to do so without adding extra sodium from those foods.

The sweet potato label lists a contribution of only 2 percent of the Daily Value for sodium. This is typical of single-ingredient foods and of those processed without added salt. In contrast, the soup label shows that the processors of the soup liberally seasoned it with salt. One serving of the soup provides a full one third of the Daily Value for sodium. At the same time, a serving of the soup provides only 3 percent of the calories for a person needing 2,000 calories a day. The rest of that day's foods will have to be very low in sodium if the person who eats this soup is not to exceed the Daily Value limit for sodium.

Percent Daily Values for vitamins and minerals other than sodium are listed under the second thick rule. A label reader can use this information to find exactly how much of a vitamin or mineral is in a serving of the food. Then, a comparison of the milligrams of a nutrient to the RDA recommendation is possible. For example, the vegetable soup provides 20 percent of the Daily Value of 1,000 RE, or 200 RE vitamin A. This amount can be compared with your own RDA for vitamin A. The same sort of comparison works as well for the other vitamins and minerals whose values are given only as percent of Daily Value on labels. The Daily Value tables on page C, inside front cover, and Appendix C provide help with these calculations.

Notice that the amount of vitamin A from beta carotene is also listed. This information is optional and may only appear on labels of foods that contribute significant beta carotene. Labels may also omit listings for nutrients present in insignificant amounts as the vegetable soup label has done for saturated fat, cholesterol, and calcium.

HEALTH CLAIMS

Both labels bear banners announcing their contribution of beta carotene because both meet the legal definition of a food that is high in that nutrient. One, though, goes on to make a claim about cancer, fruits and vegetables, and vitamin A. This is a health claim, and some of the requirements for making such a claim were described in the Checking Out Food Labels section of Chapter 6. The ones there described allowable fat, saturated fat, and cholesterol, but other requirements concern the vitamins and minerals. First, a food must contain a vegetable or fruit or be a vegetable or fruit and both these products meet that requirement. Second, the food must qualify as a "good source" of vitamin A, vitamin C, or dietary fiber. (Recall from Table 2-9 of Chapter 2 that a "good source" of a nutrient provides, per serving, at least 10 percent of the Daily Value of that nutrient.) Both the products shown here also meet this requirement. Third, a serving of the food "must not contribute any nutrient or food substance in an amount that increases the risk of a disease or health condition."[43] In the case of sodium, the cutoff point for allowing a health claim is 360 mg of sodium per serving. Of the two labels here, the one from sweet potatoes alone meets all three of these requirements and so earns the privilege to bear a health claim.

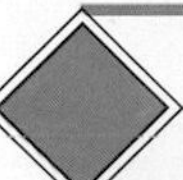

CHECKING OUT FOOD LABELS

How to Read Vitamin and Mineral Information on a Food Label *continued*

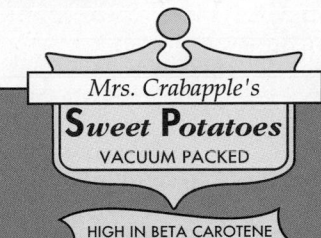

HIGH IN BETA CAROTENE

Nutrition Facts

Serving Size 1/2 cup (95 g)
Servings per Can 4

Amount per serving

Calories 92 Calories from Fat 0

	% Daily Value*
Total Fat 0g	0%
Saturated Fat 0g	0%
Cholesterol 0mg	0%
Sodium 55mg	2%
Total Carbohydrate 21g	7%
Dietary fiber 2g	8%
Sugars 5g	
Protein 2g	

Vitamin A 160% (100% as Beta Carotene) •
Vitamin C 40% • Calcium 2% • Iron 4%

*Percent Daily Values are based on a 2,000 calorie diet. Your Daily Values may be higher or lower depending on your calorie

	Calories	2,000	2,500
Total Fat	Less than	65g	80g
Sat Fat	Less than	20g	25g
Cholesterol	Less than	300mg	300mg
Sodium	Less than	2,400mg	2,400mg
Total Carbohydrate		300g	375g
Dietary Fiber		25g	30g

Calories per gram
Fat 9 • Carbohydrate 4 • Protein 4

INGREDIENTS: Sweet Potatoes

DEVELOPMENT OF CANCER DEPENDS ON MANY FACTORS. EATING A DIET LOW IN FAT AND HIGH IN FRUITS AND VEGETABLES, FOODS THAT ARE LOW IN FAT AND MAY CONTAIN VITAMIN A, VITAMIN C, AND DIETARY FIBER, MAY REDUCE YOUR RISK OF SOME CANCERS. SWEET POTATOES ARE A FOOD LOW IN FAT AND HIGH IN VITAMIN A (BETA CAROTENE).

BEDFORD FALLS

Vegetable Soup

HIGH IN BETA CAROTENE

Nutrition Facts

Serving Size 1 cup (245 g)
Servings per Can 2

Amount per serving

Calories 69 Calories from Fat 9

	% Daily Value*
Total Fat 1g	2%
Sodium 800mg	33%
Total Carbohydrate 13g	4%
Dietary fiber 4g	16%
Sugars 0g	
Protein 2g	

Vitamin A 160% (100% as Beta Carotene) •
Vitamin C 10% • Iron 2%

Not a significant source of saturated fat, cholesterol, and calcium

*Percent Daily Values are based on a 2,000 calorie diet. Your Daily Values may be higher or lower depending on your calorie needs.

	Calories	2,000	2,500
Total Fat	Less than	65g	80g
Sat Fat	Less than	20g	25g
Cholesterol	Less than	300mg	300mg
Sodium	Less than	2,400mg	2,400mg
Total Carbohydrate		300g	375g
Dietary Fiber		25g	30g

Calories per gram
Fat 9 • Carbohydrate 4 • Protein 4

INGREDIENTS: Water, potatoes, carrots, tomatoes, celery, "Italian" green beans, enriched macaroni product (enriched with niacin, ferrous sulfate, thiamine mononitrate and riboflavin), potato starch, kidney, salt, parmesan cheese (Pasteurized milk, cheese culture, salt, enzymes), dehydrated onions, monosodium glutamate, butter, spice, dehydrated garlic and dehydrated parsley.

Figure 8-9

SWEET POTATOES AND VEGETABLE SOUP

Table 8-7
The Minerals—A Summary

Mineral Name	Chief Functions in the Body	Deficiency Symptoms	Toxicity Symptoms	Significant Sources
		MAJOR MINERALS		
Calcium	The principal mineral of bones and teeth. Also acts in normal muscle contraction and relaxation, nerve functioning, blood clotting, blood pressure, and immune defenses.	Stunted growth in children; adult bone loss (osteoporosis).	Excess calcium is excreted except in hormonal imbalance states (not caused by nutritional deficiency).	Milk and milk products, oysters, small fish (with bones), tofu (bean curd), greens, legumes.
Phosphorus	Phosphorus is important in cells' genetic material, in cell membranes as phospholipids, in energy transfer, and in buffering systems.	Phosphorus deficiency unknown.	Excess phosphorus may cause calcium excretion.	All animal tissues.
Magnesium	Another factor involved in bone mineralization, the building of protein, enzyme action, normal muscular contraction, transmission of nerve impulses, and maintenance of teeth.	Weakness; confusion; depressed pancreatic hormone secretion; if extreme, convulsions, bizarre movements (especially of eyes and face), hallucinations, and difficulty in swallowing. In children, growth failure.[a]	Not known; large doses have been taken in the form of the laxative Epsom salts, without ill effects except diarrhea.	Nuts, legumes, whole grains, dark green vegetables, seafoods, chocolate, cocoa.
Sodium	Sodium, chloride, and potassium (electrolytes) maintain cells' normal fluid balance and acid-base balance in the body. Sodium is critical to nerve impulse transmission.	Muscle cramps, mental apathy, loss of appetite.	Hypertension.	Salt, soy sauce, processed foods.
Chloride	Chloride is also part of the hydrochloric acid found in the stomach, necessary for proper digestion.	Growth failure in children; muscle cramps, mental apathy, loss of appetite; can cause death (uncommon).	Normally harmless (the gas chlorine is a poison but evaporates from water); can cause vomiting.	Salt, soy sauce; moderate quantities in whole, unprocessed foods, large amounts in processed foods.

[a]A still more severe deficiency causes tetany, an extreme, prolonged contraction of the muscles similar to that caused by low blood calcium.

(continued on next page)

Table 8-7
The Minerals—A Summary (continued)

Mineral Name	Chief Functions in the Body	Deficiency Symptoms	Toxicity Symptoms	Significant Sources
		MAJOR MINERALS		
Potassium	Potassium facilitates reactions, including the making of protein; the maintenance of fluid and electrolyte balance; the support of cell integrity; the transmission of nerve impulses; and the contraction of muscles, including the heart.	Deficiency accompanies dehydration; causes muscular weakness, paralysis, and confusion; can cause death.	Causes muscular weakness; triggers vomiting; if given into a vein, can stop the heart.	All whole foods: meats, milk, fruits, vegetables, grains, legumes.
Sulfur	A component of certain amino acids; part of the vitamins biotin and thiamin and the hormone insulin; combines with toxic substances to form harmless compounds; stabilizes protein shape by forming sulfur-sulfur bridges (see Figure 6-11 in Chapter 6).	None known; protein deficiency would occur first.	Would occur only if sulfur amino acids were eaten in excess; this (in animals) depresses growth.	All protein-containing foods.
		TRACE MINERALS		
Iodine	A component of the thyroid hormone thyroxine, which helps to regulate growth, development, and metabolic rate.	Goiter, cretinism.	Depressed thyroid activity; goiter-like thyroid enlargement.	Iodized salt; seafood; bread; plants grown in most parts of the country and animals fed those plants.
Iron	Part of the protein hemoglobin, which carries oxygen in the blood; part of the protein myoglobin in muscles, which makes oxygen available for muscle contraction; necessary for the utilization of energy.	Anemia: weakness, pallor, headaches, reduced resistance to infection, inability to concentrate, lowered cold tolerance.	Iron overload: infections, liver injury, possible increased risk of heart attack, acidosis, bloody stools, shock.	Red meats, fish, poultry, shellfish, eggs, legumes, dried fruits.

(continued on next page)

Table 8-7
The Minerals—A Summary (continued)

Mineral Name	Chief Functions in the Body	Deficiency Symptoms	Toxicity Symptoms	Significant Sources
		TRACE MINERALS		
Zinc	Part of the hormone insulin and many enzymes; involved in making genetic material and proteins, immune reactions, transport of vitamin A, taste perception, wound healing, the making of sperm, and normal fetal development.	Growth failure in children, sexual retardation, loss of taste, poor wound healing.	Fever, nausea, vomiting, diarrhea, muscle incoordination, dizziness, anemia, accelerated atherosclerosis, kidney failure.	Protein-containing foods: meats, fish, shellfish, poultry, grains, vegetables.
Selenium	Part of an enzyme that breaks down reactive chemicals that harm cells; works with vitamin E.	Muscle discomfort, weakness, pancreas damage, heart disease (cardiomyopathy).	Nausea, abdominal pain, nail and hair changes, nerve damage.	Seafoods, organ meats; other meats, grains and vegetables depending on soil conditions.

Notes

1. T. Vokes, Water homeostasis, *Annual Review of Nutrition* 7 (1987): 383–406.
2. Food and Nutrition Board, *Recommended Dietary Allowances*, 10th ed. (Washington, D.C.: National Academy Press, 1989), pp. 247–261.
3. V. Lambert, Bottled water: New trends, new rules, *FDA Consumer*, June 1993, pp. 9–11.
4. G. Bellafante, Bottled water: Fads and facts, *Garbage: The Practical Journal for the Environment*, January/February 1990, pp. 46–50.
5. Bellafante, 1990.
6. V. Matkovic, Calcium metabolism and calcium requirements during skeletal modeling and consolidation of bone mass, *American Journal of Clinical Nutrition* 54 (1991): 245S–260S.
7. C. C. Arnaud and S. D. Sanchez, The role of calcium in osteoporosis, *Annual Review of Nutrition* 10 (1990): 397–414.
8. Food and Nutrition Board, 1989, pp. 174–184.
9. Food and Nutrition Board, 1989, p. 176.
10. Magnesium deficiency and ischemic heart disease, *Nutrition Reviews* 46 (1988): 311–312.
11. Low-magnesium diet may clog heart arteries, *Science News* 137 (1990): 214.
12. P. O. Webster, Magnesium, *American Journal of Clinical Nutrition* 45 (1987): 1305–1312; Food and Nutrition Board, 1989, pp. 190–191.
13. Food and Nutrition Board, 1989, p. 253.
14. H. S. Wright and coauthors, The 1987–88 Nationwide Food Consumption Survey: An update on the nutrient intake of respondents, *Nutrition Today*, May/June 1991, pp. 21–27.
15. Committee on Diet and Health, Food and Nutrition Board, *Diet and Health: Implications for Reducing Chronic Disease Risk* (Washington, D.C.: National Academy Press, 1989), pp. 99–135.
16. Food and Nutrition Board, 1989, p. 251.
17. G. R. DeLong, Effects of nutrition on brain development in humans, *American Journal of Clinical Nutrition* 57 (1993): 286S–290S.
18. J. A. Pennington, A review of iodine toxicity reports, *Journal of the American Dietetic Association* 90 (1990): 1571–1581.
19. H. C. Holt, B. J. Demott, and J. A. Bacon, The iodine concentration of market milk in Tennessee, 1981–1986, *Journal of Food Protection* 52 (1989): 115–118.
20. P. R. Dallman, Iron, in *Present Knowledge in Nutrition*, 6th ed., ed. M. L. Brown (Washington, D.C.: International Life Sciences Institute, Nutrition Foundation, 1990), pp. 241–250.
21. R. D. Baynes and T. H. Bothwell, Iron deficiency, *Annual Review of Nutrition* 10 (1990): 133–148.
22. R. Yip, The changing characteristics of childhood iron nutritional status in the United States, in *Dietary Iron: Birth to Two Years*, ed. L. J. Filer (New York: Raven Press, 1989), pp. 37–56.
23. Yip, 1989.
24. B. S. Skikne and J. D. Cook, Screening test for iron overload, *American Journal of Clinical Nutrition* 46 (1987): 840–843; V. Herbert, Everyone should be tested for iron disorders (abstract), *Journal of the American Dietetic Association* 92 (1992): 1502.
25. C. B. Gable, Hemochromatosis and dietary iron supplementation: Implications from U.S. mortality, morbidity, and health survey data, *Journal of the American Dietetic Association* 92 (1992): 208–212.
26. Gable, 1992.
27. J. T. Salonen and coauthors, High stored iron levels are associated with excess risk of myocardial infarction in Eastern Finnish men, *Circulation* 86 (1992): 803–811.
28. B. Halliwell, J. M. C. Gutteridge, and C. E. Cross, Free radicals, antioxidants, and human disease: Where are we now? *Journal of Laboratory and Clinical Medicine* 119 (1992): 598–620.
29. T. Yancy, quoting the American Association of Poison Control Centers in Parents are urged to watch for iron poisoning in children as deaths rise, *Tallahassee Democrat*, 29 September 1993.
30. R. D. Baynes and T. H. Bothwell, Iron deficiency, *Annual Review of Nutrition* 10 (1990): 133–148.
31. A. S. Prasad, Discovery of human zinc deficiency and studies in an experimental human model, *American Journal of Clinical Nutrition* 53 (1991): 403–412.
32. R. W. Crofton and coauthors, Inorganic zinc and the intestinal absorption of ferrous iron, *American Journal of Clinical Nutrition* 50 (1989): 141–144.
33. J. R. Arthur, F. Nicol, and G. J. Beckett, Selenium deficiency, thyroid hormone metabolism, and thyroid hormone deiodinases, *American Journal of Clinical Nutrition* 57 (1993): 236S–239S.
34. Food and Nutrition Board, 1989, p. 219.
35. Acute and chronic selenium toxicity (Diet Therapy/Obesity Update), *Nutrition and the M.D.*, January 1991, p. 7.
36. Food and Nutrition Board, 1989, p. 219.
37. D. Schultz, Fluoride: Cavity-fighter on tap, *FDA Consumer*, January/February 1992, pp. 34–38.
38. F. H. Nielsen, Chromium in M. E. Shils, J. A. Olson, and M. Shike, eds., *Modern Nutrition in Health and Disease* (Philadelphia: Lea & Febiger, 1994) pp. 264–268.
39. R. A. Anderson and coauthors, Supplemental-chromium effects on glucose, insulin, glucagon, and urinary chromium losses in subjects consuming controlled low-chromium diets, *American Journal of Clinical Nutrition* 54 (1991): 909–916.
40. Anderson and coauthors, 1991.
41. J. McBride, Chromium supplementation helps keep blood glucose levels in check, *Journal of the American Dietetic Association* 91 (1991): 178.
42. F. H. Nielsen, Facts and fallacies about boron, *Nutrition Today*, May/June 1992, pp. 6–12.
43. D. Farley, Look for "legit" health claims on foods, *FDA Consumer*, May 1993, pp. 14–21.

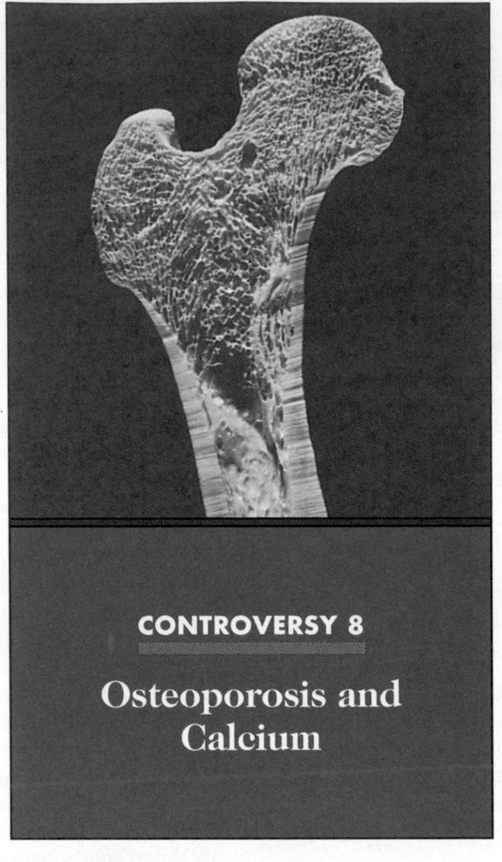

CONTROVERSY 8

Osteoporosis and Calcium

Last year well over a million people in the United States suffered bone breaks attributable to osteoporosis, making it one of the most prevalent of the degenerative diseases. Half of all women over age 45, and 90 percent of those over 75, suffer effects of osteoporosis.[1]

Osteoporosis sets in silently, producing no symptoms until late in life. As a young person, you cannot feel if you are losing bone tissue, but if you are, you may pay a high price in pain and disability later. The causes are tangled, and it is not yet proved that abundant dietary calcium can prevent or forestall osteoporosis. This Controversy addresses several questions about osteoporosis: What is it and who gets it? What factors increase the risk? What can people do to reduce their risks? And where does calcium fit into the picture?

THE PROBLEM OF OSTEOPOROSIS

Often, osteoporosis first becomes apparent when someone's hip suddenly gives way. People say, "She fell and broke her hip," but in fact the hip may have been so fragile that it broke *before* she fell. Just stepping off a curb may jar a bone enough to shatter it, if the bone is already porous from loss of minerals. The break is not clean; it is an explosion into fragments so numerous and scattered that they cannot be reassembled. To remove them is a struggle, and to replace them with an artificial joint requires major surgery. Such a fracture condemns many older people to wheelchairs for the rest of their lives. About a third die of complications within a year.

To understand how the skeleton loses minerals in later years, you must first know a few things about bones. Table C8-1 offers definitions of relevant terms. The photograph on this page shows a human leg bone sliced lengthwise, exposing the lattice of calcium-containing crystals (the **trabecular bone**) inside. These lacy crystals, part of the body's calcium bank, are tapped to raise blood calcium when the supply from the day's diet runs short; they are redeposited in bone when dietary calcium is plentiful. Invested in savings during the milk-drinking years of childhood and young adulthood, these deposits provide a nearly inexhaustible fund of calcium.

In contrast to trabecular bone, **cortical bone** is the dense, ivorylike bone that forms the exterior shell of a bone. Cortical bone also composes the shafts of the long bones, as you can easily see in the photograph. If you look closely at the ball at the top of the bone, you can also see the thin cortical shell surrounding the trabeculae. Both types of bone are crucial to overall bone strength. Cortical bone forms a sturdy outer wall and trabecular bone provides strength along the lines of stress.

The differences between the two types of bone are meaningful with regard to osteoporosis. Trabecular bone is generously supplied with blood vessels and is more metabolically active than is cortical bone. Trabecular bone is also more sensitive to hormones that govern withdrawal of calcium from day to day. Cortical bone's calcium can be withdrawn, but slowly, and at a steady pace. Trabecular bone, on the other hand, readily gives up some of its minerals whenever blood calcium needs replenishing. Losses of trabecular bone begin to be significant for men and women in their twenties, although losses can occur any time calcium withdrawals exceed calcium deposits. Cortical

Table C8-1
Osteoporosis Terms

- **trabecular** (tra-BECK-you-lar) **bone** the weblike structure composed of calcium-containing crystals inside of a bone's solid outer shell; it provides strength and acts as a calcium storage bank.
- **cortical bone** the ivorylike outer bone layer that forms a shell surrounding trabecular bone and that comprises the shaft of a long bone.
- **type I osteoporosis** osteoporosis characterized by rapid bone losses, primarily of trabecular bone.
- **type II osteoporosis** osteoporosis characterized by gradual losses of both trabecular and cortical bone.

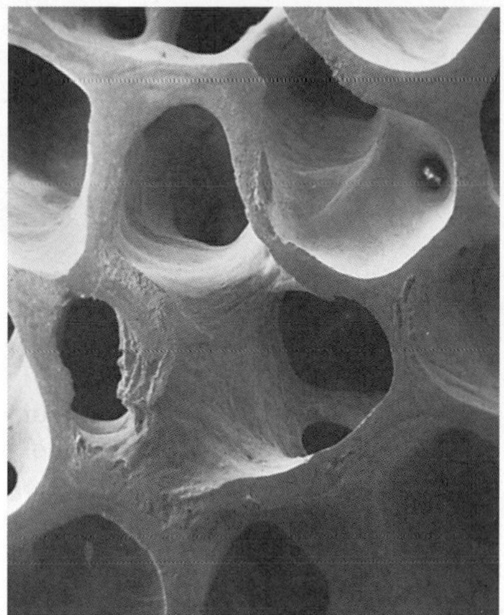
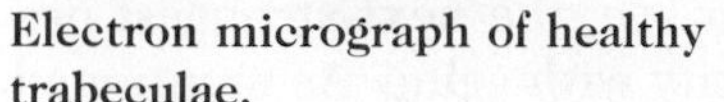

Electron micrograph of healthy trabeculae.

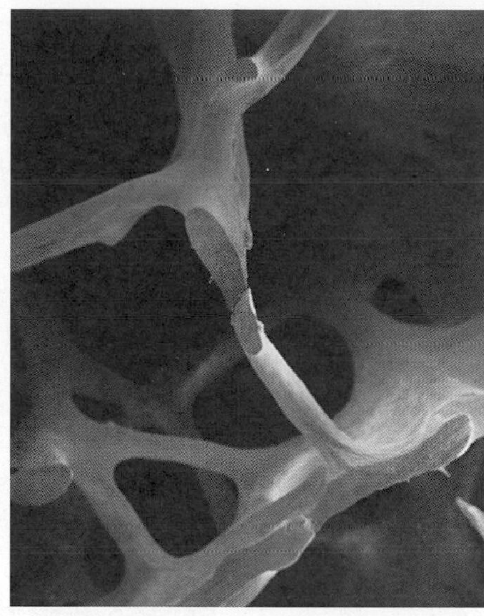

Electron micrograph of trabecular bone affected by osteoporosis.

Figure C8-1

LOSSES OF TRABECULAR BONE

bone loss begins at about age 40; bone tissue recedes steadily thereafter.

Menopause, a period in which a woman's estrogen secretion sharply declines, imposes special perils on women's bones. As hormone levels change and menstruation ceases, bone losses surge. This surge tapers off after a few years so that, once again, women's losses equal those sustained by men of the same age. Losses of bone minerals continue throughout the rest of a woman's life, but not at the free-fall pace of the menopause years.

As age advances and losses compound, the later symptoms of osteoporosis can become dramatic. Researchers have associated the losses of trabecular and cortical bone with two types of osteoporosis, types I and II, identified by the bone breaks they produce.[2] People with **type I osteoporosis** lose mostly trabecular bone (see Figure C8-1), sometimes at three times the expected rate or even faster, and bone breaks may come on suddenly when the victim passes the age of 65 years. In this condition trabecular bones become so fragile that even the body's own weight can overburden the spine; vertebrae may suddenly disintegrate and crush down, painfully pinching major nerves. Wrists may break as trabecula-rich bone ends weaken, and teeth may loosen or fall out as the trabecular bone of the jaw recedes. Women are most often the victims of type I osteoporosis, six to one over men.

In **type II osteoporosis,** the calcium of both cortical and trabecular bone is drawn out of storage, but slowly over the years. As old age approaches, the vertebrae may compress into wedge shapes, usually painlessly, forming what is often called "dowager's hump," the posture many older people assume as they "grow shorter." Figure C8-2 shows the effect of the compression of spinal bone on a woman's height and posture. Because the cortical shell as well as the trabecular interior weaken, breaks most often occur in the hip, as in the opening example. A woman is twice as likely as a man to suffer type II osteoporosis, probably due to the process set in motion years before, at menopause.

Scientists searching for ways to prevent osteoporosis must first discover its causes. So far, many findings seem to conflict with each other, and others simply lead to more questions. However, some areas of agreement have been reached concerning factors that influence osteoporosis. Whether a person develops osteoporosis seems to depend partly on heredity and partly on the environment, including nutrition. The sections that follow discuss the factors thought to be the main determinants of bone density. The first two, age and gender, are known to be major; the order of importance of the other factors is not known.

AGE AND BONE CALCIUM The bones gain strength and density all through the growing years and into

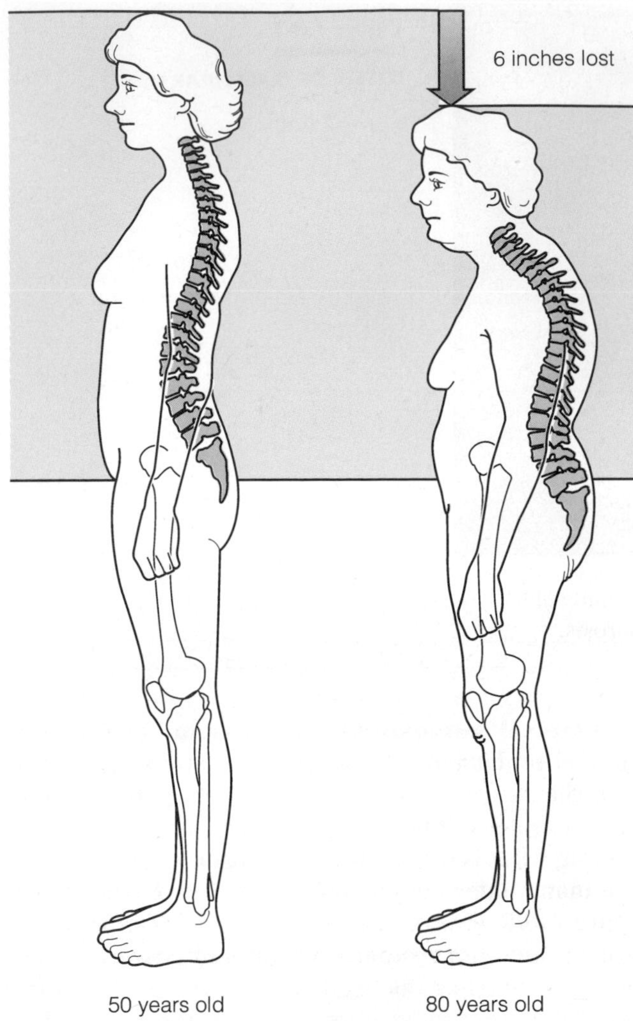

Figure C8-2

LOSS OF HEIGHT IN A WOMAN CAUSED BY OSTEOPOROSIS
The woman on the left is about 50 years old. On the right, she is 80 years old. Her legs have not grown shorter; only her back has lost length, due to collapse of her spinal bones (vertebrae). Collapsed vertebrae cannot protect the spinal nerves from pressure that causes excruciating pain.

young adulthood. As the mid-thirties approach, bones stop growing, and as years pass, bone tissue is lost, and bones lose strength and density. With advancing age, the cells that build bone gradually become less active, while those that dismantle bone continue working.

Among factors that weigh in the balance of bone withdrawal and deposition, one may be calcium nutrition in childhood and early adult life. Another factor, which becomes important in later life, is calcium absorption. Absorption declines after about the age of 70 years, probably because the kidneys do not activate vitamin D as well as they did earlier. Also, sunlight is needed to form vitamin D, and many older people fail to go outdoors into the sunshine. Some of the hormones that regulate bone maintenance and calcium metabolism also change with age and accelerate bone mineral withdrawal.*

When people reach the bone-losing years of middle age, those who formed dense bones during youth have the advantage. They simply have more bone tissue starting out and can lose more before beginning to suffer ill effects. Therefore, whatever the factors are that contribute to the building of strong bones in youth, these same factors are protective against osteoporosis much later. One of these factors may be calcium nutrition of the young.

GENDER AND HORMONES Being female and experiencing menopause is, after age, the next-strongest predictor of loss of bone density with aging. As mentioned, losses are more substantial in older women, as estrogen secretion declines, than in older men. However, cases exist in which *young* women's ovaries fail to produce enough estrogen to maintain menstruation. These young women also undergo rapid bone losses. In some, it is because diseased ovaries have had to be removed; in others, it is because the women overexercise and restrict their body weights unreasonably, developing athletic amenorrhea (discussed in Controversy 10). Estrogen taken as a prescription drug can help nonmenstruating women to prevent further bone loss, and current therapy regimens carry little risk to health. For those who take them, the drugs do indeed reduce the incidence of bone fractures.[3]

If estrogen deficiency is a major cause of osteoporosis in women, what is the case in men? Men produce only a little estrogen, yet they are normally more resistant to osteoporosis than are women. Do male sex hormones play roles in osteoporosis? Perhaps so, because men do suffer more fractures after removal of the testes (in cases of disease) or when their testes lose functional ability with aging.

Even in women, estrogen is clearly only one of several factors affecting bone. Some menstruating women may lose bone tissue in middle age before menopause, as though they were predisposed to do so.

INHERITED BONE DIFFERENCES Risks of osteoporosis run along racial lines. People of African extraction have

*Among the hormones suggested as influential are parathyroid hormone and calcitonin.

denser bones than do those of Northern European descent, and these differences are dramatically evident even before birth in x-ray images of fetuses.[4] This holds true for both sexes of all ages and expresses itself in a much lower total rate of osteoporosis among Africans. Hip fractures, for example, are reported to be about three times more likely in 80-year old North European women than in African women of the same age.

Other ethnic groups have lower bone densities than do Northern Europeans. Asians from China and Japan, Mexican-Americans, Hispanic people from Central and South America, and Inuit people from St. Lawrence Island all have lower bone density than do people with Northern European background. Knowing this might lead to the prediction that these groups would suffer more bone fractures, but the picture is not that tidy. Chinese people living in Singapore have low bone density, but have hip fracture rates among the lowest in the world. In Yugoslavia, bone fracture rates are tied to locations, despite racial similarities. There are lower fracture rates in high calcium-intake areas, and higher rates in low calcium-intake areas.

These studies of populations demonstrate that although a person's genes may lay the groundwork for a likely outcome, environmental factors influence the genes' ultimate expression. From the findings reported in Yugoslavia, it appears that calcium nutrition may be one of those environmental factors, but there are others, such as physical activity, body weight, smoking, alcohol use, and protein intake. It is worth noting that all of these factors are under people's own control.

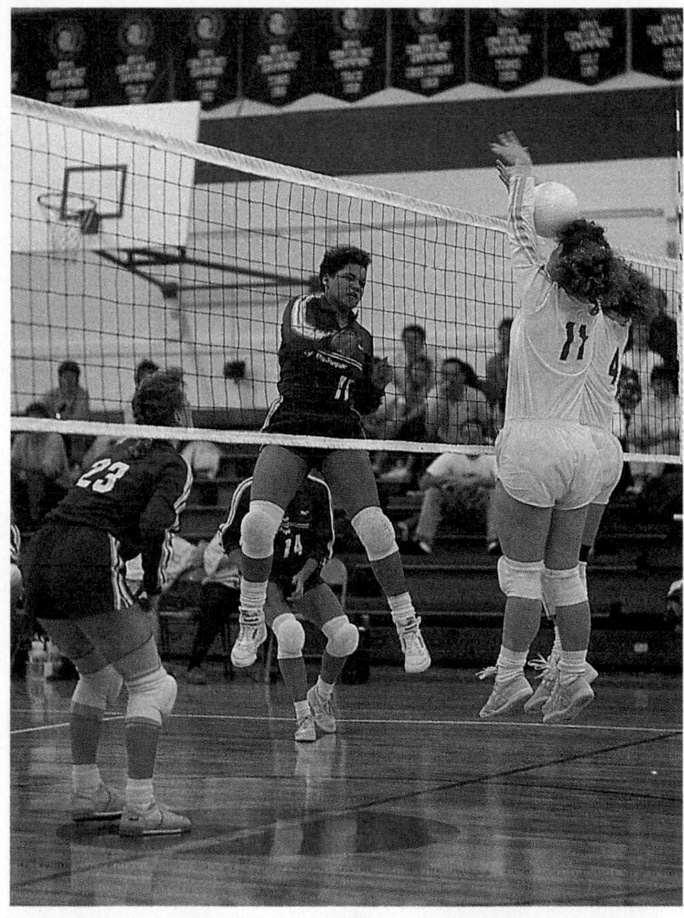
These college women are putting bone in the bank.

PHYSICAL ACTIVITY While you can't do much about your genetic inheritance, you can control your physical activity. It has long been known that when people lie idle—for example, when they are confined to bed—the bones lose strength just as the muscles do. Astronauts who live without gravity for days or weeks at a time also experience remarkably rapid and extensive bone losses.

Muscle strength and bone strength usually go together, and muscle use seems to promote bone strength. When cross sections of bones of sedentary and active people are compared, the active bones are more dense by far.[5] To keep the bones healthy, weight-bearing exercises, such as walking, dancing, jogging, sports, gardening, or calisthenics, are especially effective. Recently even swimming has been added to the list of activities that may build bone strength, although how exactly it does so is not yet known.[6] When muscles work on a regular basis, this signals that stronger bone tissue is needed. The hormones that promote synthesis of new muscle tissue also favor the building of bone.

BODY WEIGHT Heavier body weights stress bones and promote their maintenance; osteoporosis is most often associated with underweight. Slender women, especially those who diet and exercise to extremes, run greater risks of suffering from osteoporosis than do heavier women. A too-slender body size, severely restricted calorie intake, and extreme daily exercise combined with absence of menstruation reliably predict bone loss.[7] In such cases, exercise fails to protect against bone losses, even for black women.[8] Also, the type of diabetes associated with slender body structure alters the body's handling of calcium and magnesium with possible harmful effects on the health of the bones.[9]

SMOKING AND ALCOHOL Smokers experience more fractures from slight injury than do nonsmokers.

Researchers speculate that the lower body weights of smokers may be one factor; early menopause in female smokers may be another.

People who are addicted to alcohol also experience relatively more frequent fractures. It may be that because alcohol (a diuretic) causes fluid excretion, it induces excessive calcium losses through the urine. Also, women's ovaries are sensitive to the effects of alcohol, and drinking may upset the hormonal balance required for healthy bones.

Table C8-2 summarizes the risk factors covered so far and includes some others, among them, high protein and low calcium intakes, discussed next. The more risk factors that apply to you, the greater your chances of developing osteoporosis in the future and the more seriously you should take the advice offered in the last section of this Controversy.

Table C8-2
Risk and Protective Factors that Correlate with Osteoporosis

Risk Factors	Protective Factors
HIGH CORRELATION	
Advanced age	Black race
Alcoholism	Estrogens, long-term use
Chronic steroid use	
Female gender	
Rheumatoid arthritis	
Surgical removal of ovaries	
Thinness	
White race	
MODERATE CORRELATION	
Chronic thyroid hormone use	Having given birth
Cigarette smoking	High body weight
Diabetes (insulin-dependent type)	
Early menopause	
Excessive antacid use	
Low-calcium diet	
Sedentary lifestyle	
Vitamin D deficiency	
PROBABLY IMPORTANT BUT NOT YET PROVED	
Alcohol taken in moderation	High-calcium diet
Caffeine use	Regular physical activity
Family history of osteoporosis	
High-fiber diet	
High-protein diet	

Source: Adapted from C. D. Arnaud and S. D. Sanchez, The role of calcium in osteoporosis, *Annual Review of Nutrition* 10 (1990): 397–414.

A ROLE FOR PROTEIN Researchers have discovered that extra dietary protein causes the body to excrete calcium in the urine. The finding has often been repeated, leading to the suspicion that a lifetime of consuming excess dietary protein may accelerate bone loss.[10] One study showed that even when calcium intakes were very high (1,400 milligrams a day in this experiment), excess protein intake caused a negative calcium balance.

The converse is also true: that is, diets low in protein help to conserve bone density. This is seen both in laboratory animals and in strict vegetarians, who consume a lower than average amount of protein. Vegetarians who center meals on eggs and dairy products, however, have been observed to take in as much protein and to lose bone just as rapidly as do meat eaters.[11] A tentative link has been suggested between the hormone insulin, released in response to dietary protein, and increased calcium losses in the urine.[12]

There is a limit to how low the protein intake can safely be, of course. Below that limit, too little protein is as harmful as too much. Protein deprivation stimulates calcium losses.[13] These facts seem to conflict at first glance, but they really just demonstrate a sound nutrition principle—that a happy medium is best.

CALCIUM, VITAMIN D, AND FLUORIDE To return to calcium nutrition in the early years: when calcium supplies are low, or when vitamin D deficiency limits calcium absorption, the result is poor calcification of the bones. Conversely, preteen children who consume extra calcium together with adequate vitamin D lay more calcium into the structure of their bones.[14] In addition to calcium and vitamin D, fluoride taken during the bone-building years may increase bone density.*

As important as calcium intake may be, bone loss is not a calcium-deficiency disease comparable to iron-deficiency anemia. In iron-deficiency anemia, high iron intakes reliably reverse the condition. With respect to calcium balance, though, high calcium intakes alone do little or nothing to reverse bone loss. One study of over a hundred women, aged 23 to 88 years, demonstrated this. Each woman's daily calcium intake was essentially the same from day to day, but among individuals the average daily consumption ranged from as little as one third the RDA to almost three times the RDA. Despite

*In the elderly, pills of fluoride may not reliably prevent bone fractures.

the dramatic differences in intakes of calcium, the rates of loss of bone minerals were similar for all the women in the study.[15]

It is also not clear whether high calcium intakes during adulthood help prevent osteoporosis. One early report found no correlation at all between calcium intakes in adults (between 500 and 1,500 milligrams daily) and incidence of osteoporosis.[16] In direct contradiction to this, in another study, women who had attained menopause began drinking three cups of milk a day. They continued drinking this amount for two years, and showed marked improvement in calcium balance. Recently, the combination of 1,200 milligrams of calcium with a dose of vitamin D equal to that in two quarts of milk, taken daily, was found to lower the incidence of hip fractures by more than 40 percent.[17] Another study determined that women who took in less than about 400 milligrams of calcium a day lost spinal bone tissue faster than women whose intakes were close to 800 milligrams (the RDA amount for older women).[18] Still another study showed low dietary calcium to be associated with increased hip fractures in men and women, even taking into account other factors such as smoking, alcohol intake, and exercise.[19]

While researchers argue about ideal calcium intakes for bone health, most experts agree that there must certainly exist a low threshold below which bone loss accelerates. The RDA and Canadian RNI for adults are known to be set well above this minimum, although exactly what the minimum is, is a point of disagreement. Some cultures seemingly maintain calcium balance on small intakes, and these countries set their calcium recommendations much lower than does the United States or Canada. For example, WHO recommends between 400 and 500 milligrams of calcium per day. Perhaps the higher protein intakes of North Americans warrant the setting of higher calcium allowances.

CALCIUM RECOMMENDATIONS Unfortunately few girls meet the RDA for calcium during their bone-forming years.[20] (Boys obtain amounts close to the RDA because they eat more food.) This may mean that most girls start their adult lives with less than optimal bone density. As for adults, women rarely meet even the RDA of 800 to 1,200 milligrams from food within their energy allowances. Not enough firm evidence exists to justify making a recommendation to everyone, but some evidence suggests that women may benefit from taking extra calcium for at least the first ten years after menopause.[21]

And how should this calcium be obtained? Consider a bit of hard-won advice: use foods if at all possible, not supplements. People can best support their bones' health by following the recommendations of Table C8-3.

Table C8-3
A Lifetime Plan for Healthy Bones

Age	Action
0–18	Use milk as the primary beverage to meet the RDA for calcium within a balanced diet that provides all nutrients; play actively, in sports or other activities; limit television; do not start smoking or drinking alcohol; drink fluoridated water.
19–25	Choose milk as the primary beverage, or if milk causes distress, include other calcium sources to meet the RDA; commit to a lifelong program of physical activity; do not smoke or drink alcohol—if you have started, quit; drink fluoridated water.
26–50	Continue as for 19-to-25 year olds; at menopause, women should be evaluated for possible estrogen replacement therapy. Obtain the RDA for calcium from food. Take calcium and fluoride supplements only if prescribed by physician.
51 and above	Continue as for 19-to-25 year olds; continue following physician's advice concerning estrogen and supplements. Continue striving to meet the calcium RDA from diet, and continue bone-strengthening exercises.

Calcium supplements cannot equal any of the actions listed in the table. No one should be led to think that popping pills can take the place of sound food choices and other healthy habits. For those who desire details on supplements, however, a discussion follows.

A PERSPECTIVE ON CALCIUM SUPPLEMENTS Calcium supplements are part of standard therapy for already-developed osteoporosis. Taking self-prescribed calcium supplements entails problems, though. For example, two supplemental forms of calcium, calcium carbonate and calcium hydroxyapatite, interfere with iron absorption. People who take these pills with foods absorb less iron from those foods and could develop iron deficiencies. Other people develop severe constipation. People taking larger doses, in multiples of a gram, risk more serious consequences such as milk alkali syndrome, an alkalosis seen only in those taking four to 10 grams a day, and kidney stones in those with a history of forming them. Calcium supplements often contain vitamin D needed to enhance calcium absorption, but continued high intakes of vitamin D can be toxic. About 2,500 milligrams is thought to be the maximum safe dose for calcium. Don't forget that some calcium is contributed by foods and more by the supplement; the total of these two sources should fall short of the maximum safe dose.

Some calcium preparations contain hidden hazards (see Table C8-4), and it seems that the purified forms are best. Based on limited research to date, it seems that most healthy people absorb calcium equally well—and as well as from milk—from many forms listed in Table C8-4.

A way to get around the problem of nutrient interactions may be to take calcium supplements between, not with, meals, but for anyone with reduced stomach acid secretion, this is not a satisfactory solution. Only meals stimulate the secretion of enough stomach acid to permit the absorption of the calcium. (Score another point here for food sources of calcium.)

Consider another point for food. *Some* people absorb calcium better from milk and milk products than from even the most absorbable supplements named in Table C8-4.[22] Furthermore, *after* absorption the source affects the body's internal use of the nutrient. Only one study has shown this to be true of calcium, but that study shows that the body makes better use of calcium from milk than from calcium carbonate.[23]

Think one more time, then, before you commit yourself to taking supplements for calcium. The Consensus Conference on Osteoporosis recommends milk. The American Society for Bone and Mineral Research recommends foods as a source of calcium in preference to supplements.[24] Nutrition authorities Mayer and Goldberg, whose syndicated column on nutrition reaches newspaper readers nationwide, state, "We stand firmly in favor of dietary measures to meet the RDA . . . of calcium."[25] The authors of this book are so impressed with the importance of using abundant, calcium-rich foods that they have worked out ways to do so at every meal. Seldom do nutritionists agree so unanimously.

Table C8-4
Calcium Forms in Supplements

- **amino acid chelates** compounds of minerals (such as calcium) combined with amino acids in a form that favors their absorption. Absorption approximates that of calcium from milk.
- **antacids** acid-buffering agents used to counter excess acidity in the stomach. Calcium-containing preparations (such as Tums) contain calcium but reduce stomach acidity necessary for maximum calcium absorption. Antacids with aluminum or magnesium hydroxides (such as Rolaids) can even accelerate calcium losses.
- **bone meal, powdered bone** crushed or ground bone preparations intended to supply calcium to the diet. Calcium from bone is not well absorbed and is often contaminated with toxic materials.
- **calcium citrate** a calcium salt reported to have high absorbability. Other absorbable forms are calcium acetate, calcium gluconate, calcium lactate, calcium malate, and calcium phosphate dibasic.
- **dolomite** a compound of minerals (calcium magnesium carbonate) found in limestone and marble. Dolomite is powdered and is sold as a calcium-magnesium supplement, but may be contaminated with toxic minerals such as arsenic, cadmium, mercury, and lead. It is not well absorbed and adversely affects absorption of other essential minerals.
- **oyster shell** a product made from the powdered shells of oysters, sold as a calcium supplement, but not well absorbed by the digestive system.

Notes

1. National Research Council, *Diet and Health: Implications for Reducing Chronic Risk* (Washington D.C.: National Academy Press, 1991): p. 121.
2. C. Niewoehner, Calcium and osteoporosis, *Cereal Foods World* 33 (1988): 784–787; National Research Council, 1991, pp. 316–317.
3. B. L. Riggs and L. J. Melton, The prevention and treatment of osteoporosis, *New England Journal of Medicine* 327 (1992): 620–627.
4. A history of racial and ethnic differences in bone health appears in W. S. Pollitzer and J. J. B. Anderson, Ethnic and genetic differences in bone mass: A review with a hereditary vs environmental perspective, *American Journal of Clinical Nutrition* 50 (1989): 1244–1259.
5. C. N. Meridith, Exercise in the prevention of osteoporosis, in *Nutrition of the Elderly* (New York: Raven, 1992) pp. 169–175.
6. E. S. Orwoll and coauthors, The relationship of swimming exercise to bone mass in men and women, *Archives of Internal Medicine* 149 (1989): 2197–2200.
7. B. L. Drinkwater, B. Bruemner, and C. H. Chestnut III, Menstrual history as a determinant of current bone density in young athletes, *Journal of the American Medical Association* 263 (1990): 545–548.
8. O. Walden and J. DeWorth, Body size of black women who suffered a hip fracture, *Journal of Nutrition for the Elderly*, April 1988, pp. 3–8.
9. G. Saggese and coauthors, Hypomagnesemia and the parathyroid hormone-vitamin D endocrine system in children with insulin-dependent diabetes mellitus, *Journal of Pediatrics* 118 (1991): 220–225.
10. R. P. Blank and coauthors, Calcium metabolism and osteoporotic ridge resorption: A protein connection, *Journal of Prosthetic Dentistry* 58 (1987): 590–595; E. Fernandez-Repollet, P. Van Loon, and M. Martinez-Maldonado, Renal and systemic effects of short-term high protein feeding in normal rats, *American Journal of the Medical Sciences* 297 (1989): 348–354; J. C. Howe, Postprandial response of calcium metabolism in post menopausal women to meals varying in protein level/source, *Metabolism Clinical and Experimental* 39 (1990): 1246–1252.
11. R. Tesar and coauthors, Axial peripheral bone density and nutrient intakes of post menopausal vegetarian and omnivorous women, *American Journal of Clinical Nutrition* 56 (1992): 699–704.
12. Howe, 1990.
13. J. Bonjour and coauthors, Hip fracture, femoral bone mineral density, and protein supply in elderly patients, in *Nutrition of the Elderly* (New York: Raven, 1992): pp. 151–159.
14. C. C. Johnson and coauthors, Calcium supplementation and increases in bone mineral density in children, *New England Journal of Medicine* 327 (1992): 82–87; Maximizing peak bone mass: Calcium supplementation increases bone mineral density in children, *Nutrition Reviews* 50 (1992): 335–337.
15. B. L. Riggs and coauthors, Dietary calcium intakes and rates of bone loss in women, *Journal of Clinical Investigation* 80 (1987): 979–982.
16. R. W. Smith and B. Frame, Concurrent axial and appendicular osteoporosis: Its relation to calcium consumption, *New England Journal of Medicine* 273 (1965): 73–78.
17. M. C. Chapuy and coauthors, Vitamin D_3 and calcium to prevent hip fractures in elderly women, *New England Journal of Medicine* 327 (1992): 1637–1642.
18. B. Dawson-Hughes, J. Jacques, and C. Shipp, Dietary calcium intake and bone loss from the spine in healthy postmenopausal women, *American Journal of Clinical Nutrition* 46 (1987): 685–687.
19. T. L. Holbrook, E. Barrett-Connor, and D. L. Wingard, Dietary calcium and risk of hip fracture: 14-year prospective population study, *Lancet* 12 (1988): 1046–1049.
20. J. A. T. Pennington, B. E. Young, and D. B. Wilson, Nutritional elements in U.S. diets: Results from the Total Diet Study, 1982 to 1986, *Journal of the American Dietetic Association* 89 (1989): 659–664; Dietary calcium and the prevention of postmenopausal osteoporosis: Review from the National Nutrition Institute in Canada, *Nutrition Today*, May/June 1988, pp. 33–35.
21. K. J. Polley and coauthors, Effect of calcium supplementation on forearm bone mineral content in postmenopausal women: A prospective, sequential controlled study, *Journal of Nutrition* 117 (1987): 1929–1935.
22. M. S. Sheikh and coauthors, Gastrointestinal absorption of calcium from milk and calcium salts, *New England Journal of Medicine* 317 (1987): 532–536.
23. L. D. McBean, Food versus pills versus fortified foods, *Dairy Council Digest*, March-April 1987.
24. McBean, 1987.
25. J. Mayer and J. Goldberg, Sufficient calcium intake still a major problem, *Tallahassee Democrat*, 5 November 1987.

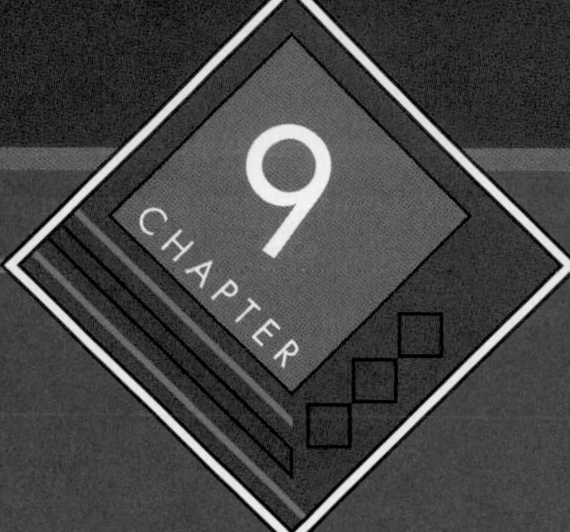

Energy Balance and Weight Control

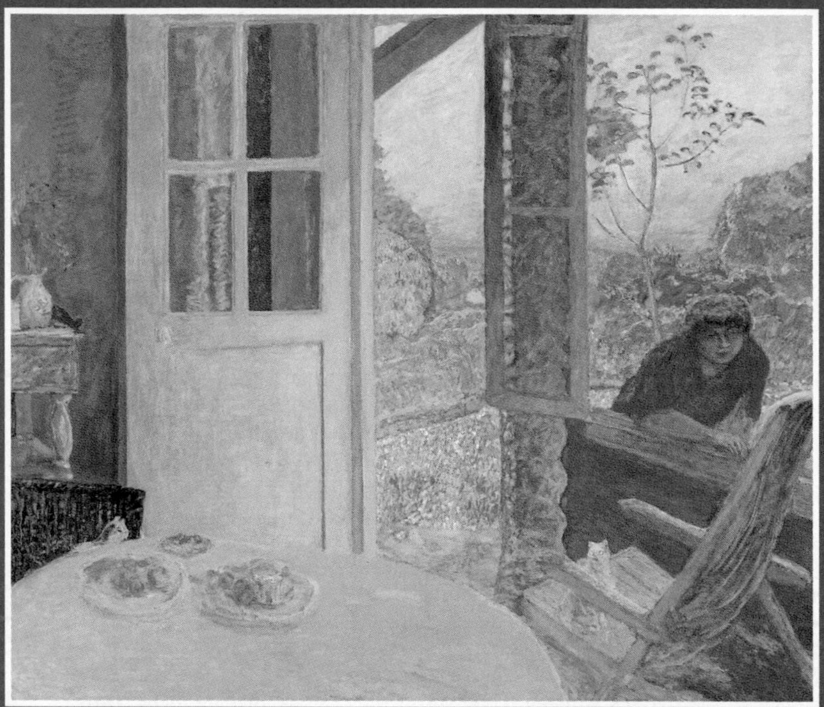

Contents

Pierre Bonnard, Dining Room in the Country, 1913, The John R. Van Derlip Fund, The Minneapolis Institute of Arts.

9

Are you pleased with your body weight? If you answered yes, you are a rare individual. Nearly all people in our society think they should weigh more or less (mostly less) than they do. Usually, their primary reason is appearance, but they often perceive, correctly, that physical health is also somehow related to weight. At the extremes, both overweight and underweight present definite health risks.

People also think of their weight as something they should control. A pair of misconceptions frustrates their efforts, however. The first is to focus on *weight;* the second is to focus on *controlling* weight. To put it simply, it isn't your weight you need to control; it's the fat in your body in proportion to the lean. And it isn't possible to control either one, directly; it is possible only to control your *behavior.* In other words, the words "Weight Control" in this chapter's title are wrong; they should be replaced with the words "Behavior to Promote Appropriate Body Composition." If the chapter bore that name, though, hardly anyone would read it.

This chapter's missions are to present the problems associated with deficient and excessive body fatness; to present strategies toward solving these problems; and to point out how appropriate body composition, once achieved, can be maintained. First, consider how the body manages its energy budget.

◆ Energy Balance

Suppose you decide that you are too fat or too thin. How did you get that way? By having an unbalanced energy budget—that is, by eating either more or less food energy than you spent.

Energy In

In Chapter 5, Figure 5-1 illustrated that excess fat enters the fat cells for storage, and that stored fat is withdrawn when energy supplies run low. A day's energy balance can therefore be stated like this:

Change in energy (fat and glycogen) stores equals food energy taken in minus energy spent on metabolism and muscle activities.

More simply:

Change in energy stores = energy in − energy out.

The energy in foods and beverages is the only contributor to the "energy in" side of the energy balance equation. Before you can decide how much food energy you need in a day, you must first become familiar with the amounts of energy in foods and beverages. One way to do this is to look up calorie amounts associated with foods and beverages in Appendix A.

Remember these average values of the energy-yielding nutrients and alcohol:

1 g carbohydrate = 4 cal.
1 g fat = 9 cal.
1 g protein = 4 cal.
1 g alcohol = 7 cal.

In addition to looking up energy values in a table, you can also estimate them using the exchange system, which classes foods by their protein, fat, and carbohydrate contents. Alcohol's calories must also be included, if alcohol is present. A later section shows you how to use the exchange system to estimate calories quickly.

As examples of the numbers of calories associated with food portions, an apple gives you 125 calories from carbohydrate; an average candy bar gives you 425 calories mostly from fat and carbohydrate. As for numbers of calories spent on activities, for a 150-pound person, brisk walking for 20 minutes costs about 100 calories; jogging for 20 minutes costs about 200 cal-

1 lb body fat = 3,500 cal.

ories. You may already know that for each 3,500 calories you eat in excess of expenditures, you store approximately 1 pound of body fat.*

KEY POINT The "energy in" side of the body's energy budget is measured in calories taken in each day in the form of foods and beverages. Calories in foods and beverages can be estimated using the exchange system or obtained from published tables.

Energy Out

While it is easy to estimate the energy present in a serving of food or in a day's meals, it is not easy to determine the energy an individual spends or needs. The U.S. Committee on Recommended Dietary Allowances (RDA) and the Canadian Department of National Health and Welfare have published recommended energy intakes for various age-sex groups in their populations. These are useful for population studies, but among individuals in a group, the range of energy needs is so broad that it is impossible to guess any individual person's need without knowing something about the person's lifestyle. The RDA for energy are based on average people. For example, the energy RDA for a woman is for a 20-year-old woman 5 feet 5 inches tall, who weighs about 128 pounds, is of average body fatness, and engages in light activity. This woman needs 2,200 calories of energy a day. The RDA for a man is for a healthy 20-year-old man who stands 5 feet 10 inches tall, weighs 160 pounds, and is lightly active. He needs 2,900 calories a day. Taller people, because of their greater surface area, need proportionately more energy and shorter people proportionately less energy to balance their energy budgets. Older people generally need less due to both slowed metabolism and reduced activity, with the number of calories diminishing by about 5 percent per decade beyond the age of 30 years.

Light activity, for both women and men, means sleeping or lying down for eight hours a day, sitting for seven hours, standing for five, walking for two, and spending two hours a day in light physical activity.

In reality, though, no one is average and people vary widely in their energy needs. In any group of 20 similar people with similar activity levels, one may expend twice as much energy per day as another. Clearly it is impossible to determine any person's energy need within such a wide range of variation without studying that person.

The energy RDA are presented in the inside front cover; Canadian energy allowances are presented in Appendix B.

One way to obtain an estimate of your energy needs is to monitor your food intake and body weight over a period of time in which your activities are typical of your lifestyle. If you keep a strictly accurate record of all the foods and beverages you consume for a week or two and if your weight has not changed during the past few months, you can conclude that your energy budget is balanced. At least a week of record keeping is necessary, though, because intakes fluctuate from day to day. (On about half the days you eat less food energy than the average; on the other half more.)

An alternative method of determining energy output is to compute the two major components of energy expenditure and then to add them together. This method leaves out a third energy component, the body's metabolic response to food, first mentioned in Controversy 5. About 5 to 10 percent of a meal's energy value is used up in stepped-up metabolism in the

*Pure fat is worth 9 calories per gram. A pound of it (450 grams), then, would store 4,050 calories. A pound of body fat is not pure fat, though; it contains water, protein, and other materials, hence the lower calorie value.

four or so hours following each meal, a category of energy expenditure called the **thermic effect of food.** This amount of energy could affect expenditures over the long run, but most experts believe its effects to be negligible.[1] For purposes here, it can be ignored.

The two major ways in which the body spends energy are: (1) to fuel its **basal metabolism** and (2) to fuel its **voluntary activities.** The basal metabolism supports the body's work that goes on all the time, without conscious awareness. The beating of the heart, the inhaling and exhaling of air, the maintenance of body temperature, and the sending of nerve and hormonal messages to direct these activities are all basal processes that maintain life.

The **basal metabolic rate (BMR)** is surprisingly fast. A person whose total energy needs are 2,000 calories a day spends as many as 1,200 to 1,400 of them to support basal metabolism. The hormone thyroxine directly controls basal metabolism—the less secreted, the lower the energy requirements for basal functions. Many other factors affect the BMR (Table 9-1).

People often want to know how they can speed up their metabolism, to promote fat loss. You cannot speed up your BMR much today. You can, however, amplify the second component of your energy expenditure, your voluntary activities. If you do this, you will spend more calories today, and if you keep doing this day after day, it will ultimately change your BMR. A way to increase your BMR to the maximum possible is to make strength-building exercise a daily habit, so that your body composition will change toward the lean. Lean tissue is more metabolically active than fat tissue, so your basal energy output will pick up the pace as well.[2] A warning: some ads for weight-loss diets claim that eating certain foods can elevate the BMR, and thus promote weight loss. This is a false claim. Any meal promotes a temporary stepped-up energy expenditure in the form of the thermic effect of food, and the differences among meals are not large enough to be worth notice.

As for fuel for voluntary activities, the amount of energy you spend in exercise depends somewhat on your personal style. For example, the heavier the weight of the body parts you move in your activity and the longer the time you invest, the more calories you spend. Are you well trained or

thermic effect of food (TEF) the body's speeded up metabolism in response to having eaten a meal. Also called *diet-induced thermogenesis.*

basal metabolism the sum total of all the involuntary activities that are necessary to sustain life, including respiration, circulation, and new tissue synthesis and excluding digestion and voluntary activities; the largest component of the average person's daily energy expenditure.

voluntary activities activities (such as walking, sitting, running) conducted by voluntary muscles.

basal metabolic rate (BMR) the rate at which the body uses energy to support its basal metabolism.

Table 9-1
Factors that Affect the BMR

Factor	Effect on BMR
Age	In youth, the BMR is higher; age brings less lean body mass and slows the BMR.
Height	Tall, thin people have higher BMRs.
Growth	Children and pregnant women have higher BMRs.
Body composition	The more lean tissue, the higher the BMR.
Fever	Fever raises the BMR.
Stress	Stress hormones raise the BMR.
Environmental temperature	Both heat and cold raise the BMR.
Fasting/starvation	Fasting/starvation hormones lower the BMR.
Malnutrition	Malnutrition lowers the BMR.
Thyroxine	The thyroid hormone thyroxine is a key BMR regulator; the more thyroxine produced, the higher is the BMR.

Table 9-2
Energy Demands of Activities

Activity	Energy per Pound of Body Weight per Minute	Body Weight (lb)				
		110	125	150	175	200
	cal/lb/min[a]	CALORIES PER MINUTE				
Aerobic dance (vigorous)	.062	6.8	7.8	9.3	10.9	12.4
Basketball (vigorous, full court)	.097	10.7	12.1	14.6	17.0	19.4
Bicycling						
13 miles per hour	.045	5.0	5.6	6.8	7.9	9.0
15 miles per hour	.049	5.4	6.1	7.4	8.6	9.8
17 miles per hour	.057	6.3	7.1	8.6	10.0	11.4
19 miles per hour	.076	8.4	9.5	11.4	13.3	15.2
21 miles per hour	.090	9.9	11.3	13.5	15.8	18.0
23 miles per hour	.109	12.0	13.6	16.4	19.0	21.8
25 miles per hour	.139	15.3	17.4	20.9	24.3	27.8
Canoeing (flat water, moderate pace)	.045	5.0	5.6	6.8	7.9	9.0
Cross-country skiing (8 miles per hour)	.104	11.4	13.0	15.6	18.2	20.8
Golf (carrying clubs)	.045	5.0	5.6	6.8	7.9	9.0
Handball	.078	8.6	9.8	11.7	13.7	15.6
Horseback riding (trot)	.052	5.7	6.5	7.8	9.1	10.4
Rowing (vigorous)	.097	10.7	12.1	14.6	17.0	19.4
Running						
5 miles per hour	.061	6.7	7.6	9.2	10.7	12.2
6 miles per hour	.074	8.1	9.2	11.1	13.0	14.8
7.5 miles per hour	.094	10.3	11.8	14.1	16.4	18.8
9 miles per hour	.103	11.3	12.9	15.5	18.0	20.6
10 miles per hour	.114	12.5	14.3	17.1	20.0	22.9
11 miles per hour	.131	14.4	16.4	19.7	22.9	26.2
Studying	.011	1.2	1.4	1.7	1.9	2.2
Soccer (vigorous)	.097	10.7	12.1	14.6	17.0	19.4
Swimming						
20 yards per minute	.032	3.5	4.0	4.8	5.6	6.4
45 yards per minute	.058	6.4	7.3	8.7	10.2	11.6
50 yards per minute	.070	7.7	8.8	10.5	12.3	14.0
Table tennis (skilled)	.045	5.0	5.6	6.8	7.9	9.0
Tennis (beginner)	.032	3.5	4.0	4.8	5.6	6.4
Walking (brisk pace)						
3.5 miles per hour	.035	3.9	4.4	5.2	6.1	7.0
4.5 miles per hour	.048	5.3	6.0	7.2	8.4	9.6

[a]Use this column if you want to calculate calories spent for your own exact body weight. Multiply cal/lb/min by your exact weight and then multiply that number by the number of minutes spent in the activity. For example, if you weigh 142 pounds, and you want to know how many calories you spent doing 30 minutes of vigorous aerobic dance: .062 × 142 = 8.8 calories per minute. 8.8 × 30 (minutes) = 264 total calories spent.

Source: Values for swimming, bicycling, and running have been adapted with permission of Ross Laboratories, Columbus, Ohio 43216, from G. P. Town and K. B. Wheeler, Nutrition concerns for the endurance athlete, *Dietetic Currents* 13 (1986): 7–12. Copyright 1986 Ross Laboratories. Values for all other activities have been adapted from *Physical Fitness for Practically Everybody: The Consumers Union Report on Exercise.* Copyright 1983 by Consumers Union of U.S., Inc., Yonkers, NY 10703–1057. Reprinted by permission from CONSUMER REPORTS BOOKS, 1983.

a novice? (The streamlined moves of an expert swimmer, for example, may seem more effortless than movements of the untrained, but the swimmer moves more muscle mass more powerfully while exercising, and so uses more energy.) These and other factors bear on how much fuel an activity will require. Table 9-2 shows the approximate numbers of calories people

Table 9-3
Activity Equivalents of Food Energy Values

Food	Calories	Activity Equivalent for a 150-Pound Person to Work Off the Calories (minutes)		
		WALK[a]	RUN[b]	WAIT[c]
Apple, large	125	24	8	75
Regular beer, 1 glass (8 oz)	100	19	6	61
Cookie, chocolate chip	50	10	3	30
Ice cream, ½ cup	175	34	11	106
Steak, T-bone (6 oz)	475	91	31	288

[a]Energy cost of walking at 3.5 mph—5.2 calories per minute.
[b]Energy cost of running at 9 miles per hour—15.5 calories per minute.
[c]Energy cost of sitting—1.65 calories per minute.

of various weights spend on activities. For fun, Table 9-3 translates some activity values into food energy terms.

Long periods of vigorous activity, engaged in frequently, can place great demands on energy supplies. During football or basketball season, a player may need 5,000 calories a day or even more to play well and to maintain weight. To avoid gaining unwanted fat after the season, it is equally important for an athlete to cut back to an energy intake that suits the off-season activity. The next section shows how to calculate an approximation of your daily energy output.

KEY POINT Two major components of the "energy out" side of the body's energy budget are basal metabolism and voluntary activities. A third component of energy expenditure is the thermic effect of food.

Estimation of Energy Needs

To estimate total energy expenditure, first estimate the two major components separately, then add them together. The first component is the energy spent in basal metabolism. Follow these steps. Use the BMR factor 1.0 calorie per kilogram of body weight per hour for men or 0.9 for women (men usually have more muscles than do women). Example (for a 150-pound man):

1. Change pounds to kilograms:

150 pounds ÷ 2.2 pounds per kilogram = 68 kilograms.

2. Multiply weight in kilograms by the BMR factor:

68 kilograms × 1 calorie per kilogram per hour = 68 calories per hour.

3. Multiply the calories used in one hour by the hours in a day:

68 calories per hour × 24 hours per day = 1,632 calories per day.

The second major component of energy expenditure is the energy spent on voluntary muscular activity. The following figures are crude approximations based on the amount of muscular work a person typically performs in a day. To select the one appropriate for you, remember to think in terms of the amount of *muscular* work performed; don't confuse being *busy* with being *active*. If you sit down most of the day and drive or ride whenever possible, use the value for a sedentary person. If you move around some of the time, as a teacher might during working hours, use the light activity values. If you do some amount of intentional exercise, such as an hour of jogging four or five times a week, or if your occupation calls for some physical work, consider yourself moderately active. A person whose job requires much physical labor, such as a roofer or a carpenter, would be in the heavy-activity range. The exceptional category is reserved for those few who spend many hours a day in intense physical training, such as professional or college athletes during their seasons. Perform calculations for both the upper and lower ends of the range of percentages given for your gender and activity level:

- Sedentary: Men 25% to 40%; women 25% to 35%.
- Light activity: Men 50% to 70%; women 40% to 60%.
- Moderate activity: Men 65% to 80%; women 50% to 70%.
- Heavy activity: Men 90% to 120%; women 80% to 100%.
- Exceptional activity: Men 130% to 145%; women 110% to 130%.*

Suppose the 150-pound man we used as an example earlier is a student who bikes about ten minutes a day and walks to classes but otherwise sits and studies. He falls into the "light activity" category, so we can estimate the range of energy he needs by multiplying his BMR calories per day by both 50 and 70 percent:

1,632 calories per day × 0.50 = 816 calories per day.
1,632 calories per day × 0.70 = 1,142 calories per day.

The man needs from 816 to 1,142 calories per day for his activities. Now total the two components. The man in our example spends, in a day:

1,632 calories per day + 816 calories per day = 2,448 calories per day.
1,632 calories per day + 1,142 calories per day = 2,774 calories per day.

Express the man's needs as a range of rounded values: 2,400 to 2,800 calories/day.

KEY POINT To estimate the energy spent on basal metabolism, use the factor (for men) 1.0 cal/kg/hr (or for women, 0.9 cal/kg/hr) for a 24-hour period. Then add an increment of this amount depending on the extent of daily muscular activity.

The Problems of Underweight and Overweight

Both deficient and excessive body fat present health risks. It has long been known that thin people will die first during a siege or in a famine. A fact not always recognized, even by health care providers, is that overly thin people are also at a disadvantage in the hospital, where they may have to go for days without food so that they can undergo tests or surgery. Under-

*Percentages derived from the RDA (1989) formula for energy expenditure, allowing a 15% to 30% range.

weight also increases the risk for any person fighting a wasting disease. In fact, people with cancer often die, not from the cancer itself, but from starvation. Thus underweight people are urged to gain body fat as an energy reserve and to acquire protective amounts of all the nutrients that can be stored.

As for excessive body fat, it is associated with increased risks of diseases. For example, it can precipitate hypertension and thus increase the risk of stroke. Often weight loss alone can normalize the blood pressure of an overfat person; some people with hypertension can tell you exactly at what weight their blood pressure begins to rise. Weight gain can also precipitate diabetes in genetically susceptible people and thus bring on its associated ills. If hypertension or diabetes runs in your family, you urgently need to attend to weight control.

The health risks of overfatness are so many that it has been declared a disease: **obesity.**[3] In addition to diabetes and hypertension already mentioned, other risks threaten obese adults. Among them are high blood lipids, cardiovascular disease, sleep apnea (abnormal ceasing of breathing during sleep), osteoarthritis, abdominal hernias, some cancers, varicose veins, gout, gallbladder disease, arthritis, respiratory problems (including Pickwickian syndrome, a breathing blockage linked with sudden death), liver malfunction, complications in pregnancy and surgery, flat feet, and even a high accident rate. Moreover, after the effects of diagnosed diseases are taken into account, the risk of death from other causes remains twice as high for people with lifelong obesity as for others. An estimated 25 percent of U.S. adults are overweight to a degree that incurs such risks.[4]

People want to know exactly how fat is too fat for health, but research results vary on this point. Some evidence indicates that being even mildly or moderately overweight increases the risk of heart disease.[5] Even lean adults who were 20 pounds or more overweight as teenagers may be at increased risk of dying of heart disease.[6] On the other hand, some obese people seem to remain healthy and live long despite their body fatness. It may be that genetics determines who among the overweight are most susceptible to diseases and who stay well. Still, the majority of obese people do develop health problems.

Even more than total fatness, fat that collects in the central abdominal area of the body may be especially dangerous with regard to the risks of diabetes, stroke, hypertension, and coronary artery disease.[7] In fact, the risk of death from all causes may be higher in those with **central obesity** than in those whose fat accumulates elsewhere in the body.[8]

The body fat collected deep in the interior of the abdominal cavity, the **intraabdominal fat,** seems especially important in disease risk (see Figure 9-1). Unlike the fat layers lying just beneath the skin (subcutaneous) of the abdomen and elsewhere, the intraabdominal fat, when mobilized, goes directly to the liver where it is made into cholesterol-carrying low-density lipoprotein (LDL). Fat from elsewhere may arrive in the liver eventually, but it takes a circuitous route that first allows other tissues the chance to pull it from circulation and metabolize it.

Some people are more prone to develop the "apple" profile of central obesity while others develop more of a "pear" profile (fat around the hips and thighs). Men of all ages and women past menopause are likely to carry more intraabdominal fat than are women in their reproductive years.[9] Some women change profile at menopause, and lifelong "pears" may suddenly face increased risks of diseases along with a change to the apple profile. Smokers,

obesity overfatness with adverse health effects. Conventionally defined as weight 20% or more above the appropriate weight for height. Obesity also can be defined by body mass index; see p. 320.

central obesity excess fat on the abdomen and around the trunk.

intraabdominal fat fat stored within the abdominal cavity in association with the internal abdominal organs, as opposed to the fat stored directly under the abdominal skin (subcutaneous fat).

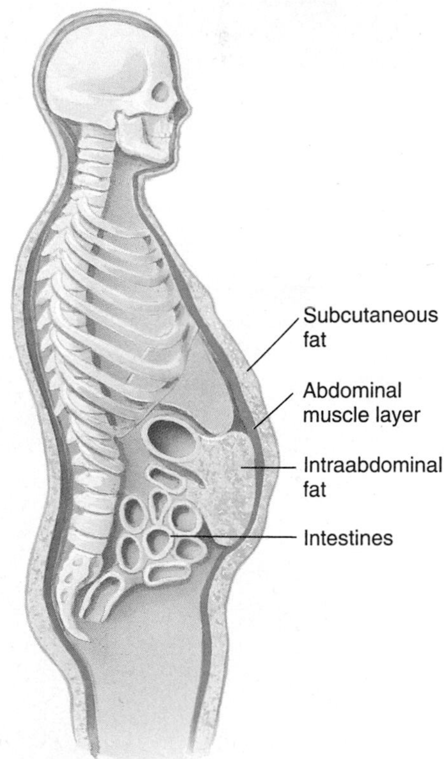

Figure 9-1

INTRAABDOMINAL FAT AND SUBCUTANEOUS FAT

The fat lying deep within the body's abdominal cavity may pose an especially high degree of risk to health.

frame size the size of a person's bones and musculature. A person with a large frame can weigh more than one the same height with a small frame before risk begins to increase.

too, may carry more of their body fat centrally. Whereas a smoker may weigh less than the average nonsmoker, the smoker's waist-to-hip ratio may be greater, leading researchers to think that smoking may directly affect body fat distribution.[10] Two other factors that may affect body fat distribution are intakes of alcohol (a positive association with central adiposity) and exercise (a negative association).

While some overfat people seem to escape health problems, no one who is fat in our society quite escapes the social and economic handicaps. Our society places enormous value on thinness, and fat people are less sought after for romance, less often hired, and less often admitted to college. They pay higher insurance premiums, and they pay more for clothing. Psychologically, too, fat people are made to feel rejected and embarrassed, and this diminishes self-esteem.

Traditional medical advice urges all obese people to reduce their weight to reduce associated risks. This advice stems from concern for the health of overweight people, and indeed may be lifesaving for some. Lately, though, experts are divided on the issue of whether this advice applies equally to all overweight people or whether some may be more at risk from the process of losing weight than from the obesity itself. This chapter's Controversy comes back to explore this debate from both points of view.

KEY POINT Both deficient and excessive body fatness present health risks, and overfatness presents social and economic handicaps as well. Central obesity may be more hazardous to health than other forms of obesity.

Definition of Healthy Weight

Once upon a time the definition of appropriate weight was simple. A person's weight could be compared with that in the "ideal weight" tables. If the actual weight was 20 percent or more above the table weight, then the person was obese; if it was 10 percent under, the person was underweight. Now (to tell a long story in a few words), the term *ideal weight* is no longer in use, and the definition of obesity is no longer simple.

Among the problems are these. Weight depends on the density and thickness of bones—a person's **frame size**—but how do you measure frame size? Body weight doesn't matter as much as body composition, and especially body fat content, but how do you evaluate body fat content? And if the location of fat on the body makes a difference to disease risk, how do you tie this to ideal weight and the definition of obesity?

The problem of using weight as an indicator of health or risk status is that body weight says so little about body composition. People tend to shrink in height and gain fat as they age, making the height and weight charts meaningless. One proposed solution is to measure height only from the ground to the knee, a measurement that doesn't change with age.[11] A person whose weight seems right according to suggested weights for heights may still carry too much of that weight as body fat, especially when lean muscle tissue is minimal due to lack of exercise. Conversely, a person who seems to weigh too much may not be too fat. A dancer or an athlete, whose muscles are well developed and whose bones are well mineralized thanks to consistent exercise, may weigh above the suggested weight range, but may be at a healthy weight. An example of incorrectly relying on height-

Table 9-4
Suggested Weights for Adults

	Weight (lb)[b]			
	19 TO 34 YEARS		35 YEARS AND OVER	
Height[a]	MIDPOINT	RANGE	MIDPOINT	RANGE
5′0"	112	97–128	123	108–138
5′1"	116	101–132	127	111–143
5′2"	120	104–137	131	115–148
5′3"	124	107–141	135	119–152
5′4"	128	111–146	140	122–157
5′5"	132	114–150	144	126–162
5′6"	136	118–155	148	130–167
5′7"	140	121–160	153	134–172
5′8"	144	125–164	158	138–178
5′9"	149	129–169	162	142–183
5′10"	153	132–174	167	146–188
5′11"	157	136–179	172	151–194
6′0"	162	140–184	177	155–199
6′1"	166	144–189	182	159–205
6′2"	171	148–195	187	164–210
6′3"	176	152–200	192	168–216
6′4"	180	156–205	197	173–222
6′5"	185	160–211	202	177–228
6′6"	190	164–216	208	182–234

The higher weights in the ranges generally apply to men, who tend to have more muscle and bone; the lower weights more often apply to women, who have less muscle and bone. The higher weights for people aged 35 and older reflects recent research that seems to indicate that people can carry a little more weight as they grow older without added risk to health.

[a]Without shoes.

[b]Without clothes.

Source: U.S. Department of Agriculture and U.S. Department of Health and Human Services, Home and Garden Bulletin No. 232, *Nutrition and Your Health: Dietary Guidelines for Americans,* 3rd ed. (Washington, D.C.: U.S. Government Printing Office, 1990).

weight tables to determine obesity occurred with a group of football players. They were rejected from the armed forces for being obese according to the table, but their *muscle* weight was actually responsible for the elevated scale weights.[12]

Table 9-4 presents a table professionals can use to look up appropriate weights for people's heights. It offers ranges of weights for every height, permits the user to exercise judgment regarding people's muscle mass, and allows for some weight gain (or height loss) in older people. Taken with a grain of salt, it is a useful table.

You may find some medical professionals still use another table—the Metropolitan Height and Weight Table—to determine "ideal" weights. For at least three reasons, the Metropolitan tables are rejected by most professionals today:

- They are based on people 25 to 29 years of age and then applied to everyone.
- They are based on people who purchased insurance in the past twelve years. Those who purchase insurance turn out to have a longer life expectancy and, on average, to weigh less than the general population.

body mass index (BMI) the weight in kilograms divided by the square of the height (in meters), an indicator of obesity.

fatfold test measurement of the thickness of a fold of skin on the back of the arm (over the triceps muscle), below the shoulder blade (subscapular), or in other places, using a caliper (depicted below). Also called *skinfold test.*

- The concept of "ideal weight" has been replaced by "healthy weight," a term that implies that a person's body composition reflects a healthy balance between lean and fat tissue.

In case you are curious, the 1983 Metropolitan tables appear on page X of the inside back cover.

Despite problems with their use the height-weight tables have three undeniable advantages in assessing obesity—they are available, cheap, and easy to use. If you choose to use the one presented in Table 9-4, be sure to use your barefoot height, and if you wear clothing while weighing, adjust the numbers. Add three pounds to the table weight for light summer clothing, five pounds for heavier winter apparel.

While weight measurements have advantages, they also have the two major drawbacks already mentioned: they fail to indicate how much of the weight is fat and where that fat is located. To find out, one must measure body composition and fat distribution. There is no easy way to look inside a person to measure bones and muscles, but some indirect approximations can reveal clues about health risks associated with overfatness or underweight.

KEY POINT The definition of ideal weight or obesity based on frame size, weight, and standard tables is beset with problems. The currently preferred weight-for-height table allows for differences in muscle mass and age.

Find Your BMI:

$$\text{BMI} = \frac{\text{weight (kilograms)}}{\text{height}^2\text{ (meters)}}$$

or

$$\text{BMI} = \frac{\text{weight (lb)}}{\text{height (in)}^2} \times 705$$

Example: A 5′10″ (70″) person weighing 150 pounds has a BMI of 21.6

$$\text{BMI} = \frac{150}{70^2} \times 705$$

$$\text{BMI} = \frac{150}{4900} \times 705$$

$$\text{BMI} = .0306 \times 705$$

$$\text{BMI} = 21.6 \text{ (rounded)}$$

Body Composition

Nutritionists today often use a more sensitive indicator of body composition than weight, the **body mass index (BMI).** BMI values can indicate underweight or overweight as Table 9-5 shows. The inside back cover of this book provides an easy way to find and evaluate BMI.

Several laboratory techniques for estimating body fatness have also been used for years. These include:

- *Anthropometry.* Measurements such as the **fatfold test,** body circumferences, and body breadths can be taken.
- *Density* (the measurement of body weight compared with volume). Lean tissue is denser than fat tissue, so the denser a person's body is, the more lean tissue it must contain. From the density, an estimate of the percentage of body fat can be derived.

Table 9-5
BMI Values for Men and Women

BMI		
MEN	WOMEN	Risk
< 20.7	< 19.1	Underweight. The lower the BMI the greater the risk
20.7 to 26.4	19.1 to 25.8	Normal, very low risk
26.4 to 27.8	25.8 to 27.3	Marginally overweight, some risk
27.8 to 31.1	27.3 to 32.2	Overweight, moderate risk
31.1 to 45.4	32.3 to 44.8	Severe overweight, high risk
> 45.4	> 44.8	Morbid obesity, very high risk

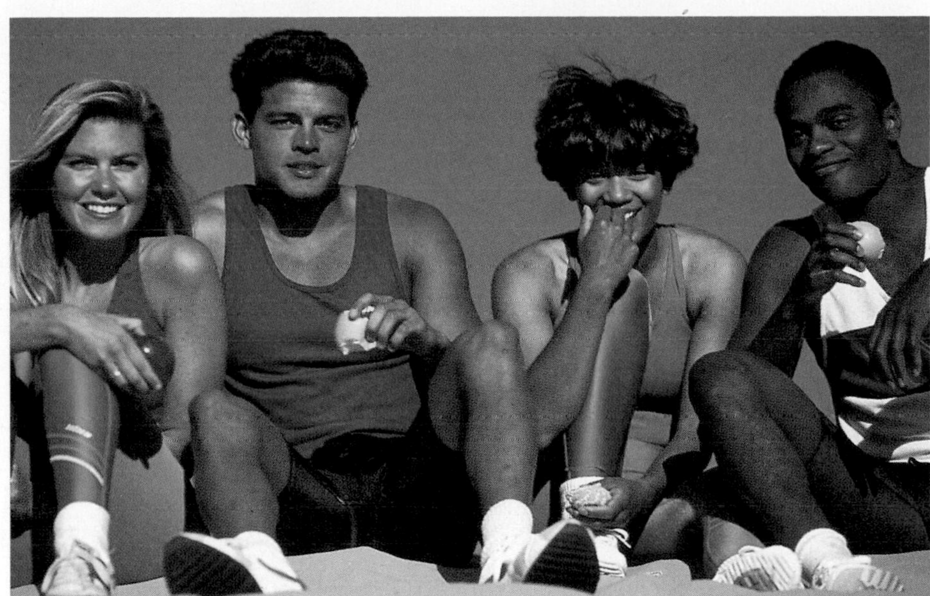

A healthy body contains enough lean tissue to support health and the right amount of fat to meet body needs.

Sophisticated techniques are available to determine these measures, and some can not only estimate lean versus fat tissue but also determine where the fat is located.* However, even these methods are not perfect in their analyses of some people. For example, the body fat of African American women may be underestimated in laboratory studies because standard methods do not account for body composition variability in ethnic groups.[13]

Fatfold measurements also do not take the fat distribution difference into account. They also often lack accuracy (see Table 9-6). For a fair indication of whether you develop fat centrally, try the simple method of comparison of waist and hip measurements presented in Figure 9-2 on the next page.

Even after you have a body fatness estimate, questions arise. What is the "ideal" amount of fat for a body to have? The question—ideal for what?—has to be answered first.

The ideal depends partly on who you are. A man of normal weight may have, on the average, 15 percent and a woman 20 percent of the body weight as fat. Special needs exist, however. For example, competitive endurance athletes need a certain minimum of body fat to provide fuel, to insulate the body, and to permit normal fat-soluble hormone activity, but not so much as to weigh them down. An Alaskan fisherman, on the other hand, needs a blanket of insulating fat to prevent excessive loss of body heat. For a woman starting pregnancy, the ideal percentage of body fat may be different again; the outcome of pregnancy is compromised if the woman begins it with too little body fat. Below a threshold for body fat content set by heredity, some individuals become infertile, develop depression or abnormal hunger regulation, or become unable to keep warm. These thresholds are not the same for each function or in all individuals, and much remains to be learned about them.

Table 9-6
Clues to Fatfold Accuracy

Look for these factors in a fatfold test:

- A trained professional with experience in measuring fatfolds. Inexperienced or untrained persons obtain inconsistent results.
- Metal calipers. Plastic calipers bend and flex, and so lose accuracy in the measurement.
- Choice of the correct sites for measuring. Measurements for men should be made on the chest, the abdomen, or thigh; for women over the triceps muscle, at the waist, or on the thigh. Other sites may not yield meaningful measurements.
- An average of at least three readings to produce a final score. Fewer than three readings provides less reliable data.

*Techniques used in research laboratories include measures of body density and volume such as underwater weighing; isotope dilution; imaging techniques such as ultrasound; measures of conductivity such as bioelectrical impedance; and dual-photon absorptiometry.

Figure 9-2

DETERMINING YOUR WAIST-TO-HIP CIRCUMFERENCE RATIO

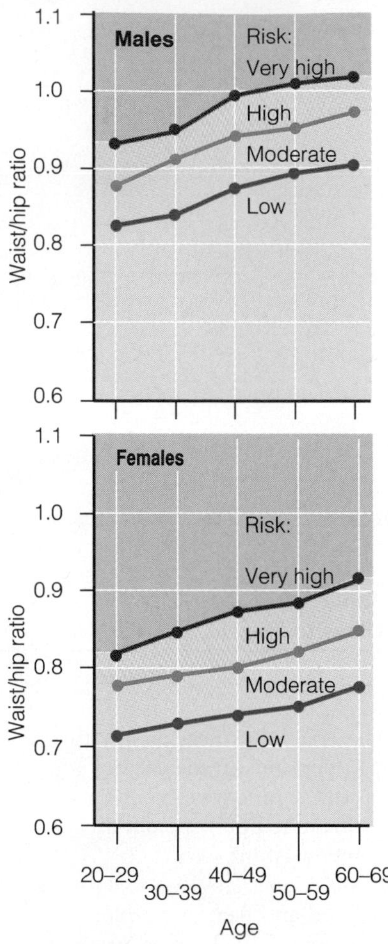

1. Measure your waist and hips with a measuring tape. For your hips, use the largest circumference you find.
2. Calculate your waist-to-hip circumference ratio:

   Waist-to-hip ratio = waist circumference ÷ hip circumference

   Example: a woman with a 28-inch waist and 38-inch hips:

   28 ÷ 38 = 0.74 ratio
3. Evaluate your ratio. A ratio over .95 for males or .80 for females indicates a need to reduce body fatness to reduce health risks. Our example woman's ratio of 0.74 is in the range considered healthy.

Source: Percentile scales from National Research Council, *Diet and Health: Implications for Reducing Chronic Disease Risks* (Washington, D.C.: National Academy Press, 1989), p. 566.

Table 9-7
Body Fat Percentage Standards

Classification	Men (ages 18 to 30)[a]	Women (ages 18 to 30)[a]
Excessively lean	< 5%	< 10%
Lean	5–12%	10–18%
Normal	13–19%	19–25%
Overfat	20–24%	26–32%
Obese	25% or higher	33% or higher

[a]If you are over 30, you can use these standards, but you can relax them a little. It is probably normal to grow a little fatter as you grow older. For many athletes, "normal" body fat percentages may be too high and the "lean" ranges listed here may be most appropriate.

Source: L. K. DeBruyne, F. S. Sizer, and E. W. Whitney, *The Fitness Triad* (St. Paul: West, 1991), p. 50.

Beyond the basic needs for body fat, you should strive to keep body fat content low. Table 9-7 presents some standards for comparison.[14] Blood pressure and other disease-risk indicators also rise and fall with body fatness—blood glucose and blood cholesterol, for example. For those in whom these signs appear with added fat, weight reduction may be critical. The most useful definition of obesity might be, "body fatness in excess of that consistent with optimal health, as determined by a reliable measure." For now, professionals are still seeking a method of pinpointing the amount of fatness that poses dangers to any individual.

The person seeking a single, authoritative answer to the question "How much should I weigh?" is bound to be disappointed. No one can tell you *exactly* how much you should weigh; but with health as a value, at least you have a starting framework. Your weight should fall within the range that supports your health. Within the range, the weight to choose is up to you. Your own priorities are important.

KEY POINT Body mass index indicates underweight or overweight. The assessor can determine the percentage of fat in a person's body by measuring fatfold thickness, body density, or other parameters. Distribution of fat can be assessed by determining the waist-to-hip ratio.

The Mystery of Obesity

Why do some people get fat? Why do some get thin? And most amazingly, why do some people stay at the same weight year after year? Is obesity due to the genetic control of inside-the-body factors or to environmental, outside-the-body influences? In general, two schools of thought attempt to explain obesity development. One attributes it to inherited metabolic causes, the other to behavioral factors. The two views are not mutually exclusive, and both are usually operating, even in the same person. Furthermore, even behavioral tendencies can have a genetic basis.

For whatever reason, the truth remains that people who are overweight must necessarily consume more food energy than they use up each day, and then store the extra as fat. The energy budget is unbalanced.

Inside-the-Body Causes of Overweight

For a person who has one parent with a weight problem, the chance of becoming obese is 60 percent; if both parents have weight problems, the probability may rise to as high as 90 percent.[15] This suggests that a person's genetic makeup may influence the tendency of the body to consume or store too much energy. One way researchers have attempted to study what makes people consume more energy (calories) than they spend is to investigate **hunger, appetite,** and satiety (see Figure 9-3 on the next page). Hunger is a drive programmed into us by our heredity. Appetite, which is learned, can teach us to ignore hunger or to overrespond to it. Hunger is physiological, while appetite is psychological, and the two do not always coincide. Satiety (feeling full) signals that it is time to stop eating, most likely the result of communication between the stomach and small intestine and the brain's hypothalamus. Some overeaters claim they never feel full.

hunger the physiological need to eat, experienced as a drive for obtaining food, an unpleasant sensation that demands relief.

appetite the psychological desire to eat, a learned motivation and a positive sensation that accompanies the sight, smell, or thought of appealing foods.

set-point theory the theory that the body tends to maintain a certain weight by means of its own internal controls.

LPL (lipoprotein lipase) an enzyme mounted on the surfaces of fat cells that splits triglycerides in the blood into fatty acids and glycerol to be absorbed into the cells for reassembly and storage.

Set-Point Theory One popular theory of why the obese person's body may store too much fat is the **set-point theory.** Researchers have noted that most people who lose weight on reducing diets later quickly regain all the lost weight.[16] This phenomenon seems to suggest that somehow the body chooses a weight that it wants to be and defends that weight by regulating eating behaviors and hormonal actions.[17] This theory is supported by research that shows that some types of obese rats defend their body overweight condition as precisely as rats who naturally stay thin.

Chapter 3 described the brain's hypothalamus.

Enzyme Theory Strong evidence also links fat storage with elevated concentrations of the enzyme that enables fat cells to store triglycerides. Concentrations of this enzyme, **LPL** or **lipoprotein lipase,** increase as cells become enlarged with fat. The more LPL, the more easily fat cells store lipid, and the more likely the body will remain obese.[18] An interesting question relating to the set-point theory just described is whether or not some people's fat cells contain elevated concentrations of LPL *before* the onset of obesity. If so, this situation might partly explain why obesity tends to run in families, for the making of all enzymes including LPL is governed by the genes.

Fat Cell Theory Another cause of obesity may be the development of excess fat cells during childhood. The amount of fat on a person's body reflects both fat cell *number* and *size.* The number of fat cells increases during the growing years and then levels off during adulthood. Fat cell number increases more rapidly in obese children than in lean children, and obese children entering their teen years may already have as many fat cells as do adults of normal weight.

A fat cell can expand eight to tenfold in size. Once a cell reaches some critical size, it may also divide. Fat cells of obese people also contain more LPL, so they are likely to reach a large size quickly.[19] Therefore, obesity reflects not only more and larger fat cells, but more efficient ones, too. With fat loss, the fat cells shrink in size, but not in number and perhaps not in their LPL concentrations, either.[20] For this reason, people with extra fat cells may encounter extra difficulty in trying to lose weight. They may also tend to regain lost weight rapidly. Prevention of obesity may be most critical during the growing years when fat cell number is increasing.

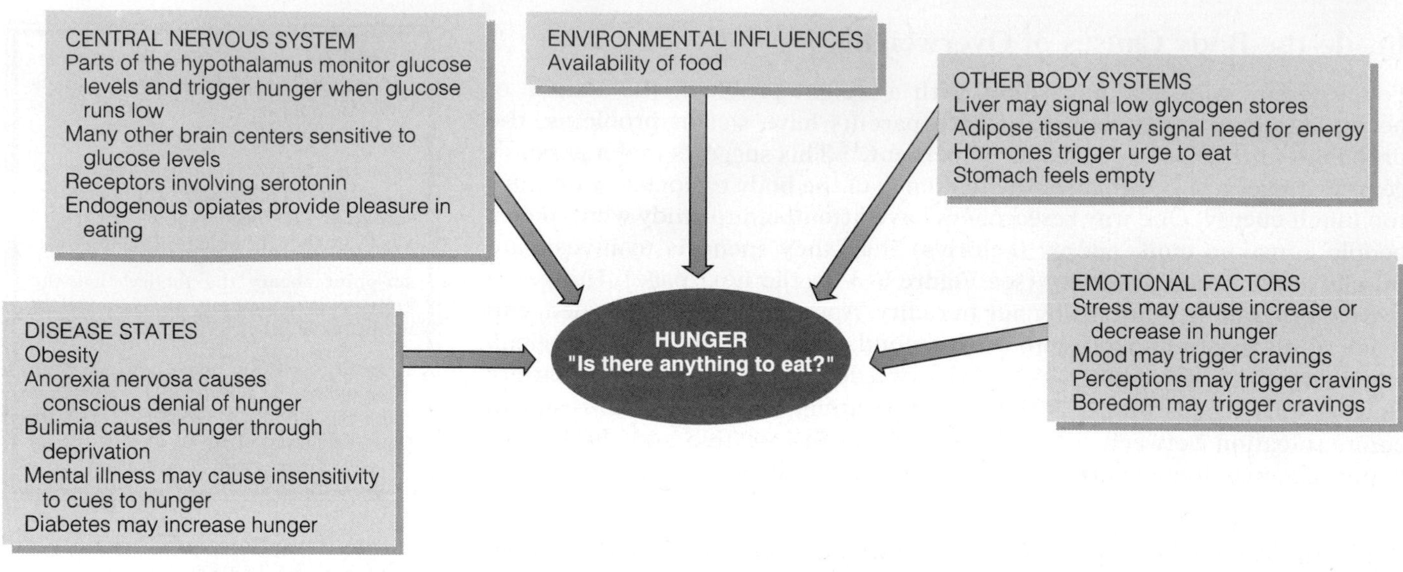

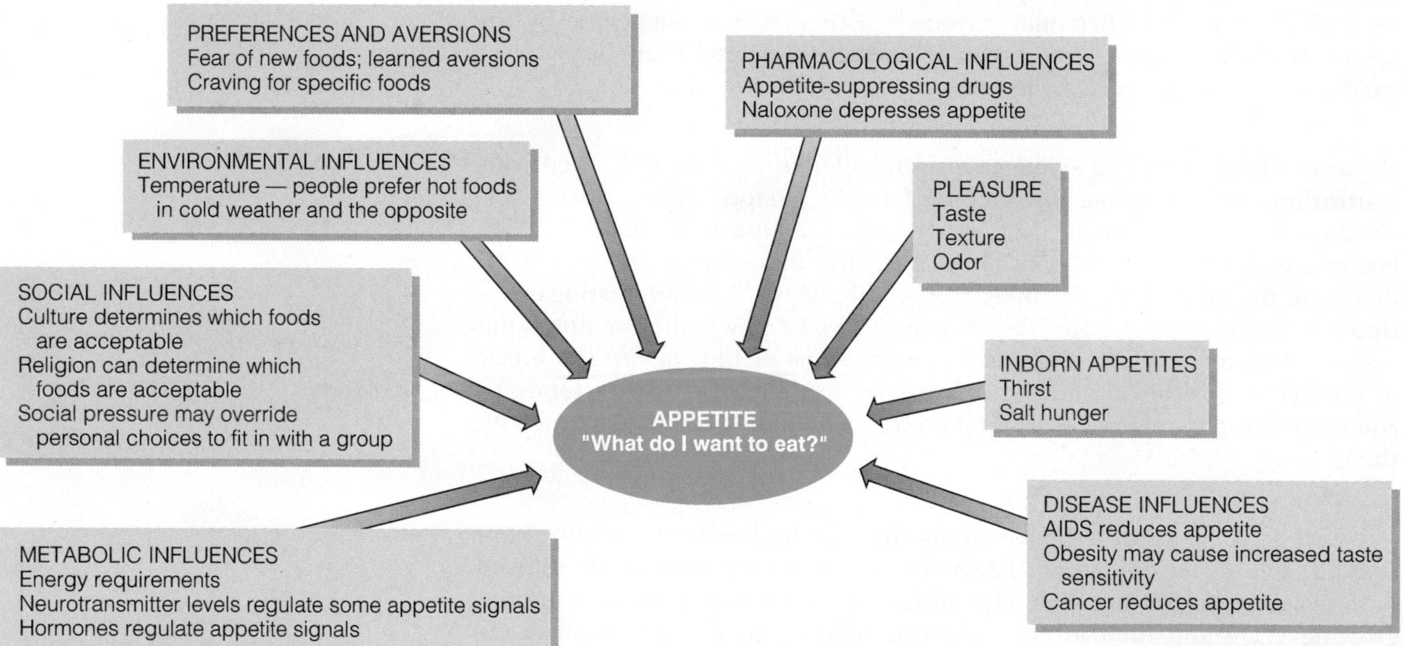

Figure 9-3

HUNGER AND APPETITE

This is a partial list of the factors that are thought to affect hunger and appetite.

Source: Adapted from T. W. Castonguay and coauthors, Hunger and appetite: Old concepts/new distinctions, *Nutrition Reviews* 41 (1983): 101–110.

The Theory of Thermogenesis A theory about the body's manufacturing of heat, **thermogenesis,** and its relation to overweight concerns a tissue that specializes in converting energy to heat—**brown fat.** Regular white fat cells store energy in fat's chemical bonds and have a slow metabolic rate; brown fat cells break those bonds and actively release their stored energy as heat. Brown fat is more abundant and more active in lean animals than in fat ones. It is theorized that a person whose brown fat burns off too little energy or a person who has less than the normal amount of brown fat would tend to store more white fat than other people store. While it is known that heredity plays a role in development of brown fat in animals, a role for brown fat's involvement in human obesity remains uncertain.[21]

thermogenesis the generation and release of body heat associated with the breakdown of body fuels.

brown fat adipose tissue abundant in hibernating animals and human infants. Brown fat cells are packed with pigmented, energy-burning enzymes that give brown fat cells a darkened appearance under a microscope.

arousal heightened activity of certain brain centers associated with excitement and anxiety.

stress eating eating in response to stress, an inappropriate response.

Thermic Effect of Food Another form of thermogenesis, the thermic effect of food (TEF) mentioned earlier, varies between obese and nonobese people. In lean people who have just eaten a meal, energy use speeds up for a while, and then drops back to normal. In many obese people no change in energy use occurs after eating. While TEF costs little energy, some researchers believe this amount of expenditure adds up over a lifetime and may contribute to leanness.

So far no one has shown conclusively that overweight people expend less energy overall than normal weight people, and in fact, the opposite seems to hold true. Overweight people seem to spend more energy each day, not less, than do people of normal weight.[22] This is probably because heavier bodies require more energy to move and to maintain themselves.

KEY POINT Inside-the-body theories about causes of obesity include abnormal regulation of food intake, the set-point theory, enzyme theory, fat cell theory, and theories centered around thermogenesis and the body's use of fuels.

Outside-the-Body Causes of Overweight

A different line of research contends that obesity is determined by behavioral responses to environmental stimuli. It asks what external forces might cause people to take in more food energy than their bodies need.

Eating behavior seems to occur not only in response to internal hunger and appetite, but also to complex human sensations such as yearning, craving, addiction, or compulsion. For an emotionally insecure person, eating when lonely may be less threatening than calling a friend and risking rejection. Often people eat to relieve boredom or depression. Some people experience food cravings when feeling down or depressed.[23] Food picks them up for a while.

Any kind of **arousal** can cause overeating, perhaps because aroused feelings are mistaken for hunger. The eating done in response to arousal is **stress eating.** However, while some people overeat in response to stress, others cannot eat at all. It is not yet known why people react differently. Obese people do not seem to be especially likely to feel anxiety or depression.

External Cue Theory Proponents of this view hold that people overeat as a response to their surroundings—foremost among them, the availability of a multitude of delectable foods.[24] This theory cannot fully explain obesity development because almost everyone, not just obese people, can be enticed to overeat when choosing from an abundance of rich and appetizing foods. A classic experiment showed that even animals respond in this way. Normal-weight rats rapidly became obese when fed "cafeteria style" on a variety of rich, palatable foods. Rats are known to precisely maintain a healthy weight when fed a standard rat-chow diet.

It may be that obese people are supersensitive to delicious tastes, and this sensitivity may lead them to consume more of whatever food they perceive as delicious. The overweight subjects of one study more often sought the foods they found most palatable and they ate them more quickly.[25] These ideas may bear on how much of which foods overweight people consume in a day.[26] One food constituent stands out among others in being perceived as palatable—fat.[27]

The Fattening Power of Fat Controversy 5 made clear that not only does fat deliver more than twice the calories, gram for gram, as protein and carbohydrate, it also seems to be stored preferentially by the body and with great efficiency. Of the three energy nutrients, fat stimulates the least energy expenditure in diet-induced thermogenesis. Carbohydrate and protein, on the other hand, stimulate much larger responses.

A high percentage of fat in a person's diet more strongly predicts a high percentage of body fat than does a high number of total calories. A person whose diet contains much fat, even when total calories are reasonable, is often one who battles against overweight.[28]

Exercise One other cause of obesity is lack of exercise. The control of hunger/appetite appears to work well in most healthy, active people; few athletes are obese. But appetite control often fails when activity falls below a certain minimum level. For many people, television-watching has all but replaced outdoor work and play as the major spare-time activity. In addition, sponsors run advertisements for delicious, high-fat (and low-nutrient) foods designed to trigger the appetites of viewers. One study showed that in children, obesity increases by 2 percent per hour of television-watching per day. Another linked elevated blood cholesterol concentrations to increased time of viewing television.[29]

Although we may have been born with the instinct to eat, we are not helpless when confronted with food. We also have the ability to override the instinct to eat delicious high-fat foods, at least most of the time. We can also reverse a sedentary lifestyle and arrange to be more physically active. Later sections of this chapter show how people can modify their behavior by changing their responses to cues in the environment and by arranging to experience consequences for their behavior.

KEY POINT Among the theories of behavioral causes of obesity are inappropriate eating in response to stress, arousal, or the sight, smell, and taste of foods. Two major contributors to obesity are believed to be the fattening power of fat in foods and the underactivity of some obese people.

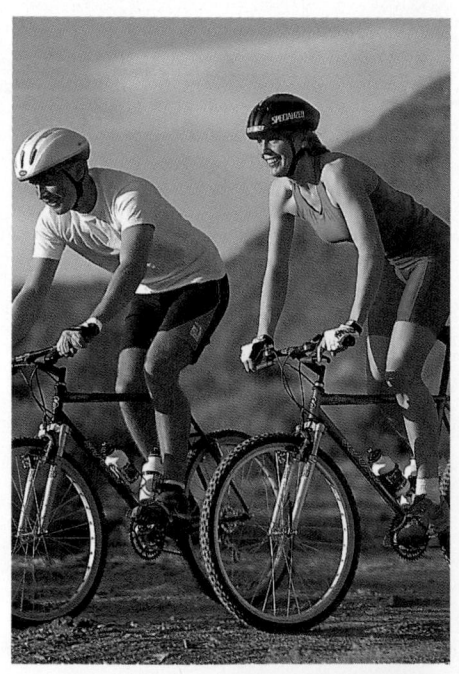

Physical activity can help to regulate the appetite.

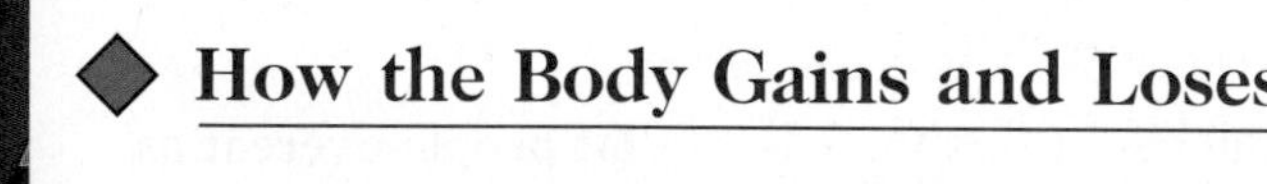

How the Body Gains and Loses Weight

The balance between the energy you take in and the energy you spend determines whether you will gain, lose, or maintain body *fat*. However, when you step on the scale and note a change in *weight* of a pound or two, this may not indicate a change in body fat. A change in weight can reflect shifts in body fluid content, in bone minerals, in lean tissues such as muscles, or in the contents of the digestive tract. It often correlates with the time of day: people generally weigh the least before breakfast. It is important for people concerned with weight control to realize that quick, large changes in weight are usually not changes in fat alone, or even at all.

A person who stands about 5 feet 10 inches tall and who weighs 150 pounds carries about 90 of those pounds as water and 30 as fat. The other 30 pounds are the so-called lean tissues— muscles; organs such as the heart, brain, and liver; and the bones of the skeleton. Stripped of water and fat, then, the person weighs only 30 pounds!* This lean tissue is vital to health. The person who seeks to lose weight wants, of course, to lose fat, not this precious lean tissue. And for someone who wants to gain weight, it is desirable to gain lean and fat in proportion, not just fat.

The type of tissue gained or lost depends on how the person goes about losing or gaining it. To lose fluid, for example, one can take a "water pill" (diuretic), causing the kidneys to siphon extra water from the blood into the urine. Or one can engage in heavy exercise while wearing thick clothing in the heat, losing abundant fluid in sweat. (Both practices are dangerous, incidentally, and are not being recommended here.) To gain water weight, a person can overconsume salt and water; for a few hours the body will then retain water until it manages to excrete the salt. (This, too, is not recommended.) Most quick weight-change schemes promote large changes in body fluids that register temporary, dramatic changes on the scale but that accomplish little weight change in the long run. It is important to stress physical activity as a means of gaining and maintaining lean tissue during weight adjustments.

Gain of Body Weight

Weight gain comes from eating more food energy than is spent. Weight may be gained as body fat or as lean tissue, depending largely upon whether the eater is also exercising. Those who begin weight training and dieting to gain lean tissue may be disappointed when body weight on the scales doesn't change much. Muscle does, however, develop quickly with the right kind of regular exercise. If muscle is growing while fat is shrinking, the desired changes are happening, regardless of what the scale says.

Chapter 10 comes back to muscle gains in response to exercise.

What happens inside the body when a person does not use up all of the food energy taken in? What does the body do with it? Previous chapters have already provided the answer; the energy-yielding nutrients contribute to body stores as follows:

- Carbohydrate (other than fiber) is broken down to sugars for absorption. In the body tissues, excesses of these may be built up to *glycogen* or converted to *fat* and stored.
- Fat is broken down to glycerol and fatty acids for absorption. Inside the body, these are especially easy for the body to store as body *fat.*
- Protein is broken down to amino acids for absorption. Inside the body, these may be used to replace lost body *protein* and, in a person who is exercising, to build new muscle and other lean tissue. This protein must be functioning protein; excess protein is not passively stored. Any excess amino acids have their nitrogen removed and are converted to *fat.*

Note that although three kinds of energy-yielding nutrients enter the body, they become only two kinds of energy stores: glycogen and fat. Glycogen stores amount to about three-fourths of a pound; fat stores can, of course, amount to many pounds. Note, too, that when excess protein is converted to fat, it cannot be recovered later as protein because the nitrogen is stripped from the amino acids and is excreted in the urine. No matter whether you are eating steak, brownies, or baked beans, then, if you eat enough of them, any excess will be turned to fat within hours.

---

*For a healthy 5 foot tall person who weighs 100 pounds, the comparable figures would be 60 pounds of water, 20 pounds of fat, 20 pounds of lean.

Alcohol also becomes fat if it isn't burned off. Alcohol may also make fat storage likely. Ethanol, the alcohol of alcoholic beverages, has been shown to slow down the body's use of fat for fuel by as much as a third, causing more fat to be stored, primarily in the intraabdominal fat tissue of the "beer-drinkers belly" and also on the thighs, legs, or anywhere the person tends to store surplus fat.[30] Alcohol therefore is fattening, both through the calories it provides and through its effects on fat metabolism.*

It is worth emphasizing these points by repeating them:

- Any food can make you fat if you eat enough of it. A net excess of energy is stored in the body as fat in fat tissue.
- Fat from food, as opposed to carbohydrate or protein, is especially easy for the body to store as fat tissue.
- Protein is not stored in the body except in response to exercise; it is present only as working tissue.** Excess protein is stored as fat.
- Alcohol both delivers calories and encourages fat storage.

KEY POINT When energy balance is positive, the three energy-yielding nutrients are converted to glycogen or fat and stored. Dietary fat is especially easy for the body to store. Protein, once converted to fat, cannot later be recovered as amino acids; only its energy value is recovered. Alcohol delivers calories and encourages fat storage.

Moderate Weight Loss vs Rapid Weight Loss

When you eat less food energy than you need, your body draws on its stored fuel to keep going. It is a great advantage to be able to eat periodically, store fuel, and then use up that fuel between meals. The between-meal interval is normally about four to six waking hours—about the length of time it takes to use up most of the available liver glycogen—or 12 to 14 hours at night, when body systems are slowed down and the need is less.

When you moderately restrict your calories and consume an otherwise balanced diet that meets your protein and carbohydrate needs, your body will be forced to use up its stored fat for energy. Gradual weight loss will occur. This is preferred to rapid weight loss because lean body mass is spared and fat is lost.

If a person doesn't eat for, say, three whole days or a week, then the body makes one adjustment after another. Soon, the liver's glycogen is essentially exhausted. Where, then, can the body obtain glucose to keep its nervous system going? Not from the muscles' glycogen because that is reserved for the muscles' own use. The underfed body must turn to the protein in its own lean tissues.

An alternative source of energy might be the abundant fat stores most people carry, but these are of no use to the nervous system. The muscles, heart, and other organs use fat as fuel, but at this stage the nervous system needs glucose. Most importantly, the body's major fuel, fat, cannot be converted to glucose—the body lacks enzymes for this conversion.*** The body

*People *addicted* to alcohol are often overly thin because of diseased organs and subsequent malnutrition.

**Amino acids are present in all body fluids, performing such functions as maintaining the acid-base balance there, and the liver is considered by some to be an amino acid storage site.

***Glycerol, 5% of fat, can yield glucose but is a negligible source.

does, however, possess enzymes that can convert *protein* to glucose. Therefore, body proteins are sacrificed to supply raw materials from which to make glucose.

ketone bodies acidic compounds derived from fat and certain amino acids; normally rare in the blood, they help to feed the brain during times when too little carbohydrate is available. Also defined in Chapter 4.

If the body were to continue to consume its lean tissue unchecked, death would ensue within about ten days. After all, not only skeletal muscle but also the blood proteins, the liver, the heart muscle, the lung tissue—all vital tissues—are being burned as fuel. (In fact, fasting or starving people remain alive only until their stores of fat are gone or until half their lean tissue is gone, whichever comes first.) To prevent this, the body that has run out of glucose plays its last ace: it begins converting fat into compounds that the nervous system can adapt to use and so forestall the end. This is ketosis, which was first mentioned in Chapter 4 as an adaptation to prolonged fasting or carbohydrate deprivation.

In early food deprivation:

The nervous system cannot use fat as fuel; it can use only glucose.

Body fat cannot be converted to glucose.

Body protein can be converted to glucose.

In ketosis, instead of breaking down fat molecules to carbon dioxide and water, as it normally does, the body takes partially broken down fat fragments and combines them to make **ketone bodies,** compounds that are normally rare in the blood. (It converts some amino acids to ketone bodies, too: those that cannot be used to make glucose.) These ketone bodies circulate in the bloodstream and help to feed the brain, since about half of the brain's cells can make the enzymes needed to use them for energy. Within about 10 days of fasting, the brain and nervous system can meet most of their energy needs using ketone bodies.[31]

Thus indirectly the nervous system begins to feed on the body's fat stores. This reduces the nervous system's need for glucose, it spares the muscle and other lean tissue from being devoured quickly, and it prolongs the starving person's life. Thanks to ketosis, a healthy person starting with average body fat content can live totally deprived of food for as long as six to eight weeks. Figure 9-4 on the next page reviews how energy is used during both feasting and fasting and in ketosis.

Fasting has been practiced as a periodic discipline by respected, wise people in many cultures. Clearly the body tolerates short-term fasting, although there is no evidence that the body becomes internally "cleansed," as some believe. Ketosis may harm the body by upsetting the acid-base balance of the blood and by promoting mineral losses in the urine. In addition, people with eating disorders (see Chapter 10's Controversy section) often report that a fast or a severely restrictive diet heralded the beginning of their loss of control over eating.

For the person who wants to lose weight, fasting is not the best way. The body's lean tissue continues to be degraded. The body is deprived of nutrients it needs to assemble new enzymes, red and white blood cells, and other vital components. The body also slows its metabolism to conserve energy. A diet only moderately restricted in calories has actually been observed to promote a greater rate of *weight* loss, a faster rate of *fat* loss, and a retention of more lean tissue than a severely restricted fast.[32]

Just how to design a low-calorie diet is the subject of a later section, but it should be mentioned that any diet too low in carbohydrate will bring about responses that are similar to fasting. Many low-carbohydrate diets have been promoted to the public in many different guises. Each diet has enjoyed a surge of popularity thanks largely to a sizable initial weight loss. These diets are designed to throw a person into ketosis. The sales pitch is that "you'll never feel hungry" and that "you'll lose weight fast—faster than you would on any ordinary diet." Both claims are true, but both are misleading. Loss of appetite accompanies any low-calorie diet. Severe calorie restriction means loss of water and lean tissue, and the water is rapidly

Names of some low-carbohydrate diets include Atkins Diet Revolution, Calories Don't Count Diet, Drinking Man's Diet, Mayo Diet, Protein-Sparing Fast, Scarsdale Diet, Simeons HCG Diet, Ski Team Diet, and Stillman Diet. New ones keep coming out under new names.

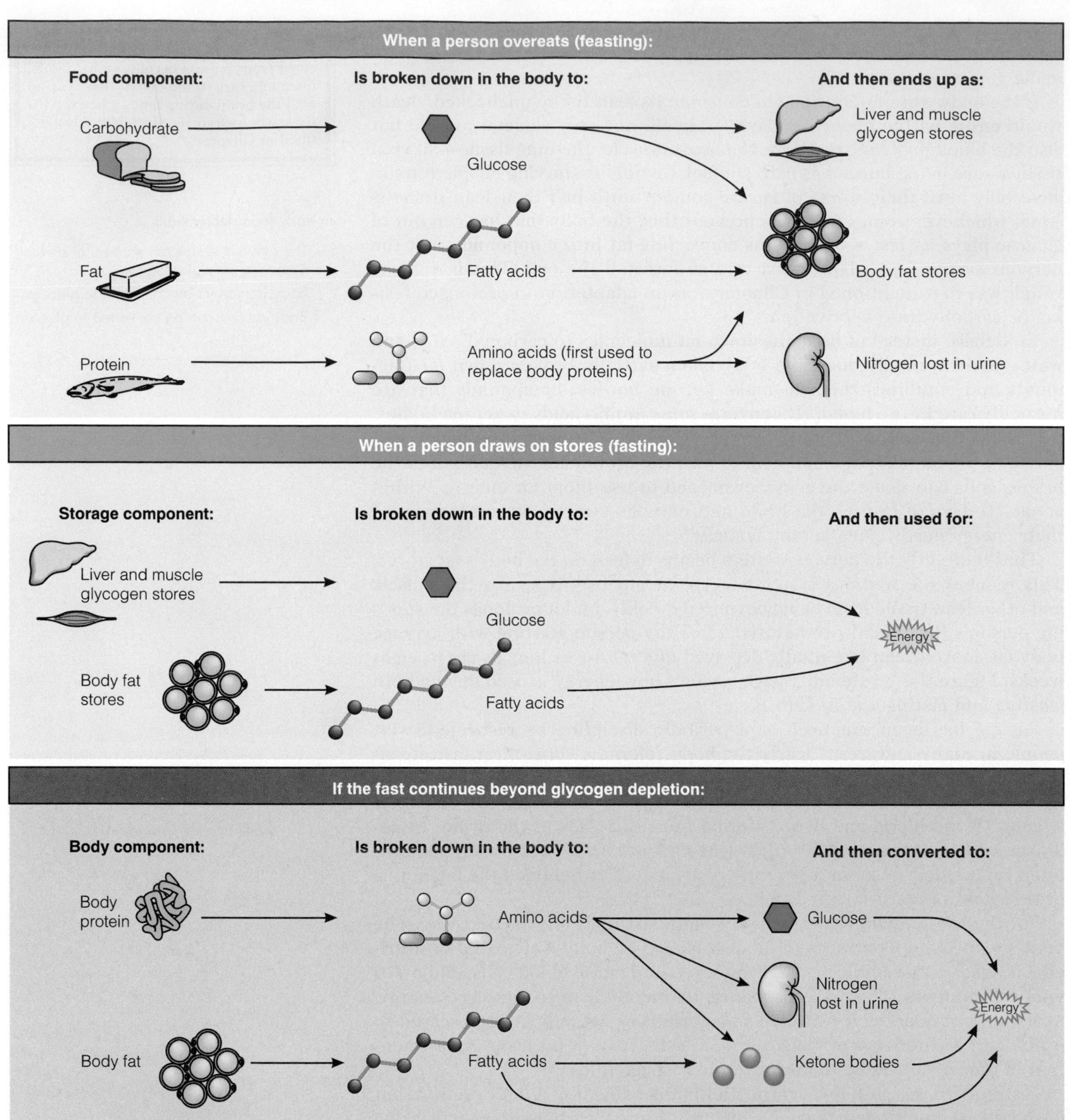

Figure 9-4

FEASTING AND FASTING

regained when people begin eating normally again. But most importantly, these diets, undertaken without medical supervision, are dangerous.

Many physiological hazards accompany low-carbohydrate diets: high blood cholesterol, hypoglycemia, mineral imbalances, and other metabolic abnormalities. Some low-carbohydrate diets, particularly those called protein-sparing fasts, have caused heart failure. These diets are never recommended by knowledgeable practitioners. Some diets that are very low in calories may be recommended by physicians to correct severe, health-threatening obesity. These are the very-low-calorie diets (VLCD) discussed in Controversy 9.

Some diet plans are sound and can assist a person who needs guidance and support. Others are ineffective or even unsafe. Table 9-8 provides a way of judging weight loss programs and diets according to standard nutrition principles.

Table 9-8
Rating Sound and Unsound Weight-Loss Schemes and Diets

Start by giving each diet or program 160 points. Subtract points as instructed, whenever a diet falls short of ideals.

Does the diet or program:

1. Provide a reasonable number of calories (not fewer than 1,200 calories for an average-size person)? If not, give it a minus 10.
2. Provide enough, but not too much, protein (at least the recommended intake or RDA, but not more than twice that much)? If no, minus 10.
3. Provide enough fat for balance but not so much fat as to go against current recommendations (about 30 percent of calories from fat)? If no, minus 10.
4. Provide enough carbohydrate to spare protein and prevent ketosis (100 grams of carbohydrate for the average size person)? Is it mostly complex carbohydrate (not more than 10 percent of the calories as concentrated sugar)? If no to either or both, minus 10.
5. Offer a balanced assortment of vitamins and minerals—that is, foods from all food groups? If it omits a food group (for example, meats), does it provide a suitable substitute? Count five food groups in all: milk/milk products, meat/fish/poultry/eggs/legumes, fruits, vegetables, and starches/grains. For *each* food group omitted and not adequately substituted for, subtract 10 points.
6. Offer variety, in the sense that different foods can be selected each day? If you'd class it as boring or monotonous, give it a minus 10.
7. Consist of ordinary foods that are available locally (for example, in the main grocery stores) at the prices people normally pay? Or does the dieter have to buy special, expensive, or unusual foods to adhere to the diet? If you would class it as "bizarre" or "requiring special foods," minus 10.
8. Promise dramatic, rapid weight loss (substantially more than 1 percent of total body weight per week)? If yes, minus 10.
9. Encourage permanent, realistic lifestyle changes, including regular exercise and the behavioral changes needed for weight maintenance? If not, minus 10.
10. Misrepresent salespeople as "counselors" supposedly qualified to give guidance in nutrition and/or general health without a profit motive, or collect large sums of money at the start, or require that clients sign contracts for expensive, long-term programs? If so, minus 10.
11. Fail to inform clients about the risks associated with weight loss in general or the specific program being promoted? If so, minus 10.
12. Promote unproven or spurious weight-loss aids such as human chorionic gonadotrophin hormone (HCG), starch blockers, diuretics, sauna belts, body wraps, passive exercise, ear stapling, acupuncture, electric muscle stimulating (EMS) devices, spirulina, amino acid supplements (e.g., arginine, ornithine), glucomannan, appetite suppressants, "unique" ingredients, and so forth? If so, minus 10.

Ineffective or dangerous weight loss gimmicks:

- Diet pills, all types
- Expanding pills
- Glucomannan, bee pollen, spirulina
- Hormones
- Laxatives
- Lipectomy and suctioning
- Massages, muscle stimulators
- Spa belts, rollers, saunas, whirlpools
- Stomach stapling, surgery, balloons

In addition to diets, weight loss gimmicks abound in the marketplace (see the margin). Most are ineffective, and some are truly dangerous. As for drugs, surgery, and stapling, each can be hazardous and all three are reserved for efforts at saving the lives of obese people at critical risk, as the Consumer Caution points out.

KEY POINT When energy balance is negative, glycogen returns glucose to the body; when glycogen runs out, body protein is called upon to do so. Fat also supplies fuel as fatty acids. In a fast, after glycogen runs out, fat supplies fuel as ketone bodies; ketone bodies may disturb the acid-base balance of the blood. Low carbohydrate diets are dangerous.

gastric bypass surgery that reroutes food from the stomach to the lower part of the small intestine, creating a chronic, lifelong state of malabsorption by preventing normal digestion and absorption of nutrients.

gastroplasty surgery involving partitioning of the stomach by stapling off a "pouch" or otherwise constricting the volume of food the stomach can accept at a meal, and thereby reducing total food intake.

Surgery and Drugs for Weight Loss

CONSUMER CAUTION People who suffer from obesity may seek help from surgery, prescription or over-the-counter pills, and other products. Medical interventions can indeed help, but only rarely.

Weight-loss help from surgery is available only to those carrying serious risks of disease and early death from severe obesity. Two surgical procedures performed today—**gastric bypass** and **gastroplasty**—seem to offer some hope.[33] Bypass surgery, the shortening of the digestive tract by joining a section of the small intestine directly to the stomach, has proved to reduce risks associated with coronary artery disease.[34] Gastroplasty, the constricting of the stomach's volume (sometimes called *stomach stapling*), can also reverse a trend toward worsening health as a result of obesity. About half of those who undergo these two procedures find long-term success, defined as five to ten years of reduced weight and lasting improvements in medical and other conditions arising from obesity.[35] The other half of surgical patients, though, fail to lose or to maintain their losses.

Surgeons carefully screen obese candidates for surgery because the risks from both the surgery and its expected consequences can be severe. During surgery, obese people face more infections, more respiratory problems, more blood clots, more difficulties in anesthesia, and slower wound healing than do normal-weight surgery patients. In addition to immediate risks of surgery, the person must accept lifelong problems of severe diarrhea, frequent vomiting, intolerance to sweets and milk, dehydration, limited dietary intake, and multiple nutrient deficiencies even with medical follow-up care.[36] Staples pull out, stomach pouches enlarge, and surgeries must sometimes be repeated with repeated risks. Lifelong medical supervision is critical for those who choose the surgical route, but for up to half of those who choose it, the benefits of weight loss have proven worth the risks.

Somewhat less risky than surgery for help in weight loss are the prescription drugs. Most prescription drugs either suppress appetite and so cause a drop in food intake or speed up energy metabolism and so cause an increased use of fat for fuel.[37] A new drug, currently under testing, acts on the small intestine's fat-digesting enzymes to prevent digestion and absorption of about a third of the fat consumed. The

Surgery and Drugs for Weight Loss *continued*

drug, tetrahydrolipostatin, now faces years of rigorous study before it can be approved by FDA. Government regulations restrict the use of prescription drugs for obesity to a three-month maximum time limit. While some drugs have proved effective in promoting initial weight loss, the long-term effects of their use are unknown.[38]

Years ago physicians routinely prescribed amphetamines (pep pills) to reduce the appetite. Not only did amphetamines prove of little value in weight loss, but also they are highly addictive. Many dieters who used them remained overweight and were left with the additional problem of getting off the drugs. Amphetamines are no longer approved by the FDA for weight loss.

One safer, more effective drug, dexfenfluramine, shows promise in laboratory tests. Dexfenfluramine is not addicting and it seems to curb the appetite in the long term.[39] The drug works by stimulating the brain to release the brain's neurotransmitter serotonin. Serotonin in turn depresses the appetite. Several other appetite-suppressing drugs are also under study and may one day prove their worth.

For most people with just a few pounds to lose, prescription drugs are not the answer. What about over-the-counter (OTC) weight-loss pills? Are they safe? Some people who have tried OTC pills that they assumed to be safe have ended up on a surgeon's table and one person died from a complication of the surgery.[40] The pills they took contained soluble fiber (guar gum) that swelled in their systems. The intent was to make them feel full and eat less, but the result was a dangerous intestinal blockage that required surgical removal. This weight-loss product and most others sold over the counter were swept from the shelves when FDA reviewed their ingredients and found them lacking both safety and effectiveness.

Only two OTC ingredients remain lawfully for sale today. One, **phenylpropanolamine (PPA)** also found in cold medications, carries a side effect of elevated blood pressure.[41] It makes some people feel jumpy because one of the drug's actions is to trigger the body's stress response. PPA does seem to cause a statistically greater weight loss in dieters, but no one yet knows why PPA has this effect. The other ingredient, the anesthetic benzocaine (usually in gum or candy form) numbs the taste buds and supposedly reduces the desire to taste food. These two drugs are still under study by FDA and could still be removed from shelves should they prove ineffective or unsafe.

As for water pills, an attractive idea is that excess water in the body is responsible for excess body weight and that taking a water pill (diuretic) can get rid of it. Temporary water retention, seen in many women around the time of the menstrual period, can account for several pounds on the scale. This is normal and is not related to the dangerous water retention associated with diseases for which diuretic treatment is intended. Taking a self-prescribed diuretic can make a person lose a few pounds for half a day or so, but it does nothing to solve a fat problem, and it threatens the taker with dehydration and mineral imbalances.

(continued on next page)

phenylpropanolamine (PPA) a stimulant of the sympathetic nervous system used as a weight-loss agent and available in over-the-counter medications.

Surgery and Drugs for Weight Loss *continued*

CONSUMER CAUTION In the end, the only means of reducing body fat is to shift the energy budget from positive to negative, to take less energy in and put more energy out. Nonprescription diet pills, diuretics, illegal hormones, and use of jiggle machines at spas are useless; they enjoy brisk sales, however, because the lifelong effort required for weight control is difficult.

Behaviors to Promote Appropriate Body Composition

At the start of this chapter, the point was made that *behavior* is the only piece of the weight control puzzle that is truly under voluntary control. The following sections therefore present a series of strategies for shaping behavior to promote a healthy body composition.

Diet Strategies for Weight Loss

Whether a person wants to lose 10 pounds or 50 pounds, the techniques of diet, physical activity, and behavior modification discussed in order here apply equally. The following sections are written in terms of advice to "you," not to put you under pressure to take it personally but to give you the illusion of listening in on a conversation in which an overweight person (with say 50 pounds to lose) is being competently counseled by someone familiar with the techniques known to be safe and effective.

Strategies for diet planning:

1. Get involved personally.
2. Adopt a realistic plan.
3. Make the diet adequate.
4. Keep track of calories and especially those from fat.
5. Emphasize high-carbohydrate, high-nutrient density foods.
6. Individualize. Use foods you like.
7. Stress dos, not don'ts.
8. Eat regular meals with no skipping—at least three a day and especially breakfast.

No particular food plan is magical, and no particular food must be either included or avoided. You are the one who will have to live with the plan, so you had better be involved in designing it. Don't think of yourself as going "on" a *diet* because then you may be tempted to go "off." Think of yourself as adopting an eating *plan* for life. It must consist of foods that you like or can learn to like, that are available to you, and that are within your means.

Choose an energy level you can live with. For the person wanting to lose weight, a deficit of 500 calories a day for seven days (3,500 calories a week) is enough to lose a pound a week of body fat. It is urgent not to try to cut calories too far for all the reasons already mentioned. A rule of thumb is that you need to eat at least 10 calories per pound of current body weight each day to lose fat efficiently while retaining lean tissue.

There is no point in hurrying. You will never go off the plan; you will only modify it slightly when you have reached your goal. Nutritional adequacy is hard to achieve on a low-calorie diet and even a small person should not try to get by on fewer than 1,200 calories (1,000 at the very least). A larger person should adjust the calories upwards; some people can lose weight steadily on diets of 1,600 calories or more. When planning meals, follow a pattern that includes at least the minimum servings suggested in the Daily Food Guide (Chapter 2) without frills. Making the diet adequate is a way of putting yourself first. For the lower calorie ranges, it is appropriate to take a balanced vitamin-mineral supplement; see Contro-

Table 9-9
A Sample Day's Balanced Weight-Loss Plan

Exchange Item	Number of Exchanges	Carbohydrate (g)	Protein (g)	Fat (g)	Energy (cal)[a]
Starch/bread	6	90	18	Trace	432
Vegetables	3	15	6	0	84
Fruits	4	60	0	0	240
Meat (lean) or alternates	4	0	28	12	220
Milk (nonfat)	2	24	16	Trace	160
Fat	3	0	0	15	135
Total		189 g	68 g	27 g	1,271 cal

This diet typifies the balance recommended for a weight-loss diet: approximately 60% of the calories are from carbohydrate, 21% from protein, and 19% from fat. This plan is high in protein because it includes the minimum servings of meat and milk required for adequacy. When the dieter returns to a maintenance plan by adding mostly carbohydrate foods, the ratio will resemble the 15% protein, 30% fat, and 55% carbohydrate recommended for almost everyone.

[a]Energy values in Tables 9-9 and 9-10 determined by applying the calorie/gram factors of 4 cal/g carbohydrate and protein, and 9 cal/g fat.

versy 7 for how to choose one. Table 9-9 presents a sample balanced low-calorie weight-loss plan.

If you plan resolutely to include a certain number of servings of food that you enjoy from each food group each day, you may be so busy making sure you get what you need that you will have little time or appetite left for high-fat or empty-calorie foods. Foods such as fruits, vegetables, and whole grains are high in carbohydrates and fiber, low in fat, and take a lot of chewing too. Crunchy, wholesome foods offer bulk and satiety for far fewer calories than smooth, refined foods. Limit your meats: an ounce of ham contains more calories than an ounce of bread, and many of them are from fat.

Counting the calories in foods is time consuming, and only the most motivated will persist at it for long. For the rest of us, some acquaintance with the exchange system (introduced in Chapter 2) provides a simpler method. Figure 9-5 offers a chance to practice estimating calories. The foods depicted there could be found one by one in Appendix A, but it is quicker to translate them into exchanges and to add up the energy values to get a rough idea of the total. With some practice you can look at any plate of food and "sense" the number of calories it represents. The energy amounts to remember are:

- One nonfat milk exchange—90 calories (for low-fat milk, 120 calories; for whole milk, 150).
- One vegetable exchange—25 calories.
- One fruit exchange—60 calories.
- One starchy vegetable/bread exchange—80 calories.
- One lean meat exchange—55 calories (for medium-fat meat, 75 calories; for high-fat meat, 100 calories). Remember, one exchange of meat is 1 *ounce.*
- One fat exchange—45 calories.
- One teaspoon sugar—20 calories.

So how many calories are in the meal in Figure 9-5? Size up the foods by exchanges and compare your total calorie amount to the answer in Figure 9-6 at the end of this chapter.

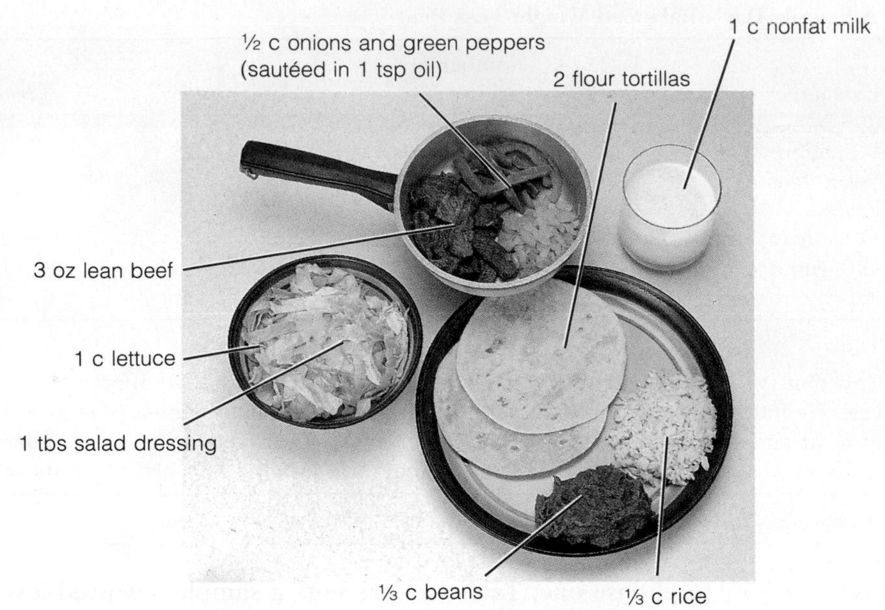
1 c nonfat milk
½ c onions and green peppers
(sautéed in 1 tsp oil)
2 flour tortillas
3 oz lean beef
1 c lettuce
1 tbs salad dressing
⅓ c beans
⅓ c rice

Figure 9-5

CALORIE QUIZ

In case you'd like to guess how many calories are in the meal depicted here, assign to each food an exchange value (see Figure 2-9 of Chapter 2). Then translate these values into numbers of calories. Add up the total. The answers are on page 343.

Especially don't lose track of the fat you add. Remember that fat calories probably contribute more to body fat stores than do carbohydrate calories, and fat has so many calories per bite that it is easy to overload quickly. Just a few bites of fatty food can provide the whole allowance of calories for a meal long before the diner feels full.

Three meals a day is standard for our society, but your lifestyle may not facilitate eating three meals. No law says you shouldn't have four or five meals—only be sure they are smaller, of course. What is important is to eat regularly and, if at all possible, to eat before you are very hungry. Make sure it is hunger, not appetite, urging you to eat. When you do decide to eat, eat the entire meal you have carefully planned for yourself. Then don't eat again until the next meal. Save "free" or favorite foods or beverages for a planned snack at the end of the day if you need insurance against late-evening hunger.

One meal you should strive to include is breakfast. Much evidence supports the health effects of breakfast, and people who eat breakfast seem to need fewer snacks and consume less fat all day long.[42]

KEY POINT People should be involved in planning their own weight-loss diets. Diet plans should be adequate, should control calories, and should be as personally pleasing as possible.

Diet Strategies for Weight Gain

Should an underweight person try to gain weight? Not necessarily: the question is whether the underweight affects health. If you are healthy at your present weight, stay there. If your physician has advised you to gain, if you are excessively tired, if you are unable to keep warm, if you are 15 percent below the expected weight, or if, for women, you have missed at least three consecutive menstrual periods, you may be in danger from a too-low body weight.

Weight gain is an individual matter. In deciding whether to undertake it, be as aware as you can be of what your body will permit and tolerate, and be willing to accept what you cannot change. Some people are unalterably thin by reasons of heredity or early physical influences. Those who wish to gain weight for appearance's sake or to improve athletic performance should be aware that a healthful weight gain can be achieved only through physical activity, particularly strength training, combined with eating a high-calorie diet. Eating more calories of food can bring about weight gain, but it will be mostly fat, and this can be as detrimental to health as being slightly underweight. In an athlete, such a weight gain can impair performance. Therefore in weight gain, as in weight loss, physical activity is an essential component of a sound plan.

As important to weight gain as exercise are the calories to support that activity—otherwise you will lose weight (body fat). If you eat just enough to fuel the activity, you will build muscle, but at the expense of body fat, that is, fat will be burned to support the muscle building. If you eat more, you will gain both muscle and fat.

It takes an excess of about 2,000 to 2,500 calories, in theory, to support the gain of a pound of pure lean tissue, and about 3,500 calories to gain a pound of fat.[43] To gain a mixture, then, which is the goal, requires about 3,000 calories. The rate at which a person can build muscle tissue also depends on the person. Both men and women have a mixture of both male and female hormones; those with more male hormones build muscle more easily than others, but it is not known what the limits are. (Chapter 10 provides cautions on the abuse of steroid hormone drugs.) Conventional advice on diet to the person building muscle is to eat about 700 to 1,000 calories a day above normal energy needs; this is enough to support both the added activity and the formation of new muscle. Table 9-10 offers one plan that provides adequate nutrients along with the calories to support weight gain.

It is as hard for a person who tends to be underweight to gain a pound as it is for a person who tends to be overweight to lose one. Like the weight

Table 9-10
A Sample Day's Balanced Weight-Gain Plan

Exchange Item	Number of Exchanges	Carbohydrate (g)	Protein (g)	Fat (g)	Energy (cal)
Starch/bread	15	225	45	Trace	1,080
Vegetables	4	25	10	0	140
Fruits	6	90	0	0	360
Meat (Medium-fat)	7	0	49	35	511
Milk (nonfat)	3	36	24	Trace	240
Fat	12	0	0	60	540
Total		376 g	128 g	95 g	2,871 cal

This plan offers 52 percent of calories from carbohydrate, 30 percent from fat, and 18 percent from protein. This plan provides sufficient calories and nutrients to promote weight gain in all but the most active people. For a diet plan for athletes, see the next chapter.

weight cycling repeated rounds of weight loss and subsequent regain, with reduced ability to lose weight with each attempt.

loser, the person who wants to gain must learn new habits and learn to like new foods. You may need to learn to eat different foods. No matter how many sticks of celery you consume, you won't gain weight very fast because celery simply doesn't offer enough calories. The person who cannot eat much volume is encouraged to use calorie-dense foods in meals (the very ones the dieter is trying to stay away from). These foods are high in fat, but if they are contributing energy that will be spent building new tissue, and if their fat is mostly unsaturated, they will not contribute to heart disease. Choose nutritious foods, but choose peanut butter instead of lean meat, avocado instead of cucumber, olives instead of pickles, whole-wheat muffins instead of whole-wheat bread, milkshakes instead of milk. When you do eat celery, stuff it with tuna salad (use oil-packed tuna); add creamer and sugar to coffee; use olive-oil or canola-oil dressings on salads, whipped toppings on fruit, margarine on potatoes, and the like. Because fat contains twice as many calories per teaspoon as sugar, it adds calories without adding much bulk, and its energy is in a form that is easy for the body to store.

Expect to feel full, sometimes even uncomfortably so. Most underweight individuals are accustomed to small quantities of food. When they begin eating significantly more food, they complain of uncomfortable fullness. This is normal, and it passes over time.

Eat more frequently. Make three sandwiches in the morning and eat them between classes in addition to the day's three regular meals. Spend time making foods appealing—the more varied and palatable the better. If you fill up fast during a meal, eat the highest calorie items first. Start with the main course or a meaty or cheese-filled appetizer. Drink between meals, not with them, to save space for higher-calorie foods. Make milkshakes to drink between meals. Always finish with dessert. Many an underweight person has simply been too busy (for months) to eat or to exercise enough to gain or to maintain weight. These strategies will help you to change this behavior pattern.

Not only diet but physical activity is important both for weight loss and weight gain. This may sound paradoxical—if physical activity supports weight loss, how can it help the person who wishes to gain? The secret seems to lie partly in the type of activity each person chooses, and partly in the ability of exercise to regulate body processes, as the following sections make clear.

KEY POINT The person who wants to gain weight must train physically and add extra calories of food to the diet, and is most likely to succeed by tailoring a weight-gain plan to personal preferences.

Physical Activity for Weight Loss

Some people hate the very idea of exercise, and obese people often, understandably, do not enjoy moving their bodies. They feel heavy, clumsy, even ridiculous. A word to reassure them: weight loss, at least to a point, is possible without exercise, but let your mind be set to take up some activity later on. Without exercise, losing and maintaining weight proves difficult.[44] You can start by simply walking instead of driving. As the pounds come off, moving your body will become a pleasure.

Those who endeavor to lose weight without exercise often become trapped in **weight cycling,** the endless repeating rounds of weight loss and regain from "yoyo" dieting. Nearly a third of all women interviewed in one poll reported themselves to be perpetual dieters who dieted at least once a month. At any one time, estimates place 25 percent of adult men and more than 40 percent of adult women on weight-loss diets, with another 25 or so percent struggling to maintain recent losses.[45]

A theory about weight cycling is that it may have detrimental effects on body composition. Evidence from rats, repeatedly placed on weight-loss diets, indicates that weight losses in later diets become slower and slower with less and less weight lost each time. The same effect sometimes shows up in human beings.[46] One proposed explanation is that weight loss reduces the body's lean tissue with each round of dieting while increasing body fatness. A recent review found little evidence to support the idea that dieting produces permanent changes in human body composition, however.[47]

Strategies for using exercise for weight control:

1. Choose active exercise.
2. Move large muscle groups.
3. Think in terms of time, not speed.
4. Exercise informally, in daily routines.

Whether or not body composition changes, a serious risk may await those who weight cycle. A recent study reported a link between repeated fluctuations in body weight and increased risks of death from heart disease and other causes.[48] No conclusions are yet possible, and previous dieters are probably not in danger, so long as they have stopped weight cycling. This is a good idea from another point of view, too, for weight cyclers face an emotionally demoralizing stream of diet "failures," as this chapter's Controversy explains. The frustration of weight cycling may even be severe enough to trigger eating disorders in some people.

People who repeatedly diet and fail should know that exercise can be of benefit in breaking the weight-cycling pattern. The effects of exercise on those who diet is well-documented. Dieters who fail to exercise may lose some weight, but not as much or as fast as those who take up walking, jogging, or other regular physical activity. Dieting or exercise alone can produce some weight loss, but the combination is more powerful.

An interesting discovery was made regarding the role of exercise in weight maintenance. At the end of a study of the effects of a low-calorie diet and exercise on weight loss, some subjects gave up exercise along with the experimental diet. The researchers continued tracking their body weights. Predictably, the subjects quickly regained all the weight they had lost. The outcome was dramatically different for subjects who continued exercising even after they gave up the experimental diet. The group kept their weight off even after abandoning the diet.[49]

Thinness is not the same as fitness. For a definition of fitness, see the next chapter.

While the results of a single study do not prove that exercise alone controls weight, a long-held nutrition truth states that physical activity is a contributor to a healthy body composition. Among the contributions that exercise makes are:

- Increased expenditure of energy.
- Long-term increase in resting metabolic rate.
- Promotion of weight loss, particularly loss of body fat.[50]
- Appetite control.
- Control of stress and stress-induced overeating or undereating.
- Increased self-esteem.

Chapter 10 provides much more information on fat and energy during activity, but a few strategies are in order here. For one thing, you must keep in mind that if exercise is to help you with weight control, it must be active exercise—voluntary moving of muscles. Being moved passively, as by a machine at a health spa or by a massage, neither increases energy expenditure nor builds muscles. The more muscles you move, the more muscle tissue you build, and the more calories you spend.

People sometimes think that workouts have to be fast paced. This is not true. For example, whether you choose to walk or to run a given distance, you will use up about the same amount of energy; walking will just take you longer.* In general, to burn up the most fat, the longer (not the faster) the better.

Another strategy is to incorporate more physical activity into your daily schedule in many simple, small-scale ways. Park the car at the far end of the parking lot; use the stairs instead of the elevator; work in a garden; work your abdominal muscles while you stand in line; tighten your buttocks each time you get up from your chair. These activities add up to only a few calories each, but over a year's time they become significant.

KEY POINT Physical activity is important in weight loss and maintenance: it favors a lean body composition. To be effective, exercise needs to be active, not passive.

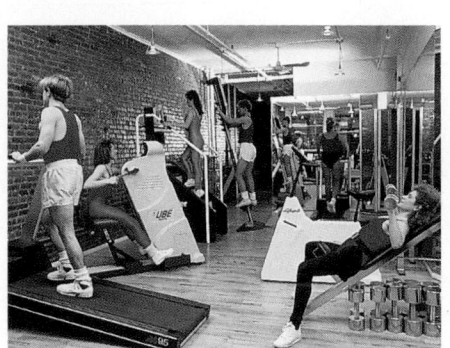

Physical activity can help overweight people lose and underweight people gain, weight.

Physical Activity for Weight Gain

Some of the principles of exercise offered to the weight-loss seeker apply to those who wish to gain as well. For one thing, no special machine that electrifies, vibrates, or moves muscles around will do anything to build them up. Such gadgets are designed to pad the wallets of their creators, most of whom don't care whether or not you gain an ounce while using them (you won't). The activities you choose must be active and undertaken regularly, at least every other day.[51] They also must be of the type that *builds* muscles.

Activity that builds muscles also changes the muscle cells, called fibers, structurally. If you could look through a powerful microscope at a muscle before and after a strength-training program you would be able to observe a thickening of the sheets of contracting proteins responsible for muscle movement. You would also see a buildup of many more white granules of stored glycogen, for intense strengthening exercises rely heavily on glucose for fuel while sparing the body's fat reserves—a benefit to those who wish to gain weight. Glycogen itself attracts and holds water and this increases the body's weight slightly, as well. The work that builds muscles is the type that involves resistance—an opposing force against which the muscles must work. Exactly which exercises help build muscles and how they do so are topics of the next chapter.

You may experience a depression of appetite when you first begin a training program. Don't be concerned—depressed appetite following exercise is normal and expected. Within a few days, your appetite will pick up and will probably exceed your normal appetite. This, of course, is desirable, and if you stay sensitive to your hunger signals, it can provide an opportunity to pack in some extra servings of food. A word about smoking and appetite is appropriate here. The drug of tobacco, nicotine, depresses the appetite and smoke-exposed taste buds and olfactory (smelling) organs become less sensitive. A person who smokes must first quit before weight gain is possible.

---

*Runners use about 10% more energy than do walkers because they push their weight up, as well as forward, with each step.

Quitters find that appetite picks up, food tastes and smells better, and the body reaps additional benefits too numerous to mention.

Also, be aware that most "weight-gain" supplements designed to add body weight are useless without exercise and confer no special benefits on the taker. Of body weight gained in a day, only a half ounce to an ounce is protein tissue, so no special protein supplements can help speed weight gain faster than an ordinary high-calorie balanced diet. Ordinary food in abundance along with exercise to work the nutrients into place support efforts to gain weight.

Once you have succeeded in changing your weight, will you maintain the change? This may be even more difficult than achieving the change in the first place, but some people do succeed. Their secrets are revealed in the next section.

More on the effects of nicotine and other drugs on nutrition in Controversy 12.

Strategies for using exercise to build up body mass:

1. Choose strength-building exercises.
2. Think in terms of exercise intensity (see next chapter).
3. Expect appetite changes; follow your hunger signals.

KEY POINT Resistance exercise can strengthen muscles, add lean tissue to the body, and increase body weight.

Weight Maintenance

"I have lost 200 pounds, but I was never more than 20 pounds overweight." Millions have experienced the frustration of winning the struggle to achieve a desired change in weight only to face the even greater frustration of seeing their hard work visibly slipping away. Whether the goal is to lose or gain, weight cycling with periodic losses and gains often becomes a lifelong pattern. What makes the difference between a successful, long-term weight control program and a temporary one?

Secrets of Success

People who maintain a weight change have some things in common.[52] Particularly, they develop social support systems; they attend support groups or create supportive relationships with others. Another key factor is physical activity. Successful weight maintainers exercise regularly. Still another factor is planning and the ability to carry a plan through. Those who maintain weight:

- Follow written diet plans and keep records.
- Eat three meals a day at planned times, and eat them at a leisurely pace.
- Follow the rule of no eating after a certain time in the evening (usually about 6:00 to 8:00 p.m.).
- Plan high-fiber foods into their diets, along with 8 glasses or more of water a day.

They also cultivate positive attitudes and beliefs and use techniques such as positive self-talk: "You can do it," "You're a success." They believe in their ability to succeed despite past diet "failures." Also important are realistic expectations regarding body size and shape. Acceptance of how much progress one can make and how long the weight-loss process takes prepares the mind for the task ahead.

Another key to success is an attitude of ownership of and responsibility for the weight loss. People who succeed in maintaining weight have a full understanding that they alone are ultimately responsible for their weight

lapse a falling back into a former condition. In weight maintenance, a temporary, expected backslide into old habits.

relapse the outcome of an uncontrolled series of lapses, such as regaining of weight after successful loss and returning to old patterns of eating.

control.[53] They realize that no other person can control their weight for them. In contrast, many unsuccessful dieters place the responsibility for their weight control outside of themselves, on weight-loss programs, on health care professionals, or on pills and potions. This attitude weakens people's self-confidence and predicts failure.

Ownership is learnable. Successful dieters report coming to a turning point—the point at which they accept responsibility for their own body weights. Only then can they develop workable solutions to barriers. The lesson is, *expect* success but also know that you alone can make it happen.

Self-acceptance predicts success, while self-hate predicts failure. When people feel disgusted with their appearance and hate themselves when they get on the scale, they erode the positive mental environment needed to maintain weight, once it is lost. A paradox of behavior change is that it takes self-acceptance (loving the overweight self) to lay the foundation for change. Self-acceptance leads to an unshakable self-worth that does not depend on body weight.

KEY POINT Many traits related to positive self-image characterize people who succeed at maintaining lost weight. The more of these a person possesses or cultivates, the more likely that person will succeed.

Lapse Management and Relapse Prevention

"I did it again," a chronic dieter confided. "I binged again after five years of dieting." Some dieters are forever frustrated by their backsliding behavior. "I feel angry, depressed, and ashamed. All of those meetings! All that therapy! All that work! Why do I still go back to old behaviors?" Disappointment, frustration and self-condemnation are common in dieters who find themselves in a **lapse** or **relapse.**[54]

The term *relapse* describes the end result of a loss of control that results in defeat for dieters. It doesn't have to happen. Many a relapse begins with just a lapse, and dieters need to understand the differences in kind and degree. Lapses can happen to people who have been dieting or maintaining weight for ten months or ten years. They are a normal part of the behavior-change process and do not indicate lack of will power.

A dieter in a lapse can take corrective action and can thus regain control. Without any action, however, a lapse can lead to relapse: weight gain due to total abandonment of the weight-control program. The dieter's responses to individual lapses determine if relapse will occur; if the dieter perceives a total loss of control, then relapse is likely.[55]

A perfectionistic "all or nothing" attitude is destructive to weight maintenance efforts and can lead people to think that a mistake means that control is totally and forever lost. If this sounds familiar, it could be that erroneous thinking is blocking your progress in weight maintenance.

When faced with a lapse into old behaviors, identify the circumstances surrounding your lapse and redouble your attention to them. For example, if after a party you find that you unexpectedly overate, you might benefit from first adopting an attitude of compassion and forgiving yourself. Then get tough with yourself and commit to specific actions to control your intake at the next party. Vow to say "no" to food when you're not hungry (to fortify against social pressure), to eat a balanced meal beforehand (to defend against hunger), and to position yourself well away from party buffets (to reduce temptation).

It helps to monitor your behavior with regard to your plan for weight maintenance. Set specific tolerance ranges for lapses, and take action should you exceed them. Look for any of the following:

- A weight gain of from 3 to 5 pounds.
- A lack of physical activity for more than four days in a row.
- A second repetition of any old destructive behavior.
- Withdrawal from support system for a period lasting more than a week.
- Failure to participate in nonfood-oriented leisure activities for more than a week.

Take action. Review the appropriate steps to behavior modification, and apply them. Improving behavior is rarely a straight-line progress; it more often follows a path of two steps forward, one step back. Lapses are inevitable, and may even be helpful: they reveal to people information about behaviors of concern. When the normal lapses occur, the healthy person can cope by saying, "Oops! I'm doing it again, but, it's okay, I do it less often now, and I'm making progress."

Behavior modification principles can work to change the behaviors of undereating as well as overeating. The person who needs to gain weight must strengthen cues to appropriate eating and exercise. The Food Feature that follows is written to assist in weight loss, but it presents tips that can help both the weight loser and gainer to reach their goals. For example, learning and practicing assertiveness is important to the person who must say no to requests that would interfere with mealtimes. The undereater might also identify and select the cues that the overeater is trying to eliminate. For example, *do* snack while watching television; make large portions of food look small; keep treats in view.

KEY POINT After achieving a weight goal, many people find maintenance a challenge. A key to maintaining desired weight is distinguishing lapses from relapse. Lapses offer opportunities to practice needed recovery skills; they are part of success, not of failure.

Did you guess the answer to Figure 9-5's Quiz? Our answer is in Figure 9-6, in the margin.

Figure 9-6

ANSWERS TO CALORIE QUIZ

Using the exchange system, we figure about 690 calories. A computer diet analysis provided a total of 715. Any estimate within 10 to 20 percent is reasonable.

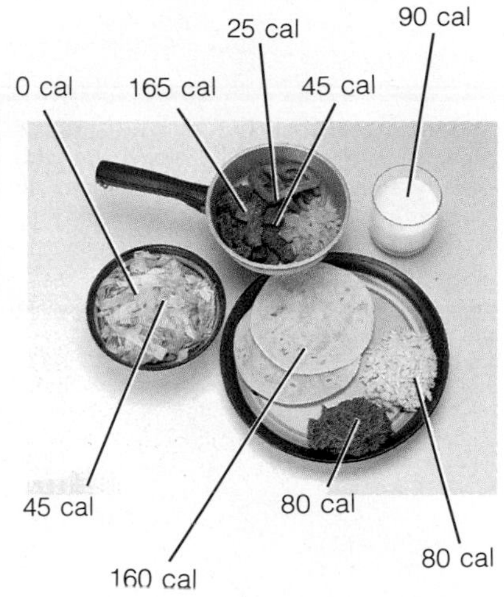

Food (exchange)	cal/ exchange[a]	Total cal
2 flour tortillas		
2 (starch/bread)	× 80 cal =	160
⅓ c beans		
1 (starch/bread)	×80 cal =	80
⅓ c rice		
1 (starch/bread)	× 80 cal =	80
3 oz lean beef		
3 (lean meat)	× 55 cal =	165
½ c onions and green peppers		
1 (vegetable)	× 25 cal =	25
1 tsp oil		
1 (fat)	× 45 cal =	45
1 c lettuce		
(free)		—
1 tbs salad dressing		
1 (fat)	× 45 cal =	45
1 c nonfat milk		
1 (nonfat milk)	× 90 cal =	90
	Total	690

[a]Exchange system energy values.

FOOD FEATURE

Behavior Modification for Weight Control

behavior modification alteration of behavior using methods based on the theory that holds that actions can be controlled by controlling the environmental factors that cue, or trigger, the actions.

Supporting both diet and exercise is the technique of **behavior modification.** Behavior modification works to cement into place all the behaviors that lead to and perpetuate the desired body composition.

An important concept is that habits direct behaviors. Suppose a friend informs you of a new shortcut to school. All that is required is that you make a left-hand turn at a corner where you now turn right. You may decide to try the shortcut right away, but the next day, when you arrive at the familiar corner, you turn right, as always. Not until you arrive at school do you realize that you failed to turn left as planned. You can learn to turn left, of course, but it takes an effort of will to remember to do so at first. After a while, the new behavior will become as automatic as the earlier one was. Habits are like the "auto pilot" feature of a plane—they'll always take you somewhere, but to arrive at your desired destination, you must consciously plan the route ahead of time. This Food Feature applies behavior modification principles to helping you plan and adjust your habits concerning diet and exercise.

The six elements of behavior modification to change eating habits are:

1. Eliminate inappropriate eating cues.
2. Suppress the cues you cannot eliminate.
3. Strengthen cues to appropriate eating and exercise.
4. Repeat the desired eating and exercise behaviors.
5. Arrange or emphasize negative consequences of inappropriate eating.
6. Arrange or emphasize positive consequences of appropriate eating and exercise behaviors.

Six behavior modification strategies for weight change:

1. Eliminate inappropriate eating cues.

Before you begin to apply strategies that employ the six principles above, establish a baseline, a record of your present eating behaviors against which to measure future progress. Keep a diary so that you can learn what particular eating stimuli, or cues, affect you.

To begin, set about eliminating or suppressing the cues that prompt you to eat inappropriately. There may be many such cues in an overeater's life: watching television, talking on the telephone, entering a convenience store, being offered food, and many more. Resolve to respond no longer to such cues by eating. Respond only to one set of cues designed by you: one particular place in one particular room. Also:

- Don't buy problem foods.
- Shop when you aren't hungry.
- Serve only low-calorie sauces and toppings and avoid rich ones.
- Let spouse and children buy, store, and serve their own sweets (monitor children's total intake).
- Change channels or look away when food commercials appear on the television screen.
- Shop only from a list.
- Carry appropriate snacks, and avoid vending machines.
- Prepare only as much food as you have planned to eat.

If some cues to inappropriate eating behavior can't be eliminated, suppress them:

2. Suppress the cues you cannot eliminate.

- Minimize contact with excessive food.
- Serve individual plates, don't put serving dishes on the table, and leave or clear the table when finished.
- Have family members scrape their plates directly into the garbage.
- Create obstacles to the eating of problem foods. For example, make it necessary to unwrap, cook, and serve each one separately.
- Make small portions look large by spreading them out and serving them on small plates.
- Control deprivation so that you will not overeat to compensate. Plan and eat regular meals; don't skip meals.
- Avoid getting overtired and avoid boredom by keeping cues to interesting activities in plain sight.

Next, to strengthen the cues to appropriate eating and activity:

3. Strengthen cues to appropriate behaviors.

- Encourage others to eat appropriate foods with you.
- Keep your favorite appropriate foods in the front of the refrigerator.
- Learn appropriate portion sizes.
- Save permitted foods from meals for snacks; these should be your only snacks.
- Prepare permitted foods attractively.
- Keep your ski poles (walking shoes, tennis racket) by the door.

A way to alter the response itself is to repeat the desired behavior:

4. Repeat the desired behaviors.

- Slow down by pausing for two to three minutes—put down utensils, and swallow before reloading the fork.
- Always use utensils.
- Leave some food on the plate.
- Move more—shake a leg, pace, fidget, stretch your muscles.
- Join in and cultivate fitness with a group of active people.

Arrange to have negative consequences follow inappropriate eating behavior and activity. Scolding is *not* a negative consequence (it is a form of attention-giving, which is positive), so don't ask to be scolded:

5. Arrange negative consequences for negative behaviors.

- Have others nearby when you eat.
- Ask that others respond neutrally to your deviations (make no comment). This is a negative consequence because it withholds attention.
- If you slip, don't punish yourself.

Consider the last item. If you ate an extra 1,000 calories yesterday, don't try to eat 1,000 fewer calories today. Just go back to your plan. On the other hand, you can plan ahead and budget for special occasions. If you want to celebrate your birthday with cake and ice cream, cut a few calories from your bread and milk allowance each day for several days *beforehand.* Your weight loss will be as smooth as if you had stayed with the daily plan.

6. Reward yourself. Make rewards personal and immediate.

Make sure, also, that positive consequences, including material rewards, follow the desired behaviors. Rewards should be personal—they should give *you* pleasure; and they should be immediate (see Table 9-12 for specific suggestions):

- Update records of food intake, exercise, and weight change regularly.
- Arrange for material reinforcement—rewards (other than food) for each unit of behavior change or weight loss.
- Provide social reinforcement (ask to be encouraged).
- Take well-spaced weighings to avoid discouragement.

If you stop making progress, you may have to get tough with yourself. Ask yourself honestly, "What am I doing wrong?" (no one is listening in). Seldom does an unpredicted weight plateau of any duration have no explanation in the dieter's own choices.

Also, if you stop making progress, be aware that this may be a good time to stop. Your weight may be at a point that you are willing to accept, at least for the present. In fact, you may have come to realize that your original goal weight was unrealistic or not worth the effort it would take to get there. You may decide to join the ranks of people who have rejected the magazine-cover physical ideal and opt to work on other facets of your life leading to self-acceptance. Hold your head high and take the attitude, "This is the way I am."

Also:
Learn and practice assertiveness.

Should you choose to continue weight-loss efforts, you may find help in a group such as TOPS or Weight Watchers. Or you may benefit from individual nutrition counseling with a registered dietitian (RD). RDs are trained to assist with food behavior change. It may also help to obtain some assertiveness training. Learning to say "No, thank you" might be one of your first objectives. Learning not to "clean your plate" might be another.

Table 9-11
Activities and Rewards to Substitute for Eating

Exercise or sports	Shopping
Attending sporting events	Naps
Reading	Relaxation exercises
Telephoning	New clothes
Hobbies and crafts	Weekend trips
Listening to music	Movie or theater trips
Gardening or yardwork	Saving money for future use
Recreation	Self-praise
Household chores	Praise by significant others
Bathing	Token rewards (stars, stickers)

Adapted from B. B. Hollie, Using behavior modification in nutrition counseling, *Journal of the American Dietetic Association* 88 (1988): 1530–1538.

From all the available behavior changes, you choose the ones to begin with. Don't try to master them all at once. No one who attempts too many changes at one time is successful. Set your own priorities. Pick one behavior you can handle, start with that, and practice it until it is habitual and automatic. Then select another.

As you progress in physical activity and behavior modification, enjoy your new, emerging self. Get in touch with—reach out your hand to—your fit and healthy self, and help that self to feel welcome in the light of day.

Use small-step modification.

Notes

1. Food and Nutrition Board, *Recommended Dietary Allowances*, 10th ed. (Washington, D.C.: National Academy of Sciences, 1989), pp. 29–30; Y. Schutz and E. Jéquier, Energy needs: Assessment and requirements, in M. E. Shils, J. A. Olson, and M. Shike, eds., *Modern Nutrition in Health and Disease* (Philadelphia: Lea & Febiger, 1994), pp. 101–111.
2. J. P. Flatt, The biochemistry of energy expenditure, in P. Björntorp and B. N. Brodoff (eds.), *Obesity* (Philadelphia: Lippincott, 1992), pp. 100–116.
3. F. X. Pi-Sunyer, Health implications of obesity, *American Journal of Clinical Nutrition* 53 (1991): 1595S–1603S.
4. R. J. Kuczmarski, Prevalence of overweight and weight gain in the United States, *American Journal of Clinical Nutrition* 55 (1992): 4955–5025.
5. J. E. Manson and coauthors, A prospective study of obesity and risk of coronary heart disease in women, *New England Journal of Medicine* 322 (1990): 882–889.
6. A. Must and coauthors, Long-term morbidity and mortality of overweight adolescents, *New England Journal of Medicine* 327 (1992): 1350–1355; G. A. Bray, Adolescent overweight may be tempting fate, *New England Journal of Medicine* 327 (1992): 1378–1380.
7. Pi-Sunyer, 1991.
8. National Research Council, *Diet and Health: Implications for Reducing Chronic Disease Risk* (Washington, D.C.: National Academy Press, 1989), p. 117.
9. C. Ley, B. Lees, and J. C. Stevenson, Sex- and menopause-associated changes in body fat distribution, *American Journal of Clinical Nutrition* 55 (1992): 950–954.
10. R. J. Troisi, Cigarette smoking, dietary intake, and physical activity: Effects on body fat distribution—The Normative Aging study, *American Journal of Clinical Nutrition* 53 (1991): 1104–1111.
11. R. Roubenoff and P. W. F. Wilson, Advantage of knee height over height as an index of stature in expression of body composition in adults, *American Journal of Clinical Nutrition* 57 (1993): 609–613.
12. A. Frisancho, Nutritional anthropometry, *Journal of the American Dietetic Association* 88 (1988): 553–555.
13. O. Ortiz and coauthors, Differences in skeletal muscle and bone mineral mass between black and white females and their relevance to estimates of body composition, *American Journal of Clinical Nutrition* 55 (1992): 8–13.
14. G. A. Bray, Obesity: Classification of subtypes, an address presented at the North American Association for the Study of Obesity and Emory University School of Medicine conference, Obesity Update: Pathophysiology, Clinical Consequences, and Therapeutic Options, Atlanta, Georgia, August 31–September 2, 1992.
15. C. Bouchard and L. Pérusse, Genetics of obesity, *Annual Review of Nutrition* 13 (1993): 337–354 lends an in-depth perspective on the topic.
16. Failure to maintain weight loss: Permissive role of lipoprotein lipase, *Nutrition Reviews*, October 1989, pp. 328–331.
17. A. J. Stunkard, Body weight regulation, an address presented at the conference, Obesity Update, 1992.
18. R. H. Eckel, Lipoprotein lipase, *New England Journal of Medicine* 320 (1989): 1060–1068; P. Lönnroth and U. Smith, Intermediary metabolism with an emphasis on lipid metabolism, adipose tissue, and fat cell metabolism, in P. Björntorp and B. N. Brodoff, eds., *Obesity* (Philadelphia: Lippincott, 1992), pp. 3–14.
19. R. H. Eckel, Lipoprotein lipase regulation in obesity and after weight loss, an address given at the conference, Obesity Update, 1992.
20. Lönnroth and Smith, 1992.
21. G. Ailhaud, P. Grimaldi, and R. Négrel, Cellular and molecular aspects of adipose tissue development, *Annual Review of Nutrition* 12 (1992): 207–233.
22. S. Welle and coauthors, Energy expenditure under free-living conditions in normal-weight and overweight women, *American Journal of Clinical Nutrition* 55 (1992): 14–21.
23. A. J. Hill, C. F. Weaver, and J. E. Blundell, Food craving, dietary restraint and mood, *Appetite* 17 (1991): 187–197.
24. P. J. Rogers, Why a palatability construct is needed, *Appetite* 14 (1990): 159–161.
25. T. A. Spiegel, E. E. Shrager, and E. Stellar, Responses of lean and obese subjects to preloads, deprivation, and palatability, *Appetite* 13 (1989): 45–69.
26. M. S. Westerterp-Plantenga, L. Wouters, and F. ten-Hoor, Restrained eating, obesity, and cumulative food intake curves during four-course meals, *Appetite* 16 (1991): 149–158; J. Rodin, Determinants of food intake regulation in obesity, in P. Björntorp

and B. N. Brodoff, eds., *Obesity* (Philadelphia: Lippincott, 1992): pp. 220–230.
27. D. J. Mela and D. A. Sacchetti, Sensory preferences for fats: Relationships with diet and body composition, *American Journal of Clinical Nutrition* 53 (1991): 908–915.
28. W. C. Miller and coauthors, Diet composition, energy intake, and exercise in relation to body fat in men and women, *American Journal of Clinical Nutrition* 52 (1990): 426–430; B. J. Rolls and D. J. Shide, The influence of dietary fat on food intake and body weight, *Nutrition Reviews* 50 (1992): 283–290.
29. L. A. Tucker and M. Bagwell, Relationship between serum cholesterol levels and television viewing in 11,947 employed adults, *American Journal of Health Promotion* 6 (1992): 437–442.
30. P. M. Suter, Y. Schutz, and E. Jéquier, The effect of ethanol on fat storage in healthy subjects, *New England Journal of Medicine* 326 (1992): 983–985.
31. M. C. Linder, Nutrition and metabolism of proteins, in *Nutrition, Biochemistry and Metabolism*, M. C. Linder, ed. (New York: Elsevier, 1991), pp. 87–109.
32. M. E. Sweeny and coauthors, Severe vs moderate energy restriction with and without exercise in the treatment of obesity: Efficiency of weight loss, *American Journal of Clinical Nutrition* 57 (1993): 127–134.
33. J. G. Kral, L. V. Sjöström, and M. B. E. Sullivan, Assessment of quality of life before and after surgery for severe obesity, *American Journal of Clinical Nutrition* 55 (1992): 611S–614S.
34. J. J. Gleysteen, J. J. Barboriak, and E. A. Sasse, Sustained coronary-risk-factor reduction after bypass for morbid obesity, *American Journal of Clinical Nutrition* 51 (1990): 774–778.
35. F. Pollner, Obesity surgery regaining favor, *Medical World News*, May 1991, p. 37, a report of the NIH Symposium *Gastrointestinal Surgery for Severe Obesity*, March 1991.
36. J. D. Halverson, Metabolic risk of obesity surgery and long-term follow-up, *American Journal of Clinical Nutrition* 55 (1992): 602S–605S.
37. G. A. Bray, Drug treatment of obesity, *American Journal of Clinical Nutrition* 55 (1992): 538S–544S; A. Astrup and coauthors, The effect of ephedrine/caffeine mixture on energy expenditure and body composition in obese women, *Metabolism: Clinical and Experimental* 41 (1992): 686–688.
38. R. L. Atkinson, Treatment of obesity (editorial), *Nutrition Reviews* (1992): 338–345.
39. N. Finer, F. Finer, and P. Naoumova, Drug therapy after very-low-calorie diets, *American Journal of Clinical Nutrition* 56 (1992): 195S–198S.
40. T. Cramer, Cal-Ban banned, *FDA Consumer*, June 1992, pp. 39–40.
41. S. Alger and coauthors, Effect of phenylpropanolanine on energy expenditure and weight loss in overweight women, *American Journal of Clinical Nutrition* 57 (1993): 120–126.
42. D. G. Schlundt and coauthors, The role of breakfast in the treatment of obesity: A randomized clinical trial, *American Journal of Clinical Nutrition* 55 (1992): 645–651.
43. W. D. McArdle, F. I. Katch, and V. L. Katch, *Exercise Physiology: Energy, Nutrition, and Human Performance*, 3rd ed. (Philadelphia: Lea & Febiger, 1991), pp. 651–652.
44. S. D. Phinney, Exercise during and after very-low-calorie dieting, *American Journal of Clinical Nutrition* 56 (1992): 1905–1945.
45. NIH Technology Assessment Conference Panel, Methods for vountary weight loss and control, *Annals of Internal Medicine* 116 (1992): 942–949.
46. G. L. Blackburn and coauthors, Weight cycling: The experience of human dieters, *American Journal of Clinical Nutrition* 49 (1989): 1105–1109.
47. A. M. Prentice and coauthors, Effects of weight cycling on body composition, *American Journal of Clinical Nutrition* 56 (1992): 2095–2165.
48. L. Lissner and coauthors, Variability of body weight and health outcomes in the Framingham population, *New England Journal of Medicine* 324 (1991): 1839–1844; L. Lissner and K. D. Brownell, Weight cycling, mortality, and cardiovascular disease: a review of epidemiologic findings, in P. Björntorp and B. N. Brodoff, eds., *Obesity* (Philadelphia: Lippincott, 1992), pp. 653–661.
49. K. N. Pavlou, S. Krey, and W. P. Steffee, Exercise as an adjunct to weight loss and maintenance in moderately obese subjects, *American Journal of Clinical Nutrition* 49 (1989): 1115–1123.
50. K. N. Pavlou and coauthors, Physical activity as a supplement to a weight-loss dietary regimen, *American Journal of Clinical Nutrition* 49 (1989): 1110–1114.
51. Experts release new recommendation to fight America's epidemic of physical inactivity (news release), *American College of Sports Medicine*, 29 July 1993.
52. L. Pauley and W. J. Wyatt, Big losers: A compilation of success characteristics, *The Bariatrician*, Fall 1987, pp. 23–27.
53. You can lose weight and keep it off, *Tufts University Diet and Nutrition Letter*, March 1989, pp. 1–2.
54. L. W. Turner, Weight maintenance and relapse prevention, *Nutrition Clinics*, January/February, 1990.
55. C. L. Rock and A. Coulston, Preventing relapse in dieters, *Nutrition and the M.D.*, January 1989, p. 7.

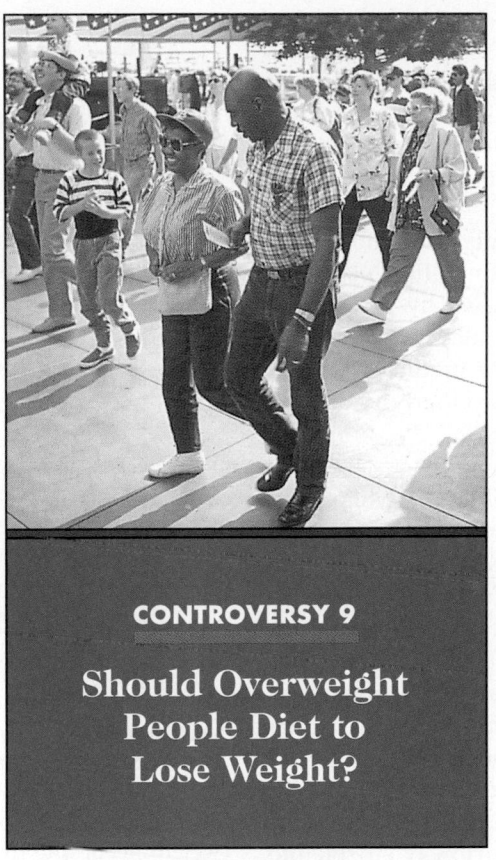

CONTROVERSY 9

Should Overweight People Diet to Lose Weight?

Recently, leaders in obesity research have gathered at symposiums around the country to address a growing controversy in nutrition science.[1] These great minds from many specialties are sharing their experiences in treating obese clients and some are questioning the very foundations of obesity treatment. The issues dividing the experts center on how, when, or even whether to advise weight-loss programs for overweight clients.

Do all obese clients benefit from routine advice to reduce weight? The question comes on the heels of research that suggests that diets almost always fail in the long term and that weight cycling may be hazardous. Right away, it should be said that weight loss is possible and that techniques explained in Chapter 9 are valid. The chapter also made clear, however, that controlling weight is a lifelong effort. A problem can occur when overweight people "go on a diet," lose weight, but then return to old eating patterns and sedentary lifestyles. Another problem is unrealistic expectations. Hardly any dieter can end up looking like a model despite sales pitches from diet programs. A more attainable and sustainable goal would be losing enough weight to regain health. This Controversy centers on the question who, exactly, should lose weight for health's sake; it also introduces an alternative for healthy overweight people: self-acceptance.

THE DECISION TO TREAT OBESITY Those in favor of aggressive treatment of obesity are still in the majority. All major government dietary guidelines mention weight control as a health-supporting ideal. The experts cite many studies showing that with obesity come increased disease risks.[2] What good would it do to treat a person's diabetes, say researchers, without treating the obesity underlying the disorder? The treatment may reduce the ravages of the present symptoms, but more symptoms will surely develop unless truly effective and lasting treatment for the predisposing condition is offered.

The opposing view points out that, in science, correlation is not cause. Yes, obesity is often found in those who suffer from the conditions just mentioned, but this does not demonstrate that obesity causes those conditions. It is as likely that a high-fat diet, excess caloric intake, or lack of exercise cause both the diseases and obesity. Or it may be that a hereditary factor predisposes people to developing both the diseases and the obesity (some evidence exists to support this idea). To say that obesity is a direct cause of disease, and that it must be reversed to prevent disease, may be to disobey the laws of scientific reasoning.

Other medical authorities counter these arguments by pointing to proved benefits from even 10 to 20 pounds of weight loss in obese patients. They report rapid improvement in many of the complications of obesity such as glucose tolerance and insulin resistance, hypertension, hyperlipidemia, and sleep apnea. The practical effects accompanying weight loss in the obese who suffer these conditions are proved beneficial and, whether they are brought about by reduction in body fatness or adoption of healthy lifestyle habits seems immaterial.

A larger question may be whether the weight loss and benefit correlation holds true in a linear fashion for people who are less dramatically overweight. Obese people may carry 80, 100, or even more pounds of excess weight and suffer health hazards, but is a seemingly healthy person who carries 30 or 40 extra pounds also inviting those hazards? Should such a person be advised by medical and nutrition experts to lose weight? A blanket weight-loss recommendation to all overweight people, based on health, may not be warranted.

The fallacy in making such a blanket recommendation is seen also in the case of diabetes and obesity. True, many more obese than thin people suffer from diabetes (the noninsulin dependent type), but it is thin people who develop diabetes (the insulin-dependent type) that carry the greater risk of severe effects. The critics who raise this point ask, "Should we recommend that all thin people gain weight to reduce risks of dying of diabetes?" The answer, of course, is no. The point is that just as all thin people do not suffer excess risks of diabetes, all overweight people do not suffer health risks, either. People therefore should not be urged to either gain or lose weight without an individual evaluation of risks.

Obesity treatment benefits not only individuals but also society, some argue. Almost $40 billion could be saved in health care costs annually, just by preventing and reversing obesity.[3] Fewer sick days taken from work, fewer visits to physicians, fewer medications and medical procedures, and increased productivity add up to the total.

THE PROBLEM OF OBESITY ASSESSMENT Chapter 9 pointed out that methods of assessing obesity are not perfect. Many health care professionals still use the Metropolitan Insurance Corporation's height-weight tables to define obesity and the tables are commonly on display in physicians' offices and clinics, but these tables may be flawed in design. The data from which the tables were made included only people rich enough to purchase insurance, and this left out the large population of people of modest means in the United States. Much of the information was recorded from telephone conversations with the subjects, a notoriously unreliable data-collection method. Also, insurance companies charge extra high prices for policies sold to people who are overweight. This means that any obese people represented in the tables were especially motivated to purchase insurance, even at high cost. Such people might have believed themselves ill or likely to become ill, and so considered the insurance to be worth the asking price. These biases in the height-weight tables are thought by some to render them unsuitable for defining obesity or for identifying its accompanying health risks.

The table data have been interpreted to imply that fat people die younger than thin people but this may not be true. Information refuting the idea came from a study of the population of Norway.[4] Almost all (1.8 million) of the adult citizens of that country were given physical examinations and then tracked for mortality for 10 years. Figure C9-1 shows that, in Norwegians, the thinnest members of both sexes carried high risks of early death. The extremely obese people's lives were also cut short. The longest life expectancies in this study, though, coincided with what would be considered an "overweight" condition by U.S. standards—up to a body mass index of 27 kg/m^2.

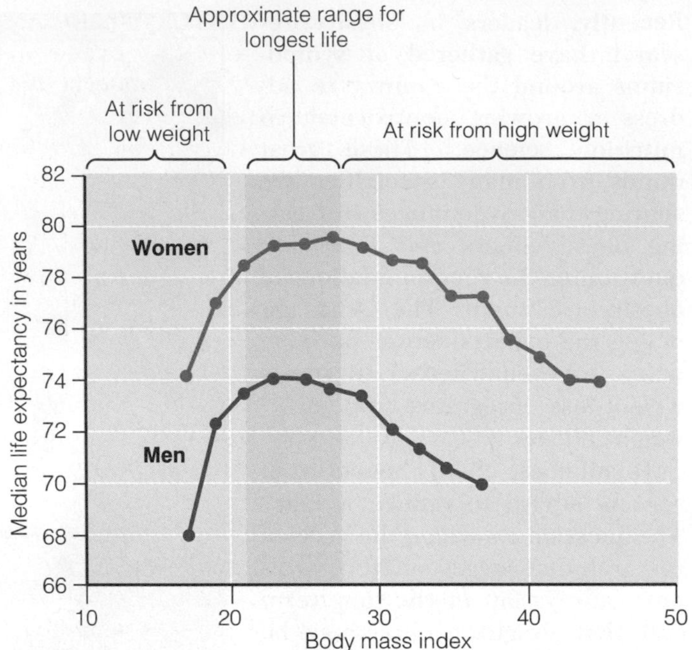

Figure C9-1

BODY WEIGHT AND LIFE EXPECTANCY IN NORWAY

Median life expectancies are shown here for Norwegian men and women according to body mass index. The "ideal" weight according to the height-weight tables would fall at about the "21" mark on the BMI scale (horizontal axis). In fact people may live longest when their BMI fall within the shaded range between 21 and 26.

Source: Adapted from P. Ernsberger, Obesity is hazardous to your health: Negative, *Debates in Medicine* 2 (1989): 102–137.

Notice on the left-hand side of both curves of the figure that even a small deficit in body weight dramatically shortens life, whereas the same number of pounds of overweight produces only a slight decline in longevity. The severe effect of underweight may reflect other hazards that occur along with underweight. A number of the underweight people in the study may have been suffering from wasting diseases such as cancer, or addictions to alcohol, tobacco, or other drugs that cause both weight loss and early death. People who are naturally slender are probably not in danger, so long as their weight is stable.

So far, this discussion has asked whether risks always accompany obesity. Now, what about the risks that may accompany weight-loss efforts?

DIET SAFETY—PROVED OR JUST IMPLIED? When consumers are offered a medical treatment, they expect to be fully informed of any risks involved in undertaking it. This expectation is reasonable because FDA requires proof that treatments such as medicines and surgery not only work, but are safe. This is not true of many diets, which carry risks but do not inform users about them, a practice that many believe to be unethical. An expert witness to a Senate subcommittee investigating weight-loss fraud said that, overall, "the unregulated multibillion dollar weight-loss industry is placing our citizens at significant health risk."[5]

The risks associated with weight loss are more serious than most dieters would suspect. Linked with fluctuations in body weight, but not specific to any one mode of achieving weight loss, is an increased risk of death from heart disease.[6] The authors of the study that put forth this finding point out weight cycling as especially dangerous. Also, anyone who undertakes to restrict caloric intake also invites the risk of losing control of dieting and developing an eating disorder such as anorexia nervosa or bulimia. (More about this link in Controversy 10.)

Some people think that all risks associated with diets should be explained to potential clients, along with honest predictions of success in the long term. New York City has adopted a "Truth-in-Dieting" regulation that calls for voluntary steps on the part of the weight-loss businesses in that great city to disclose safety risks to clients before they sign up. The regulation resulted from an undercover investigation of diet programs by New York City's Department of Consumer Affairs. The investigators found that weight-loss centers intentionally hid risks and costs associated with the programs while exaggerating their efficacy. What is true of weight-loss businesses in New York City is probably true across the country, and the Federal Trade Commission is working to establish guidelines concerning advertising of weight-loss programs. Table C9-1 reprints the "Consumer Bill of Rights" that the New York regulation asks weight-loss establishments to post. As of this writing Weight Watchers alone had complied with the request.

If most diet programs are unsafe, very-low-calorie diets (VLCD) can be even more so, even when medically supervised. The fewer the calories a diet provides or the more out of balance it is, the greater the risks it presents. In an effort to find a diet to promote rapid weight loss safely, many commercially prepared VLCD formulas were developed in the 1980s. Most VLCD formulas provide about 400 to 800 calories per day and are available by prescription only. They provide the RDA of all vitamins and minerals but fall short of providing the minimum for fiber and energy-yielding nutrients.

At first, these plans appealed to millions of people who wanted to lose 10 or 20 pounds. Many hospitals and clinics met this need by establishing centers to administer VLCD and to monitor their use. The diets were designed to give dieters a sort of jump-start on weight loss by producing large initial losses quickly. This sounds logical, but the body's metabolism responds to the severe calorie deficit as if the person were starving—it begins to *conserve* energy, guarding every calorie. The body also sacrifices tissue protein to supply glucose to the brain, as Chapter 9 explained. Today, some clinics and hospitals have stopped using VLCD except in cases of extreme, life-threatening obesity because, although the diets successfully produce large initial weight losses, the long-term outlook for those who use

Table C9-1
Weight Loss Consumer Bill of Rights

1. WARNING: Rapid weight loss may cause serious health problems. (Rapid weight loss is weight loss of more than 1½ to 2 pounds per week or weight loss of more than 1% of body weight per week after the second week of participation in a weight loss program.)
2. Only permanent lifestyle changes—such as making healthful food choices and increasing physical activity—promote long-term weight loss.
3. Consult your personal physician before starting any weight loss program.
4. Qualifications of this provider's staff are available on request.
5. You have a right to:
   i. ask questions about the potential health risks of this program, its nutrition content, and its psychological-support and educational component;
   ii. know the price of treatment including the prices of any extra products, services, supplements and laboratory tests; and
   iii. know the program duration that is being recommended for you.

Source: Adopted in May 1992 by the New York City Department of Consumer Affairs, Mark Green, Commissioner.

them is bleak. More than 90 percent of clients who lost weight using the diets alone regained all of it, and many ended up fatter than before they started. The only people who succeed may be those with the highest initial weights: One study showed that they lost the most weight and kept it off for at least a year.[7] Other studies link success to effective long-term social and professional support, such as skills training for relapse prevention, physical activity groups, self-help groups, and behavior modification.[8]

Along with high failure rates, many physical risks accompany the use of VLCD (see Table C9-2). This makes them inappropriate for most overweight people. For people with diabetes whose obesity has aggravated their symptoms, however, VLCD may be deemed appropriate, since even a temporary improvement in diabetes may forestall serious consequences.

MEDICAL ETHICS, WEIGHT LOSS, AND PROFITS Officially, obesity is a disease. Most physicians feel compelled by medical ethics to offer treatment for all diseases. One conscientious weight-control expert believes obesity to carry medical risks so severe that for a physician to delay offering treatment would be a form of malpractice.[9] Not only do obese people who lose weight experience reversal of disease risks, he says, but they often discover a new sense of self-esteem and improved quality of life. Certainly to deprive people of the opportunity to achieve these benefits would be unethical.

Besides, weight-loss advocates argue, if doctors withdraw their medical support for weight control, quacks will rush to fill the void in the multibillion dollar diet industry. Physicians may not be able to dictate to society or even to individuals what an ideal weight should be but they should stay involved with weight control and strive to guide their clients toward healthy habits.

While no one could argue against treating a disease that causes misery and illness, questioners point out that weight-loss efforts involving dietary changes are not effective—they almost always fail to produce long-term results.[10] This makes promoting them as effective treatments unethical and misleading to patients. If the Food and Drug Administration (FDA) was asked to approve the sale of a medical drug with the failure record of weight-loss schemes, the FDA would declare the drug ineffective and would disallow or severely restrict its use. If obesity is treated as a medical problem, shouldn't prescribed treatments be required to meet the criteria that other treatments must meet?

Unquestionably, profits drive many programs.[11] An estimated 30 to 40 percent of all adult U.S. women (and 20 to 25 percent of U.S. men) are trying to lose weight at any given time, spending up to $30 to $40 billion each year to do so. Income potentials as high as these are bound to attract an army of "get-rich-quick" scam artists. In fact, FDA names weight-loss schemes as one of the leading forms of fraud in the United States. "Even if one's chances of losing and keeping off weight are better than one's chances of winning the lottery, the motivation is much the same: winning promises transformation."[12] People have learned to attach so many unproved benefits to weight loss that they are willing to risk huge sums for the slightest chance of success. These factors—a hard-to-change condition, a willingness to believe in unproved benefits, and the ability to pay—create a fertile field for profiteers who continue, year after year, to rake in huge sums while hiding the reality of improbable odds of success.[13]

ATTITUDES TOWARD OVERWEIGHT People in this country value slenderness highly. The image of successful, healthy, well-adjusted people almost invariably includes a slender body form. Irrationally, many people equate slenderness with happiness, intelligence, psychological stability, harmony in relationships, success in the workplace, and many other valued attributes that have little if anything to do with body size or weight. Some claim we place emphasis on a slender appearance, especially for women, not for the sake of their health, but for other people's viewing pleasure.

A widespread misconception holds that obese people are to blame for their overfatness; they face rejection from unspoken accusations of laziness, slothfulness, and self-indulgence. This amounts to a prejudice and discrimination against overweight people, and especially overweight women, that causes them great psychological stress. Overweight people in our society readily assume the burden of responsibility for their fatness and feel guilty when weight-loss diets fail to produce promised results.[14]

Especially damaging are the attitudes of some physicians toward the overweight. Many have come to accept overfatness as the primary cause of most of the medical problems that bother people today. Some even overlook sound techniques that could solve medical problems because they believe that the "cure" for such problems is weight loss. A story is told of a woman who had this problem:

Table C9-2
Possible Physical Consequences of Very-Low-Calorie Diets

Blood	Immunity
■ Blood carotene concentrations increase ■ Blood cholesterol concentrations increase ■ Blood urea concentrations increase	■ Immune response diminishes ■ White blood cells decrease in number
Cardiovascular/respiratory	**Metabolic**
■ Blood pressure declines ■ Carbon dioxide production declines ■ Cardiac output declines ■ Heart muscle atrophies ■ Heartbeat becomes irregular ■ Low blood pressure develops ■ Oxygen consumption declines ■ Pulse rate declines ■ Respiratory rate declines	■ Basal metabolism declines ■ Bone mineral content shifts ■ Cold intolerance occurs ■ Dehydration may occur ■ Gout may occur ■ Ketosis develops ■ Lean body tissues are lost ■ Mineral and electrolyte imbalances occur ■ Nitrogen balance becomes negative
Digestive	**Other**
■ Gallstones and kidney stones form ■ GI tract motility declines ■ Liver inflammation and fibrosis develop ■ Nausea, vomiting, diarrhea, abdominal discomfort, and constipation occur	■ Body and breath odor (from ketone excretion) may become apparent ■ Hair falls out ■ Headaches occur ■ Lethargy, fatigue, and loss of stamina set in ■ Skin dries out ■ Sleeplessness may occur ■ Sudden death becomes possible
Hormonal	
■ Menstrual irregularity develops ■ Sex drive is lost	

Sources: Evidence on metabolic rate, lean body tissue, liver, gallstone, heartbeat, bones, nitrogen balance, from various authors in *American Journal of Clinical Nutrition* 56 (1992): supplement; immune failure reported in C. J. Field, R. Gougeon, and E. B. Marliss, *American Journal of Clinical Nutrition* 54 (1991): 123–129; reduced oxygen consumption reported in K. N. Pavlou and coauthors, Exercise as an adjunct to weight loss and maintenance in moderately obese subjects, *American Journal of Clinical Nutrition* 49 (1989): 1115–1123; low blood pressure, headache, atrophy of heart muscle, and hormonal effects from R. L. Atkinson, Low calorie diets and obesity, in D. D. Bills and S. D. Kung, *Biotechnology and Nutrition* (Boston: Butterworth-Heinemann, 1992), pp. 29–45.

The woman had complained to her family physician for years about her indigestion and diarrhea. He always reminded her that she was overweight and if she wouldn't eat so much, her digestion would be fine. Finally, she was diagnosed by a specialist as having a gluten [wheat] intolerance. Although her health is better today, she is still overweight and is embarrassed to see her family doctor for her regular checkup.[15]

Not just physicians, but even dietitians who run weight-loss clinics can be moralistic in their approach to the obese.[16] They present weight loss as an easily achievable goal, a grossly misleading attitude. They may consider those who do not become slender as "deviant" and as failures. Most people who are exposed to these attitudes willingly accept the blame, and believe that failure to lose weight is proof of their inadequacy. In reality, such people are among the overwhelming majority who have repeatedly proved that weight-loss diet schemes are failures.

TOWARD DEVELOPING ANSWERS In searching for appropriate future solutions to the problem of obesity, researchers have looked back 100 years to the population of the time. In those days, significantly fewer people were overweight and dieting was practically unknown. Physical activity was necessarily a part of life, for elevators, automobiles, and other labor-saving devices were yet to be invented.

Perhaps one significant clue to the effortless weight control of a century ago is that the general diet of the time closely followed recommendations made for diets of today. In those days, meat, eggs, and dairy products were consumed in much smaller quantities, and cereals and grains were central to most people's meals. This created a diet low in fat, high in carbohydrate, much like the diet the guidelines suggest. With passing years and with discovery of the importance of protein to human health people all but abandoned high-carbohydrate foods. They falsely believed them to be low in nutrients and began eating meat with every meal. Of course, along with the protein of meat comes a lot of fat. Later, the advent of fast foods with their greasy commercial-grade hamburger, fried potatoes, and ice cream shakes cemented into place our current high-fat diet.

At the same time these dietary changes were taking place, obesity was gaining prevalence in the population. As mentioned once before, a leading obesity expert has suggested that, to prevent or reverse obesity, "the single most important thing you can do is to get the fat out of the diet."[17] It is known that adopting a low-fat, high-carbohydrate eating plan *for life* can significantly change body composition toward the lean. Equally important, though, is a lifestyle that includes regular physical activity. Our forebears lived actively.

Beyond cutting fat intake and living actively, should some people make further efforts to lose weight? Should they turn to surgery, very-low-calorie diets, and prescription drugs, for which success rates are below 50 percent? Those who suffer from severe obesity and experience the brunt of its related health hazards would be well advised to take whatever measures are possible to reduce disease risks. However, overweight people who lack markers of obesity-related diseases should seriously consider the risks and benefits they can reasonably expect. A key point of consensus, even among the most unwavering supporters of aggressive treatment for obesity, is that a large subset of the obese population, termed "the healthy obese," is not at increased risk of disease. For these people, the risks associated with weight-loss dieting far outweigh any health benefits they can expect from weight loss.

Others should seriously consider their ideals. People who hold to thin ideals do not see the danger to their own and others' self-esteem and well-being. Fashion models whose careers depend on body shape often develop eating disorders. Teenaged girls across the country feel compelled to diet, ignorant of their peril. To break free from these dangerous ideals requires that people revamp old ways of thinking and accept themselves and others regardless of body weight. Table C9-3 lists tips offered to people who are working to accept their body weights rather than to change them.

A safe option exists for those who would like to promote a lean body composition, however. The low-fat, adequate diet advocated by the Dietary Guidelines and the Daily Food Guide can make a difference for those who are accustomed to eating high-fat diets. Taken with a routine of behavior modification and physical activity as described in Chapter 9, the change can produce a leaner body composition, while removing the issue of weight from the realm of success or failure. This course of action is not only life-changing for the people who adopt it, but it also sends an important message of self-acceptance to a younger generation.

Table C9-3
Tips for Accepting a Healthy Body Weight

- Adopt a new value system. Value yourself and others for human attributes other than body weight. Realize that prejudging people by weight is as harmful as prejudging them by race, religion, or gender.
- Accept that no magic diet can help anyone lose weight, and that it is *diets* that fail, not people who try to employ them.
- Stop dieting to lose weight. Adopt healthy eating and exercise habits.
- Memorize and employ the Daily Food Guide and the Exchange System calorie values. Never restrict calories beyond the minimum levels that meet nutrient needs.
- Become a physically active person. Use all the tips suggested in the next chapter for doing so.
- Seek support from loved ones. Explain what you have learned about the mysteries of why people become overweight. Tell them of your plan for a healthy life in the body you have been given.
- Seek professional counseling, *not* from a weight-loss counselor, but from someone who can help you make gains in self-esteem without weight as a factor.
- Join with others to fight weight discrimination. (Search your local paper, or see the Appendix of Addresses at the back of this book for names of groups.)
- Become politically active. Tell your representative that you support efforts to end the misleading and false claims made by the weight-loss industry. Ask them to lobby for full disclosure by diet peddlers of the risks of dieting. Write to the FDA telling them to establish safety and effectiveness criteria for diets and weight-loss programs.

Notes

1. A combined effort by the North American Association for the Study of Obesity and Emory University School of Medicine brought about one such conference, the Obesity Update: Pathophysiology, Clinical Consequences, and Therapeutic Options in Atlanta, Georgia, August 31–September 2, 1992.
2. F. X. Pi-Sunyer, Health implications of obesity, *American Journal of Clinical Nutrition* 53 (1991): 1595S–1603S.
3. G. A. Colditz, Economic costs of obesity, *American Journal of Clinical Nutrition* 55 (1992): 503S–507S.
4. P. Ernsberger, Obesity is hazardous to your health: Negative, *Debates in Medicine* 2 (1989): 102–137.
5. A. Gott, relating 1989 findings of the Michigan Health Council, in *Deception and Fraud in the Diet Industry*, Part I, serial no. 101–50 (Washington, D.C.: Government Printing Office, 1990), p. 2.
6. L. Lissner and coauthors, Variability of body weight and health outcomes in Framingham population, *New England Journal of Medicine* 324 (1991): 1839–1844.
7. T. A. Wadden and coauthors, Clinical correlates of short- and long-term weight loss, *American Journal of Clinical Nutrition* 56 (1992): 271S–274S.
8. M. G. Perri, S. F. Sears, and J. E. Clark, Strategies for improving maintenance of weight loss: Toward a continuous care model of obesity management, *Diabetes Care* 16 (1993): 200–209.
9. G. L. Blackburn, Treatment of obesity is imperative: Physicians can make a difference, an address presented at the conference, Obesity Update, 1992.
10. T. A. Wadden and coauthors, Treatment of obesity by very low calorie diet, behavior therapy, and their combination: A five year perspective, *International Journal of Obesity* 13 (1989): 39–46.
11. F. X. Pi-Sunyer, The role of very-low-calorie diets in obesity, *American Journal of Clinical Nutrition* 56 (1992): 2405–2435.
12. S. C. Wooley and D. M. Garner, Obesity treatment: The high cost of false hope, *Journal of the American Dietetic Association* 91 (1991): 1248–1251.
13. D. M. Garner, Positive alternatives to weight loss in selected patients, an address presented at the conference, Obesity Update, 1992.
14. Wooley and Garner, 1991.
15. E. S. Parham, Applying a philosophy of nutrition education to weight control, *Journal of Nutrition Education* 22 (1990): 194–197.
16. Parham, 1990.
17. R. L. Atkinson, Role of diet in obesity treatment, an address presented at the conference, Obesity Update, 1992.

Nutrition and Physical Activity

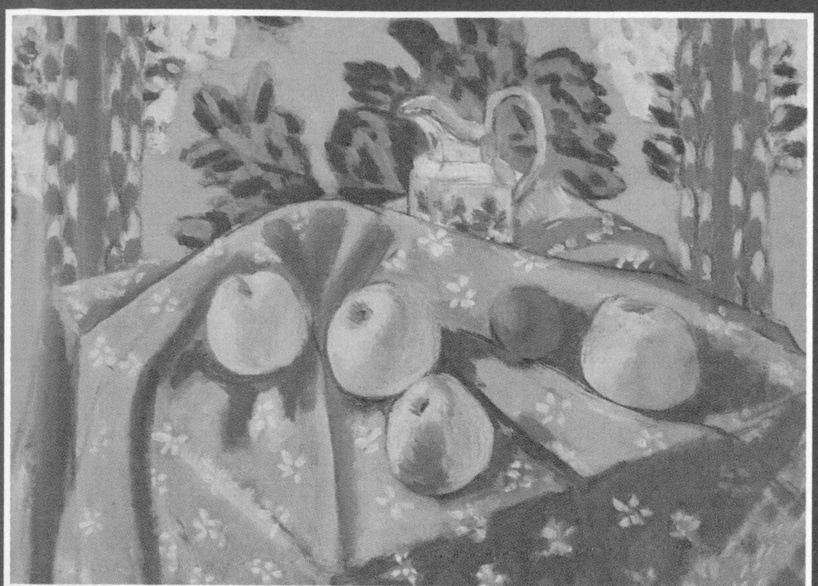

Contents

Thomas Eakins, The Biglin Brothers Racing; National Gallery of Art, Washington; Gift of Mr. and Mrs. Cornelius Vanderbilt Whitney.

10

In the body, nutrition and physical activity go hand in hand. The working body demands energy-yielding nutrients to fuel activity, and it needs protein and a host of supporting nutrients with which to build lean tissue. In addition, it needs stores of fuel in the form of fat and glycogen for exercise. Exercise uses up fat and stimulates the deposit of lean tissue, and so pushes body composition toward the lean, a change considered beneficial to health.

A certain amount of physical activity correlates with a healthy body. The American College of Sports Medicine specifies that people should spend an accumulated minimum of 30 minutes in some sort of physical activity on most days of each week.[1] The activity need not be sports. A few minutes walking up stairs, another few spent pulling weeds, and several more spent walking the dog all contribute to the day's total. Some people recall an earlier recommendation to obtain at least 20 minutes of sustained moderate-intensity activity at least four days a week. This recommendation still stands because it produces superb results in terms of health, and it improves the heart's capacity to do its work. People who meet this requirement can rest assured that they have well covered their bodies' activity needs.

A sedentary lifestyle is as powerful a risk factor as smoking, obesity, or hypertension for developing the major killer diseases of our time—cardiovascular disease, some forms of cancer, stroke, diabetes, and hypertension.[2] People who regularly engage in just moderate physical activity live longer on average than those who fail to exercise.[3] Exercisers may also receive these benefits:

- Improved mental outlook and capacity.
- Feeling of vigor.
- Feeling of belonging—the fun and companionship of sports.
- Improved self-image and self-confidence.
- Reduced fatness and increased lean body tissue.
- Greater bone density (better protection against osteoporosis).
- Improved circulation, heart capacity, and lung function.
- Sound, beneficial sleep.
- A youthful appearance; healthy skin; improved muscle tone.
- Reduced risk of cardiovascular disease.
- Reduced low-density lipoprotein (LDL) cholesterol; raised high-density lipoprotein (HDL), indicators of low heart-disease risk.
- Normalized blood pressure and slowed resting pulse rate, indicators of a healthy cardiovascular system.
- Reduced risk of stroke (even in oral contraceptive users, who have an increased risk).
- Improvement of symptoms of diabetes.
- Reduced risk of constipation and colon disorders, including cancer.
- Fast wound healing.
- Improvement or elimination of menstrual cramps.
- Improved resistance to colds and infections.

Science cannot promise that you will receive all of these benefits if you exercise, but almost everyone who is physically active reaps at least some of them. If even half of these rewards were yours for the asking, wouldn't you step up to claim them? Despite evidence of the benefits, not even a

Ways to include physical activity in a day.

Join a fitness club.
Make friends with people who help one another stay fit.
Play a sport.
Get credit hours for classes in dancing, sports, conditioning, or swimming.
Hike, bike, or walk to nearby stores.
Park a block from your destination and walk.
Take the stairs, not the elevator.
Give two labor-saving devices to charity.
Stretch often during the day.
Lift small hand weights when talking on the phone or viewing TV.
Garden.
Play with children.
Walk a dog.
Coach a sport.
Mow, trim, and rake by hand.
Wash your car with extra vigor, or bend and stretch to wash your toes in the bath.
Be imaginative.

training regular practice of an activity, which leads to physical adaptations of the body, with improvements in flexibility, strength, or endurance.

flexibility the ability to bend without injury, which depends on the elasticity of muscles, tendons, and ligaments and on the condition of the joints.

strength the ability of muscles to work against resistance.

endurance the ability to sustain an effort for a long time.

muscle endurance the ability of a muscle to contract repeatedly within a given time without becoming exhausted.

cardiovascular endurance the ability of the cardiovascular system to sustain effort over a period of time.

overload an extra physical demand placed on the body; an increase in the frequency, duration, or intensity of an exercise. A principle of training is that for a body system to improve, it must be worked at frequencies, durations, or intensities that increase by increments.

hypertrophy (high-PURR-tro-fee) an increase in size (for example, of a muscle) in response to use.

atrophy (AT-tro-fee) a decrease in size of a muscle because of disuse.

myoglobin the muscles' iron-containing protein that stores and releases oxygen in response to muscles' energy needs.

quarter of the population of the United States exercises regularly. Perhaps this is because they think of exercise as another task to add to their already work-filled days. We'd like them to think, instead, in terms of physical activities, that is, fun and leisure activities that meet people's needs for both relaxation and the maintenance of a fit body.

This chapter is written for "you," whoever you are—the athlete, the health seeker, the sports player, the weight-loss seeker, or the person who has yet to begin exercising. To understand the interactions between physical activity and nutrition, you must first know a few things about **training.**

KEY POINT Physical activity benefits people's physical, psychological, and social well-being and improves their resistance to disease. A certain minimum amount of physical activity is necessary to produce these benefits.

◆ The Essentials of Training

Training doesn't require that you develop a Ms. Olympia or Mr. Universe body; rather, you need to develop your own potential along several lines. You need to achieve enough of the four components of fitness—**flexibility, strength, muscle endurance,** and **cardiovascular endurance**—to allow you to meet the everyday demands of life, plus some to spare.

The Body's Response to Activity People shape their bodies by what they do and by what they choose not to do. Muscle cells and tissues respond to an **overload** of exercise by gaining strength and size, a response called **hypertrophy.** The opposite is also true: if not called on to perform, muscles **atrophy.** Thus cyclists often have well-developed legs but little arm or chest strength; a tennis player may have one arm that is superbly strong, while the other is just average. A variety of physical activities will produce the most uniform overall fitness. To obtain a balance of activity, people are told to work different muscle groups from day to day. For balanced fitness, stretching enhances flexibility, weight training and calisthenics develop muscle strength and endurance, and aerobic activity improves cardiovascular endurance. It makes sense to give muscles a rest, too, because it takes a day or two to replenish muscle fuel supplies and to repair any slight damage incurred through exercise.

Periodic rest also gives muscles time to adapt to an activity by building more of the equipment required to perform it. The muscle cells of a superbly trained weightlifter, for example, store extra granules of glycogen, build up strong connective tissues, and add bulk to the special proteins that contract the muscle, thereby increasing the muscle's ability to perform.* In the same way, the muscle cells of a distance swimmer develop huge stocks of **myoglobin,** the muscle's version of hemoglobin, and other equipment needed to burn fat and to sustain prolonged exertion. This means that people who wish to play a sport should train mainly by playing that sport, to develop in their muscles the specific equipment most needed in the chosen

*All muscles contain a variety of muscle fibers, but there are two main types—slow-twitch (also called *red fibers*) and fast-twitch (also called *white fibers*). Slow-twitch fibers contain extra metabolic equipment to perform fat-burning aerobic work, while the fast-twitch type store extra glycogen for anaerobic work. Muscle fibers of one type take on some of the characteristics of the other as an adaption to exercise.

activity. Keep in mind that while everyone's muscles adapt to exercise to some degree, true champions are born with the genetic potential to excel while others are not. This fact cannot be changed even through hard work.

aerobic (air-ROE-bic) requiring oxygen.

anaerobic (AN-air-ROE-bic) not requiring oxygen.

stroke volume the amount of blood ejected from the heart toward body tissues at each beat.

Aerobic Activity and the Heart Aerobic activity builds cardiovascular endurance: a healthy condition of the heart and arteries. With cardiovascular endurance, the total blood volume and number of red blood cells increase, so that the blood can carry more oxygen. The heart muscle becomes stronger and larger, and each beat empties the heart's chambers more completely, so that the heart pumps more blood per beat. This makes fewer beats necessary, so the pulse rate falls. The muscles that inflate and deflate the lungs gain strength and endurance and this allows breathing to become more efficient. Blood moves easily through the blood vessels because the muscles of the heart contract powerfully, and contraction of the skeletal muscles pushes the blood through the veins. Such improvements keep resting blood pressure normal because vessel resistance diminishes. They also raise blood HDL, the beneficial lipoprotein. Figure 10-1 shows the major relationships between the heart, lungs, and muscles.

The importance of HDL to heart health is a topic of the next chapter.

What sorts of activities produce these beneficial changes? Recall from page 357 that the advice for a healthy body was to spend 30 *collective* minutes on each of several days a week in various activities. In contrast, training for cardiovascular endurance requires *sustained* activity—that is, activity performed for certain time periods. Effective activities are those that elevate the heart rate, that are sustained for longer than 20 minutes, and that use most of the large muscle groups of the body (legs, buttocks, and abdomen). Examples are swimming, cross-country skiing, rowing, fast walking, jogging, fast bicycling, soccer, hockey, basketball, water polo, lacrosse, and rugby.

An informal pulse check can give you some indication of how conditioned your heart is. The average resting pulse rate for adults is around 70 beats per minute, but the rate can be higher or lower. Active people can have resting pulse rates of 50 or even lower. To take your pulse, place your finger over a pulse point (under the jawbone at the side of the adam's apple of the throat, for instance) and count the number of beats in 30 seconds. Multiply by two to get beats per minute.

Cardiovascular endurance is characterized by:

- Increased blood volume and oxygen delivery.
- Increased heart strength and **stroke volume.**
- Slowed resting pulse.
- Increased breathing efficiency.
- Improved circulation.
- Reduced blood pressure.

In contrast to aerobic activity, **anaerobic** activity generally brings about less cardiovascular conditioning but superbly develops strength and bulk of muscles. It involves sudden, all-out exertions of muscles that last for fewer than 90 seconds. This form of exercise develops lean tissue and so improves overall body composition. Examples include sprinting (100 meter dash), serving a tennis ball, jumping a fence, doing pushups, or lifting weights.

After learning the ways activity affects the body, people often want to know where their own activity levels stand in relation to body needs. Complex ways of finding this out are available, but a group of researchers devised a quicker way. They asked this single question: "Do you currently participate in any regular activity or program (either on your own or in a formal class) designed to improve or maintain your physical fitness?" The researchers discovered that positive answers correlated closely with healthy body mass index, high blood HDL, and efficient use of oxygen, all indicators of physical activity levels.[4] If your honest answer to their question is "yes," chances are good that you are physically active enough to favorably influence your own health.

The person who would develop a fit body for health or sports performance must also master nutrition. The rest of this chapter provides detailed

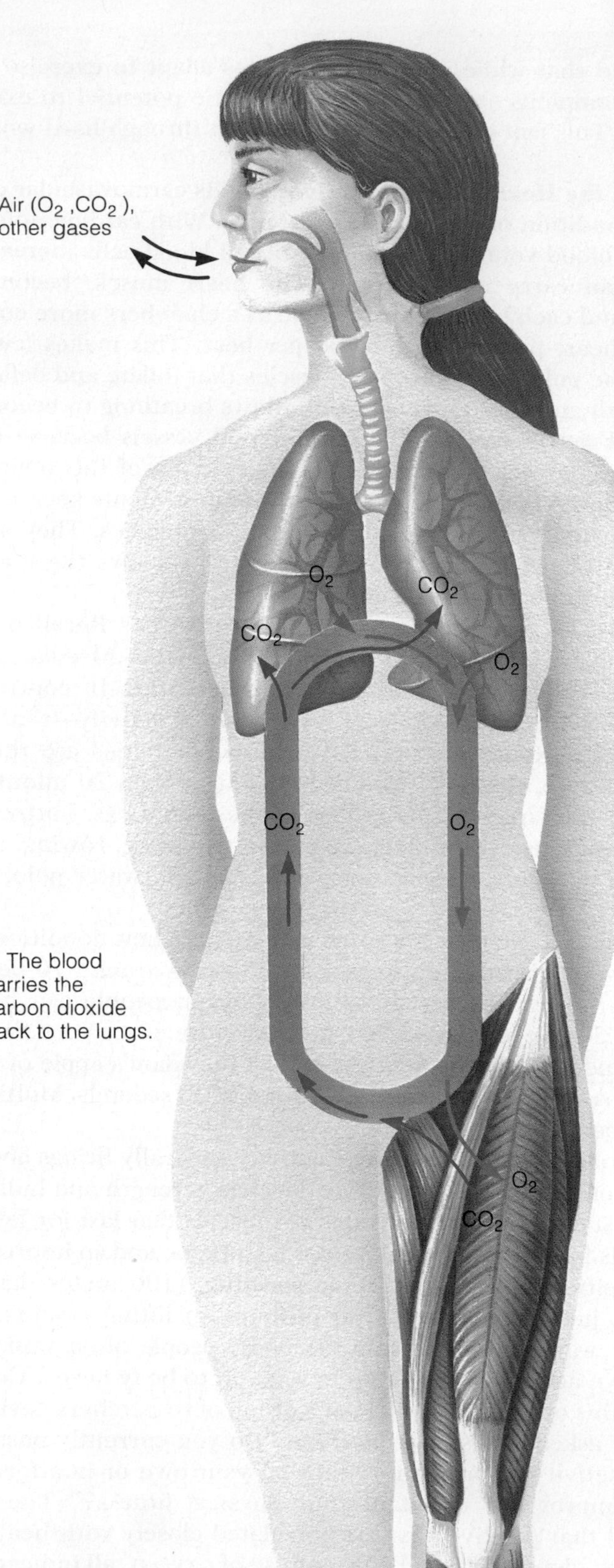

Figure 10-1

DELIVERY OF OXYGEN BY THE HEART AND LUNGS TO THE MUSCLES

The more fit a muscle is, the more oxygen it draws from the blood. This oxygen comes from the lungs, so the person with more fit muscles extracts oxygen from inhaled air more efficiently than a person with less fit muscles. The cardiovascular system responds to increased demand for oxygen by building up its capacity to deliver oxygen. Researchers can measure cardiovascular fitness by measuring the amount of oxygen a person consumes per minute while working out. This measure of fitness is called **VO_2 max.**

VO_2 max the maximum rate of oxygen consumption by an individual at sea level.

descriptions of interactions between nutrients and physical activity. Nutrition alone cannot endow you with fitness or athletic ability, but along with the right mental attitude, it can complement the effort you put forth to obtain them. Conversely, unwise food selections can stand in your way.

KEY POINT To build fitness, whose components are flexibility, strength, muscle endurance, and cardiovascular endurance, a person must engage in physical activity. Muscles adapt to activities they are called upon to perform.

Using Glucose to Fuel Activity

The exercising body responds to physical activity by adjusting its fuel mix. During rest, the body derives a little more than half of its energy from fatty acids, most of the rest from glucose, and a little from amino acids. Of the fuels mentioned, carbohydrate is of major interest to exercisers. The stored glucose of muscle glycogen is a major fuel for exercise. In the early minutes of an activity, muscle glycogen alone provides the energy the muscles use to go into action. As exercise continues, hormones, including the hormone epinephrine and the neurotransmitter norepinephrine, flow into the bloodstream to signal the liver and fat cells to liberate their stored energy nutrients, primarily fatty acids and glucose. Thus hormones set the table for the muscles' energy feast, and the muscles help themselves to the fuels passing by in the blood.

Glucose Use and Storage

Both liver and muscles store glucose as glycogen, a fuel considered vital for physical activity; the liver can also make glucose from fragments of other nutrients. It has been said that muscles hoard their glycogen stores—they do not release their glucose into the bloodstream to share with other body tissues, as the liver does. This is fortunate. A muscle that shared its glycogen reserves with other tissues might lack glucose at critical times, say, when running from danger. A muscle that conserves its glycogen is prepared to act in emergencies because muscle glucose is essential to quick action. Later on, as activity continues, glucose from the liver and digestive tract also become important sources of fuel for muscle activity.

Muscle glycogen also supports long-duration endurance exercise; and the more glycogen muscles store, the longer the stores will last to support this exercise. A classic report compared fuel use during exercise among three groups of runners, each on a different diet.[5] For several days before testing, one of the groups consumed a normal mixed diet (55 percent of calories from carbohydrate); a second group consumed a high-carbohydrate diet (83 percent of calories from carbohydrate); and the third group consumed a high-fat diet (94 percent of calories from fat). Figure 10-2 shows that the high-carbohydrate diet allowed the athletes to work longer before exhaustion. This study and many others that followed established that a high-carbohydrate diet enhances an athlete's endurance by ensuring ample glycogen stores.

When a high-carbohydrate diet is consumed, glycogen storage is speeded up, as is the body's use of carbohydrate for fuel.[6] These two actions are especially important because the body has such limited carbohydrate storage capacity. The body stores what glucose it can as glycogen and uses up

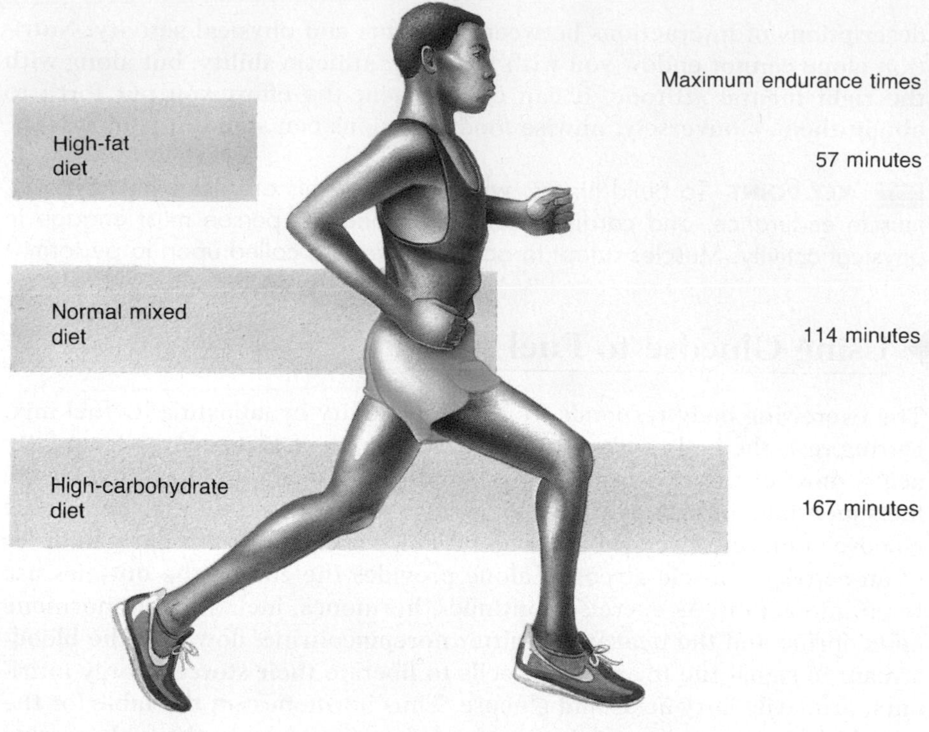

Figure 10-2

THE EFFECT OF DIET ON PHYSICAL ENDURANCE

A high-carbohydrate diet can triple an athlete's endurance.

Source: Data from P. Astrand, Something old and something new . . . very new, *Nutrition Today*, June 1968, pp. 9–11.

much of the remainder as fuel. Any excess must be converted to fat before storage, an inefficient process.

Not only diet but also training affects the amount of glycogen that muscles use and store. When muscles work hard enough to deplete their glycogen stores, they adapt to store more glycogen in the future.

KEY POINT Glucose is supplied by dietary carbohydrate or made by the liver. It is stored in both liver and muscle tissue as glycogen. Total glycogen stores affect an athlete's endurance. Both storage and use of glycogen increase with increasing carbohydrate intakes. Glycogen-depleting exercise also stimulates increased glycogen storage.

Exercise Intensity, Glucose Use, and Glycogen Stores

Muscle and liver glycogen is limited when compared with the body's fat. A person with 30 pounds of body fat to spare may have only a pound or so of glycogen to draw on. How long an exercising person's glycogen will last depends not only on diet but also partly on the intensity of the exercise. The more intense the activity, the more glycogen is needed to support it. The less intense the activity, the more conservative of glycogen. Thus, competitive athletes place large demands on their glycogen stores, while casual joggers demand less from their stores. Even joggers still use glycogen, however, and eventually they can run out of it. Glycogen depletion usually occurs after about two hours of vigorous exercise.*

*"Vigorous exercise," here, means exercise at 75 percent VO_2 max.

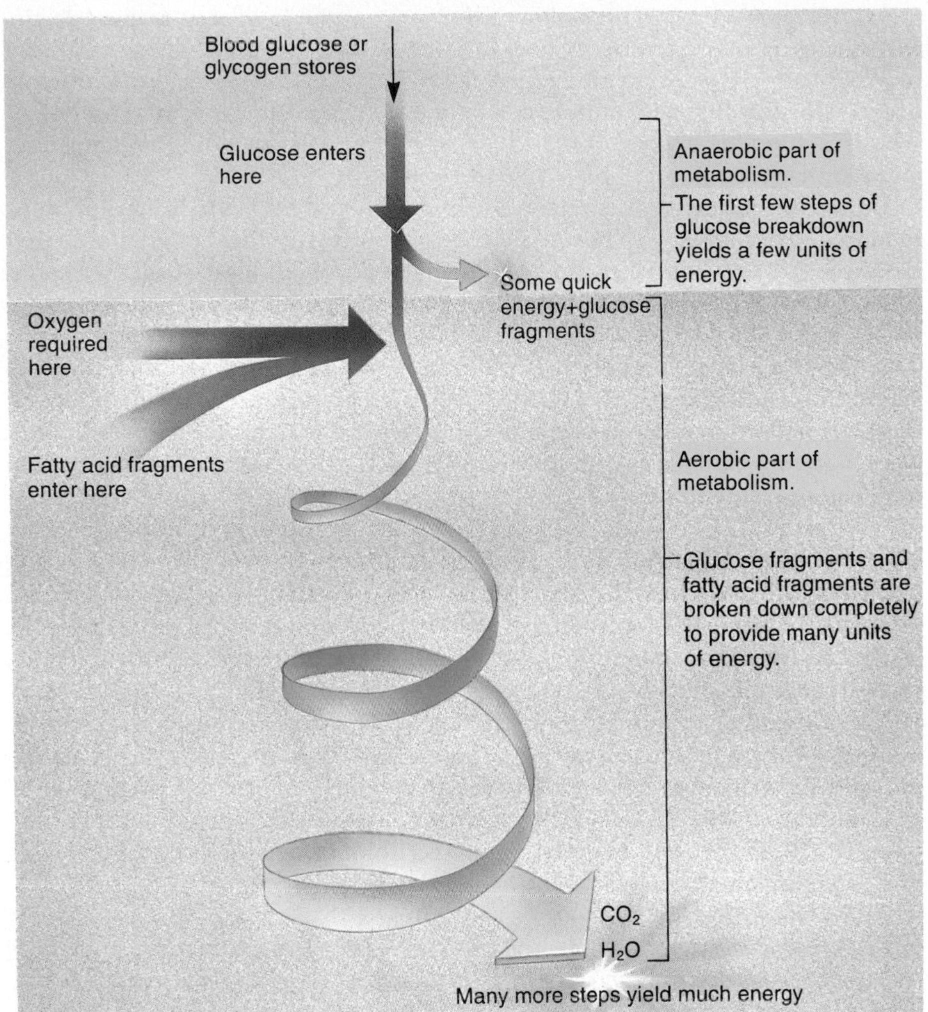

Figure 10-3

GLUCOSE AND FATTY ACIDS IN THEIR ENERGY-RELEASING PATHWAYS

Glucose is partially broken down under anaerobic conditions to yield some quick energy. The fragments of glucose molecules are then broken down completely in aerobic conditions, a process that yields carbon dioxide, water, and energy. Fat can enter the energy cycle only in the presence of oxygen.

In moderate exercise, glucose contributes to the fuel used to support activity. Oxygen plays a key role. With ample oxygen, muscles can extract all available energy from glucose and fat. During *moderate* aerobic exercise the exerciser breathes deeply and easily, and the lungs and circulatory system meet the muscles' need for oxygen with ease. Figure 10-3 shows that in aerobic metabolism muscles extract all the energy they can from both glucose and fatty acids when both are present together with oxygen. In this way, a little glucose helps to metabolize a lot of fat. Fat yields a lot of energy, so moderate aerobic exercise conserves glycogen stores.

Intense exercise presents a different picture. The heart and lungs can provide only so much oxygen only so fast. When muscle exertion is so great that the demand for energy outstrips the oxygen supply, aerobic metabolism cannot sufficiently meet energy needs. This means that fat cannot be used, because aerobic breakdown is its only option. It also means that glucose cannot be broken down as fully, or yield as much energy, as when oxygen is freely available. Muscles must instead rely more heavily on glucose which can be partially broken down *anaerobically*. Thus the muscles must draw more heavily on their limited glycogen supply.

The upper portion of Figure 10-3 shows that glucose can yield some energy in anaerobic metabolism, but not nearly as efficiently as in aerobic

oxygen debt a deficit of oxygen built up during anaerobic exercise; the debt must be repaid by rapid breathing after the activity slows down or stops. Also called *recovery oxygen consumption.*

lactic acid an incomplete-breakdown product produced from glucose during anaerobic metabolism. When oxygen becomes available, lactic acid can be completely broken down for energy or converted back to glucose.

metabolism. Anaerobic breakdown of glycogen yields energy to muscle tissue during times when energy demands are so large as to outstrip the ability to provide energy aerobically. Examples of such times are periods of intense exercise or the first few minutes of moderate exercise. Thus anaerobic metabolism supplies energy, but it does so by lavishly spending the muscles' glycogen reserves.

During intense exercise, anaerobic metabolism builds up an **oxygen debt** in an exerciser's body.[7] The classic theory about why this occurs holds that rapid partial breakdown of glucose during anaerobic metabolism is responsible. Anaerobic glucose breakdown produces fragments of glucose molecules, **lactic acid,** that accumulate in the tissues and blood. The nervous and hormonal systems detect these fragments in the blood, and they respond by speeding up the heart and lungs to draw in more oxygen and break the fragments down. However, a point comes at which the heart and lungs can't keep up and lactic acid accumulates. If you exercise intensely, you may have to slow down or even stop to "catch your breath" (replenish your oxygen supply). When you do, your body begins relying on aerobic metabolism once more. At this point lactic acid is burned for fuel or used by the liver to generate glucose. (That is why this physiological state is called a *debt;* oxygen can be "repaid" later.) Other ideas about oxygen debt exist, and state that hormonal, circulatory, and other adjustments made by the body in recovery from exercise may be the cause.

Lactic acid causes burning muscle pain with a type of muscle fatigue that follows within seconds. A strategy for dealing with lactic acid is to relax the muscles at every opportunity during activity so that the circulating blood can carry away the lactic acid and bring in oxygen to support aerobic metabolism. This is what mountaineers are doing when they relax their leg muscles at each step (the "mountain rest step").

KEY POINT The more intense an activity, the more demanding of glucose is that activity. The body in anaerobic metabolism spends glucose rapidly, accumulates lactic acid, and builds up an oxygen debt.

The mountain rest step permits muscles to relax and recover even during strenuous hikes.

Exercise Duration, Glucose Use, and Glycogen Stores

Glucose use during exercise depends not only on the *intensity* but also on the *duration* of the exercise. In the first 10 minutes or so of an activity, the active muscles rely almost completely on their own stores of glycogen. Within the first 20 minutes or so of moderate exercise, a person uses up about one fifth of the available glycogen. As the muscles devour their own glycogen, they become ravenous for more glucose and increase their uptake of blood glucose 30-fold or more.[8] If you tested a person's blood glucose during moderate exercise, you would see it decline slightly, reflecting the muscles' use of the glucose supplied to the blood by the liver.

A person who continues exercising moderately for longer than 20 minutes begins to use less glucose and more fat for fuel. Still, glucose use continues, and if the exercise goes on for long enough and at high enough intensity, muscle and liver glycogen stores will run out almost completely (see Figure 10-4). Physical activity can continue for a short time thereafter only because the liver scrambles to produce some glucose from available lactic acid and certain amino acids.[9] This minimum amount of glucose may briefly forestall exhaustion but when hypoglycemia accompanies glycogen depletion, it brings nervous system function almost to a halt, making exercise impossible. This is what "hitting the wall" means to athletes in a marathon.[10]

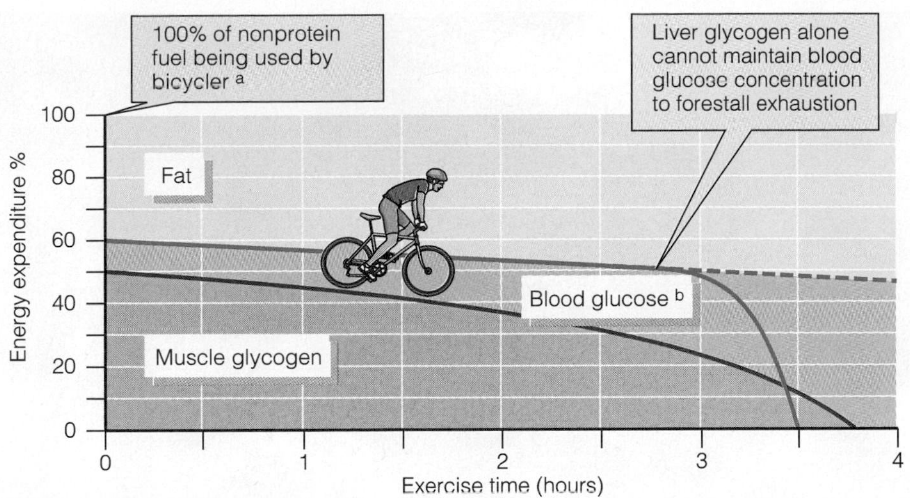

Figure 10-4

GLYCOGEN DEPLETION IN CYCLISTS

After three and a half hours of constant cycling, muscle glycogen is used up but the demand for glucose fuel declines only slightly. Fat remains abundant, but it cannot support exercise without a minimum amount of carbohydrate.

Source: Adapted from E. F. Coyle and S. J. Montain, Carbohydrate and fluid ingestion during exercise: Are there trade-offs? *Medicine and Science in Sports and Exercise* 24 (1992): 671–678.

To avoid exhaustion, endurance athletes must try to maintain their blood glucose concentrations for as long as they can. Three dietary strategies and one exercise strategy may help maintain glucose concentrations. One diet strategy is to eat a high-carbohydrate diet on a day-to-day basis (see this chapter's Food Feature). Another is to take in some glucose during the exercise, usually in fluid (see below). The third is to eat carbohydrate-rich foods following exercise to boost the storage of glycogen. As for exercise, the strategy involves training the muscles to store as much glycogen as they can, while supplying all the dietary glucose they need to do so (carbohydrate loading, as described in the next section).

During a long-duration competition, as glycogen runs low, glucose ingested before or during the event may assist the working body. Glucose seems to make its way from the digestive tract to the exercising muscles to augment the glucose from the muscle and liver glycogen stores. The glucose from carbohydrate-containing drinks can supplement the body's own glucose to support continued activity.[11] Athletes competing in games such as soccer or hockey, which last for hours and demand repeated bouts of intense activity, may also benefit from carbohydrate ingestion during the game.

Four strategies can help to maintain blood glucose to support sports performance (for *endurance* athletes only):

1. Eat a high-carbohydrate diet regularly.
2. Take glucose during activity performance.
3. Eat carbohydrate-rich foods after performance.
4. Train the muscles to maximize glycogen stores.

Before concluding that sugar might be good for your own performance, consider first whether you engage in *endurance* activity. That is, do you run, swim, bike, or ski nonstop at a rapid pace for more than 1½ hours at a time or do you compete in games lasting for hours? If not, the sugar picture changes. For an everyday jog or swim lasting less than 90 minutes, sugar probably won't help performance, because such exercise is not limited by carbohydrate availability. The body's glycogen stores are sufficient, so more will not be better. Extra sugar simply means extra empty calories the body must store, leaving less room for nutrient-dense foods that the body needs. Even among athletes, extra carbohydrate does not benefit those who engage in sports in which fatigue is unrelated to blood glucose, such as 100-meter sprinting, baseball, easy basketball, and weight-lifting.[12]

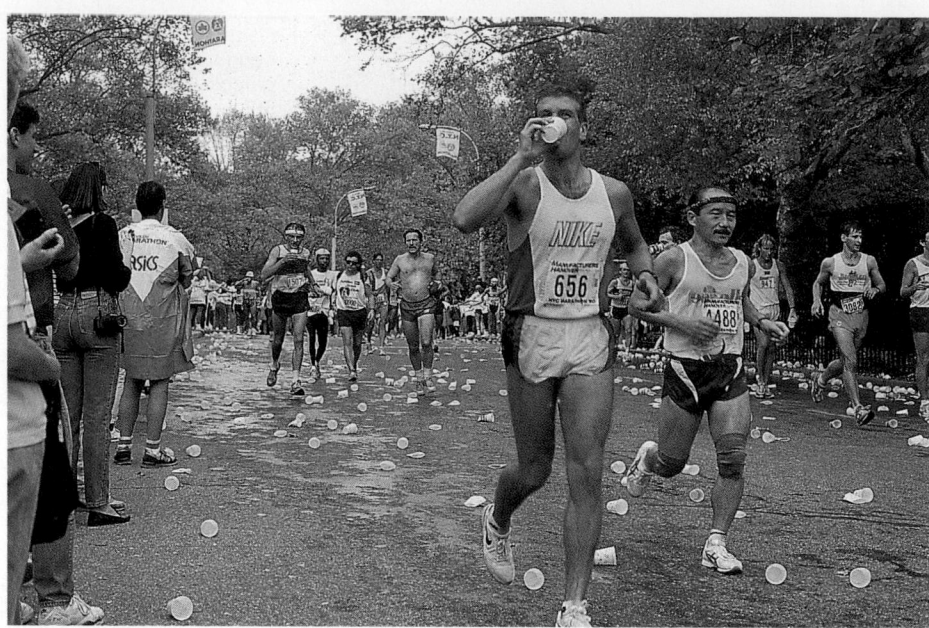

Those who compete in endurance activities require fluid and carbohydrate fuel.

carbohydrate loading a regimen of exhaustive exercise, followed by consuming a high-carbohydrate diet, that enables muscles to store glycogen beyond their normal capacity; also called *glycogen loading* or *glycogen supercompensation.*

Casual exercisers who believe that small amounts of sugary foods or beverages help them in their workouts probably do themselves no harm in partaking of them. It may be true that different people react differently to exercise and to sugar. Some specific recommendations for athletes concerning carbohydrate intakes before, during, and after exercise appear later on.

KEY POINT Exercise of long duration places demands on the body's glycogen stores. Carbohydrate ingested before and during long-duration activity may help to forestall hypoglycemia and fatigue. Sugar taken during short-duration exercise provides no benefits, and may displace nutrient-dense foods from the diet.

Carbohydrate Loading

Athletes whose sport exhausts their glycogen stores sometimes use a technique called **carbohydrate loading** to trick their muscles into storing extra glycogen before a competition.

First, the athlete increases exercise intensity without restricting carbohydrates. Next, during the week before competition, the athlete gradually cuts back on exercise, rests completely the day before, and eats a very high-carbohydrate diet for a few days before competition. In this plan an athlete never restricts carbohydrate intake; to do so incurs serious side effects, such as abnormal heartbeats and swollen muscles. By manipulating exercise and packing in carbohydrate, the athlete gains extra glycogen to fuel exercise lasting 90 minutes or longer at a stretch. Those whose work is of shorter duration need only eat a regular high-carbohydrate diet. In a hot climate, extra stored glycogen confers an additional advantage on the endurance athlete: as glycogen breaks down, it releases water, which helps to meet the athlete's fluid needs.

For people who would not make the effort of carbohydrate loading but still wish to have full glycogen stores, a simpler measure is possible. It appears that a high-carbohydrate meal within two hours after physical activity accelerates the rate of glycogen storage by 300 percent.[13] Eating the meal after two hours has passed reduces the glycogen synthesis rate by almost half. So after each workout, an exerciser might want to relax with a glass of orange juice and some crackers or other carbohydrate-rich snack.

To make glycogen, muscles need carbohydrate, but they also need rest. Vary daily exercise routines to work different muscles on different days.

KEY POINT Carbohydrate loading is a regime of exercise and diet that enables an athlete's muscles to store larger-than-normal amounts of glycogen to extend exercise endurance.

Degree of Training and Carbohydrate Use

One more factor that affects glycogen use during exercise is the degree of training of the muscles. A person trained to do the exercise at hand can work at high intensities longer than a less-trained person. Trained muscles can burn more fat at higher intensities than untrained muscles, and they require less glucose to perform the same amount of work. A person first attempting an activity uses up much more glucose per minute than an athlete who is trained to perform it. Oxygen delivery to the muscles by the heart and lungs plays a role in this effect, but equally importantly, untrained muscles have not developed extra enzymes to facilitate aerobic work and so depend heavily on the anaerobic breakdown of glucose, even when the exercise is just moderate.

Factors that affect glucose use in exercise:

- Carbohydrate intake.
- Intensity and duration of exercise.
- Degree of training.

People with diabetes should know that the moderating effect of exercise training on glucose metabolism may have implications for them. Those who must take insulin or insulin-eliciting drugs sometimes find that as their muscles adapt to exercise, they can reduce their daily drug doses. Another benefit to those with diabetes: exercise helps in loss of excess body fat, and this also helps to improve type II diabetes.

Chapter 4 described the action of insulin on blood sugar.

KEY POINT Highly trained muscles use less glucose than do untrained muscles to perform the same work. The changes in glucose metabolism that come with training are of benefit to those with diabetes.

◆ Using Fat and Fatty Acids to Fuel Activity

If a person should regularly eat mostly fat and protein with little measurable carbohydrate, that person would burn more fat than normal during exercise. However, that person would also sacrifice athletic performance, as Figure 10-2 showed, and could incur a major risk of cardiovascular disease. Not even exercisers are immune to heart attacks and strokes, so it is no wonder that every reliable source speaks out against high-fat diets for athletes.

Body fat stores are more important as fuel for exercise than is fat in the diet. Unlike the body's glycogen stores, which are limited, fat stores can fuel hours of exercise without running out; body fat is (theoretically) an unlimited source of energy. Even the lean bodies of elite runners carry enough fat to fuel several marathon runs.

Early in exercise, muscles begin to draw on fatty acids from two sources—fats stored within the working muscles and fats from fat depots such as the fat under the skin. Areas that have the most fat to spare donate the greatest amounts of fatty acids to the blood (although they may not be the areas that appear to you as the most fatty). This is why "spot reducing" doesn't work: muscles do not own the fat that surrounds them. Fat cells release fatty acids into the blood for all the muscles to share. Proof of this is found in a tennis player's arms: the fatfolds measure the same in both arms, even though the muscles of one arm are better developed than those of the other.

At the start of exercise blood fatty acid concentrations fall, but a few minutes into an activity, the neurotransmitter norepinephrine signals the fat cells to break apart their stored triglycerides and to liberate fatty acids into the blood. After about 20 minutes of exercise, the blood fatty acid concentration rises and surpasses the normal resting concentration. It is during this phase of sustained, submaximal exercise, beyond the first 20 minutes, that the fat cells begin to shrink in size as they empty out their fat stores.

The *intensity* of the exercise partly determines the percentage of energy contributed by fat. Figure 10-3 showed that fat can be broken down for energy in only one way, by aerobic metabolism. When intensity of exercise is so great as to incur oxygen debt, the body cannot burn more fat. Instead, it burns more glucose. Also, low-intensity exercise uses up more fat in proportion to the effort of the exerciser.

The *duration* of exercise also matters to fat use. The longer the duration, the greater the percentage of energy contributed by fat. The person who wishes to burn fat by exercising should know that patient, persistent, consistent training, such as fast walking, is the road to maximum use of fat and conservation of glycogen. Remember, aerobically trained muscles develop more fat-burning equipment, and so burn fat more readily than do untrained muscles. An old rule of thumb states that to burn fat, you should exercise at an intensity at which you can talk but not sing. If you can sing, speed up; if you can't talk, you are incurring oxygen debt and should slow down.

Factors that affect fat use in exercise:

- Fat intake.
- Intensity and duration of the exercise.
- Degree of training.

KEY POINT Body fat stores are more important to use as fuel during exercise than dietary fat. Norepinephrine stimulates fat cells to release fatty acids for use by exercising muscles. Fatty acids generate energy aerobically during low- to moderate-intensity activity.

Using Protein and Amino Acids for Building Muscles and to Fuel Activity

If a high-fat diet is ill advised for athletes, what about a high-protein diet? People who exercise need protein to build muscle and other lean tissue structures and, to some extent, for fuel.

Protein for Building Muscle Tissue

In the hours of rest that follow physical activity, muscles speed up their rate of protein synthesis—they build the proteins they need to perform the activity. Additionally, whenever the body rebuilds a part of itself, it must tear down the old structures to make way for the new ones. Exercise, with just a slight overload, calls into action both the protein-dismantling and protein-synthesizing equipment of each muscle cell.

Dietary protein provides the needed amino acids for synthesis of new muscle proteins. The true director of synthesis of muscle protein, however, is physical activity itself. Exercise sends the signal to the muscle cells' genetic material to begin producing proteins needed to perform the work at hand.[14]

The genetic protein-making equipment inside the nuclei of muscle cells seems to "know" when proteins are needed. Furthermore, it knows *which* proteins are needed to support each type of physical activity. The key communicator seems to be the exercise itself—muscle contractions initiate signals that inform the muscles' genetic material of the intensity and pattern of muscular contractions. The genetic material synthesizes muscle proteins accordingly. Thus, the genes of muscle cells respond specifically to the type of exercise performed.[15] For example, a weight lifter's workout sends the information that muscle fibers need added bulk for strength and more enzymes for making glycogen and for breaking down glucose anaerobically. A jogger's workout stimulates production of proteins involved in the aerobic oxidation of fat and glucose. (Joggers can usually remember a time when their activity "suddenly" became easier to perform.) Muscle cells are exquisitely responsive to the need for proteins, and they build them conservatively.

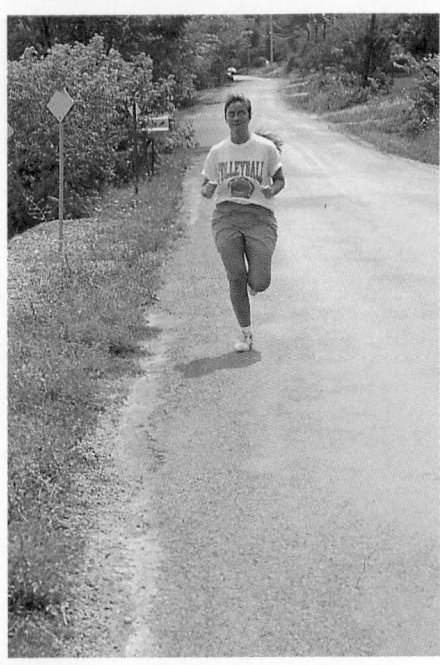

Exercise itself controls the building of muscle protein.

Finally, after muscle cells have made all the decisions about when to build proteins and which proteins are needed, protein nutrition comes into play. On the mandate from exercise, the muscle cells draw on the available amino acids to build the needed structures.

During active muscle-building phases of training, a weight lifter might add to existing muscle mass between ¼ ounce and 1 ounce (between 7 and 28 grams) of protein each day.[16] This happens only during periods of *building* muscle, and not during maintenance. Muscle cells that lack needed amino acids cannot build additional muscle proteins.

KEY POINT Exercise stimulates muscle cell protein break down and synthesis, resulting in muscle adaptation to exercise.

Protein Used for Fuel

Not only do athletes retain more protein; they also use a little more protein as fuel.[17] Studies of nitrogen balance show that an exercising body speeds up its use of amino acids for energy, just as it speeds up the use of glucose and fatty acids. Still, protein is not a major source of energy. It is estimated to contribute an average of 10 percent of the total fuel used, both during exercise and during rest. Endurance athletes use up enormous amounts of all energy fuels during performance, so they break down more protein. Moderate exercisers use less. However, all who eat enough total calories of a balanced, high-carbohydrate diet also consume enough protein.

The factors that regulate how much protein is used during activity seem to be the same three that regulate the use of glucose and fat. One factor is diet. Athletes who consume diets rich in carbohydrate use less protein than those who eat protein-rich or fat-rich diets.[18] This could be related to the protein-sparing effect of carbohydrate first discussed in Chapter 6. Some amino acids can be converted into glucose. Others, the **branched-chain**

branched-chain amino acids amino acids that, unlike the others, can directly provide energy to muscle tissue: leucine, isoleucine, and valine.

Factors that affect protein use in exercise:

- Amount of *carbohydrate* in the diet.
- Intensity and duration of exercise.
- Degree of training.

amino acids, take the place of glucose in energy pathways. If the diet is low in carbohydrate, much more protein will be used for fuel in place of glucose.

A second factor, the intensity and duration of the exercise, also modifies protein use.[19] Casual exercisers, those who exercise moderately for less than an hour, seem to show no increased need for protein. Athletes who train intensely for many hours during each session demand more protein to support their activities. In any case, those wishing to develop muscles for activity should plan workouts carefully and avoid overwork. The effects of overwork on muscle protein are negative—overworked muscles sustain damage to protein-containing structures and suffer leakage of enzymes from ruptured muscle cells.[20]

A third factor also modifies use of protein—the degree of training. The better trained the athlete, the less protein used during exercise at a given intensity.

How much protein should an athlete consume? A joint position paper from the American Dietetic Association (ADA) and the Canadian Dietetic Association (CDA) recommends: 1 to 1.5 grams protein per kilogram of body weight each day, an amount somewhat higher than the 0.8 g/kg/day recommended for sedentary people.[21] Other experts disagree with the ADA and recommend higher protein intakes. For example, one group of researchers found that 2 grams of protein per kilogram per day effectively maintained positive nitrogen balance during early training and prevented the drop in blood hemoglobin concentrations observed at lower protein intakes.[22] Another authority suggests different protein intakes for different athletes.[23] Table 10-1 lists some recommendations and translates them into daily intakes for an athlete who weighs 70 kilograms (154 pounds).

After considering these recommendations, an athlete might still wonder what level is best and how the recommendations translate into diet. Before drawing conclusions, read the Food Feature, where questions about choosing a performance diet are answered. Meanwhile, relax. Most athletes' protein intakes are already within the highest ranges recommended by any knowledgeable source.[24] Those with questions concerning their own protein intakes should keep diet records so that they can compare their actual intakes with recommendations. Chances are excellent that the diet already contains more than enough protein.

Table 10-1
Total Daily Protein Needs of a 70-Kilogram Athlete

Authority	Recommendation (g/kg/day)	Protein/ Day (g)
Food and Nutrition Board (RDA)	0.8	56
ADA/CDA	1.0–1.5	70–105
Lemon, P. W. R. (endurance athletes)	1.2–1.4	70–84
Lemon, P. W. R. (strength-speed athletes)	1.2–1.7	91–112
Yoshimura (early training)	2.0	140

Sources: Position of the American Dietetic Association and the Canadian Dietetic Association: Nutrition for physical fitness and athletic performance for adults, *Journal of the American Dietetic Association* 93 (1993): 691–695; P. W. R. Lemon, Effect of exercise protein requirements in C. Williams and J. T. Devlin, *Foods, Nutrition and Sports Performance: An International Scientific Consensus* (London: E & FN Spon, 1992), pp. 65–86; P. W. R. Lemon, Protein and exercise: Update 1987, *Medicine and Science in Sports and Exercise* 19 (1987): S179–S188; H. Yoshimura and coauthors, Anemia during hard physical training (sports anemia) and its causal mechanism with special reference to protein nutrition, *World Review of Nutrition and Dietetics* 35 (1980): 1–86.

KEY POINT Athletes use some protein both for building muscle tissue and for energy, but they need not strive to consume more protein than is present in the average U.S. diet.

◆ Vitamins and Minerals—Keys to Performance

Vitamin C is needed for the formation of collagen, a protein that forms the linings of the joints and other connective tissues. Folate supports the building of red blood cells that carry oxygen to the working muscles. Calcium and magnesium help make muscles contract, and so on. Do active people need extra nutrients to support their work? Do they need supplements?

Vitamins and Performance

An estimated 84 percent of world-class athletes take nutrient supplements. Many other athletes and even casual exercisers also take supplements in the belief that doing so will support their efforts in activity. Science, however, indicates otherwise.[25]

Thiamin Failure to obtain enough of any of four vitamins, thiamin, riboflavin, vitamin B_6, and vitamin C, has been shown to reduce aerobic power and cause blood lactic acid to accumulate during exercise.[26] Scientists have also studied the effects of thiamin supplements in athletes and have concluded that extra thiamin does not benefit performance. An adequate diet supplies all the thiamin a person needs, even an athlete doing heavy work. Almost any kind of nutrient-dense food supplies thiamin. Athletes, with their greater energy needs, eat more food, so most athletes' diets are adequate in thiamin.

The summary tables listing functions of vitamins and minerals begin on pages 249 and 298.

This does not mean that thiamin or any other vitamin is not important. The words *adequate diet* are weighty in this regard. To meet athletes' nutrient needs means that the athletes' extra energy must come from nutrient-dense foods, not fats, sweets, or highly refined foods. Anyone who consumes a "junk" diet of relatively empty-calorie foods risks becoming thiamin deficient.

Riboflavin Riboflavin, another B vitamin, also plays a role in energy release. To try to answer the question of whether extra riboflavin assists athletic performance, researchers studied groups of sedentary middle-aged women who began an exercise regimen.[27] One group of women consumed a diet containing the RDA of riboflavin while the other group's diet contained almost twice the RDA. Blood tests to evaluate riboflavin activity seemed to indicate a deficiency in the group that consumed the RDA amount. Even so, the aerobic capacity of both groups increased similarly; extra riboflavin provided no competitive advantage. To fully answer questions about riboflavin requirements during exercise will require more research.

The food sources of nutrients are shown in the vitamin and mineral snapshots of Chapters 7 and 8.

Niacin Excess niacin may affect performance adversely: it suppresses the release of fatty acids and thus forces muscles to use extra glycogen during exercise. This may shorten the time to glycogen depletion and may make the work seem more difficult to the exerciser. More niacin than the RDA could hinder performance.

Vitamin B_6 Vitamin B_6 plays key roles in the release of energy from nutrients, in the liberation of glucose from glycogen, and in the formation of hemoglobin. Thus sellers of supplements claim that vitamin B_6 in amounts greater than the RDA promotes extra aerobic endurance. However, research shows that supplemental vitamin B_6 does not improve aerobic performance. To ensure that the diet is adequate in vitamin B_6, a person need only include some green leafy vegetables, meats, fish, legumes, fruits, and whole grains. Megadoses of vitamin B_6 can do no more.

Nutrients necessary to ward off anemias include vitamins A, B_6, B_{12}, and folate and the minerals zinc, copper, and magnesium along with protein—in short, the perfect mix of nutrients that occurs naturally in whole, nutrient-dense foods.

Vitamin B_{12} The belief that vitamin B_{12} supplementation will enhance performance stems from its role in the production of red blood cells. Anemias of all kinds reduce the number and impair the function of circulating red blood cells, and rob the blood of its oxygen-carrying capacity. Vitamin B_{12} deficiency causes anemia, but so do iron and folate deficiencies (and others, see margin). Chances are, a diet low enough in vitamin B_{12} to bring on anemia will be low in other nutrients as well. A person with so poor a diet does not need to take pills; more importantly, the person needs to eat right. For a well-nourished athlete, any perceived benefits from vitamin B_{12} supplements or shots taken before competition are based on psychology, not physiology.

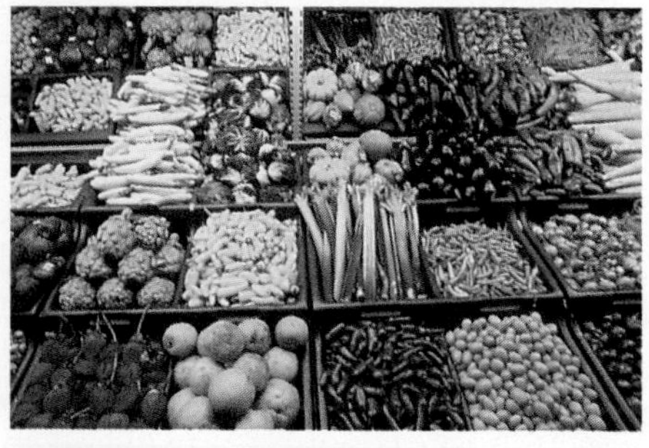

Vitamins in abundance.

Vitamin C Years ago evidence that exercise caused increased excretion of vitamin C led some to think that two to three times the RDA of vitamin C might best serve the needs of the athlete. Since that time the great bulk of work designed to explore this theory has disproved it.[28] In one study, even severe restriction of vitamin C intakes caused no measurable changes in athlete's health or aerobic power.[29]* Most experiments show that athletes perform no better when taking vitamin C supplements than when they receive the RDA from food. Even so, athletes are often told by "advisors" in health food stores to ingest huge quantities of vitamin C, measured in multiples of a gram.

For people who eat a reasonable diet, it is almost impossible *not* to receive two to three times the RDA for vitamin C. A person who drinks a small glass of orange juice and eats a baked potato and a serving of broccoli in a day receives about five times the RDA for vitamin C from these foods alone. When shown the full array of values for vitamins and minerals, including vitamin C, in foods such as these, people have been known to throw away their pills and to learn to cook broccoli.

Vitamins A, D, and E Of the fat-soluble vitamins, supplemental A and D have been shown not to benefit athletic performance, and they are toxic in excess. Vitamin E, however, is important, especially to endurance athletes.

*Aerobic power was measured by onset of blood lactate accumulation (OBLA).

During an endurance event, the cells use great quantities of oxygen to process fuels, and vitamin E vigorously defends the cell membranes against oxidative damage.[30] Vitamin E may also protect a part of the metabolic equipment involved in aerobic metabolism.* However, an athlete's muscles have no more vitamin E in them than do the muscles of a sedentary person.[31]

Another kind of muscle cell damage was mentioned earlier—the cell damage that occurs when muscles overwork. This damage seems unrelated to the oxidative damage that vitamin E prevents, and vitamin E does not seem effective in preventing it.[32]

Researchers have also investigated the possibility that vitamin E may enhance athletic performance. Most such studies were performed on swimmers, and most conclude that vitamin E supplements are useless for enhancing performance beyond the level attained through training alone.

So far, then, research does not support the idea that athletes need supplements of vitamins to perform their best. Athletes need only to meet the RDA for nutrients from food—and they certainly can do so. In fact, some young male Finnish athletes who met their energy needs with nutritious foods were seen to meet and exceed by far the RDA for three vitamins and four minerals.[33] Those who are trying to comply with weight requirements may consume so little food that they fail to obtain all the nutrients they need. For them, a single daily multivitamin and mineral tablet that provides no more than the RDA of nutrients may be beneficial.

Controversy 7 can guide an athlete in selecting an appropriate supplement.

Stringent weight requirements pose a risk of developing eating disorders, as this chapter's Controversy shows.

KEY POINT Vitamins are essential for releasing the energy trapped in energy-yielding nutrients and for other functions that support exercise. Active people can probably meet their vitamin needs with ordinary diets of nutrient-dense foods sufficient to meet their energy needs.

Exercise and Bone Loss

Osteoporosis, the condition of reduced bone mass, increases susceptibility to bone damage, including **stress fractures.** Controversy 8 pointed out that moderate exercise and adequate calcium intakes protect against bone loss. Extremes in exercise, however, may be detrimental to bone health, at least in some young women and especially in adolescent girls. A side effect of overzealous endurance training in women is **athletic amenorrhea,** characterized by low estrogen concentrations, infertility, and increased calcium losses.

Some evidence implicates low body-fat content along with amenorrhea in loss of bone calcium. A study of ballet dancers found that those with extremely low body-fat content and who suffered from amenorrhea incurred more bone injuries than did those with a more normal percentage of body fat.[34] Some athletes and dancers in their twenties have been seen to have bone densities as low as those of women in their seventies. No amount of calcium can protect against bone loss in this condition, but athletes who

stress fracture bone damage or breaks caused by the stress of exercise on bone surfaces.

athletic amenorrhea cessation of menstruation associated with low body fat and strenuous athletic training.

*The molecule believed to be protected is coenzyme Q.

suffer these disturbances and who take in too little calcium suffer the greatest bone losses. Overtraining threatens women with irregular menstruation, bone loss, and eating disorders. Controversy 10 comes back to the topic of eating disorders in athletes.

KEY POINT Women who have too little body fatness and amenorrhea are especially susceptible to stress fractures and osteoporosis. For others, moderate exercise strengthens the bones.

Iron and Performance

Endurance athletes, and especially women athletes, are prone to iron deficiency. Iron status might be affected by exercise in any of several ways. One possibility is that iron lost in sweat creates the deficiency, although the sweat of trained athletes contains less iron than the sweat of others (an adaptation to conditioning). Still, athletes sweat more copiously. Another possible route to iron loss is red blood cell destruction; blood cells are squashed when body tissues (such as the soles of the feet) make high-impact contact with an unyielding surface (such as the ground). Perhaps more significant than losses is reduced iron absorption in some athletes and increased iron demands by muscles to make the iron-containing molecules of aerobic metabolism. In addition, exercise may cause small blood losses through the digestive tract, at least in some athletes.

Studies often find women athletes to have low iron intakes. Of adolescent girl gymnasts, a study found 95 percent to have iron intakes below the RDA.[35] Habitually low intakes of iron-rich foods as well as increased losses may contribute to iron deficiency in young women athletes.[36] Vegetarian women athletes may be especially at risk for iron insufficiency.[37]

Iron deficiency impairs performance because iron is crucial to the body's handling of oxygen. One consequence of iron-deficiency anemia is impaired oxygen transport. This reduces aerobic work capacity, so that the person tires easily. Whether marginal deficiency without clinical signs of anemia impairs physical performance is a point of debate among researchers.[38]

Early in training, athletes may develop low blood hemoglobin for a while. This condition, sometimes called "sports anemia," probably reflects a normal adaptation to exercise. Aerobic exercise training promotes increases in the fluid of the blood; with more fluid, red blood cell count in a unit of blood drops. True iron-deficiency anemia requires treatment with prescribed iron supplements, but this temporary reduced red blood cell count goes away by itself with continued training.

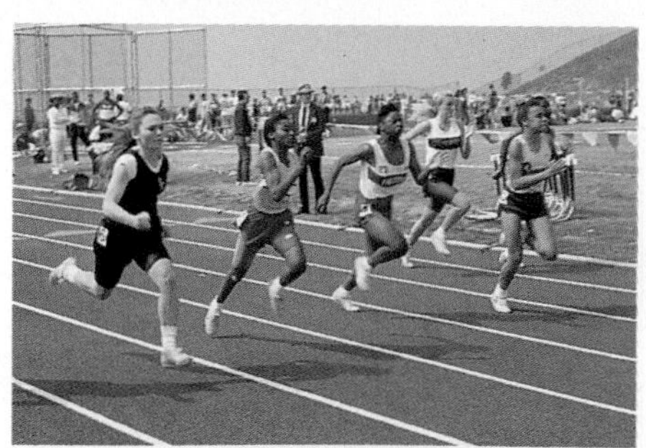

Woman athletes may be at special risk of iron deficiency.

The best strategy concerning iron may be to try to determine individual needs. Many menstruating women probably border on iron deficiency even without the additional iron losses incurred through exercise.[39] Teens of both sexes, because they are growing, have high iron needs, too. Especially for women and teens, then, prescribed supplements may be needed to correct a deficiency of iron as determined by medical testing. (Medical testing is needed to eliminate nondietary causes of anemia, such as internal bleeding or cancer.)

KEY POINT Iron-deficiency anemia impairs physical performance because iron is the blood's oxygen handler. Sports anemia is probably a harmless temporary stage of adaptation to exercise.

Other Minerals

Other minerals are also affected by training. Three trace minerals—chromium, zinc, and copper—are of current scientific interest. Each of these minerals has specific roles in physical activity and all are excreted in larger amounts when people exercise than when they are sedentary.[40] So far it is too early to say whether their excretion is meaningful in terms of active people's nutrition.

Electrolytes, the minerals sodium, potassium, chloride, and magnesium, are lost from the body in sweat. Beginners lose electrolytes to a much greater extent than do trained athletes. As the body adapts to exercise, it becomes better at conserving most electrolytes.

An exception is magnesium. Its losses in sweat are about the same for trained and untrained individuals. One study found magnesium levels in the blood serum to be lower in exercising people than in others; the effect remained even three months after the exercise program began.[41] This could mean that a magnesium deficiency was coming on, or it could mean that the magnesium had moved out of the blood and into the tissues in response to training. In any case, anyone interested in building muscle should plan to get enough magnesium in the diet, because a deficiency has been shown to cut in half the muscle gains associated with a given amount of training.[42] Magnesium is abundant in leafy vegetables, legumes, and whole-wheat products. Other foods offer small but significant amounts. Convenience and snack foods lack magnesium.

As for potassium, it usually remains safely inside the cells where it does its work. However, in prolonged dehydration from profuse sweating, it may migrate outside of cells, and it may be lost by excretion in the urine. Even so, it is easily replaced with just a few servings of fresh fruits and vegetables. Avoid potassium supplements unless prescribed by a physician because while they improve some conditions, they worsen others. Most times athletes need not make a special effort to replenish lost electrolytes; a regular diet supplies all the electrolytes they need.

Athletes constitute a huge and favorable market for the supplement industry and they stand out as one of the groups most often victimized by frauds. The following Consumer Caution touches on a few of the most common schemes aimed at athletes and warns of the dangers faced by athletes who use steroid and other drugs.

KEY POINT Adequate mineral intake is critical to exercise.

Steroids and "Ergogenic" Aids

CONSUMER CAUTION Athletes can be sitting ducks for an endless list of scams aimed at them: protein supplements, vitamin or mineral supplements, steroid replacers, "muscle-building" powders, electrolyte pills, and many other so-called **ergogenic** aids. Some athletes take dangerous, illegal drugs to try to gain a competitive edge. Others use sodium bicarbonate, caffeine, or other products (see Table 10-2). The

(continued on next page)

ergogenic the term implies "energy giving," but, in fact, no products impart such a quality (*ergo* means "work"; *genic* means "gives rise to").

Steroids and "Ergogenic" Aids *continued*

CONSUMER CAUTION term *ergogenic* implies that such products have special work-enhancing powers, but no food or supplement is really ergogenic.

An athlete who takes a nutrient supplement to improve performance cannot be sure that it will deliver on its verbal promises. Supplements are not required to be tested for safety or effectiveness because they are a special case.

FDA does not regulate supplements as it regulates drugs (see Controversy 7). FDA could question claims made by a drug manufacturer that their product "rams the body into turbo charge" or that it "deposits slabs of muscle bulk," yet such claims for supplements shout from the pages of magazines that appeal to athletes. If the products were drugs, FDA would require clinical evidence of those turbocharged bodies and muscle slabs and would also require proof of safety.

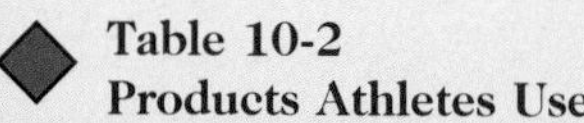

Table 10-2
Products Athletes Use

- **bee pollen** a product consisting of bee saliva, plant nectar, and pollen that confers no benefit on athletes and may cause an allergic reaction in individuals sensitive to it.
- **blood doping** the process of injecting red blood cells to enhance the blood's oxygen-carrying ability. Risks include dangerous blood clotting, especially in athletes who become dehydrated, infections from nonsterile equipment, transfusion reactions, and dangers of improperly transferred blood. Blood doping is banned in Olympic competitions.
- **branched-chain amino acids** see text, page 370.
- **caffeine** a stimulant that in small amounts may produce alertness and reduced reaction time in some people, but that also creates fluid losses. Overdoses cause headaches, trembling, an abnormally fast heart rate, and other undesirable effects. More about caffeine appears later in this chapter and in Controversy 12.
- **calcium pangamate** a compound once thought to enhance aerobic metabolism, now known to have no such effect.
- **cell salts** a mineral preparation supposedly prepared from living cells.
- **coenzyme Q10** a lipid found in cells (mitochondria) shown to improve exercise performance in heart-disease patients, but not effective in improving performance of healthy athletes.
- **DNA** and **RNA** (**deoxyribonucleic acid** and **ribonucleic acid**) the genetic materials of cells necessary in protein synthesis, falsely promoted as ergogenic aids.
- **glycine** a nonessential amino acid, promoted as an ergogenic aid because it is a precursor of the high-energy compound phosphocreatine. Other amino acids commonly packaged for athletes and that are equally useless include ornithine, arginine, lysine, and the branched-chain amino acids.
- **growth hormone releasers** herbs or pills falsely promoted for enhancing athletic performance.
- **inosine** an organic chemical which is falsely said to "activate cells, produce energy, and facilitate exercise," but which has been shown actually to reduce the endurance of runners.
- **octacosanol** an alcohol extracted from wheat germ, often falsely promoted to enhance athletic performance.
- **phosphate salt** a salt that has been demonstrated to raise the concentration of a metabolically important compound (diphosphoglycerate) in red blood cells and enhance the cells' potential to deliver oxygen to muscle cells; the salts may cause calcium losses from the bones if taken in excess.
- **plant sterols** lipid extracts of plants, called *ferulic acid, oryzanol, phytosterols,* or *"adaptogens,"* marketed with false claims that they contain hormones or enhance hormonal activity.
- **royal jelly** a substance produced by worker bees and fed to the queen bee, often falsely promoted as enhancing athletic performance.
- **sodium bicarbonate** baking soda; an alkaline salt believed to neutralize blood lactic acid and thereby reduce pain and enhance possible workload. Some studies show that sodium bicarbonate in recommended doses can enhance performance of high-intensity exercise (in 1 to 5 minute exercise sessions) but its effects on endurance exercise is unknown; "soda loading" may cause intestinal bloating and diarrhea.

Steroids and "Ergogenic" Aids *continued*

Someone considering using illegally obtained drugs such as steroids should be aware that illegal drugs can contain anything, even poisons, because no one tests them. Among the most dangerous products sold to athletes are steroid drugs, other hormones, amphetamines, cocaine, muscle relaxants, tranquilizers, barbiturates, diuretics, and even veterinary drugs.

Of the hormones, anabolic steroids are made naturally by the testes and adrenal cortex in men and by the adrenal cortex in women. The steroid drugs some athletes take are synthetic varieties that combine the masculinizing effects of male hormones and growth stimulation of the adrenal steroids. In the body, the steroids produce accelerated muscle bulking in response to exercise in both men and women. Injections of these hormones produce muscle size and strength far beyond that attainable by training alone, but at the price of great risks to health as Figure 10-5 on the next page demonstrates.

growth hormone a hormone produced by the brain's pituitary gland that regulates normal growth and development. Also called *somatotropin*.

While not a steroid, **growth hormone** can induce huge body size and it is less readily detected than steroids in drug tests. A syndrome resulting from its abuse includes a widened jawline, a widened nose, a protruding brow, buck teeth, weakened heart walls, and an increased likelihood of death before the age of 50 years, a condition known as acromegaly. Athletes who have faced the consequences of hormone abuse, even some for whom the drugs made careers in sports possible, have come forward to warn young athletes away from growth hormones. They say that the price of using drugs is too dear, even for the rewards of success in sports.

Growth hormone "stimulators," such as the amino acids ornithine and arginine, are useless in the form sold to athletes. In laboratory studies, huge doses of these amino acids do stimulate growth hormone release, but the effective dose would be dangerous to an athlete. There are safe ways to maximize growth hormone production, however. One is rest. Growth hormone is released during sleep, so getting enough rest is important. Exercise itself also triggers the release of growth hormone during the period of sleep that follows, so adequate training is also effective. These steps, unlike single amino acid supplements, are safe and effective in evoking the body's release of growth hormone.

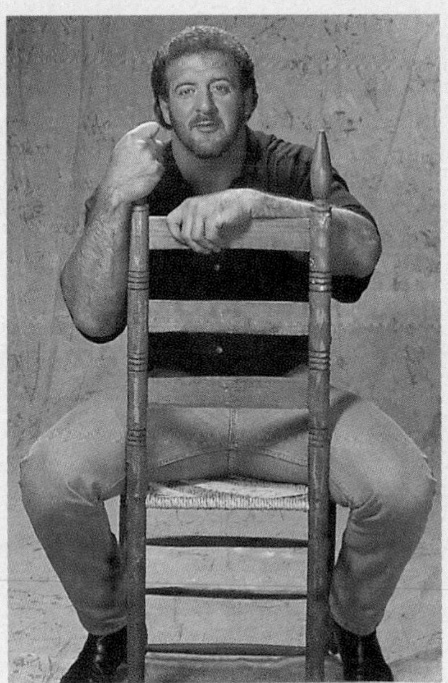

"I lied to a lot of people for a lot of years when I said I didn't use steroids. . . . If you're on steroids or human growth hormone, stop. I should have." Lyle Alzado, former NFL football player who died of cancer in May of 1992; as quoted by S. Smith, I'm sick and I'm scared, *Sports Illustrated*, 8 July 1991, pp. 21–25.

Extracted herb and insect sterols are hawked as legal substitutes for steroid drugs.[43] Sellers falsely claim that these substances contain hormones or that they enhance the body's natural ability to make anabolic hormones. In some cases, the substances may actually contain some amount of a plant or insect sterol but even so, the body cannot convert herbal or insect compounds to human anabolic steroids.[44] None of these products has any proven anabolic activity, nor can they strengthen muscles, but they may contain natural toxins. Don't make the mistake of equating "natural" with "harmless."

It bears repeating that amino acid supplements can be dangerous (see the Consumer Caution of Chapter 6). They are never needed by

Steroids and "Ergogenic" Aids *continued*

CONSUMER CAUTION healthy athletes. Advertisers point to research that identifies the branched-chain amino acids as a source of fuel for the exercising body. What the advertisers leave out is that compared with glucose and fatty acids, branched-chain amino acids provide only minuscule amounts of fuel and that when amino acids are needed, the muscles have plenty on hand. The person concerned about branched-chain amino acids should know that a diet too low in carbohydrate or calories seems to activate or assist an enzyme that breaks down branched-chain amino acids for energy.[45] In the presence of sufficient energy and adequate carbohydrate fuel, the enzyme shuts down its activity, and limits the amount of branched-chain amino acid breakdown, conserving the body's protein. The athlete who wants the

Figure 10-5

PHYSICAL RISKS OF TAKING EXCESS STEROID HORMONE DRUGS

Sources: K. L. Ropp, No-win situation for athletes, *FDA Consumer*, December 1992, pp. 8–12; National Academy of Sports Medicine policy statement and position paper; Anabolic androgenic steroids, growth hormones, stimulants, ergogenics, and drug use in sports, in B. Goldman and R. Klatz, *Death in the Locker Room II: Drugs and Sports* (Chicago: Elite Sports Medicine Publications, 1992), pp. 328–373.

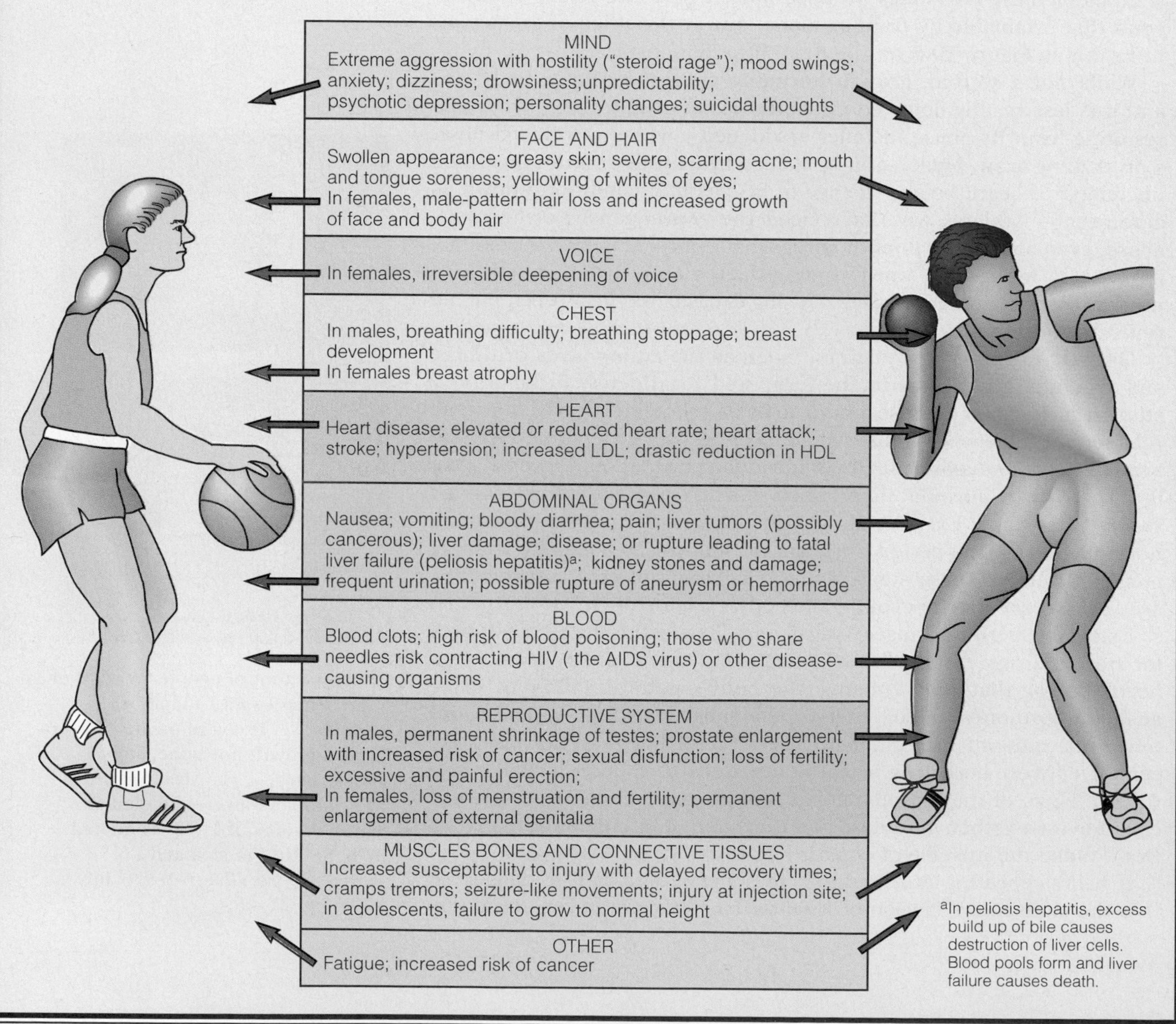
MIND
Extreme aggression with hostility ("steroid rage"); mood swings; anxiety; dizziness; drowsiness;unpredictability; psychotic depression; personality changes; suicidal thoughts
FACE AND HAIR
Swollen appearance; greasy skin; severe, scarring acne; mouth and tongue soreness; yellowing of whites of eyes;
In females, male-pattern hair loss and increased growth of face and body hair
VOICE
In females, irreversible deepening of voice
CHEST
In males, breathing difficulty; breathing stoppage; breast development
In females breast atrophy
HEART
Heart disease; elevated or reduced heart rate; heart attack; stroke; hypertension; increased LDL; drastic reduction in HDL
ABDOMINAL ORGANS
Nausea; vomiting; bloody diarrhea; pain; liver tumors (possibly cancerous); liver damage; disease; or rupture leading to fatal liver failure (peliosis hepatitis)a; kidney stones and damage; frequent urination; possible rupture of aneurysm or hemorrhage
BLOOD
Blood clots; high risk of blood poisoning; those who share needles risk contracting HIV (the AIDS virus) or other disease-causing organisms
REPRODUCTIVE SYSTEM
In males, permanent shrinkage of testes; prostate enlargement with increased risk of cancer; sexual disfunction; loss of fertility; excessive and painful erection;
In females, loss of menstruation and fertility; permanent enlargement of external genitalia
MUSCLES BONES AND CONNECTIVE TISSUES
Increased susceptability to injury with delayed recovery times; cramps tremors; seizure-like movements; injury at injection site; in adolescents, failure to grow to normal height
OTHER
Fatigue; increased risk of cancer
aIn peliosis hepatitis, excess build up of bile causes destruction of liver cells. Blood pools form and liver failure causes death.

benefits conferred by amino acids needs no supplements, but only needs to make the diet adequate in carbohydrate and in total energy.

The overwhelming majority of potions touted for athletes are frauds. The placebo effect works strongly in athletes. When you hear reports of a performance boost from a new concoction, give it time. Chances are that the effect was simply the power of the mind over the body. Incidentally, don't discount that power, since it is formidable. You can use it by visualizing yourself as a winner in your sport. You don't have to rely on magic for an extra edge because you already have a real one—your mind.

More about amino acid supplements in the Consumer Caution of Chapter 6.

*If you have questions about a fitness product, book, or program, write to the American College of Sports Medicine at their address in Appendix E.

Fluids and Temperature Regulation in Exercise

The body's need for water far surpasses that for any other nutrient. Should the body lose too much water, as in dehydration, its life-supporting chemistry would become compromised. Exercisers can be prone to dehydration.

The body loses water primarily via sweat; second to that, breathing costs water, exhaled as vapor. In exercise, both routes can be significant, and dehydration is a real threat. The first symptom of dehydration is fatigue. A rapid water loss equal to 5 percent of body weight can reduce muscular work capacity by 20 to 30 percent. The athlete who arrives at an event even slightly dehydrated arrives with a disadvantage.

Temperature Regulation

Sweat is the body's coolant. Working muscles produce heat as a by-product of energy release. To rid itself of the excessive heat that builds up during exercise, the body routes its blood supply through the capillaries just under the skin. At the same time; the skin secretes sweat, and the water in sweat evaporates, cooling the skin and the underlying blood. Cooled blood then flows back to cool the body's core.

In humid, hot weather, sweat doesn't evaporate well because the surrounding air is already laden with water. Body heat builds up and triggers maximum sweating, the body's only defense against excess heat. Still, without sweat evaporation, little cooling takes place. In such conditions active people must take precautions to prevent thermal injuries—**heat exhaustion** or its more severe cousin **heat stroke.** Heat stroke is an especially dangerous accumulation of body heat with accompanying loss of body fluid. The only way to prevent heat stroke is to drink enough fluid before and during the activity, to rest in the shade when tired, and to wear light-weight clothing that encourages evaporation. (Hence the rubber or heavy suits sold with promises of weight loss during exercise are dangerous, because they promote profuse sweating, prevent sweat evaporation, and invite heat stroke.) If you experience any of the symptoms of heat exhaustion or heat stroke listed in the margin, stop your activity, sip fluids, seek shade, and ask for help. The condition can be fatal and demands medical attention.

Symptoms of heat exhaustion: weak, rapid pulse, low blood pressure, sweating, headache, dizziness, weakness, and somewhat elevated body temperature.

Symptoms of heat stroke: headache, nausea, dizziness, clumsiness, stumbling, sudden cessation of sweating (hot, dry skin), internal (rectal) temperature above 104° Fahrenheit, and confusion or loss of consciousness.

heat exhaustion a fluid-depleted state with slightly elevated body temperature (below 104° Fahrenheit) that, while not usually dangerous, requires intake of fluid and rest in a cool place to avoid heat stroke.

heat stroke an acute and dangerous reaction to heat buildup in the body.

hypothermia a below-normal body temperature.

In cold weather, **hypothermia,** or loss of body heat, can pose as serious a threat as heat stroke. During exercise in cold or wet, chilly weather, the body still sweats and needs fluids, but the fluids should be warm or at room temperature, not cold. Dress in layers so clothing may be adjusted as body temperature changes.

KEY POINT Evaporation of sweat cools the body. Heat exhaustion and heat stroke are common threats to exercisers in hot humid weather. Hypothermia threatens those who exercise in the cold.

Fluid Needs During Exercise

Athletes can lose 2 to 4 quarts of fluid in every hour of heavy exercise, and the digestive system can absorb only about a quart or so an hour.[46] Hence the athlete must hydrate before and rehydrate during and after exercise to replace it all. Even then, in hot weather the digestive tract may not be able to absorb enough water fast enough to keep up with an athlete's sweating losses, and some degree of dehydration becomes inevitable. Wise athletes preparing for competition drink extra fluids in the few days of training before the event. The extra fluid is not stored in the body, but drinking extra ensures maximum tissue hydration at the start of the event. Any coach or athlete who withholds fluids during practice for any reason takes a great risk.

Casual exercisers should be aware that exercise blunts the thirst mechanism. Exercisers who rely on thirst to govern fluid intake can easily become dehydrated. During exercise thirst becomes detectable only after fluid stores are depleted. Don't wait to feel thirsty before drinking. Table 10-3 presents one schedule of hydration for exercise. To find out how much water you need to replenish losses, weigh yourself before and after the activity. The difference is all water. Two cups of fluid weigh about a pound.

What is the best fluid for most exercising bodies? Surprisingly, the best drink is just plain cool water, at least for most people, for two reasons: (1) because it rapidly leaves the digestive tract to enter the tissues, and (2) because it cools the body from the inside out.[47] Many good-tasting drinks are marketed for active people. Manufacturers reason that if a drink tastes good, people will drink more, thereby ensuring adequate hydration. The drinks also can provide a psychological edge to people who equate the drinks with success in sports. Keep in mind that while you may hear much promotion of these drinks from their manufacturers, no company is likely to run ads about any possible advantages of water because they aren't selling water.

Table 10-3
Schedule of Hydration Before and During Exercise

When to Drink	Total Amount of Fluid (Consume in 1 c Servings)
2 hr before exercise	About 3 c
10 to 15 min before exercise	About 2 c
Every 15 to 30 min during exercise	4–8 oz (about 1 qt in 60 to 90 min)
After exercise	Replace each pound of body weight lost with 2 c fluid

What about drinks or candylike sport bars claiming to provide "complete" nutrition? These mixtures of carbohydrate, protein (usually amino acids), fat, some fiber, and certain vitamins and minerals usually taste good and provide additional food energy before a game or for those needing to gain weight. However, they fall short of providing "complete" nutrition, since they lack many of real food's nutrients and the nonnutrients that benefit health. These products provide no special advantage for active people except one—convenience. They are an easy way to obtain some extra energy, some fluid, and the carbohydrate needed in the hours before a competition. However, they are expensive. A milkshake of nonfat milk and ice milk blended with flavorings can do the same thing, and less expensively. Don't drop a raw egg in the blender, though, because raw eggs often carry bacteria that cause food poisoning.[48]

KEY POINT Exercisers lose fluids and must replace them to avoid dehydration. Thirst is an unreliable indicator of water loss.

Sports Drinks

Exercisers sweat. Sweat contains minerals. So do exercisers need special mineral-containing drinks to replace those lost in sweat? Most authorities agree that exercisers and athletes normally need not replace minerals lost in sweat until after the exercise when they resume eating normal food.

In strenuous world-class competitions lasting for many hot, humid days, heavy sweating coupled with consumption of large amounts of plain water has been reported to dangerously dilute the blood concentration of sodium. If an athlete works up a drenching sweat, exceeding 5 to 10 pounds a day (or 3 percent of body weight) for several consecutive days, electrolyte replacement is advised. Athletes who *compete* for longer than six to eight hours each day also should make an effort to replace sodium.[49]

Sports drinks supply glucose. A beverage that supplies glucose in some form can be useful during endurance activity lasting longer than 90 minutes or during prolonged competitive games that demand repeated intermittent exercise. This advantage must be sought carefully, however, because a solution of greater than 10-percent glucose can delay fluid emptying from the stomach, and this could slow down the delivery of water to the tissues. Furthermore, ingesting a carbohydrate beverage during exercise has been shown to alter the body's hormonal response to exercise, with unknown effects on the exerciser.[50] Still, the drinks have been well-studied and so widely used for so many years that discoveries of new serious adverse effects stemming from their use are unlikely.

No evidence supports the old idea that electrolytes taken during activity prevent muscle cramping, but the small amounts of sodium in sports drinks seem to accelerate water and glucose absorption from the digestive tract. Sodium also encourages fluid retention after exercise, an effect that may or may not be of value to exercisers who replenish their fluids after exercising.

Equally as effective as commercial sports drinks but much less expensive is a homemade mixture of one-third teaspoon of salt (sodium chloride) and 1 cup of sugar-sweetened fruit juice to provide potassium and carbohydrate added to each quart of water.* Avoid electrolyte or salt tablets; they in-

*Large quantities of pure fruit juice contain enough fructose to upset the stomach, but most people can tolerate small amounts. Should fruit juice pose a problem when used this way, substitute 1 cup flavored punch.

glucose polymers compounds that supply glucose, not as single molecules, but linked in chains somewhat as in starch. The less-sweet taste of glucose polymers may appeal to those who would avoid sweet-tasting drinks.

crease potassium losses, can irritate the stomach, cause vomiting, and always cause water to flow out of the tissues into the digestive tract at first.

Some drinks contain glucose in the form of starchlike **glucose polymers** in hopes of improving fluid availability, and these, in concentrations of up to 7½ percent, seem to empty from the stomach as well as water does. Drinks with glucose concentrations higher than 10 percent, even glucose polymer drinks, have been proved to inhibit fluid absorption and could pose a serious threat for those who use them during prolonged exercise in hot, humid conditions.[51]

Some drinks, such as iced tea, deliver caffeine along with fluid. Moderate doses of caffeine (2 milligrams per pound of body weight or about 2 cups of coffee) one hour prior to exercise seem to assist some people's athletic performance while having no effect on others.[52] Theoretically, caffeine may stimulate the body's release of fatty acids into the blood early in exercise, thus conserving glycogen. Better than caffeine for this purpose is a warm-up activity. Light exercise before a workout stimulates fat release and also warms the muscles and connective tissues, making them flexible and resistant to injury. Caffeine produces no such beneficial effects.

Controversy 12 provides a discussion of caffeine's effects and sources.

Caffeine also has adverse effects, including stomach upset, nervousness, sleeplessness, irritability, headaches, and diarrhea. It has been shown to constrict the arteries and raise some exercisers' blood pressure above normal.[53] Caffeine's constriction of the arteries makes the heart work harder to circulate blood to exercising muscles, an effect detrimental to sports performance. Exercise also slows the excretion of caffeine, prolonging its effects.[54] Its diuretic effect is potentially hazardous for exercisers in a hot environment. Caffeine-containing beverages should be used, if at all, in moderation and in addition to other fluids, not as a substitute for them. In college, national, and international athletic competitions, the use of caffeine is forbidden in amounts greater than about 800 milligrams, the equivalent of 5 or 6 cups of strong, brewed coffee drunk within an hour or two. Urine tests that detect excess caffeine disqualify Olympic athletes from international competition.

Beer facts:

- *Beer is not carbohydrate rich.* (Beer is *calorie* rich, but only ⅓ of its calories are from carbohydrates. The other ⅔ are from alcohol.)
- *Beer is mineral poor.* (Beer contains a few minerals, but to replace those lost in sweat, athletes need good sources such as fruit juices.)
- *Beer is vitamin poor.* (Beer contains tiny traces of some B vitamins, but it cannot compete with rich food sources.)
- *Beer causes fluid losses.* (Beer is a fluid, but alcohol is a diuretic and causes the body to lose more fluid in urine than is provided by the beer.)

Athletes, like others, sometimes drink beverages that contain alcohol, but these beverages are inappropriate as fluid replacements. Like caffeine, alcohol is a diuretic. Both substances promote the excretion of water; of vitamins such as thiamin, riboflavin, and folate; and of minerals such as calcium, magnesium, and potassium—exactly the wrong effects for fluid balance and nutrition. It is hard to overstate alcohol's detrimental effects on physical activity. Its diuretic effect impairs temperature regulation, making hypothermia or heat stroke much more likely. It alters perceptions and slows reaction time. It depletes strength and endurance, and deprives people of their judgment, thereby compromising their safety in sports. Many sports-related fatalities and injuries each year involve alcohol or other drugs.

KEY POINT Electrolytes are lost during exercise but most do not require replacement during activity. Glucose intake may be useful during endurance activities.

Read about alcohol's effects on the brain in Controversy 11.

FOOD FEATURE

Choosing a Performance Diet

No particular diet supports an athlete's performance perfectly; many different diets can be excellent for athletes. However, food choices must be made within the framework of rules for diet planning.

Nutrient Density First, athletes need a diet composed mostly of nutrient-dense foods, the kind that supply a maximum of vitamins and minerals for the energy they provide. When athletes eat mostly refined, processed foods that have suffered nutrient losses and that contain added sugar and fat, nutrition status suffers.[55] Even if foods are fortified or enriched, manufacturers cannot replace the whole range of nutrients and nonnutrients lost in refining. Consider, for example, that manufacturers mill out much of a food's original magnesium and chromium but do not replace them. This doesn't mean that athletes can *never* choose a white bread, bologna, and mayonnaise sandwich but only that later they should eat a large, fresh salad or big portions of vegetables and whole grains and drink a glass of milk to compensate. That way the nutrient-dense foods provide most of the needed nutrients, including magnesium and chromium; the bologna sandwich provided extra energy, mostly from fat.

Balance Athletes must eat for energy, and energy needs may be immense. They need full glycogen stores, and they need to strive to prevent heart disease and cancer by limiting fats. Simply stated, a diet that is high in carbohydrate (60 to 70 percent of total calories), low in fat (20 to 25 percent), and adequate in protein (10 to 15 percent) is best for all these purposes. Even if the athlete does not compete in glycogen-depleting events, such a diet will help control weight and provide adequate fiber while supplying abundant nutrients and energy.

With these principles in mind, compare the two 500-calorie sandwich meals in the margin. The trick to getting enough carbohydrate energy is easy, at least in theory: just reduce the amount of fat and meat in a meal and let carbohydrate-rich foods fill in for them.

Adding carbohydrate-rich foods is a sound and reasonable option for increasing energy intake, up to a point. The point at which it becomes unreasonable is when the person's energy needs outstrip the capacity to eat enough food to provide them. At that point the person can add more food energy to the diet by using refined sugars and fats or liquid meals. Still, these energy-rich additions must be superimposed on nutrient-rich choices; energy alone is not enough.

Protein In addition to carbohydrate, athletes need protein. What quantities of what kinds of foods supply enough protein to meet the needs of athletes? The exchange lists, of course, point out rich protein sources, and meats and milk head the list. To suggest that athletes eat more than the recommended servings of meat would be short-sighted advice for many reasons. Athletes must protect themselves from heart disease, and even lean meats contain fat, much of it saturated fat. Besides, the extra servings of carbohydrate-rich foods that an athlete needs to meet energy requirements also boost protein intakes.

Compare and decide which best meets your needs:

1 sandwich of:
- 2 slices bologna, 2 slices white bread, 2 tbsp mayonnaise
  - (525 calories, 9% protein, 23% carbohydrate, 69% fat)

OR

2 sandwiches of:
- 2 slices lean ham, 4 slices whole wheat bread, 2 tsp mayonnaise
  - (503 calories, 20% protein, 51% carbohydrate, 29% fat)

Small daily choices, when made consistently, make a difference to an athlete's nutrition.

(continued on the next page)

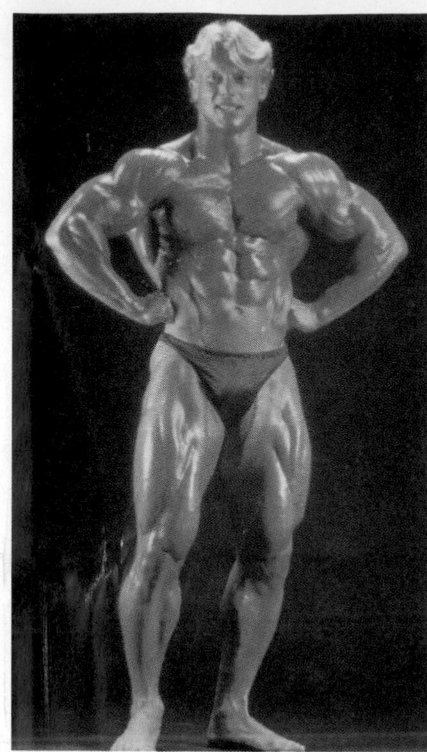

This is a body that vegetables built: Andreas Cahling, a vegetarian.

Earlier in this chapter Table 10-1 showed some possible protein intakes for a 70-kilogram athlete based on recommendations of various authorities. It is likely that an athlete weighing 70 kilograms who exercises vigorously on a daily basis could require 3,000 to 5,000 calories per day. To meet such an energy requirement, an athlete could select from a variety of nutrient-dense foods. Figure 10-6 provides one example; it itemizes foods that provide the extra nutrients an athlete needs beyond regular meal selections to attain a 3,000-calorie diet. These meals supply 124 grams of protein, an amount greater than all but the highest recommended level of 140 grams per day for such a person. For those with reasonable diets, protein is rarely a problem.

The meals in Figure 10-6 provide 61 percent of their calories from carbohydrate. Athletes who train exhaustively for endurance events may want to aim for somewhat higher carbohydrate levels—from 65 to 75 percent—and they can use the exchange system as demonstrated in Chapter 2 to alter the meals accordingly.[56] Notice that breakfast, while light in fat, is filling and hearty. Current thinking supports the idea that athletes benefit from such a morning start.[57] If you train early in the morning, try splitting breakfast into two parts. An hour or so before training eat just some toast, juice, and fruit. Later, after your workout, come back for the cereal and milk.

Planning an Athlete's Meals Table 10-4 shows some sample food intake patterns for athletes who wish to increase their energy and carbohydrate intakes. These plans are effective only if the user chooses foods to provide nutrients as well as energy—extra milk for calcium and riboflavin, many servings of fruit for folate and vitamin C, energy-rich vegetables such as sweet potatoes, peas, and legumes, modest portions of lean meat, and especially red meat for iron and other vitamins and minerals, and whole grains for B vitamins, magnesium, zinc, and chromium. In addition, these foods provide plenty of electrolytes.

Table 10-4
High-Carbohydrate Food Patterns for Athletes

	Number of Exchanges					
	ENERGY LEVEL (CALORIES)					
FOOD GROUP	1,500	2,000	2,500	3,000	3,500	4,000[a]
Milk	3	3	4	4	4	4
Fruit	5	6	7	9	10	12
Vegetable	3	3	3	5	6	7
Grain	7	11	16	18	20	24
Fat	2	3	5	6	8	10
Meat	5	5	5	5	6	6
Percent carbohydrate:	58%	58%	63%	64%	60%	62%

[a]A way to add more energy to the diet without adding much bulk is to include snacks of milkshakes or "complete meal" liquid supplements (see text).

Figure 10-6

AN ATHLETE'S MEALS

This figure shows how to modify regular meals to meet an athlete's needs.

Regular Meals

Modifications

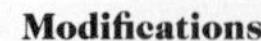

Athlete's Meals

The regular breakfast *plus:*

- 2 pieces whole-wheat toast
- 4 tsp jelly
- ½ c orange juice
- 2 tsp brown sugar on the oatmeal
- low-fat milk instead of nonfat

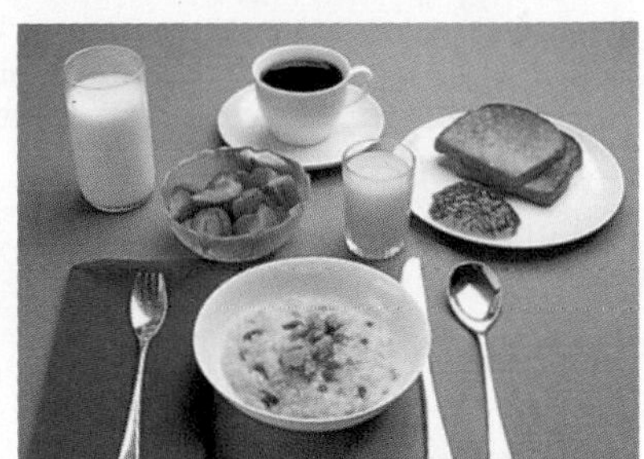

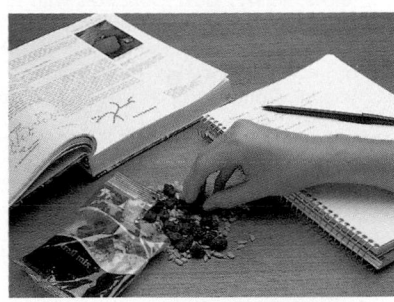

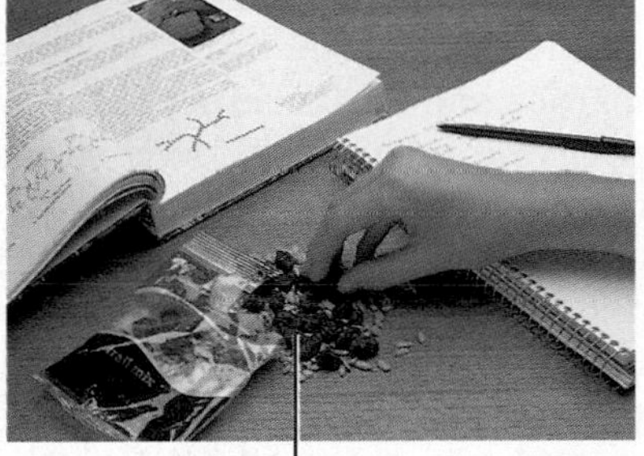

The regular morning snack

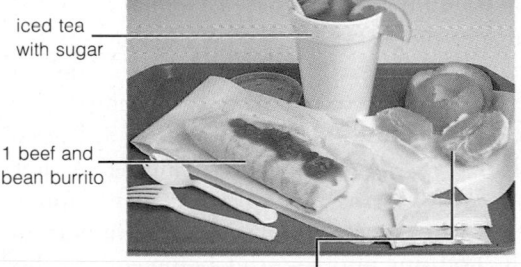

The regular lunch *plus:*

- 1 beef and bean burrito
- 1 banana

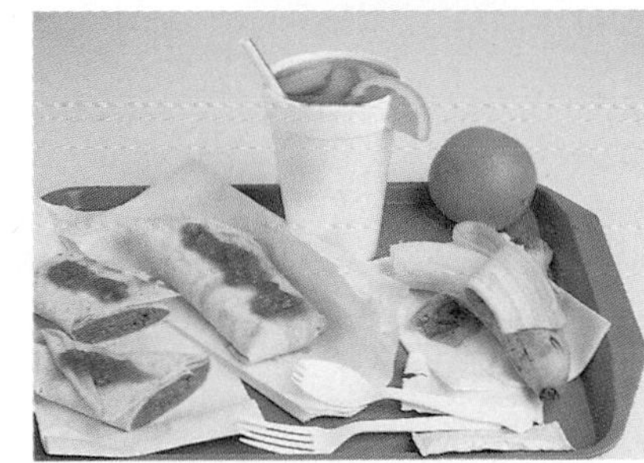

Plus an afternoon snack:

- 1 c low-fat milk
- 1 piece angel-food cake

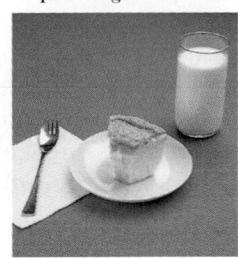

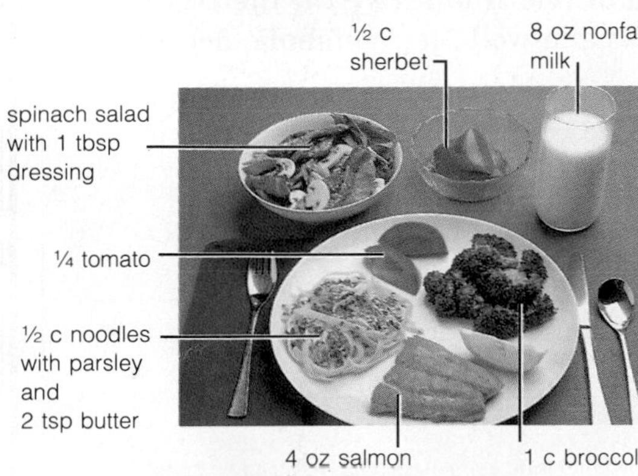

The regular dinner *plus:*

- 1 dinner roll
- 2 tsp butter
- ¼ c noodles
- ½ c sherbet
- low-fat milk instead of nonfat

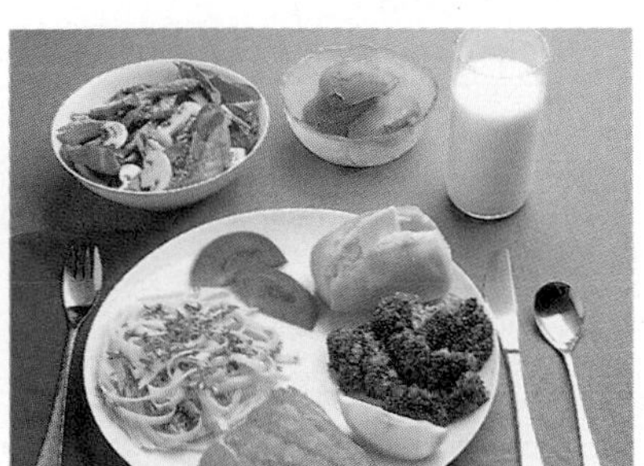

Total cal: 1,759
57% cal from carbohydrate
24% cal from fat
19% cal from protein

Total cal: 3,119
61% cal from carbohydrate
24% cal from fat
15% cal from protein

pregame meal a meal eaten three to four hours before athletic competition.

Good choices for pregame meals:
Apricot nectar, pineapple juice, grape juice, jello, sherbet, popsicles, jams, jellies, honey, toast, pancakes with syrup, baked white or sweet potatoes, pasta with steamed vegetables, lentils or other peas or beans, raisins, figs, dates, frozen yogurt, graham crackers, sponge cake, angel-food cake.

Not recommended:
Stuffing, muffins, biscuits, croissants, french fries, onion rings, potato chips, meats, cheese, pies, ice cream, eggnog, creams, nuts, butter, gravy, mayonnaise, salad dressing, frosted cakes.

A trick used by professional sports nutritionists to maximize athletes' intakes of energy and carbohydrates is to make sure that vegetable and fruit choices are as dense as possible in both nutrients and energy. Iceberg lettuce supplies few calories or nutrients in a whole cupful, but a half-cup portion of cooked sweet potatoes is a powerhouse of vitamins, minerals, and carbohydrate energy. Similarly, it takes a whole cup of cubed melon to equal the calories and carbohydrate in a half cup of canned fruit. Small choices like these, made consistently, can make a big difference to total energy and carbohydrate intakes. As a rule of thumb, endurance athletes should aim for an intake of 50 calories per kilogram (2.2 pounds) of body weight, on average.[58]

Athletes may eat particular foods or practice rituals before competition that convey psychological advantages. One eats steak the night before; another spoons up honey at the start of the event. As long as these foods or rituals remain harmless, they should be respected. Still, science has recommendations for the **pregame meal.** The foods should be carbohydrate rich and the meal light (300 to 1,000 calories). It should be easy to digest and should contain fluids. Some evidence suggests that foods such as lentils or beans which release glucose slowly might provide glucose to the athlete over time while blunting the insulin response.[59] Beans can cause gas, though, so don't wait until a game day to try them out, for the first time. The competitor should finish eating three to four hours before competition to allow time for the stomach to empty before exertion, because digestion interferes with muscle work. Some athletes prefer easy-to-digest commercial liquid meals for their pregame fare. Table 10-5 demonstrates that there is no point in paying high prices for fancy name-brand drinks. Homemade shakes are inexpensive, easy to prepare, and perform every bit as well as do commercial products.

The person who wants to excel physically will apply the most accurate nutrition knowledge along with dedication to rigorous training. A diet that provides ample fluid and consists of a variety of nutrient-dense foods in quantities to meet energy needs will not only enhance athletic performance but overall health as well. Training and genetics being equal, who would win a competition—the person who habitually consumes less than the amounts of nutrients needed or one who arrives at the event with a long history of full nutrient stores and well-met metabolic needs?

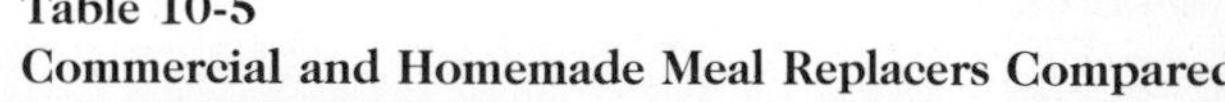

Table 10-5
Commercial and Homemade Meal Replacers Compared

	Energy (cal)	Protein (g)	Carbohydrate (g)	Fat (g)
12-ounce commercial liquid meal replacer[a] Cost: about $2 per serving	360	15 (17% of calories)	55 (61%)	9 (22%)
12-ounce homemade milkshake[b] Cost: about 50¢ per serving	330	15 (18% of calories)	53 (63%)	7 (19%)

[a]Average values for three commercial formulas.

[b]Home recipe: 8 oz nonfat milk, 4 oz ice milk, 3 heaping tsp malted milk powder. For even higher carbohydrate and calorie values, blend in ½ mashed banana or ½ c other fruit. For athletes with lactose intolerance, use lactose-reduced or soy milk and chocolate or other flavored syrup, with mashed banana or other fruit blended in.

Notes

1. U.S. Centers for Disease Control and Prevention and American College of Sports Medicine, Summary statement: Workshop on physical activity and public health, 29 July 1993.
2. S. N. Blair, as quoted by American College of Sports Medicine, Experts release new recommendation to fight America's epidemic of physical inactivity (news release), 29 July 1993.
3. S. N. Blair and coauthors, Physical fitness and all-cause mortality, *Journal of the American Medical Association* 262 (1989): 2395–2401.
4. K. B. Schechtman and coauthors, Measuring physical activity with a single question, *American Journal of Public Health* 81 (1991): 771–773.
5. P. Astrand, Something old and something new . . . very new, *Nutrition Today*, June 1968, pp. 9–11.
6. W. G. H. Abbott and coauthors, Short-term energy balance: Relationship with protein, carbohydrate, and fat balances, *American Journal of Physiology* 255 (1988): E332–E337.
7. W. D. McArdle, F. I. Katch, and V. L. Katch, *Exercise Physiology: Energy, Nutrition, and Human Performance* (Philadelphia: Lea & Febiger, 1991), pp. 133–141.
8. M. Hargreaves, Carbohydrate and exercise, in C. Williams and J. T. Devlin, eds., *Foods, Nutrition and Sports Performance: An International Scientific Consensus* (London: E & FN Spon, 1992), pp. 19–33.
9. L. J. Hoffer, Cori cycle contribution to plasma glucose appearance in man, *Journal of Parenteral and Enteral Nutrition* 14 (1990): 646–648.
10. D. C. Nieman, *Fitness and Sports Medicine* (Palo Alto: Bull, 1990) p. 231.
11. E. F. Coyle, Timing and method of increased carbohydrate intake to cope with heavy training, competition, and recovery, in Willaims and Devlin, 1992, pp. 35–63; J. M. Davis and coauthors, Carbohydrate-electrolyte drinks: Effects on endurance cycling in the heat, *American Journal of Clinical Nutrition* 48 (1988): 1023–1030.
12. Coyle, 1992.
13. J. L. Ivy and coauthors, Muscle glycogen synthesis after exercise: Effect of time of carbohydrate ingestion, *Journal of Applied Physiology* 64 (1988): 1480–1485.
14. P. Babij and F. W. Booth, Biochemistry of exercise: Advances in molecular biology relevant to adaptation of muscle to exercise, *Sports Medicine* 5 (1988): 137–143.
15. Babij and Booth, 1988.
16. J. R. Brotherhood, Nutrition and sports performance, *Sports Medicine* 1 (1984): 350–389.
17. P. W. R. Lemon, Effect of exercise protein requirements in Williams and Devlin, 1992, pp. 65–86.
18. P. W. R. Lemon, Protein and exercise: Update 1987, *Medicine and Science in Sports and Exercise* 19 (1987): S179–S188.
19. Lemon, 1987.
20. Lemon, 1992.
21. Position of the American Dietetic Association and the Canadian Dietetic Association: Nutrition for physical fitness and athletic performance in adults, *Journal of the American Dietetic Association* (1993): 691–695.
22. H. Yoshimura and coauthors, Anemia during hard physical training (sports anemia) and its causal mechanism with special reference to protein nutrition, *World Review of Nutrition and Dietetics* 35 (1980): 1–86.
23. Lemon, 1992.
24. J. R. Berring and S. N. Steen, *Sports Nutrition for the 90s: The Health Professional's Handbook* (Gaithersburg, Md.: Aspen, 1991), pp. 8–9.
25. A. Singh, F. M. Moses, and P. A. Deuster, Chronic multivitamin-mineral supplementation does not enhance physical performance, *Medicine and Science in Sports and Exercise* 24 (1992): 726–732.
26. W. van Dokkum, Vitamin restriction and functional performance in man (abstract), *American Journal of Clinical Nutrition* 49 (1989): 1138–1139.
27. L. R. Trebler Winters and coauthors, Riboflavin requirements and exercise adaptation in older women, *American Journal of Clinical Nutrition* 56 (1992): 526–532.
28. E. J. van der Beek, Vitamin supplementation and physical exercise performance, in Williams and Devlin, 1992, pp. 95–112.
29. E. J. van der Beeck and coauthors, Controlled vitamin C restriction and physical performance in volunteers, *Journal of the American College of Nutrition* 9 (1990): 332–339.
30. I. Gillam, S. Skinner, and R. Telford, Effect of antioxidant supplements on indices of muscle damage and regeneration (abstract), *Medicine and Science in Sports and Exercise* 24 (1992): S17; W. Sullivan, T. M. Manos, and B. Gutin, Plasma volume shifts in trained and untrained men cycling at similar relative intensities (abstract), *Medicine and Science in Sports and Exercise* 24 (1992): S16.
31. K. Gohil and coauthors, Effect of exercise training on tissue vitamin E and ubiquinone content, *Journal of Applied Physiology* 63 (1987): 1638–1641.
32. J. D. Robertson and coauthors, Influence of vitamin E supplementation on muscle damage following endurance exercise, *International Journal for Vitamin and Nutrition Research* 60 (1990): 171–172.
33. G. M. Fogelholm, Dietary and biochemical indices of nutritional status in male athletes, *Journal of the American College of Nutrition* 11 (1992): 181–191.
34. J. E. Benson and coauthors, Relationship between nutrient intake, body mass index, menstrual function, and ballet injury, *Journal of the American Dietetic Association* 89 (1989): 58–63.
35. D. Benardot, M. Schwartz, and D. Heller, Nutrient intake in young, highly competitive gymnasts, *Journal of the American Dietetic Association* 89 (1989): 401–403.
36. P. M. Clarkson, Minerals: Exercise performance and supplementation in athletes, in Williams and Devlin, 1992, pp. 113–146.
37. A. C. Snyder, L. L. Dvorak, and J. B. Roepke, Influence of dietary iron source on measures of iron status amoung female runners, *Medicine and Science in Sports and Exercise* 21 (1989): 7–10.
38. W. B. Strong and coauthors, The effect of iron therapy on the exercise capacity of nonanemic iron-deficient adolescent runners, *American Journal of Diseases of Children* 142 (1988): 165–169.
39. Food and Nutrition Board, *Recommended Dietary Allowances*, 10th ed. (Washington, D.C.: National Academy of Sciences, 1989), p. 200.
40. W. W. Campbell and R. A. Anderson, Effects of aerobic exercise and training on the trace minerals chromium, zinc, and copper, *Sports Medicine* 4 (1987): 9–18.
41. G. Stendig-Lindberg, Changes in serum magnesium concentration after strenuous exercise, *Journal of the American College of Nutrition* 6 (1987): 35–40.
42. L. R. Brilla and T. F. Haley, Effect of magnesium supplementation on strength training in humans, *Journal of the American College of Nutrition* 11 (1992): 326–329.

43. K. L. Ropp, No-win situation for athletes, *FDA Consumer*, December 1992, pp. 8–12.
44. V. E. Tyler, "Bodybuilding" herbs, *Nutrition Forum* (Philadelphia, Pa.: Stickley), March 1988, p. 23.
45. A. J. M. Wagenmakers, J. H. Coakley, and R. H. T. Edwards, Metabolism of branched-chain amino acids and ammonia during exercise: Clues from McArdle's disease, *International Journal of Sports Medicine* 11 (1990): S101–S113.
46. E. F. Coyle and S. J. Montain, Carbohydrate and fluid ingestion during exercise: Are there trade-offs? *Medicine and Science in Sports and Exercise* 24 (1992): 671–678.
47. American College of Sports Medicine, Position statement on prevention of heat injuries during distance running, *Medicine and Science in Sports and Exercise* 16 (1984): ix–xiv.
48. M. St. Louis and coauthors, The emergence of grade A eggs as a major source of *Salmonella enteritidis* infections, *Journal of the American Medical Association* 259 (1988): 2103–2107.
49. N. Clark, J. Tobin, and C. Ellis, Feeding the ultraendurance athlete: Practical tips and a case study, *Journal of the American Dietetic Association* 92 (1992): 1258–1262.
50. P. A. Deuster and coauthors, Hormonal responses to ingesting water or a carbohydrate beverage during a 2 h run, *Medicine and Science in Sports and Exercise* 24 (1992): 72–79.
51. R. J. Maughn, Fluid and electrolyte loss and replacement in exercise, in Williams and Devlin, 1992, pp. 147–178.
52. N. Clark, Revving up with sugar and caffeine, *Physician and Sports Medicine*, November 1991, pp. 15–16.
53. B. H. Sung and coauthors, Effects of caffeine on blood pressure response during exercise in normotensive healthy young men, *American Journal of Cardiology* 65 (1990): 909–913.
54. J. M. Duthel and coauthors, Caffeine and sport: Role of physical exercise upon elimination, *Medicine and Science in Sports and Exercise* 23 (1991): 980–985.
55. S. A. Tilgner and M. R. Schiller, Dietary intakes of female college athletes: The need for nutrition education, *Journal of the American Dietetic Association* 89 (1989): 967–969; D. R. Green and coauthors, An evaluation of dietary intakes of triathletes: Are RDA's being met? *Journal of the American Dietetic Association* 89 (1989): 1653–1654.
56. C. J. Hoffman and E. Coleman, An eating plan and update on recommended dietary practices for the endurance athlete, *Journal of the American Dietetic Association* 91 (1991): 325–330.
57. N. Clark, Breakfast *is* for champions, *Physician and Sports Medicine*, July 1992, pp. 29–30.
58. L. Houtkooper, as quoted in Sports nutrition expert shares secrets of success, *Journal of the American Dietetic Association* 92 (1992): 420.
59. D. E. Thomas, J. R. Brotherhood, and J. C. Brand, Carbohydrate feeding before exercise: Effect of glycemic index, *International Journal of Sports Medicine* 12 (1991): 180–186.

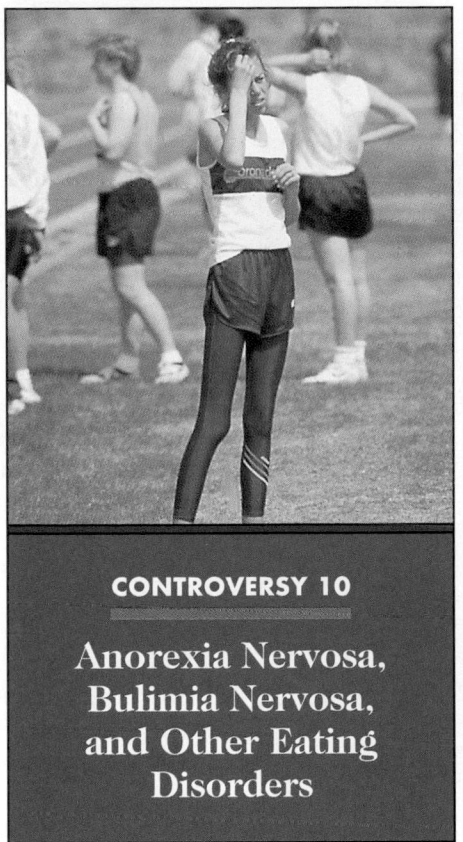

CONTROVERSY 10

Anorexia Nervosa, Bulimia Nervosa, and Other Eating Disorders

An estimated 2 million people in the United States, primarily girls and women, suffer from the **eating disorders, anorexia nervosa** and **bulimia nervosa.** Many more suffer from related conditions that do not meet the strict criteria for anorexia nervosa or bulimia nervosa but that still imperil sufferers' well-being. This category of eating disorders is known among psychologists as **unspecified eating disorders.**[1] Beyond these people, some evidence indicates that certain characteristics of disordered eating such as restrained eating, binge eating, purging, fear of fatness, and distortion of body image may be extraordinarily common among young middle-class girls.[2] Table C10-1 defines some eating disorder terms.

Athletes are among those who seem to be at special risk for eating disorders. To succeed in competition, athletes must often meet stringent weight requirements. Many athletes report that they engage in behaviors that are typical of people with eating disorders. Female competitors often report being terrified of becoming fat, being obsessed with food, and using laxatives in attempting to control weight. They judge themselves to have suffered anorexia at some time.[3] Ballet dancers, jockeys, wrestlers, distance runners, gymnasts, and others whose body weight and appearance are frequently judged in comparison with an "ideal," are especially prone to develop problems. Also, people with eating disorders often pursue athletics as a means of ridding the body of energy from food. As many as one third of ballet dancers and almost two thirds of female distance runners who also fail to menstruate report attitudes and behaviors consistent with eating disorders.[4]

Why do so many people in our society suffer from these disorders? One factor, excessive pressure to be thin, is at least partly to blame. When low body weight becomes an important goal, people begin to view normal healthy body weight as being too fat, and they take unhealthy actions to lose weight. Any severe restriction of energy intake may lead to binging, and set in motion a pattern of repeated weight losses and gains—weight cycling. The reason for this is unknown but the disorders are most likely multifactorial: sociocultural, neurochemical, and psychological. Treatment ideally addresses a multitude of needs and includes the person's entire family.[5]

ANOREXIA NERVOSA Julie is 18 years old. She is a superachiever in school and a fine ballet dancer. She watches her diet with great care, and she exercises and practices ballet daily, maintaining a heroic schedule of self-discipline. She is thin, but she is determined to lose more weight. She is 5 feet 6 inches tall and weighs 85 pounds. She has anorexia nervosa.

Julie is unaware that she is undernourished, and she sees no need to obtain treatment. She stopped menstruating (developed amenorrhea) several months ago and is moody and chronically depressed. She insists that she is too fat, although her eyes are sunk in deep hollows in her face. She has recently been told by her dance master that her performance is not up to her potential; she blames this on a slow-healing stress fracture.[6] Although she is close to physical exhaustion, she no longer sleeps easily. Her family is concerned, and although reluctant to push her, they have finally insisted that she see a psychiatrist. Julie's psychiatrist has diagnosed anorexia nervosa and has prescribed group therapy as a start, but warns that if Julie does not begin to gain weight soon, she will need to be hospitalized.

Most anorexia nervosa victims come from middle- or upper-class families. Men account for only about 1 in 20 cases in the general population, but eating disorders among male athletes and dancers are much more common, possibly equaling the incidence among female peers.[7] Male teenagers normally average about 15 percent of body weight as fat, but some high-school athletes strive to carry only 5 percent or so of their body weight as fat.

Certain attitudes among coaches, trainers, and especially parents contribute to eating disorders.[8] Such

Table C10-1
Eating Disorder Terms

- **anorexia nervosa** a disorder involving self-starvation to the extreme, seen (usually) in teenaged girls and young women (*anorexia* means "without appetite"; *nervos* means "of nervous origin").
- **binge eating disorder** a proposed new eating disorder whose criteria are still under study but may be similar to those of bulimia nervosa, excluding only purging or other compensatory behaviors.
- **bulimia** (byoo-LEEM-ee-uh) **nervosa** recurring binge eating combined with a morbid fear of becoming fat, sometimes followed by self-induced vomiting or purging.
- **cathartic** a strong laxative.
- **compulsive overeating** an eating disorder characterized by uncontrolled chronic episodes of overeating without other symptoms of eating disorders.
- **eating disorder** a disturbance in eating behavior that jeopardizes a person's physical or psychological health.
- **emetic** (em-ETT-ic) an agent that causes vomiting.
- **endogenous opiates, endorphins** compounds made in the brain whose actions mimic those of opiate drugs (morphine, heroin) in reducing pain and stimulating pleasure.
- **limbic system** a group of tissues at the center of the brain responsible for feelings of pleasure and involved in the addiction process.
- **naloxone** a drug used in the treatment of narcotic addictions.
- **neurotransmitter** a substance released from the end of a nerve cell in response to a nerve impulse. The neurotransmitter diffuses across the gap to the next nerve cell, and alters that cell's membrane to make the cell more or less likely to fire.
- **unspecified eating disorders** eating disorders that do not meet the criteria for specific eating disorders previously defined. See Table C10-5.

authority figures are likely to be critical and to overvalue outward appearances while undervaluing inner self-esteem. Family patterns often include parents who oppose one another's authority, and who vacillate between defending the anorexic child's behavior and condemning it, confusing the child and disrupting normal parental control.[9] In the extreme, parents may even be abusive. Julie is a perfectionist, and her parents expect perfection: she identifies so strongly with her parents' ideals and goals that she cannot get in touch with her own identity. She sometimes feels like a robot, and she may act that way, too: polite but controlled, rigid, and unspontaneous. For Julie, rejecting food means gaining control. While some of her behaviors appear out of control, they are a part of her plan. She smokes cigarettes and drinks coffee incessantly because she believes these substances reduce her sensations of starvation.

How can a person as thin as Julie continue to starve herself? Julie uses tremendous discipline against her hunger to strictly limit her portions of low-calorie foods. She will deny her hunger, saying she is full after having eaten only a half-dozen carrot sticks. She can recite the calorie contents of dozens of foods and the calorie costs of as many exercises. If she feels that she has gained an ounce of weight, she runs or jumps rope until she is sure she has exercised it off. If she fears that the food she has eaten outweighs the exercise she has done, she takes laxatives to hasten the passage of food from her system. Her other methods of staying thin are so effective that she is unaware that laxatives have no effect on body fat. She is desperately hungry. In fact she is starving, but she doesn't eat because her need for self-control dominates.

Many people, on learning of this disorder, say they wish they had "a touch" of it to get thin. They mistakenly think that people with anorexia feel no hunger. They also fail to recognize the pain of the associated psychological and physical trauma.

Central to the diagnosis of anorexia nervosa is a distorted body image that overestimates body fatness.[10] When Julie looks at herself in the mirror, she sees her 85-pound body as fat. The more Julie overestimates her body size, the more resistant she is to treatment, and the more unwilling to examine her faulty values and misconceptions. Malnutrition itself is known to affect brain functioning and judgment in this way. Table C10-2 shows the criteria that professionals use to diagnose anorexia nervosa (anorexia nervosa cannot be self-diagnosed).

Anorexia nervosa damages the body much as starvation does. Victims are dying to be thin, quite literally. In young people, growth ceases and normal development falters. They lose so much lean tissue that basal metabolic rate slows, an effect that may remain even after treatment and regain of weight.[11] In athletes, the loss of lean tissue affects physical performance unfavorably. Hormonal changes and nutrient deprivation compromise bone density and lead to stress fractures.[12] Losses of bone density are especially pronounced in female athletes who cease menstruating because of overtraining. In fact, eating disorders, premature bone loss,

Table C10-2
Criteria for Diagnosis of Anorexia Nervosa

A person with anorexia nervosa demonstrates the following:

A. Refusal to maintain body weight at or above a minimal normal weight for age and height, e.g., weight loss leading to maintenance of body weight less than 85% of that expected; or failure to make expected weight gain during period of growth, leading to body weight less than 85% of that expected.
B. Intense fear of gaining weight or becoming fat, even though underweight.
C. Disturbance in the way in which one's body weight or shape is experienced; undue influence of body weight or shape on self-evaluation, or denial of the seriousness of the current low body weight.
D. In females past puberty, amenorrhea, i.e., the absence of at least three consecutive menstrual cycles. (A woman is considered to have amenorrhea if her periods occur only following hormone, e.g., estrogen, administration.)

Two types:
Restricting type: During the episode of anorexia nervosa, the person does not regularly engage in binge eating or purging behavior (i.e., self-induced vomiting or the misuse of laxatives or diuretics).
Binge eating/purging type: During the episode of anorexia nervosa, the person regularly engages in binge eating or purging behavior (i.e., self-induced vomiting or the misuse of laxatives or diuretics).

Source: Reprinted with permission from the *DSM-IV Draft Criteria* (Washington, D.C.: American Psychiatric Association, 1993), p. P:1. Copyright 1993 American Psychiatric Association.

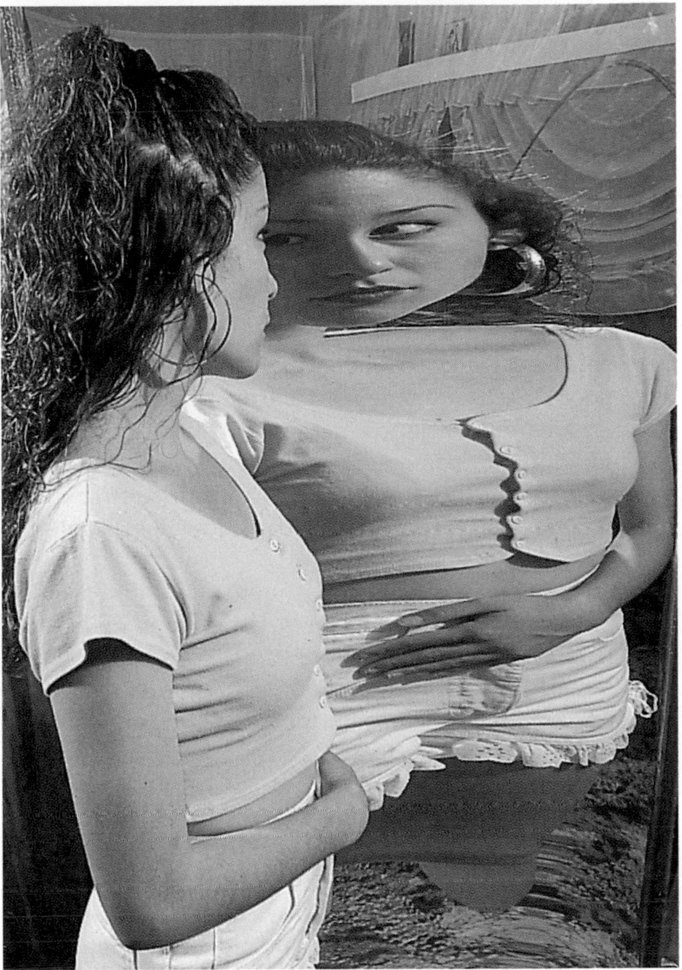

Women with anorexia nervosa see themselves as fat, even when they are dangerously underweight.

and irregular menstruation are seen as a triple threat to overtrained female athletes.[13] Additionally, the heart pumps inefficiently and irregularly, the heart muscle becomes weak and thin, the chambers diminish in size, and the blood pressure falls. Electrolytes that help to regulate heartbeat become unbalanced. Many deaths in people with anorexia are due to heart failure.

Starvation brings other physical consequences as well: impaired immune response, anemia, and a loss of digestive functions that worsens malnutrition. Digestive functioning becomes sluggish, the stomach empties slowly, and the lining of the intestinal tract shrinks. The ailing digestive tract fails to provide sufficient digestion of any food the victim may eat. The pancreas slows its production of digestive enzymes. The person may suffer from diarrhea, further worsening malnutrition.

Starvation also brings altered blood lipids, high concentrations of vitamin A and vitamin E in the blood, low blood proteins, dry skin, abnormal nerve functioning, low body temperature, and the development of fine body hair (the body's attempt to keep warm). The electrical activity of the brain becomes abnormal, and insomnia is common. Both women and men lose their sex drives.

Treatment artfully combines medical, psychosocial, and dietary facets to initiate and sustain weight gain with psychological techniques to resolve personal and family problems. Teams of physicians, nurses, psychiatrists, family therapists, and dietitians work together to treat people with anorexia nervosa. Appropriate diet is crucial and must be tailored individually to each client's needs. Seldom are clients willing to eat for themselves,

but if they are, chances are they can recover without other interventions.

High-risk clients may require hospitalization and may need to be force-fed by tube at first to forestall death. This step causes psychological trauma.[14] Drugs are commonly prescribed, but to date, they play a limited role in treatment.[15]

Denial runs high among those with anorexia nervosa. Few seek treatment on their own. Almost half of the women who are treated can maintain their body weight within 15 percent of a healthy weight; at that weight, many of them begin menstruating again. The other half have poor or fair outcomes of treatment, and two thirds of those treated continue a mental battle with recurring morbid thoughts about food and body weight.[16] Many relapse into abnormal eating behaviors to some extent. About 5 percent die during treatment, 1 percent by suicide.

Before drawing conclusions about someone who is extremely thin or who eats very little, remember that diagnosis of anorexia nervosa requires professional assessment. People who are seeking help with anorexia nervosa, either for themselves or for others, can call the National Anorexic Aid Society hotline for information.*

BULIMIA NERVOSA Sophia is a charming, intelligent, 20-year-old airline stewardess of normal weight who thinks constantly about food. She alternately starves herself and then secretly binges; when she has eaten too much, she vomits. Few people would fail to recognize these symptoms as those of bulimia nervosa.

Bulimia nervosa is distinct from anorexia nervosa and is more prevalent, although the true incidence is difficult to establish because denial runs high in people with bulimia nervosa.[17] More men suffer from bulimia nervosa than from anorexia nervosa; but bulimia nervosa is still most common in women. The secretive nature of bulimic behaviors makes recognition of the problem difficult, but once it is recognized, diagnosis is based on the criteria listed in Table C10-3.

Table C10-3
Criteria for Diagnosis of Bulimia Nervosa

A person with bulimia nervosa demonstrates the following:

A. Recurrent episodes of binge eating. An episode of binge eating is characterized by both of the following:
   (1) eating, in a discrete period of time (e.g., within any two hour period), an amount of food that is definitely larger than most people would eat during a similar period of time and under similar circumstances, and,
   (2) a sense of lack of control over eating during the episode (e.g., a feeling that one cannot stop eating or control what or how much one is eating).

B. Recurrent inappropriate compensatory behavior in order to prevent weight gain, such as: self-induced vomiting; misuse of laxatives, diuretics, or other medications; fasting; or excessive exercise.

C. Binge eating and inappropriate compensatory behaviors that both occur, on average, at least twice a week for three months.

D. Self-evaluation unduly influenced by body shape and weight.

E. The disturbance does not occur exclusively during episodes of anorexia nervosa.

Two types:

Purging type: the person regularly engages in self-induced vomiting or the misuse of laxatives or diuretics.

Nonpurging type: the person uses other inappropriate compensatory behaviors, such as fasting or excessive exercise, but does not regularly engage in self-induced vomiting or the misuse of laxatives or diuretics.

Source: Reprinted with permission from the *DSM-IV Draft Criteria* (Washington, D.C.: American Psychiatric Association, 1993), pp. P:1–P:2. Copyright 1993 American Psychiatric Association.

Families of bulimic people often establish unusually close emotional ties between members, and they may be over controlling and intermeshed in ways that stifle individual growth and development.[18] Should the member with bulimia nervosa begin taking steps toward recovery, others in the family may feel threatened. Any changes in the familiar structure, even if such change would greatly benefit the person with bulimia nervosa, often meet with resistance. Additionally, the family may have "secrets" that are hidden from outsiders. Many bulimic women report having been abused sexually or physically by family members or family friends.

Like the typical person with bulimia nervosa, Sophia is single, female, and white. She is well educated and close to her ideal body weight, although her weight fluctuates over a range of 10 pounds or so over a few weeks. As a flight attendant, she is required to "make weight," that is, to weigh no more than a certain cut-off weight slightly below the weight that her body maintains naturally.

*Phone numbers and addresses are in Appendix E.

Sophia seldom lets her bulimia nervosa interfere with her work or other activities, although a third of all bingers do so. From early childhood she has been a high achiever, emotionally dependent on her parents. As a young teen, Sophia cycled on and off crash diets. Sophia feels anxious at social events and cannot easily establish close relationships. She is sometimes depressed, is often impulsive, and she has not yet developed a personal identity.

A bulimic binge is unlike normal eating, and the food is not consumed for its nutritional value. During a binge, Sophia's eating is accelerated by her hunger from previous calorie restriction. She may take in anywhere from 1,000 to many thousands of calories of easy-to-eat, low-fiber, smooth-textured, high-fat, and, especially, high-carbohydrate foods. Typically, she chooses cookies, cakes, and ice cream; and she eats the entire bag of cookies, the whole cake, and every spoonful in a carton of ice cream.

The binge is a compulsion and usually occurs in several stages: "anticipation and planning, anxiety, urgency to begin, rapid and uncontrollable consumption of food, relief and relaxation, disappointment, and finally shame or disgust."[19] Then, to purge the food from her body, she may use a **cathartic**—a strong laxative that can injure the lower intestinal tract. Or she may induce vomiting, using an **emetic**—a drug intended as first aid for poisoning. After the binge she pays the price with hands scraped raw against the teeth during induced vomiting, swollen neck glands and reddened eyes from straining to vomit, with bloating, fatigue, headache, nausea, and pain that follow.

On first glance, purging seems to offer a quick and easy solution to the problems of unwanted calories and body weight. Many people perceive such behavior as neutral or even positive, when, in fact, binging and purging have serious physical consequences.[20] Fluid and electrolyte imbalances caused by vomiting or diarrhea can lead to abnormal heart rhythms and injury to the kidneys. Urinary tract infections can lead to kidney failure. Vomiting causes irritation and infection of the pharynx, esophagus, and salivary glands; erosion of the teeth; and dental caries. The esophagus may rupture or tear, as may the stomach. Overuse of emetics can lead to death by heart failure.

Unlike Julie, Sophia is aware that her behavior is abnormal, and she is deeply ashamed of it. She wants to recover, and this makes recovery more likely for her than for Julie, who clings to denial. Feeling inadequate ("I can't even control my eating"), Sophia tends to be passive and to look to others, primarily men, for con-

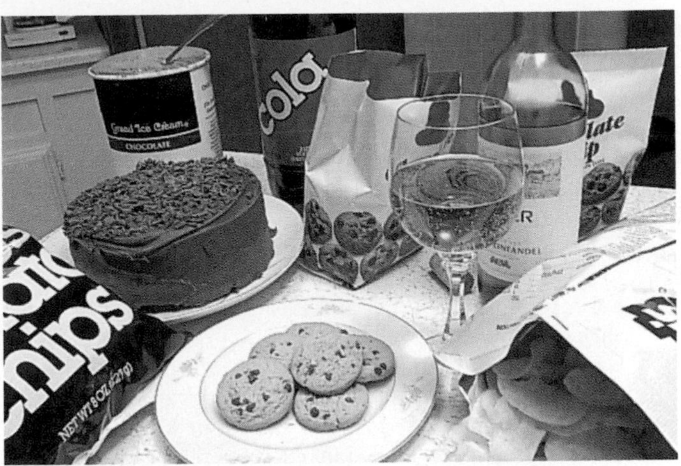

A person may consume up to 10,000 calories during an eating binge.

firmation of her sense of worth. When she experiences rejection, either in reality or in her imagination, her bulimia nervosa becomes worse. If Sophia's depression deepens, she may seek solace in drug or alcohol abuse.

To help clients gain control over food and establish regular eating patterns requires adherence to a structured eating plan. Restrictive weight-loss dieting almost always precedes and may even trigger binging. Weight maintenance, rather than cyclic gains and losses, is the goal for the person who has recovered. Many a former bulimia nervosa victim has taken a major step toward recovery by learning to eat enough food to satisfy hunger needs (at least 1,600 calories a day). Table C10-4 offers some ways to begin correcting the eating problems of bulimia nervosa.

Anorexia nervosa and bulimia nervosa are distinct eating disorders, each having a specific set of diagnostic criteria and medical complications. Yet they also sometimes overlap. Anorexia victims may purge, and victims of both conditions share an overconcern with body weight and the tendency to drastically undereat. The two disorders can also appear in the same person, or one can lead to the other.

OTHER EATING DISORDERS Many people with eating disorders fall short of the diagnostic criteria for either anorexia nervosa or bulimia nervosa, and may have an "unspecified" eating disorder. Disordered eating, fear of body fatness, distorted body image, purging, or binging may place them at risk of the same consequences that the more well-defined eating disorders present. About one third of obese people regularly engage in binge eating. Evidence is mounting to support the creation of a

Table C10-4
Diet Strategies for Combatting Bulimia Nervosa

- Avoid finger foods; eat foods that require the use of utensils.
- Enhance satiety by eating warm foods.
- Include vegetables, salad, and/or fruit at meals to prolong eating time.
- Choose whole-grain and high-fiber breads and cereals to maximize bulk.
- Eat a well-balanced diet and meals consisting of a variety of foods.
- Use foods that are naturally divided into portions, such as potatoes (rather than rice or pasta); 4- and 8-oz. containers of yogurt, ice cream, or cottage cheese; precut steak or chicken parts; and frozen entrees.
- Include foods containing ample complex carbohydrates (for satiety) and some fat (to slow gastric emptying).
- Eat meals and snacks sitting down.
- Plan meals and snacks, and record plans in a food diary prior to eating.

Source: Adapted from C. L. Rock and J. Yager, Nutrition and eating disorders: A primer for clinicians, *International Journal of Eating Disorders* 6 (1987): 276, as cited in *Nutrition and the M. D.,* July 1988, with permission. Reprinted with permission of John Wiley & Sons, Inc., copyright 1987.

Table C10-5
Unspecified Eating Disorders—Some Examples

Many people have eating disorders but do not meet all the criteria to be classified as having anorexia nervosa or bulimia nervosa. Some examples include those who:

A. Meet all of the criteria for anorexia nervosa, except irregular menses.
B. Meet all of the criteria for anorexia nervosa, except that their weights fall within the normal ranges.
C. Meet all of the criteria for bulimia nervosa, except that binges occur less frequently than stated in the criteria.
D. Are of normal body weight and who compensate inappropriately for eating small amounts of food (example: self-induced vomiting after eating two cookies).
E. Repeatedly chew food, but spit it out without swallowing.
F. Have recurrent episodes of binge eating but who do not compensate as do those with bulimia nervosa.

Source: Data from task force on DSM-IV, 307.50 Eating Disorder Not Otherwise Specified, *DSM-IV Draft Criteria* (Washington, D.C.: American Psychiatric Association, 1993), p. P:2.

third category of eating disorder, called **binge eating disorder** to include obese people who binge. Table C10-5 lists other examples of unspecified eating disorders.

Clinicians note differences between people with bulimia nervosa and those with binge eating disorder.[21] For example, binge eaters rarely purge or excessively restrict eating during dieting. Similarities also exist, including feeling out of control, feeling disgusted, depressed, embarrassed or guilty, and feeling distress caused by binging.[22]

Treatment of binge eating is a helpful complement to weight control programs. It also improves physical health, mental health, and the chances of success in breaking the cycle of rapid weight losses and gains.

EATING DISORDERS, ADDICTIONS, AND DEPRESSION

Researchers believe that anorexia nervosa and substance addictions may be based on the same brain chemistry. Anorexia improves when treated with **naloxone,** a drug that controls heroin addiction. Given to an addict, the drug can block the craving for heroin; given to people with bulimia nervosa, it can abolish their compulsive drive to binge, probably by diminishing the brain's pleasure response to sweet tastes.[23] A similar drug has no effect on other people's taste perceptions.[24] Naloxone also blocks the thrill sensations that arise when people listen to well-loved music. These seemingly unrelated effects may actually be connected. All such feelings of thrill likely arise from the same set of brain chemicals, namely, the **endogenous opiates,** or **endorphins,** which kill pain and induce feelings of pleasure, including sexual pleasure. Any drug use or other behavior that stimulates the **limbic system** of the brain (the site where these chemicals originate) is likely to be repeated, sometimes irresistibly. Naloxone interferes with this system, thus eliminating the repetition of behaviors.

Some of the brain's endorphins have also been implicated as playing direct roles in appetite regulation. The concentrations of these endorphins in women with bulimia nervosa may differ from those in women who eat normally.[25] Researchers found that the plasma concentration of one of the endorphins was depressed in bulimic women and that the relationship was linear—the lower the endorphin, the worse the bulimia nervosa. This finding was taken to imply that too-low levels of endorphins might trigger bulimia nervosa. However, the reverse could also be true—that starvation leading to binging somehow depresses certain brain endorphins.

The vomiting that can follow bulimic binges also may stimulate the brain's endorphin release.[26] ("Purging the soul" by intense crying—catharsis—may do the same thing.) In addition, pain sensitivity seems reduced after vomiting, a feeling of peacefulness and relief ensues, and depression reportedly lifts, suggesting that vomiting stimulates the release of endorphins. Obviously the links of endorphins to eating disorders warrant further investigation.

The **neurotransmitter** serotonin is also implicated in bulimia. Almost 90 percent of people who first seek help for bulimia are subsequently found to be clinically depressed.[27] Feelings of depression can result from low serotonin in the brain, and serotonin plays roles in the regulation of food intake, particularly the intake of carbohydrate-rich food (see Controversy 13).

In general, mood is depressed when people are hungry, as it is when they lack sleep or have to work too hard for too long. In some people, when severe depression occurs it disturbs both their diets and their sleep patterns. Psychiatrists describe the relationship between depression and eating behavior as robust. Connections to the mood-regulating neurotransmitter serotonin are under study.

Even after recovery, some people with bulimia nervosa have lower than normal levels of a serotonin product in their brains. Certain subgroups of depressed people also share this abnormality. It is believed that in bulimic people, this may impair their ability to experience satiety after eating a reasonable amount of food. Depression, in fact, is an invariable accompaniment to bulimia nervosa, and altered serotonin synthesis may turn out to be of major significance in mediating the prominent clinical symptoms in bulimia nervosa.

Antidepressant medications given to depressed bulimia sufferers have been found to lift depression, reduce bulimic tendencies, and restore normal appetite.[28] Today many drugs used to treat psychological disorders are being tried in the treatment of bulimia. Also being tested are drugs derived from the neurotransmitters themselves, which may help correct the imbalances that disrupt appetite.

A word of caution: while science has hinted of connections between addictions and eating disorders, this realm is largely unexplored, and the relationships are not simple. No one should be led to believe that individual foods might be addictive. Claims that sugar, flour, fat, or other food components can lead to addiction are false. They are also dangerous, because they can mislead victims of eating disorders down a path of quackery and so can delay their recovery. People with eating disorders need treatment by teams of professionals that include psychologists and dietitians. Even excellent treatment does not ensure recovery, but without it, the chances for recovery are especially slim.

PREVENTING EATING DISORDERS IN ATHLETES To prevent eating disorders in athletes and dancers, both the performers and their coaches must be educated about links between inappropriate body-weight ideals, improper weight-loss techniques, eating disorder development, proper nutrition, and safe weight-control methods. It has been suggested that weight standards, which work fairly well for most people, are invalid for athletes. Athletes are heavier for their heights (they have more healthy muscle and bone tissue), and they are taller than others. When athletes consult weight standards designed for sedentary people, they can easily be led to believe, wrongly, that they are too fat. Underwater weighing and other body composition measures are more appropriate for them. When presented with a false assessment of too much body fat, many athletes resort to bulimic techniques in an attempt to lose weight and to solve an imaginary problem.[29]

Coaches and dance instructors should never encourage unhealthy weight loss to qualify for competition or to conform with distorted artistic ideals. Frequent weighings can push young people who are striving to lose weight into a cycle of starving to confront the scale, then binging uncontrollably afterwards. The erosion of self-esteem that accompanies these events can interfere with the normal identity development of the teen years and set the stage for serious problems later on.

Athletes and dancers can achieve stable, healthy weights through sound nutrition practices, but only if they are willing to accept that this is a lifelong task. This can be more difficult than it sounds. For a dancer like Julie, it may mean accepting that her healthy body is not right for performance of certain roles as they have been traditionally interpreted. Such interpretations have recently been changing to include fewer stereotypes, but slowly. For a wrestler, it may mean competing with opponents of higher weights or embarking on a lifelong weight-control regimen. Perhaps the time has come to question old standards that involve appearance or body weight and to replace them with more performance-based standards. Meanwhile, athletes and dancers need to protect themselves against developing eating disorders. Table C10-6 provides some suggestions.

EATING DISORDERS IN SOCIETY Eating disorders seem to have complex causes. Some people may be genetically predisposed to them. Some disorders have psychological components that develop within the context of society. Proof that society plays a role in eating disorders is found in their demographic distribution: they are known only in developed nations, and they become more prevalent as wealth increases and food becomes plentiful.

A food-centered society that favors thinness puts people in a bind. Families may encourage hearty eating and socializing around the dinner table. Party hosts take pride in the delicacies they serve, and guests are obliged to indulge. A child raised in such a setting may see little alternative but to celebrate with the family; indulge in vast quantities of food; and then vomit, crash diet, or fast to "undo" possible weight gain. Then, starving and guilty, the child may begin binging in secret to relieve a desperate hunger.

There is no doubt that our society sets unrealistic ideals for body weight, especially in women, and devalues those who do not conform to them. Even professionals, including physicians and dietitians, are prone to praise people for losing weight and to suggest weight loss to people who do not need to reduce for health's sake. As a result, at so tender an age as 11 or 12, beautifully growing, normal-weight girls are already worried that they are too fat. Most are "on diets," and many are poorly nourished. Some eat too little food to support normal growth; thus they miss out on their adolescent growth spurts and may never catch up.[30]

Perhaps a young person's best defense against these disorders is to learn to appreciate his or her own uniqueness. When people discover and honor the body's real needs, they become unwilling to sacrifice health for conformity. The author Eda LeShan, once a slave to bulimic behavior, achieved this inner ideal and described her recovery from overeating: "Deep inside there had always been a small child begging for my attention. . . . All I gave her was food. Now I give her love."[31]

Table C10-6
Tips for Combatting Eating Disorders

General Guidelines
■ Never restrict food servings to below the numbers suggested for adequacy by the Daily Food Guide.
■ Eat frequently. People often do not eat frequent meals because of time constraints, but eating can be incorporated into other activities, such as snacking while studying or commuting. The person who eats frequently never gets so hungry as to allow hunger to dictate food choices.
■ Establish a reasonable weight goal based on a healthy body composition. (Chapter 9 provides help in doing so.)
■ Allow a reasonable time to achieve the goal. A reasonable loss of excess fat can be achieved at the rate of one-half to one pound per week, not faster.
■ Establish a weight-maintenance support group with people who share interests.
Specific Guidelines For Athletes and Dancers
■ Remember that eating disorders impair physical performance. Obtain confidential help in obtaining treatment if needed.
■ Restrict weight-loss activities to the off season.
■ Focus on proper nutrition as an important facet of your training, as important as proper technique.

Notes

1. Task force on DSM-IV, 307.50 Eating Disorder Not Otherwise Specified, *DSM-IV Draft Criteria* (Washington, D.C.: American Psychiatric Association, 1993), p. P:2.
2. L. M. Mellin, C. E. Irwin, and S. Scully, Prevalence of disordered eating in girls: A survey of middle-class children, *Journal of the American Dietetic Association* 92 (1992): 851–853.
3. J. L. Walbery and C. S. Johnston, Menstrual function and eating behavior in female recreational weight lifters and competitive body builders, *Medicine and Science in Sports and Exercise* 23 (1991): 30–36.
4. J. H. Wilmore, Eating and weight disorders in female athletes, *Sports Medicine Digest*, June 1990, p. 4.
5. D. B. Woodside and L. Shekter-Wolfson, eds., *Family Approaches in Treatment of Eating Disorders* (Washington, D.C.: American Psychiatric Press, 1991), pp. xi-xvi.
6. N. T. Frusztajer and coauthors, Nutrition and the incidence of stress fractures in ballet dancers, *American Journal of Clinical Nutrition* 51 (1990): 779–783.
7. "Anorexia athletica," Special report on nutrition and the athlete, *Sports Medicine Digest*, 1989, p. 10; S. N. Steen and K. D. Brownell, Patterns of weight loss and regain in wrestlers: Has the tradition changed? *Medicine and Science in Sports and Exercise* 22 (1990): 762–768.
8. B. J. Larson, Relationship of family communication patterns to Eating Disorder Inventory scores in adolescent girls, *Journal of the American Dietetic Association* 91 (1991): 1065–1067.
9. G. Szmukler and C. Dare, Family therapy of early-onset, short-history anorexia nervosa, in Woodside and Shekter-Wolfson, 1991, pp. 25–47.
10. A. E. Andersen, Anorexia nervosa: Who are you? Where are you? (editorial), *Mayo Clinic Proceedings* 63 (1988): 511–513.
11. R. C. Casper and coauthors, Total daily energy expenditure and activity level in anorexia nervosa, *American Journal of Clinical Nutrition* 53 (1991): 1143–1150; L. Scalfi and coauthors, Bioimpedance analysis and resting energy expenditure in under nourished and refed anorectic patients, *European Journal of Clinical Nutrition* 47 (1993): 61–67.
12. R. B. Mazess, H. S. Barden, and E. S. Ohlrich, Skeletal and body-composition effects of anorexia nervosa, *American Journal of Clinical Nutrition* 52 (1990): 438–441; L. K. Bachrach and coauthors, Decreased bone density in adolescent girls with anorexia nervosa, *Pediatrics* 86 (1990): 440–447.
13. R. C. Henderson, Bone health in adolescence: Anorexia and athletic amenorrhea, *Nutrition Today*, March/April 1991, pp. 25–29; F. Munnings, Tackling women's health issues, *Physician and Sportsmedicine*, September 1992, p. 33.
14. B. R. Carruth, Adolescence, in *Present Knowledge in Nutrition*, ed. M. L. Brown (Washington, D.C.: International Life Sciences Institute, 1990), pp. 325–332.
15. L. G. Tolstoi, The role of pharmacotherapy in anorexia nervosa and bulimia, *Journal of the American Dietetic Association* 89 (1989): 1640–1646.
16. American Psychiatric Association Workgroup on Eating Disorders, Practice guidelines for eating disorders, I. Disease definition, epidemiology, and natural history, *American Journal of Psychiatry* 150 (1993): 212–228.
17. D. M. Stein, The prevalence of bulimia: A review of empirical research, *Journal of Nutrition Education* 23 (1991): 205–213.
18. L. G. Roberto, Impasses in the family treatment of bulimia, in Woodside and Shekter-Wolfson, 1991, pp. 69–85.
19. M. A. Balaa and D. A. Drossman, *Anorexia Nervosa and Bulimia: The Eating Disorders, Disease a Month* (Chicago: Year Book Medical Publishers, June 1985), pp. 1–52.
20. P. W. Meilman, F. A. von Hippel, and M. S. Gaylor, Self-induced vomiting in college women: Its relation to eating, alcohol use, and Greek life, *College Health* 40 (1991): 39–41.
21. G. T. Wilson, Do obese patients have eating disorders? An address presented at the North American Association for the Study of Obesity and Emory University School of Medicine conference on Obesity Update: Pathophysiology, Clinical Consequences, and Therapeutic Options, Atlanta, Georgia, August 31–September 2, 1992.
22. R. L. Spitzer and coauthors, Binge eating disorder: A multisite field trial of the diagnostic criteria, *International Journal of Eating Disorders* 11 (1992): 191–203.
23. A. Drewnowski and coauthors, Taste responses and preferences for sweet high-fat foods: Evidence for opioid involvement, *Physiology and Behavior* 51 (1992): 371–379.
24. M. M. Hetherington and coauthors, Failure of naltrexone to affect the pleasantness or intake of food, *Pharmacology, Biochemistry, and Behavior* 40 (1991): 185–190.
25. Drewnowski and coauthors, 1992; J. Rodin and coauthors, Bulimia and taste: Possible interactions, *Journal of Abnormal Psychology* 99 (1990): 32–39.
26. H. D. Abraham and A. B. Joseph, Bulimic vomiting alters pain tolerance and mood, *International Journal of Psychiatry in Medicine* 16 (1986): 311–316.
27. J. D. Killen and coauthors, Depressive symptoms and substance use among adolescent binge eaters and purgers: A defined population study, *American Journal of Public Health* 77 (1987): 1539–1541.
28. D. B. Herzog and P. M. Copeland, Bulimia nervosa—psyche and satiety, *New England Journal of Medicine* 319 (1988): 716–718; Tolstoi, 1989.
29. P. K. Welch and coauthors, Nutrition education, body composition, and dietary intake of female athletes, *Physician and Sportsmedicine*, January 1987, pp. 63–64, 67–69, 73–74.
30. F. Lifshitz and N. Moses, Nutritional dwarfing: Growth, dieting, and fear of obesity, *Journal of the American College of Nutrition* 7 (1988): 367–376.
31. E. LeShan, *Winning the Losing Game: Why I Will Never Be Fat Again* (New York: Crowell, 1979).

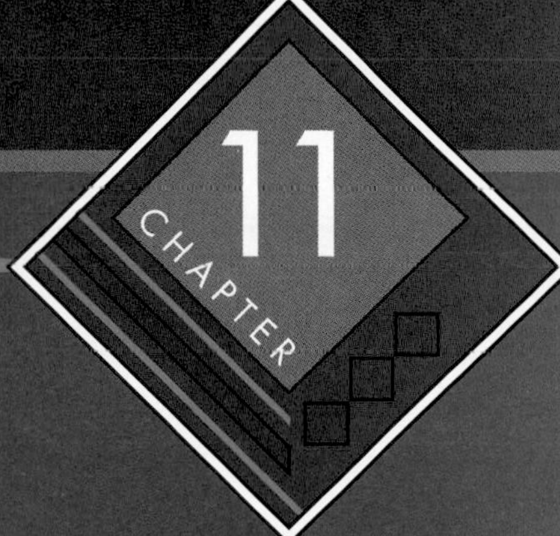

Nutrition and Disease Prevention

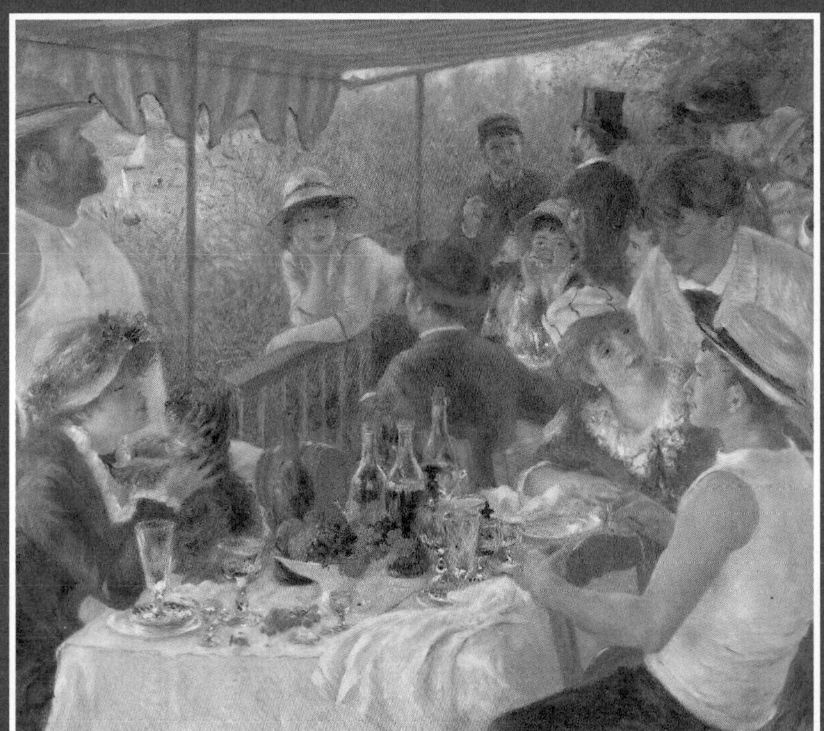

Contents

Renoir, The Luncheon of the Boating Party, © The Phillips Collection, Washington, D.C.

degenerative diseases chronic, irreversible diseases characterized by degeneration of the body organs due in part to such personal lifestyle elements as poor food choices, smoking, alcohol use, and lack of physical activity. Examples are diabetes, cancer, heart disease, and osteoporosis.

AIDS *A*cquired *I*mmune *D*eficiency *S*yndrome, caused by infection with HIV, a virus that is transmitted primarily by sexual contact, by contact with infected blood, by needles shared among drug users, or by the transmission of the virus to a fetus or infant by an infected mother.

11

Throughout history our ancestors have feared infectious diseases, such as tuberculosis, smallpox, and polio, that claimed many lives and curtailed the average life expectancy. Today medical research has bestowed upon us both preventions and cures for many infectious diseases. Our water supply is disinfected to prevent the spread of many infections. Immunizations protect us from many others. Consequently today's average life expectancy for those living in developed countries is considerably longer than that of 100 years ago. Despite these advances, though, infectious diseases still make people sick, and even with medical treatments, they can kill or lead to consequences that last a lifetime. While it is too much to claim that nutrition alone can prevent infectious diseases, it is true that a healthy, well-nourished immune system can often prevent minor infections from becoming major problems.

While a few infectious diseases remain serious threats, the diseases we most often face are not infectious, but are of a different nature. Figure 11-1 shows the top eleven killer diseases of today. Of these, six are **degenerative diseases:** heart disease, cancers, strokes, lung diseases, diabetes, and liver disease. Four are associated directly with poor nutrition, and four others are associated with excessive alcohol intake, which affects nutrition indirectly. Taken together, these eight conditions account for about three fourths of the nation's 2 million deaths each year. The other three major killers are chronic obstructive lung disease, which is most often related to smoking, pneumonia/influenza, which strikes old people and infants whose defenses are weak, and **AIDS,** attributable to the transmission of the virus known as HIV.

This chapter's main goal, then, is to present what is now known of nutrition's role in the prevention of degenerative diseases.[1] It does so by following the guidelines presented in Chapter 1 on evaluating research, and it presents mostly concepts supported by a great weight of evidence, with some single-study results to spark interest. First, however, this chapter takes a brief look at how nutrition helps to support the immune system and strengthens the body against infectious diseases. While nutrition is powerless to prevent or cure HIV infection or AIDS, those living with HIV or AIDS do benefit from proper nutrition and a special section addresses their needs.

Figure 11-1

ELEVEN LEADING CAUSES OF DEATH

The causes listed in bold are topics of this chapter; liver disease and cirrhosis are associated with alcoholism and are topics of Controversy 11.

Source: Centers for Disease Control, Mortality patterns—United States, 1989, *Morbidity and Mortality Weekly Report* 41 (1992): 121–125.

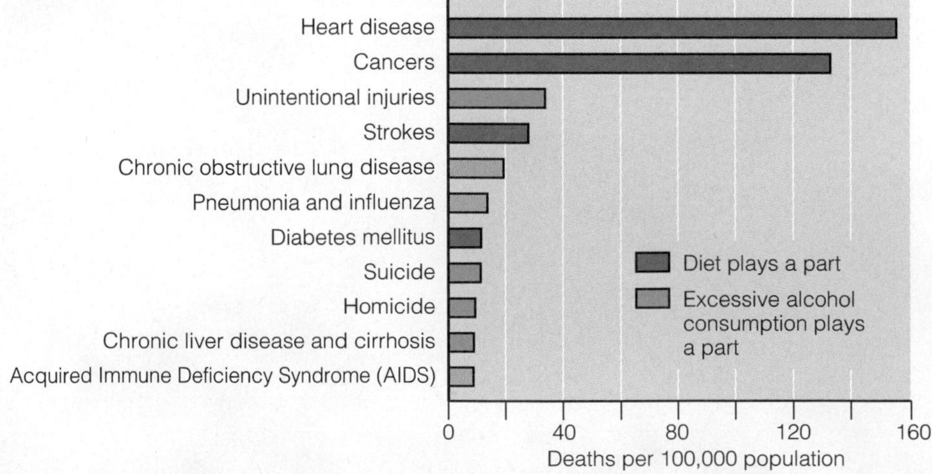

◆ Nutrition and Immunity

Without your awareness, your immune system guards continuously against thousands of enemy attacks mounted against you by microorganisms and cancer cells. If your immune system falters, you become vulnerable to disease-causing agents and disease invariably follows.

Nutrients and the Immune System

Among the body's systems, the immune system responds most sensitively to subtle changes in nutrition status. When people do not eat well, for whatever reason, malnutrition often sets in, compromising immunity. Impaired immunity opens the way for diseases, diseases reduce food intake, and nutrition status suffers further. Thus disease and poor nutrition together form a downward spiral that must be broken for recovery to occur (see Figure 11-2).

People most likely to be caught in the downward path to malnutrition and weakened immunity are those who:

- Suffer from PEM (protein-energy malnutrition).
- Are hospital patients.
- Live in poverty in large inner-city populations.
- Diet for weight loss.

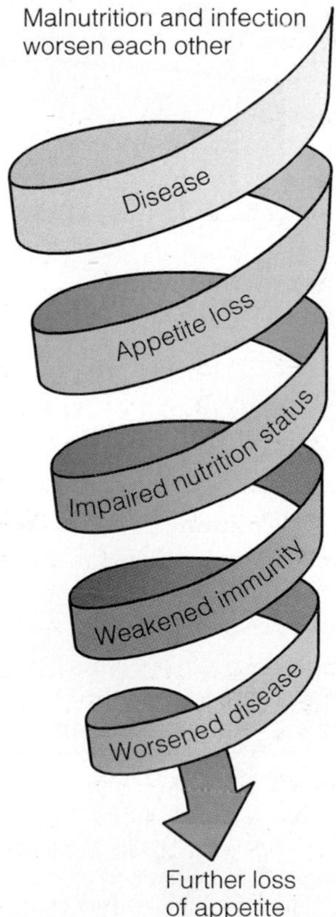

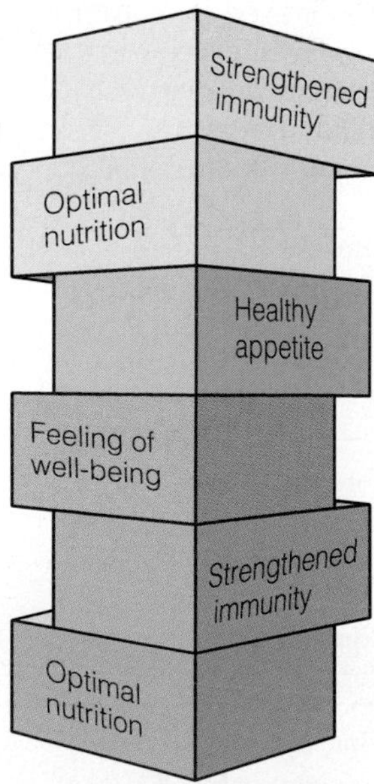

Figure 11-2

NUTRITION AND IMMUNITY

- Restrict food intake for any reason.[2]
- Are elderly.[3]

A deficiency of even a single nutrient can weaken the body's defenses considerably. While this area of nutrition research is still in its infancy, some preliminary findings are gathered into Table 11-1, not to memorize as facts carved in stone, but to give an impression of the overall importance of proper diet to the immune response.

Chapter 3 pointed out that a deficiency of any nutrient is likely to weaken the immune system. The chapters on vitamins and minerals listed toxicity symptoms from nutrient overdoses, and many of these can damage immunity. The trick of planning a diet to support the immune system is to meet

Table 11-1
Evidence on Dietary Factors and Immunity

Factor	Effect
Protein/energy deficiency	Weakens immunity
Energy excess	May impair the immune response, but this point is debated
Vitamin A deficiency	Weakens body linings, weakens antibody and immune cell response
Vitamin A excess	Weakens immunity
Vitamin D deficiency (rickets)	Predisposes to infections, but link to immunity not proved
Vitamin D excess	Unknown
Vitamin E deficiency	Weakens immunity
Vitamin E excess	Evidence conflicts; may stimulate immune response at first, then depress it
Thiamin deficiency	Weakens immunity
Thiamin excess	Unknown
Riboflavin deficiency	Weakens immunity
Riboflavin excess	Unknown
Folate deficiency[a]	Reduces capacity of immune cells to kill infection
Folate excess	Unknown
Vitamin B_{12} deficiency	Changes immune cell characteristics; possible delays immune response
Vitamin B_{12} excess	Unknown
Vitamin B_6 deficiency	Weakens immunity
Vitamin B_6 excess	Unknown
Vitamin C deficiency	Weakens immunity, reduces white blood cell killing power
Vitamin C excess	See accompanying Consumer Caution
Zinc deficiency	Reduces number of immune cells; depresses immunity
Zinc excess	Changes immune cell characteristics; exerts unknown effect on immunity
Copper deficiency	Reduces immune cell number; impairs immunity
Copper excess	Reduces immune cell number; impairs immunity

[a]Even mild folate deficiency produces weakened killing ability.

Sources: Data from P. M. Newberne and M. Lockniskar, Nutrition and immune status, in I. R. Rowland (ed.), *Nutrition, Toxicity, and Cancer* (Boca Raton, Fla.: CRC Press, 1991), pp. 301–378; M. C. Goldschmidt, Reduced bactericidal activity in neutrophils from scorbutic animals and the effect of ascorbic acid on these target bacteria in vivo and in vitro, *American Journal of Clinical Nutrition* 54 (1991): 1214S–1220S; R. A. Jacob and coauthors, Immunocompetence and oxidant defense during ascorbate depletion in healthy men, *American Journal of Clinical Nutrition* 54 (1991): 1302S–1309S.

Table 11-2
Effects of Protein-Energy Malnutrition on the Body's Defense Systems

System Component	Effects of Malnutrition
Skin	Thinned, with less connective tissue to serve as a barrier for protection of underlying tissues; delayed skin sensitivity reaction to antigens
Digestive tract and other body linings	Antibody secretions and immune cell number reduced
Lymph tissues	Thymus gland, lymph nodes, and spleen reduced in size; cells of immune defense depleted
General response	Invader kill time delayed; circulating immune cells reduced; antibody response impaired

Source: Data on immune response and cells from R. K. Chandra, Nutrition and immunity in the elderly, *Nutrition Reviews* 50 (1992): 367–371.

the minimum need for each nutrient while not ingesting a dose that would cause harm.

Protein-energy malnutrition (PEM) is especially destructive to various immune-system organs and tissues. Table 11-2 shows its effects. Listed first are the body's initial barriers to infection—the skin and the mucous membranes. The digestive system is especially active in this regard. The mucous membranes of the digestive system are heavily laced with active immune tissues. These tissues may work at the absorptive site or they may form cells that travel to other organs, such as the liver, pancreas, mammary glands, and uterus.[4] During PEM, these precious cells dwindle in size and number, opening the whole body to infection. Also the skin becomes thinner with less connective tissue, and so becomes less of a barrier to agents of disease. The antibody concentration normally present in secretions of the lungs and digestive tract becomes depressed and this may help explain why malnourished children have repeated lung and digestive tract infections. Normally barred from the body, infectious agents are allowed to enter, and the attack against them, once they are inside, is weak.

KEY POINT Adequate nutrition is a key player in maintaining a healthy immune system to defend against infectious diseases.

When speaking of nutrition and immunity, people often ask whether supplements of vitamin C can help the body fight off the viruses that cause colds and flu. The following Consumer Caution presents some current scientific thought on the topic.

Vitamin C and the Common Cold

CONSUMER CAUTION Over past years, vitamin C has been rated the most-often-taken single vitamin supplement. What is it about vitamin C that people seek? Most who take it believe that the vitamin helps defend against viral illnesses, specifically colds and flu.[5] While many takers have adhered to their beliefs with an almost religious zeal,

(continued on next page)

Vitamin C and the Common Cold *continued*

CONSUMER CAUTION most scientists have dismissed the idea that doses of vitamin C can benefit people in this way.[6] Today, though, some are seriously discussing the possibility that vitamin C may actually be effective.

The idea that taking vitamin C supplements reduces the severity and duration of colds was put forth in 1970 by a respected physicist, Dr. Linus Pauling.[7] A spate of studies followed, and in 1975 a physician reviewed many of them.[8] He found that, statistically, takers of vitamin C did indeed suffer fewer and milder colds than takers of placebos. The difference averaged one-tenth of one cold per year, and one tenth of one day per cold in favor of the vitamin C-takers. While such a measurable difference is cause for great excitement among laboratory scientists, a person hearing about it wouldn't think the gain worth considering.

Statistics may, however, pool together all of the results and report only the average occurrence. The statistics just mentioned might give the impression that every single subject taking vitamin C who also caught a cold suffered exactly 2½ hours fewer than control subjects receiving no vitamin C. This is not the case, however. In human terms, some vitamin C takers probably suffered just as long and some even longer than the controls; others probably found relief much sooner. The average worked out to be slight, but for *individuals* the results might have been dramatic. It could also be true that some individuals began the study in a vitamin-C deprived state, and that, of these people, the ones who received the lacking vitamin enjoyed a greatly boosted immune response, changing the average for the group. While all these things are possible, none are proven. The point here is that early studies remain inconclusive.

One certainty is that the placebo effect is always at work. A questionnaire given at the end of one study revealed that a number of the subjects had made guesses concerning the contents of their capsules. Subjects who had actually received the placebo, but who believed they were receiving vitamin C, experienced *fewer* colds than the group who had received the vitamin but believed they had received the placebo.

As of the early 1990s, researchers have found other connections. A study found that a single gram dose of vitamin C elevated subjects' body temperatures and reduced their serum iron, two metabolic responses that normally occur with infections.[9] Gram doses of vitamin C are many times the RDA and are not being recommended here. While the two effects observed are related to immune function, no conclusion may be drawn about whether the effects protect against infection.

In another study using an even larger two-gram vitamin C dose, researchers observed an involvement of the body's immune system. The researchers measured a 40 percent increase in blood histamine after administration of the supplement.[10] Histamine assists in fighting off local invasion of the body's tissues by increasing blood flow to the area. Thus, this study seems to support the idea that vitamin C supplements boost immunity.

One more study is worth mentioning, this one involving ultramarathon runners. Such athletes have been observed to suffer increased

Vitamin C and the Common Cold *continued*

rates of upper respiratory infections. In the study, athletes who were given daily supplements of 600 milligrams of vitamin C suffered less than half the number of upper respiratory infections after a race than runners given a placebo.[11] Those of the supplemented group who did contract infections had, on average, milder symptoms that cleared up more quickly than in the control group.

These studies do not make a strong case for saying that vitamin C can prevent or shorten colds or flu, but they provide promising directions for future research. This uncertainty leaves the person who takes vitamin C supplements as cold preventives in a predicament. No scientific authority would refute the importance of adequate vitamin C in the body's immunity, nor would they advise gram doses of the vitamin for its benefit. High doses place some people at risk of iron overload, a dangerous toxicity state, and vitamin C supplements have been declared dangerous for such people.[12] Still, many people are convinced, through personal experience, that they suffer fewer colds when taking vitamin C supplements. Some day science may reveal some underlying reason for this effect. Until then takers of vitamin C should treat the supplements as drugs, keep close tabs on their blood iron concentrations, and avoid doses larger than 2,000 milligrams. Most people seem able to tolerate some supplemental vitamin C, but megadoses can harm health.

Nutrition in the Treatment of AIDS

More and more people are finding that someone they know has been diagnosed with HIV infection or AIDS. Adequate nutrition, while offering nothing in the way of cure, can enhance strength, provide comfort, and generally improve life's quality. A well-nourished person with AIDS can often remain independent longer than if nutrition had not been optimal.[13]

Severe malnutrition resembling PEM with wasting of lean body tissue is common in people with AIDS.[14] This wasting appears to be related to poor food intake, increased nutrient requirements, poor nutrient absorption, and especially the losses of fluids and nutrients associated with persistent diarrhea.[15] This loss of lean body mass may begin even before an HIV infected person comes down with AIDS.[16] While it is unknown whether nutrition can prevent these early changes, it can't hurt for people who test positive for the HIV virus to tend carefully to their nutrient intakes and exercise habits. AIDS strips its victims of their immune defenses, compounding the effects of malnutrition.[17] An individual with both AIDS and malnutrition is extremely vulnerable to other infections and cancers that often prove fatal.

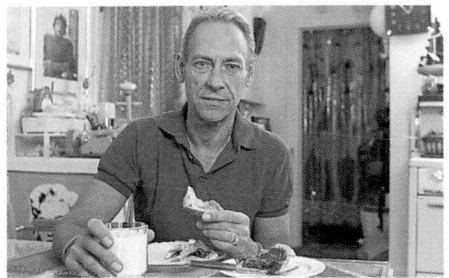
Nutrition can make the difference between living independently and being confined to a nursing home or hospital.

People wishing to offer help to someone with AIDS can do no better than to tend intelligently to the person's nutrition, which is often overlooked in medical treatment. People with AIDS suffer anorexia and so may refuse food. They may more readily accept small frequent meals, such as an assortment of nutritious snacks and juices, rather than three large meals. A valid goal is to meet the criteria of the Daily Food Guide to ensure adequacy of nutrient intake. In addition to food, a supplement containing the RDA amounts of vitamins and minerals can be helpful and will not cause harm. Some liquid meal supplements are fortified with vitamins and minerals, and

risk factors factors known to be related to (or correlated with) a disease but not proven to be causal.

they provide the carbohydrate, fat, and protein that the AIDS patient needs for energy and building materials. They also taste good and are easy to swallow.

Whatever foods are served, primary attention must be paid to food safety. A common bacterium in food, *Salmonella*, can cause a deadly infection in people with compromised immunity.[18] Cleanliness and thorough cooking are protective. Should AIDS complications progress, the person's diet may become more prescriptive, dictated by therapy and guided by a dietitian's advice.[19] Still, the caring attitude shown through attention to nutrition can lend emotional support to the sick person, a powerful medicine in itself.

Family, friends, and victims may, out of desperation, try special diet regimens or supplements in hopes of finding a cure or adding days to life. In the case of AIDS, no diet or nutrient regimen has been shown helpful beyond providing the nutrients needed for the body's defenses. However, to extinguish hope would serve no purpose, and, while not all agree, unproved dietary "remedies" may best be allowed as long as they do no harm.

HIV infections are often preventable. The authors urge you to seek out information about AIDS prevention and to heed it.

KEY POINT Adequate nutrition cannot prevent or cure AIDS, but can bolster the quality of life for the person with AIDS.

Lifestyle Choices and Risks of Disease

In contrast to the infectious diseases, each of which has a distinct microbial cause such as a bacterium or virus, the degenerative diseases of adulthood tend to have clusters of suspected causes known as **risk factors.** Among them are environmental, behavioral, social, and genetic factors that tend to occur in clusters and interact with each other. In many cases one disease or condition intensifies the risk of another.

People's behaviors, including food behaviors, underlie many risk factors. The choice to eat a high-fat diet, for example, is a choice to increase the probabilities of becoming obese and of contracting cancer, hypertension, diabetes, atherosclerosis, diverticulosis, or other diseases. Figure 11-3 on page 408 shows the interrelationships of some of the risk factors associated with today's major degenerative diseases and highlights the diet-related behaviors that contribute to them.

The exact contribution diet makes to each disease is hard to estimate. Many experts believe that diet accounts for about a third of all cases of coronary heart disease, but they argue that it may cause from one tenth to nine tenths of all cases of cancer.* Diet is largely under an individual's own control. If a dietary change can't hurt and might help, why not make it?

To make such choices is doubtless more important for some people than for others, since some people are genetically predisposed to certain diseases. To begin deciding whether certain diet recommendations are especially important to you, you should consider your family's medical history to see which diseases are common to your forebears. Any condition that shows up in several close blood relatives may be a special concern for you. Another

*Other important risk factors for cancer development include use of tobacco, overconsumption of alcohol, exposure to radiation, exposure to environmental and other contamination, and advanced age.

Table 11-3
Lifestyle Risk Factors and Priorities in Nutrition

Nutrition Changes Recommended for All People	This Is Especially Important If Your Family History Indicates:	And/Or If Your Medical History Indicates:
Reduce consumption of fat (especially saturated fat) and cholesterol. Achieve and maintain a desirable body weight. Increase consumption of complex carbohydrates and fiber.	Diabetes, obesity, cancer, or any form of cardiovascular disease (atherosclerosis, hypertension, heart attacks, strokes)	Glucose intolerance, high blood cholesterol or triglycerides, hypertension
Salt/sodium: Reduce intake of salt/sodium.	Hypertension, diabetes, or any form of cardiovascular disease (atherosclerosis, hypertension, heart attacks, strokes)	Hypertension
Alcohol: To reduce the risk of chronic disease, take alcohol only in moderation, if at all.	Liver disease (cirrhosis), cancer, any form of cardiovascular disease (atherosclerosis, hypertension, heart attacks, strokes), osteoporosis	Glucose intolerance, high blood cholesterol or triglycerides, hypertension, any sign of adult bone loss

Source: Adapted from *The Surgeon General's Report on Nutrition and Health: Summary and Recommendations,* DHHS (PHS) publication no. 88-50211, (Washington, D.C.: Government Printing Office, 1988), Table 1, p. 3.

piece of advice about what lifestyle changes to make is to find out, after your next physical examination, which test results are out of line. The two together are powerful predictors of disease. Table 11-3 presents a summary of the signs to watch for in both categories.

Table 11-3 points to the places where you can make the personal investments that will bring the greatest probable rewards. Accepting that you have certain unchangeable "givens," you can look to the things you can change and choose the most influential among them. For example, a person whose parents, grandparents, or other close blood relatives suffered with diabetes and heart disease is urgently advised to avoid becoming obese. A person who has hypertension is urged to control weight, to exercise regularly, to eat a nutritious diet, and to not smoke. The guidelines presented in this chapter can benefit most people, while presenting the smallest possible risk to health.[20]

Diabetes is related to the major killer diseases as shown in Figure 11-3. The progression of degenerative diseases is hastened by both diabetes and obesity, and each of these two conditions worsens the other.[21] Thus although other conditions may appear to be more threatening, diabetes and obesity may be the two that are most important to prevent.

See Chapter 4 for a review of diabetes and its relationship to obesity.

KEY POINT Diet and lifestyle risk factors associated with one degenerative disease may contribute to others as well; some degenerative diseases themselves contribute to some of the others.

Nutrition and Atherosclerosis

For decades our major cause of death has been disease of the heart and blood vessels **(cardiovascular disease,** or **CVD).** CVD accounts for more of

Figure 11-3

DIET/LIFESTYLE RISK FACTORS AND DEGENERATIVE DISEASES

The chart at the top shows that the same risk factors affect many chronic conditions. For example, genetic risk factors and high-fat diets affect many diseases; smoking affects fewer; and environmental contaminants affect fewer still. This does not mean that people who smoke or are exposed to environmental contaminants become less often or less severely ill than those who eat a high-fat diet, but just that the fat-eaters may become ill from a larger variety of conditions.

The flow chart at the bottom shows that some of the conditions are themselves risk factors for other conditions. For example, atherosclerosis and hypertension are known to worsen each other.

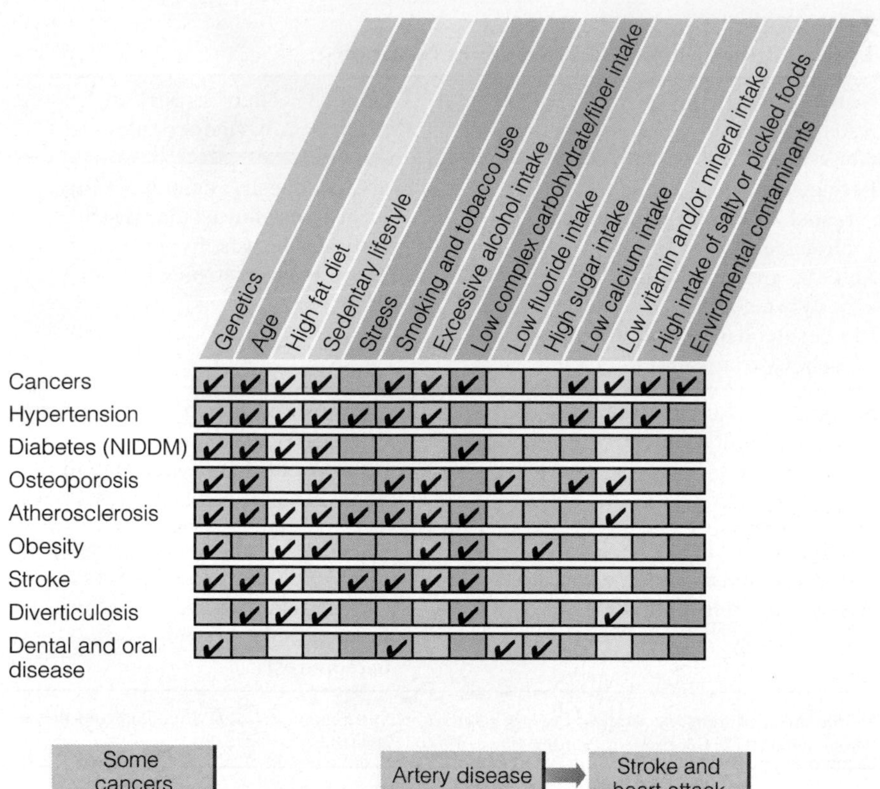

	Genetics	Age	High fat diet	Sedentary lifestyle	Stress	Smoking and tobacco use	Excessive alcohol intake	Low complex carbohydrate/fiber intake	Low fluoride intake	High sugar intake	Low calcium intake	Low vitamin and/or mineral intake	High intake of salty or pickled foods	Enviromental contaminants
Cancers	✓	✓	✓	✓		✓	✓	✓			✓	✓	✓	✓
Hypertension	✓	✓	✓	✓	✓	✓	✓				✓	✓	✓	
Diabetes (NIDDM)	✓	✓	✓	✓				✓						
Osteoporosis	✓	✓		✓		✓	✓		✓		✓	✓		
Atherosclerosis	✓	✓	✓	✓	✓	✓	✓	✓				✓		
Obesity	✓		✓	✓			✓	✓		✓				
Stroke	✓	✓	✓		✓	✓	✓	✓						
Diverticulosis		✓	✓	✓				✓				✓		
Dental and oral disease	✓					✓			✓	✓				

CVD (cardiovascular disease) a general term for all diseases of the heart and blood vessels. Atherosclerosis is the main form of CVD. Also called *coronary heart disease* or *CHD.*

atherosclerosis(ath-er-oh-scler-OH-sis) the most common form of artery disease, characterized by plaques along the inner walls of the arteries. (The related term *arteriosclerosis* means *all* forms of hardening of the arteries and includes some rare diseases. *Athero* means "porridge" or "soft"; *scleros* means "hard"; *osis* means "too much.")

hypertension high blood pressure (see the next major section of this chapter).

the nation's deaths each year than any other single cause, mostly by way of heart attacks and strokes. Efforts to fight CVD have led to valuable discoveries and public education. We now know that smoking, high blood pressure, and high blood cholesterol are the three major risk factors for CVD, and many people have changed their lifestyles accordingly. Many have quit smoking or have refrained from starting. Many have been willing to change their diets, consuming less food energy, less fat, less cholesterol, less salt, and more fiber. Many are exercising more. The rate of CVD has fallen somewhat since 1950, but it still remains high. How can people minimize their risks? How can we improve our chances of leading long and healthy lives?

The twin demons that lead to most CVD are **atherosclerosis** and **hypertension.** Atherosclerosis is the common form of hardening of the arteries; hypertension is high blood pressure; and each makes the other worse.

How Atherosclerosis Develops

No one is free of atherosclerosis. The question is not whether you have it but how far advanced it is and what you can do to retard or to reverse it.

It usually begins with the accumulation of soft, fatty streaks along the inner walls of the arteries, especially at branch points. These gradually enlarge and become hardened **plaques,** making the artery walls lose their elasticity and narrowing the passage through them (see Figure 11-4). Most people have well-developed plaques by the time they reach age 30.

plaques (PLACKS) mounds of lipid material, mixed with smooth muscle cells and calcium, which develop in the artery walls in atherosclerosis. (The same word is also used to describe the accumulation of a different kind of deposits on teeth, which promotes dental caries. *Placken* means "patch.")

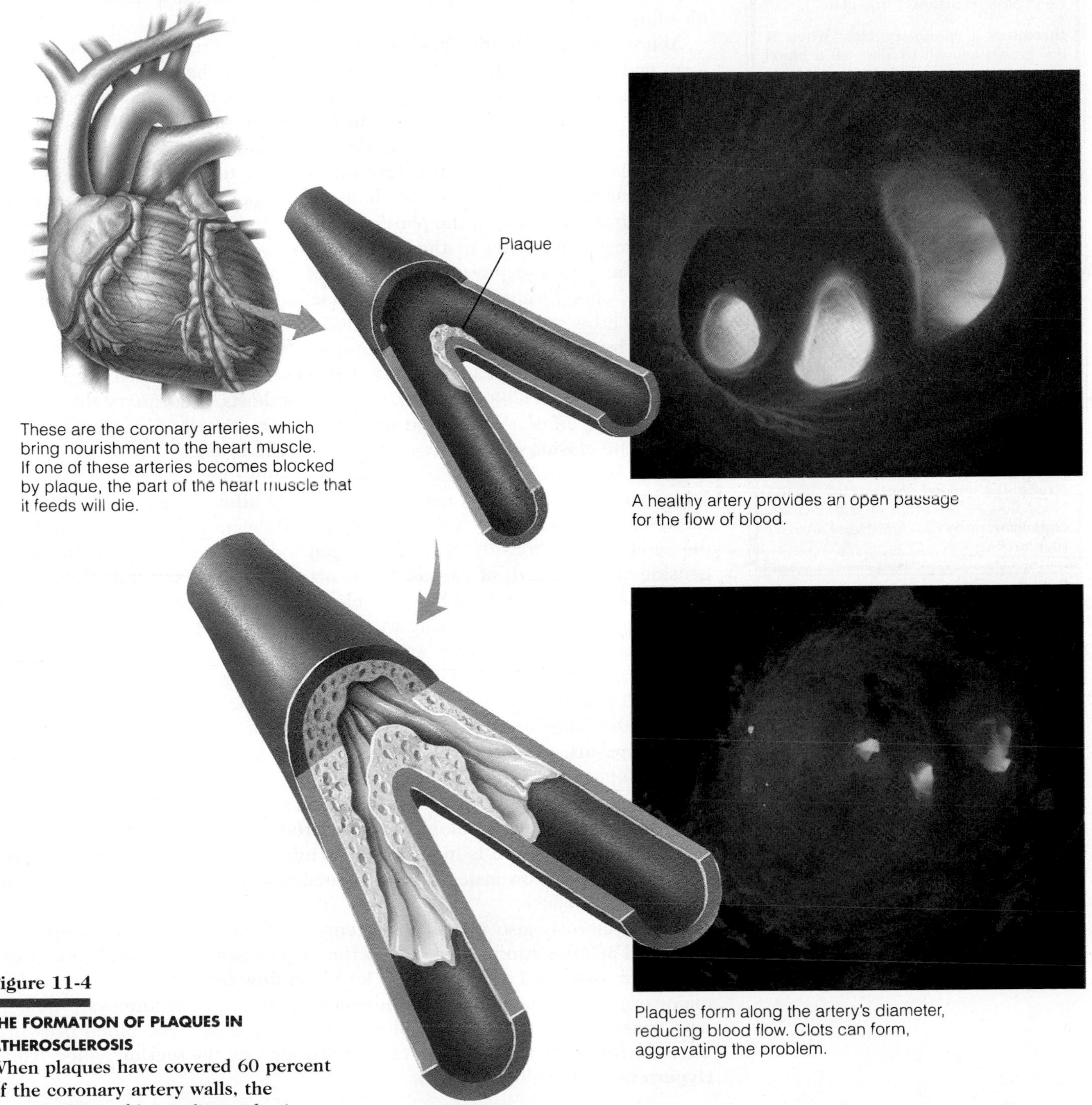

Plaque
These are the coronary arteries, which bring nourishment to the heart muscle. If one of these arteries becomes blocked by plaque, the part of the heart muscle that it feeds will die.
A healthy artery provides an open passage for the flow of blood.
Plaques form along the artery's diameter, reducing blood flow. Clots can form, aggravating the problem.

Figure 11-4

THE FORMATION OF PLAQUES IN ATHEROSCLEROSIS

When plaques have covered 60 percent of the coronary artery walls, the critical phase of heart disease begins.

aneurysm (AN-you-rism) the ballooning out of an artery wall at a point where it has been weakened by deterioration.

aorta (ay-OR-tuh) the large, primary artery that conducts blood from the heart to the body's smaller arteries.

platelets tiny cell-like fragments in the blood, important in blood clot formation (*platelet* means "little plate").

thrombus a stationary clot. When it has grown enough to close off a blood vessel, it is a *thrombosis.* A *coronary thrombosis* is the closing off of a vessel that feeds the heart muscle. A *cerebral thrombosis* is the closing off of a vessel that feeds the brain [*coronary* means "crowning" (the heart); *thrombo* means "clot"; the *cerebrum* is part of the brain].

embolus (EM-boh-luss) a thrombus that breaks loose. When it causes sudden closure of a blood vessel, it is an *embolism* (*embol* means "to insert").

heart attack the event in which the vessels that feed the heart muscle become closed off by an embolism, thrombus, or other cause with resulting sudden tissue death. A heart attack is also called a *myocardial infarction* (*myo* means "muscle"; *cardial* means "of the heart"; *infarct* means "tissue death").

stroke the sudden shutting off of the blood flow to the brain by a thrombus, embolism, or by the bursting of a vessel (hemorrhage).

Omega-6 and omega-3 fatty acids were described in Chapter 5.

Normally the arteries expand with each heartbeat to accommodate the pulses of blood that flow through them. Arteries hardened and narrowed by plaques cannot expand, so the blood pressure rises. The increased pressure damages the artery walls further and puts a strain on the heart. At damaged points, plaques are especially likely to form; thus the development of atherosclerosis is a self-perpetuating process.

As pressure builds up in an artery, the arterial wall may become weakened and balloon out, forming an **aneurysm.** An aneurysm can burst, and when this happens in a major artery such as the **aorta,** it leads to massive bleeding and death.

Abnormal blood clotting also contributes to life-threatening events. Clots form and dissolve in the blood all the time, and the balance between these processes ensures that clots do no harm. That balance is disturbed in atherosclerosis. Small, cell-like bodies in the blood, known as **platelets,** normally cause clots to form whenever they encounter injuries in blood vessels. In atherosclerosis, the platelets respond this way to plaques and form clots when none are needed. Active products of omega-6 and omega-3 fatty acids help control the action of the platelets, and an imbalance among these compounds may contribute to the formation of clots. Substances released by platelets also may aggravate the growth of plaques.

A clot, once formed, may remain attached to a plaque in an artery and gradually grow until it shuts off the blood supply of that portion of the tissue supplied by the artery. That tissue may die slowly and be replaced by scar tissue. The stationary clot is called a **thrombus.** When it has grown large enough to close off a blood vessel, it is a thrombosis. A coronary thrombosis is the closing off of a vessel that feeds the heart muscle. A cerebral thrombosis is the closing off of a vessel that feeds the brain.

A clot can also break loose, becoming an **embolus,** and travel along the system until it reaches an artery too small to allow its passage. Then the tissues fed by this artery will be robbed of oxygen and nutrients and will die suddenly (embolism). Such a clot can lodge in an artery of the heart, causing sudden death of part of the heart muscle; we say that the person has had a **heart attack.** When the clot lodges in an artery of the brain, killing a portion of brain tissue, we call the event a **stroke.**

On many occasions heart attacks and strokes occur with no apparent blockage. An artery may go into spasms, restricting or cutting off the blood supply to a portion of the heart muscle or brain. Much research today is devoted to finding out what causes plaques to form, what causes arteries to go into spasms, what governs the activities of platelets, and why the body allows clots to form unopposed by clot-dissolving cleanup activity.

Hypertension makes atherosclerosis worse. A stiffened artery, already strained by each pulse of blood surging through it, is more greatly stressed if the internal pressure is high. Lesions (injured places) develop more frequently, plaques grow faster, and weakened vessels are more likely to burst, causing hemorrhage.

Atherosclerosis also makes hypertension worse. As already mentioned, hardened arteries cannot expand, so the heart's beats raise the blood pressure. Also, hardened arteries fail to let blood flow freely through the body's major organs in charge of controlling blood pressure—the kidneys. The kidneys sense the reduced flow of blood and respond as if the blood pressure were too low; they take steps to raise it further (see the section called "How Hypertension Develops," later).

KEY POINT Plaques of atherosclerosis induce hypertension and trigger abnormal blood clotting, leading to heart attacks or strokes. Heart attacks and strokes can also be caused by abnormal vessel spasms.

Risk Factors for CVD

Risk Factors for CVD:

- Smoking
- Hypertension
- High blood cholesterol, high LDL, and/or low HDL
- Obesity, especially central obesity, as described in Chapter 9
- Glucose intolerance (diabetes)
- Lack of exercise
- Stress
- Heredity (history of CVD in family members younger than 55 years of age)
- Gender (being male)
- Menopause in women

The risk factors for CVD are listed in the margin. It befits a nutrition book to focus on dietary strategies to reduce them. It should be noted, though, that diet is not the only, and perhaps not even the most important, factor in the causation of CVD. In fact, among the many controversies over diet and nutrition in recent years, one of the noisiest ones has been over the questions of how important diet is in heart disease; whether changes in diet can reduce the risk; and if so, whether such changes should be advocated for everyone or just for selected high-risk individuals.

The big *diet-related* risk factors for CVD are glucose intolerance and obesity, high blood cholesterol (to be discussed here), and hypertension (the subject of the next section). The standards by which these and other risk factors are evaluated are shown in Table 11-4 on the next page. Table 11-4 divides cholesterol and LDL cholesterol values into three groups: desirable, borderline high, and high. Almost half of all deaths from CVD occur among men with blood cholesterol in the borderline-high range, so it would be a serious mistake to consider all but the highest values as "safe." Generally, cholesterol carried in LDL correlates *directly* with risk of heart disease, whereas that carried in HDL correlates *inversely* with risk (see Figure 11-5).[22] Even in young men, high cholesterol values seem to correlate strongly with a high risk of heart disease as they get older.[23] As for the triglyceride value listed in the table, this measurement is often elevated in people with CVD. By themselves, elevated triglycerides are not considered causal in CVD, but high triglycerides may increase atherosclerosis and clotting activity while decreasing clot destruction in the blood. To people with other risk factors for CVD, such as diabetes, central obesity, artery disease, hypertension, or kidney disease, triglyceride measures become more meaningful.[24]

Other factors now beginning to take on importance in CVD research are the antioxidant nutrients and nonnutrients in foods. Information about these, along with a few other lifestyle factors appear later in this section.

Figure 11-5

HDL AND LDL RATIO AND RISK OF HEART DISEASE

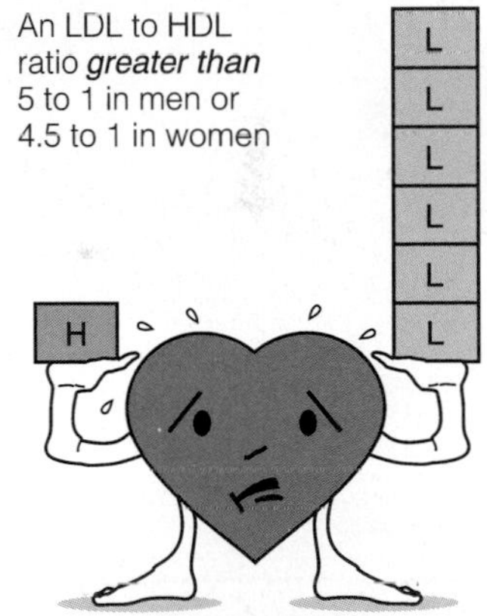

Increased risk of heart disease

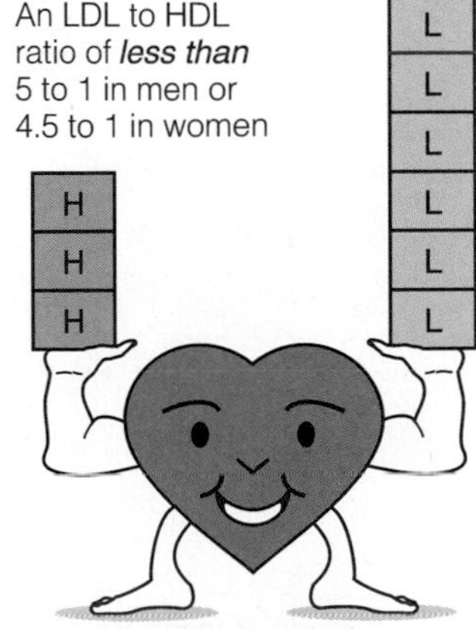

Reduced risk of heart disease

Blood Cholesterol High *blood* cholesterol, particularly when the ratio of LDL to HDL is high, predicts CVD. A population with average blood cholesterol 10 percent lower than another will suffer one-third less CVD; a 30-percent difference in blood cholesterol predicts a rate of CVD that is lower by four times.[25] Now, how does *diet* relate to high blood cholesterol? The currently accepted hypothesis has two parts: (1) that high blood cholesterol is at least partly caused by a diet high in saturated fat; and (2) that reducing the saturated fat in the diet will lower blood cholesterol and will reduce the rate of CVD.

Both parts of this hypothesis have some strong support. Regarding the first part, wherever in the world diets are high in saturated fat, blood cholesterol is high and heart disease takes a great toll on health and life.[26] Conversely, wherever dietary fat consists mostly of monounsaturated fats, blood cholesterol and the rate of death from heart disease are low.

The second part of the hypothesis, that lowering saturated fat intakes will lead to lower blood cholesterol and reduced heart disease risks, is well-

Table 11-4
Standards for CVD Risk Factors

Blood Pressure	Obesity
Diastolic pressure[a]: 85 or lower = normal. 85 to 89 = high normal. 90 to 99 = mild hypertension. 100 to 109 = moderate hypertension. 110 to 119 = severe hypertension. 120 or higher = very severe hypertension.	Body mass index: Men: greater than 27.8 Women: greater than 27.3.
Total Cholesterol	**Lipid Profile and Ratio**
Below 200 mg/dL = desirable.[b] 200 to 239 mg/dL = borderline high. 240 mg/dL or higher = high.	HDL: 35 mg/dL or lower indicates risk.[c] LDL to HDL ratio > 5 for men, or 4.5 for women indicates risk.
LDL Cholesterol	**Triglycerides (Fasting)[d]**
Below 130 mg/dL = desirable. 130 to 159 mg/dL = borderline high. 160 mg/dL or higher = high.	> 200 mg/dL may indicate risk in those with other risk factors (see text).

[a]The diastolic pressure is the lower of the two numbers in the blood pressure reading—for example, the 70 in 105/70.

[b]210–215 = average (U.S.).

[c]According to the 1993 NIH consensus conference on triglyceride, high-density lipoprotein, and CHD, this value may be too low for women; no alternative value has yet been proposed.

[d]High triglycerides do not normally indicate direct risk, but may reflect lipoprotein abnormalities associated with CVD. High triglycerides also occur in conditions such as kidney disease and diabetes, which suggest a high CVD risk.

Source: Blood lipid standards adapted from summary of the second report of the National Cholesterol Education Program (NCEP), Expert Panel on Detection, Evaluation, and Treatment of High Blood Cholesterol in Adults (Adult Treatment Panel), *Journal of the American Medical Association* 269 (1993): 3015–3023. Hypertension standards adapted from the fifth report of the Joint National Committee on Detection, Evaluation, and Treatment of High Blood Pressure, National High Blood Pressure Education Program, National Heart, Lung, and Blood Institute, National Institutes of Health, October 30, 1992, p. 5.

accepted by most authorities, and is supported by the bulk of research.[27] Most agree that for people living in the United States and Canada, the percentage of calories from saturated fat in the diet should be not more than 10 percent.[28]

Recommendations for U.S. and Canadian citizens also urge that *total* fat be held to no more than 30 percent of calories, and that the cholesterol intake from food be limited to 300 milligrams a day. These measures may be important for some people; but perhaps not for all. The links between total fat and dietary cholesterol on the one hand, and blood cholesterol (and CVD) on the other, are not as firm as those between saturated fat, blood cholesterol, and CVD. Data on the people of Greece, France, and other Mediterranean countries illustrate that diets high in total fat can coexist with low rates of heart disease. The key difference between their high-fat diets and those of U.S. and Canadian people's high-fat diets seems to be that theirs are high in monounsaturated, rather than saturated, fats.

More about the Mediterranean diets in Controversy 2.

A valid question is whether Mediterranean peoples may be more naturally resistant to heart disease, but research has shown that this is not the case. People who move from one place to another and who adopt the dietary habits of the new location demonstrate heart disease rates typical of people born in the new location.[29] Other factors may, however, explain the Mediterranean people's low heart disease rates. They are more physically active than people in the United States and Canada. They also consume more fruits and vegetables, less meat and animal fat, more olive oil, and a greater percentage of each day's calories early in the day. Don't discount the effects of meal timing on heart disease risk, by the way. A small but significant improvement in blood lipids is seen in those with a meal pattern of taking frequent small meals each day, rather than the standard few large meals.[30]

Other dietary factors that can lower blood cholesterol, already mentioned in previous chapters, are soluble fiber and omega-3 fatty acids. Exercise also helps.

Many aspects of life probably affect heart health. But blood cholesterol was supposed to be this section's topic. To return to the main points: (1) high blood cholesterol indicates a risk of heart disease, and (2) it is possible to lower blood cholesterol, in part, by controlling dietary saturated fat. Theoretically, if people lower their blood cholesterol, they will reduce their risks of heart disease.

foam cells immune cells that contain scavenged oxidized LDL cholesterol, and which are believed to stimulate plaque formation and the development of atherosclerosis.

Antioxidant Nutrients and Nonnutrients Some recent findings suggest that the antioxidant nutrients, including vitamins C and E, beta carotene (the vitamin A precursor), and the mineral selenium, may play direct roles in defending the body against CVD. Researchers are searching for the mechanism by which antioxidants may act. To date, their findings linking antioxidants and CVD are interesting, although tentative and preliminary.

Chapter 7 presents more information about antioxidant nutrients.

A connection between oxidation of body compounds and CVD seems to center on the long-known heart molesters, LDL. When oxygen attacks the LDL, their cholesterol becomes oxidized and is scavenged by the immune system's white blood cells.* Once full of oxidized cholesterol, the cells are known as **foam cells.** Foam cells stick to the internal linings of the arteries, the first step in the formation of arterial plaques.[31]

In theory, if LDL are protected from oxidation, fewer foam cells will form, less injury of arterial walls will occur, and fewer plaques will result. Vitamin E is a well-known player in protecting body lipids from oxidation, and selenium works by its side on the task. Research suggests similar cooperation between vitamins E and C.

Regardless of mechanism, evidence suggests a negative correlation between vitamin E, vitamin C, and beta carotene levels in the blood and incidences of heart disease.[32] The lower the intakes of the vitamins, the higher the risks of heart disease. Studies of thousands of people all over the world follow this trend: when diets are rich in vegetables and fruits, life expectancies are long and heart disease incidence is low. One study considered 16 European regions in which rates of death from heart disease varied sixfold—the lowest rate was just one-sixth as high as the highest rate. They measured blood vitamin E and cholesterol, and the blood pressures of men from each region. Those men with the lowest vitamin E concentrations in their blood had the highest rates of death from heart disease. A study of 90,000 U.S. female nurses and a related study of 40,000 male health care

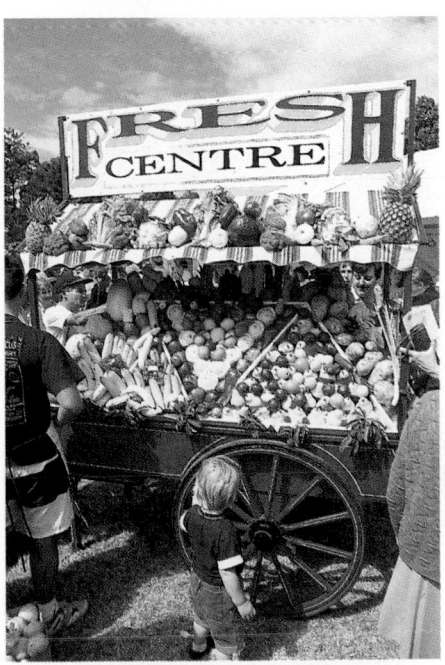

When diets are rich in vegetables and fruits, life expectancies are long.

*The white blood cells that scavenge oxidized LDL are macrophages.

professionals were already mentioned in Chapter 7. They found that daily consumption of self-chosen vitamin E capsules over two years cut heart disease risks by 40 percent compared to controls.[33] Another report suggests that stroke victims with high serum vitamin A concentrations may be less likely to die or to suffer lasting consequences of stroke than those with lower values.[34] All of these studies are of one kind—epidemiological studies—whose results are strictly limited to correlations. They can never show cause and effect. As you read this sentence, laboratories across the globe are working on placebo-controlled studies to provide confirmation of the idea that antioxidant vitamins are protective.

Experts are also calling for long-term effectiveness and safety studies so that valid recommendations concerning supplement use in disease prevention may be possible.[35] Their findings are anxiously awaited.

As for selenium, many studies implicate low blood levels of a selenium-containing enzyme in risk of atherosclerosis.[36] The enzyme is active against the oxidation of lipids thought to be instrumental in heart disease. A form of heart disease is prevalent in areas of the world where selenium is lacking in the soil and diet, and other links exist between low selenium in the blood and heart-disease risks. Selenium is toxic at intakes of just twice the RDA, so supplements of selenium are not recommended. People in the United States probably receive more than enough selenium.

For those tempted to think in terms of supplements for disease prevention, a word of caution: stay conscious of the preliminary nature of these findings and give science the time it needs to prove or refute them. Even if the nutrients are proved effective against heart disease, supplements may not turn out to be the best way to obtain vitamin E and other antioxidant nutrients.

Chemicals other than nutrients in foods, the nonnutrients first introduced in Chapter 1, oftentimes act as drugs in the body. In foods, the chemicals may impart flavor or color, but in the body they have physiological effects. Technically, the definition of a drug is "a substance with a physiological effect," so these compounds in food can be considered to be drugs. This is true even though, in many cases, their individual identities are not known and they make their presence apparent only as "something in the food." For example, garlic and related plants contain a substance thought to exert an anticlotting effect on the blood; hot peppers contain another such substance. More research into these effects is needed. Some other nonnutrients also may be linked to cancer prevention, as discussed later in the section "How Cancer Develops."

Other Strategies for Reducing Risk of CVD In addition to diet, some types of exercise are effective in lowering LDL and in raising HDL concentrations. Particularly *aerobic* exercise, when combined with a low-fat diet, may help to reverse atherosclerosis. There is some evidence to suggest that some forms of weight training also may elevate blood HDL concentrations somewhat, if undertaken regularly.[37] Even light exercise, such as walking and gardening at intervals throughout the day improves the odds against heart disease considerably if consistently pursued. The beneficial effects of exercise on HDL are twofold. Both exercise itself and the weight loss it induces raise HDL concentrations, and the effects of these two factors are *additive.* And when exercise brings about reduction of central obesity, it is especially beneficial. Central obesity is considered by many experts to be the most important single determinant of CVD risk.[38]

Central obesity reflects accumulation of fat in the abdominal region. See Chapter 9 for details.

People ask whether moderate intakes of alcohol may reduce CVD risk. Some studies from the late 1980s compared moderate drinkers with alcohol abstainers and seemed to show that moderate alcohol consumption correlated with significantly reduced heart disease incidence. Moderate alcohol intakes have also been shown to elevate a form of HDL in the blood. Questions have been raised since that time, though, in a report by the World Health Organization.[39] The report asserts that the association between CVD risk and abstinence from alcohol "can be partly or wholly explained by the inclusion in the group of abstainers, or ex-drinkers, who had stopped drinking for health reasons." In other words, people who had sustained damage to the body from alcoholism and a lifetime of heavy drinking were included in the "non-drinkers" data, and may have skewed the average by being counted as abstainers. Heavy alcohol use and abuse is known to elevate blood pressure, to damage the heart muscle, and to have many other deleterious effects on the body's organs. More details about all of these effects are in this chapter's Controversy.

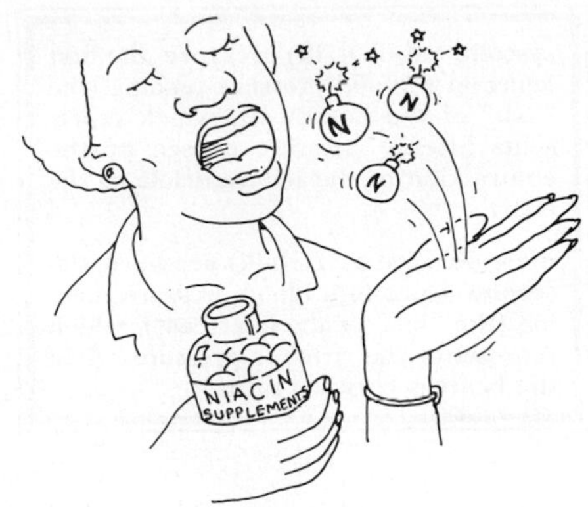

High doses of niacin may cause unexpected side effects.

Periodically, the media repopularize the idea that the vitamin niacin can lower blood cholesterol. Experimentally, pharmaceutical doses of a form of niacin act like a drug in lowering blood cholesterol and prolonging life, but other drugs are also effective for this purpose and have fewer side effects.[40] Regular niacin supplements are useless in lowering blood cholesterol, and in high doses may cause side effects in some people such as skin flushing, abnormal liver function, and some symptoms of diabetes.

While diet and exercise are not the easy route to heart health that everyone hopes for, the combination will do a lot for health in general. Weight control may not reduce blood cholesterol, but it may reduce blood pressure (see next section). So will eating a low-fat, restricted-cholesterol, high complex-carbohydrate diet.[41] * And even if the high-complex-carbohydrate diet does not help by way of lowering cholesterol or blood pressure, it will help by normalizing blood glucose (diabetes). Remember, diabetes is itself a major risk factor for CVD. Meals of low-fat fish may also help by favoring the right fatty acid balance so that clot formation is unlikely. The pattern of protection from the recommended diet and exercise regimen becomes clear—the effects of each small choice add to the beneficial whole. While you are at it, don't smoke. Relax. Meditate or pray. Play. Happy people have lower blood cholesterol levels.

KEY POINT Dietary measures to reduce saturated fat and cholesterol intakes are the first line of treatment for high blood cholesterol. Antioxidant nutrients are also important; so are exercise, moderate alcohol intakes, and a healthy diet in general.

◆ Nutrition and Hypertension

Anyone concerned with the risk of cardiovascular disease that atherosclerosis presents must also be concerned about high blood pressure. The two together are a threatening combination. You cannot tell if you have high blood pressure; it presents no symptoms you can feel. But if you do have it, it threatens to impair the quality of your life and even strike you down

*Dr. Ornish, cited here, reports some success with a comprehensive on-site plan combining an extremely low-fat (<10% of calories) vegan diet, no cigarette smoking, stress management training, and moderate exercise for reversing established heart disease without drugs.

systolic (sis-TOL-ik) **pressure** the first figure in a blood pressure reading (the "dub" of the heartbeat), which represents arterial pressure caused by the contraction of the left ventricle of the heart.

diastolic (dye-as-TOL-ik) **pressure** the second figure in a blood pressure reading (the "lub" of the heartbeat), which represents the arterial pressure when the heart is between beats.

before your time. Chronic high blood pressure, or hypertension, is the most prevalent form of cardiovascular disease, believed to affect some 60 million people in the United States—more than a third of the entire adult population.[42] It contributes to half a million strokes and to over a million heart attacks each year. The higher above normal the blood pressure, the greater the risk of heart disease. Except in extreme cases, low blood pressure is generally a sign of long life expectancy and low heart disease risk.

The most effective single step you can take toward protecting yourself from hypertension is to find out whether you have it. At checkup time, a health care professional can give you an accurate resting blood pressure reading. Self-test machines in drugstores and other places are often inaccurate. If your resting blood pressure is above normal, the reading should be repeated before confirming the diagnosis of hypertension. Thereafter it should be checked at regular intervals. When blood pressure is measured, two numbers are important: the pressure during contraction of the heart's ventricles (large pumping chambers) and the pressure during ventricular relaxation. The numbers are given as a fraction, with the top number representing the **systolic pressure** (ventricular contraction) and the bottom number the **diastolic pressure** (ventricular relaxation). Return to Table 11-4 to see how to interpret your resting diastolic pressure.

Resting blood pressure should ideally be 120 over 80 or lower. However, it is generally considered normal if it is less than 140 over 90. Above this level the risks of heart attacks and strokes increase in direct proportion to increasing diastolic blood pressure.

KEY POINT Hypertension is silent, progressively worsens atherosclerosis, and makes heart attacks and strokes likely. All adults should know their blood pressure.

How Hypertension Develops

Blood pressure is vital to life. It pushes the blood through the major arteries into smaller arteries and finally into tiny capillaries whose thin walls permit exchange of fluids between the blood and the tissues (see Figure 11-6). When the pressure is right, the cells receive a constant supply of nutrients and oxygen and are relieved of their wastes.

The kidneys depend on the blood pressure to help them filter waste materials out of the blood into the urine. (The pressure has to be high enough to force the blood's fluid out of the capillaries into the kidney's filtering networks.) If the blood pressure is too low, the kidneys set in motion actions to increase it; they release hormones into the bloodstream to constrict the peripheral blood vessels and to lead to the retention of water and salt in the body.

When dehydration sets these actions in motion, they are beneficial, because when the blood volume is low, higher blood pressure is needed to deliver substances to the tissues. By constricting the blood vessels and conserving water and sodium, the kidneys ensure that normal blood pressure is maintained until the dehydrated person can drink water. Atherosclerosis also sets this process in motion, however, and this is not beneficial. Atherosclerosis, by obstructing blood vessels, fools the kidneys: they react as if there were a water deficiency. The kidneys raise the blood pressure high enough so that they will get the blood they need, but in the process they may make the pressure too high for the arteries and heart to withstand. As

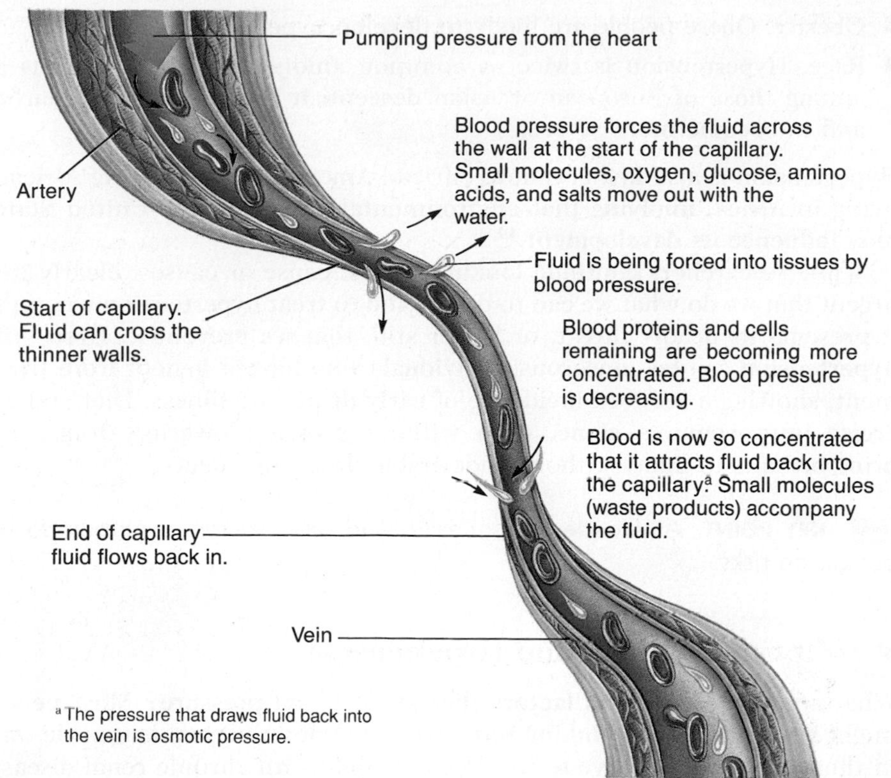
Pumping pressure from the heart
Blood pressure forces the fluid across the wall at the start of the capillary. Small molecules, oxygen, glucose, amino acids, and salts move out with the water.
Artery
Fluid is being forced into tissues by blood pressure.
Start of capillary. Fluid can cross the thinner walls.
Blood proteins and cells remaining are becoming more concentrated. Blood pressure is decreasing.
Blood is now so concentrated that it attracts fluid back into the capillary.[a] Small molecules (waste products) accompany the fluid.
End of capillary fluid flows back in.
Vein
[a] The pressure that draws fluid back into the vein is osmotic pressure.

Figure 11-6

THE BLOOD PRESSURE

Three major factors contribute to the pressure inside an artery. One is that the heart pushes blood into the artery. Another is that the small-diameter arteries and capillaries at the other end resist the blood's flow (peripheral resistance). The third determining factor is the volume of fluid in the circulatory system, which depends in turn on the number of dissolved particles in that fluid.

mentioned earlier, hypertension aggravates atherosclerosis by mechanically injuring the artery linings, making plaques likely to form; plaques block blood flow to the kidneys; this may raise the blood pressure still further; and the problem snowballs.

Obesity makes hypertension still worse. Added adipose tissue means miles of extra capillaries through which the blood must be pumped. The threatening combination of hypertension, atherosclerosis, obesity, and insulin resistance so frequently occurs together that the group is considered to be a distinct condition in itself.* Called "the soil from which both type II diabetes and cardiovascular disease spring," the condition puts a severe strain on the heart and arteries, leading to many forms of cardiovascular disease and often to death.[43] Strain on the heart's pump, the left ventricle, can enlarge and weaken it, until finally it fails (heart failure). Pressure in the aorta may cause it to balloon out and burst (aneurysm). Pressure in the small arteries of the brain may make them burst and bleed (hemorrhage, a form of stroke). The kidneys can also be damaged when the heart is unable to adequately pump blood through them (kidney failure).

Epidemiological studies have identified several risk factors that predict the development of hypertension, including:

- Age. Blood pressure levels increase with age; most people who develop hypertension do so in their 50s and 60s.
- Family background. A family history of hypertension and heart disease raises the risk of developing hypertension two to five times.

*The combination of hypertension, atherosclerosis, obesity, and insulin resistance is sometimes referred to as "Syndrome X."

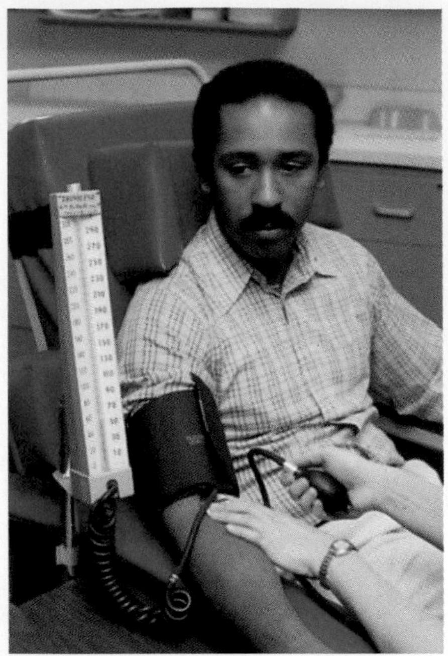

The most effective single step you can take against hypertension is to learn your own blood pressure.

- Obesity. Obese people are likely to develop hypertension.
- Race. Hypertension is twice as common among African Americans as among those of European or Asian descent; it tends to develop earlier and to become more severe.

Hypertension is also higher among African Americans than among Africans living in Africa, implying that environmental factors in the United States may influence its development.[44]

While researchers continue looking for the cause or causes, clearly it is urgent that we do what we can to detect and to treat hypertension wherever it presents its deadly threat, or better still, that we prevent it. Even mild hypertension can be dangerous; individuals who have it benefit from treatment, showing a reduced incidence of early death and illness. Diet and exercise improvements alone, even without pressure-lowering drugs, can bring benefits to many without undesirable drug side effects.

KEY POINT Atherosclerosis, obesity, and other factors contribute to hypertension risks.

Weight Control, Diet, and Hypertension

What are the diet-related factors that affect blood pressure? Most people might respond "salt" (thinking sodium), but sodium plays a large role only in those who are sensitive to its effects. People with chronic renal disease, those whose parents (one or both) have hypertension, African Americans, and persons over 50 years of age are most likely to be sodium or salt sensitive, and for them, salt avoidance prevents hypertension. For others—the majority of people with hypertension—it may be ineffective. Salt restriction fails to lower the blood pressure in about half of the hypertensive people in whom it is tried. It is important to look further to see what other dietary factors might be relevant. Many other factors are suspect, and among them, two are weighty—obesity and alcohol intake. A sedentary lifestyle and some nutrients other than sodium also play roles.

Details concerning sodium, salt, and hypertension were presented in Chapter 8.

Weight Control and Physical Activity Evidence supports a positive link between obesity and hypertension. For people who are obese and hypertensive, even a loss of just 10 pounds may significantly lower blood pressure.[45] Those who are using drugs to control their blood pressure can often reduce or discontinue use of them if they lose weight. Weight loss alone may be one of the most effective nondrug treatments for hypertension. Moderate physical activity of the right kind helps in weight loss and also helps to reduce hypertension directly. Although blood pressure rises temporarily at each bout of exercise, the effect in the long run is to lower the resting blood pressure significantly.[46]

The "right kind" of activity is the same kind observed to increase blood HDL and lower LDL, that is, the kind recommended for cardiovascular endurance (Chapter 10 provides details). Physical activity also changes the hormonal climate in which the body does its work. It alters stress hormone secretion and lowers blood pressure. It redistributes body water, and it eases transit of the blood through the peripheral arteries. Physical activity may also stimulate development of new arteries to nourish the heart muscle, and this may be a factor in the excellent recovery seen in some heart attack victims who exercise.

Alcohol In moderate doses, alcohol initially reduces pressure in the peripheral arteries and so reduces blood pressure, but high doses clearly raise blood pressure. Hypertension is common in people with alcoholism. The hypertension is apparently caused directly by the alcohol, and it leads to cardiovascular disease, the same as hypertension caused by any other factor. Furthermore, alcohol causes strokes—even *without* hypertension. The Surgeon General's advice on alcohol use is straightforward: if you drink, do so in moderation. *Moderation* means 1 to 2 drinks a day, not more. The current *Dietary Guidelines* do not recommend the use of alcohol at all; for those who do drink, the *Guidelines* recommend limiting daily intake to 1 ounce of pure alcohol, the equivalent of 2 drinks.

Potassium Some authorities believe that adequate potassium might help both to prevent and to treat hypertension.* Even in people without high blood pressure, potassium added to the diet in amounts equivalent to that in a serving or two of fruits and vegetables has been associated with reduced risk of stroke, so potassium in the diet seems worthy of attention.[47] People who eat many foods high in salt often happen to be eating fewer potassium-containing foods at the same time. Table 8-5 in Chapter 8 showed that as the *same* food goes through several processing steps, it loses potassium and gains sodium, so that its potassium-to-sodium ratio falls dramatically. Sodium avoidance may help in two ways, by reducing blood pressure in salt-sensitive individuals and by indirectly raising potassium intakes in people who replace processed foods with whole foods. As the next paragraphs show, calcium helps in a similar way.

Calcium Several surveys report that people with hypertension consume less calcium than those with normal blood pressure.[48] Researchers estimate that people with the lowest calcium intakes (below 300 milligrams per day) have a two to three times greater risk of developing hypertension than people with the highest calcium intakes (1,200 milligrams per day).

Calcium may be important in both prevention and treatment of hypertension. One study showed that a calcium-rich diet reduced blood pressure, even in some people with normal blood pressure. It is recommended, therefore, that people with hypertension or those who are at risk of developing it *at least* meet the current RDA for calcium—800 to 1,200 milligrams a day for adults. Milk products are recommended because they provide not only calcium but potassium and magnesium, which may also help keep blood pressure normal. Low-fat or nonfat milk products are most beneficial because the saturated fat of whole milk may worsen atherosclerosis, a risk factor for hypertension.

Salt The role of salt in *treatment* of hypertension is not questioned. For the salt-sensitive person, it is effective to reduce salt intake. As for diet in *prevention* of hypertension, there is less agreement, but many professionals and agencies believe that enough evidence is available to warrant a recommendation to the general public to moderately restrict salt intake (the Chapter 8 Food Feature showed how). They reason that, at worst, such a diet cannot be harmful. The Food Feature of this chapter provides more detail on dietary measures that help support normal blood pressure.

---

*People using diuretics to control hypertension should know that some cause potassium excretion and can induce a deficiency. Those using these drugs must be particularly careful to include rich sources of potassium in their daily diets.

cancer a disease in which cells multiply out of control and disrupt normal functioning of one or more organs.

carcinogen (car-SIN-oh-jen) a cancer-causing substance (*carcin* means "cancer"; *gen* means "gives rise to").

initiation an event, probably in the cell's genetic material, caused by radiation or by a chemical carcinogen that can give rise to cancer.

promoters factors that do not initiate cancer but that favor its development once the initiating event has taken place.

Other Factors Research is continuing to reveal relationships of other factors to hypertension. For example, adequate (but not excessive) magnesium seems to protect against it. Magnesium deficiency may make the walls of arteries and capillaries more likely to constrict, thus raising blood pressure.[49] Since hypertension may also be an insulin-resistant state, it is possible that measures to prevent diabetes can also protect against hypertension. Other substances may affect blood pressure in one way or another: roles for cadmium, selenium, lead, caffeine, protein, fat, and, as mentioned, the hormone insulin are currently under study.

KEY POINT For most people, weight reduction, exercise, restricted alcohol use, and a diet that provides adequate nutrients work to keep blood pressure normal. For some, salt restriction is also required.

Nutrition and Cancer

In this country, one out of every four people will eventually contract **cancer;** estimates state that up to 40 percent of cancers in men, and up to 60 percent in women are attributable to diet.[50] Dietary fat is thought to be especially important in relation to cancer, but diet relates to cancer in several ways. It is important to get them all in perspective. Constituents in foods may be cancer causing, cancer promoting, or protective against cancer. Also, for the person who has cancer, diet can make a crucial difference in recovery.

Of course nondiet factors are also important in relation to cancer. A very few cancers are genetic and will appear regardless of lifestyle choices. For other cancers, environmental factors other than diet are involved, including smoking, sun exposure, and water and air pollution. The emphasis here is on diet, of course.

How Cancer Develops

The steps in cancer development are thought to be as follows:

1. Exposure to a **carcinogen.**
2. Entry of the carcinogen into a cell.
3. **Initiation,** probably by the carcinogen's somehow altering the cellular genetic material.
4. Enhancement of cancer development by **promoters,** probably involving several more steps before the cell begins to multiply out of control.
5. Disruption of normal body functions.

Researchers think that the first three steps, which culminate with initiation, are the key ones, so people have the idea that they should therefore learn to avoid eating foods that contain carcinogens. This would be an impossible feat, considering that most carcinogens are natural food constituents found in minute amounts among thousands of other chemicals and nutrients the body needs. Luckily, the body is well equipped to deal with the tiny levels of naturally-occurring carcinogens in foods. Many people suspect food additives of being carcinogenic. However, food additives are held to such strict standards concerning carcinogenic properties that no additive legally in food has any proven ability to cause cancer. (Details concerning saccharin are found in Controversy 4.) Contaminants that enter foods by accident, on the other hand, may be powerful carcinogens, or they may be converted to carcinogens by the body's attempts to metabolize them.[51]

Chapter 14 comes back to the topics of accidental industrial contamination of foods, but you should know now that legal pesticides, when used according to established guidelines, are believed to pose few health risks to healthy adult consumers.[52] The most likely role for food itself in the causation of cancer is not that of initiation, but of promotion. Prudence dictates, however, that consumers should wash produce thoroughly before cooking or eating it.

The incidence of certain cancers varies both by geographical area and by racial group. For example, Japanese people living in Japan develop more stomach cancers and fewer colon cancers than people in the United States. However, when Japanese people come to the United States, their children develop both stomach and colon cancers at rates like those of native-born U.S. citizens. Japan and the United States are both industrial countries, and their environmental pollution rates are similar. However, something in the environment must account for the changed cancer pattern in immigrants, and an obvious candidate is diet. The traditional Japanese diet is rich in vegetables and low in fat, two characteristics of diets associated with low colon-cancer rates. The Japanese diet also contains numerous salted and pickled foods associated with stomach cancer. Traditional Japanese foods are not widely available in the United States, however, so immigrants shift their diets to those more typical of U.S. choices. This is probably how they incur the U.S. cancer-risk profile.

Another finding is that vegetarians have lower mortality rates from cancer than the rest of the population, even when cancers linked to smoking and alcohol are taken out of the picture. In general, studies of populations have suggested that low cancer rates correlate with high vegetable and grain intakes. Case-control studies, in which researchers can control some of the variables, have supported the population studies, and they implicate fat in cancer causation.

Selected naturally occurring chemicals and carcinogens in breakfast foods:

Coffee:
acetaldehyde, acetic acid, acetone, atractylosides, butanol, cafestol palmitate, chlorogenic acid, dimethyl sulfide, ethanol, furfural, furan, guaiacol, hydrogen sulfide, isoprene, kahweal palmitate, methanol, methyl butanol, methyl formate, methyl glyoxal, propionaldehyde, pyridine, 1,3,7-trimethylxanthine.

Toast and coffee cake:
acetone, acetic acid, butyric acid, caprionic acid, ethyl acetate, ethyl ketone, ethyl lactate, methyl ethyl ketone, propionic acid, valeric acid.

Note: While some of the chemicals listed here are known carcinogens, the body is equipped to handle them safely, so consuming coffee, toast, and coffee cake does not elevate a person's risk of developing cancer.

Cancer and Foods

From the evidence presented so far, it appears likely that diet affects cancer rates in the world's people. The paragraphs that follow describe what is known about the effects of food constituents on cancer development.

Fat and Fatty Acids Laboratory studies using animals confirm suspicions that high fat intakes correlate with cancer. In human beings, diets high in fat and cholesterol have been positively associated with lung cancer risk.[53] Fat does not initiate the cancers, however. To get the tumors started, an experimenter has to expose the animals to a known carcinogen. After that exposure, the high-fat diet makes more cancers develop and makes them develop earlier than do low-fat diets. Thus fat appears to be a cancer promoter rather than an initiator. A high-fat diet may promote cancer in any of a number of ways:

- By causing the body to secrete more of certain hormones, thus creating a climate favorable to the development of certain cancers.
- By promoting the secretion of bile into the intestine. Bile may then be converted by organisms in the colon into compounds that cause cancer.
- By being incorporated into cell membranes and changing them so that they offer less defense against cancer-causing invaders.

It may not be fat in general but certain forms of fat that have these effects but the details from research can be hard to follow. For example, some findings point to linoleic acid, the essential omega-6 fatty acid of vegetable

Chapter 5's Food Feature presents details of cutting fat from the diet, and Figure 5-6 shows the fatty acid breakdown of common fats.

oils, as particularly implicated in promotion of cancer.[54] At the same time, a modified form of linoleic acid found only in food from animal sources seems protective against cancers.[55] * Importantly, it seems that omega-3 fatty acids and monounsaturated fatty acids may not promote cancer, and some preliminary evidence suggests possible protective effects.[56] Meanwhile, moderation remains a sound principle concerning fat intakes.

Alcohol and Smoked Foods Cancers of the head and neck seem to correlate best with the combination of alcohol and tobacco use and with low intakes of green and yellow fruits and vegetables. Alcohol intake alone is associated with cancers of the mouth and throat, and alcoholism often damages the liver and increases the risk of liver cancer. Controversy 11 comes back to the topic of alcoholic beverages and cancer risks.

Smoke generated from burning charcoal, just like smoke from burning tobacco, is made up of a multitude of chemical substances, some of which are carcinogens.** The carcinogens from smoke settle on food during cooking, and more form when fat such as meat drippings or oily marinades land on the coals and vaporize, and then rise to stick to the cooking food. Carcinogens also form when foods are charbroiled over an open flame. Eating the food introduces the carcinogens into the body, but once inside, the compounds are captured and detoxified by the body's competent detoxifying system. No studies to date link the eating of smoked or grilled foods with increased cancer risk.[57] This is probably because the body's detoxifying system steps up its activity in people who eat charcoal-broiled foods and so, successfully defends them against the kinds of carcinogens such foods contain.[58]

Calcium Some evidence suggests that a high-calcium diet may be linked to prevention of colon cancer. In a large, long-term study, people who developed colon cancer consumed slightly less calcium and vitamin D than people who did not develop the cancer. Other studies attempting to confirm the finding have obtained mixed results, but when calcium intakes of populations are compared, the trend becomes apparent. Populations consuming more calcium are seen to develop less colon cancer when researchers account for the effects of dietary fat in the analysis.[59] In animal studies, calcium seems to protect the colon lining from some of the effects of a high-fat diet. These studies are not yet sufficient to conclude that dietary calcium prevents colon cancer, but with all the other points in calcium's favor, prudence dictates that everyone should arrange to meet calcium needs each day.

Fiber A diet containing foods high in fiber also helps protect against some forms of cancer.[60] It may do so by promoting the excretion of bile from the body, by absorbing toxins and carrying them out of the body, or by generating beneficial acidic fragments within the colon. Whereas fiber is especially important for preventing cancers of the colon and rectum, some features of a high-fiber diet other than fiber itself may help fight other forms of cancer.[61] High-fiber diets that are also high in both fat and calories often show no protection against cancer risks.

It may be that the source of fiber may also play a role. In a critical review of studies on high-fiber diets and colon cancer, one research group deter-

---

*The linoleic compound referred to here is known by the acronym CLA for *Conjugated [dienoic derivatives of] Linoleic Acid.*

**The carcinogens of most concern are members of the group known as polycyclic aromatic hydrocarbons.

mined that colon cancer risk was reduced by 40 percent in people with high intakes of grains and vegetables.[62] Researchers are now exploring compounds in these foods other than fiber, and are finding statistical associations with cancer risks; these are described next.

If a fat-rich diet is implicated in causation of certain cancers and if a vegetable-rich diet is associated with prevention, then vegetarians should have a lower incidence of those cancers. They do, as the many studies cited in Controversy 6 have shown.

Folate Cervical cancer is by far the most common cancer among U.S. women, and is also a major health threat for women in the developing world.[63] In this country, 50,000 new cases of cervical cancer are diagnosed each year and even more cases of early cancerous changes known as cell dysplasia are treated each year. The underlying cause of this ailment is an often symptomless sexually transmitted virus, human papilloma virus (HPV). Inadequate folate seems to permit activation of the virus. For this reason alone all sexually active women should attend to their folate needs. Many other reasons were evident in previous chapters.

Antioxidant Nutrients Over 100 studies now concur that plant foods play special roles in cancer resistance. Almost without exception, studies find that infrequent use of green and yellow fruits and vegetables and citrus fruits correlates with cancers of many types.[64] Specifically, infrequent use of cabbage, broccoli, and brussels sprouts is common in colon cancer victims. Stomach cancer, too, correlates with low intakes of vegetables: in one study, vegetables in general; in another, fresh vegetables; in others, lettuce and other fresh greens or vegetables containing vitamin C.

Frequent consumption of green and yellow fruits and vegetables seems protective against cancer of the:

- bladder
- breast
- cervix
- lung
- mouth and throat
- ovaries
- prostate
- stomach.

Antioxidant vitamins are implicated as protective against cancers of the head, neck, lungs, cervix, pancreas, stomach, rectum, colon, ovary, endometrium, breast, and bladder. Fruits and vegetables that contribute beta carotene (the vitamin A precursor) and vitamin E seem to be especially active in this regard.[65]

Oxidation of body compounds was mentioned earlier in relation to atherosclerosis, but its role in cancer causation is a topic of intense study, too. Much research today is focused on the theory that beta carotene, vitamin C, vitamin E, and the mineral selenium can destroy oxygen-derived free radicals and thereby help prevent cells from undergoing cancer-causing changes in their genetic material.[66] The antioxidant nutrients absorb the brunt of oxygen's attack by offering themselves for oxidation, thus sparing the cells any genetic damage.

Antioxidants may play other roles in cancer prevention as well. Vitamin A regulates aspects of cell division and communication that go awry in cancer. It and beta carotene also help to maintain the immune system.[67] Immunity can work even after cancerous changes are under way. Lung cancer incidence can be dramatically lower in people with high beta carotene intakes than in those with low intakes. In Japan, a study of about 300,000 people showed lung cancer rates to be 20 to 30 percent lower in smokers who ate yellow or green vegetables daily than in those who did not.

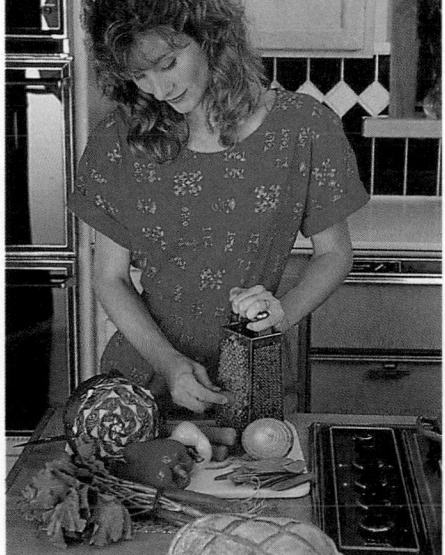

The cook who uses these vegetables and fruits generously is helping to guard against disease.

More work is needed to completely understand these relationships, but many experts are urging everyone to take action now to obtain the recommended five servings of fruits and vegetables daily, and to choose several yellow, orange, or dark green vegetables and fruits each day. Anyone who might be tempted to think that pills containing vitamin A or carotene might provide the same benefit as green and orange vegetables should remember

antipromoters compounds in foods that act in several ways to oppose the formation of cancer.

cruciferous vegetables a group of vegetables named for their cross-shaped blossoms. They have been shown to protect against cancer in laboratory animals. Examples are cauliflower, cabbage, brussels sprouts, broccoli, turnips, and rutabagas.

indoles a family of compounds with a structure resembling that of the amino acid tryptophan, mentioned here because they have anticancer activity.

dithiolthiones a class of compounds, important in connection with diet and cancer because some are found in plant foods and seem to exhibit anticancer activity.

protease inhibitors compounds that inhibit the action of protein-digesting enzymes.

Table 11-5
Cruciferous Vegetables and Carotene-Rich Fruits and Vegetables

Cruciferous Vegetables		Carotene-rich Fruits and Vegetables	
Broccoli	Kale	Apricots	Mango
Brussels sprouts	Kohlrabi	Asparagus	Oriental cabbages
Cabbage (all varieties)	Rutabaga	Broccoli	Papaya
Cauliflower	Turnip roots	Cantaloupe	Parsley
Greens (collards, mustards, turnips)		Carrots	Spinach
		Green onions	Squash (hard, winter)
		Greens (all varieties)	Sweet potato
		Lettuce (dark green)	

the other protective effects of vegetables beyond those of interest here. Other nutrients in vegetables are also cited as possible antipromoters: vitamin B_6, folate, pantothenic acid, vitamin B_{12}, iron, zinc, and more, along with many nonnutrients. The idea that vitamin supplements can provide all the benefits of vegetables is erroneous.

Nonnutrients It seems clear that food contains **antipromoters,** substances that oppose cancer. These nonnutrient, anticancer compounds are worth a moment's attention. Best-known are those in vegetables of the cabbage family—the so-called **cruciferous vegetables.** In these vegetables, **indoles, dithiolthiones** and other chemicals activate enzymes that destroy carcinogens.* The body's toxin-destroying system must be stimulated continually in order to be ready for the day when dangerous agents arrive. In theory, the role of many nonnutrients in cancer prevention may be to stimulate the body's detoxifying system to keep it fine tuned, so to speak, while themselves presenting no hazard to the body.[68] Table 11-5 lists cruciferous vegetables and carotene-rich fruits and vegetables. The photo shows foods rich in antioxidant nutrients and possibly cancer-preventing nonnutrients.

Foods possessing nonnutrient effects under study for disease prevention:
apricots, asparagus, barley, basil, berries, broccoli, brown rice, brussels sprouts, cabbages, cantaloupe, carrots, cauliflower, celery, chives, citrus, cucumber, flax seed, garlic, ginger, green onions, greens, kale, kohlrabi, lettuce (dark), mango, oats, onions, papaya, parsley, parsnips, potatoes, rutabaga, soybeans, spinach, squash (winter), sweet potato, tarragon, tea, thyme, turmeric, turnips, whole wheat.

Another class of possible anticancer compounds occurs in soybeans, chick peas, lima beans, and potatoes. These are **protease inhibitors,** and they are thought to inhibit enzymes associated with the spreading of tumors. Still another nonnutrient of soybeans is believed to block the development of the new blood vessels cancer tissue needs to grow.[69] The pharmaceutical properties of nonnutrients are still theoretical and require much more research to establish solid evidence of their benefits. The margin lists foods of interest with regard to nonnutrients and cancer prevention.[70]

The anticancer constituents of vegetables and fruits are so widespread

*Another such compound, called sulphoraphane, was recently identified in broccoli.

among plants that to try to single out *the* food or two to choose is impossible. The single most valuable application of the information obtained to date is *not* to eat cabbages or soybeans in particular but to eat a wide variety of vegetables and fruits in generous quantities every day.

KEY POINT A high-fat diet is associated with the development of cancer. Fiber; vitamin C; the vitamin A precursor carotene; many other vitamins and minerals; and the nonnutrients found in cruciferous vegetables, greens, and other vegetables are thought to be protective.

FOOD FEATURE

Diet for Disease Prevention

This chapter began with infectious diseases, went on to the major diseases affecting the heart and blood vessels, and concluded with cancer—three apparently dissimilar conditions with apparently distinct sets of causes. Yet all are responsive to diet, and in some ways the responses are similar. Dietary excesses increase the likelihood of all of them: overdoses of vitamins and minerals harm immune function and invite infection; and excess food energy and fat intakes set the stage for heart disease and cancer. Likewise, dietary deficiencies increase the likelihood of all of them, particularly deficiencies in vitamin, mineral, and fiber intakes. Not all diet recommendations apply equally to all of the diseases (salt has a special relationship with hypertension, for example), but fortunately for the consumer, the dietary recommendations to help prevent individual diseases do not contradict each other.

For those who choose to change their diets, the pointers relevant to atherosclerosis in the *Dietary Guidelines* cited in Chapter 2 are repeated here:

- Reduce total fat intake to 30 percent or less of calories. Reduce saturated fat intake to less than 10 percent of calories and the intake of cholesterol to less than 300 milligrams daily.
- Every day eat five or more one-half cup servings of a combination of vegetables and fruits, especially green and yellow vegetables and citrus fruits. Also increase intake of starches and other complex carbohydrates by eating six or more daily servings of a combination of breads, cereals, and legumes. Carbohydrates should total more than 55 percent of calories.
- Maintain protein intake at moderate levels, that is, approximately the current RDA for protein but not exceeding twice that amount or 1.6 grams per kilogram of body weight for adults.
- Balance food intake and physical activity to maintain appropriate body weight.

To keep total fat down, select low-fat foods. If the percentage of calories from fat is to be less than 30 percent, then it is especially important to limit pure fat foods such as sour cream, butter, and margarine; high-fat foods such as mayonnaise, cheese and cream cheese; and foods high in hidden fat such as convenience foods with sauces, fried foods, fat-marbled meat cuts, sausages, ground beef, whole milk, and the many others identified in Chapter 5. For each 1,000 calories of food, 33 grams of fat should be the maximum allowed. Shop for foods whose labels indicate no more than 3 grams of fat per 100 calories.

When you must add fat, use olive oil or canola oil, since these are high in monounsaturated fatty acids, but use them, like all fat, sparingly. Eat meals of fish regularly, especially fatty fish such as salmon, to balance your intakes of omega-6 fatty acids with the omega-3 type. Consult Appendix A, the columns showing fat breakdown, for further details on the fatty acid contents of your favorite foods.

As far as cholesterol is concerned, use eggs in moderation (three to four per week); but unless medically advised to do so, do not shun them altogether. They are an inexpensive source of high-quality protein, and while their yolks are high in cholesterol, they are not as high as was once thought, and they are not high in saturated fat. Feel free to use shellfish occasionally; they are not as high in cholesterol as has been believed, they are low in fat (if not fried), and they do contain beneficial fatty acids. And to help lower blood cholesterol, choose foods high in soluble fiber, such as oats, oat bran, barley, and legumes, as well as fruits and vegetables.

Standard advice to those who wish to correct high blood pressure through diet is to eat less salt. Probably, though, the person wishing to avoid hypertension would benefit from all the recommendations relevant to atherosclerosis and from a serious program of weight control. Expend energy, so as to earn the right to eat more nutrient-dense foods. In other words, be physically active. (If that benefit doesn't motivate you, then exercise to improve your circulation, to reduce your weight, to improve your morale, or to make friends—but do exercise.) Eat foods high in potassium (whole foods), high in calcium and magnesium (milk products and appropriate substitutes), low in fat, and high in fiber (whole grains, legumes, vegetables, fruits). Vary your diet, because not all the factors that affect blood pressure have been studied yet. Use moderation with respect to alcohol.

Many of the dietary guidelines for cancer prevention are identical to those given for CVD prevention, in that they recommend controlling energy and fat intakes, increasing intakes of fruits and vegetables, and limiting intakes of salt-cured products. Two, though, are especially pertinent to cancer prevention—notably those numbered 4 and 6 below:

1. Control total food energy intake.
2. Reduce the consumption of both saturated and unsaturated fats.
3. Include fruits (especially citrus fruits), vegetables (particularly carotene-rich and cruciferous vegetables), and whole-grain products in the daily diet.
4. Do not eat spoiled or moldy food or food that smells or appears old.
5. Consume only moderate amounts of alcohol, if any.
6. Consult your public officials to discover how your drinking water rates for toxic substances. Take action, if necessary, to ensure that your drinking water is safe.

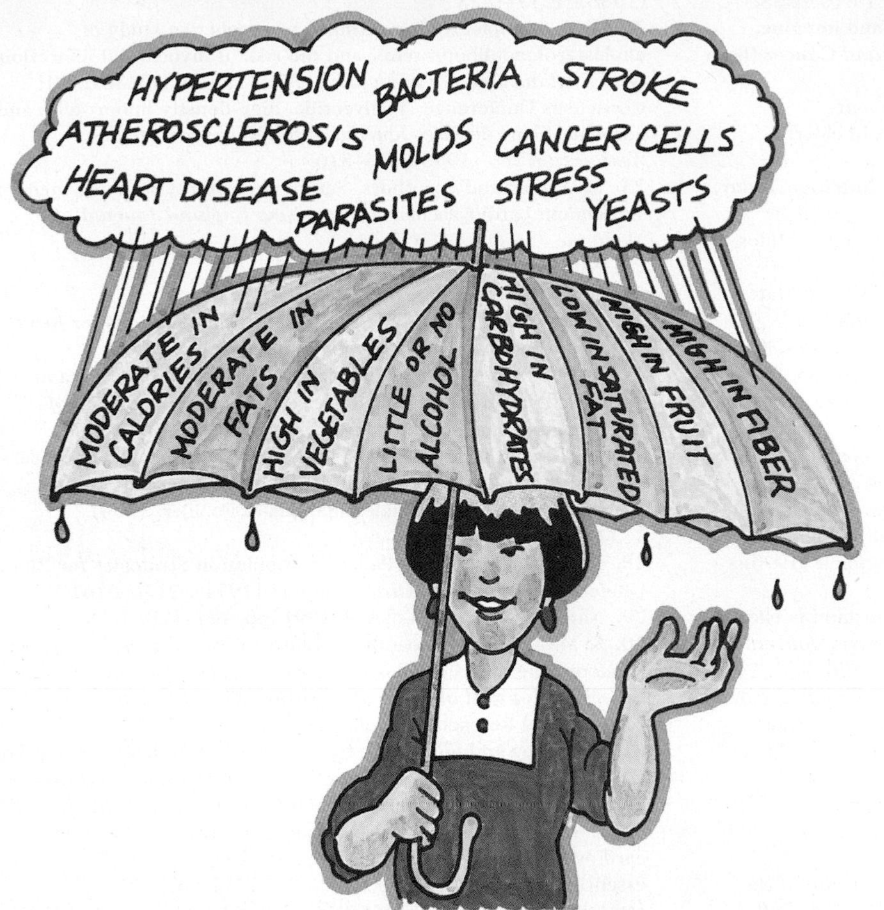

Figure 11-7

PROPER NUTRITION HELPS PROTECT AGAINST DISEASES

A well-nourished, fully functional immune system is best able to ward off infections and cancer, and a well-nourished cardiovascular system often stays healthy when others fail.

Source: Adapted from an idea in R. K. Chandra, 1990 McCollum Award Lecture: Nutrition and immunity: lessons from the past and new insights into the future, *American Journal of Clinical Nutrition* 53 (1991): 1087–1101.

To the recommendations made in these guidelines, we would add one other already mentioned for hypertension: vary your choices. Don't let your diet become monotonous. This last suggestion is based on an important concept in the prevention of cancer initiation—dilution. Whenever you switch from food to food, you are diluting whatever is in one food with what is in the others. It is safe to eat *some* salt-cured foods, or smoked or grilled meats, but don't eat them all the time. If you include fruits, vegetables, and high-fiber grains and reduce your fat intake, you have every reason to feel confident that you are providing your body with the best nutrition at the lowest possible risk. Remember also to exercise.

It is worth repeating a remark by the Surgeon General, that for the two out of three Americans who do not smoke or drink excessively, "your choice of diet can influence your long-term health prospects more than any other action you might take."[71] Indeed, healthy young adults today are a privileged group: they are the first generation in history with the opportunity to lay the foundation for healthy later years through a lifetime of proper nutrition. Figure 11-7 illustrates this point.

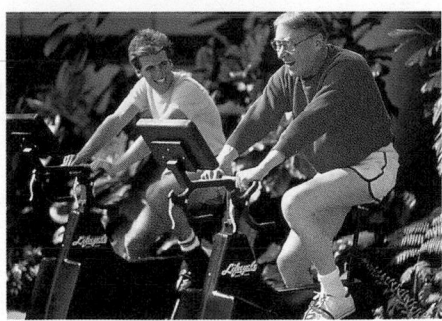

Exercise regularly, all your life.

Notes

1. WHO Study Group, Diet, nutrition, and the prevention of chronic diseases, *World Health Organization Technical Report Series 797* (Geneva: WHO Office of Publications, 1990), p. 55.
2. P. M. Newberne and M. Lockniskar, Nutrition and immune status, in I. R. Rowland, ed., *Nutrition, Toxicity, and Cancer* (Boca Raton, Fla.: CRC Press, 1991), pp. 301–378.
3. R. K. Chandra, Effect of vitamin and trace-element supplemention on immune response and infection in elderly subjects, *Lancet* 340 (1992): 1124–1127.
4. Immune function of the gastrointestinal tract, *Nutrition Today*, September/October 1991, p. 5.
5. Use of vitamin and mineral supplements in the United States, *Nutrition Reviews* 48 (1990): 161–162.
6. Use of vitamin and mineral supplements in the United States, 1990; D. M. Medeiros and coauthors, Vitamin and mineral supplementation practices of adults in seven western states, *Journal of the American Dietetic Association* 89 (1989): 383–386.
7. L. C. Pauling, *Vitamin C and the Common Cold* (San Francisco: W. H. Freeman, 1970).
8. T. C. Chalmers, Effects of ascorbic acid on the common cold, *American Journal of Medicine* 58 (1975): 532–536.
9. C. S. Johnston, Effect of a single oral dose of ascorbic acid on body temperature and trace mineral fluxes in healthy men and women, *Journal of the American College of Nutrition* 9 (1990): 150–154.
10. C. S. Johnston, L. J. Martin, and X. Cai, Antihistamine effect of supplemental ascorbic acid and neutrophil chemotaxis, *Journal of the American College of Nutrition* 11 (1992): 172–176.
11. E. M. Peters and coauthors, Vitamin C supplementation reduces the incidence of postrace symptoms of upper-respiratory-tract infection in ultramarathon runners, *American Journal of Clinical Nutrition* 57 (1993): 170–174.
12. R. F. Labbe, Dangers of iron and vitamin C supplements (letter), *Journal of the American Dietetic Association* 93 (1993): 526.
13. S. S. Resler, Nutrition care of AIDS patients, *Journal of the American Dietetic Association* 88 (1988): 828–832; P. A. Cuff, Acquired immunodeficiency syndrome and malnutrition: Role of gastrointestinal pathology, *Nutrition in Clinical Practice* 5 (1990): 43–53.
14. D. P. Kotler, Protein-energy malnutrition in AIDS, *Nutrition in Clinical Practice* 5 (1990): 41–42.
15. R. Ullrich and coauthors, Small intestinal structure and function in patients infected with human immunodeficiency virus (HIV): Evidence for HIV-induced enteropathy, *Annals of Internal Medicine* 111 (1990): 15–21.
16. M. Ott and coauthors, Early changes of body composition in human immunodeficiency virus-infected patients: Tetrapolar body impedance analysis indicates significant malnutrition, *American Journal of Clinical Nutrition* 57 (1993): 15–19.
17. R. K. Chandra, Nutrition and immunity: Lessons from the past and new insights into the future, *American Journal of Clinical Nutrition* 53 (1991): 1087–1101.
18. D. Farley, Food safety crucial for people with lowered immunity, *FDA Consumer*, July/August 1990, pp. 7–9.
19. J. T. Dwyer and coauthors, Unproven nutrition therapies for AIDS: What is the evidence? *Nutrition Today*, March/April 1988, pp. 25–33.
20. National Research Council, *Diet and Health: Implications for Reducing Chronic Disease Risk* (Washington, D.C.: National Academy Press, 1989), pp. 665–710.
21. S. Lillioja and coauthors, Impaired glucose tolerance as a disorder of insulin action, *New England Journal of Medicine* 318 (1988): 1217–1225.
22. M. J. Stampfer and coauthors, A prospective study of cholesterol, apolipoproteins, and the risk of myocardial infarction, *New England Journal of Medicine* 325 (1991): 373–381; NIH Consensus Conference, Triglyceride, high-density lipoprotein, and coronary heart disease, *Journal of the American Medical Association* 269 (1993): 505–510.
23. M. J. Klag and coauthors, Serum cholesterol in young men and subsequent cardiovascular disease, *New England Journal of Medicine* 328 (1993): 313–318.
24. NIH Consensus Conference, 1993.
25. WHO Study Group, 1990, p. 55.
26. D. Krombout, Dietary fats: Long-term implications for health, *Nutrition Reviews* 50 (1992): 49–53.
27. D. M. Hegsted, Dietary fatty acids, serum cholesterol, and coronary heart disease in G. J. Nelson, ed., *Health Effects of Dietary Fatty Acids* (Champaign, Ill: American Oil Chemists' Society, 1991), pp. 50–68; D. J. McNamara, Cardiovascular disease, in M. E. Shils, J. A. Olson, and M. Shike, *Modern Nutrition in Health and Disease* (Philadelphia: Lea & Febiger, 1994): 1533–1544.
28. Report of the Expert Panel on Population Strategies for Blood Cholesterol Reduction, *Circulation* 83 (1991): 2156–2161.
29. National Research Council, 1991, pp. 177–178.
30. L. M. Arnold and coauthors, Effect of isoenergetic intake of three or nine meals on plasma lipoproteins and glucose metabolism, *American Journal of Clinical Nutrition* 57 (1993): 446–451.
31. National Reseach Council, 1991, pp. 176–177.
32. K. F. Gey and coauthors, Inverse correlation between plasma vitamin E and mortality from ischemic heart disease in cross-cultural epidemiology, *American Journal of Clinical Nutrition* 53 (1991): 326–334; K. F. Gey and coauthors, Increased risk of cardiovascular disease at suboptimal plasma concentrations of essential antioxidants: An epidemiological update with special attention to carotene and vitamin C, *American Journal of Clinical Nutrition* 57 (1993): 787S–798S.
33. M. J. Stampfer and coauthors, Vitamin E consumption and the risk of coronary disease in women, *New England Journal of Medicine* 328 (1993): 1444–1449; E. B. Rimm and coauthors, Vitamin E consumption and the risk of coronary heart disease in men, *New England Journal of Medicine* 328 (1993): 1450–1456.
34. J. Dekeyser and coauthors, Serum concentrations of vitamins A and E and early outcome after Ischaemic stroke, *Lancet* 339 (1992): 1562–1565.
35. D. Steinberg, Antioxidant vitamins and coronary heart disease, *New England Journal of Medicine* 328 (1993): 1487–1489.
36. Selenium deficiency and heart disease, *Nutrition and the M.D.*, June 1993, pp. 1, 6.
37. I. H. Ullrich, C. M. Reid, and R. A. Yeater, Increased HDL-cholesterol levels with a weight lifting program, *Southern Medical Journal* 80 (1987): 328–331.
38. R. R. Wing and coauthors, Change in waist-hip ratio with weight loss and its association with change in cardiovascular risk factors, *American Journal of Clinical Nutrition* 55 (1992): 1086–1092; C. Bouchard, G. A. Bray, and V. S. Hubbard, Basic and clinical aspects of regional fat distribution, *American Journal of Clinical Nutrition* 52 (1990): 946–950; G. A. Bray, Obesity, in *Present Knowledge in Nutrition*, 6th ed., ed. M. L. Brown (Washington, D.C.: International Life Sciences Institute, 1990), pp. 23–38.

39. WHO Study Group, 1990, pp. 57–58.
40. J. R. DiPalma and W. S. Thayer, Use of niacin as a drug, *Annual Review of Nutrition* 11 (1991): 169–187.
41. D. Ornish and coauthors, Can lifestyle changes reverse coronary heart disease? The Lifestyle Heart Trial, *Lancet* 336 (1990): 129–133; D. C. Goff and coauthors, Does body fatness modify the association between dietary cholesterol and risk of coronary death? *Arteriosclerosis and Thrombosis* 12 (1992): 755–761.
42. D. Farley, High blood pressure: Controlling the silent killer, *FDA Consumer*, December 1991, pp. 28–33.
43. From presentations at the American Heart Association's Scientific Sessions, 1992, as reported in Syndrome X: Insulin resistance, hypertension, dyslipidemia, obesity, and CAD, *Nutrition Close-Up*, vol. 9, no. 4, 1992.
44. R. F. Murray, Skin color and blood pressure: Genetics or environment, *Journal of the American Medical Association* 266 (1991): 2049.
45. S. A. Corrigan and coauthors, Weight reduction in the prevention and treatment of hypertension: A review of representative clinical trials, *American Journal of Health Promotion* 5 (1991): 208–214.
46. M. H. Keleman and coauthors, Exercise training combined with antihypertensive drug therapy: Effects on blood lipids, blood pressure, and left ventricular mass, *Journal of the American Medical Association* 263 (1990): 2766–2771.
47. K. T. Khaw and E. Barrett-Connor, Dietary potassium and stroke-associated mortality: A 12-year prospective population study, *New England Journal of Medicine* 316 (1987): 235–240.
48. D. A. McCarron and coauthors, Dietary calcium and blood pressure: Modifying factors in specific populations, *American Journal of Clinical Nutrition* (supplement) 54 (1991): 215–219.
49. M. R. Joffres, D. M. Reed, and K. Yano, Relationship of magnesium intake and other dietary factors to blood pressure: The Honolulu heart study, *American Journal of Clinical Nutrition* 45 (1987): 469–475.
50. WHO Study Group, 1990, p. 62.
51. K. E. Anderson and A. Kappas, Dietary regulation of cytochrome P450, *Annual Review of Nutrition* 11 (1991), pp. 141–167.
52. American Medical Association's Council on Scientific Affairs, Diet and cancer: where do matters stand? *Archives of Internal Medicine* 153 (1993): 50–56.
53. WHO Study Group, 1990, p. 65.
54. R. A. Karmall, Fatty acid metabolism and biochemical mechanisms in cancer, in *Health Effects of Dietary Fatty Acids*, ed. G. J. Nelson (Champaign, Ill.: American Oil Chemists Society, 1991), pp. 150–156.
55. S. F. Chin and coauthors, Dietary sources of CLA (conjugated dienoic isomers of linoleic acid), a newly recognized class of anticarcinogens, *Journal of Food Composition* 5 (1992): 185–197.
56. L. A. Sauer, R. T. Cauchy, and A. S. Hurtubise, Effects of omega-6 and omega-3 fatty acids on the rate of 3H-thymidine incorporation (^{3}H-TI) in hepatoma 7288CTC perfused in situ, *FASEB Journal* 43 (1990): A508; K. K. Carroll, Nutrition and cancer: Fat, in Rowland, 1991, pp. 439–453.
57. National Research Council, 1991, p. 481.
58. Anderson and Kappas, 1991.
59. National Research Council, 1991, pp. 356–357.
60. J. Dwyer, Dietary fiber and colorectal cancer risk, *Nutrition Reviews* 51 (1993): 147–148.
61. D. Kritchevsky, Dietary fiber and colon cancer, in Rowland, 1991, pp. 481–489.
62. B. J. Trock, E. Lanza, and P. Greenwald, High-fiber diet and colon cancer: A critical review, *Recent Progress in Research on Nutrition and Cancer* (New York: Wiley-Liss, 1990), pp. 145–157.
63. C. S. Muir as cited by C. E. Butterworth and coauthors, Folate deficiency and cervical dysplasia, *Journal of the American Medical Association* 267 (1992): 528–533.
64. J. H. Weisburger, Nutritional approach to cancer prevention with emphasis on vitamins, antioxidants, and carotenoids, *American Journal of Clinical Nutrition* (supplement) 53 (1991): 226–237; R. G. Ziegler, Vegetables, fruits, and carotenoids and the risk of cancer, *American Journal of Clinical Nutrition* (supplement) 53 (1991): 251–259.
65. G. Block, The data support a role for antioxidants in reducing cancer risk, *Nutrition Reviews* 50 (1992): 207–213.
66. A. T. Diplock, Antioxidant nutrients and disease prevention: An overview, *American Journal of Clinical Nutrition* (supplement) 53 (1991): 189–193; K. Smigel, Vitamin E moves on stage in cancer prevention studies, *Journal of the Institute of Cancer* 84 (1992): pp. 996–997; Various articles in Ascorbic acid: Biologic functions and relation to cancer, *American Journal of Clinical Nutrition* (supplement) December 1991; Block, 1992; P. Knekt and coauthors, Serum selenium and subsequent risk of cancer among Finnish men and women, *Journal of the National Cancer Institute* 82 (1990): 864–868.
67. R. R. Watson and coauthors, Effect of beta-carotene on lymphocyte subpopulations in elderly humans: Evidence for a dose-response relationship, *American Journal of Clinical Nutrition* 53 (1990): 90–94.
68. J. D. Potter and K. L. Graves, Diet and cancer: Evidence and mechanisms—An adaptation argument, in Rowland, 1991, pp. 379–412.
69. L. Schweigerer and J. Fotis, Genistein, a dietary-derived inhibitor of in vitro angiogenesis, *Proceedings of the National Academy of Sciences*, 90 (1993): 2690–2694.
70. A. B. Caragay, Cancer preventive foods and ingredients, *Food Technology*, April 1992, pp. 65–79.
71. *The Surgeon General's report on Nutrition and Health, Summary and Recommendations* (Washington, D.C.: DHHS [PHS] publication no. 88-50211, 1988).

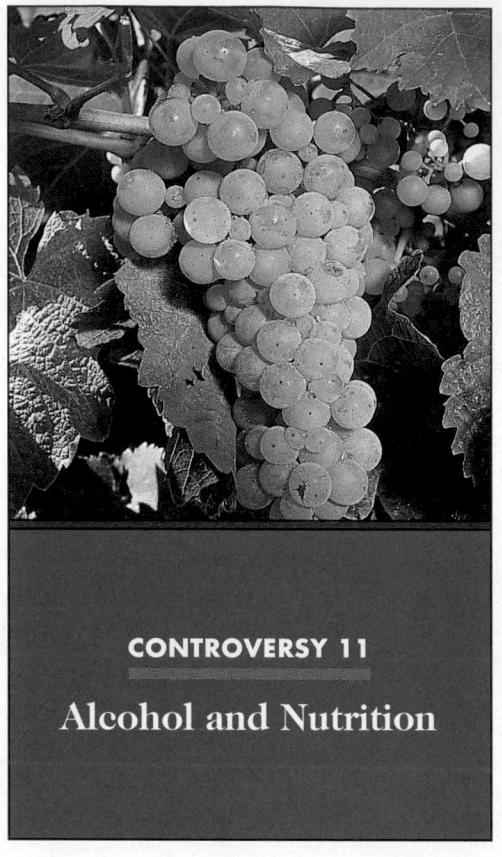

CONTROVERSY 11

Alcohol and Nutrition

People naturally congregate to enjoy conversation and companionship, and it is natural, too, to offer beverages to companions. All beverages ease conversation, whether or not they contain alcohol. Still, in most of the world's cultures, some people choose alcohol over cola, juice, milk, or coffee. For most, alcohol is a pleasant accompaniment to a meal, a drink of celebration, or a way to relax with friends. For others, alcohol becomes a life-shattering addiction, **alcoholism,** that leads to severe malnutrition, physical illness, and demoralizing erosion of self esteem. (Alcohol terms are defined in Table C11-1.)

A serving of alcohol is called a **drink,** and delivers ½ ounce pure ethanol:

3 to 4 ounces wine.

10 ounces wine cooler.

12 ounces beer.

1 ounce hard liquor (whiskey, gin, brandy, rum, vodka).

However, the serving that some people consider one drink may be more than the standard drink. The percentage of alcohol in distilled liquor is stated as *proof:* 100-proof liquor is 50 percent alcohol; 90-proof is 45 percent, and so forth. Compared with hard liquor, beer and wine have relatively low percentages of alcohol.

BENEFITS OF MODERATE ALCOHOL USE Taken in moderation, alcohol relaxes people, reduces their inhibitions, and encourages social interactions. Today's nonalcoholic beers and wines seem to do the same thing, a fact that bears testimony to the placebo effect at work.

The term *moderation* is important in the statement just made. Just what is moderation in the use of alcohol? No single amount of alcohol per day is appropriate for everyone because people differ in their tolerances to alcohol. But authorities have attempted to set limits that are appropriate for most healthy people: not more than two drinks a day for the average-sized, healthy man; not more than one drink a day for the average-sized, healthy woman. This amount is supposed to be enough to produce an elevation of mood without incurring any long-term harm to health. Doubtless some people could consume slightly more; others, especially those prone to alcohol addiction, could definitely not handle nearly so much without significant risk. If you think your own drinking might not be moderate or normal or has caused problems in your life, or if you feel guilty about your drinking, you may want to seek a professional evaluation.*

Alcohol in any beverage has the same mood effects. In addition, wine in particular is credited with some special effects. The high potassium content of grape juice is beneficial to people with high blood pressure, and when the grape juice is made into wine, this effect carries over. In fact, since alcohol raises blood pressure, the grape juice is more suitable than wine for people with hypertension. Dealcoholized wine also increases the absorption of potassium, calcium, phosphorus, magnesium, and zinc. So does wine, but the alcohol in it promotes the *excretion* of these minerals, so again the dealcoholized version is preferred.

Alcoholic beverages affect the appetite. Usually they reduce it, making people unaware that they are hungry. But in people who are tense and unable to eat, small doses of wine taken 20 minutes before meals improve the appetite. Certain acid compounds in the wine, known as **congeners,** are credited with this effect. For undernourished people and for people with severely depressed appetites, wine may facilitate eating even when psychotherapy fails to do so. Congeners are also involved in producing a hangover, as a later section notes.

An interesting correlation has been noted between consumption of alcoholic beverages and the development of the dangerous viral liver disease hepatitis.[1]

*National Clearinghouse for Alcohol and Drug Information: 1-800-729-6686.

Hepatitis can be transmitted by way of eating raw oysters. During a recent hepatitis outbreak, researchers noted that people who ate contaminated oysters and who also took one drink of liquor, such as whiskey, or one glass of wine were 70 percent less likely to develop the infection. More alcohol did not diminish the likelihood further, and intakes of less than a drink, or a drink of beer, did not correlate with reduced risk. In no way does this prove that eating raw seafood can be made a safe practice by way of drinking liquor. Hepatitis is too serious an illness to take any chances. It does serve as a reminder that alcohol is a disinfectant and that it effectively destroys some microorganisms.

As mentioned in the preceding chapter, research shows an association between moderate alcohol consumption, especially consumption of red wine, increased blood HDL, and a reduced risk of heart disease.[2] Red wine contains chemicals known as phenols, and these may act as nonnutrient antioxidants in the body. The blood lipid response varies widely from individual to individual, and no authority recommends that nondrinkers begin drinking wine or other alcoholic beverages to obtain these uncertain effects. The association between moderate alcohol consumption and strokes is less clear. Moderate alcohol consumption in one study of women lowered the risk of one type of stroke but increased the risk of a different type. Some researchers argue that the concept that moderate alcohol consumption is protective against heart disease ignores the abundant evidence showing a relationship between alcohol consumption and poor health.[3]

Another example of the beneficial use of alcohol is provided by research showing that moderate use of wine in later life improves morale, stimulates social interaction, and promotes restful sleep. In nursing homes, improved patient and staff relations have been attributed to greater self-esteem among elderly patients who drink moderate amounts of wine. Researchers hypothesize that chronic fatigue may be responsible for some behaviors associated with old age. The positive effects of wine on sleep may alleviate the fatigue, permitting more social interactions. Alcohol, used responsibly and in moderation, can bring some benefits. For those who choose to drink, a valid goal is learning to drink moderately. The next sections address the physical effects of alcohol on the body.

Table C11-1
Alcohol Terms

- **acetaldehyde** (ass-et-AL-deh-hide) a substance to which ethanol is metabolized on its way to becoming harmless waste products that can be excreted.
- **alcohol dehydrogenase** an enzyme system that breaks down alcohol.
- **alcoholism** a dependency on alcohol marked by compulsive uncontrollable drinking with negative effects on physical health, family relationships, and social health.
- **antidiuretic hormone (ADH)** a hormone produced by the pituitary gland in response to dehydration (or a high sodium concentration in the blood); it stimulates the kidneys to reabsorb more water and so to excrete less. (This hormone should not be confused with alcohol dehydrogenase, which is sometimes also abbreviated ADH.)
- **cirrhosis** (seer-OH-sis) advanced liver disease, often associated with alcoholism in which liver cells have died, hardened, turned an orange color, and have permanently lost their function.
- **congeners** (CON-jen-ers) chemical substances other than alcohol that account for the physiological effects, such as taste and after effects, that are unique to different alcoholic beverages.
- **drink** a dose of any alcoholic beverage that delivers ½ ounce of pure ethanol.
- **fatty liver** an early stage of liver deterioration seen in several diseases, including kwashiorkor and alcoholic liver disease. Fatty liver is characterized by accumulation of fat in the liver cells.
- **fibrosis** (fye-BROH-sis) an intermediate stage of alcoholic liver deterioration in which liver cells lose their function and assume the characteristics of connective tissue cells (fibers).
- **formaldehyde** a substance to which methanol is metabolized on the way to being converted to harmless waste products that can be excreted.
- **gout** (GOWT) accumulation of uric acid crystals in the joints.
- **MEOS** (microsomal ethanol oxidizing system) a system of enzymes in the liver that oxidize not only alcohol but also several classes of drugs.
- **methanol** an alcohol produced in the body continually by all cells.

ALCOHOL ENTERS THE BODY From the moment an alcoholic beverage is swallowed, the body pays special attention to it. Unlike foods, which require digestion before they can be absorbed, the tiny alcohol molecules can diffuse right through the walls of an empty stomach and reach the brain within a minute. Ethanol is a toxin, and a too-high dose of alcohol triggers one of the body's

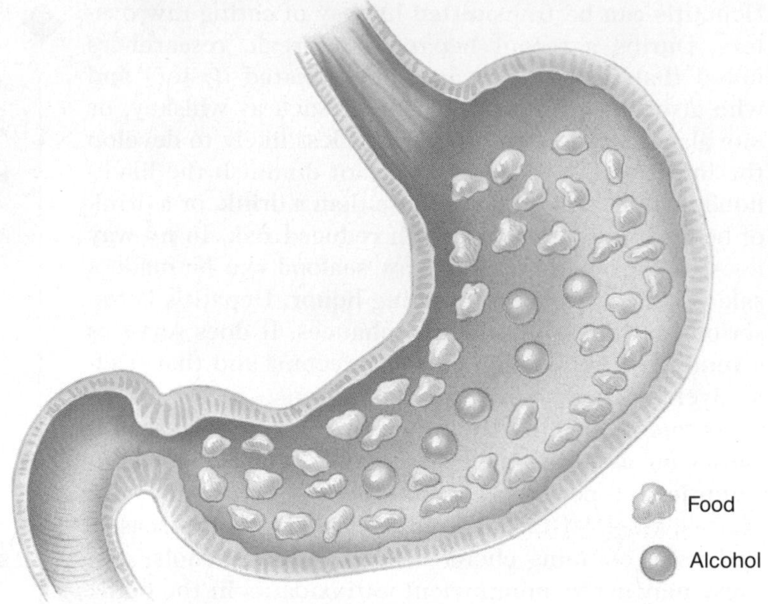

Figure C11-1

FOOD SLOWS ALCOHOL'S ABSORPTION
The alcohol in a stomach filled with food has a low probability of touching the walls and diffusing through. Food also traps alcohol in the stomach longer.

primary defenses against poison—vomiting. Many times, alcohol arrives gradually and in the form of dilute enough beverages so that the vomiting reflex is delayed and the alcohol is absorbed.

A person can become intoxicated almost immediately when drinking, especially if the person's stomach is empty. When the stomach is full of food, molecules of alcohol have less chance of touching the stomach walls and diffusing through, so alcohol affects the brain a little less immediately (see Figure C11-1). By the time the stomach contents are emptied into the small intestine, the presence of food makes no difference: alcohol is absorbed rapidly whether or not food is present.

A practical pointer derives from this information. If a person wants to drink socially and not become intoxicated, the person should eat the snacks provided by the host (avoid the salty ones; they make you thirstier). Carbohydrate snacks are best suited for slowing alcohol absorption. High-fat snacks help too because they slow peristalsis, keeping the alcohol in the stomach longer. Other tips include adding ice or water to drinks to dilute them, and choosing nonalcoholic beverages every other round to quench thirst.

If one drinks slowly enough, the alcohol, after absorption, will be collected into the liver and processed without much affecting other parts of the body. If one drinks more rapidly, however, some of the alcohol bypasses the liver and flows for a while through the rest of the body and the brain.

ALCOHOL ARRIVES IN THE BRAIN Some people use alcohol as a kind of social anesthetic to help them relax or to relieve anxiety. One drink relieves inhibitions, and this gives people the impression that alcohol is a stimulant. Actually the way it gives this impression is by sedating *inhibitory* nerves, allowing excitatory nerves to take over. This is temporary. Ultimately alcohol acts as a depressant and sedates all the nerve cells. Figure C11-2 describes alcohol's effects on the brain.

It is lucky that the brain centers respond to rising blood alcohol in the order shown, because a person usually passes out before managing to drink a lethal dose. It is possible, though, for a person to drink fast enough so that the effects of alcohol continue to accelerate after the person has gone to sleep. The yearly deaths that take place during drinking contests are attributed to this effect. The drinker drinks fast enough, before passing out, to receive a lethal dose. Table C11-2 (page 434) shows the blood alcohol levels that correspond with progressively greater intoxication and Table C11-3 (page 434) shows the brain responses that occur at these blood levels.

Brain cells are particularly sensitive to excessive exposure to alcohol. The brain shrinks, even in people who drink only moderately. The extent of the shrinkage is proportional to the amount drunk. Abstinence, together with good nutrition, reverses some of the brain damage, and possibly all of it, if heavy drinking has not continued for more than a few years. However, pro-

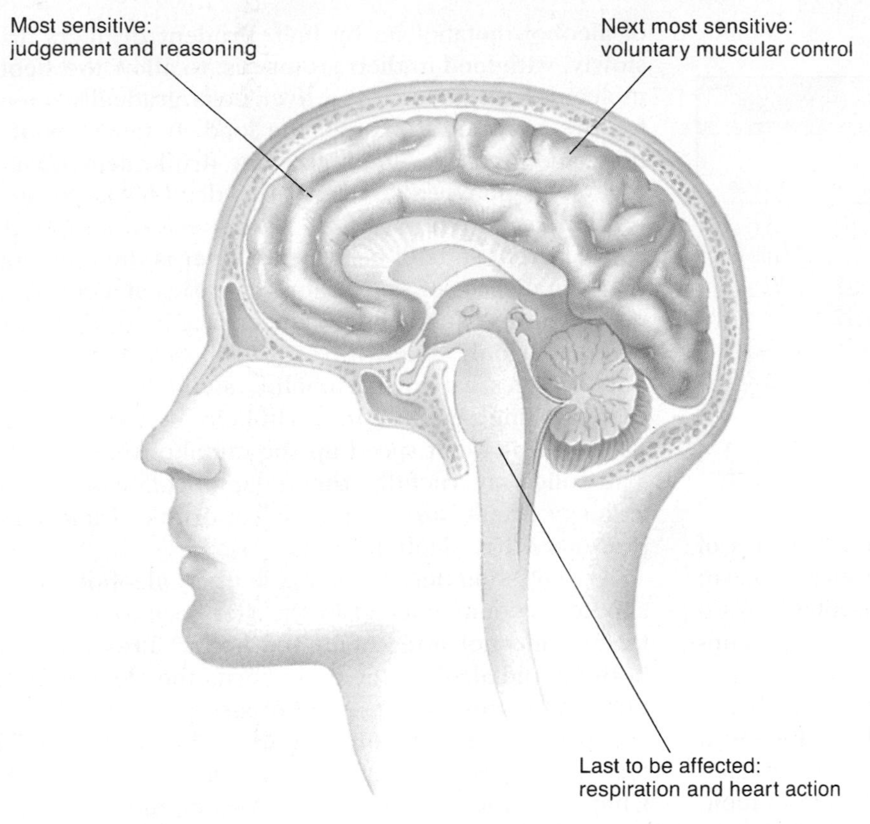

Figure C11-2

ALCOHOL'S EFFECTS ON THE BRAIN
When alcohol flows to the brain, it first sedates the frontal lobe, the reasoning part. As the alcohol molecules diffuse into the cells of this lobe, they interfere with reasoning and judgment. With continued drinking, the speech and vision centers of the brain become sedated, and the area that governs reasoning becomes more incapacitated. Still more drinking affects the cells of the brain responsible for large-muscle control; at this point people under the influence stagger or weave when they try to walk. Finally the conscious brain becomes completely subdued, and the person passes out. Now the person can drink no more. This is fortunate because a higher dose would anesthetize the deepest brain centers that control breathing and heartbeat, causing death.

longed drinking beyond an individual's capacity to recover can cause severe and irreversible effects on vision, memory, learning ability, and other functions.

Anyone who has had an alcoholic drink knows that alcohol increases urine output. This is because alcohol depresses the brain's production of **antidiuretic hormone.** Loss of body water leads to thirst. The only fluid that will relieve dehydration is water, but if alcoholic beverages are the only drinks available, each drink may worsen the thirst. The smart drinker, then, alternates alcoholic beverages with nonalcoholic choices and when thirsty chooses the latter.

The water loss caused by hormone depression involves loss of more than just water. The water takes with it important minerals, such as magnesium, potassium, calcium, and zinc, depleting the body's reserves. These minerals are vital to the maintenance of fluid balance and to nerve and muscle action and coordination. Each time they are lost from the body, they must be replaced the next day if deficiencies are not to cause harm.

ALCOHOL ARRIVES IN THE LIVER The capillaries that surround the digestive tract merge into veins that carry the alcohol-laden blood to the liver. Here the veins branch and rebranch into capillaries that touch every liver cell. The liver cells make nearly all of the body's alcohol-processing machinery, and the routing of blood through the liver allows the cells to go right to work on the alcohol. The liver's location at this point along the circulatory system enables it to remove toxic substances before they reach other body organs such as the heart and brain.

The liver makes and maintains two sets of equipment for metabolizing alcohol. One is an enzyme that removes hydrogens from alcohol to break it down; the name, **alcohol dehydrogenase (ADH),** almost says what it does.* This enzyme handles about 80 percent or more of the alcohol in the body. The other alcohol-metabolizing equipment is a chain of enzymes (known as the **MEOS**) thought to handle about 10 to 20 percent of the alcohol.

The amount of alcohol a person's body can process in a given time is limited by the number of ADH

*There are actually two ADH enzymes, each performing a specific task in alcohol breakdown.

Table C11-2
Alcohol Doses and Blood Levels

	Percent Blood Alcohol by Body Weight				
NUMBER OF DRINKS[a]	100 lb	120 lb	150 lb	180 lb	200 lb
2	0.08	0.06	0.05	0.04	0.04
4	0.15	0.13	0.10	0.08	0.08
6	0.23	0.19	0.15	0.13	0.11
8	0.30	0.25	0.20	0.17	0.15
12	0.45	0.36	0.30	0.25	0.23
14	0.52	0.42	0.35	0.34	0.27

[a]Taken within an hour or so; each drink equal to ½ ounce pure ethanol.

enzymes that reside in the liver. If more molecules of alcohol arrive at the liver cells than the enzymes can handle, the extra alcohol must wait. It circulates again and again through the brain, liver, and other organs until enzymes are available to degrade it.

Some ADH enzymes reside in the stomach and break down some alcohol before it enters the blood. Research shows that people with alcoholism make less stomach ADH than others, and that women make less than men. Women may absorb about one-third more alcohol than men, even when they are the same size and drink the same amount of alcoholic beverage.[4]

The number of ADH enzymes present is also affected by whether or not a person eats. Fasting for as little as a day causes degradation of body proteins, including the ADH enzymes in the liver, and this can reduce the rate of alcohol metabolism by half. Prudent drinkers drink slowly, with food in their stomachs, to allow the alcohol molecules to move to the liver cells gradually enough for the enzymes to handle the load. It takes about an hour and a half to metabolize one drink, depending on a person's body size, on previous drinking experience, on how recently the person has eaten, and on the person's current state of health. The liver is the only organ that can dispose of significant quantities of alcohol, and its maximum rate of alcohol clearance is fixed. This explains why only time will restore sobriety. Walking will not; muscles cannot metabolize alcohol. It is a myth that drinking a cup of coffee will help. Caffeine is a stimulant, but it won't speed up the metabolism of alcohol. The police say, ruefully, that a cup of coffee only makes a sleepy drunk into a wide-awake drunk. Table C11-4 presents other alcohol myths.

A suggestion has been made that alcohol calories should be counted as fat in the diet because of the way fat and alcohol interact in the body.[5] Presented with both fat and alcohol, the body burns the alcohol for energy and stores the fat. Alcohol also promotes fat storage in the central abdominal area—the "beer belly" effect whose risks to the heart were already described in Chapter 9. Alcohol yields 7 calories of energy per gram to the body, so many alcoholic drinks are much more fattening than their non-alcoholic counterparts.

Upon exposure to alcohol, the liver speeds up its synthesis of fatty acids. Fat accumulation has been observed in the livers of young men after a single night of heavy drinking. The condition persists for more than a day. **Fatty liver,** the first stage of liver deterioration seen in heavy drinkers, interferes with the distribution of nutrients and oxygen to the liver cells. If the condition lasts long enough, fibrous scar tissue invades the liver. This is the second stage of liver deterioration, called **fibrosis.** Fibrosis is reversible with good nutrition and abstinence from alcohol, but the next (last) stage, **cirrhosis,** is not. In cirrhosis, the liver cells harden, turn orange, and lose function forever as they die. All of this points to the importance of moderation in the use of alcohol.

The presence of alcohol alters amino acid metabolism in the liver cells. Synthesis of some proteins important in the immune system slows down, weakening the body's defenses against infection. Synthesis of lipoproteins speeds up, increasing blood triglyceride and HDL levels. In addition, excessive alcohol increases the body's acid burden and interferes with normal uric acid metabolism, causing symptoms like those of **gout.**

Table C11-3
Alcohol Blood Levels and Brain Responses

Blood Level (%)	Brain Response
0.05	Judgment impaired
0.10[a]	Emotional control impaired
0.15	Muscle coordination and reflexes impaired
0.20	Vision impaired
0.30	Drunk, totally out of control
0.35	Stupor
0.50–0.60	Total loss of consciousness, finally death

[a]The legal limit for intoxication according to most states' highway safety ordinances; driving ability is, however, already impaired at blood alcohol levels lower than 0.10 percent.

Table C11-4
Myths and Truths Concerning Alcohol

Myth:	Alcohol is legal, and therefore not a drug.
Truth:	Alcohol is legal, but it alters one or more of the body's functions and is medically defined as a depressant drug.
Myth:	A shot of alcohol warms you up.
Truth:	Alcohol diverts blood flow to the skin making you *feel* warmer, but it actually cools the body.
Myth:	Wine and beer are mild; they do not lead to addiction.
Truth:	Wine and beer drinkers worldwide have high rates of death from alcohol-related illnesses. It's not what you drink, but how much, that makes the difference.
Myth:	Mixing drinks is what gives you a hangover.
Truth:	Too much alcohol in any form produces a hangover.
Myth:	Alcohol is a stimulant.
Truth:	Alcohol depresses the activity of the brain.

Liver metabolism clears most of the alcohol from the blood. However, about 10 percent is excreted through the breath and in the urine. This fact is the basis for the breathalyzer test that law enforcement officers administer when they suspect someone of driving under the influence of alcohol: the alcohol in the breath is directly proportional to the alcohol in the blood.

THE HANGOVER The hangover—the awful feeling of headache pain, unpleasant sensations in the mouth, and nausea that one has the morning after drinking too much—is a mild form of drug withdrawal. The worse form is a delirium with severe tremors that warns of a danger of death and demands medical management. Hangovers are caused by several factors. One is the toxic effects of congeners, already mentioned, that accompany the alcohol in alcoholic beverages. The congeners in gin are different from those in vodka, which in turn are different from those in bourbon or rye whiskey. One particular kind of liquor may produce a hangover and another may not. However, this is only one of several factors that produce hangovers, and mixing or switching drinks will not prevent them if too much is drunk.

Dehydration of the brain is a second factor: alcohol not only causes the body to lose water, but actually reduces the brain cells' water content. When they rehydrate the morning after, nerve pain accompanies their swelling back to their normal size. Another contributor to the hangover is **formaldehyde,** the same chemical that medical laboratories use to preserve dead animals. Formaldehyde comes from **methanol,** an alcohol produced constantly by normal chemical processes in all the cells. Normally, a set of liver enzymes converts this methanol to formaldehyde and then a second set immediately converts the formaldehyde to carbon dioxide and water, harmless waste products that can be excreted. But the same two sets of liver enzymes that do this are needed to process ethanol to its own intermediate waste product, **acetaldehyde,** and then to carbon dioxide and water. The enzymes prefer ethanol 20 times over methanol. Both alcohols are metabolized without delay until the load of acetaldehyde becomes too great for its enzyme to handle; at that point, formaldehyde starts accumulating and the hangover begins.

Time alone is the cure for a hangover. Simple-minded remedies clearly will not work: vitamins, tranquilizers, aspirin, drinking more alcohol, breathing pure oxygen, exercising, eating, or drinking something awful. The headache pain, unpleasantness in the mouth, and nausea of a hangover come simply from drinking too much.

ALCOHOL'S LONG-TERM EFFECTS By far the longest term effects of alcohol are those felt by the child of a woman who drinks during pregnancy. When a pregnant woman takes a drink, her fetus takes the same drink within minutes and its body is defenseless against the effects. This is a topic so important that it is given a space of its own in Chapter 12, where the recommendation is made that pregnant women should not drink at all. For nonpregnant adults, however, what are the effects of alcohol over the long term?

A couple of drinks sets into motion many destructive processes in the body, but the next day's abstinence may reverse most of them. As long as the doses taken are moderate, the time between them is ample, and nutrition is adequate meanwhile, recovery is probably complete.

If the doses of alcohol are heavy, however, and if the time between them is short, complete recovery cannot take place, and repeated onslaughts of alcohol gradually take a toll on the body. For example, alcohol is directly toxic to skeletal and cardiac muscle, causing weakness and deterioration in a dose-related manner.[6] Alcoholism makes heart disease more likely probably because chronic alcohol use raises the blood pressure.[7] At autopsy, the heart of a person with alcoholism appears bloated and weighs twice as much as a normal heart.

Alcohol attacks brain cells directly, and alcoholism causes irreversible brain disorders that cost society an estimated $90 billion in medical services, lost wages, criminal costs, and other losses.[8] Cirrhosis of the liver also develops after 10 to 20 years of addiction from the cumulative effects of frequent heavy episodes of drinking.

Alcohol abuse also leads to cancers of the mouth, throat, esophagus, rectum, and lungs. A reliable source tentatively ranks daily human exposure to ethanol high among possible carcinogenic hazards.[9]

A debated point is whether moderate alcohol intakes over many years increase cancer risks. Some studies link moderate alcohol intakes with breast cancer, but these results have been challenged by later studies. Cancer of the rectum occurs more often in people who drink more than 15 ounces of beer each day.[10] It is unknown whether cancer's association with beer results from alcohol itself or from other compounds formed during brewing. The FDA is now reviewing studies to determine the long-term health effects of a compound, urethane, often found in some alcoholic beverages, especially flavored imported brandy. Urethane is known to cause cancer in animals, but the risk to human beings is unknown.[11]

Other long-term effects of alcohol abuse include:

- Diabetes (noninsulin dependent).[12]
- Ulcers of the stomach and intestines.
- Severe psychological depression.
- Kidney, bladder, prostate gland, and pancreas damage.
- Skin rashes and sores.
- Impaired immune response.
- Deterioration in the testicles and adrenal glands, leading to feminization and sexual impotence in men.
- Central nervous system damage.
- Malnutrition.
- Bone deterioration and osteoporosis.
- Increased risk of violent death.

This list is by no means all-inclusive. Alcohol has direct toxic effects on all body organs.

Alcohol also does damage indirectly, via malnutrition. The more alcohol a person drinks, the less likely that he or she will eat enough food to obtain adequate nutrients. Alcohol is empty calories, like pure sugar and pure fat; it displaces nutrients. In a sense, each 150 calories of alcohol are spent on a luxury item: the drinker receives no nutritional value in return. The more calories spent this way, the fewer are left to spend on nutritious foods. Table C11-5 shows the calorie amounts of typical alcoholic beverages.

Alcohol abuse not only displaces nutrients from the diet but also affects every tissue's metabolism of nutrients. Alcohol causes stomach cells to oversecrete both acid and an agent of the immune system, histamine, that produces inflammation. Beer particularly can irritate the stomach by stimulating it to release extra acid into its interior.[13] These changes make the stomach and esophagus linings vulnerable to ulcer formation. Intestinal cells fail to absorb thiamin, folate, vitamin B_6, and others. Liver cells lose efficiency in activating vitamin D and alter their production and excretion of bile. Rod cells in the retina, which normally process vitamin A alcohol (retinol) to the form needed in vision, find themselves processing drinking alcohol instead. The kidneys excrete magnesium, calcium, potassium, and zinc.

Alcohol's intermediate products interfere with metabolism too. They dislodge vitamin B_6 from its protective binding protein so that it is destroyed, causing a vitamin B_6 deficiency and thereby reducing production of red blood cells.

Most dramatic is alcohol's effect on folate. When alcohol is present, the body actively expels folate from all its sites of action and storage. The liver, which normally contains enough folate to meet all needs, releases its folate into the blood. As the blood folate concentration rises, the kidneys are deceived into excreting it, as if it were in excess. The intestine normally releases and retrieves folate continuously, but it becomes damaged by folate deficiency and alcohol toxicity, so it fails to retrieve its own folate and misses out on any that may trickle in from food as well. Alcohol also interferes with

Table C11-5
Calories in Alcoholic Beverages and Mixers

Beverage	Amount (oz)	Energy (cal)
Beer	12	150
Light beer	12	100
Gin, rum, vodka, whiskey (86 proof)	1½	105
Dessert wine	3½	140
Table wine	3½	85
Tonic, ginger ale, other sweetened carbonated waters	8	80
Cola, root beer	8	100
Fruit-flavored soda, Tom Collins mix	8	115
Club soda, plain seltzer, diet drinks	8	1

the action of what little folate is left. This inhibits the production of new cells, especially the rapidly dividing cells of the intestine and the blood.

Nutrient deficiencies are thus a virtually inevitable consequence of alcohol abuse, not only because alcohol displaces food but also because alcohol directly interferes with the body's use of nutrients, making them ineffective even if they are present. Over a lifetime, excessive drinking brings about deficits of all the nutrients. People treated for alcohol addiction often also need nutrition therapy to reverse deficiency diseases rarely seen in others: night blindness, beriberi, pellagra, scurvy, and protein-energy malnutrition.

This discussion has touched on some of the ways alcohol affects health and nutrition. In contrast to some possible benefits of moderate alcohol consumption, the potential for harm is great with excessive alcohol consumption. In addition to deaths from health problems, about 20,000 people die each year in alcohol-related traffic accidents.[14] While this number is decreasing, it is still unacceptably high. The best way to escape the harmful effects of alcohol is, of course, to refuse alcohol altogether. If you do drink, do so with care, and in moderation.

Notes

1. J. A. Desenclos and coauthors, The protective effect of alcohol on the occurrence of epidemic oyster-borne Hepatitis-A, *Epidemiology* 3 (1992): 371–374.
2. H. Koyama and coauthors, Positive association between serum zinc and apolipoprotein A-II concentrations in middle-aged males who regularly consume alcohol, *American Journal of Clinical Nutrition* 57 (1993): 657–661.
3. A. G. Shaper, G. Wannamethee, and M. Walker, Alcohol and mortality: The myth of the U-shaped curve, *Lancet* 2 (1988): 1267–1273.
4. M. Frezza and coauthors, High blood alcohol levels in women: The role of decreased gastric alcohol dehydrogenase activity and first-pass metabolism, *New England Journal of Medicine* 322 (1990): 95–99.
5. J. P. Flatt, Body weight, fat storage, and alcohol metabolism, *Nutrition Reviews* 50 (1992): 267–270.
6. A. Urbano-Marquez and coauthors, The effects of alcoholism on skeletal and cardiac muscle, *New England Journal of Medicine* 320 (1989): 409–415.
7. M. Russell and coauthors, Alcohol drinking patterns and blood pressure, *American Journal of Public Health* 81 (1991): 452–457.
8. R. J. Rubin and coauthors, *The Cost of Disorders of the Brain* (Washington, D.C.: National Foundation for Brain Research, 1992), pp. 45–49.
9. B. N. Ames, R. Magaw, and L. S. Gold, Ranking possible carcinogenic hazards, *Science* 236 (1987): 271–280.
10. H. K. Seitz and U. A. Simoonowski, Alcohol and carcinogenesis, *Annual Review of Nutrition* 8 (1988): 99–119.
11. J. E. Foulke, Urethane in alcoholic beverages under investigation, *FDA Consumer*, January–February 1993, pp. 19–23.
12. T. L. Holbrook, E. Barrett-Connor, and D. L. Wingard, A prospective population-based study of alcohol use and non-insulin-dependent diabetes mellitus, *American Journal of Epidemiology* 132 (1990): 902–909.
13. M. V. Singer, S. Teyssen, and V. E. Eysselein, Action of beer and its ingredients on gastric acid secretion and release of gastrin in humans, *Gastroenterology* 10 (1991): 935–942.
14. Alcohol-related traffic fatalities, *FDA Consumer*, March 1993, p. 26.

pregnant women more often suffer gestational diabetes, hypertension, and infections after the birth than do women of healthy weight. The birth itself may be more likely to require drugs to induce labor or to require surgical intervention. An appropriate goal for the obese woman who wishes to become pregnant is to attain a body weight low enough to minimize her medical risks.

A major reason why the mother's nutrition before pregnancy is so crucial is that it determines whether her **uterus** will be able to grow a healthy **placenta** during the first month of pregnancy. If the placenta works perfectly, the fetus wants for nothing; if it doesn't, however, no alternative source of sustenance is available and the fetus will fail to thrive.[6] The placenta is shown in Figure 12-1; it is a sort of cushion of tissue in which the mother's and baby's blood vessels intertwine and exchange materials. The two bloods never mix, but nutrients and oxygen cross from the mother's into the baby's blood while wastes move out of the baby's blood, to be ultimately excreted by the mother. The **amniotic sac** forms to house the baby, cushioning it with fluids.

Far from being passive in its transport of molecules, the placenta is a highly metabolic organ with some 60 sets of enzymes of its own. It actively gathers up hormones, nutrients, and protein molecules such as antibodies and transfers them into the fetal bloodstream. It also produces hormones that maintain pregnancy and prepare the mother's breasts for **lactation.**

If the mother's nutrient stores are inadequate during the period when the body is preparing to develop the placenta, then the placenta will never develop properly. As a consequence, no matter how well she eats later, the woman's unborn baby will not receive optimal nourishment. The infant is likely to be a low-birthweight baby with all of the associated risks. After getting such a poor start on life, a girl child may be ill equipped, even as an adult, to store sufficient nutrients, and so she may also be unable to grow an adequate placenta. In turn, she may bear an infant who is unable to

uterus (YOO-ter-us) the womb, the muscular organ within which the infant develops before birth.

placenta (pla-SEN-tuh) the organ that develops inside the uterus in early pregnancy in which the mother's and fetus's circulatory systems intertwine and in which exchange of materials between maternal and fetal blood takes place. The fetus receives nutrients and oxygen across the placenta; the mother's blood picks up carbon dioxide and other waste materials to be excreted via her lungs and kidneys.

amniotic (am-nee-OTT-ic) **sac** the "bag of water" in the uterus, in which the fetus floats.

lactation production and secretion of breast milk for the purpose of nourishing an infant.

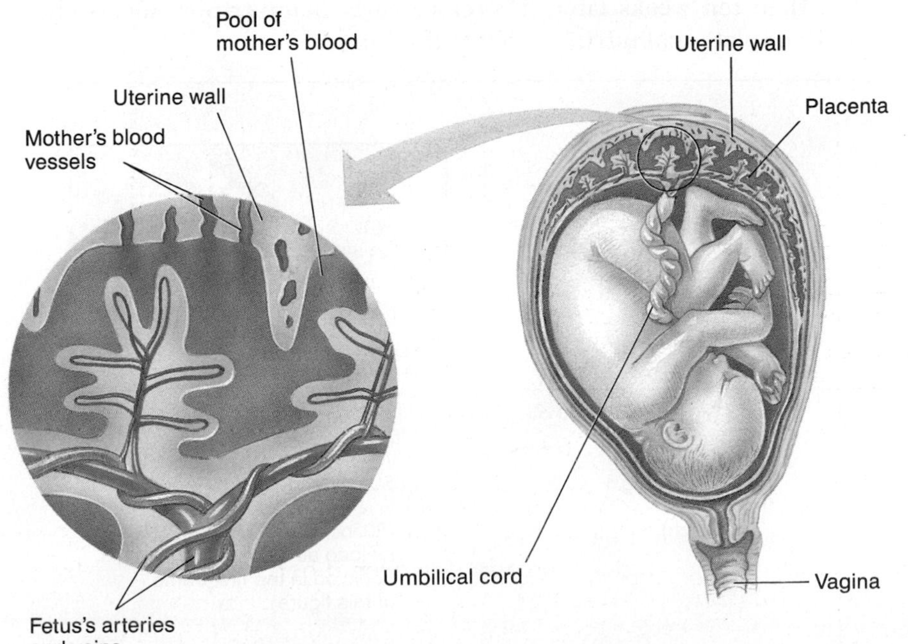

Figure 12-1

THE PLACENTA

The placenta is a sort of pillow of tissue in which maternal blood vessels lie side by side with fetal blood vessels entering it through the umbilical cord. This close association between the two circulatory systems permits the mother's bloodstream to deliver nutrients and oxygen to the fetus and to carry away fetal waste products.

implantation the stage of development, during the first two weeks after conception, in which the fertilized egg embeds itself in the wall of the uterus and begins to develop.

ovum the egg, produced by the mother, that unites with a sperm from the father to produce a new individual.

zygote (ZYE-goat) the term that describes the product of the union of ovum and sperm during the first two weeks after fertilization.

critical period a finite period during development in which certain events may occur that will have irreversible effects on later developmental stages. A critical period is usually a period of cell division in a body organ.

embryo (EM-bree-oh) the stage of human gestation from the third to eighth week after conception.

fetus (FEET-us) the stage of human gestation from eight weeks after conception until birth of an infant.

reach full potential. The effect may even extend to the *next* generation: the poor nutrition of a woman during her early pregnancy can have an impact on the health of her *grandchild*, even after that child has become an *adult*.

Not all cases of low birthweight reflect poor nutrition. Other factors that are associated with low birthweight are heredity, disease conditions, smoking, and drug (including alcohol) use during pregnancy. Even with optimal nutrition and health during pregnancy, some women give birth to small infants for reasons unknown. Still, poor nutrition is the major factor in low birthweight, and, ideally, an avoidable one as later sections make clear.

KEY POINT Adequate nutrition before pregnancy establishes physical status and food habits that best support fetal growth. Babies who weigh less than 5½ pounds at birth face greater health risks than normal-weight babies.

The Events of Pregnancy

On **implantation** of the newly fertilized **ovum** (or **zygote**) in the uterine wall, the uterus begins to grow a placenta. During the two weeks following fertilization, the zygote divides into many cells, and these cells sort themselves into three layers. Minimal growth in size takes place at this time, but it is a **critical period** developmentally. Adverse influences such as smoking, drug abuse, and malnutrition at this time lead to failure to implant or to abnormalities that can cause loss of the zygote, possibly even before the woman knows she is pregnant. Both mother and child will benefit most from an optimal supply of nutrients uncontaminated by other materials.

The next six weeks of the development of the **embryo** register astonishing physical changes (see Figure 12-2). At eight weeks, the **fetus** has a complete central nervous system, a beating heart, a fully formed digestive system, and the beginnings of facial features.

The growth of each organ and tissue type has its own characteristic pattern and timing. Each organ is most dependent on an adequate supply of nutrients during its own intensive growth period. For example, the fetus's heart and brain are well developed at 14 weeks; the lungs do not mature until more than ten weeks later. Therefore early malnutrition affects the heart and brain; late malnutrition affects the lungs.

Figure 12-2

STAGES OF EMBRYONIC AND FETAL DEVELOPMENT

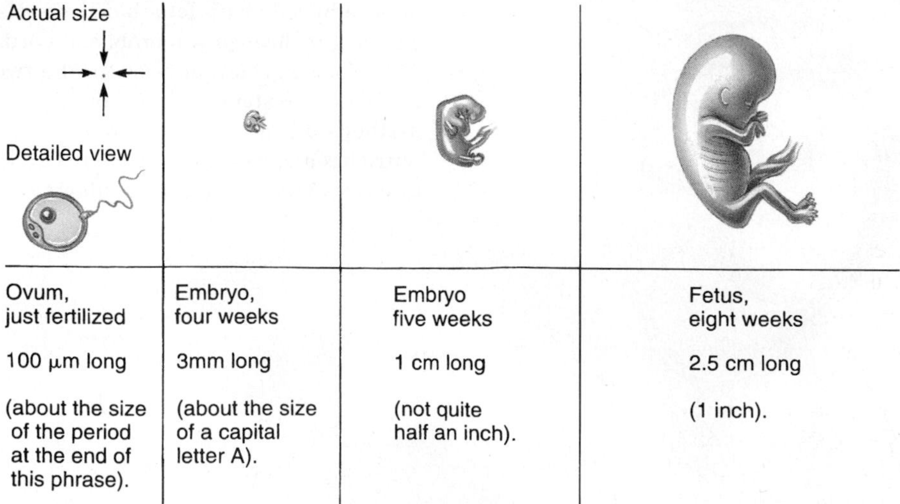

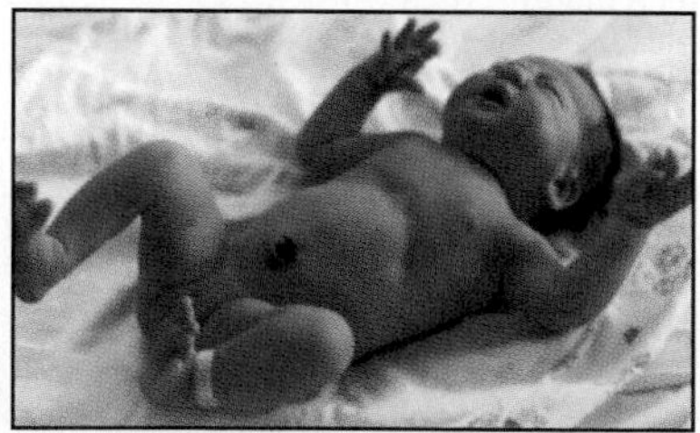

Newborn, nine months

50 cm long

(20 inches, 5,000 times as long as the ovum, depicted in the first frame of this figure).

Events during a critical period can occur only at that time and at no other. Whatever nutrients and other environmental conditions are necessary during this period must be supplied on time if the organ is to reach its full potential. If the development of an organ is limited during a critical period, recovery is impossible. Thus early malnutrition often has irreversible damaging effects, although they may not become fully apparent until maturity and may never be attributed to events of pregnancy. Table 12-1 provides a list of factors that make nutrient deficiencies likely during pregnancy. Notice that young age heads the list; a later section explains why pregnant adolescents are especially prone to malnutrition.

gestation the period from conception to birth, the term of a pregnancy.

The effects of malnutrition during critical periods are seen in neural tube defects of the nervous system (explained later), in the short height of people who were undernourished in their early years, and in the poor dental health of children whose mothers were malnourished during pregnancy. Even when they reach adulthood, people having such a poor start on life may be vulnerable to infections and some may have high risks of stroke or heart disease.[7] These examples demonstrate that the effects of malnutrition during critical periods are irreversible. There is no second chance to provide nutrients. No matter how abundant and nourishing the food, if it is fed after the critical time, it fails to remedy the harm done during the critical period.

Neural tube defects were first defined in Controversy 7.

The last seven months of pregnancy, the fetal period, bring about a tremendous increase in the size of the fetus. Critical periods of cell division and development occur in organ after organ. The amniotic sac fills with fluid to cushion the infant. The mother's body changes greatly, too. The uterus and its supporting muscles increase greatly in size, the breasts may become tender and full, the nipples may darken in preparation for lactation, and the mother's blood volume increases by half to accommodate the added load of materials it must carry. The **gestation** period, which lasts approximately 40 weeks, ends with the birth of the infant.

KEY POINT Maternal nutrition before and during pregnancy affects both present and future development of the infant. Placental development, implantation, and early critical periods depend on nutrient supply and in turn affect future growth and developmental events.

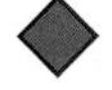

Table 12-1
Factors Placing Pregnant Women at Nutritional Risk

Women likely to develop nutrient deficiencies include those who:

- Are young (adolescents).
- Have had many recent previous pregnancies. (This depletes maternal nutrient stores, but may not affect infant birthweight.)
- Lack nutrition knowledge, have too little money to purchase adequate food, or have too little family support.
- Ordinarily consume an inadequate diet due to food faddism, preferences, weight-loss "dieting," uniformed vegetarianism, other limited food choices, or other reasons.
- Smoke cigarettes or abuse alcohol or illicit drugs.
- Are lactose intolerant or suffer chronic health conditions requiring special diets.
- Are underweight or overweight at conception.
- Are carrying twins or triplets.
- Gain insufficient or excessive weight during pregnancy.
- Have a low level of education.

Increased Nutrient Needs

Nutrient needs during periods of intensive growth are greater than at any other time and are greater for certain nutrients than for others. The nutrient needs of pregnancy are shown in Figure 12-3.

Energy, Protein, and Fat One of the smallest increases recommended is for energy: pregnancy requires only 300 extra calories per day above the allowance for nonpregnant women.[8] The greatest need for energy begins about week 10 and lasts about five months, with needs tapering off in pregnancy's final weeks.[9] A pregnant teenager or a physically active pregnant woman may require more. In each case, enough calories are needed to spare protein for its all-important tissue-building work.

The increase in the recommendation for protein is greater than for energy: from about 45 to 50 grams in a nonpregnant woman to about 60 grams per day for a pregnant woman. Many women in the United States exceed the recommended protein intake for pregnancy even when they are not pregnant, and so need not add protein-rich foods to their diets. Excessive protein may have adverse effects.

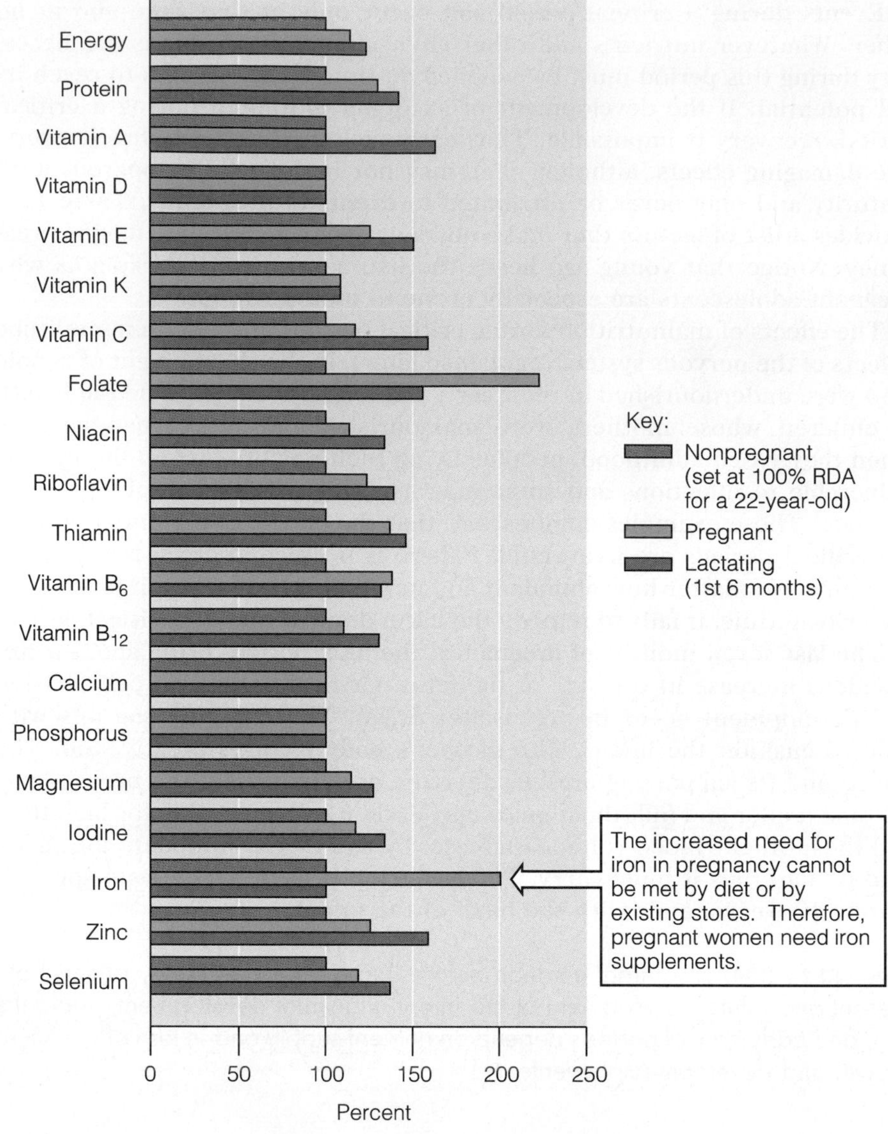

Figure 12-3

COMPARISON OF NUTRIENT RDA OF NONPREGNANT, PREGNANT, AND LACTATING WOMEN

For actual values, turn to the RDA tables on the inside front cover.

Recommended protein intake: 60 grams/day.

Recommended carbohydrate intake: about 50 percent of energy intake. In a 2,000 calorie/day intake, this represents 1,000 calories of carbohydrate, or about 250 grams.

Some vegetarian women limit or omit protein-rich meats, eggs, and dairy products from their diets. For them, meeting the RDA for food energy each day and including several generous servings of plant-protein foods such as legumes, whole grains, nuts, and seeds are imperative steps. All pregnant women need generous amounts of carbohydrate-rich foods to spare their protein and to provide energy.

The high nutrient requirements of pregnancy leave little room in the diet for added purified fats such as oil, margarine, and butter. Some lipids, especially the essential fatty acids, are important to the growth of the fetus, and are regarded by some as "essential nutrients in early human development."[10] The brain is largely made of lipid material, and it depends heavily on products of both omega-3 and omega-6 fatty acids for its growth, function, and structure. A mother-to-be who regularly eats seafood supplies a balance of the essential fatty acids and their derivatives both during pregnancy and afterward in her milk.[11] Supplements of fish oil are not recommended, however, both because they may carry concentrated toxins and

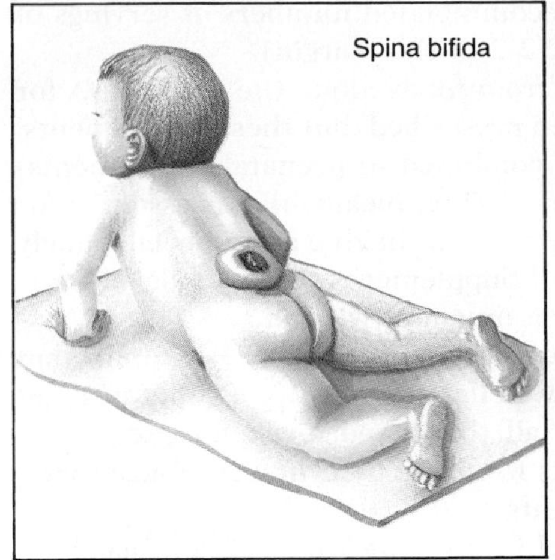

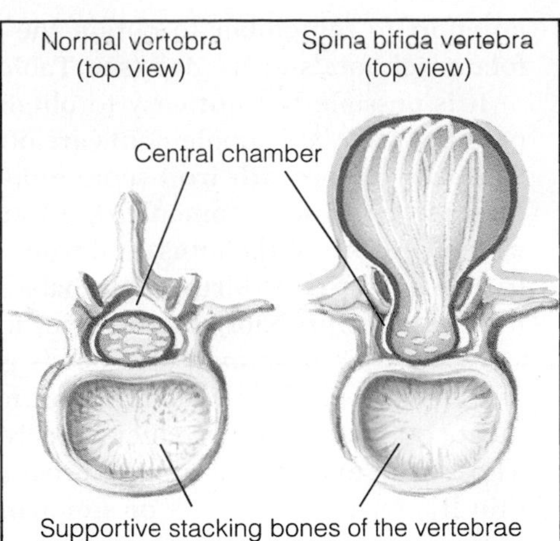

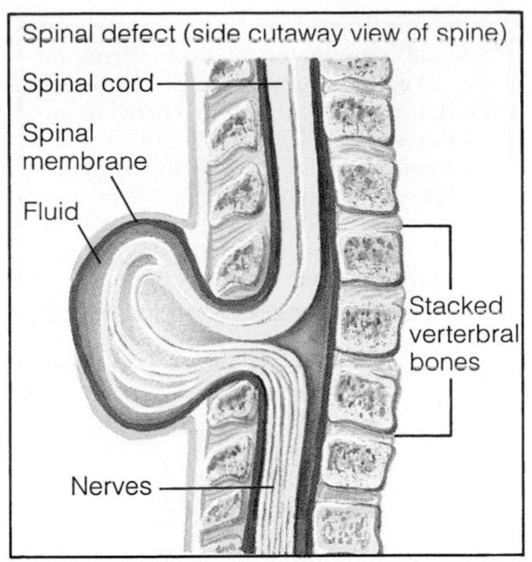

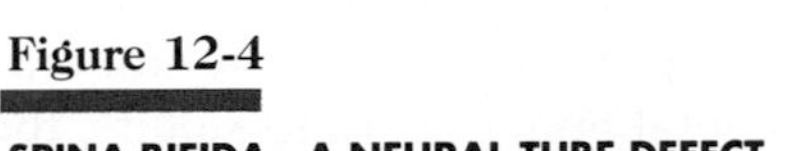

Figure 12-4

SPINA BIFIDA—A NEURAL TUBE DEFECT

Normally, the bony central chamber closes fully to encase the spinal cord and its surrounding membranes and fluid. In spina bifida, the two halves of the slender bones that should complete the casement of the cord fail to join.

In the serious form shown here, membranes and fluid have bulged through the gap and nerves are exposed, invariably leading to some degree of paralysis and often to mental retardation.

because high fish oil intakes have been seen to alter the course of pregnancy and labor with unknown effects.[12] A wiser course is to eat fish or seafood two or three times per week.

Vitamins and Minerals The growing fetus, the altered hormonal activity, and the increased protein metabolism of pregnancy increase the metabolic demand for vitamin B_6. A vitamin B_6 shift occurs during pregnancy, shunting the vitamin from the woman's blood to the tissues of pregnancy where it is needed. This shift causes most pregnant women to test low in blood indicators of vitamin B_6. While this might seem to indicate that supplements are needed, no one knows if this would harm or help. The depressed blood vitamin B_6 in the woman seems not to be harmful, and excess vitamin B_6 taken by her might be forced into the fetal tissue, causing a build-up with unknown consequences. No benefit has been consistently shown to result from supplements of vitamin B_6 in amounts greater than the RDA.

The pregnant woman's RDA for folate is twice that of the nonpregnant woman due to the great increase in her blood volume and the rapid growth of the fetus. Controversy 7 has already described one consequence of entering pregnancy without adequate folate stores and the precedent-setting doubling of the folate recommendation for reproductive-aged women. In review, nearly 400,000 infants each year are born with **neural tube defects,** and half of these are believed to be related to inadequate maternal folate during the earliest weeks of pregnancy. These early weeks are a critical period for the **neural tube,** an open tube of tissue that will later develop to form the brain and spinal cord, and will close, sealing itself off from the body and the outside. By the time a woman suspects she is pregnant, usually around the sixth week, the embryo's neural tube is supposed to have undergone this transformation and closed. If folate is inadequate before pregnancy, however, the tube may not close fully, and **spina bifida** may result (see Figure 12-4 above). Worse, the brain may fail to develop at all, a condition called **anencephaly.** Not every folate-deficient woman will give birth to a child with neural tube defects. Some will, however, so all fertile women of childbearing age who would avoid these devastating effects should make

neural tube the embryonic tissue that later forms the brain and spinal cord.

neural tube defects a group of nervous system abnormalities caused by interruption of the normal early development of the neural tube.

spina bifida (SPEE-na BIFF-ih-duh) a type of neural tube defect in which infants are born with gaps in the bones of the spine, leaving the spinal cord protected only by a sheath of skin in those spots, or with no protection at all. The wall of the spinal cord may bulge and protrude through the gaps in the vertebral column.

anencephaly (an-en-SEFF-ah-lee) a severe neural tube defect in which an infant is born without a formed brain; such infants usually die soon after birth.

The general functions of folate appear in Chapter 7; more about folate supplements appears in Controversy 7.

Special Supplemental Food Program for Women, Infants, and Children (WIC) a USDA program to provide nutrition support to low-income women who are pregnant or who have infants or preschool children. WIC offers coupons redeemable for specific foods to supply the nutrients deemed most needed for growth and development.

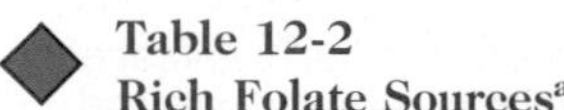

Table 12-2
Rich Folate Sources[a]

Asparagus	Liver
Beets	Orange juice
Fortified cereals	Oranges
Legumes	Spinach and other leafy greens

[a]Folate amounts for these and 1,700 other foods are listed in Appendix A.

Ordinarily a hemoglobin level below 13 grams/100 milliliters is considered low for a woman. In pregnancy, values of 12 grams are not unusual, and 11 grams is where the line defining "too low" is often drawn.

Table 12-3
Nutrient Supplements for Pregnancy

Nutrient	Amount
Folate	300 µg
Vitamin B_6	2 mg
Vitamin C	50 mg
Vitamin D	5 µg
Calcium	250 mg
Copper	2 mg
Iron	30 mg
Zinc	15 mg

Source: Reprinted with permission from *Nutrition During Pregnancy* c. 1990 by the National Academy of Sciences. Published by National Academy Press, Washington, D.C.

an effort to remember to obtain the recommended numbers of servings of folate-rich foods every day (see Table 12-2 in the margin).

It is possible but not easy to obtain from foods alone the folate RDA for pregnancy. Folate supplements are often prescribed, but these supplements, especially those with iron (commonly combined in prenatal supplements) may compromise a woman's zinc status.[13] Zinc, meanwhile, is essential for normal growth of the fetus, and women deficient in zinc are especially likely to give birth to low-birthweight babies.[14] Supplements that include all three nutrients are probably the best bet for a pregnant woman.

The pregnant woman also needs greater amounts of the B vitamin that assists folate in the manufacture of new cells, vitamin B_{12}. People who eat meat, eggs, or dairy products receive all they need, even for pregnancy. Those who exclude all animal products from the diet, however, need vitamin B_{12}-fortified soy milk or supplements.

Among the minerals, those involved in building the skeleton, calcium, phosphorus, and magnesium, are in great demand during pregnancy. Intestinal absorption of calcium doubles early in pregnancy, and the mineral is stored in the mother's bones. Later, as the fetal bones begin to calcify, there is a dramatic shift of calcium across the placenta, and the mother's bone stores are drawn upon. Women's diets are notoriously low in calcium while pregnancy and breastfeeding draw on women's skeletal reserves; thus the increases required for pregnancy may be large. Recommendations for calcium and phosphorus are 1,200 mg per day. Magnesium, needed for bone and tissue growth, is needed in amounts slightly higher than the RDA for nonpregnant women.

The body conserves iron even more than usual during pregnancy. Menstruation ceases, and absorption of iron increases up to threefold. Despite these conservation measures, iron stores dwindle because the developing fetus draws on its mother's iron stores to create stores of its own to carry it through the first three to six months of life. In addition, maternal blood volume increases by as much as 50 percent, and this can give the blood the appearance of anemia in blood tests. The same amount of iron is still in the blood, but it has been diluted. Add to these factors that few women enter pregnancy with adequate stores to meet pregnancy demands, and the wisdom of the committee on RDA becomes evident in their recommendation that women take prescribed iron supplements throughout pregnancy. Supplements for pregnancy include iron along with other needed nutrients (see Table 12-3). Ideally, supplements plus food intakes will cover the needs of all pregnant women, even pregnant vegetarians who most often lack iron.

Pregnancy is clearly a time of increased nutrient needs. A woman of limited financial means may need help in obtaining the needed food and counseling that women of greater means can afford. At the federal level, an underprivileged woman can turn to the **Special Supplemental Food Program for Women, Infants, and Children (WIC)** to receive nutrition counseling and coupons redeemable for nutritious foods. Federal food stamps can also help to stretch her grocery dollars. Her own community may provide educational services and materials, including nutrition, food budgeting, and shopping information, through the local agricultural extension service. Organizations such as the American Diabetes Association and local hospitals may also provide nutrition information.

KEY POINT Pregnancy induces maternal physiological adjustments that demand increases in intakes of energy and even greater increases in intakes of nutrients.

Weight Gain

The pregnant woman must gain a certain amount of weight during pregnancy as a defense against bearing a low-birthweight baby.[15] Ideally she will have begun her pregnancy at the appropriate weight for her height, but even more importantly, she will gain enough weight based on her prepregnancy body mass index (BMI; Table 12-4). The ideal pattern is thought to be about 2 to 4 pounds during the first three months and a pound per week thereafter.

Dieting during pregnancy is not recommended. Even an obese woman should gain about 15 pounds for the best chances of delivering a healthy infant.[16] Weight gain standards must be adjusted primarily to a woman's BMI, as mentioned. Weight gain must be especially generous to meet the needs of a teenager who is still growing herself, and to support women who are carrying twins or triplets. Women have been known to exceed or undershoot the recommended limits in pregnancy without ill effects but the best chances of health are predicted by recommended weight gains. A *sudden*, large weight gain is always a danger signal: it may indicate the onset of pregnancy-induced hypertension. See the section entitled "Troubleshooting" below.

The weight the pregnant woman puts on is nearly all lean tissue: placenta, uterus, blood, milk-producing glands, and, of course, the baby itself (see Table 12-5). The fat she gains is needed later for lactation. Some weight is lost at delivery, but many women retain a pound or two from each pregnancy.

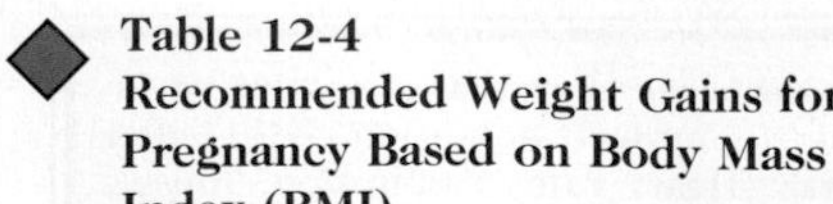

Table 12-4
Recommended Weight Gains for Pregnancy Based on Body Mass Index (BMI)

BMI	Recommended Gain (lb)[a]
<19.8	28–40
19.8–26.0	25–35
26.0–29.0	16–25

[a]Teens should strive to gain the maximum pounds in their ranges; short women (less than 62 inches tall) should strive for the minimum. Weight gain varies widely and these values are suggested only as guidelines for identifying individuals whose weights may be too high or low for health.

Source: National Academy of Sciences, Food and Nutrition Board, *Nutrition During Pregnancy* (Washington, D.C.: National Academy Press, 1990).

KEY POINT Weight gain is critical for a healthy pregnancy. A woman's prepregnancy BMI, her own nutrient needs, and whether or not she is carrying multiple fetuses help to determine an appropriate weight gain.

Exercise

Exercise is important to the pregnant woman, not only to help her carry the extra weight of pregnancy without strain, but also to help ease her upcoming childbirth. In the old days pregnant women were admonished to "stay off their feet," and to "take it easy." However, research indicates that

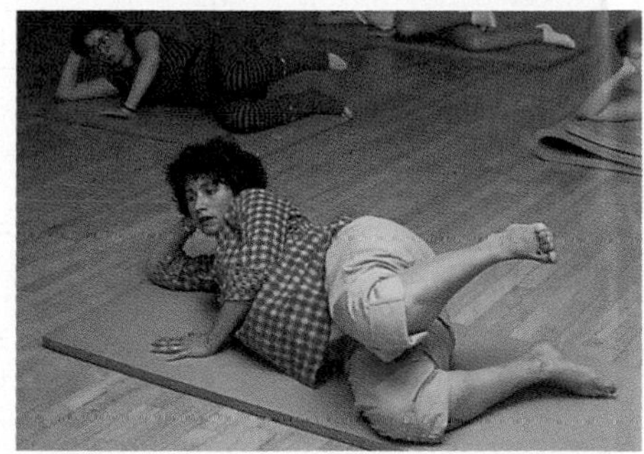

Pregnant women can enjoy the benefits of exercise.

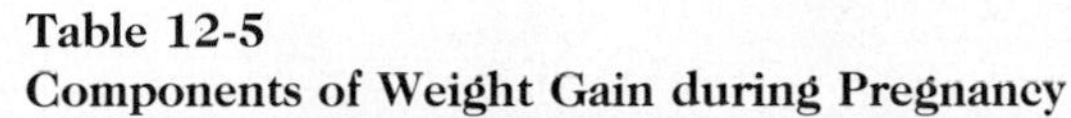

Table 12-5
Components of Weight Gain during Pregnancy

Development	Weight Gain (lb)
Infant at birth	7½
Placenta	1½
Extra blood volume	4
Extra fluid volume	4
Increase in size of uterus	2
Increase in size of breasts	2
Amniotic fluid	2
Mother's fat stores	7
Total	30

Source: The American College of Obstetricians and Gynecologists, *ACOG Guide to Planning for Pregnancy, Birth, and Beyond* (Washington, D.C.: The American College of Obstetricians and Gynecologists, 1990), p. 109.

taking it too easy may be as detrimental to a pregnant woman and her fetus as overexertion. A balanced, 45-minute exercise session three days per week has been associated with more robust babies, fewer surgical births, higher **Apgar scores,** and shorter hospital stays after birth.[17] All pregnant women should consult with their health care providers before taking on any exercise program and should follow the rules listed in the margin.

Apgar score a system of scoring an infant's physical condition right after birth. Heart rate, respiration, muscle tone, response to stimuli, and color are ranked 0, 1, or 2. A low score indicates that medical attention is required to facilitate survival.

Rules for exercising during pregnancy:

- Stop exercising if you feel overheated.
- Drink plenty of fluids before you exercise.
- Avoid exercising in hot, humid weather; do not sit in saunas, steam rooms, or hot tubs.
- Protect the abdomen, especially in games such as baseball or basketball, in which jarring contacts and injuries are likely.
- Discontinue any exercise that causes discomfort.
- After about the fourth month, do not exercise while lying on your back.
- Do not allow your heart rate to exceed 140 beats per minute.

KEY POINT Weight gain is essential to a healthy pregnancy. The pregnant woman should gain from 15 to 40 pounds (25 to 35 pounds for average-weight women) by eating balanced diets of nutrient-dense foods.

Teen Pregnancy

A teen pregnancy presents a special case of intense nutrient needs.[18] Each year one out of every ten teenaged girls becomes pregnant. Of these, 1 million, about half, give birth. Even when not pregnant, a teenaged girl is hard put to meet her own nutrient needs, but when pregnant, a teenaged girl is likely to be deficient in many vitamins and minerals, including vitamins A and C, niacin, iron, and chromium. Nourishing a growing fetus adds to her burden. Her own high nutrient requirements can compete with those of her fetus, especially if she is going through her most rapid growth phase. To support the needs of both mother and fetus, a pregnant teenager with a body mass index in the normal range is encouraged to gain 35 pounds or so. Teenagers who gain less have smaller newborns with associated risks. Complications are common in pregnant teenagers. The greatest risk of a teen pregnancy is death of the infant. The infant mortality rate for mothers under the age of 20 years is high, and mothers under 15 years of age have the highest rate of all age groups.

Little information is available on the specific nutrient needs of pregnant adolescents. Estimates of their nutrient needs are usually made by adding to the RDA for nonpregnant girls 15 to 18 years of age the same amounts of recommended nutrients as are added for pregnant adult women. A pregnant teenager's needs for many nutrients increase greatly, although her energy allowance increases by only a few percent. If a young woman starts pregnancy already malnourished or lacks education, resources, and support, she may develop serious nutrient deficiencies. Table 12-6 provides a guide to the number of food servings recommended to provide nutrients needed

Table 12-6
Daily Food Guide for Teenagers, Pregnant and Lactating Teenagers, and Adult Pregnant and Lactating Women

	Number of Servings[a]		
Food Group	TEENAGERS	PREGNANT OR LACTATING TEENAGERS	PREGNANT OR LACTATING WOMEN
Meat and meat alternates	2 to 3	3	3
Milk and milk products	3	4	3 to 4
Vegetables	3 to 5	4 to 5	4 to 5
Fruits	2 to 4	3 to 4	3 to 4
Breads and cereals	6 to 11	9 to 12	7 to 11

[a]Figure 2-4 provided details concerning serving sizes and foods within the groups listed here.

by teenagers, by pregnant and lactating teenagers, and by pregnant or lactating adult women according to the Daily Food Guide.

Teens are notorious for their poor eating habits. They skip meals, snack on chips and colas, or grab doughnuts for breakfast, and many continue on this path to malnutrition even after becoming pregnant.[19] Luckily, some make at least some effort to eat well, but even those with the best intentions usually fall short of obtaining RDA amounts of at least some nutrients.[20]

Teens' psychological development may affect their nutrition. It is an important developmental task for each teenager to develop an individual identity.[21] The search for identity, while critical to later emotional health, can cause pregnant teens to reject most advice, including nutrition advice, from adult authorities. Most teens do care about their future infants' health, and they may accept advice from respected school coaches or counselors or other people they trust.

KEY POINT Of all the population groups, pregnant teenaged girls have the highest nutrient needs.

Food Choices and Cravings

Because energy needs increase less than nutrient needs, the pregnant woman must select foods of high nutrient density. Appropriate choices include nonfat milk, lean meats, legumes, eggs, liver, dark green vegetables, fruits, and whole-grain breads and cereals. Vitamin C-rich foods at every meal will ensure maximum iron absorption from other foods.

Does pregnancy give a woman the right to nudge her mate out of bed at 2 A.M. to fetch her some pickles and ice cream? Perhaps not for nutrition's sake, but he may choose to humor her anyway. Food cravings and also aversions during and after pregnancy, while common, do not seem to reflect real physiological needs.[22] In other words, a woman who craves pickles is not likely in need of salt. Food cravings and aversions that arise during pregnancy are usually due to changes in taste and smell sensitivities, and they quickly disappear after the baby's birth.

Sometimes cravings may occur in women with nutrient-poor diets. A pregnant woman who is deficient in certain nutrients may crave and eat clay, ice, cornstarch, and other nonnutritious substances, but this does not prove cause and effect. The practice is pica (first mentioned in Chapter 8). Such cravings are not adaptive; the substances she craves do not deliver the nutrients she needs. In fact, clay and other substances can cling to the intestinal wall and form a barrier that interferes with normal nutrient absorption.

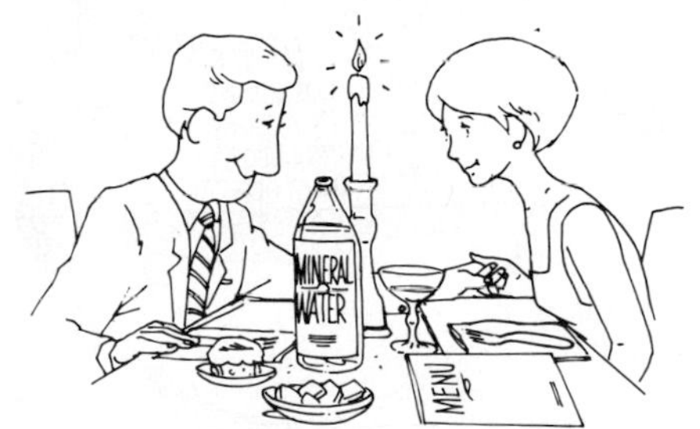

To plan a healthy pregnancy, both parents must make wise choices in advance.

KEY POINT Careful food choices can ensure optimal nutrition during pregnancy. Food cravings usually do not reflect physiological needs and some may interfere with nutrition.

Practices to Avoid

Some substances in a woman's diet and environment can be harmful, and their potential impact is too great to ignore. Of these, alcohol is most ubiquitous and is the topic of the next section. A few others also deserve some discussion.

A clearly harmful practice is smoking. Smoking restricts the blood supply to the growing fetus and so limits the delivery of oxygen and nutrients and the removal of wastes. It slows growth, thus retarding physical development in the uterus; and it causes behavioral problems later on.[23] Constituents of cigarette smoke such as nicotine, cyanide, and others pose a danger to the fetus. One study found the incidence of cancer and leukemia in children of women who continued smoking while pregnant to be twice as high as in nonsmokers. Growing evidence also links smoking with sudden infant death syndrome (SIDS), the unexplained deaths that sometimes occur in otherwise healthy infants.[24] The link to SIDS is true both when the pregnant woman smokes, and when someone smokes in the household of the newborn. The Surgeon General has warned that parental smoking can be lethal to an otherwise normal fetus or newborn.

Fetal effects of abused drugs:

- Amphetamines: Suspected nervous system damage; behavioral abnormalities.
- Barbiturates: Drug withdrawal symptoms in the newborn, lasting up to six months.
- Cocaine: Uncontrolled jerking motions; paralysis; permanent mental and physical damage.
- Marijuana: Short-term irritability at birth.
- Opiates (including heroin): Drug withdrawal symptoms in the newborn, permanent learning disability (attention deficit disorder).

Other drugs taken during pregnancy can cause serious birth defects. The use of drugs not prescribed by a physician, even over-the-counter drugs or high dose vitamin supplements, is inadvisable. Research shows that mothers who abuse drugs such as marijuana and cocaine during pregnancy inflict serious health consequences, including nervous system disorders, on their future infants.[25] Crack and other forms of cocaine pose hazards to infants who may face low birthweight complications, heartbeat abnormalities, and increased risks of death or the pain of withdrawal as they first experience life outside the womb.[26] Some effects of other drugs of abuse on the fetus are listed in the margin.

Among vitamins, a single massive dose of vitamin A (100 times the RDA) has caused birth defects. Experts urge pregnant women not to exceed daily intakes of three times the RDA of vitamin A. Other poisons also injure fetuses, including household insecticides and solvents, lead or other heavy metals from any source, and many other toxins.

Dieting, even for short periods, is also hazardous during pregnancy. Low-carbohydrate diets or fasts that cause ketosis deprive the growing brain of needed glucose and may impair its development. Such diets are also likely to be deficient in other nutrients vital to fetal growth. Energy restriction during pregnancy is dangerous, regardless of the woman's prepregnancy weight or the amount of weight gained in the previous month.

Caffeine crosses the placenta, and the fetus has only a limited ability to metabolize it. No firm limit for caffeine intake is yet available. Intakes of up to the amount in three or four cups of coffee or tea spaced throughout a day are generally thought to be safe.[27] (Caffeine amounts in food and beverages are listed in this chapter's Controversy.)

KEY POINT Abstinence from smoking and other drugs, avoiding dieting, and moderation in the use of caffeine are recommended during pregnancy.

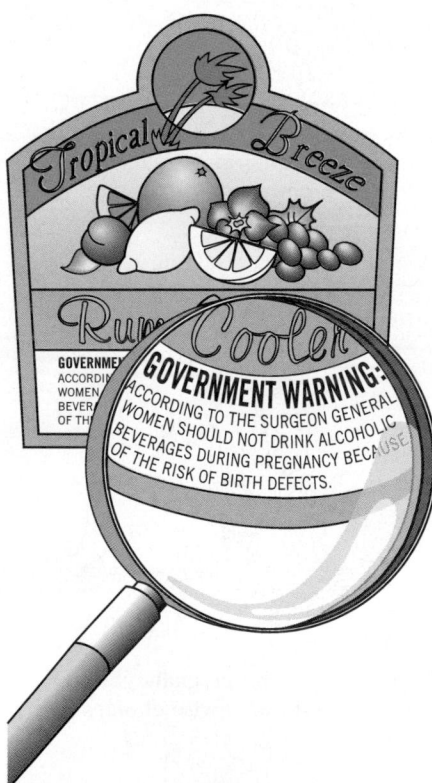

Figure 12-5

MIXED MESSAGES IN ALCOHOL ADVERTISEMENTS
Labels on alcoholic beverages often display "healthy" images, but their warnings tell the truth.

◆ Drinking during Pregnancy

Alcohol is arguably the most hazardous drug to future generations because it is legally available, heavily promoted, and widely abused. Society often sends mixed messages concerning alcohol. Companies promote an image of drinkers as wealthy, healthy, young, and active while health authorities warn that alcohol may have adverse effects, especially during pregnancy (see Figure 12-5). Every container of beer, wine, or liquor for sale in the United States is now required to warn pregnant women of the danger of drinking during pregnancy. In the past, many women who would have ceased drinking during pregnancy, had they known the danger, unwittingly damaged their infants. Women of childbearing age need to know about alcohol's effects.

Alcohol's Effects

As mentioned, oxygen is indispensable on a minute-to-minute basis to the development of the fetus's central nervous system. A sudden dose of alcohol can halt the delivery of oxygen through the umbilical cord. Alcohol also slows cell division, reducing the number of cells produced and inflicting abnormalities on those that are produced.[28] During the first month of pregnancy, even a few minutes of alcohol exposure can exert a major effect on the fetal brain, which at that time is growing at the rate of 100,000 new brain cells a minute. Alcohol also interferes with placental transport of nutrients to the fetus and can cause malnutrition in the mother; then all of malnutrition's harmful effects compound the effects of the alcohol.[29]

KEY POINT Alcohol limits oxygen delivery to the fetus, slows cell division, and reduces the number of cells organs produce. Alcoholic beverages must bear warnings to pregnant women.

fetal alcohol syndrome (FAS) the cluster of symptoms seen in an infant or child whose mother consumed excess alcohol during her pregnancy. FAS includes but is not limited to brain damage, growth retardation, mental retardation, and facial abnormalities.

fetal alcohol effect (FAE) partial abnormalities from prenatal alcohol exposure, not sufficient for diagnosis with FAS, but disruptive and impairing to the child. Also called *alcohol-related birth defects (ARBD)* or *subclinical FAS.*

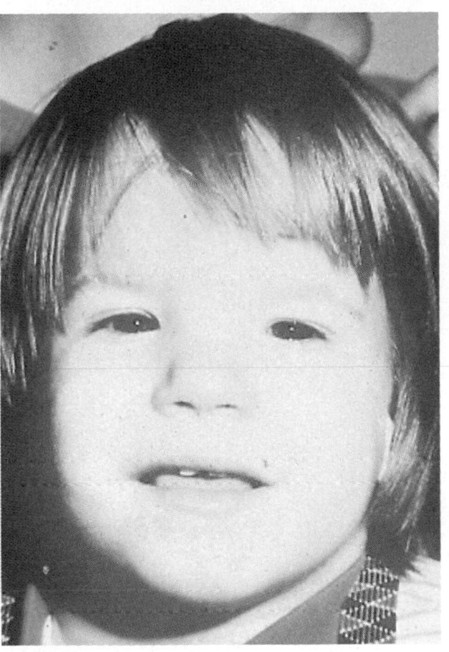

A child with FAS.

Controversy 11 defined "a drink" as:

- 3 to 4 ounces wine
- 10 ounces wine cooler
- 12 ounces beer
- 1 ounce hard liquor

Fetal Alcohol Syndrome

Drinking alcohol during pregnancy threatens the fetus with irreversible brain damage, growth retardation, mental retardation, facial abnormalities, and more than 40 identifiable health problems, a cluster of symptoms known as **fetal alcohol syndrome** or **FAS.**[30] The fetal brain is extremely vulnerable to a glucose or oxygen deficit, and alcohol causes both. In addition, alcohol itself crosses the placenta freely and is directly toxic to the defenseless fetal brain and nervous system. The result is permanent brain damage and life-long mental retardation. FAS is not curable, only preventable by limiting alcohol intake during pregnancy. For women who want to drink during their pregnancies, then, the important question is how much alcohol is too much.

Clearly, 3 ounces of alcohol (about 6 drinks) a day is too much early in pregnancy, even if the woman stops drinking immediately after she learns that she is pregnant. Birth defects have been observed in the children of some women who drank 2 ounces (4 drinks) of alcohol daily during pregnancy. Low birthweight has been observed in infants born to some women who drank 1 ounce (2 drinks) per day during pregnancy. At that level of alcohol intake, a sizable and significant increase occurs in the rate of spontaneous abortions, perhaps by poisoning the fetus or perhaps by causing the placenta to detach. FAS is also known to occur with as few as 2 drinks a day.

In all studies of alcohol doses and damage to the fetus, it is important to take into account that the pattern of drinking, even more than the average alcohol intake, may play an important role. For example, a woman whose average intake was only 1 ounce of alcohol a day might not drink at all during the week, but then might have 14 drinks each weekend. Thus the fetus might be exposed, intermittently, to high alcohol levels.[31] For all intake levels and patterns, the most severe impact is likely to occur in the first month, before the woman may be aware that she is pregnant.

Research using animals shows that one fifth of the amount of alcohol needed to produce major, outwardly visible defects will surely produce learning impairment in the offspring, a condition known as **fetal alcohol**

Figure 12-6

TYPICAL FACIAL CHARACTERISTICS OF FAS

The severe facial abnormalities shown here are just outward signs of the severe mental impairments within. The internal organs also suffer irreversible damage that, while hidden, may create major problems to a child's health.

Source: Adapted from J. O. Beattie, Alcohol exposure and the fetus, *European Journal of Clinical Nutrition* 46 (1992): S7–S17.

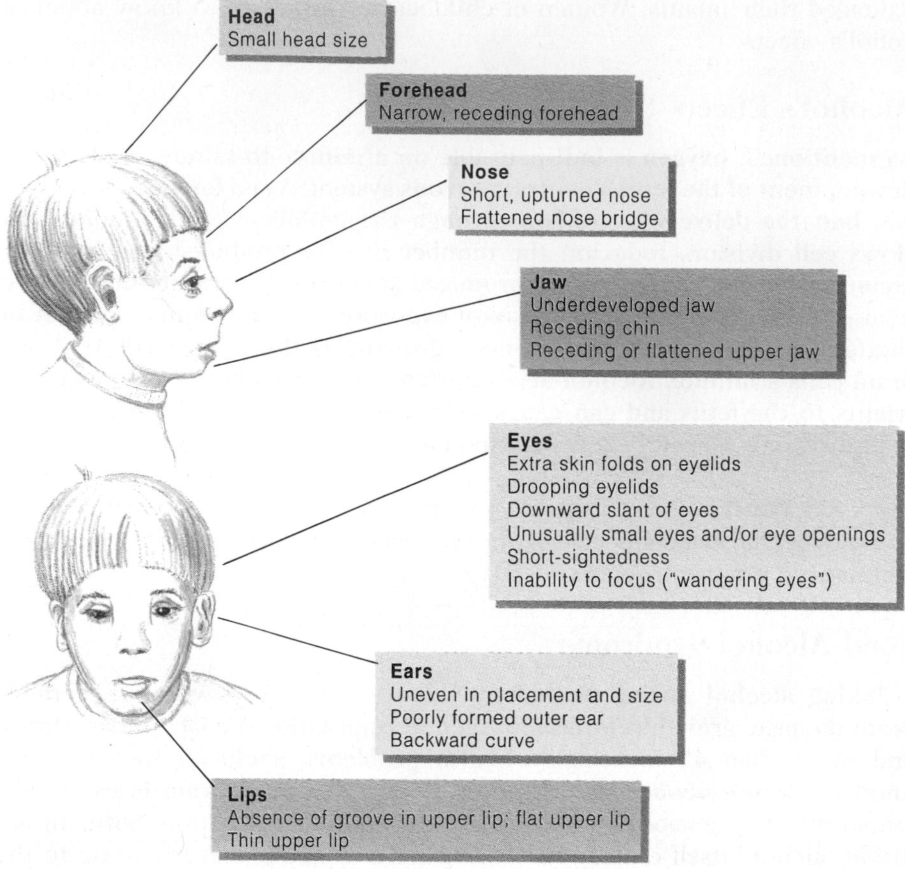

effect (FAE). Some children bear no outward sign of the impairment, but the damage is there on the inside. Others may be short in stature or display minor facial abnormalities. Most perform poorly in school and in social interactions and suffer a subtle form of brain damage. An individual exposed to alcohol before birth may respond differently to it, and also to certain drugs, in adulthood than if no exposure had occurred. Even before fertilization, alcohol may damage the ovum or sperm in the mother or father-to-be, and so lead to abnormalities in children.[32]

Although the syndrome was named for damage evident at birth, it has been shown that children born with it remain damaged. They may live, but they never fully recover. Figure 12-6 shows the facial abnormalities of FAS, because they are easy to depict. A visual picture of the internal harm is impossible, but it is that damage that virtually seals the fate of the child for life. About 3 in every 1,000 children are victims of this preventable damage, making FAS the leading known cause of mental retardation in the world.[33] Moreover, for every baby diagnosed with FAS, 3 or 4 with FAE may go undiagnosed until problems develop later in the preschool years.[34] Upon reaching adulthood, such children are ill equipped for employment, relationships, and the other facets of life most adults take for granted.

KEY POINT The birth defects of fetal alcohol syndrome arise from severe damage to the fetus caused by alcohol. A lesser condition, fetal alcohol effect, may be harder to diagnose but also robs the child of a normal life.

Experts' Advice

The American Academy of Pediatrics takes the position that women should stop drinking as soon as they *plan* to become pregnant.[35] As mentioned, this step is important for fathers-to-be as well. It is important to know, though, that if a woman has drunk heavily during the first two thirds of her pregnancy, she can still prevent some organ damage by stopping heavy drinking during the third trimester.

Not everyone has always agreed that women need to abstain totally from using alcohol during pregnancy. Researchers looking for a "safe" intake limit have come full circle to conceding that abstinence from alcohol is the best policy for pregnant women.[36] The authors of this book do, too. It is a personal choice, but if we had it to make, we would opt for the healthy baby. We would give up even the pleasure of wine with meals "for the duration." After the birth of our healthy baby, we would celebrate, if at all, with one glass of the finest champagne.

KEY POINT Abstinence from or strict restriction of alcohol is critical to prevent irreversible damage to the fetus.

Troubleshooting

Some additional measures can help women to avoid the most common problems encountered during pregnancy. Pregnancy precipitates the onset of **gestational diabetes** in some women. Without proper management, diabetes can lead to fetal or infant sickness and death. Properly managed, it will cause no harm at all. It is therefore recommended that all pregnant women be screened for diabetes at about the sixth month. Thereafter, at every checkup, routine testing of urine for ketone bodies is in order.

A certain degree of **edema** is to be expected in late pregnancy, but in some women it is part of a larger problem known as **pregnancy-induced hypertension (PIH).** Preexisting hypertension and PIH are the most common medical complications of pregnancy. They can cause maternal death, infant death, retarded growth, lung problems, and other birth defects. It is important to keep track of maternal blood pressure throughout pregnancy and if PIH is diagnosed, to initiate treatment promptly. Treatment is medical; salt restriction is not usually part of the treatment.

The nausea of "morning" (actually, anytime) sickness seems unavoidable because it arises from the hormonal changes of early pregnancy. Nausea can often be alleviated by sipping water and nibbling soda crackers or other bland, carbohydrate-rich food before getting out of bed. Carbonated beverages also may help, as may eating small frequent meals throughout the day. Should morning sickness interfere with normal eating for more than a week or two, the woman should seek medical treatment to prevent nutrient deficiencies.

Later, as the hormones of pregnancy alter her muscle tone and the thriving fetus crowds her intestinal organs, an expectant mother may complain of heartburn or constipation. Many women find that, to remedy nighttime heartburn, raising the head of the bed with two or three pillows helps. A high-fiber diet and a plentiful water intake help relieve constipation. Exercise may also help, and it should be a daily practice. The woman should use laxatives or heartburn medication only if her physician prescribes them.

gestational diabetes abnormal glucose tolerance appearing during pregnancy, with subsequent return to normal after the end of pregnancy.

edema accumulation of fluid in the tissues (also defined in Chapter 6).

pregnancy-induced hypertension (PIH) a cluster of symptoms seen in pregnancy, including edema, hypertension, kidney complications, and in severe cases, coma.

Warning signs of PIH:

- Headaches
- Swelling, especially facial swelling
- Dizziness
- Blurred vision
- Sudden weight gain.

The normal edema of pregnancy is a response to gravity: fluid from blood pools in the ankles. The edema of PIH causes swelling of the face and hands as well as of the feet and ankles.

Pregnancy is a time of adjustment to major changes, physical, social, emotional, and financial. The couple who are expecting a baby will have to change their lifestyles as they take on the responsibility of caring for a child. Ideally the mother will start developing this sense of responsibility by caring for herself during pregnancy. The expectant parents need support in thinking of themselves as important people with a new and challenging task that they can and will perform well.

KEY POINT Common medical problems associated with pregnancy are gestational diabetes and pregnancy-induced hypertension (PIH). These should be managed to minimize associated risks.

Breastfeeding

As the time of childbirth nears, a woman must decide whether she will feed her baby breast milk or formula. Before she makes this choice, she should be aware of some things about breastfeeding. For more than ten years, the American Academy of Pediatrics (AAP) has strongly recommended breastfeeding for full-term infants, except in the few cases where contraindications exist. Today, the AAP states that, "Human milk is the best source of nutrition for full-term infants during the first months of life."[37] The American Dietetic Association advocates breastfeeding for the nutritional health it confers on the infant as well as for the physiological, social, economic, and other benefits it gives to the mother.[38] All other legitimate nutrition authorities share this view, but some makers of baby formula would like women to believe otherwise, as the Consumer Caution that follows the next section points out.

Breast Milk

alpha-lactalbumin (lact-AL-byoo-min) the chief protein in human breast milk. The chief protein in cow's milk is *casein* (CAY-seen).

lactoferrin (lak-toe-FERR-in) a factor in breast milk that binds iron and keeps it from supporting the growth of the infant's intestinal bacteria.

Breast milk is tailor-made to meet the nutrient needs of the human infant. Its carbohydrate is lactose, and its fat provides a generous portion of the essential omega-6 fatty acid linoleic acid and its products. In addition, a mother who consumes food rich in omega-3 fatty acids will pass these beneficial nutrients on to her child through her milk. Breast milk contains fat-digesting enzymes that help ensure efficient fat absorption by the infant.[39] Breast milk also conveys information to the infant's body about its environment by way of antibodies, whole proteins, and other constituents. Breast milk even changes in composition, from early milk for the newborn to later milk to feed the older infant. Milk from the mother of a premature infant is different still, and meets the developmental needs of a preterm infant in ways that full-term mother's milk cannot match. For example, the milk for a premature infant provides more protein in less volume, just the right mix to support the rapid growth required to help a premature infant survive its first critical weeks. It may also provide the preterm infant an as-yet-unidentified advantage over formula-fed preterm infants to develop greater intelligence in later childhood.[40]

The protein in breast milk is largely **alpha-lactalbumin,** a protein the human infant can easily digest. Another protein of breast milk, **lactoferrin,** indirectly benefits the baby's iron nutrition and at the same time acts as an antibacterial agent. Lactoferrin is an iron-gathering compound that keeps intestinal bacteria from getting enough iron to grow out of control, helps absorb iron into the infant's bloodstream, and also works directly to kill some bacteria.

The vitamin content of the breast milk of a well-nourished mother is ample. Even vitamin C, for which cow's milk is a poor source, is supplied generously by the breast milk of a mother whose diet is adequate. The concentration of vitamin D in breast milk is low, but this is not a threat to light-skinned infants who are taken out into the sunshine regularly. The dark-skinned infant, or one who has little exposure to sunlight, however, may not make enough vitamin D to prevent rickets. Because so many variables exist regarding vitamin D and sunlight exposure, the American Academy of Pediatrics (AAP) recommends vitamin D supplementation (400 IU per day) beginning at birth for breastfed babies.

colostrum (co-LAHS-trum) a milklike secretion from the breast, rich in protective factors, present during the first day or so after delivery, before milk appears.

As for minerals, the 2-to-1 calcium-to-phosphorus ratio of breast milk is ideal for the absorption of calcium, and both of these minerals, along with magnesium, are present in amounts appropriate for the rate of growth expected in a human infant. Breast milk is also low in sodium. The limited amount of iron in breast milk is highly absorbable, and its zinc, too, is absorbed better than from cow's milk, thanks to the presence of a zinc-binding protein. Given the nutrient composition of breast milk, supplements are not necessary, with the possible exceptions of vitamin D, fluoride, and, after a few months, iron.

If the baby lives in an area with very low concentrations of fluoride in the water, then the pediatrician is likely to prescribe fluoride supplements too. Fluoride concentrations in breast milk appear to remain constant even when the mother's fluoride supply increases somewhat. Infants who consume formula that is mixed with fluoridated water do not need additional fluoride. In areas of nonfluoridated water, continued fluoride supplementation is favored through young life.

As for iron, it seems desirable to begin feeding the breastfed infant iron-fortified cereals by about six months. Before four months, iron is unnecessary because babies are born with enough iron in their livers to last about half a year. Iron deficiency is rarely seen in very young infants.

Breast milk also offers the infant unsurpassed protection against infection. This protection includes antiviral and antibacterial agents and infection inhibitors. Some of these immune molecules are proteins that the infant absorbs whole. The greatest protection offered by these factors, however, may occur in the milk itself where they interfere with growth of bacteria that could otherwise attack the infant's vulnerable digestive tract linings.[41]

During the first two or three days of lactation, the breasts produce **colostrum,** a premilk substance containing antibodies and white cells from the mother's blood. Colostrum is relatively free of bacteria as it leaves the breast, and the baby cannot contract a bacterial infection from it even if the mother has one. Because it contains immunity factors, colostrum helps protect the newborn infant from those infections against which the mother has developed immunity, precisely those in the environment likely to infect the infant. Maternal antibodies from colostrum inactivate harmful bacteria within the infant's digestive tract. Later, breast milk also delivers antibodies, although not as many as colostrum. The degree to which antibodies are delivered in milk depends partly on how well nourished the woman is herself.[42] Malnourished women often have abnormal immune responses, so they do not have enough antibodies to share.

The effects of malnutrition on immunity were presented in Chapter 11.

Certain factors in colostrum and breast milk favor the growth of "friendly" bacteria in the infant's digestive tract, so that other, harmful bacteria cannot grow there.* Another factor present in colostrum and breast milk stimulates the development of the infant's digestive tract. Worn cells in the infant's digestive tract are promptly replaced, facilitating the tract's functioning.

Other factors in breast milk include several enzymes, several hormones, and lipids, all of which protect the infant against infection. Prolonged breastfeeding (six months or more) may reduce the incidence of allergic or autoimmune disease in babies with family histories of such diseases. Much remains to be learned about the composition and characteristics of human milk. Clearly it is a very special substance.

KEY POINT Breast milk is normally the ideal food for infants. It contains not only the needed nutrients in the right proportions but also protective factors. It is especially valuable for premature infants.

*The "friendly" bacteria are the *Lactobacillus bifidus* type.

Formula's Advertising Advantage

CONSUMER CAUTION Most women know that breastfeeding has advantages, yet a third more women chose bottle feeding in 1990 than in 1980.[43] Why, when every legitimate nutrition authority strongly recommends breastfeeding, do so many women who could breastfeed choose formula?

Certainly, most women are free to choose whatever feeding method best suits their needs. For only a few is breastfeeding prohibited for medical reasons. Many women, though, are influenced by formula advertisements leading them to believe that formula is just as good for infants as human milk.

Advertisers of infant formulas often strive to create the illusion that formula is *identical* to human milk. In reality no formula can match the nutrients, agents of immunity, and environmental information conveyed to infants through human milk. The ads are convincing, though: "Like mother's milk, our formula provides complete nutrition" or "Why trust anything but our brand? It's scientifically formulated to meet your baby's needs." These ads imply, falsely, that breast milk is "unscientific," unknown, and therefore untrustworthy.

To augment their market share, formula sellers give new mothers coupons for free formula. After childbirth, women receive "goodie bags" with coupons to tempt them to go and receive their "gifts." Later, drug stores dispense more coupons whenever computerized cash registers ring up items related to breastfeeding, such as pads that protect clothing from milk. Still more coupons may arrive by mail three months later, when some women give up breastfeeding, even though authorities urge continued breastfeeding for several more months.[44]

The U.S. Surgeon General set a goal that 75 percent of new mothers should be breastfeeding on discharge from the hospital in 1990. In 1990 the actual number of women breastfeeding at the time of leaving the hospital was barely over 50 percent, and the government-

Formula's Advertising Advantage *continued*

sponsored WIC program was providing almost half a billion dollars in free formula each year to impoverished new mothers.[45]

Contrary to appearances, the WIC program is not passing off baby formula on new mothers. The registered dietitians who advise WIC mothers promote breastfeeding at every opportunity. Many mothers who seek help from WIC have already begun to feed formula but cannot afford its price. Once a mother starts feeding her infant formula, her own milk dries up. Then she must continue feeding formula. At this point WIC has no choice but to supply her baby with the formula it needs.

A problem can occur if the mother's income goes up slightly. She may lose WIC support but still not earn enough to purchase expensive formula each week. In the past, impoverished women of developing countries who received free formula at first, just long enough to dry up their milk, were in the same bind. To save money, they tried to stretch the formula by adding extra usually polluted, water; or they made a dangerous early switch to regular cow's milk. Many babies died from infection as a result. Most developing nations now wisely ban free formula gimmicks within their borders. Meanwhile, in the United States, no one knows how many impoverished women resort to measures similar to those that third-world women have used and injure the health of their infants.

Formula-fed infants in the United States are generally healthier than those of third-world countries, and they usually grow normally on formula, but they do miss out on the breastfeeding advantages pointed out in the text. Women should of course be free to choose between breast and bottle, but the decision is important and should be made by carefully weighing true, unslanted facts. The choice should not be influenced by sophisticated advertising ploys created by an industry that profits from formula sales.

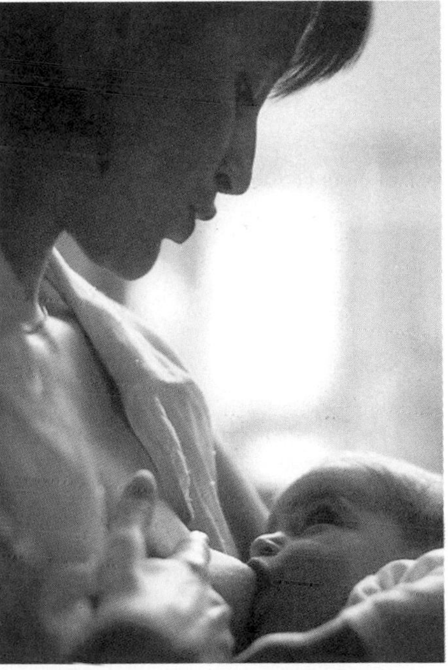

Breastfeeding goes most smoothly for the woman who prepares.

Concerns for the Breastfeeding Mother

Toward the end of her pregnancy, a woman who plans to breastfeed her baby should begin to prepare. No elaborate or expensive preparations are needed, but the expectant mother might want to read at least one of the many handbooks available on breastfeeding.* Among the preparations is to learn what dietary changes are needed. Adequate nutrition is essential to successful lactation; without it, lactation may falter.

A nursing mother produces about 25 ounces of milk a day (more in early lactation, less later on when the baby begins eating other foods). Producing this milk costs a woman almost 650 calories per day. About 500 calories of

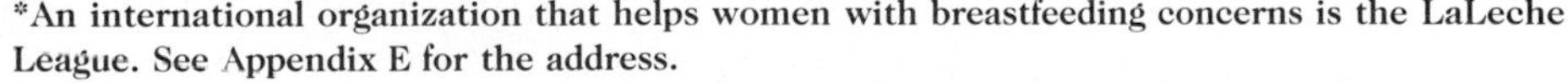

*An international organization that helps women with breastfeeding concerns is the LaLeche League. See Appendix E for the address.

this energy should be provided by the diet. The other 150 calories may be drawn from the fat stores the woman accumulated during pregnancy.

The food energy consumed by the nursing mother should carry with it abundant nutrients, especially those needed to make milk, such as calcium, protein, magnesium, zinc, and enough fluid to prevent dehydration. Figure 12-3 showed the differences between a lactating woman's nutrient needs and those of a nonpregnant woman, and Table 12-6 suggested a food pattern that meets them.

Breast-milk volume depends not on how much fluid the mother drinks but on how much milk the baby demands.[46] The nursing mother is nevertheless advised to drink at least 2 quarts of liquids each day to protect herself from dehydration. To help themselves remember to drink enough liquid, many women make a habit of drinking a glass of milk, juice, or water each time the baby nurses as well as at mealtimes.

People often ask about the old adage "beer makes good milk." Beer does seem to stimulate prolactin, a hormone important to lactation. However, the alcohol in beer enters breast milk and can easily overwhelm an infant's immature alcohol-degrading system. A woman's hormones need no external assistance to perform perfectly, and even beer should be strictly limited to an occasional one serving. Even this amount may alter the taste of the milk to the disapproval of the nursing infant, who may, in protest, drink less milk than normal.[47] Similarly, excess caffeine can make a baby jittery and wakeful. Other drugs have worse effects.

Infants may be sensitive to foods such as cow's milk, onions, or garlic in the mother's diet, and they may become uncomfortable when she eats them. However, while a few babies may be sensitive to certain foods, not all nursing mothers need to avoid them. A mother who is nursing her baby is advised to eat whatever nutritious foods she chooses. Then, if she suspects a particular food of causing the infant discomfort, she can try eliminating that food from her diet for a few days and see if the problem goes away.

Another question often raised is whether a mother's milk may lack a nutrient if she fails to get enough in her diet. The answer differs from one nutrient to the next, but in general, the effect of nutritional deprivation of the mother is to reduce the *quantity*, not the *quality*, of her milk. For protein, carbohydrate, and most minerals, the milk of a healthy mother has a fairly constant composition. Any excess water-soluble vitamins the mother takes in are excreted in the urine; the body does not release them into the milk. The amounts of fat-soluble vitamins in human milk are affected, however, by the mother's excessive or deficient intakes. For example, large doses of vitamin A correspondingly raise the concentration of this vitamin in breast milk.[48] Vitamin supplementation of *undernourished* women appears to help normalize the vitamin concentrations in their milk and may be beneficial.

If a mother does not breastfeed, she may find it hard to lose the fat she gained during pregnancy.[49] This does not mean that a breastfeeding woman can eat unlimited food and still effortlessly return to prepregnancy weight. Breastfeeding costs energy, true, but carefully chosen programs of diet and exercise are still the cornerstones of weight control. A gradual weight loss (1 pound per week) is safe and has no effect on milk output. However, too large an energy deficit, especially soon after birth, will inhibit lactation. A new mother's exercise program is contingent on her physician's approval.

KEY POINT The lactating woman needs extra fluid and enough energy and nutrients to make 30 ounces of milk a day. Malnutrition most often diminishes the quantity of the milk produced, without altering quality. Lactation facilitates loss of the extra fat gained during pregnancy.

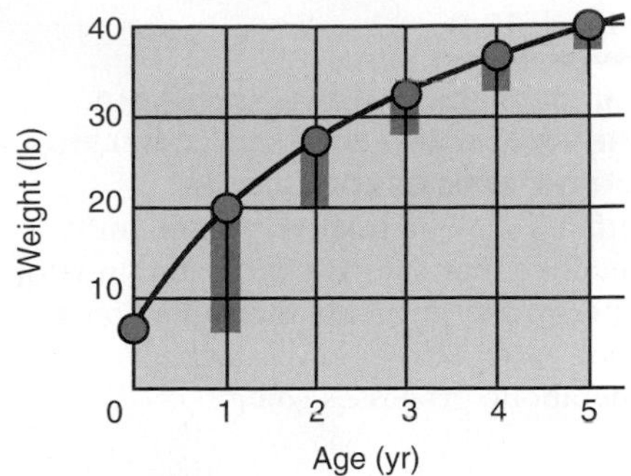

Figure 12-7

WEIGHT GAIN OF HUMAN INFANTS IN THE FIRST FIVE YEARS OF LIFE

The colored vertical bars show how the yearly increase in weight gain diminishes over the years.

Feeding the Infant

For a while the infant drinks only breast milk or formula, but later it becomes able to handle other foods. Early nutrition affects later development, and early feedings establish eating habits that influence nutrition throughout life.

Trends change and experts argue the fine points, but nourishing a baby is relatively simple. Common sense in the selection of infant foods and a nurturing, relaxed environment go far to promote the infant's well-being.

Nutrient Needs

A baby grows faster during the first year of life than ever again, as Figure 12-7 shows. Pediatricians carefully monitor the growth of infants and children, since growth is an important reflection of nutrition status. The birthweight doubles around four months of age and triples by the age of one year. (If a 150-pound adult were to do this, the person's weight would increase to 450 pounds in a single year.) By the end of the first year, the growth rate slows considerably, so that between the first and second birthdays, the weight gained amounts to less than 10 pounds.

The rapid growth and metabolism of the infant demand an ample supply of all the nutrients. However, the energy nutrients and those vitamins and minerals critical to the growth process, such as vitamin A, vitamin D, calcium, and iron, have special importance during infancy.

Babies, because they are small, need smaller total amounts of these nutrients than adults do; but as a percentage of body weight, babies need over twice as much of most nutrients. Figure 12-8 compares a three-month-old baby's needs (per unit of body weight) with those of an adult man. As you can see, some of the differences are extraordinary. Sometime around six months of age, energy needs increase less rapidly as the growth rate begins to slow down, but some of the energy saved by slower growth is spent in increased activity. When their growth slows, infants spontaneously reduce their energy intakes. This means that parents should expect their babies to adjust their food intakes downwards when appropriate, and they should not force or coax them to eat more.

The most important nutrient of all, for infants as for everyone, is the one easiest to forget: water. The younger a child the greater the percentage of the body weight is water, and the more rapid is the turnover. Proportionately more of the infant's body water than the adult's is between the cells and in the vascular space, and this water is easy to lose. Conditions that cause fluid loss, such as vomiting, diarrhea, or sweating, can rapidly propel an infant into life-threatening dehydration. In early infancy, breast milk or infant formula normally provides enough water for a healthy infant to replace water losses from the skin, lungs, feces, and urine. When the child starts eating solid foods, additional water is required. If an infant is exposed

Figure 12-8

NUTRIENT RDA OF A FIVE-MONTH-OLD INFANT AND AN ADULT MALE COMPARED ON THE BASIS OF BODY WEIGHT

Infants may be relatively small and inactive, but they use large amounts of energy and nutrients in proportion to their body size to keep all their metabolic processes going.

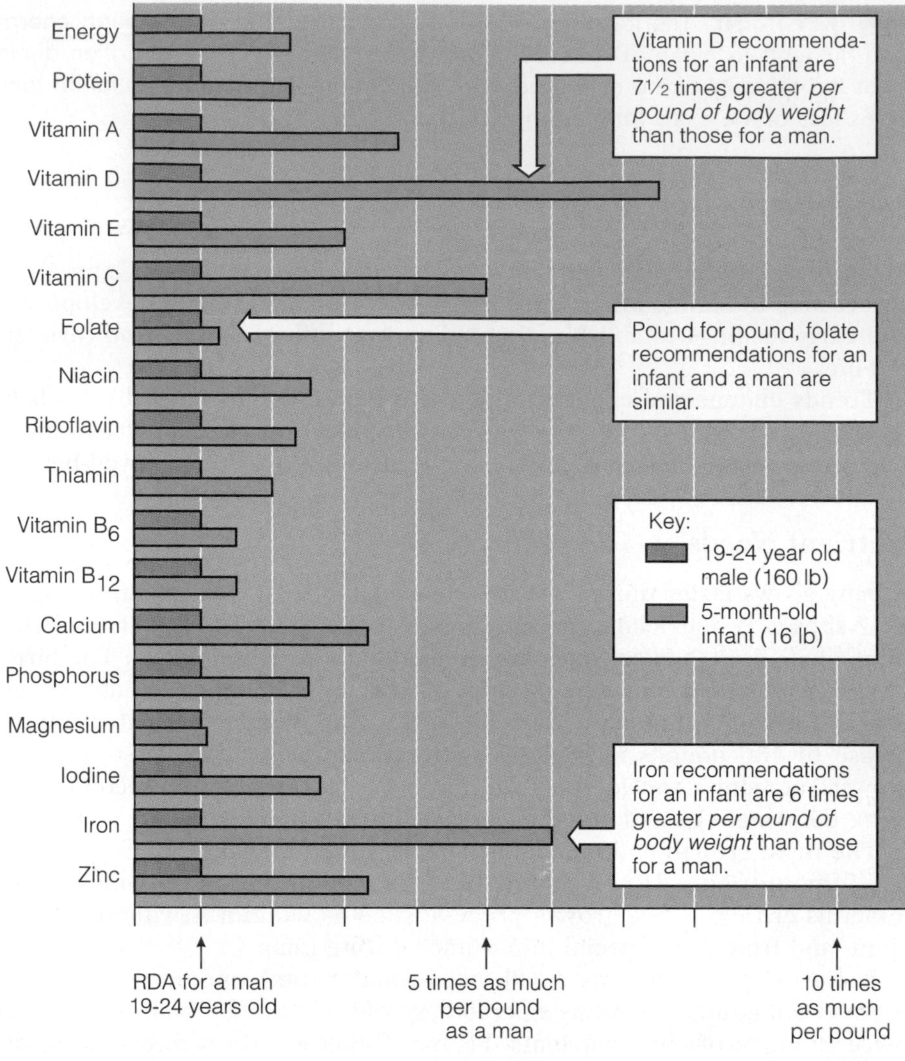

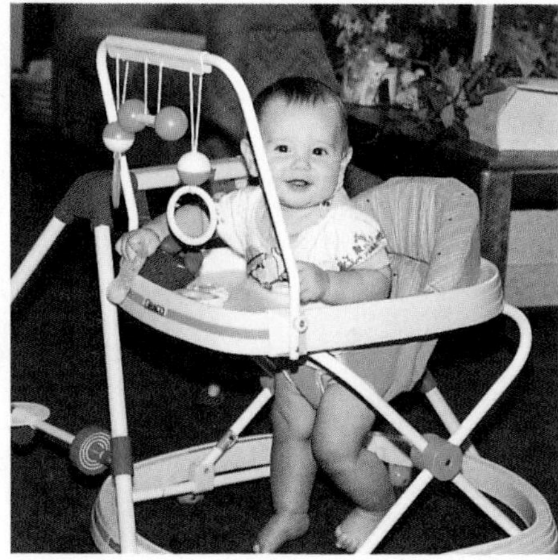

After age six months, energy saved by the slowing of growth is spent on increasing activity.

to hot weather or is ill with diarrhea or persistent vomiting, supplemental water is needed to prevent dehydration. If the weather is hot and the mother is thirsty, her infant probably is, too. Should a dangerous dehydration set in, a physician must decide whether to give a special rehydrating solution containing sodium by mouth or to administer the needed solution intravenously. Infants cannot tell you what they are crying for; remember that they may need plain water, and let them drink it until they quench their thirst.

The type of milk the infant receives and the age at which solid foods are introduced are major areas of concern in infant nutrition research. Under most circumstances a woman can freely choose to feed breast milk or formula, knowing that either will meet the infant's nutrient needs. However, if the family has a low income or if other factors threaten the baby's health, then the advantages of breast milk tip the balance in favor of breastfeeding.

KEY POINT Infants' rapid growth and development depend heavily on adequate nutrient supplies. Adequate water is also crucial.

When Not to Breastfeed

If a woman has an ordinary cold, she can go on nursing without worry. The infant will probably catch it from her anyway, and thanks to immunological protection, a breastfed baby may be less susceptible than a formula-fed baby would be. If a woman has a communicable disease such as tuberculosis or hepatitis that could threaten the infant's health, then mother and baby have to be separated. Breastfeeding may be continued by pumping the mother's breasts several times a day and letting the baby drink the milk from a bottle (see margin). The virus responsible for causing AIDS (HIV) can be passed from an infected mother to her infant during pregnancy, at birth, or through breastfeeding, so women who have tested positive for HIV should not breastfeed.

For safe breast milk storage:

- Wash hands thoroughly before pumping.
- Clean pumping equipment according to manufacturer's directions.
- Sterilize bottles, nipples, and rings before using.
- Refrigerate milk to be fed within 48 hours. Freeze milk to be stored longer than 48 hours.
- Thaw milk gently on defrost cycle of microwave or in refrigerator.
- Do not refreeze thawed milk.

Similarly, if a nursing mother must take medication that is secreted in breast milk and that is known to affect the infant, then breastfeeding is contraindicated. Many prescription drugs do not reach nursing infants in sufficient quantities to affect them adversely. Some, however, do. As a precaution, a nursing mother should consult with the prescribing physician prior to ingesting any drug. Many women wonder about using oral contraceptives during lactation. One type that combines the hormones estrogen and progestin seems to suppress milk output, lower the nitrogen content of the milk, and shorten the duration of breastfeeding. In contrast, progestin-only pills have been shown to have no effect on breast milk or breastfeeding and so are considered appropriate for lactating women.[50] Drug addicts, including alcohol abusers, are capable of taking such high doses that their infants can become addicts by way of breast milk; in these cases, too, breastfeeding is contraindicated.

A woman sometimes hesitates to breastfeed because she has heard that environmental contaminants may enter breast milk and harm her infant. While some contaminants do enter breast milk, others may be filtered out of the milk. Formula-fed infants consume a great deal of tap water because formula is made with water, and so they receive directly whatever contaminants may appear in the water supply. The decision whether to breastfeed on this basis might best be made after consultation with a physician or dietitian familiar with the local circumstances.

For more about contaminants and nutrition, turn to Chapter 14.

KEY POINT Most ordinary infections such as colds have no effect on breastfeeding. Breastfeeding may be inadvisable if milk is contaminated with drugs or environmental pollutants.

Formula Feeding and Weaning to Milk

The substitution of formula feeding for breastfeeding involves striving to copy nature as closely as possible. Human and cow's milks differ; cow's milk is significantly higher in protein, calcium, and phosphorus, for example, to support the calf's faster growth rate. A formula can be prepared from cow's milk that does not differ significantly from human milk in these respects; the formula makers first dilute the milk and then add carbohydrate and nutrients to make the proportions comparable to those of human milk. Still, some evidence seems to indicate that formula-fed infants attain larger size at an earlier age than do breastfed infants. It is unknown what, if any, long-term effects early feeding choices may have on children's later growth, or whether this extra growth harms or benefits health or is just neutral.

Formula preparation:

- Liquid concentrate (inexpensive, relatively easy)—mix with equal part water.
- Powdered formula (cheapest, lightest for travel)—read label directions.
- Ready-to-feed (easiest, most expensive)—pour directly into clean bottles.
- Whole milk—do not use before 12 months of age.

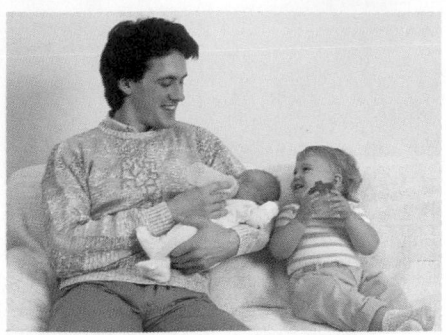

Bottle feeding lets other family members in on the fun.

Formula feeding offers a major advantage to the mother whose attempts at breastfeeding have met with frustration. Nourishment for the infant from formula is adequate, and a mother can choose this course with confidence. Other advantages are that parents can see that the baby is getting enough milk during feedings. Also, other family members can enjoy participating in feeding sessions, offering them a chance to develop the special closeness that feeding fosters, and freeing the mother to give time to her other children or to herself. Mothers who resume employment early after giving birth may choose formula for their infants, but they have another option. Breast milk can be pumped into bottles and given to the baby in day care. At home, mothers may breastfeed as usual. Many mothers use both methods—they breastfeed at first but wean to formula within the first six months.

Table 12-7 compares the composition of human milk with typical formulas. For infants with special problems, formulas can be adapted to meet their special needs (adjusted protein ratio, lower linoleic acid, lower minerals). For premature babies, special premature formulas are available. For infants of strict vegetarians or for those allergic to milk protein, special formulas based on soy protein are available. For infants with lactose intolerance, formulas with the lactose replaced can be used. For infants with other special needs, many other variations are available.

For as long as formula or breast milk is the baby's major food, ordinary milk is an inappropriate replacement, primarily because cow's milk provides insufficient vitamin C, essential fatty acids, and iron. Once the baby is obtaining at least two-thirds of the total daily food energy from a balanced mixture of cereals, vegetables, fruits, and other foods (usually after twelve months of age), then whole cow's milk in any form, fortified with vitamins A and D, is acceptable as an accompanying beverage.

The AAP and many pediatricians advise continued use of infant formula and not cow's milk throughout the first year because formula provides more nutrients, particularly iron, and is more suited to an infant's needs.[51] Plain, unmodified cow's milk (including whole, skim, low-fat, or evaporated milk) is not recommended before 12 months. The infant's digestive tract may be sensitive to the protein content and, if so, may bleed and worsen iron de-

Table 12-7
Human Milk Compared with Infant Formula for Selected Nutrients

Content	Mature Human Milk	Fortified Infant Formula
Energy (cal/100 ml)	64	67
Protein (% of cal)	6	9
Fat (% of cal)	40–50	50
Carbohydrate (% of cal)	41	42
Iron (mg/L)	0.5	1.5–12
Vitamin A (μg/L)	675	660
Niacin (mg/L)	1.5	7.5
Vitamin D (μg/L)	2.2	41
Inositol (mg/L)	149	32

Sources: Data from K. J. Motil, Breast-feeding: Public health and clinical overview, in *Pediatric Nutrition,* eds. R. J. Grand, J. L. Sutphen, and W. H. Dietz (Stoneham, Mass.: Butterworths, 1987), pp. 251–263; L. A. Barness, ed., Committee on Nutrition, American Academy of Pediatrics, *Pediatric Nutrition Handbook* (Elk Grove, Ill.: American Academy of Pediatrics, 1993), Appendix E.

Table 12-8
Milk Terms

- **casein or sodium caseinate** the principal protein of cow's milk. Other milk proteins, found in a higher percentage in human milk, include **lactalbumin**, found in the milk's **whey.**
- **condensed milk** evaporated milk to which a large amount of sugar (sucrose) is added during processing, intended for making desserts, not for feeding babies. Accidental use of condensed milk in preparation of infant formula can cause dehydration.
- **evaporated milk** milk concentrated to half volume by evaporation. Adding water reconstitutes the milk; the taste, however, is altered by the processing.
- **evaporated milk formula** formula made at home from evaporated milk, sugar, and water, seldom used today and not recommended.
- **fortified** (with respect to milk) milk to which vitamins A and D have been added.
- **homogenized milk** milk treated to mix the fat evenly with the watery part (fat ordinarily floats to the top as cream). Heated milk is forced under high pressure through small openings to emulsify the fat.
- **lactalbumin** see *casein.*
- **pasteurized milk** milk that is heat treated to eliminate disease-causing microbes and to reduce its total bacterial count to an acceptable level.
- **powdered milk** dehydrated milk solids. Some powdered milks rehydrate easily (instant milk); others require extensive blending. Both whole and nonfat milk can be powdered.
- **whey** the liquid that remains after milk has coagulated (see also *casein*).
- **whole milk** full-fat cow's milk.

ficiency. A lasting allergy to cow's milk may develop. Also, the infant's immature kidneys are stressed by plain cow's milk. Table 12-8 defines some terms applied to types of milk.

KEY POINT Infant formulas are designed to resemble breast milk and must meet an AAP standard for nutrient composition. Special formulas are available for premature babies, allergic babies, and others. Formula should be replaced with milk only after the baby is eating a balanced assortment of foods, no earlier than at six months; a year is preferred.

First Foods

Foods can be introduced into a baby's diet as the baby becomes physically ready to handle them. This readiness develops in stages. A newborn baby can swallow only liquids that are well back in the throat. Later (at four months or so) the baby's tongue can move against the palate to swallow semisolid food such as hot cereal. Still later, the first teeth erupt, but it is not until sometime during the second year that a baby can begin to handle chewy food. The stomach and intestines are immature at first; they can digest milk sugar (lactose) but not starch. At about four months, most babies can begin to digest starchy foods.

The baby's kidneys are unable to concentrate waste efficiently, so a baby must excrete relatively more water than an adult to carry off a comparable amount of waste. This means that the risk of dehydration is higher for infants than for adults, and it becomes even greater once solid foods are

milk anemia iron-deficiency anemia caused by drinking so much milk that iron-rich foods are displaced from the diet.

introduced. Water and other fluids take on added importance to prevent dehydration.

Iron deficiency is prevalent in children between the ages of six months and three years due to their rapid growth rate and the significant place that milk has in their diets. This can lead to iron-deficiency anemia, popularly called **milk anemia.**

Iron ranks highest on the list of nutrients most needing attention in infant nutrition. A baby's stored iron supply from before birth runs out after the birthweight doubles, so formula with iron, then iron-fortified cereals, and then meat or meat alternates are recommended. By the end of the first year, half or more of all infants are receiving less than the RDA for iron, and one fourth are receiving less than two thirds of the RDA. Six-month-old infants who are weaned to cow's milk have lower blood-iron measures than those who remain on formula.[52] While iron is of primary importance, vitamin C is also important.

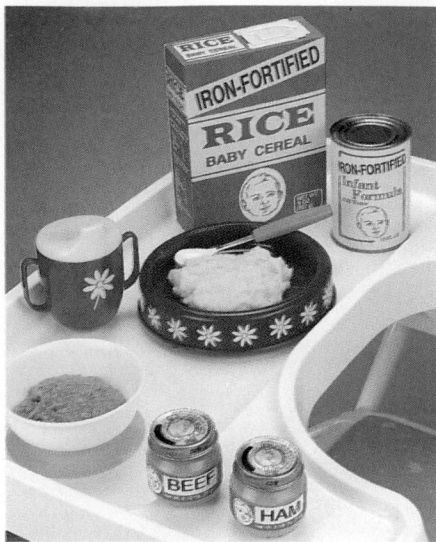

Foods such as iron-fortified cereals and formulas, mashed legumes, and strained meats provide iron.

The timing for adding solid foods to a baby's diet depends on several factors. Formula or breast milk alone is sufficient until age four to six months. Babies who are ready for solid foods thrive when they receive them, and they develop new skills through handling foods in their diets. Any of the following indicates readiness:

- When the infant can sit with support and can control its head movements.
- When the birthweight has doubled.
- When the infant is about six months old.

All babies develop according to their own schedules, and while Table 12-9 presents a suggested sequence, individuality is important. Three considerations are relevant: the baby's nutrient needs, the baby's physical readiness to handle different forms of foods, and the need to detect and control allergic reactions.

Table 12-9
First Foods for the Infant

Age (Months)	Addition
0–4	Breast milk or formula only—no advantage gained from supplemental foods
4–6	Iron-fortified rice cereal, followed by other cereals (for iron; baby can swallow and can digest starch now)[a]
5–7	Strained vegetables and/or fruits and their juices,[b] one by one (perhaps vegetables before fruits, so the baby will learn to like their less sweet flavors)
6–8	Soft or strained protein foods (cheese, yogurt, tofu, cooked beans, meat, fish, chicken, egg yolk)
8–10	Finely chopped meat (baby can chew now), toast, teething crackers (for emerging teeth) and soft table foods (start slowly)
10–12	Whole egg (allergies are less likely now), whole milk (at 12 months), more table foods

[a]Later you can change cereals, but don't forget to keep on using the iron-fortified varieties.

[b]All baby juices are fortified with vitamin C. Orange juice causes allergies in some babies; apple juice is often recommended.

stroyed the tyramine from the cheese and wine. Tyramine built up in the woman's body to levels that caused the potentially fatal reaction.

These three examples involved legal medicines' interactions with nutrients. Table C12-1 gives some examples of other possible drug-nutrient interactions, including both prescription and OTC medications.

OTC drugs are readily available and widely used in the United States and can harm people's nutrition status, especially when they are misused. For example, people who use laxatives daily for weeks or months may find that their intestines can no longer function without them. Laxative dependence can lead to malnutrition, since laxatives can cause nutrients to travel so rapidly through the intestines that many vitamins do not have time to be absorbed. The laxative mineral oil can rob a person of fat-soluble vitamins because they dissolve in the indigestible oil and are excreted. Vitamin D deficiencies can occur this way; calcium, too, may be excreted with the oil, accelerating adult bone loss.

Advertisers promote antacids as a panacea for those who overindulge themselves in rich food and drink, but people with recurrent stomach pain should be checked by a physician. Such pain can indicate a serious condition such as an ulcer. Antacids containing calcium are also promoted as mineral supplements, but taking antacids every day can cause an iron deficiency as already mentioned. Similarly, the presence of aluminum hydroxide in an antacid can inhibit the absorption of phosphorus.[2] Phosphorus is necessary for bone mineralization, and chronic use of some antacids can eventually impair bone health. One elderly woman had to be admitted to the hospital because the pain in her legs had gotten so bad that she could barely stand up or walk unassisted. During this same period of time she had more than doubled her consumption of antacids. Once she stopped taking the antacids, the pain in her legs subsided.

Many people take large quantities of aspirin, easily 10 to 12 tablets each day, to relieve the pain of arthritis, backaches, and headaches. This much aspirin can speed up blood loss from the stomach by as much as ten times, enough to cause iron-deficiency anemia in some people.[3] People who take aspirin regularly should make sure they eat iron-rich foods regularly as well.

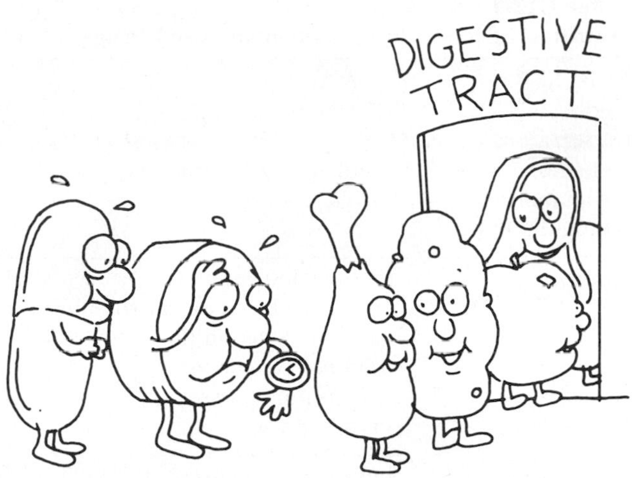

Foods can slow down the absorption of drugs in the digestive tract.

ORAL CONTRACEPTIVES AND ESTROGEN REPLACEMENT THERAPY Millions of women use **oral contraceptives,** daily doses of hormones that prevent pregnancy by creating a hormonal climate similar to that of pregnancy itself. After a 30-year history, oral contraceptives have become the most studied drugs in the United States. The identification of a number of risk factors has prompted changes in the dosages and formulations to produce effective contraceptives with wide margins of safety. The many effects of oral contraceptives illustrate that interactions between just one drug and nutrients can be complex.

Women past menopause may take **estrogens** to protect their bones from excessive calcium losses and to minimize their risks of developing heart disease. Estrogen replacement therapy also brings some alterations of metabolism, including nutrient interactions.

Oral contraceptives clearly do alter the concentrations of nutrients in the blood. One of their most significant health effects is to alter blood lipids, possibly raising the risk of cardiovascular disease.[4] This effect poses very little risk for young, healthy women who do not smoke.[5] Beyond about age 35, however, most oral contraceptives raise total cholesterol and triglyceride concentrations and lower HDL, amplifying the risk of stroke and heart disease. Fewer than 5 percent of women using oral contraceptives also experience mild hypertension. A leading expert in contraceptive technology puts these risks in perspective, however, by comparing the risk to life of a woman who both smokes and uses oral contraceptives with risks from other activities. A ride in a power boat or a drive in a car are more than twice as risky to life, and a motorcycle ride carries 16 times the risk.[6]

Each nutrient responds differently to oral contraceptive use. Oral contraceptives depress tissue concentra-

Table C12-1
Nutrition Effects of Some Commonly Used Drugs

Medicines and Caffeine	Effects on Absorption	Effects on Excretion	Effects on Metabolism
Antacids (aluminum containing)	Reduce iron absorption	Increase calcium and phosphorus excretion	May accelerate destruction of thiamin
Antibiotics	Reduce absorption of fats, amino acids, folate, fat-soluble vitamins, vitamin B_{12}, calcium, copper, iron, magnesium, potassium, phosphate, zinc	Increase excretion of folate, niacin, potassium, riboflavin, vitamin C	Interfere with synthesis of vitamin K
Aspirin	Lower blood concentration of folate	Increase excretion of thiamin, vitamin C, vitamin K; causes iron and potassium losses through blood loss	
Caffeine		Increase excretion of calcium and magnesium	In large doses, may elevate blood cholesterol
Diuretics		Raise blood calcium and zinc; lower blood folate, chloride, magnesium, phosphorus, potassium, vitamin B_{12}; increase excretion of calcium, sodium, thiamin, potassium, chloride, magnesium	Interfere with storage of zinc
Laxatives	Reduce absorption of glucose, fat, carotene, vitamin D, other fat-soluble vitamins, calcium, phosphate, potassium	Increase excretion of all unabsorbed nutrients	
Oral Contraceptives	Reduce absorption of folate, may improve absorption of calcium	Cause sodium retention	Raise blood vitamin A, copper, iron; may lower blood folate, riboflavin, vitamin B_6, vitamin B_{12}, vitamin C; may elevate requirements for riboflavin and vitamin B_6
Estrogen Replacement Therapy	May reduce absorption of folate	Cause sodium retention	May raise blood glucose, triglycerides, vitamin A, vitamin E, copper, and iron; may lower blood vitamin C, folate, vitamin B_6, riboflavin, calcium, magnesium, and zinc

Sources: J. J. Murray and M. D. Healy, Drug-mineral interactions: A new responsibility for the hospital dietitian, *Journal of the American Dietetic Association* 91 (1991): 66–70, 73; S. Landvik, Drug and food interactions: The antioxidant nutrients, *RD* 1 (1990): 1, 48; J. E. Henningfield and coauthors, Drinking coffee and carbonated beverages blocks absorption of nicotine from nicotine polacrilex gum, *Journal of the American Medical Association* 264 (1990): 1560–1564; D. E. Powers and A. O. Moore, *Food Medication Interactions* (Phoenix: Food Medication Interactions, 1988).

tions of folate and blood concentrations of vitamin C, vitamin B_6, and zinc, while they raise blood concentrations of vitamin A, vitamin K, iron, and copper. At first glance this might seem to indicate that women using them may be on their way to suffering deficiencies of the first four nutrients named and may have somehow enlarged their body stores of the last four. The research in the area has yielded conflicting results, however, so any such assumptions would be premature. Research suggests that the changed blood concentrations of some nutrients may reflect a redistribution of the nutrients within the body and not a changed total-body content of the nutrients.

Take vitamin A, for example. The higher-than-usual vitamin A blood concentrations in oral contraceptive users appear to be due to the release of extra vitamin A from storage in the liver. Knowing this, researchers became concerned that this might deplete vitamin A in the liver and lead to deficiency.[7] They found otherwise. Oral contraceptives do not appear to deplete liver vitamin A or cause deficiency.

Oral contraceptive users also have higher blood concentration of iron. In this case, unlike that of vitamin A, the drugs seem to have brought about enhanced conservation of iron by the body. Oral contraceptive use brings about both less blood loss in menstruation and greater absorption of iron in the intestine. However, iron in the blood of oral contraceptive users stays well within the normal range.

The vitamin B_6 status of oral contraceptive users has been extensively studied. Research shows that some oral contraceptive users have low blood concentrations of vitamin B_6. Since vitamin B_6 assists in the body's handling of the amino acid tryptophan, this pathway is impaired. Because other vitamin B_6-dependent functions remain normal, confusion persists about whether oral contraceptive users require more vitamin B_6 than nonusers. Excess vitamin B_6 can be toxic (see Chapter 7), so oral contraceptive users are generally advised to rely on vitamin rich, nutrient-dense foods to replenish their supply and to avoid supplements.

Some women feel that taking oral contraceptives makes them gain or lose weight. Indeed, approximately as many women lose as gain weight when taking oral contraceptives, and some may gain 20 pounds or more, especially those who retain fluid.[8] Some of the gain is from fat deposited in hips, thighs, and breasts. Some may be lean tissue deposited in response to an androgenic (steroid) effect of the pills. Sometimes a switch to another form of pill can normalize body weight.

estrogen a female sex hormone that regulates the ovulatory cycle and has widespread effects on other body tissues.

oral contraceptives pills containing synthetic hormones that disrupt the female menstrual cycle and prevent ovulation; used to prevent conception, often called birth control pills.

over-the-counter (OTC) drug a drug legally available without a prescription.

prescription drug a drug available only with a physician's order.

As with oral contraceptives, women's responses to estrogen replacement drugs must be assessed individually. Some women may suffer edema, because estrogen promotes sodium conservation by the kidneys. This requires sodium restrictions for its correction.[9] Others may develop abnormally low blood concentrations of folate or vitamin B_6, indicating a need to include more vitamin-rich, nutrient-dense foods in the diet. All women taking estrogen should be aware that vitamin C doses of a gram or more may elevate serum estrogen and falsely indicate the need for a reduced dose.[10]

If a woman who uses oral contraceptives or estrogen replacement therapy thinks she may have a nutrient deficiency, she should refrain from taking individual supplements and seek testing and a diagnosis from a health care professional to rule out other causes of her symptoms. For most women a nutritious diet is all that is needed. However, if a woman feels compelled to take a supplement, a multivitamin-mineral supplement that does not exceed the RDA is probably harmless, as long as it is in addition to a well-balanced diet and not a replacement for such a diet. Controversy 7 showed how to select a supplement.

CAFFEINE The well-known "wake-up" effect of caffeine is the primary reason why people in every society use it in some form. Compared with the drugs discussed so far, though, caffeine's interactions with foods and nutrients are subtle. And yet in one important way caffeine's relationship to nutrition is more notable. People usually ingest caffeine by way of foods and beverages, and they may even be unaware that they are consuming it at all. Many OTC cold and headache remedies also contain caffeine because it perks up even sick people and relieves the headache caused by caffeine withdrawal that no other pain reliever can touch.[11] Table C12-2 lists the caffeine contents of beverages and foods.

Caffeine is a true stimulant drug. Like all stimulants, it increases the respiration rate, heart rate, blood pres-

Table C12-2
Caffeine Content of Beverages and Foods

Drinks and Foods	Average (mg)	Range (mg)
Coffee (5-oz cup)		
Brewed, drip method	130	110–150
Brewed, percolator	94	64–124
Instant	74	40–108
Instant "lite"	30	no data
Decaffeinated, brewed or instant	3	1–5
Tea (5-oz cup)		
Brewed, major U.S. brands	40	20–90
Brewed, imported brands	60	25–110
Instant	30	25–50
Iced (12-oz glass)	70	67–76
Herb teas (caffeine-free)	0	0
Soft drinks (12-oz can)		
Dr. Pepper		40
Colas and cherry colas:		
Regular		30–46
Diet		2–58
Clear and caffeine free		0–trace
Extra caffeine (Jolt)		75–100
Mountain Dew, Mello Yello		52
Big Red		38
Fresca, 7–Up, Sprite, Squirt, Sunkist Orange, seltzers, root beers		0
Cocoa beverage (5-oz cup)	4	2–20
Chocolate milk beverage (8 oz)	5	2–7
Milk chocolate candy (1 oz)	6	1–15
Dark chocolate, semisweet (1 oz)	20	5–35
Baker's chocolate (1 oz)	26	26
Chocolate-flavored syrup (1 oz)	4	4
Carob	0	0

Note: Many over-the-counter medications such as pain relievers and cold medicines also contain caffeine. Their labels must list the milligram amounts of caffeine per dose of medicine. Read medicine labels carefully.

sure, and secretion of stress and other hormones. It stimulates the digestive tract, promoting efficient elimination, and promotes water loss from the body as well.

Caffeine is the most popular and widely consumed drug in the United States.[12] One in three people in the United States consumes about 200 milligrams of caffeine per day (the amount in 2 small cups of coffee), but many others consume amounts that could be harmful.[13] Children are especially sensitive to caffeine's effects because they are small and, at first, not adapted to its use. Parents should stay aware of the caffeine in items their children favor such as chocolate bars, colas, and other soft drinks.

Despite caffeine's tremendous popularity, many people today are cutting their use of it because they fear it will harm them. Research in the last decade has yielded sporadic reports linking caffeine to health problems such as hypertension, fibrocystic breast disease, birth defects, clinical anxiety, and cancer, to name a few.[14] However, much other research refutes these findings. For example, the weight of evidence now seems to suggest no link between caffeine and cancer or birth defects.[15] Increased caffeine intake seems to accompany advanced age, higher body weight, and more cigarette and alcohol use.[16]

Results of another study suggest that moderate caffeine intakes may speed up metabolic energy expenditures.[17] As little as 100 milligrams of caffeine noticeably raised the metabolic rates of both lean and previously obese people for several hours after consumption.

Caffeine seems relatively harmless when used in moderation (the equivalent of fewer than, say, 2 to 4 average-sized cups of coffee a day). In amounts greater than this, caffeine can cause symptoms associated with anxiety: sweating, tenseness, and inability to concentrate. Caffeine is even suspected but not proved to raise heart disease and heart attack risks.[18] Caffeine may also contribute to painful but benign fibrocystic breast disease.

If you like consuming caffeine-containing foods or beverages, the most reasonable approach may be to limit your intake to the equivalent of about 2 small cups of coffee per day. For most people this is enough to produce the desired effects of reduced drowsiness and keener awareness of tasks at hand without paying too high a price. Pregnant women, especially, should exercise moderation in using caffeine, and parents should monitor and control their children's intakes.

TOBACCO Cigarette and other smoking is a pervasive health problem causing thousands of people to suffer from cancer and diseases of the cardiovascular, digestive, and respiratory systems. These effects are beyond the scope of nutrition, but smoking does influence hunger, body weight, and nutrient status. Links between smoking's nutrition effects and lung cancer are also known.

Smoking a cigarette eases feelings of hunger. A smoker who receives a hunger signal can quiet it with a cigarette instead of food. Such behavior ignores body signals and postpones energy and nutrient intake. Thus smokers tend to weigh less than nonsmokers and to gain weight upon cessation of smoking.[19] Weight gain is often a concern for people contemplating giving up cigarettes, but researchers are beginning to view the effect as a temporary and helpful compensation mechanism that brings weight regulation back to normal.[20] The message to smokers wanting to quit is to adjust diet and exercise habits to maintain weight during and after cessation.

Nutrient intakes of smokers and nonsmokers differ.[21] Smokers have lower intakes of dietary fiber, vitamins, and minerals, even when their energy intakes are quite similar to those of nonsmokers. The association between smoking and low vitamin intake may be noteworthy, considering the altered metabolism of vitamin C in smokers, their lowered blood levels of beta carotene, and the possible protective effect of antioxidant vitamins against lung cancer. Research on beta carotene and faulty immunity of smokers is just beginning, but much is known about vitamin C.[22]

Research shows that the vitamin C requirement of smokers exceeds that of nonsmokers.[23] Smokers break down vitamin C faster, and so must take in more vitamin C-containing foods to achieve steady body pools comparable to those of nonsmokers. It is estimated that the vitamin C requirement of smokers may be twice as high as that of nonsmokers. The evidence for this is so strong that it is reflected in the vitamin C RDA, set at 100 milligrams per day for smokers compared to 60 for nonsmokers.[24]

ILLICIT DRUGS People know that illicit drugs are harmful, but in spite of the risks, many choose to abuse them anyway. Like OTC and prescription drugs, illegal drugs modify body functions. They are unlike medicines, however, in that no watchdog agency such as the FDA monitors them for safety, effectiveness, or even for purity. Drugs purchased on the street are likely to contain impurities or to be mixed with cheaper drugs to maximize profits for the pushers. The risks of using illicit drugs are many and diverse, ranging from health risks to imprisonment to early death. Marijuana and cocaine are probably the best known illicit drugs.

Smoking a marijuana cigarette has several characteristic effects on the body, altering, among other things, the sense of taste. Among the apparent taste changes induced by marijuana is an enhanced enjoyment of eating, especially of sweets, commonly known as "the munchies." Why or how this effect occurs is not known. Despite increased food intakes, marijuana abusers often consume fewer nutrients than do nonabusers. This is probably because the extra foods they choose are usually high-calorie, low-nutrient snack foods. In addition to the effects on nutrition, regular marijuana users may face the same risk of lung cancer as people who smoke a pack of cigarettes a day.[25]

Cocaine elicits effects such as intense euphoria, restlessness, heightened self-confidence, irritability, insomnia, and loss of appetite. Weight loss is a common side effect, and cocaine abusers often develop eating disorders. Repeated use can cause a rapid heart rate, irregular heartbeats, heart attacks, and even death. Cocaine use continues to escalate as cheaper and more dangerous forms of the drug become available. Cocaine in its smokable form, crack, is more addicting than any other drug. The addictive power of the drug is overwhelming and frightening. One former crack addict tells the story of holding a gun to his brother's head to steal money for his next crack purchase.

Unlike marijuana use, cocaine use brings serious nutritional consequences. Notably, the craving for the drug replaces hunger; the stronger the craving for cocaine, the less a drug abuser wants nutritious food. Rats given unlimited access to cocaine will choose the drug over food until they die of starvation.

The effects of other addictive drugs vary in degree but are similar in kind to those of cocaine. A few are listed in Table C12-3. Drug abusers face multiple problems that impinge on nutrition:

- They spend money for drugs that could be spent on food.
- They lose interest in food during "high" times.
- Some drugs induce at least a temporary depression of appetite.
- Their lifestyle often lacks the regularity and routine that promote good eating habits.
- They may contract hepatitis, a viral liver disease spread via infected needles, which causes taste changes, loss of appetite, and loss of weight. (They risk contracting AIDS in the same way.)
- Their nutrition status may be altered by treatments and medicines.
- Those who become ill with infectious diseases develop increased needs for nutrients.

During withdrawal from drugs, an important aspect of treatment is the identification and correction of nutrition problems.

PEOPLE AT RISK Not all the interactions discussed here occur every time a person takes a drug. Some

Table C12-3
Nutrition Effects of Four Nonmedical Drugs

Drug of Abuse	Possible Effects on Nutrition Status
Cocaine	Reduces intakes of nutritious foods; increases intakes of alcohol, coffee, and fat; may increase incidence of eating disorders
Heroin	Heightens and delays insulin response to glucose; reduces intakes of nutritious foods
Marijuana	Increases food intakes, especially sweets; may cause weight gain
Nicotine	Reduces intakes of sweet foods and water; increases intakes of fat; reduces fetal weight in pregnant women; lowers blood concentration of beta carotene

Sources: Data from M. E. Mohs, R. R. Watson, and T. Leonard-Green, Nutritional effects of marijuana, heroin, cocaine, and nicotine, *Journal of the American Dietetic Association* 90 (1990): 1261–1267; G. van Poppel, S. Spanhaak, and T. Ockhuizen, Effects of beta carotene on immunological indexes in healthy male smokers, *American Journal of Clinical Nutrition* 57 (1993): 402–407.

people are more vulnerable than others to drug-nutrient interactions. The potential for undesirable drug-nutrient interactions is greatest for those who:

- Take medication or any drug for a long period of time.
- Take two or more drugs at the same time.
- Are not well nourished to begin with or are not eating adequate diets.

In conclusion, when you need to take a medicine, do so wisely. Ask your health care provider for specific instructions about the doses and when to take them—for example, with meals or on an empty stomach. If you notice new symptoms or if the drug does not seem to be working well, consult your health care provider. The only instruction people need about illicit drugs is to avoid them altogether for countless reasons. As for smoking and chewing tobacco, the same advice applies: don't take these habits up, or if you already have, take steps to quit. For drugs with lesser consequences to health, such as caffeine, use moderation.

Try to live life in a way that requires less chemical assistance. If sleepy, try a 15-minute nap or meditation instead of a 15-minute coffee break. The coffee will stimulate your nerves for an hour, but the alternatives will refresh your attitude for the rest of the day. If you suffer constipation, try getting enough exercise, fiber, and water for a few days. Chances are that a laxative will be unnecessary. The strategy being suggested here is to take control of your body, allowing your reliable, self-healing nature to make fine adjustments in functioning without overriding them with chemicals. Bodies have few requests: adequate nutrition, rest, exercise, and hygiene. Give yours what it needs, and let it function naturally, without interference from drugs on a day-to-day basis.

Notes

1. J. E. Henningfield and coauthors, Drinking coffee and carbonated beverages blocks absorption of nicotine from nicotine polacrilex gum, *Journal of the American Medical Association* 264 (1990): 1560–1564.
2. J. J. Murray and M. D. Healy, Drug-mineral interactions: A new responsibility for the hospital dietitian, *Journal of the American Dietetic Association* 91 (1991): 66–70, 73.
3. Why food and medicine don't always make a good mix, *Tufts University Diet and Nutrition Letter*, July 1989, pp. 3–6.
4. E. L. Marut, Oral contraceptives—Who, which, when, and why? *Postgraduate Medicine* 82 (1987): 66–70.
5. R. A. Hatcher and coauthors, *Contraceptive Technology* (New York: Irvington, 1992), pp. 240–241.
6. Hatcher, 1992, p. 146.
7. K. Amatayakul and coauthors, Oral contraceptives: Effect of long-term use on liver vitamin A storage assessed by the relative dose response test, *American Journal of Clinical Nutrition* 49 (1989): 845–848.
8. Hatcher, 1992, pp. 284–285.
9. Murray and Healy, 1991.
10. D. E. Powers and A. O. Moore, *Food Medication Interactions* (Pheonix: Food Medication Interactions, 1988), p. 102.
11. K. Silverman and coauthors, Withdrawal syndrome after the double-blind cessation of caffeine consumption, *New England Journal of Medicine* 327 (1992): 1109–1114.
12. T. K. Leonard, R. R. Watson, and M. E. Mohs, The effects of caffeine on various body systems: A review, *Journal of the American Dietetic Association* 87 (1987): 1048–1053.
13. R. Watson, Caffeine: Is it dangerous to health? *American Journal of Health Promotion* Spring 1988, pp. 13–22.
14. Watson, 1988.
15. Grounds for breaking the coffee habit? *Tufts University Diet and Nutrition Letter*, February 1990, pp. 3–6.
16. M. R. Joesoef and coauthors, Are caffeinated beverages risk factors for delayed conception? *Lancet* 335 (1990): 136–137.
17. A. G. Dulloo and coauthors, Normal caffeine consumption:

Influence on thermogenesis and daily energy expenditure in lean and postobese human volunteers, *American Journal of Clinical Nutrition* 49 (1989): 44–50.
18. L. Rosenberg and coauthors, Coffee drinking and nonfatal myocardial infarction in men under 55 years of age, *American Journal of Epidemiology* 128 (1988): 570–578; A. L. Klatsky, G. D. Friedman, and M. A. Armstrong, Coffee use prior to myocardial infarction restudied, *American Journal of Epidemiology* 132 (1990): 479–488.
19. M. E. Mohs, R. R. Watson, and T. Leonard-Green, Nutritional effects of marijuana, heroin, cocaine, and nicotine, *Journal of the American Dietetic Association* 90 (1990): 1261–1267; D. F. Williamson and coauthors, Smoking cessation and severity of weight gain in a national cohort, *New England Journal of Medicine* 324 (1991): 739–745.
20. S. R. Schwid, M. D. Hivonen, and R. E. Keesey, Nicotine effects on body weight: A regulatory perspective, *American Journal of Clinical Nutrition* 55 (1992): 878–884.
21. A. F. Subar, L. C. Harlan, and M. E. Mattson, Food and nutrient intake differences between smokers and nonsmokers in the U.S., *American Journal of Public Health* 80 (1990): 1323–1329.
22. G. van Poppel, S. Spanhaak, and T. Ockhuizen, Effects of beta carotene on immunological indexes in healthy male smokers, *American Journal of Clinical Nutrition* 57 (1993): 402–407.
23. G. Schectman, J. C. Byrd, and H. W. Gruchow, The influence of smoking on vitamin C status in adults, *American Journal of Public Health* 79 (1989): 158–162.
24. Food and Nutrition Board, Committee on Dietary Allowances, *Recommended Dietary Allowances*, 10th ed. (Washington, D.C.: National Academy of Sciences, 1989), pp. 115–124.
25. T. C. Wu and coauthors, Pulmonary hazards of smoking marijuana as compared with tobacco, *New England Journal of Medicine* 318 (1988): 347–351.

Child, Teen, and Older Adult

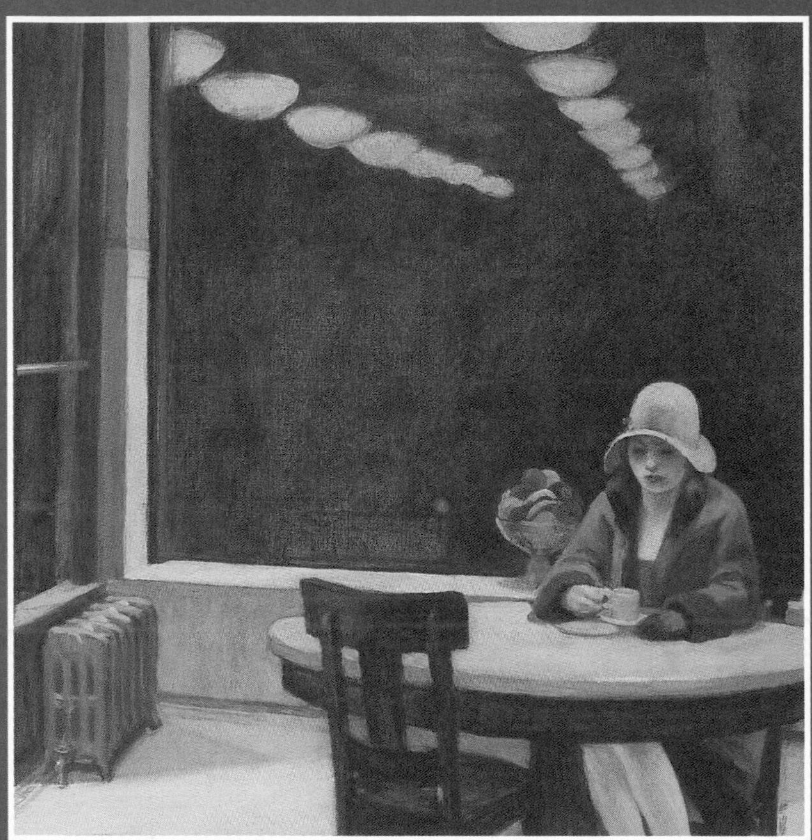

Contents

Edward Hopper, Automat, Des Moines Art Center Permanent Collection, purchased with funds from the Edmundson Art Foundation, Inc., 1958.2.

13

Parents look forward to being proud of strong, healthy, competent, and happy sons and daughters. To grow and to function well in the adult world, children need a solid background of sound eating habits. These habits begin at babyhood with the introduction of solid foods, as shown in the last chapter. But at that point nutrition has just begun; the plot thickens. Nutrient needs change steadily throughout life into old age, depending on the rate of growth, gender, activities, and many other factors. Nutrient needs also vary from individual to individual, but generalizations are possible and useful.

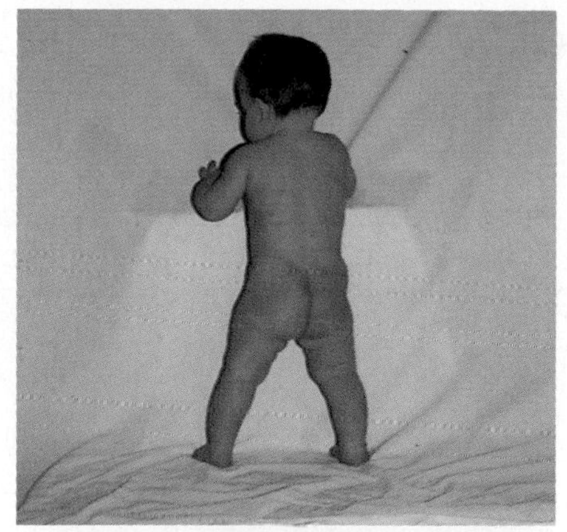

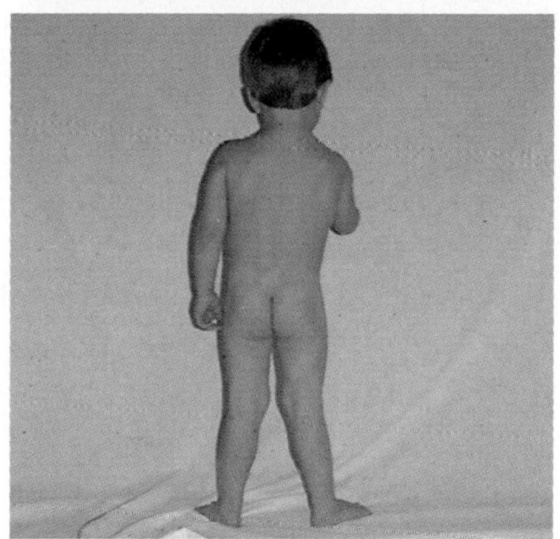

The body shape of a one-year-old (above) changes dramatically by age two (below). The two-year-old has lost much of the baby fat; the muscles (especially in the back, buttocks, and legs) have firmed and strengthened; and the leg bones have lengthened.

Early and Middle Childhood

After the age of one year, a child's growth rate slows; but the body continues to change dramatically. At age one, infants have just learned to stand and toddle; by two years they can take long strides with solid confidence and are learning to run, jump, and climb. These new accomplishments are possible thanks to the accumulation of a larger mass and greater density of bone and muscle tissue. Thereafter the same trend, a lengthening of the long bones and an increase in musculature, continues, unevenly and more slowly, until adolescence.

Growth and Nutrient Needs of Young Children

An infant's appetite decreases markedly near the first birthday, in line with the great reduction in growth rate. Thereafter the appetite fluctuates. At times children seem to be insatiable, and at other times they seem to live on air and water. Parents need not worry about this: a child will need and demand more food during periods of rapid growth than during slow periods. The perfection of appetite regulation in children of normal weight guarantees that their food energy intakes will be right for each stage of growth.[1] One caution: some children may eat in response to external cues, disregarding appetite signals and so inviting the development of obesity.

A one-year-old child needs perhaps 1,000 calories a day; a three-year-old needs only 300 calories more. At age ten a child needs only about 2,000 calories a day. Thus even though total energy needs have doubled by age ten, the child's energy need per pound of body weight has steadily declined. More active children of any age need more energy because they spend more, and an inactive child can become obese even when eating less than average.

Growth enlarges the demand for all the nutrients per pound of body weight. On this basis, a five-year-old's need for, say, vitamin A is about double the need of an adult man (see margin). Before the adolescent growth spurt, children accumulate stores of nutrients that they will need in the years ahead. Then, when they take off on that growth spurt, there comes a time during which their nutrient intakes cannot meet the demands of rapid growth, and they draw on the nutrients they stored earlier. This is especially true of calcium; the denser the bones are in childhood, the better prepared they will be to support teen growth and still withstand the inevitable bone losses of later life. Following the Daily Food Guide is a tried and true means of providing these nutrients; the recommendations for children are shown in Table 13-1.

Example: A 174-pound adult male needs 1,000 RE vitamin A. That is 5.75 RE per pound. A 44-pound 5-year-old needs 500 RE vitamin A. That is 11.4 RE per pound.

Careful food selection is essential to ensure that a child receives the right amounts of nutrients. When a child skips breakfast or is allowed to choose

Table 13-1
Daily Food Guide for Children

Food Group	Servings per Day[a]	Serving Sizes by Age Group		
		1 TO 3 YEARS	4 TO 6 YEARS	7 TO 12 YEARS
Bread and cereals (whole grain or enriched)	6 or more	½ slice	1 slice	1 to 2 slices
Vegetables	3 or more	2–4 tbs or ½ c juice	¼–½ c or ½ c juice	½–¾ c or ½ c juice
Fruits	2 or more	2–4 tbs or ½ c juice	¼–½ c or ½ c juice	½–¾ c or ½ c juice
Meat and meat alternates	2 or more	1–2 oz	1–2 oz	2–3 oz
Milk and milk products	3 to 4	½–¾ c	¾ c	¾–1 c

[a]For details, see Figure 2-4 in Chapter 2.

Source: Serving sizes from P. M. Queen and R. R. Henry, Growth and nutrient requirements of children, in *Pediatric Nutrition,* eds. R. J. Grand, Jr., L. Sophen, and W. H. Dietz, Jr. (Boston: Butterworth, 1987), p. 347.

sugary foods (candy or marshmallows) in place of nourishing ones (whole-grain cereals), it is virtually certain that the child will fail to get enough of several nutrients. The nutrients missed from a skipped breakfast won't be "made up" at lunch and dinner but will be completely left out that day. A child can't be trusted to choose nutritious foods on the basis of taste alone; the preference for sweets is inborn, as Figure 3-7 of Chapter 3 made clear.

Active, normal-weight children may enjoy occasional treats of high-calorie but nutritious foods such as ice cream or pudding from the milk group, whole-grain or enriched cakes, cookies, and even doughnuts from the bread group in addition to a balanced diet. These foods are made from milk and grain, they carry valuable nutrients, and they encourage a child to learn, appropriately, that eating is fun. However, should a child eat large quantities of these or less nourishing treats such as candy or cola, the only possible outcomes are nutrient deficiencies, obesity, or both. Parents of wandering elementary school children should be aware that they may be spending pocket money at nearby stores and filling up on sweets.[2]

While it is important to teach children nutrition principles that can help to avoid obesity, it is also important to use sensitivity in teaching. Children are impressionable and can easily get the idea that their worthiness or lovability is somehow tied to body weight. Some parents fail to realize that society's ideal of slimness can be perilously close to starvation and that a child encouraged to "diet" cannot obtain the nutrients required for normal growth and development. Even healthy children without diagnosable eating disorders have been observed to dwarf their own growth through "dieting."[3] Weight gain in truly overweight children can be controlled safely without compromising growth, but should be overseen by a registered dietitian.

Some appropriate weight-control principles to teach children are to relax while eating, to pause and enjoy their table companions, and to stop eating when they are full. Parents can assist further by not exceeding recommended serving sizes of food except as needed. Healthy snacks such as milk, crackers, and fruit rather than colas and snack chips, set a pattern for healthy choices later on. The next section presents more tips for feeding children.

KEY POINT Children's nutrient needs reflect their stage of growth. Positive parental guidance and encouragement can help establish food patterns that provide adequate nourishment for growth while not encouraging obesity.

Mealtimes and Snacking

The childhood years are a parent's last chance to influence food choices. Healthy eating habits and a healthy relationship with food ensure positive development during growth and also help future adults maintain healthy weights and reduced risks of degenerative diseases in later life.

Children naturally like nutritious foods in all the food groups, with one exception—vegetables, which some young children frequently refuse. Here the presentation may be the key. Try to imagine how you felt when first offered a cup of chicken soup, a serving of runny greens or spinach, or a pile of mixed vegetables. If the soup burned your tongue, it may have been years before you were willing to try it again. As for the bowl of greens or spinach, it was suspiciously murky looking. (Who could tell what might be lurking in that ugly, dark-green liquid?) The mixed vegetables troubled your sense of order. Before you could eat them, you felt compelled to sort the peas into one pile on the plate, the carrots into another, the corn and lima beans into still others. Then you had to separate into a reject pile all those that got mashed in the process or "contaminated" with gravy from the potatoes. Only then might you be willing to eat the intact, clean vegetable bits one by one, perhaps with your fingers, since the peas, especially, kept rolling off the fork.

Many children prefer vegetables that are mild flavored, slightly undercooked and crunchy, bright in color, and easy to eat. Cooked foods should be served warm, not hot, because a child's mouth is much more sensitive than an adult's. The mild flavors of carrots, peas, and corn are preferred because a child has more taste buds, and smooth foods such as grits, oatmeal, mashed potatoes, or pea soup should have no lumps in them. Children prefer foods that are familiar to them, and fear of unfamiliar foods is practically universal among children. Suggesting, rather than commanding, that the child try small amounts of new foods at the beginning of the meal, when the child is hungry, seems to work best.[4]

When feeding children, parents must always be alert to the dangers of choking. A child may make no sound when choking, so an adult should always be nearby when children are eating. Encouraging the child to sit when eating is a good practice; choking is more likely when a child is running or reclining.[5] Round foods such as grapes, nuts, hard candies, and hotdog pieces can easily become lodged in a child's small windpipe. Other potentially dangerous foods include tough meat, popcorn, and chips.

Little children like to eat at little tables and to be served little portions of food. If a child is offered large portions, chances are excellent that the child will fill up on favorite foods while ignoring less preferred items. In fact, toddlers may go on food jags during which they will eat nothing but one or two favored foods. The best response to food jags lasting a week or so is no response, since attention is a reward the two-year-old strives for. After two weeks of indulging the jag, try serving tiny portions of many foods, including the favored items. Distract the child with friends at meals, and make other foods as attractive as possible.

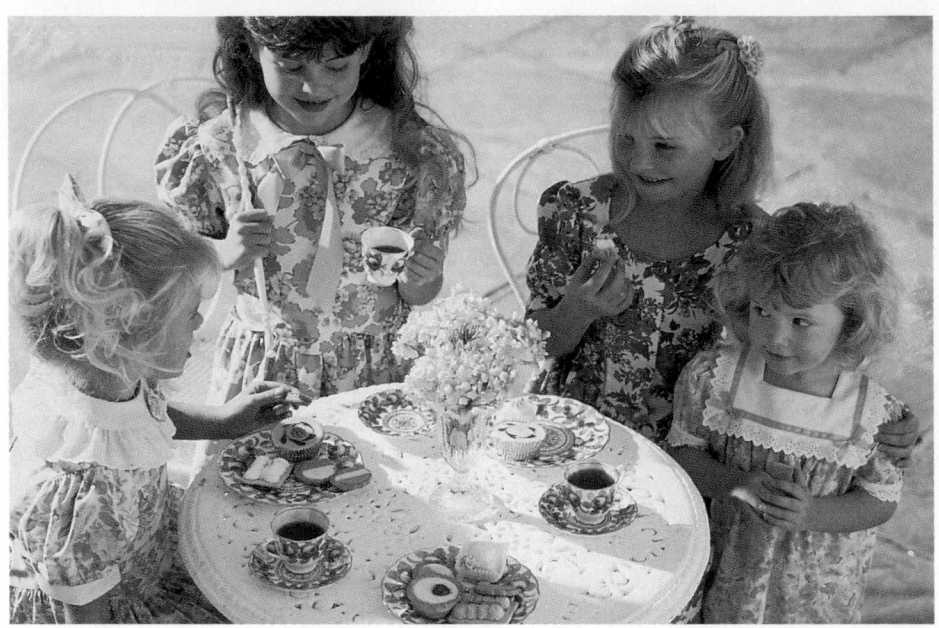

Little children like little tables and little portions.

Remember, too, that parents have likes and dislikes to which they feel entitled. A child who genuinely and consistently rejects a food should be offered the same privilege. The "clean-your-plate" dictum should be stamped out for all time. Children who are forced to override their own satiety signals are essentially in training to develop obesity. Encourage children to stop eating when they are full and to listen to their bodies. Also, do not make an issue of food acceptance. The parent is responsible for *what* the child is offered to eat, but the child is responsible for *how much* and even *whether* to eat.

Parents may find that their children often snack so much that they are not very hungry at mealtimes. This need not be a problem as long as children know *how* to snack. Snacks that are as nutritious as the foods served at mealtime become like small meals as far as nutrition is concerned. Keep them simple and readily available. Milk, cheese, fruit, yogurt, peanut butter sandwiches, and cereal are all beloved snacks that help meet nutrient needs.

A bright, unhurried atmosphere free of conflict is conducive to good appetite. Parents who serve meals in a relaxed and casual manner, without anxiety, provide the climate in which a child can learn to enjoy eating. Parents who beg, cajole, and demand that their children eat set up a power struggle that worsens the problem. A child confronted with a barrage of meal-time accusations—"Susie, your hands are filthy . . . your report card . . . and clean your plate!" may find mealtimes unbearable. Her stomach recoils as her body and mind both react to stress of this kind.

Children love to be included in activities surrounding meal preparation. Children as young as two years old can develop new skills by helping out. Importantly, positive experiences for the child are most likely when the tasks fit the child's developmental abilities, and when they are offered in a spirit of enthusiasm and enjoyment of the tasks, not one of criticism or drudgery. Praise for a job well done (or at least well-attempted) expands a child's sense of pride while developing skills and positive associations with meals. Children are also likely to eat the foods they helped to prepare.

Many parents may overlook perhaps the single most important influence on their child's food habits—their own habits. Parents who don't prepare, serve, and eat carrots shouldn't be surprised when their child refuses to eat carrots. A child learns much through imitation. Parents set an irresistible example by enjoying nutritious foods at meals and snacks.

While preparing, serving, and enjoying food, caretakers can promote not only physical but also emotional growth at every stage of a child's life. It is important for parents to help Joey or Susie to remember that they are good kids. What they *do* may sometimes be unacceptable; but what they *are* on the inside are normal, healthy, growing, fine human beings.

KEY POINT Healthy eating habits and a healthy relationship with food are learned in childhood. Parents train children in attitudes about food by their actions and by example.

Nutrient Deficiencies and Behavior

A child who suffers from nutrient deficiencies exhibits physical and behavioral symptoms: the child is sick and out of sorts. The connections between diet and behavior are of keen interest to caretakers who not only feed children but also must live with them.

Deficiencies of protein, energy, vitamin A, iron, and zinc plague the children of many countries of the world. In developing nations, such deficiencies cause or contribute to nearly half the deaths of children under four years old, and inflict blindness, stunted growth, and high susceptibility to infections on countless millions more.

In developed countries such as the United States and Canada, most deficiencies are more subtle in their effects. This point was illustrated by a study of British children. Many of the children studied, about 40 percent of them, were found to have intakes of less than half the RDA of folate, vitamin D, calcium, iron, magnesium, selenium, zinc, and many other minerals.[6] The researchers gave multinutrient supplements to some of the children and then administered intelligence tests to all of them. Those who had received the supplements scored significantly higher on the tests than did the others. The researchers took the findings to mean that while children may be well-nourished in terms of protein and some vitamins, the functioning of the brain may be sensitive to borderline deficiency states of many other nutrients, a contention supported by many previous findings.

Iron deficiency is the most common nutrient deficiency in children and adolescents, and reducing its incidence should be a top priority according to U.S. nutritionists.[7] Besides carrying the blood's oxygen, iron transports that oxygen within cells, where it works as part of large molecules to release energy. A lack of iron not only causes an energy crisis but also directly affects behavior, mood, attention span, and learning ability. Iron also plays key roles in many molecules of the brain and nervous system. Deficiencies of iron produced experimentally in animals have caused abnormal metabolism of neurotransmitters, notably those that regulate the ability to pay attention, which is crucial to learning.

Iron deficiency is usually diagnosed by a deficit of iron in the *blood*, after anemia has developed. A child's *brain*, however, is sensitive to slightly lowered iron concentrations long before the blood effects appear. It is difficult to distinguish the effects of iron deficiency from those of other factors in

Controversy 13 details the mental symptoms of anemia.

Table 13-2
Iron-Rich Foods Kids Like[a]

Breads, Cereals, and Grains
Canned macaroni (½ c)
Canned spaghetti (½ c)
Cream of wheat (¼ c)
Fortified dry cereals (1 oz)[b]
Noodles, rice, or barley (½ c)
Tortillas (1 flour, 2 corn)
Whole-wheat, enriched, or fortified bread (1 slice)
Vegetables
Baked flavored potato skins (½ skin)
Cooked mushrooms (½ c)
Cooked mung bean sprouts or snow peas (½ c)
Green peas (½ c)
Mixed vegetable juice (1 c)
Fruits
Apple juice (1 c)
Canned plums (3 plums)
Cooked dried apricots (¼ c)
Dried peaches (4 halves)
Raisins (1 tbsp)
Meats and Legumes
Bean dip (¼ c)
Canned pork and beans (⅓ c)
Mild chili or other bean/meat dishes (¼ c)
Liverwurst (½ oz)
Meat casseroles (½ c)
Peanut butter and jelly sandwich (½ sandwich)
Lean roast beef or cooked ground beef (1 oz)
Sloppy joes (½ sandwich)

[a]Each serving provides at least 1 mg iron, or one tenth of a child's RDA for iron. Vitamin C-rich foods included with these snacks increase iron absorption.

[b]Some fortified breakfast cereals contain more than 10 mg iron per half-cup serving (read the labels).

Source: Many of these ideas reflect data in A. A. Hertzler, Children's food patterns—A review: I. Food preferences and feeding problems, *Journal of the American Dietetic Association* 83 (1983): 551–554.

children's lives, but studies have found connections between iron and behavior. Iron deficiency seems to manifest itself in a lowering of the motivation to persist in intellectually challenging tasks, a shortening of the attention span, and a reduction of overall intellectual performance.[8] A child with such symptoms might be irritable, aggressive, and disagreeable or sad and withdrawn. One might label such a child "hyperactive," "depressed," or "unlikable," but these traits may not be purely psychological; they may arise from malnutrition. Inspection of a disruptive or apathetic child's diet by a qualified health care professional can identify these reversible problems, and additions to the diet can correct them. Table 13-2 lists some iron-rich foods kids like to eat. Only a health care provider should make the decision to give iron supplements, of course, and if used, supplements should be kept out of children's reach.

KEY POINT The detrimental effects of nutrient deficiencies in children of developed nations can be subtle. Iron deficiency is the most widespread nutrition problem of children and causes abnormalities in both physical health and behavior.

The Problem of Lead

Malnutrition is often a complex condition involving multiple nutrients and other factors. One such factor is lead poisoning, which can cause iron-deficiency anemia. Conversely, iron deficiency impairs the body's defenses against lead. A child with iron-deficiency anemia is three times as likely to have elevated blood-lead concentrations as a child with normal iron status.[9]

In their early years, normal-appearing babies can be silently building up toxic concentrations of lead in their bodies through normal baby activities. Babies like to explore, and they put everything into their mouths, including things that may harm them, such as chips of old paint, pieces of metal, and other unlikely substances. Not until much later, after lead toxicity has set in, do caretakers notice unusual symptoms.

Joey was such a child. This normal-appearing baby grew up in an inner city, where dust from heavily traveled streets settled on his playthings, sprinkling lead from old gasoline deposits into his environment. He loved to taste everything: table legs, toys, the spindles of flaky paint railings—whatever was within his reach. And his mother often mixed his morning formula with the first water from the tap, water that had spent the night absorbing lead from the old building's lead pipes. Figure 13-1 shows the origins of lead in children's environments.

Joey grew into a cautious, quiet preschooler who clung to stair railings with both hands as he slowly climbed up and down. Joey was late in walking, small for his age, seldom played as vigorously as other children, and was prone to small health disturbances, such as diarrhea, irritability, and lethargy. While his health quietly deteriorated, his parents shrugged off subtle symptoms as normal variations in children. They explained away his small size, awkward stair climbing, lack of fine motor coordination, hearing difficulties, and slowness in learning. Finally, a pediatrician detected that lead toxicity was present in young Joey, and started treating him with lead-scavenging drugs.[10] Except for persistent, minor learning disabilities, Joey is now growing normally and playing vigorously.

For kids like Joey, the truth can easily come too late, since even one year of lead exposure can permanently impair the brain, nervous system,

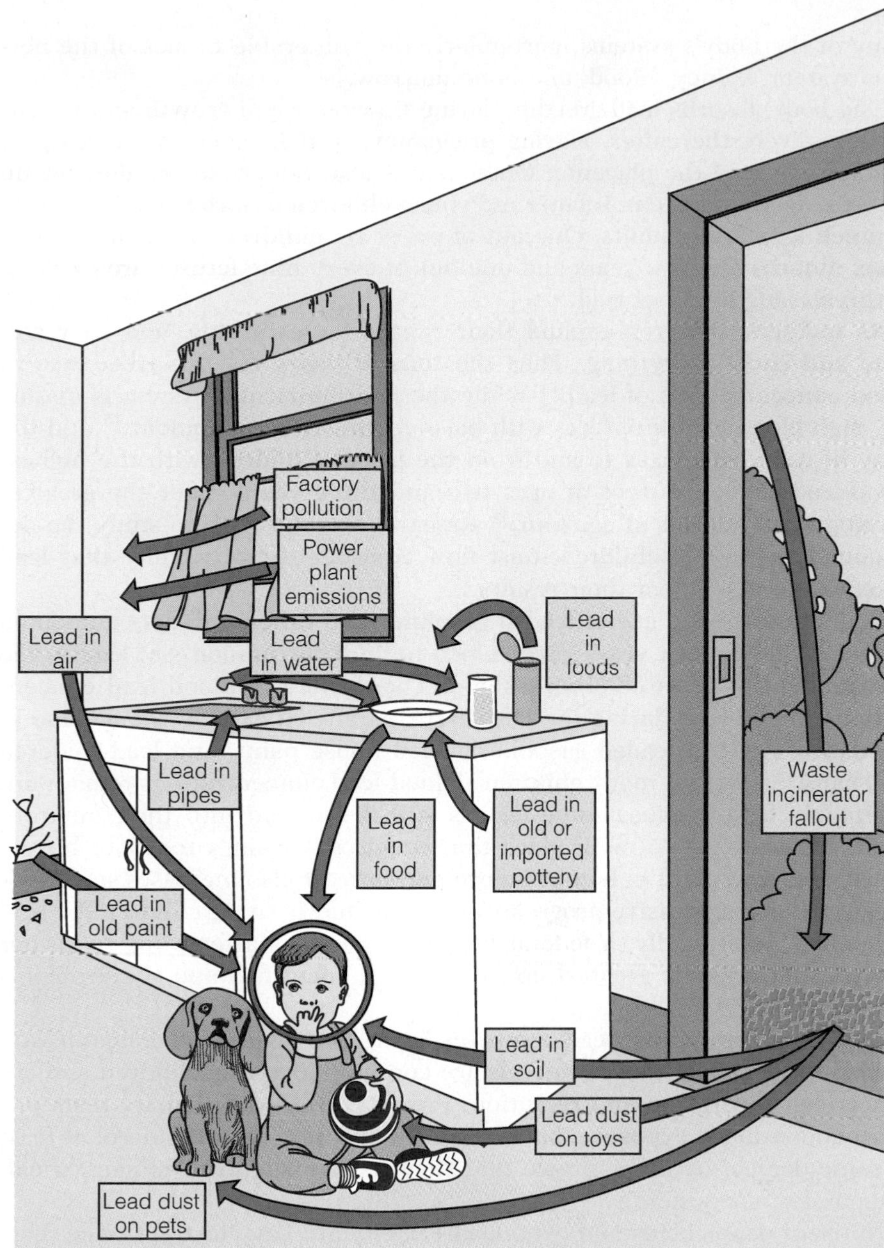

Figure 13-1

OUR CHILDREN'S DAILY LEAD

Lead finds its way into the bodies of children when they ingest lead-containing foods, water, dust, or paint chips, or when they breathe lead-laden air.

Title Source: Title borrowed from M. A. Wessel and A. Dominski, Our children's daily lead, *American Scientist* 65 (1977): 294–298.

and psychological functioning.[11] Furthermore, recent experiments have shown that the effects occur with lower doses than has been thought in the past. The Centers for Disease Control have recently lowered the blood lead level officially considered to be the poisoning threshold and have called for universal screening of children's blood.[12] The Public Health Service has singled out lead poisoning as the most serious environmental threat children face today.

The Environmental Protection Agency (EPA) provides this toll-free hotline for lead information: 1-800-LEAD-FYI (1-800-532-3394).

Lead is an indestructible metal; the body chemistry cannot alter it. Similar chemically to nutrient minerals like iron, calcium, and zinc, lead displaces these minerals from the body. Then lead is unable to perform the biological functions of these minerals. Consequently lead interferes with

allergy an immune reaction to a foreign substance (such as some components of food). Also called *hypersensitivity* by researchers.

many of the body's systems, particularly the vulnerable tissues of the nervous system, kidney, blood, and bone marrow.

The body absorbs lead greedily during times of rapid growth and hoards it possessively thereafter. During pregnancy, lead invades the developing fetus by crossing the placenta. Once inside, lead inflicts severe damage on the fetal nervous system. Infants and young children absorb five to ten times as much lead as do adults. One out of every six children between the ages of six months and five years and one out of every nine fetuses are exposed to threatening levels of lead.[13]

As toddlers, children expand their ranges for exploring, and they still taste and chew everything. Thus the toddler years see a marked rise in blood concentrations of lead.[14] While the neuromuscular system is maturing, high blood lead interferes with balance, motor development,[15] and the relay of nerve messages to and from the brain. Children with the highest blood-lead concentrations at ages two and three years suffer the greatest developmental delays at age four.[16] Researchers who wish to study the development of young children must now consider the possibility that lead intoxication may affect their results.[17]

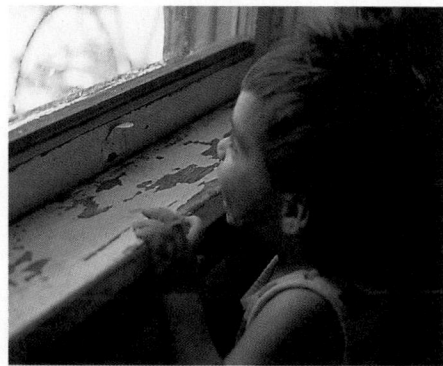

Paint is the primary source of lead in children's lives.

Reductions in the use of leaded gasolines and other products mandated by federal law in past years have helped to limit the amounts of lead in the environment—and in children's blood. The decline in blood lead concentrations in children during the late 1970s paralleled exactly the decline in the nation's use of leaded gasoline, leaded house paint, and lead-soldered food cans.[18] Even so, many children's blood-lead concentrations remain unacceptably high because some lead is still discharged into their environment. Legislation is now in place that requires warnings to home buyers concerning lead paint in houses before purchase. It also increases state budgets to pay for aggressive programs of testing and treating children for lead poisoning. Additionally, a federal tracking system is attempting to gather data so that areas of greatest concern can be identified and the problems corrected.

As mentioned earlier, lead competes in the body with iron, calcium, and zinc. Deficiencies of these minerals are common in young children and enhance lead absorption and retention. Prevention of lead toxicity rests primarily on reduced exposure, but parents can protect their children, at least to some degree, by making sure that they receive adequate intakes of calcium and other minerals.

Nutrient deficiencies and even lead toxicity are easy to treat once diagnosed; the trick is in identifying these conditions early, before too much damage has set in. Sometimes abnormal behavior is the only observable sign of poor nutrition.

Alternative agricultural and industrial processes discussed in Chapter 15 can help to reduce environmental lead and other contaminants.

KEY POINT Lead poisoning remains a serious environmental threat to children. It can inflict severe, irreparable damage on developing body systems. Environmental lead levels have declined in recent years but not enough to safeguard children's health.

Food Allergy, Intolerance, and Aversion

Food **allergy** is frequently blamed for physical and behavioral abnormalities in children. A true food allergy occurs when a whole food protein or other large molecule enters the body tissues. Recall that most large molecules of food are normally dismantled in the digestive tract to smaller ones before absorption. The body's immune system reacts to a food protein or other large molecules as it does to an **antigen,** by releasing **antibodies, histamine,** or other defensive agents. A problem not involving the immune system that results from exposure to food substances is known as a **food intolerance.**

Allergies may have one or two components. They always involve antibodies; they may or may not involve symptoms. A person may produce antibodies *without* having any symptoms or may produce antibodies *and* have symptoms. Symptoms without antibody production are *not* due to allergy. This means that allergies cannot be diagnosed from symptoms alone; they have to be diagnosed by testing for antibodies.

A food allergy can exhibit many different symptoms. In the digestive tract it may cause cramping, bloating, nausea, diarrhea, or vomiting; in the skin it may cause hives, swelling, and rashes; in the lungs it can cause asthma; it can also cause a runny nose or irritated, reddened eyes. A severe, dangerous, generalized reaction is **anaphylactic shock.**

Allergic reactions to food can occur with different timings; the appearance of symptoms may come within minutes or after up to 24 hours. Identifying a food that causes an immediate allergic reaction is easy because symptoms correlate closely with the time of eating the food. If the reaction is delayed, though, identifying the offending food is more difficult because by the time the symptoms have appeared, many other foods will have been eaten. Many people are allergic to just one food, but some are allergic to many.

Almost 75 percent of allergic reactions are caused by just three foods: eggs, peanuts, and milk.[19] The other 25 percent are caused by a variety of foods from almonds to yeast breads. The life-threatening reaction of anaphylactic shock is most often caused by peanuts, nuts, fish, and shellfish.[20]

A number of tests and food challenges are required to identify a true food allergy. However, the tests are time consuming and expensive. Often, people, and even physicians, try to guess the cause of an adverse reaction and use the term *food allergy* loosely. A parent whose child has any kind of discomfort after eating, such as stomachache, headache, pain, rapid pulse rate, nausea, wheezing, hives, bronchial irritation, cough, or any other, may decide that an allergy is responsible, when in fact the cause is something else entirely. Only careful, skilled testing by a physician can distinguish the many possibilities, and such testing is seldom done.

Because reliable food-allergy tests are inconvenient and expensive, people are tempted to believe quacks bearing sophisticated-sounding, but quick and easy laboratory work. For example, "cytotoxic testing" involves mixing blood with foods to see what blood cells "react" to. As you might guess, this test is invalid for detecting allergy because isolated blood cells are cut off from the body's immune system, which produces the allergic response. Other terms relating to allergy quackery are *brain allergy, metabolic rejectivity syndrome,* and the term *ecology* when applied to body functions.

A **food aversion,** an intense dislike of a food, may be a biological response to a food that once caused trouble. Children's food aversions may be the result of nature's efforts to protect them from allergic or other adverse reactions. Parents are advised to watch for signs of food dislikes and to take them seriously. Such a dislike may turn out to be a whim or fancy, but it should be respected. Although many cases of suspected allergies turn out to be something else, real allergies do exist, as do other valid reasons to avoid certain foods. Don't prejudge, in any case. Test. Then if an important staple food must be excluded from the diet, find other foods to provide the omitted nutrients to ensure the child's continued good nutrition.

antigen a substance foreign to the body that elicits the formation of antibodies or an inflammation reaction from immune system cells. Food antigens are usually glycoproteins (large proteins with glucose molecules attached).

antibodies large protein molecules produced in response to antigens that inactivate the antigens.

histamine a substance produced by cells of the immune system as part of a local immune reaction to an antigen; participates in causing inflammation.

food intolerance an adverse effect of a food or food additive not involving the immune response.

anaphylactic (an-AFF-ill-LAC-tic) **shock** a life-threatening whole-body allergic reaction to an offending substance.

food aversion an intense dislike of a food, possibly biological in nature, resulting from an illness or other negative association with that food.

Warning signs of allergic anaphylactic shock: itching tongue and tightness in the throat, abdominal pain, itchy and blotchy skin, nausea, vomiting, diarrhea, inflamed nasal membranes, chest pain, swelling, low blood pressure, shock, and respiratory arrest.

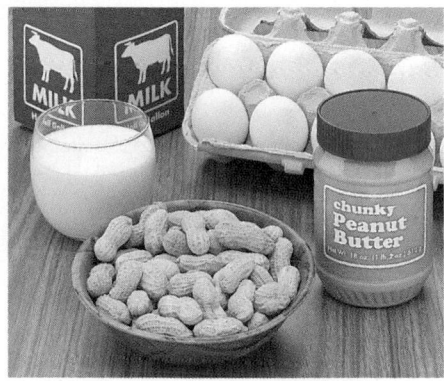

These normally wholesome foods are most likely to induce symptoms in people with allergy.

hyperactivity (in children) a syndrome characterized by inattention, impulsiveness, and excess motor activity. Usually occurs before age seven, lasts six months or more, and does not entail mental illness or mental retardation. Also called *attention deficit disorder* or *hyperkinesis* and may be associated with minimal brain damage.

learning disability an altered ability to learn basic cognitive skills such as reading, writing, and mathematics.

Allergies are often blamed when behavior problems arise. While a child who is sick from any cause is likely to be cranky, evidence does not support the hypothesis that allergy can cause misbehavior without other symptoms. The next section shows that **hyperactivity** does express itself in misbehavior—but is not caused by foods.

KEY POINT Food allergies cause illness, but diagnosis is difficult. To determine whether allergy exists, tests are imperative. Food aversions can be related to food allergies or to adverse reactions to foods.

Hyperactivity, "Hyper" Behavior, and Diet

Hyperactivity, one kind of **learning disability,** occurs in 5 to 10 percent of young, school-aged children, that is, in 2 or 3 in every classroom of 30 children. It can lead to academic failure and major behavioral problems. Parents and teachers need to deal effectively with it wherever it appears, to avert the grief that can otherwise result.

Food allergies have been blamed for hyperactivity. Research to date does not support the idea that food allergies or intolerances cause hyperactivity in children, but studies continue.

Physicians often diagnose hyperactivity by conducting trials with stimulant drugs. Stimulants normally speed up people's activity, but they have a paradoxical effect in children with hyperactivity: the drugs calm them. (Perhaps they stimulate centers in the brain that control behavior.) *In children who are responsive,* prescription medication should at least be considered as the treatment of choice for hyperactivity.

The placebo effect was defined earlier. It is the healing effect produced by faith in a treatment, rather than by the treatment itself.

Many parents, resistant to the idea of drugs for hyperactive children, hope that altering children's diets might improve their behavior. While optimal nutrition is critical to mental and physical health, appealing-sounding but unfounded dietary "treatments" may serve only to delay effective medical help. Such treatments may seem to help for a while due to the placebo effect, but they fail to provide a lasting cure.

Controversy 12 presented a table of caffeine contents of some foods and beverages.

Hyperactivity is not the same as "hyper" behavior, or excitability and anxiety in children. This kind of behavior is sometimes linked to diet through excess caffeine, which can overstimulate children. A 12-ounce cola, for example, contains as much as 50 milligrams caffeine; two or more such beverages are equivalent in the body of a 60-pound child to the caffeine in 8 cups of coffee for a 175-pound man. Large caffeine intakes bring on sleeplessness, restlessness, irregular heartbeats, and general misery. Almost 80 percent of one sample of U.S. children consumed caffeine.[21] Children cannot be expected to resist tempting colas and candy bars. It is the task of concerned adults to limit their access to such foods. Eventually children develop self-control, but it will develop within limits they encountered while young.

Without any magical answers, parents still have to deal with excitable, rambunctious, and unruly children. Common sense says that all children at times get wild and "hyper." There are many normal, everyday causes of such behavior:

- Desire for attention.
- Lack of sleep.
- Overstimulation.

- Too much television.
- Lack of exercise.

A child who often fills up on cookies, misses lunch, becomes too cranky to nap, misses out on outdoor play, and spends hours in front of a television suffers stresses that trigger chronic patterns of crankiness. This so-called tension-fatigue syndrome resolves itself when the caretakers begin giving more consistent care to the child's welfare. It helps especially to insist on regular hours of sleep, regular mealtimes, and regular outdoor exercise.

KEY POINT Hyperactivity is not caused by poor nutrition, but "hyper" behavior may reflect excess caffeine consumption or inconsistent care. A wise parent will limit children's caffeine intakes and meet their needs for structure to prevent tension and fatigue.

dental caries decay of the teeth (*caries* means "rottenness").

Television and Children's Nutrition

In addition to its contribution to tension-fatigue syndrome, television has adverse effects on children's nutrition. On the average, children in the United States spend as much time watching television as they do attending school; almost a quarter of children play outside only seldom; and 80 percent watch television each day after school and on Saturdays.[22] Watching television affects children's nutritional health adversely in several ways. First, television viewing requires no energy and seems to reduce the metabolic rate to levels below that of rest, requiring even less energy than day dreaming. The effect may be most pronounced in obese children.[23] Second, it contributes to physical inactivity by consuming time that could be spent in more vigorous activities. Third, watching television correlates with between-meal snacking and with buying and eating the calorically dense foods most heavily advertised on children's programs.

Much research has found obesity in children to correlate strongly with television viewing. This view was called into question by a recent study of adolescent girls in California in which researchers found only a weak association between body fat, physical activity, and television viewing times.[24] The design of this study was challenged, however, because while the researchers objectively measured the girls' body weights and BMIs they only estimated television viewing time and physical activity from self-reports, a data-collection method known for its high error rate. Researchers who conducted the earlier and much larger studies hold strongly to their original contention that ". . . 29 percent of the cases of obesity could be prevented by reducing television viewing to 0 to 1 hours per week."[25]

Children who watch more than two hours of television per day may also have higher serum cholesterol levels than do more active children.[26] Only a few children have elevated plasma cholesterol independently of obesity, but some children with elevated cholesterol may face an increased risk of heart disease in adult life. While some experts recommend regular cholesterol screening for all children, others find such measures unjustified and favor testing only those whose parents or grandparents developed cardiovascular disease.[27] No harm can come to children over the age of two who are encouraged to eat a variety of foods, to reach or maintain a desirable weight, and within reason, to limit fat and cholesterol intakes.[28]

Children who watch hours of television a day are also prone to frequent snacking on high-sugar foods, a major factor in **dental caries** development.

Sticky, high-carbohydrate snack foods cling to the teeth and provide an ideal environment for the growth of mouth bacteria that cause caries. What child can resist the delicious-looking, fun foods, full of sugar, that dance across their television screens? Television commercials aimed at children are intended only to promote purchase and consumption of sugary foods—they have no stake in promoting dental health. Parents must combat this influence by teaching children to do the following:

- Restrict between-meal snacking.
- Brush and floss daily, and brush or rinse after eating snacks.
- Choose foods that are swallowed quickly, not those that stick to teeth.
- Snack on crisp or fibrous foods to stimulate the rinsing action of the salivary glands.

Table 13-3 lists foods that promote dental health and those that require speedy removal from the teeth.

Table 13-3
Dietary Recommendations for Controlling Dental Caries

Food Group	Low Caries Potential	High Caries Potential[a]
Dairy	Milk, cheese, plain yogurt	Chocolate milk, ice cream, ice milk, milk shakes, fruited yogurt
Meat/meat alternates	Lean meat, fish, poultry; eggs; legumes	Peanut butter with added sugar, lunch meats with added sugar, meats with sugared glazes
Fruits	Fresh or packed in water	Dried (raisins, figs, dates), packed in syrup or juice, jams, jellies, preserves, fruit juices or drinks
Vegetables	Salad greens, cauliflower, cucumbers, radishes, carrots, celery	Candied sweet potatoes, glazed carrots
Bread/cereal	Popcorn, toast, hard rolls, pretzels, pizza, bagels	Cookies, sweet rolls, pies, doughnuts, muffins, cakes, potato chips, oatmeal,[b] oatmeal cookies,[b] puffed oat cereal,[b] dry ready-to-eat sugared cereals, snack crackers, granola bars, sandwich cookies, peanut butter crackers
Other	Sugarless gum	Sugared soft drinks, candy, fudge, caramels, honey, creme-filled cakes, sugars, syrups, jelly beans

[a]Brush and rinse the teeth especially well and quickly after eating these foods.

[b]The soluble fiber in oats makes this grain particularly sticky and therefore cariogenic.

Evidence from many points of view supports links between television and children's health. It seems prudent, therefore, to advise parents to limit children's average television viewing time to one or two hours a day.

KEY POINT Television viewing can contribute to obesity through lack of exercise and overconsumption of snacks. Television advertising of sugary foods promotes sugar consumption and tooth decay.

The Importance of Breakfast

While parents are doing what they can to establish favorable eating behaviors for children, grade school exposes children to foods prepared and served by outsiders. The U.S. government funds several programs to provide nutritious, high-quality meals, including breakfast, to children at school.

Children who eat no breakfast perform poorly in tasks of concentration, their attention spans are shorter, they achieve lower test scores, and they are tardy or absent more often than their well-fed peers.[29] Common sense tells us that it is unreasonable to expect anyone to learn and to perform work when no fuel has been provided. Even children who have eaten breakfast suffer from distracting hunger by late morning. Unfed children suffer all the more. Schools that begin to participate in the federal school breakfast program observe higher achievement test scores and lower tardiness and absence rates.[30] The improvements may be due to being fed at the day's start, but evidence suggests that nutrients consumed at breakfast also affect a child's overall nutrition profile.[31] That is, kids who miss out on breakfast don't make up for the loss of nutrients during the day; they are more poorly nourished overall than those who eat breakfast. A Canadian study found an astonishing 15 to 20 percent of children attended school once or more each week without eating breakfast, and just 30 percent consumed adequate daily servings from all food groups.[32]

Breakfast ideas for rushed mornings:

- Make ahead and freeze 5 sandwiches to thaw and serve with juice. Fillings may include peanut butter, low-fat cream cheese, other cheeses, jams, fruit slices, or meats. Or use flour tortillas with cheese, roll up, wrap, and freeze for later heating in a toaster oven or microwave oven.
- Teach school-aged children to help themselves to dry cereals, milk, and juice. Keep plastic bowls, spoons, and cups in low cupboards and keep milk and juice in small plastic pitchers on a low refrigerator shelf.
- Keep a bowl of fresh fruit and small containers of shelled nuts, trail mix (the kind without candy), or roasted peanuts for grabbing. Granola or other grain cereal poured into an 8-ounce yogurt tub is easy to eat on the run.
- Untraditional choices are often acceptable. Purchase or make ahead enough carrot sticks to divide among several containers; serve with yogurt or bean dip. Leftover casseroles, stews, or pasta dishes are nutritious choices that can be eaten hot or cold.

KEY POINT Breakfast is critical to school performance. Not all children start the day with an adequate breakfast, but school breakfast programs help to fill the need for some.

Lunches at School

Lunches served at school are designed to meet certain requirements. They must include specified servings of milk, protein-rich foods (meat, poultry, fish, cheese, eggs, legumes, or peanut butter), vegetables, fruits, and breads or other grain foods. The design is intended to provide at least a third of the RDA for each of the nutrients. Table 13-4 shows school lunch patterns for different ages.

Many parents rely on school lunches to meet a significant part of their children's nutrient needs on school days. Indeed, students who participate in the school lunch program have higher intakes of energy and nutrients than students who do not. Children don't always like what they are served, and school lunch programs must strike a balance between what children want to eat and what will nourish them.

In keeping with dietary guidelines concerning fat and cholesterol consumption, some schools offer low-fat (chocolate or white) or nonfat milk as alternatives to whole milk. Some also serve beans and fish entrees more

Table 13-4
School Lunch Patterns for Different Ages

Food Group	Preschool (Age)		Grade School through High School (Grade)		
	1 TO 2	3 TO 4	K TO 3	4 TO 6	7 TO 12
Meat or Meat Alternate					
1 serving:					
Lean meat, poultry, or fish	1 oz	1½ oz	1½ oz	2 oz	3 oz
Cheese	1 oz	1½ oz	1½ oz	2 oz	3 oz
Large egg(s)	½	¾	¾	1	1½
Cooked dry beans or peas	¼ c	⅜ c	⅜ c	½ c	¾ c
Peanut butter	2 tbsp	3 tbsp	3 tbsp	4 tbsp	6 tbsp
Peanuts, soynuts, treenuts, or seeds[a]	½ oz	¾ oz	¾ oz	1 oz	1½ oz
Vegetable and/or Fruit					
2 or more servings, both to total	½ c	½ c	½ c	¾ c	¾ c
Bread or Bread Alternate					
Servings[b]	5 per week	8 per week	8 per week	8 per week	10 per week
Milk					
1 serving of fluid milk[c]	¾ c	¾ c	1 c	1 c	1 c

[a]These foods may meet no more than one-half a serving of meat and must be accompanied by other meat or alternate in the meal.
[b]A serving is 1 slice of whole-grain or enriched bread; a whole-grain or enriched biscuit, roll, muffin, or the like; or ½ c cooked rice, pasta, or other grain.
[c]Whole milk and unflavored low-fat milk must be offered; flavored milks or nonfat milk may also be offered.

often. Such steps are gaining recognition as part of a plan to improve children's future cardiovascular health.[33]

School officials trying to lower the fat in school lunches often run into problems. For one thing, U.S. children develop a taste for fat and salt early in life and thus may reject some foods that are low in fat and high in nutrient density.[34] Should children drop out of the school's lunch program, the funding of the program may be reduced, so administrators often feel trapped by conflicts between children's tastes and their nutritional needs.

One ambitious project to reduce fat and sodium in elementary schools in Minnesota employed a nutrition information campaign for parents and students while reducing the fat contents of the children's lunches.[35] The officials developed a promotional logo, printed posters, distributed kitchen magnets, and organized games and activities "to create awareness and to encourage an atmosphere of fun and excitement for the students and staff." Their efforts paid off handsomely in terms of reduced fat and calorie intakes for the children and in a high level of lunch participation for the school. Other effective tactics include gradually reducing the fat in a few foods over several months to allow children's tastes to adjust, and monitoring plate waste to determine which foods are acceptable and which are not.

Some children face the option of choosing soft drinks and high-fat, high-sugar treats from vending machines located around some schools. The administrators of the school lunch program have tried to outlaw such machines on school grounds, but their efforts have been defeated by powerful lobby groups of industries that reap profits from children's pocket money. When given a choice, many children choose nutritious snacks, such as yogurt, milk, or fruit, when these choices are also made available in vending machines.

KEY POINT School lunches are designed to meet at least a third of the daily nutrients needed by growing children. Schools are challenged to appeal to children's food preferences while providing foods of high nutrient density. Vending machines tempt children with sweet treats.

Nutrition Education

Coincident with the school lunch program is a program of nutrition education and training (NET program) in all public schools. Evidence shows that children are indeed learning basic nutrition facts at school.[36] As children grow, they will need this knowledge of nutrition to enable them to make healthy food choices as these choices become theirs to make.

KEY POINT Schools share with families the responsibility of offering nutrition education to children.

The Teen Years

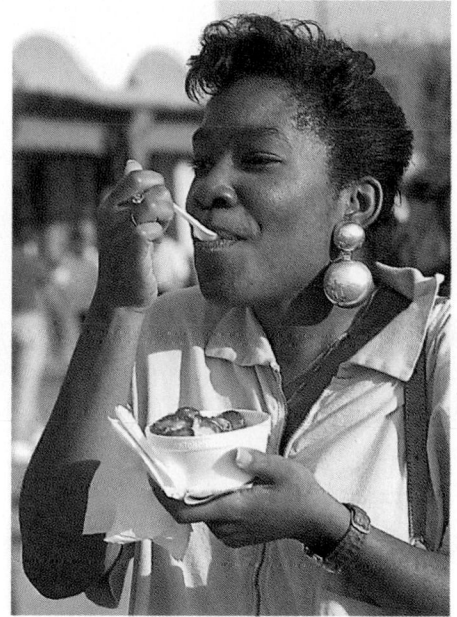

Nutritious snacks play an important role in an active teen's diet.

Teenagers are not fed; they eat. Self-directed food choices play a natural part in the search for an identity, acquired largely by trial and error, apart from the guidance of adult advice. Teens face tremendous pressures from peers and the media, especially regarding body image. Many teens readily adopt fads and scams offering promises of slenderness, developed muscles, freedom from acne, or control over symptoms that may accompany menstruation. At the same time, nutrient needs are high. Choices made during the teen years profoundly affect health, both now and in the future.

Growth and Nutrient Needs of Teenagers

With the onset of adolescence, needs for all nutrients become greater than at any other time of life except during pregnancy and lactation. The need for iron is especially great to support menstruation in girls and to develop lean body mass in boys.

Adolescence is a crucial time for bone development. The requirement for calcium reaches its peak during these years.[37] Low calcium intakes during the adolescent growth spurt, especially if paired with physical inactivity, may compromise the development of peak bone mass. The attainment of maximal bone mass during the young years is considered the best protection against age-related bone loss and fractures in later life.[38] Teenagers who choose soft drinks instead of milk take in too little calcium at the time when their needs for the mineral are greatest.[39]

Food sources of iron and calcium are listed in Chapter 8.

As they grow to adults, girls develop a somewhat higher percentage of body fat than do boys. This intensive growth period brings hormonal changes that profoundly affect every organ of the body (including the brain).

Teenagers' rates and patterns of growth vary tremendously. A growth spurt begins at the age of 10 or 11 years in girls and reaches its peak at about 12 years. A boy's growth spurt begins at 12 or 13 years and peaks at about 14 years, slowing down at about 19. Growth charts used for children don't fit teens very well, but height and weight charts meant for adults fit even less well. Two boys of the same age may vary in height by a foot, but if both have been growing steadily, each is fulfilling his genetic destiny according to an inborn schedule of events. Parents should watch only for

puberty the period in life when a person develops sexual maturity and the ability to reproduce.

gatekeeper with respect to nutrition, a key person who controls other people's access to foods and thereby has a profound impact on their nutrition; examples are the spouse who buys and cooks the food, the parent who feeds the children, and the caretaker in a day-care center.

reasonably smooth progress; to apply external standards that a child cannot "live up to" is to invite a lasting diminished self-image. The only way to be sure that a teenager is growing satisfactorily is to compare his or her height and weight with previous measures taken at intervals. Health care providers also compare measures of the changes of **puberty** with standard rating scales.[40]

The energy needs of adolescents vary tremendously. An active, rapidly growing boy of 15 may need 4,000 calories or more a day just to maintain his weight. An inactive girl of the same age, however, whose growth is nearly at a standstill may need fewer than 2,000 calories if she is to avoid becoming obese. Teen athletes are especially in need of energy and nutrients, and the nutrition advice to athletes in Chapter 10 is especially important for them. The insidious problem of obesity may first become apparent in adolescence, mostly in girls, and may last a lifetime.

KEY POINT The nutrient needs of teens can be enormous, especially for energy to support growth. Growth patterns and energy needs vary widely.

Eating Patterns and Food Choices

Teenagers come and go as they choose and eat what they want whenever they have time. With a multitude of after-school, social, and job activities, they almost inevitably fall into irregular eating habits. The adult becomes a **gatekeeper,** controlling the availability but not the consumption of food in the teenager's environment. Teens typically turn a deaf ear to adults' attempts at coercion or persuasion to eat particular foods. Wise gatekeepers will set examples to follow, and will provide access to nutritious foods that are low in sugar and fat. They welcome their teenaged sons and daughters and their friends into the kitchen with the invitation, "Help yourselves! There's plenty of food in the refrigerator" (meats and peanut butter for sandwiches, raw vegetables, milk, fruit juices) "and more on the table" (breads, fruits, nuts, popcorn, cereals).

On the average, about a fourth of a teenager's total daily energy intake comes from snacks. This is one way that teens with irregular schedules can receive substantial amounts of protein, thiamin, riboflavin, vitamin B_6, magnesium, and zinc. Their calcium intakes may fall short unless they snack on dairy products, and they often fail to obtain enough iron and vitamin A. For iron, a teen might snack on iron-containing hard-cooked eggs, low-fat bran muffins, or tortillas with spicy bean spread along with a glass of orange juice to help maximize the iron's absorption. For vitamin A, why not carrot sticks, mixed vegetable juice, cantaloupe, or some dried apricots?

Inevitably teenagers do a lot of eating away from home. A fast-food lunch of a hamburger, a chocolate shake, and french fries supplies nutrients in the amounts shown in Table 13-5 at a calorie cost of 820. With the exceptions of vitamins C, A, and folate, these are substantial percentages of recommended intakes at an energy cost some teenagers can afford. Depending on how they adjust their breakfast and dinner choices, lean, active teenagers may meet their nutrient needs more than adequately with this sort of lunch. They need only select fruits and vegetables for vitamins A, C, and folate; good fiber sources; and more good iron and zinc sources at their other meals. For those who tend to gain weight, such a meal is ill advised. Figure 5-18 of Chapter 5 offered alternatives.

Table 13-5
Selected Nutrients in a Hamburger, Chocolate Shake, and Fries

	Percentage of RDA[a]	
Nutrient	MALE	FEMALE
Energy	28	36
Protein	48	60
Calcium	38	38
Iron	36	24
Zinc	16	20
Vitamin A	8	10
Thiamin	38	49
Riboflavin	39	50
Niacin	33	42
Folate	18	20
Vitamin C	7	7

[a]RDA for an 18-year-old, moderately active person of average height and weight.

The nutritive values of selected fast foods are presented in Appendix A.

Teenagers are intensely involved in day-to-day life with their peers and in preparation for their future lives as adults. The gatekeeper can set an example, provide an environment with plenty of nutritious foods, and stand by with reliable nutrition information and advice, but the rest is up to the teens themselves. Ultimately they make the choices.

KEY POINT With planning, the gatekeeper can encourage teens to meet nutrient requirements by providing nutritious snacks.

Acne

No one knows why some people get **acne** while others do not, but heredity plays a role—acne runs in families.[41] The hormones of adolescence also play a role by stimulating the glands in the skin. The skin's natural oil is made in deep glands and is supposed to flow out through tiny ducts to the skin's surface. In acne, the ducts become clogged, and oily secretions cannot escape; they build up under the surface of the skin.

One medical treatment for acne is to apply a vitamin A relative, retinoic acid or Retin A, directly to the skin. This loosens the plugs that form in the ducts, allowing the oil to flow normally. But care is necessary because the acid may burn the skin and may cause pimples to form, making the acne look worse at first. Prescribed antibiotic pills and ointments work for some, and antibiotic ointments do not burn the skin. The oral prescription medicine Accutane is synthesized from vitamin A but is much more powerful than the vitamin itself, and it is effective against the deep lesions of cystic acne. Accutane is highly toxic and causes serious birth defects in the infants of women who have taken it during their pregnancies. Women with acne who wish to use Accutane are well advised to use an effective form of contraception before beginning treatment and for a time after treatment has ceased.

While it is true that medicines made from vitamin A are successful in treating acne, vitamin A itself has no effect, and supplements of the vitamin can be toxic. Quacks remain undaunted by these facts, though, and market vitamin A supplements to people hoping to cure acne. Enough vitamin A is essential for healthy skin but too much can damage the body.

Among foods charged with aggravating acne are chocolate, cola beverages, fatty or greasy foods, milk, nuts, sugar, and foods or salt containing iodine. None of these factors has been proved to worsen acne, and two, chocolate and sugar, have been shown not to worsen it. Stress, though, clearly worsens acne. Vacations from school often bring acne relief. Sun and swimming also help, perhaps because they are relaxing and also because the sun's rays kill bacteria and water cleanses the skin. Too much sun exposure in a teen may make skin cancer likely in later life, however.

One remedy always works: time. While waiting, attend to basic needs. Petal-smooth, healthy skin reflects a tended, cared-for body whose owner provides it with nutrients and fluids to sustain it, exercise to stimulate it, and rest to restore its cells.

KEY POINT While foods are not proven to aggravate acne, stress can worsen it. Supplements are useless against acne, but sunlight and proved medications can help.

acne a chronic inflammation of the skin's follicles and oil-producing glands, which leads to an accumulation of oils inside the ducts that surround hairs, usually associated with the maturation of young adults.

premenstrual syndrome (PMS) a cluster of symptoms, including both physical and emotional pain, that some women experience prior to and during menstruation.

prostaglandins hormonelike compounds (eicosanoids) related to and derived from polyunsaturated fatty acids (*prostagland* because the first such compound discovered was from the prostate gland).

Nutrition and the Menstrual Cycle

One of the many changes girls face as they become women is the onset of menstruation. The hormones that regulate the menstrual cycle are powerful, and they affect more than just the uterus and the ovaries. They alter the metabolic rate, glucose tolerance, appetite, food intake, mood, and behavior. Most women live easily with the cyclic rhythm of the menstrual cycle, but some are afflicted with physical and emotional pain prior to menstruation, a condition called **premenstrual syndrome, or PMS.**

Two things are believed to happen during the two weeks prior to menstruation:

- The basal metabolic rate during sleep speeds up, although the daytime rate may not change.[42]
- Appetite and calorie intakes may increase.[43]

Many women indicate, when asked, that their appetites increase before menstruation. Other women may eat more during this time without being aware that they do. One report found no significant changes in total energy intakes before menstruation but noted that premenstrual women increased their consumption of sugar-containing beverages.[44] Most studies seem to indicate that women take in an average of 300 calories a day more during the ten days prior to menstruation than during the ten days after.

At least one application of these findings seems obvious at first glance. Many women attempt to restrict their calories, sometimes severely, in the effort to control their weight. During the two weeks following menstruation, they may find this relatively easy to do, but during the two weeks before the next menstruation, they may find it hard because they are fighting a natural, hormone-governed increase in sleeping metabolic rate, an enlarged appetite, and possibly even a built-in craving for carbohydrate.

For women who suffer from physical pain before and during the menstrual period, it is important to know that it can have a wide variety of causes, some of which should clearly *not* be labeled PMS. Inflammation or infection of the lining of the uterus, a potentially dangerous condition, can cause symptoms like those ascribed to PMS but a diagnosis and treatment are imperative. Muscular abnormalities of the uterus and its opening (the cervix) can cause cramping during menstruation and again, treatment depends on diagnosis. Once these causes are ruled out, cases remain that are, at least for the present, grouped together as PMS.

A woman suffering from PMS may complain of any or all of the following symptoms: cramps and aches in the abdomen, back pain, headaches, acne, swelling of face and limbs associated with water retention, food cravings (especially for sweets), abnormal thirst, pain and lumps in the breasts, diarrhea, and mood changes, including both nervousness and depression. Some researchers are attempting to define clusters of these symptoms in hopes of assigning each cluster to a different cause.

Among the candidates for causes of PMS are abnormal secretion of **prostaglandins** and altered secretion of the two major regulatory hormones of the menstrual cycle, estrogen and progesterone. Other possibilities include an abnormality of the muscle tissue or lack of exercise. Many sedentary women find that taking up regular exercise greatly reduces menstrual discomfort. For some a brisk walk can relieve the symptoms completely.

Do emotional problems contribute to PMS? Researchers believe that at least some PMS may be psychological in origin, but it is hard to tell. After all, people are suggestible, and PMS is something of a fad. As for nutrition-related causes, this chapter devotes a Consumer Caution to them.

One thing seems clear: the woman with PMS should look to her total lifestyle, diet being only part of it. She may not have complete control over her condition, but many aspects of her lifestyle *are* under her control. If she has any nutrient deficiencies, these are best corrected by applying the nutrition principles of the earlier chapters. She should also be sure to get adequate sleep. Physical activity helps too; she should exercise regularly. She should be sensible about her intakes of sugar, caffeine, salt, alcohol, and any other abusable substances. She should watch out for snake-oil salespeople selling PMS "cures"—there are a lot of them out there.

KEY POINT The menstrual cycle may affect women's metabolism and appetites in a cyclic fashion. Premenstrual syndrome (PMS) is probably a diverse set of conditions with no single cause. A sound diet without extremes is part of the recommended lifestyle to reduce symptoms of PMS.

Nutrition and PMS

CONSUMER CAUTION Among possible nutrition-related causes of PMS, one is sodium retention, with the water retention that accompanies it. Some doctors prescribe diuretics to get rid of the excess sodium and water, with mixed results. The placebo effect is extraordinarily powerful in PMS, so much so that even an agent that appears to relieve PMS symptoms for several months may not in the long run prove to be a cure.[45] Diuretic therapy has been criticized on the basis that it may cause losses of needed minerals such as potassium, possibly making PMS symptoms worse. Also, if women do retain sodium and water just before menstruation, it may be a normal and desirable state.

Another nutrient that may have some connection with PMS is magnesium. When magnesium status was studied in "normal" and PMS subjects, the PMS group had lower concentrations of this mineral in their red blood cells. The naive reader might jump to the conclusion that people with PMS need more magnesium, but students of nutrition know to ask more questions first. Were the subjects' diets studied, so that researchers could tell whether they had a dietary deficiency, were absorbing less, or were excreting more magnesium? Had the women's total body contents of magnesium remained the same while the magnesium had shifted from the red blood cells into some other body compartment? On the basis of one finding it is impossible to say whether women with PMS need more magnesium in their diets.

One nutrient heavily researched with regard to PMS is vitamin B_6. The logic of ascribing PMS to a vitamin B_6 deficiency is that women with PMS may have abnormal levels of hormones that require vitamin B_6 for their action. One of the symptoms of PMS is depression, a disorder of mood that many people, both male and female, experience under a wide variety of conditions, including vitamin B_6 deficiency.

(continued on next page)

Nutrition and PMS *continued*

CONSUMER CAUTION Trials of vitamin B_6 in PMS have not proved conclusive. Typical is one study in which the researchers attempted to use vitamin B_6 to relieve premenstrual depression. These researchers found a dramatic positive response in only 1 of 13 women and a slight positive response in 4—balanced by a positive response in 5 women on placebo medication, no response in 2, and a strong *negative* response in 1! A follow-up study found that PMS improved in women who increased intakes of vitamin B_6 but that the improvement was not statistically significant.[46]

We might conclude from this that vitamin B_6 is not effective in PMS, but it may occasionally be just what is needed—witness the one woman who did respond positively. Confirming this, another pair of researchers tested a particular woman who claimed to be responsive to vitamin B_6. They gave her the vitamin (50 milligrams/day) and a placebo in alternate months for six months without telling her, and also without knowing themselves, which was which until the end of the study (a double-blind experiment). She experienced relief from her symptoms consistently with the vitamin and not with the placebo, showing clearly that in her case PMS was related to vitamin B_6. It is possible that "the cause" of PMS is not the same in all women. For some women a relative or absolute vitamin B_6 deficiency may aggravate or even cause PMS, whereas for others it might have no relation to the syndrome. No need exists for megadoses of vitamin B_6, and the hazards associated with such doses are well documented (see Table 7-4 of Chapter 7).

Vitamin E deficiency is another candidate for contributor to PMS. One research study, a double-blind, placebo-controlled study of 75 women, suggested that supplemental vitamin E brought relief from sore breasts associated with PMS, while the placebo did not. However, some women *without* PMS also have sore breasts that can sometimes be relieved by vitamin E. In another study of 41 women, vitamin E improved symptoms of PMS in many categories, such as nervousness, breast pain, edema, headaches, cravings, and others.[47] Possibly the correct logic is that vitamin E deficiency can worsen symptoms associated with the menstrual period, but not that vitamin E deficiency causes PMS.

One recent study pointed to tea consumption as strongly related to PMS.[48] Women who drank the most tea seemed to have the worst symptoms. Which component of tea, the caffeine, the pigments, or other substances, was not determined, but a later look at caffeine's relationship to PMS seemed to indicate a role for caffeine. Data from questionnaires administered to over 800 women correlated caffeine intakes with PMS in a linear fashion: the more caffeine the women reported consuming, up to 10 cups of caffeinated beverage per day, the more symptoms of PMS they reported suffering.[49] Even one cup of caffeinated beverage a day accompanied slight increases in PMS symptoms. So any woman who finds menstrual symptoms troublesome may freely try a caffeine-free lifestyle for a while and see if symptoms improve.

Before we can really know what to recommend to women who suffer with PMS, several kinds of studies are needed. One type of study will have to answer the question, "How do the diets of women with PMS differ from those of women unaffected by PMS?" Without such studies, we cannot really know what the typical nutrition status of PMS women is. It seems far too early for any woman who thinks she suffers from PMS to leap to the conclusion that she needs a particular supplement.

◆ The Later Years

This looks like a section about older people, but it is relevant even if the reader is only 20 years old. How you live and think at 20 years of age can profoundly affect the quality of your life at 60 or 80 years. Most people, without realizing it, hold a stereotype, largely negative, of what it is like to be old—and then, later, they become that way. An old saying has it that "as the twig is bent, so grows the tree." However, unlike a tree, you can bend your own twig.

Before you will adopt nutrition behaviors that will enhance your health in old age, you must accept on a personal level that you yourself are aging. People who fear age try to deny that it is happening to them by distancing themselves from the older generations. But, of course, everyone ages, so people who are prejudiced against older people are therefore prejudiced against *everyone*, including their own future selves. (Another form of prejudice is to view all old people as good, generous, and kind, when, in fact, thieves and crooks age too.) To learn what negative and positive views you hold about aging, try answering the questions in the margin. Your answers reveal not only what you think of older people now but also what will probably become of you. You may wish to review some of the reasons for your answers and, if they are not supported by science, to change your beliefs.

The majority of the U.S. population is now middle-aged. As that group ages, the ratio of old people to young people is growing larger. The fastest growing age group is people over 85 years old.[50]

In the United States, the **life expectancy** at birth is 79 years for women and 72 years for men, up from about 50 years in 1900.[51] Once a person survives the perils of youth and reaches age 65, the average person's life expectancy jumps to 83 years. Advances in medical science, including antibiotics and other treatments, are largely responsible for almost doubling the life expectancy in this century. Still, the biological schedule that we call aging cuts off life at a genetically fixed point in time. The **life span** (the maximum length of life possible for a species) of human beings, 115 years, has not changed over the years and is probably the upper limit of human **longevity.**

Nutrition and other lifestyle habits work together in the aging of the body. In a classic study, researchers in California studied nearly 7,000 adults and noticed that some were young for their ages, others old for their

life expectancy the average number of years lived by people in a given society.

life span the maximum number of years of life attainable by a member of a species.

longevity long duration of life.

How Will You Age?

- In what ways do you expect your appearance to change as you age?
- What physical activities do you see yourself engaging in at age 70?
- What will be your financial status? Will you be independent?
- What will your sex life be like? Will others see you as sexy?
- How many friends will you have? What will you do together?
- Will you be happy? Cheerful? Curious? Depressed? Uninterested in life or new things?

Table 13-6
Changes with Age You Probably Must Accept

These changes are probably beyond your control:
Graying of hair
Balding
Some drying and wrinkling of skin
Impairment of near vision
Some loss of hearing
Reduced taste and smell sensitivity
Reduced touch sensitivity
Slowed reactions (reflexes)
Slowed mental function
Diminished visual memory
Menopause (women)
Loss of fertility (men)
Loss of joint elasticity

ages.[52] To find out what made the difference, the researchers focused on health habits and identified six factors that affect physiological age. Three of the six factors were related to nutrition: abstinence from, or moderation in, alcohol use; regularity of meals; and weight control. (The others were regular, adequate sleep; abstinence from smoking; and regular physical activity.) The physical health of those who reported all six positive health practices was comparable to that of people *30 years younger* who followed few or none. Numerous studies have confirmed the benefits of these six factors. The findings suggest that even though people cannot alter the years of their births, they can alter the probable lengths and quality of their lives. The pair of tables in the margin, Tables 13-6 and 13-7, list some changes of aging that are unpreventable and also some that may yield to lifestyle influences.

KEY POINT Life expectancy for people in the United States has increased in the last century. The lifestyle factors that can make a difference in aging are: limited or no alcohol use, regular balanced meals, weight control, adequate sleep, abstinence from smoking, and regular physical activity.

Nutrition and Longevity

Throughout history, human beings have sought ways to prolong youth and life. The search is as relentless today as it has ever been. Scientists who study the aging process have found no specific diet or nutrient supplement that will prolong life, but they have discovered several links to nutrition.

Table 13-7
Changes with Age You Probably Can Slow or Prevent

By exercising, eating an adequate diet, reducing stress, and planning ahead, you may be able to slow or prevent:
Wrinkling of skin due to sun damage
Some forms of mental confusion
Raised blood pressure
Speeded-up resting heart rate
Reduce breathing capacity and oxygen uptake
Increased body fatness
Raised blood cholesterol
Slowed energy metabolism
Decreased maximum work rate
Loss of sexual functioning
Loss of joint flexibility
Oral health: loss of teeth, gum disease
Bone loss
Digestive problems, constipation

The first evidence that diet might extend life came more than half a century ago from experiments on rats.[53] Researchers fed young rats diets adequate in all nutrients but short in energy. The rats stopped growing. Then the researchers increased the energy, and growth resumed. Meanwhile, control rats were allowed to eat and grow normally. Many of the rats in the energy-deficient group died young from the effects of malnutrition. A few survivors, however, lived an extraordinarily long time and they developed the diseases of old age later in life, even though they suffered malformations and stunting that did not improve with normal feed. Still, the rats were alive far beyond the normal life span for such animals.

In the study just described, food restriction was begun as soon as the animals were weaned (at three weeks). Food restriction later in life seems to prolong survival, too, without incurring such severe physical malformations. Other studies have shown that even short-term food restriction in adult rats can extend their lives.[54] In view of the importance of nutrition during critical growth periods, it is not surprising that animals allowed to grow normally in youth best survive food restriction later on.

Several mechanisms to explain how energy restriction prolongs life in rats have been proposed but not proven. Research suggests that food restriction may extend the life span by delaying age-related diseases, retarding growth and development, reducing body fat, slowing the metabolic rate, controlling blood glucose, and preventing lipid oxidation.[55] Researchers hope that by discovering how food restriction slows aging in animals, they may come to understand better how aging occurs in people and how best to slow its effects. From what is known now, nutrition in the later years plays a key role in maintaining health into old age.

KEY POINT In rats, food energy deprivation may lengthen the lives of individuals who survive the treatment.

Nutrition in the Later Years

Knowledge of nutrition in aging is limited. There are no RDA for older age groups. Everyone over 50 years of age is grouped together, even though needs change as aging progresses. Too few studies exist on the effects of aging on nutrition for experts to formulate a meaningful set of standards for older groups.[56] Also, nutrient needs become more individual with age, depending on genetics and individual medical history. For example, one person may need more iron because that person's stomach acid secretion, which helps in iron absorption, has declined. Another person may excrete more folate due to past liver disease and thus need to obtain more. Despite their shortcomings, the RDA still present a gauge against which nutrient intakes may be compared, and despite individual differences, health-promoting lifestyle choices may avert some of the problems facing the elderly.

KEY POINT No special RDA exist for groups past 50 years old, even though nutrient needs change. Individual histories strongly influence older people's nutrient needs.

Energy and Exercise

Energy needs often decrease with advancing age. For one thing, the number of active cells in each organ decreases, reducing the body's overall metabolic rate (although much of this loss may not be inevitable). For another, older people usually reduce their physical activity and so their lean tissue diminishes. After about the age of 50 years, the RDA for energy assumes about a 5 percent per decade reduction in energy output (see inside front cover). For those who must limit energy there is little leeway for low-nutrient-density foods such as sugars, fats, oils, and, of course, alcohol.[57] Current thinking, however, seems to refute the idea that declining energy needs are unavoidable. Physical activity probably holds the key not only to maintaining energy needs but to upholding many other functions as well.

A respected expert on aging made these opening remarks concerning the importance of exercise to the elderly in a symposium on nutrition and aging:

> *We now know that physically active elders can build and rebuild muscle mass. Even the frail elderly can improve function by a remarkable 200 percent on a short, focused exercise regimen. No single feature of aging can more dramatically affect basal metabolism, insulin sensitivity, calorie intake, appetite, breathing, ambulation, mobility, and independence than muscle mass.*[58]

Even frail, institutionalized people in their *nineties* have been able to gain muscle bulk and strength and to put some pep in their walking steps after just eight weeks of weight training.[59] Training not only improves muscles but also increases the blood flow to the brain. Besides, a person spending energy in physical activity can afford to eat more food, and with it comes more nutrients. Any exercise, even a ten-minute walk a day, provides a benefit. Older people can feel free to exercise in their own way, at their

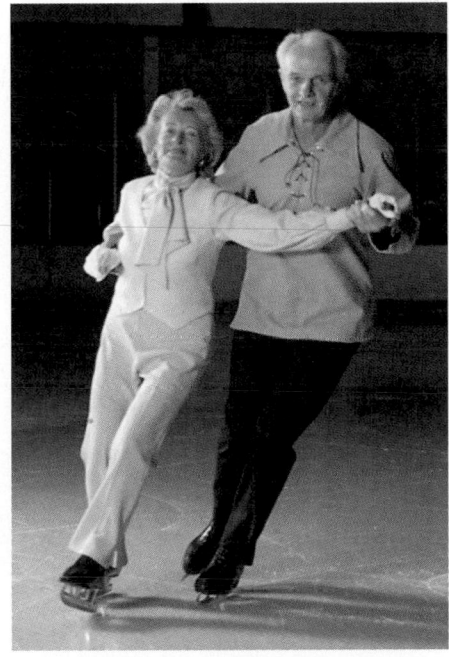

Energy like this requires continued physical activities and all the nutrients to support it.

arthritis a usually painful inflammation of a joint caused by many conditions, including infections, metabolic disturbances, or injury; usually with altered joint structure and loss of function.

gout a painful form of arthritis resulting from a metabolic abnormality in which excessive amounts of the waste product uric acid collect in the blood. Uric acid salt is deposited as crystals in the joints. Also defined in Controversy 11.

own pace. They should not hold themselves to standards set in younger days because aging necessarily brings a lessened capacity to perform exercise.[60]

KEY POINT Energy needs decrease with age, but exercise burns off excess fuel and brings benefits.

Carbohydrates and Fiber

The recommendation to obtain 6 to 11 servings of breads, grains, or pasta is appropriate for older people. It is especially wise to choose the majority of those servings from whole grains. With age, fiber takes on extra importance for its role against constipation, a common complaint among older adults and especially among nursing home residents. Older adults generally do not obtain the recommended daily 27 to 40 grams of fiber.[61] When low fiber intakes are combined with low fluid intakes, inadequate exercise, and constipating medications, constipation becomes almost inevitable.

KEY POINT Generous carbohydrate intakes are recommended for older adults. Including fiber in the diet is important to avoid constipation.

Fats and Arthritis

Fats should be limited in the diet of older adults for many reasons. Foods low in fat are often rich in vitamins and minerals. Diets constricted from such foods may help retard the development of cancer, atherosclerosis, obesity, and other diseases.

Fat in the diet is under surveillance for a possible role in causing **arthritis,** the painful deterioration and swelling of the joints that troubles many older people. During movement, the ends of normal bones are protected by small sacs of fluid that act as a lubricant. With arthritis, the sacs erode, cartilage and bone ends disintegrate, and joints become malformed and painful to move.

Dietary fat may affect the pain of rheumatoid arthritis, a severe form of arthritis that is seen to improve in many people when they adopt a low-fat diet. When these people resume eating fats and oils (except fish oils), their symptoms recur. One explanation is that the active products of both omega-6 and omega-3 fatty acids are involved in regulating pain-producing inflammation, and may be responsible for the effect. According to this theory, omega-6 fatty acids worsen the pain while the omega-3 acids relieve it. Researchers tested the theory by administering high doses of fish oil to arthritis sufferers. Those who took fish oil reported marked relief from their pain and stiffness, although the disease continued advancing.[62]

Another fat-arthritis connection may be that low-fat diets cause loss of body fat, with resultant improvements. Sufficient lean body mass may be important to reduce arthritis symptoms, as well.[63]

One form of arthritis known as **gout** worsens when sufferers consume foods that are high in purines, compounds that cause crystals of uric acid to form in the joints. Some of the best sources of omega-3 fatty acids, such as sardines, herring, anchovies, mackerel, and other fish and shellfish, are also the highest in purines. This makes attempts at self-diagnosis and treatment of arthritis especially unwise. While some with arthritis may benefit from increased fish intakes, others may make themselves worse.

Not effective as cures for arthritis:

- Alfalfa tea
- *Aloe vera* liquid
- Any of the amino acids
- Burdock root
- Calcium
- Celery juice
- Copper or copper complexes
- Dimethyl sulfoxide (DMSO)
- Fasting
- Fresh fruit
- Honey
- Inositol
- Kelp
- Lecithin
- Para-aminobenzoic acid (PABA)
- Raw liver
- Selenium
- Superoxide dismutase (SOD)
- Vitamins D, E, C, or any B vitamin supplements
- Watercress
- Yeast
- Zinc
- 100 other substances

Other connections between diet and arthritis include fasting, vegetarianism, vitamin E,[64] other antioxidant nutrients, and elimination diets. No one universally effective diet for arthritis relief is known. Many *ineffective* "cures" are sold, however, as the margin list (facing page) shows. The safest bet for those with arthritis is to obtain a medical diagnosis and treatment.

cataracts (CAT-uh-racts) thickening of the lens of the eye that can lead to blindness. Cataracts can be caused by injury, viral infection, toxic substances, genetic disorders, and possibly by some nutrient deficiencies or imbalances.

KEY POINT A low-fat diet may improve some symptoms of arthritis. Omega-3 fatty acids may also have a positive effect. Foods high in purines can worsen the arthritis of gout.

Protein

Protein needs of older people seem to remain about the same as for the young adult years. The decision of which protein-containing foods to choose takes on extra importance, however. Some older people have lost their teeth, and this makes chewing tough meats next to impossible. They need soft or chopped foods. Individuals with chronic constipation, heart disease, or diabetes may receive benefits from fiber-rich low-fat vegetable protein sources, such as legumes and grains. Such foods are easy to chew and can help stretch limited budgets as well.

KEY POINT Protein needs remain about the same through adult life, but choosing low-fat fiber-rich protein sources may help control other health problems.

Vitamins

Among the vitamins, vitamin A stands alone, in that its absorption appears to increase with aging.[65] For this reason researchers have proposed lowering the vitamin A RDA for aged populations. Some resist such a change, though, because vitamin A and its precursor beta carotene are active in prevention of oxidative damage to body tissues, an effect described in Chapter 7.

Older adults face a greater risk of vitamin D deficiency than younger people do. Many older adults drink little or no vitamin D-fortified milk, and many go day after day with no exposure to sunlight, especially if they reside in nursing homes. Additionally, as people age, vitamin D synthesis declines, setting the stage for deficiency. These age-related changes have inspired the suggestion that a higher RDA value for vitamin D for the elderly is needed, but a more effective approach would be to ensure that every elderly person obtain the RDA amount of vitamin D and get outside more often or even just sit by an open window some of the time.[66]

Adequate vitamin intakes can be ensured by following the Daily Food Guide presented in Chapter 2. Older people who are on limited budgets, or whose tastes have changed often omit foods of the vegetable group.[67] About one fifth of older people report eating no vegetables at all. Fruit is also lacking from many diets, and people who omit foods of both groups are almost sure to develop nutrient deficiencies. Some older adults shun whole-grain breads and cereals, and so miss out on the many B vitamins and trace minerals these foods provide.

Controversy 13 discusses the importance of some vitamins and minerals to the brain.

Of particular interest is the theory that links low antioxidant vitamin intakes with an age-related change in the lens of the eye: **cataracts.** A cataract is a thickening of the lens that impairs vision and ultimately leads to blindness. Cataracts can occur even in well-nourished individuals due to injury or other trauma, but most cataracts are vaguely called senile cataracts, meaning "caused by aging." Close to 400,000 new cataract cases are diagnosed in the United States each year.[68] Scientists have observed several possible (and, it should be emphasized, highly tentative) dietary links: to protein, fat, or sugar excess; to excess food energy intake (in people with diabetes); to excess intakes of milk sugar in those genetically unable to metabolize it; to deficiencies of riboflavin, of the antioxidant nutrients, or of the mineral zinc. Among these, the idea currently gaining support states that people who consume diets low in fruits and vegetables obtain too little of vitamins A, C, E, and beta carotene and that this puts them at risk of developing cataracts.[69] This is because the lens of the eye is vulnerable to damage by oxygen, and such damage is believed to underlie the formation of some kinds of cataracts. The amounts of nutrients that seem to be protective are easily provided by several servings a day of the vegetables, fruits, and other foods that contain them.

KEY POINT Vitamin A absorption increases with aging. Older people suffer from vitamin D deficiency more than young people do. Cataracts may be most likely to occur in those with low vitamin intakes.

Water and the Minerals

Dehydration is a major risk for older adults, who may not notice or pay attention to their thirst. With age, the thirst mechanism may become imprecise, and older people may go for long periods without drinking fluids.[70] The kidneys also gradually lose the ability to efficiently recapture water before it is lost as urine.[71] This causes some problems and worsens others, such as dehydration, constipation, and other intestinal problems. Even muscle weakness and mental confusion can result. Regardless of age, adults need to drink six to eight glasses of water each day.

A person we know uses this trick to ensure getting enough water: he keeps six inexpensive 8-ounce cups in the cupboard. Through the day he uses each one to drink water only once and then collects them in the dish drain. In the afternoon he checks the cupboard and makes sure to drink from any remaining cups. For him, drinking water has become a habit, and seldom are there cups left in the cupboard after supper.

Among the minerals, iron deserves mention. Iron-deficiency anemia is not as common in older adults as it is in younger people, and in fact, iron status generally improves in later life, especially for women whose iron losses greatly diminish when menstruation ceases.[72] Iron deficiency still occurs in some elderly people, however, especially in those with low food-energy intakes. Aside from diet, other factors in many older people's lives make iron deficiency likely:

- Chronic blood loss from ulcers, hemorrhoids, or the like.
- Poor iron absorption due to reduced stomach acid secretion.
- Antacid use, which interferes with iron absorption.
- Use of medicines that cause blood loss, including anticoagulants, aspirin, and arthritis medicines.

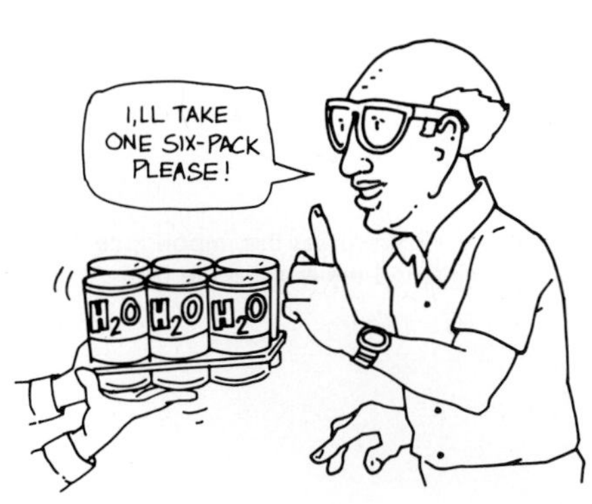

Adults of all ages need six to eight glasses of water each day.

Table 13-8
Summary of Nutrient Concerns in Aging

Nutrient	Effect of Aging	Comments
Energy	Need decreases	Physical activity moderates the decline
Fiber	Increased likelihood of constipation with low intakes	Inadequate water intakes and physical activity, along with some medications, compound the problem
Protein	Needs stay the same	Choices of low-fat, high-fiber legumes and grains meet both protein needs and other needs
Vitamin A	Absorption increases	
Vitamin D	Increased likelihood of inadequate intake, skin synthesis declines	Daily limited sunlight exposure may be of benefit
Water	Lack of thirst and increased urine output make dehydration likely	Mild dehydration is a common cause of confusion
Iron	In women, status improves after menopause, deficiencies linked to chronic blood losses and low stomach acid output	Adequate stomach acid required for absorption; antacid or other medicine use may aggravate iron deficiency; vitamin C and meat increase absorption
Zinc	Often inadequate intakes and reduced absorption; but needs may also decrease	Medications interfere with absorption, deficiency may depress appetite and sense of taste
Calcium	Intakes may be low; osteoporosis common	Lactose intolerance commonly prevents milk intake; substitutes are needed

Older people take more medicines than others, and nutrition effects are common.

Zinc deficiencies are common in older people. As many as 95 percent of older adults may not get the zinc they need, and many miss the mark by more than half.[73] Zinc deficiency, in turn, may lead to a depressed appetite and a diminished sense of taste that leads in turn to lower food intakes and worsened zinc status.

These foods provide iron and zinc together: Meat, poultry, liver, oysters, whole grains, fortified breakfast cereals, and legumes.

Some research suggests that older adults absorb zinc less efficiently than younger people do.[74] Many medications interfere with the body's absorption or use of zinc, and elderly people often need more medicines than when they were younger.[75] The bright side of the zinc story is that some healthy older adults may need less than they did when they were younger.

Abundant dietary calcium throughout life is important to protect against osteoporosis, which can set in during later life. Controversy 8 took up the question of what intake of calcium is appropriate for older adults. While researchers attempt to reach agreement about the calcium requirements of older adults, especially those of women, one aspect of calcium nutrition is not controversial: the calcium intakes of many people, especially women, in the United States are well below the RDA. If fresh milk causes stomach discomfort, as the majority of older people report, then lactose-modified milk or other calcium-rich foods should take its place.

These foods provide calcium and zinc together: Milk, yogurt, canned fish with bones, and oysters. A few dry cereals are fortified with both calcium and zinc (read the labels).

Calcium-rich foods are listed in Chapter 8.

A summary of the effects of aging on nutrient needs is located in Table 13-8. As people live longer lives, attention to nutrition concerns can help to ensure the best possible quality of life.

KEY POINT Aging brings changed vitamin and mineral needs. Some needs are increased, some decreased.

Table 13-9
Predictors of Malnutrition in the Elderly

- Recent weight loss or gain of more than 6 pounds
- Physical disabilities
- Lack of sunlight exposure
- Bereavement, depression, loneliness
- Confusion
- Alcohol abuse
- Multiple medicines
- Long-term medicine use
- Low food or fluid intake
- Rejection of food
- No or little food kept at home
- Rejection of fruits and vegetables
- Too little money for food
- Too little nutrition knowledge

Source: Adapted from L. Davies, Practical aspects of nutrition of the elderly at home, in H. Munro and G. Schlierf, eds., *Nutrition of the Elderly* (New York: Raven Press, 1992), pp. 203–209.

Food Choices of Older Adults

Results of national surveys give some indication of what older adults are eating. Many older people seem to have heard and heeded nutrition messages and have cut down on saturated fats in dairy foods and meats, and increased slightly their intakes of vegetables and whole-grain breads.[76] Smart marketers appeal to this growing group, many of whom are willing and able to spend more money on food than are people of other ages. Store shelves now prominently display good-tasting, low-fat, nutritious foods in easy-to-open, single-serving packages with labels that are easy to read. Many nutrient supplements are marketed for older adults. Whether to take a supplement is a personal choice, but evidence supports the idea that a single low-dose multivitamin and mineral tablet a day can improve resistance to disease in the elderly.[77]

The food choices and eating habits of older adults are affected not just by preference but by the changing circumstances that surround the experience of aging in society. Those who live alone, with others, and in institutions all eat differently.[78] Some life circumstances seem to make older people vulnerable to malnutrition (see Table 13-9). Men living alone are likely to consume poorer-quality diets than those living with spouses.[79] Some older people suffer medical conditions that affect nutrition. They may have difficulty chewing, or they may have lost a form of taste-induced satiety so that they no longer seek a wide variety of foods.[80] They may also take medications that interact with nutrients, depress the appetite, or alter the perception of taste.

In addition, some older people may simply lack funds to buy nutritious foods. For them, federal programs can be of at least some help. One is the Supplemental Security Income program, intended to assist the very poor by increasing their income to the defined poverty level. Another is the Title IIIC Older Americans Act of 1965, still in effect today, that provides for nutrition for the elderly. The program provides nutritious meals, social interaction, education and shopping assistance, counseling and referral to other needed services, and transportation. Many people look forward to the shared midday meals this program provides as the high point of their day. They gather with friends to enjoy conversation and a nutritious meal. For the homebound, Meals on Wheels volunteers deliver the meals to the door, a benefit even though the recipients miss out on the social event of the congregate program.

Nutritionists are wise not to focus solely on nutrients and food intakes of the elderly, because social interactions may be as important. A professor of psychiatry wrote perceptively of many elderly people, using the pronoun "he" to mean a typical elderly person:

> *It is not* what *the older person eats but* with whom *that will be the deciding factor in proper care for him. The oft-repeated complaint of the older patient that he has little incentive to prepare food for only himself is not merely a statement of fact but also a rebuke to the questioner for failing to perceive his isolation and aloneness and to realize that food . . . for one's self lacks the condiment of another's presence which can transform the simplest fare to the ceremonial act with all its shared meaning.*[81]

The need for companionship surrounding meals is as great today as it was when these words were written.

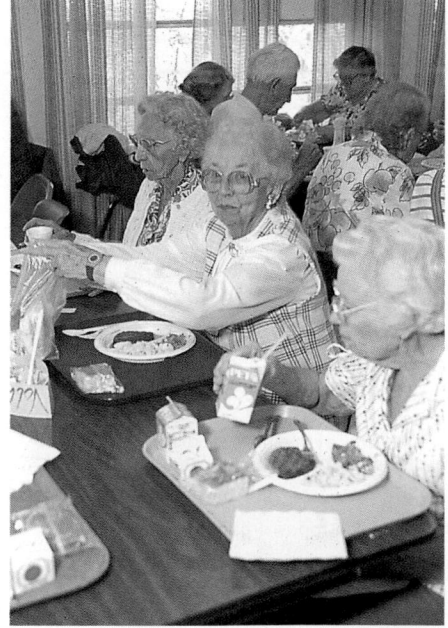

Shared meals can be the high point of the day.

Nutrition knowledge meets health in the real world of cooking, cleaning, and shopping, but many older people, even able-bodied ones with financial resources, find themselves unable to perform these tasks. For anyone living alone and for those of advanced age especially, it is important to work through the problems that food preparation presents. This chapter's Food Feature presents some ideas.

Sources of support for the elderly:

- Social Security
- Food Stamps
- Supplemental Security Income program
- Title IIIC of the Older Americans Act
- Meals on Wheels

KEY POINT Food choices in the elderly are affected by many factors. Assistance programs directly improve nutrition status; some are aimed at helping to relieve financial problems. Social stimulation is important.

In a developed society, people depend to a great degree on others to bring foods to the table. As this chapter has shown, the more people rely on others to produce and process their food, the more discerning they must become to choose among alternatives for those that best support health. In the future such decisions must also take into account the effects of new food technologies, which are described in Controversy 14.

FOOD FEATURE

Single Survival

Singles of all ages face problems concerning the purchasing, storing, and preparing of food. Whether the person is a student in a college dormitory, an elderly person in a retirement apartment, or a professional in an efficiency apartment, the problems of preparing nourishing meals are the same. Many college students live in dormitories, most without kitchens and freezers, and for them, purchasing and storage problems are compounded. Following is a collection of ideas gathered from single people who have devised answers to some of these problems.

Large packages of meat and vegetables are often suitable for a family of four or more, and even a head of lettuce can spoil before one person can use it all. Buy only what you will use. Don't be timid about asking the grocer to break open a family-sized package of wrapped meat or fresh vegetables. Look for bags of prepared salad greens to take the place of lettuce in both salads and sandwiches. Small-sized containers of food may be expensive, but it is also expensive to let the unused portion of a large-sized container spoil. Buy only three pieces of each kind of fresh fruit: a ripe one, a medium-ripe one, and a green one. Eat the first right away and the second soon, and let the last one ripen to eat days later.

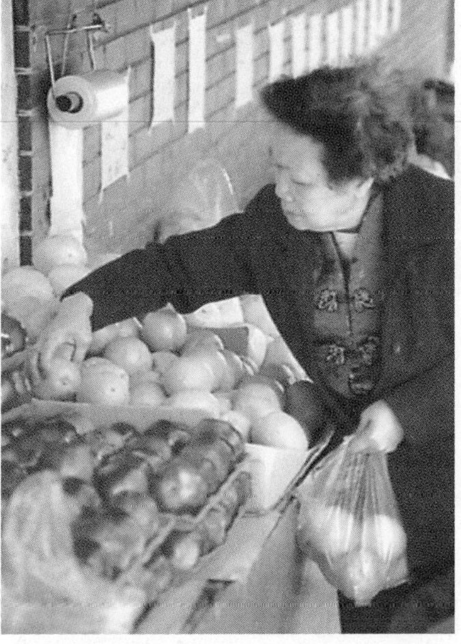

Buy only what you will use.

Think up a variety of ways to use a vegetable when you must buy it in large quantity. For example, you can divide a head of cauliflower into thirds. Cook one third and eat it as a hot vegetable. Toss another third into a salad dressing marinade for use as an appetizer. Save the rest to use raw in salad. Make mixtures using what you have on hand. A thick stew prepared from any leftover vegetables and bits of meat, with some added onion, pepper, celery, and potatoes, makes a complete and balanced meal, except for milk. If you like creamed gravy, add nonfat dry milk to your stew.

Buy fresh milk in the sizes best suited for you. If your grocer doesn't carry pints or quarts of milk, try a nearby convenience store. If you eat lunch in a cafeteria, try buying two pints of milk—one to drink and one to take home and store.

Design a space for rows of glass jars containing shelf-stable items that you can't buy in single-serving quantities—items such as rice, tapioca, lentils and other dry beans, flour, cornmeal, dry nonfat milk, and cereal, to name only a few possibilities. Cut the directions-for-use label from the package of each item and store it in the jar. Place each jar, tightly sealed, in a freezer for a few days to kill any eggs or organisms before storing it on the shelf. Then the jars will keep bugs out of the foods indefinitely. The jars make an attractive display and will remind you of possibilities for variety in your menus.

Light destroys riboflavin, so use opaque jars for enriched pasta and dry milk.

Experiment with stir-fried foods. Use a frying pan if you don't have a wok. A variety of vegetables and meats can be enjoyed this way; inexpensive vegetables such as cabbage and celery are delicious when crisp cooked in a little oil with soy sauce or lemon added. Interesting frozen mixtures of vegetables are available in the larger grocery stores. Cooked, leftover vegetables can be dropped in at the last minute. A bonus of a stir-fried meal is that you'll have only one pan to wash.

If you can afford a microwave oven, buy one. It will eliminate the need for most pots and pans and allow you to freeze or refrigerate meals in microwavable containers so that you can reheat them at your convenience. Many frozen, single-serving meals come in microwave containers that you can reuse one time. Place extra servings of home-cooked foods in them to use later on.

Depending on your freezer space, make a regular-sized recipe of a dish that takes time to prepare: a casserole, vegetable pie, or meat loaf. Freeze individual portions in containers that can be microwaved or oven heated for serving later as just described. Be sure to date these so you will use the oldest first.

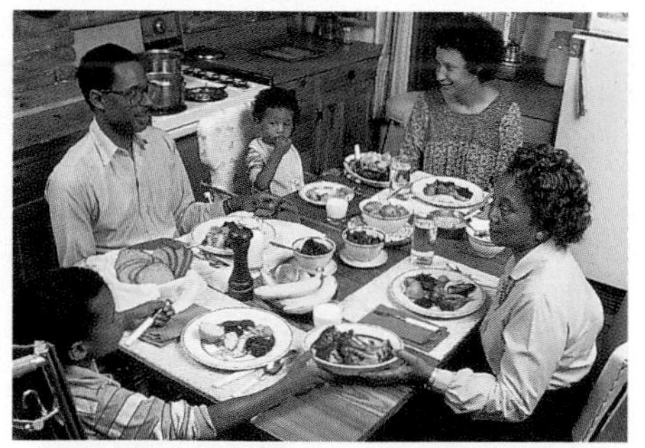

Invite guests to share a meal.

Buy a loaf of bread and immediately store half, well wrapped, in the freezer (not the refrigerator, which will make it stale). Buy frozen vegetables in a bag, toss in a variety of herbs, and divide among single-serving containers. Vary your choices to prevent boredom.

For nutrition's sake, it is important to attend to loneliness at mealtimes; the person who is living alone must learn to connect food with socializing. Cook for yourself with the idea that you will invite guests, and make enough food so that you will have some left for a later meal. If you know an older person who eats alone, you can bet that person would love to join you for a meal now and then. Invite the person often.

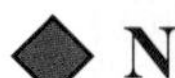

Notes

1. S. Shea and coauthors, Variability and self regulation of energy intake in young children in their everyday environment, *Pediatrics* 90 (1992): 542–546.

2. R. E. Klesges and coauthors, Parental influence on food selection in young children and its relationships to childhood obesity, *American Journal of Clinical Nutrition* 53 (1991): 859–864.

3. F. Lifshitz and N. Moses, Nutritional dwarfing: Growth, dieting, and fear of obesity, *Journal of the American College of Nutrition* 7 (1988): 367–376.

4. M. L. Burroughs and R. D. Terry, Parents' perspectives toward their children's eating behavior, *Topics in Clinical Nutrition* 8 (1992): 45–52.

5. American Red Cross Standard First Aid Workbook (American National Red Cross, 1991), p. 28.
6. D. Benton and G. Roberts, Effect of vitamin and mineral supplementation on intelligence of a sample of schoolchildren, *Lancet*, 23 January 1988, pp. 140–143.
7. P. L. Splett and M. Story, Child nutrition: Objectives for the decade, *Journal of the American Dietetic Association* 91 (1991): 665–668; N. S. Scrimshaw, Iron deficiency, *Scientific American*, October 1991, pp. 46–52.
8. J. D. Haas and M. W. Fairchild, Summary and conclusions of the International Conference on Iron Deficiency and Behavioral Development, October 10–12, 1988, *American Journal of Clinical Nutrition* 50 (1989): 703–705.
9. M. Clark, J. Royal, and R. Seeler, Interaction of iron deficiency and lead and the hematologic findings in children with lead poisoning, *Pediatrics* 81 (1988): 247–254.
10. D. E. Glotzer and H. Bauchner, Management of childhood lead poisoning: A survey, *Pediatrics* 89 (1992): 614–618.
11. H. L. Needleman and coauthors, The long-term effects of exposure to low doses of lead in childhood: An 11-year follow-up report, *New England Journal of Medicine* 322 (1990): 83–88.
12. Centers for Disease Control, as cited by H. Pearson, Stepped-up lead screenings urged, *AAP News*, April 1993, p. 1, 8.
13. R. W. Miller, The metal in our mettle, *FDA Consumer*, December 1988-January 1989, pp. 24–27.
14. J. Raloff, Lead effects show in child's balance, *Science News* 135 (1989): 54.
15. K. N. Dietrich, O. G. Berger, and P. A. Succop, Lead exposure and the motor development status of urban six-year-old children in Cincinnati, Prospective study, *Pediatrics* 91 (1993): 301–307.
16. A. J. McMichael and coauthors, Port Pirie cohort study: Environmental exposure to lead and children's abilities at the age of four years, *New England Journal of Medicine* 319 (1988): 468–475.
17. Environmental exposure to lead and cognitive deficits in children, *New England Journal of Medicine* 320 (1989): 595–596.
18. E. Yetley, Nutritional applications of the Health and Nutrition Examination Surveys (HANES), *Annual Review of Nutrition* 7 (1987): 441–463; Miller, 1989.
19. S. A. Bock and F. M. Atkins, Patterns of food hypersensitivity during sixteen years of double-blind, placebo-controlled food challenges, *Journal of Pediatrics* 117 (1990): 561–567.
20. H. A. Sampson and D. D. Metcalfe, Food allergies, *Journal of the American Medical Association* 268 (1992): 2840–2844.
21. M. L. Arbeit and coauthors, Caffeine intakes of children from a biracial population: The Bogalusa Heart Study, *Journal of the American Dietetic Association* 88 (1988): 466–471.
22. Kids get up and go—not! International Food Information Council, Press Release, 11 August 1992.
23. R. C. Klesges, M. L. Shelton, and L. M. Klesges, Effects of television on metabolic rate: Potential implications for childhood obesity, *Pediatrics* 91 (1993): 281–286.
24. T. N. Robinson and coauthors, Does television viewing increase obesity and reduce physical activity? *Pediatrics* 91 (1993): 273–280.
25. W. H. Dietz and S. L. Gortmaker, TV or not TV: Fat is the question, *Pediatrics* 91 (1993): 499–501.
26. N. D. Wong and coauthors, Television viewing and pediatric hypercholesterolemia, *Pediatrics* 90 (1992): 75–79.
27. Timely statement on NCEP report on children and adolescents, *Journal of the American Dietetic Association* 91 (1991): 983; N. A. Holtzman, The great god cholesterol, *Pediatrics* 87 (1991): 943–945.
28. Report of the Expert Panel on Blood Cholesterol Levels in Children and Adolescents, *Pediatrics* 89 (1992): entire supplement.
29. M. Weitzman, as quoted by J. Raloff in In-school breakfasts improve test scores, *Science News*, 14 October 1989, p. 247.
30. A. F. Meyers and coauthors, School breakfast program and school performance, *American Journal of Diseases of Children* 143 (1989): 1234–1239.
31. T. A. Nicklas and coauthors, Breakfast consumption affects adequacy of total daily intakes in children, *Journal of the American Dietetic Association* 93 (1993): 886–891.
32. B. A. Bidgood and C. Gameron, Meal/snack missing and dietary adequacy of primary school children, *Journal of the Canadian Dietetic Association* 53 (1992): 164–168.
33. L. Snetselaar and R. M. Lauer, Childhood, diet, and the atherosclerotic process, *Nutrition Today*, January/February 1992, pp. 22–28.
34. L. L. Birch, Children's preferences for high-fat foods, *Nutrition Reviews* 50 (1992): 249–255.
35. Birch, 1992.
36. Kids make the nutritional grade, *IFIC Review*, October 1992.
37. S. M. Ott, Bone density in adolescents, *New England Journal of Medicine* 325 (1991): 1646–1647.
38. V. Matkovic, Diet, genetics, and peak bone mass of adolescent girls, *Nutrition Today*, March–April 1991, pp. 21–24.
39. Matkovic, 1991; P. M. Guenther, Beverages in the diets of American teenagers, *Journal of the American Dietetic Association* 86 (1986): 493–499.
40. L. E. Underwood, Normal adolescent growth and development, *Nutrition Today*, March/April, 1991, pp. 11–16.
41. S. Snider, Acne: Taming that age-old adolescent affliction, *FDA Consumer*, October 1990, pp. 16–19.
42. G. A. L. Meijer and coauthors, Sleeping metabolic rate in relation to body composition and the menstrual cycle, *American Journal of Clinical Nutrition* 55 (1992): 637–640; M. Tai and coauthors, Resting metabolic rate during four phases of the menstrual cycle (abstract), *American Journal of Clinical Nutrition* 56 (1992): 101.
43. V. Tarasuk and G. H. Beaton, Menstrual-cycle patterns in energy and macronutrient intake, *American Journal of Clinical Nutrition* 53 (1991): 442–447; E. J. Gong, D. Garrel, and D. H. Calloway, Menstrual cycle and voluntary food intake, *American Journal of Clinical Nutrition* 49 (1989): 252–258.
44. A. K. H. Fong and M. J. Kretsch, Changes in dietary intake, urinary nitrogen, and urinary volume across the menstrual cycle, *American Journal of Clinical Nutrition* 57 (1993): 43–46.
45. R. S. London, L. Bradley, and N. Y. Chiamori, Effect of a nutritional supplement on premenstrual syndrome: A double-blind longitudinal study, *Journal of the American College of Nutrition* 10 (1991): 494–499.
46. M. K. Berman, M. L. Taylor, and E. Freeman, Vitamin B_6 in premenstrual syndrome, *Journal of the American Dietetic Association* 90 (1990): 859–861.
47. R. S. London and coauthors, Efficacy of alpha-tocopherol in the treatment of the premenstrual syndrome; *Journal of Reproductive Medicine* 32 (1987): 400–404.
48. A. Rossignol and coauthors, Tea and premenstrual syndrome in the People's Republic of China, *American Journal of Public Health* 79 (1989): 67–69.
49. A. M. Rossignol and H. Bonnlander, Caffeine-containing beverages, total fluid consumption, and premenstrual syndrome, *American Journal of Public Health* 80 (1990): 1106–1110.
50. R. Chernoff, Demographics of aging, in *Geriatric Nutrition: The Health Professional's Handbook*, ed. R. Chernoff (Gaithersburg, Md.: Aspen Publishers, 1991), pp. 1–9.
51. K. G. Kinsella, Changes in life expectancy 1900–1990, *American Journal of Clinical Nutrition* 55 (1992): 1196S–1202S.

52. N. B. Belloc and L. Breslow, Relationship of physical health status and health practices, *Preventive Medicine* 1 (1972): 409–421.
53. Curtailing calories may lengthen life, *FDA Consumer*, February 1989, pp. 3–4; E. J. Masoro, Food restriction in rodents: An evaluation of its role in the study of aging, *Journal of Gerontology* 43 (1988): B59–64.
54. Masoro, 1988.
55. E. J. Masoro, Assessment of nutritional components in prolongation of life and health by diet, *Proceedings of the Society for Experimental Biology and Medicine* 193 (1990): 31–34; Energy intake restriction and oxidant defense, *Nutrition Reviews* 49 (1991): 278–280.
56. H. Smicklas-Wright, Aging, in *Present Knowledge in Nutrition*, ed. M. L. Brown (Washington, D.C.: International Life Sciences Institute—Nutrition Foundation, 1990), pp. 333–340.
57. E. T. Poehlman and E. S. Horton, Regulation of energy expenditure in aging humans, *Annual Review of Nutrition* 10 (1990): 255–275.
58. I. H. Rosenberg, Nutrition in the elderly, *Nutrition Reviews* 50 (1992): 349–350.
59. M. A. Fiatrone and coauthors, High-intensity strength training in nonagenarians, *Journal of the American Medical Association* 263 (1990): 3029–3034.
60. J. V. G. A. Durnin, Energy metabolism in the elderly, in H. Munro and G. Schlierf, *Nutrition of the Elderly* (New York: Raven Press, 1992), pp. 51–63.
61. WHO Study Group on Diet, Nutrition, and Prevention of Noncommunicable Diseases, Diet, nutrition, and the prevention of chronic diseases, *Nutrition Reviews* 49 (1991): 291–301.
62. J. M. Kremer and coauthors, Fish-oil fatty acid supplementation in active rheumatoid arthritis, *Annals of Internal Medicine* 106 (1987): 497–503.
63. R. Roubenoff and L. C. Rall, Humoral mediation of changing body composition during aging and chronic inflammation, *Nutrition Reviews* 51 (1993): 1–11.
64. P. Merry and coauthors, Oxidative damage to lipids within the inflamed human joint provides evidence of radical-mediated hypoxic-reperfusion injury, *American Journal of Clinical Nutrition* 53 (1991): 362S–369S.
65. P. J. Garry and coauthors, Vitamin A intake and plasma retinol levels in healthy elderly men and women, *American Journal of Clinical Nutrition* 46 (1987): 989–994; Processing of dietary retinoids is slowed in the elderly, *Nutrition Reviews* 49 (1991): 116–118.
66. E. E. Delvin, A. Imbach, and M. Copti, Vitamin D nutritional status and related biochemical indices in an autonomous elderly population, *American Journal of Clinical Nutrition* 48 (1988): 373–378; H. Payette and K. Gray-Donald, Dietary intake and biochemical indices of nutritional status in an elderly population with estimates of the precision of the 7-day food record, *American Journal of Clinical Nutrition* 54 (1991): 478–488.
67. V. Holt, J. Nordstrom, and M. B. Kohrs, Food preferences of older adults (abstract), *Journal of the American Dietetic Association* 87 (1987): 1597.
68. G. E. Bunce and J. L. Hess, Cataract—What is the role of nutrition in lens health? *Nutrition Today*, December 1988, pp. 6–8.
69. G. E. Bunce, J. Kinoshita, and J. Horwitz, Nutritional factors in cataract, *Annual Review of Nutrition* 10 (1990): 233–254; S. D. Varma, Scientific basis for medical therapy of cataracts by antioxidants, *American Journal of Clinical Nutrition* 53 (1991): 335S–345S; P. F. Jacques and L. T. Chylack, Epidemiologic evidence of a role for the antioxidant vitamins and carotenoids in cataract prevention, *American Journal of Clinical Nutrition* 53 (1991): 352S–355S; J. M. Robertson, A. P. Donner, and J. R. Trevithick, A possible role for vitamins C and E in cataract prevention, *American Journal of Clinical Nutrition* 53 (1991): 346S–351S.
70. B. J. Rolls and P. A. Phillips, Aging and disturbances of thirst and fluid balance, *Nutrition Reviews* 48 (1990): 137–144.
71. H. Sato, T. Saito, and K. Yoshinaga, Renal function and histopathology in the elderly, in *Nutrition of the Elderly* (New York: Raven Press, 1992), pp. 29–36.
72. W. Mertz, Trace elements in aging, in H. Munro and G. Schlierf, *Nutrition of the Elderly* (New York: Raven Press, 1992), pp. 145–149.
73. C. A. Swanson and coauthors, Zinc status of elderly adults: Response to supplement, *American Journal of Clinical Nutrition* 48 (1988): 343–349.
74. R. J. Cousins and J. M. Hempe, Zinc, in *Present Knowledge in Nutrition*, 6th ed., ed. M. L. Brown (Washington, D.C.: International Life Science Institute, 1990), pp. 251–260.
75. G. J. Fosmire, Trace mineral requirements, in *Geriatric Nutrition: The Health Professional's Handbook*, ed. R. Chernoff (Gaithersburg, Md.: Aspen Publishers, 1991), pp. 77–105.
76. A. Sorenson, N. Chapman, and D. N. Sundwall, Health promotion and disease prevention in the elderly, in *Geriatric Nutrition: The Health Professional's Handbook*, ed. R. Chernoff (Gaithersburg, Md.: Aspen Publishers, 1991), pp. 449–483; Are older Americans making better food choices to meet diet and health recommendations? *Nutrition Reviews* 51 (1993): 20–23.
77. R. K. Chandra, Effect of vitamin and trace-element supplementation on immune responses and infection in elderly subjects, *Lancet* 340 (1992): 1124–1127.
78. J. V. White and coauthors, Consensus of the Nutrition Screening Initiative: Risk factors and indicators of poor nutritional status in older Americans, *Journal of the American Dietetic Association* 91 (1991): 783–787.
79. M. A. Davis and coauthors, Living arrangements and dietary quality of older U.S. adults, *Journal of the American Dietetic Association* 90 (1990): 1667–1672.
80. B. J. Rolls and T. M. McDermott, Effects of age on sensory-specific satiety, *American Journal of Clinical Nutrition* 54 (1991): 988–996.
81. J. Weinberg, Psychologic implications of the nutritional needs of the elderly, *Journal of the American Dietetic Association* 60 (1972): 293–296.

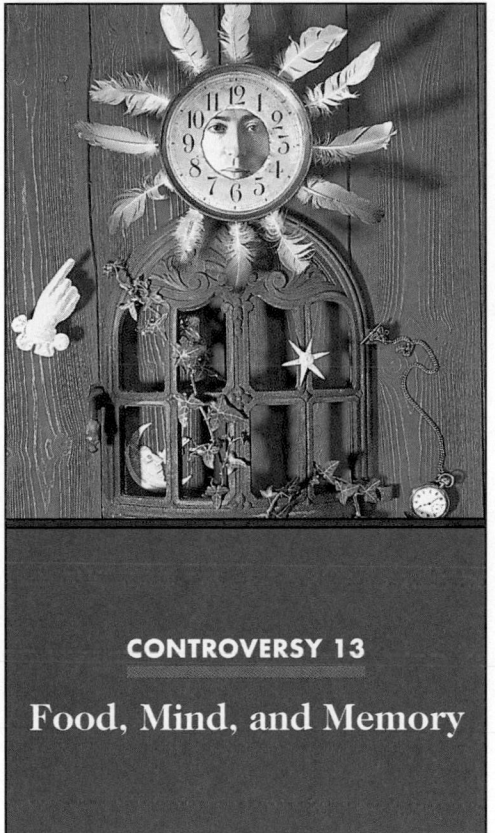

CONTROVERSY 13

Food, Mind, and Memory

Why do you feel like eating a steak at one meal and a doughnut at another? Why do you feel sleepy after lunch and not after dinner? Do some foods help you to think or to remember? Human behavior and the workings of the brain are still largely mysterious territory, and research reveals layer upon layer of complexity. Still, researchers no longer doubt that intakes of food and nutrients affect the mind and memory, and they are beginning to understand how and why. As one researcher put it, "The neurosciences are the wave of the future."[1]

THE BRAIN AND ITS NEUROTRANSMITTERS The brain has special needs. Encased in its protective skull, a hard, bony, inelastic helmet, the brain cannot expand and contract as can, say, the liver or adipose tissue. It cannot store its own reserve supply of glycogen, fat, or other molecules because those molecules take up space. It cannot store oxygen with which to oxidize those fuels. Therefore the brain must depend on the passing blood supply for both its fuels and oxygen. Furthermore, its needs for those substances are extraordinary. It comprises only 2 percent of the adult's body weight, but at any given time the brain contains 15 percent of the body's blood, and it devours 20 to 30 percent of the fuels that support the basal metabolism. Should the blood deliver too little oxygen or glucose, the brain's cells would cease communicating with each other (see Figure C13-1) and coma would occur within minutes. Should the blood supply be interrupted altogether, coma would ensue within 10 seconds.[2]

Nutrients of all kinds are crucial to brain function, and the blood supply must deliver these, too. The brain requires amino acids to make its messenger molecules, some 30 to 40 **neurotransmitters** and related compounds (see Table C13-1). The brain also needs electrically charged minerals to help transmit its electrical impulses, vitamins and other minerals to facilitate these processes, lipids to repair its cell membranes, and water to maintain an environment in which chemical processes may take place.

The brain is extremely sensitive to fluctuations in its internal chemical composition. To keep its internal environment constant, it has its own molecular sieve to filter from the blood the fluid and chemicals it needs. The blood vessels that feed the brain differ from those that feed other organs in that they are lined with highly selective cells. These cells form a barrier known as the **blood-brain barrier,** which allows desired constituents to enter the brain tissue while restricting others. When the environment outside the body fluctuates widely in temperature, humidity, and chemical composition, the body's blood changes a little in response. But the brain's internal milieu hardly fluctuates at all.

Because of its dependence on the blood's chemistry the brain monitors it closely and sends messages to other organs to signal the need for their help in regulating it. At one time the brain may need glucose; at another, amino acids. If body stores are inadequate to supply the amounts needed, the brain can even direct a person's eating behavior to obtain carbohydrate at one time and protein at another, depending on its needs. Animals regulate their intakes of protein and carbohydrate, each proportional to the other. People probably do this too, even without being aware that they are doing so. The brain can tell what it needs based on its own supply of a few nutrients that can enter the brain and change its functioning.

Scientists exploring the effects of nutrients on the brain are especially interested in these associations:

- Some dietary fats are taken into the brain and are incorporated directly into structural components of brain cells.
- Vitamins and minerals assist enzymes in the syntheses of neurotransmitters.
- Some amino acids serve as the starting material from which some neurotransmitters are built.[3]

Figure C13-1

COMMUNICATION WITHIN THE BRAIN

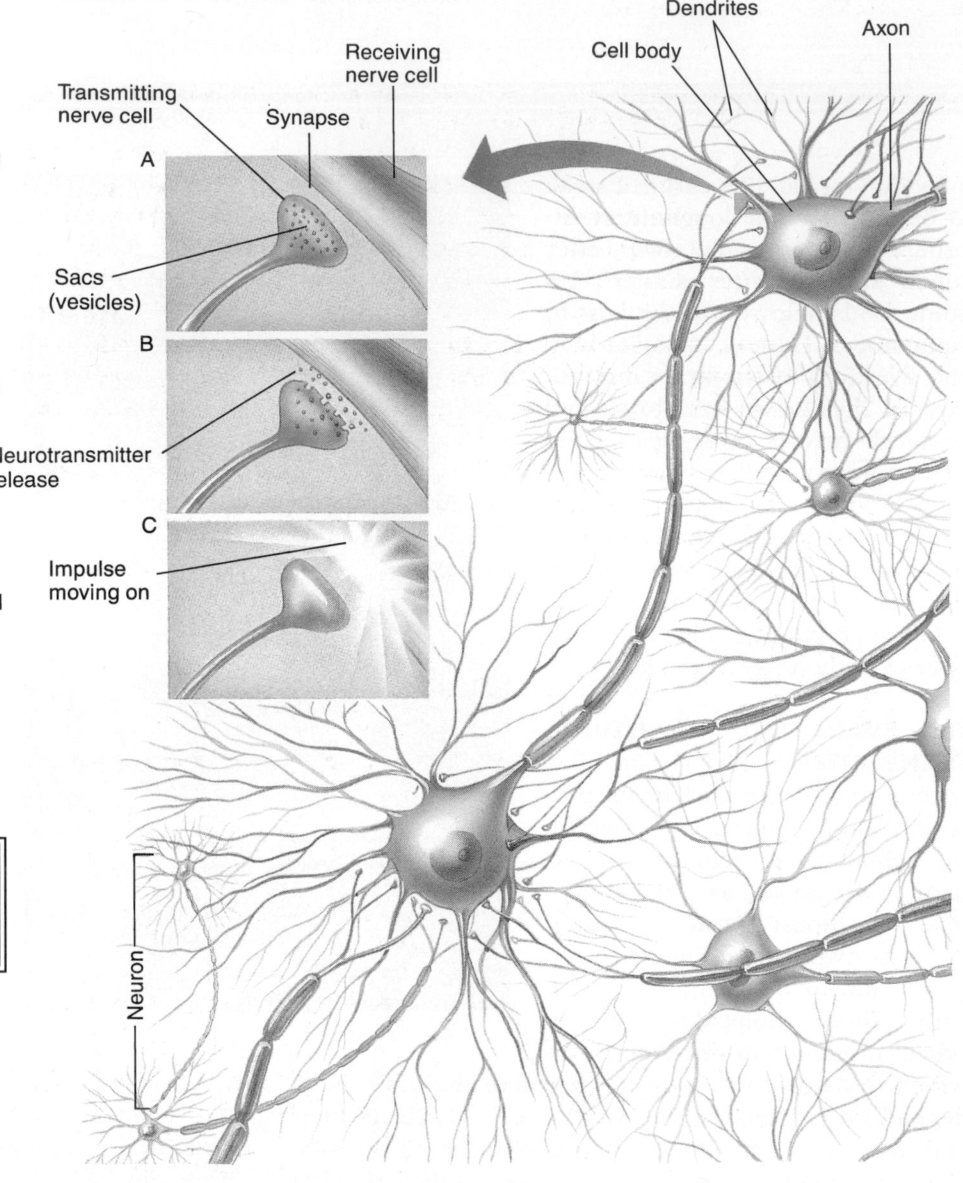
A. The nerve impulse arrives at the end of the first nerve cell. Clustered just inside the nerve cell ending are a multitude of little sacs (vescicles) filled with the neurotransmitter.
B. The vesicles fuse with the nerve cell membrane, releasing the neurotransmitter into the gap (synapse) between two cells.
C. The neurotransmitter arrives at receptor sites on the receiver cell and (in this instance) stimulates it to generate a nerve impulse that will travel along its length. Simultaneously, the receiver cell destroys the molecules of neurotransmitter at its membrane, or the releasing cell takes them up again to reuse them. Total elapsed time: a fraction of a second.
Transmitting nerve cell
Synapse
Receiving nerve cell
A
Sacs (vesicles)
B
Neurotransmitter release
C
Impulse moving on
Dendrites
Cell body
Axon
Neuron

axon the transmitting end of a neuron.

dendrites the branched, impulse-receiving structures of a neuron.

A day's intakes of fats, vitamins, and minerals are unlikely to affect the brain's functioning immediately, although they probably do affect it over time. Amino acids, in contrast, are used to form neurotransmitters within the day they are eaten, and their effects are seen within minutes or hours of ingestion.[4]

Certain amino acids help regulate the brain's function and these are given special privileges. To affect the brain, a nutrient must be free to come and go as it pleases. Its concentration must not be tightly controlled in the blood or brain, but must fluctuate. The brain's regulatory amino acids are unlike most others which never exceed a given level in the brain no matter how much of them is consumed. Amino acids that are the precursors from which neurotransmitters are made cross the blood-brain barrier freely, and their concentrations in the brain can be altered by the composition of the bloodstream. Thus the food a person eats can influence the brain chemistry by producing high or low concentrations of the precursor nutrients. Furthermore, once in the brain, these precursor nutrients exert **precursor control,** that is, the brain responds to larger or smaller amounts of them by making larger or smaller amounts of neurotransmitters from them. These facts link eating directly to brain chemistry and, as you will see in a moment, to mood and other sensations.

One neurotransmitter whose brain concentration is especially sensitive to changes in precursor supply has been studied in depth: **serotonin,** made from its precursor, the amino acid tryptophan. Another set, the **catecholamines,** similarly depends on the availability of the amino acid tyrosine. The discussion that follows centers on serotonin because more details about it are known.

Tryptophan to Serotonin Ordinary meals of the kind people eat every day raise or lower the concentration of serotonin in the brain, depending on the meal's protein and carbohydrate content.[5] Serotonin release in turn affects sensations and mood, so the ingredients of meals may have real effects on how people feel afterwards. A lack of tryptophan flowing into the brain can manifest itself in wakefulness, a tendency to startle, and an enhanced sensitivity to pain. Animals that have been made tryptophan deficient startle easily and they have a lowered threshold for pain. When they are given tryptophan, they become less easily startled and their pain thresholds return to normal as their brain serotonin is restored.[6] Tests of pain perception in people conclude similarly: tryptophan reduces sensitivity to pain.[7]

The amount of tryptophan that enters the brain depends not only on the amount of tryptophan the person eats but also on the total protein *and carbohydrate* the person eats. If tryptophan is consumed by itself, as a single amino acid, then brain serotonin increases proportionately. But normally whole proteins, not just tryptophan, are eaten. In this case some of the other large amino acids in the proteins compete with tryptophan for entry into the brain because they use the same transport mechanism to get across the blood-brain barrier. In this situation tryptophan fails to enter the brain in increased quantities and so does not effectively enhance brain serotonin synthesis.

If carbohydrate is fed along with protein, however, it can "help" the protein to deliver tryptophan to the brain because it elicits the secretion of the hormone insulin. Insulin drives the other amino acids, but not tryptophan, into *body* cells, leaving the tryptophan free to enter the brain without competition. Thus, paradoxically, a meal high in carbohydrate, but not one high in protein, eases tryptophan's transport into the brain and so promotes serotonin synthesis. It is not the total amount of tryptophan, then, but the amount relative to the competing amino acids that affects the brain's serotonin level, and this relationship is determined largely by the effect of dietary carbohydrate just described.

Table C13-1
Brain Terms

- **blood-brain barrier** a barrier composed of the cells lining the blood vessels in the brain, which are so tightly glued to each other that substances can only get through the lining by crossing the cell bodies themselves. Thus the cells, using all their sophisticated equipment, can be highly selective in permitting entry.
- **catecholamines** neurotransmitters made from the amino acid tyrosine: dopamine, epinephrine, and norepinephrine.
- **neurotransmitter** a chemical messenger released at the end of one nerve cell when a nerve impulse arrives there, which diffuses across the gap to the next nerve cell and alters the membrane of that cell in such a way that it becomes either less or more likely to fire (or does fire).
- **precursor control** control of a compound's synthesis by the availability of that compound's precursor. (The more precursor there is, the more of the compound is made.)
- **serotonin** A compound related in structure to (and made from) the amino acid tryptophan; it serves as one of the brain's principal neurotransmitters.

Serotonin and Appetite An understanding of the absorption of tryptophan by the brain may help explain how animals and human beings may know what kinds of foods they have eaten last and what foods to choose next time to ensure balance. According to one theory, a high-carbohydrate meal raises brain serotonin by increasing tryptophan uptake; this satisfies the desire for carbohydrate and so reduces the urge to eat carbohydrate-containing foods. A person or animal who has eaten plenty of carbohydrate therefore will seek out more protein at the next meal. A high-protein meal creates a serotonin deficit, awakens the carbohydrate craving, and once again leads to the consumption of carbohydrate-containing foods.[8]

While not everyone agrees, one chief appeal of this theory is that it seems to account for what is observed to happen often with low-carbohydrate diets. The more dieters try to restrict carbohydrate the more they seem to crave it. The effect is accentuated if they are insulin resistant, as is likely if they are obese. When an insulin-resistant person eats carbohydrate, insulin's normal actions do not follow and the cells continue to be hungry for glucose. Furthermore, brain serotonin does not rise, and so the carbohydrate craving is intensified.

Another theory links serotonin to obesity. The theory gains support from evidence that serotonin concentrations are often below average in the brains of obese people and of normal-weight people who report craving carbohydrate-rich food.[9] While direct cause-and-effect conclusions are not yet possible, the authors suggest that high-carbohydrate weight-loss diets are most successful because they work with many people's brain chemistry rather than against it.

Some evidence, however, weakens the theory that links serotonin to the appetite for carbohydrate. For example, under some circumstances when animals eat tryptophan, they then eat *less* protein. This cannot be explained by changes in blood tryptophan, brain tryptophan, or brain serotonin levels. When animals were injected with tryptophan, which should stimulate protein intake according to the theory, no preference for protein or carbohydrate was observed.[10] Ongoing research should ultimately help to untangle this problem, but chances are that it will first become more knotty.

Serotonin, Mood, and Sleep Some people describe themselves as anxious, tense, and somewhat depressed before eating carbohydrate and peaceful or relaxed afterward. The amino acid tryptophan given by itself seems to have similar effects, consistent with the notion that it is the indirect agent of carbohydrate's effect. When tryptophan is restricted in the diet, people report depressed feelings. When tryptophan is restored, depressed feelings lift, but in their place come drowsiness, clumsiness, and mental slowing.[11] Some reports exist of disturbances of serotonin metabolism in those with major depression, but it would be a vast oversimplification to suggest that tryptophan may be an effective antidepressant drug. Major depressive disorders are much more complex than everyday mood swings.

Another effect of carbohydrate or tryptophan is to induce fatigue or sleepiness. The effect of tryptophan in inducing sleep is particularly well known; 43 studies have demonstrated it in people and animals.[12] Carbohydrate or tryptophan can also increase the error rate in performance tests.[13] Elevated brain serotonin is known to reduce aggression in rats, and it may have that effect on people, too.[14]

Tyrosine Effects The case for a role for brain tyrosine concentrations in directing food choices is not well established, but the available evidence is suggestive. A meal high in protein, and therefore high in tyrosine, increases the production of the neurotransmitters known as catecholamines: dopamine, epinephrine, and norepinephrine. One of these, norepinephrine, is suspected of stimulating the appetite for carbohydrate at the next meal. Research on this effect is ongoing.[15]

Tyrosine, when given to animals, reverses some of the observed effects of stress. Tyrosine may also affect people's mental and physical responses to environmental stress. Normally, high altitude and exposure to cold impair mental and physical performance. Army recruits were exposed to a cold temperature for over four hours at a simulated high altitude. Those who received tyrosine experienced fewer headaches and less coldness, muscle pain, sleepiness, and dizziness while their thinking skills remained sharp.[16]

Such studies demonstrate clearly that single amino acids when administered alone act somewhat like drugs in the body. These effects are interesting, but they mean that people should not dose themselves with amino acids. The Consumer Caution of Chapter 6 warned that to do so is to imperil health.

VITAMINS, TRACE MINERALS, AND THE BRAIN This discussion thus far has focused only on the energy-yielding nutrients, particularly carbohydrate and protein. However, in the synthesis of neurotransmitters, other nutrients are involved. Iron is needed in one of the first steps of neurotransmitter synthesis. Vitamin B_6 and riboflavin are needed in later steps. These nutrients are but three among many; deficiencies of them are reflected in depressed or otherwise disturbed mood.[17] Deficiencies of many nutrients also cause anemia, which produces mental symptoms of its own (see Table C13-2). Some mental effects of nutrient deficiencies become apparent only in severe deficiency states, but others such as fatigue or depressed mood can be among the first symptoms of a developing deficiency. Some nutrient deficiencies cause mental symptoms as follows:

- Protein-energy deficiency causes apathy, fretfulness, lack of energy, and lack of interest in food.
- Thiamin deficiency causes confusion, uncoordinated movements, depressed appetite, irritability, insomnia, fatigue, personality changes, memory and cognition impairment, shortened attention span, impaired ability to work or learn, and depression.
- Riboflavin deficiency causes depression, hysteria, psychopathic behavior, lethargy, and hypochondria evident before clinical deficiency is detected.
- Niacin deficiency causes irritability, agitated depression, headaches, sleeplessness, memory loss, emotional instability (these are early signs of pellagra onset), and mental confusion progressing to psychosis or delirium.
- Vitamin B_6 deficiency impairs neurotransmitter synthesis,[18] causes irritability, insomnia, weakness, depression, abnormal brainwave patterns, convulsions, the mental symptoms of anemia (see Table C13-2), fatigue, and headaches.
- Folate deficiency causes the mental symptoms of anemia (see Table C13-2), tiredness, apathy, weakness, forgetfulness, mild depression, abnormal nerve

Table C13-2
The Mental Symptoms of Anemia

Apathy, listlessness
Behavior disturbances
Clumsiness
Hyperactivity
Irritability
Lack of appetite
Learning disorders (vocabulary, perception)
Low scores on latency and associative reactions
Lowered IQ
Reduced physical work capacity
Repetitive hand and foot movements
Shortened attention span

Note: These symptoms are not caused by anemia itself but by iron deficiency in the brain. Children with much more severe anemias from other causes, such as sickle-cell anemia and thalassemia, show no reduction in IQ when compared with children without anemia.

function, irritability, headache, disorientation, confusion, and inability to perform simple calculations.

- Vitamin B_{12} deficiency causes degeneration of the peripheral nervous system, anemia, and neuropsychiatric damage.[19]
- Vitamin C deficiency causes hysteria, depression, listlessness, lassitude, weakness, an aversion to work, hypochondria, social introversion, possible anemia, and fatigue.
- Vitamin A deficiency causes anemia.
- Iron deficiency causes fatigue, weakness, headaches, pallor, listlessness, irritability, and the mental symptoms of anemia (see Table C13-2).
- Magnesium deficiency causes apathy, personality changes, and hyperirritability.
- Copper deficiency causes iron-deficiency anemia (see Table C13-2).
- Zinc deficiency causes poor appetite, failure to grow, iron-deficiency anemia (see Table C13-2), irritability, emotional disorders, and mental lethargy.

Nutrients affect brain function in many other ways, but this list should suffice to show how dramatically the ways people eat can affect how they feel. Apparently the saying "You are what you eat" is true not only physically but also emotionally. It should go without saying, however, that self diagnosis or self-prescribed nutrient supplements could easily worsen the problem. Mental disturbances which persist even when the diet is adequate may require medical diagnosis and therapy.

"SMART" FOODS AND NUTRIENTS If severe deficiencies of nutrients can cause mental disturbances, can extra amounts of some nutrients cause the brain's functioning to excel? The idea has appeal, especially to business people, students, authors, medical workers, and others who must remain alert despite long hours, little sleep, or international travel. "Smart pills" are the topic of books and magazine articles, while establishments selling "smart cocktails" have sprung up on many urban streets.

Purveyors of "smart" drugs and drinks say they can speed thinking and learning, jump-start a failing memory, and reverse the processes of aging. Some of the drugs are prescription drugs under testing for reversal of the mental deterioration common in old age. Other drugs must be ordered from foreign countries because they are not approved for use in the United States. The drinks, also promoted as a legal high (euphoria) to those too young to buy alcohol, are made mostly of amino acids, vitamins, choline, and lecithin. In reality, no known nutrient supplement produces euphoria but the placebo effect can do so.

Users tell convincing stories about the effects of these drugs and drinks, but testimonials are not proof of effectiveness, and none of the products has been proved effective for improving intelligence in clinical trials. Researchers who attempt to measure people's feelings of being smart, witty, energetic, and able to remember run into problems even in the controlled laboratory setting. Measurements of this sort are always clouded by the placebo effect and wishful thinking.

Another confounding problem in such tests is one of prior nutrient status. A person with slight deficiencies of any of the nutrients listed in the earlier section might well respond favorably to a potion containing the lacking nutrients. Some years ago, a study of more than 200 healthy adults over 60 years of age revealed that low blood vitamin C or vitamin B_{12} impaired performance of tests of short-term memory and problem solving.[20] Those with low blood riboflavin or folate also scored poorly on a problem-solving test. Should those people suddenly receive supplemental nutrients, say in a smart drink, their perceptions of being "smarter" might be born out by test results.

An expert in the field of the neurobiology of learning and memory commented recently on smart drugs: "I think they are silly." He called the claims being made for their efficacy "scientific mumbo jumbo."[21] Experts at the FDA have warned that many of the smart drugs carry well-known side effects such as gastrointestinal distress, headaches, ulcers of the nasal cavity, and insomnia. They warn that long-term effects are not known.[22] The Federation of American Societies for Experimental Biology has warned that even amino acid supplements, often the basis for the mixtures, are not safe, and that they should not be taken without medical supervision.[23]

A few of the smart drugs may some day prove useful in treating people with the degenerative brain disease known as Alzheimer's. Such developments would be welcomed.

SENILE DEMENTIA—ALZHEIMER'S DISEASE As the population ages, more and more people fall victim to severe memory losses and cognitive impairments, all-too-common afflictions that rob many people of productive life in their later years. The findings on possible relationships between dementia and nutrition are tentative. More research is needed, and quickly, to find solutions.

In Alzheimer's disease, the brain deteriorates abnormally. Alzheimer's may affect as many as 5 percent of U.S. adults by the age of 65 years and 20 percent of those over 80 years.[24] Diagnosis depends on a cluster of symptoms: losses of memory and reasoning power; loss of the ability to communicate; loss of physical capabilities; and, eventually, loss of life.

The true cause of Alzheimer's disease is not yet known, although it appears that heredity is involved. Without a known cause, prevention is out of reach and a cure remains elusive. At present, treatment involves providing care for the person with Alzheimer's and support to the family. One drug (trade-named Tacrine) seems to slow the advancement of the disease in about 20 percent of those who use it, but it does not reverse the damage already done. Meanwhile, some drugs seem to favorably influence the ability to remember and so hold future promise for improving the lives of those with Alzheimer's disease.

Nutrition is important with regard to the aging brain and possesses some tentative links to Alzheimer's. For example, normally, as blood flow to the brain diminishes with age, the brain compensates by absorbing more glucose and oxygen. In Alzheimer's, no such compensation occurs, and concentrations of glucose and oxygen fall. Whether the brain's diminished concentrations of glucose and oxygen precede Alzheimer's or result from it remains unclear.

Another difference between the normal brain and that of a person with Alzheimer's is an extremely low concentration of an enzyme that synthesizes the neurotransmitter acetylcholine from choline. Acetylcholine is essential to memory. Experimental administration of acetylcholine-blocking drugs leads normal people to perform poorly on memory tests. Conversely, when subjects are given drugs that enhance concentrations of acetylcholine in the brain, they perform well on the same tests.[25] To date, taking oral supplements of choline or lecithin (which contains choline, first mentioned in this regard in Chapter 7) have had no effect on memory or on the progression of Alzheimer's, but researchers are still collecting data that may reveal a connection.[26] Recent trials of lecithin given in combination with certain drugs do show some improvement in limited areas of cognitive deficiencies.[27]

Most people have heard of an association between the mineral aluminum and Alzheimer's disease. A causal connection, however, seems unlikely. Brain concentrations of aluminum in people with Alzheimer's exceed normal brain concentrations by some 10 to 30 times. Still, blood and hair levels remain normal, indicating that the accumulation is caused by something in the brain itself, not by an overload of aluminum in the body. Thus the high brain aluminum must be at least partly a result, rather than a cause, of the disease.

Environmental aluminum may, however, make Alzheimer's disease progress faster. An epidemiological survey found that the risk of developing the condition was 1½ times greater in areas where water aluminum concentrations were high compared with areas where concentrations were low.[28] Still open is the question of whether aluminum cookware, which slightly increases the aluminum content of foods, can be suspected of the same connection. These data are far from proof that aluminum *causes* Alzheimer's, but they do provide pointers for research directions.

Finally, nutrient deficiencies, and especially those that continue over many years, may contribute to losses of memory and thinking ability that some older adults experience. Such deficiencies are not believed to cause Alzheimer's disease, and they can be largely reversed with diet.

With all of its mysteries and secrets, the human brain remains fascinating to researchers. Some recent inquiries have suggested a role for intakes of dietary carbohydrate (but not for blood glucose levels) on the formation of memory.[29] An interesting debate concerns the possibility that blood lipids may affect aggression and negative emotions.[30] These ideas and others like them will provide future researchers with plenty of grist for their mills for years to come. Even today, though, we know much more than 30 years ago. We certainly know that a person's nutrition status affects the health and functioning of the person's mind. Luckily, the brain

draws all the nutrients it needs from the same healthy diet that best nourishes the rest of the body. Thus the effort spent in planning to obtain adequate nutrients is well spent, in light of the vast rewards of human achievement and joyful living that are made possible by a well-fed mind.

Notes

1. T. W. Castonguay and J. S. Stern, Hunger and appetite, in M. L. Brown, ed., *Present Knowledge in Nutrition*, 6th ed. (Washington, D.C.: International Life Sciences Institute—Nutrition Foundation, 1990), pp. 13-22.
2. M. B. Krassner, Diet and brain function, *Nutrition Reviews/ Supplement*, May 1986, pp. 12–15.
3. C. E. Greenwood and R. E. A. Craig, Dietary influences on brain function: Implications during periods of neuronal maturation, in D. K. Rassin, B. Haber, and B. Drujan, eds., *Basic and Clinical Aspects of Nutrition and Brain Development* (New York: Alan R. Liss, 1987), pp. 160–161.
4. Greenwood and Craig, 1987.
5. P. Norton, G. Falciglia, and D. Gist, Physiologic control of food intake by neural and chemical mechanisms, *Journal of the American Dietetic Association* 93 (1993): 450–454.
6. B. Spring, Effects of food and nutrients on the behavior of normal individuals, in R. J. Wurtman and J. J. Wurtman, eds., *Nutrition and the Brain* 7 (New York: Raven Press, 1986), pp. 1–47.
7. Spring, 1986.
8. J. D. Fernstrom, Acute and chronic effects of protein and carbohydrate ingestion on brain tryptophan levels and serotonin synthesis, *Nutrition Reviews/Supplement*, May 1986, pp. 25–36.
9. I. Blum and coauthors, Food preferences, body weight, and platelet-poor plasma serotonin and catecholamines, *American Journal of Clinical Nutrition* 57 (1993): 486–489.
10. Brain neurochemistry and macronutrient selection: A role for serotonin feedback? *Nutrition Reviews* 50 (1992): 21–22.
11. Blum and coauthors, 1993.
12. E. L. Hartmann, Effect of L-tryptophan and other amino acids on sleep, *Nutrition Reviews/Supplement*, May 1986, pp. 70–73.
13. R. J. Wurtman, Ways that foods can affect the brain, *Nutrition Reviews/Supplement*, May 1986, pp. 2–6.
14. S. N. Young, The effect on aggression and mood of altering tryptophan levels, *Nutrition Reviews/Supplement*, May 1986, pp. 112–122; C. Greenwood, The role of diet in modulating brain metabolism and behavior, *Contemporary Nutrition* 14 (1989), whole issue.
15. G. H. Anderson, Metabolic regulation of food intake, in M. E. Shils and V. R. Young, eds., *Modern Nutrition in Health and Disease* (Philadelphia: Lea & Febiger, 1988), pp. 557–569.
16. D. E. Danford and coauthors, Report on the fourth conference for federally supported human nutrition research units and centers, *American Journal of Clinical Nutrition* 54 (1991): 164–168.
17. All of the listed symptoms can be found in R. S. Goodhart and M. E. Shils, eds., *Modern Nutrition in Health and Disease*, 7th ed. (Philadelphia: Lea and Febiger, 1988) or in M. L. Brown, ed., *Present Knowledge In Nutrition* (Washington, D.C.: International Life Sciences—Nutrition Foundation, 1990).
18. Greenwood, 1989.
19. M. W. P. Carney, Vitamin deficiencies and excesses: Behavioral consequences in adults, in J. R. Galler, ed., *Nutrition and Behavior* (New York: Plenum Press, 1984), pp. 193–222.
20. J. S. Goodwin, J. M. Goodwin, and P. J. Garry, Association between nutritional status and cognitive functioning in a healthy elderly population, *Journal of the American Medical Association* 249 (1983): 2917–2921.
21. Dr. James McGaugh, director of the center for neurobiology and memory at the University of California at Irvine as quoted in Ultra think fast, A. Purvis, *Time*, 8 June 1992, p. 80.
22. V. Lambert, Using 'smart' drugs and drinks may not be smart, *FDA Consumer*, April 1993, pp. 24–26.
23. S. A. Anderson and D. J. Raiten, eds., Safety of amino acids used as dietary supplements, *FASEB Report for Center of Food Safety and Applied Nutrition* (Bethesda, Md.: Federation of American Societies for Experimental Biology, 1992).
24. M. S. Claggett, Nutritional factors relevant to Alzheimer's disease, *Journal of the American Dietetic Association* 89 (1989): 392–396.
25. D. Drachman of the University of Massachusetts, as reported by R. Wurtman in Food and mood, *Nutrition Action Healthletter*, September 1992, pp. 1, 5–7.
26. R. Wurtman, in Food and mood, an interview by *Nutrition Action Healthletter*, September 1992, pp. 1, 5–7.
27. S. Gauthier and coauthors, Progress report on the Canadian multicentre trial of tetrahydroaminoacridine with lecithin in Alzheimer's disease, *Canadian Journal of Neurological Sciences* 16 (1989): S543–S546.
28. C. N. Martyn and coauthors, Geographical relation between Alzheimer's disease and aluminum in drinking water, *Lancet* 1 (1989): 59–62.
29. Sweet remembrances, *Science News*, 22 September 1990, p. 189; S. E. Gowans and H. P. Weingarten, Elevations of plasma glucose do not support taste-to-postingestive consequences of learning, *American Journal of Physiology* 261 (1991): 1407–1409.
30. G. Weidner and coauthors, Improvements in hostility and depression in relation to dietary change and cholesterol lowering, *Annals of Internal Medicine* 117 (1992): 820–823.

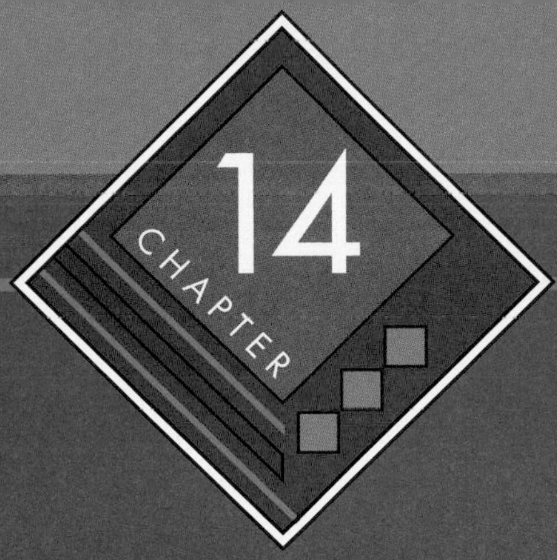

Food Technology and Food Safety

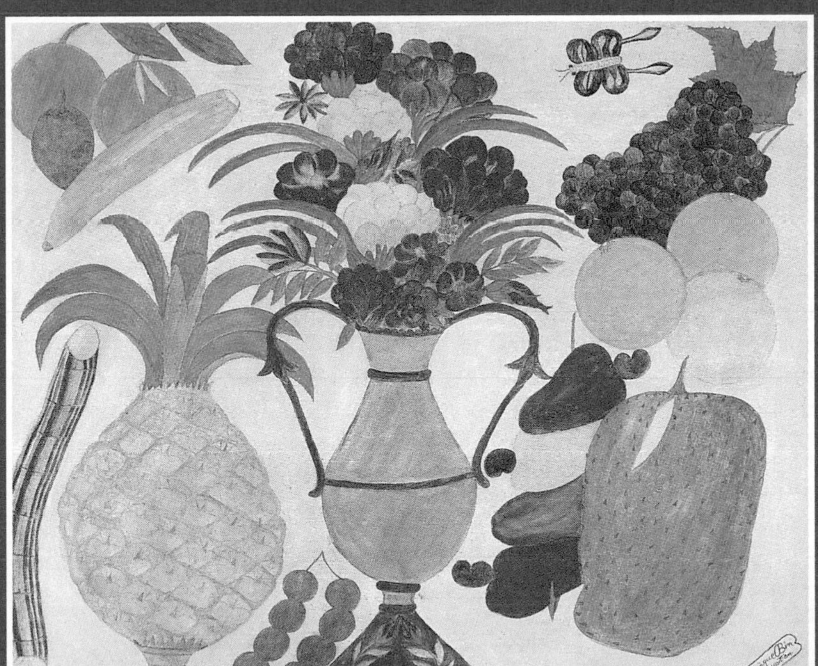

Contents

Milwaukee Art Museum, Gift of Richard and Erna Flagg

14

Consumers have questions about their food. Are today's food products nutritious? Are they pure and free from contamination? Are the additives in them safe? And who is looking out for these consumer concerns?

The Food and Drug Administration (FDA) is a major agency charged with monitoring the food supply. Other agencies are listed in Table 14-1. The FDA has identified the hazards in our food supply. The one listed first, microbial food poisoning, is the largest cluster of concerns. The one listed last, food additives, is of least concern. The others fall somewhere in between:

1. Microbial food poisoning. This affects the most people every year.
2. Natural toxins in foods. These constitute a hazard whenever people turn to consuming single foods either by choice (fad diets) or by necessity (poverty).
3. Residues in food.
   a. Environmental contaminants (other than pesticides) such as household and industrial chemicals. These are increasing yearly in number and concentration and their consequences are difficult to foresee and to forestall.
   b. Pesticides. These are a subclass of environmental contaminants, but are listed separately because they are applied intentionally to foods and so, in theory, can be controlled.
   c. Animal drugs.
4. The nutrient contents of foods. These require close attention as more and more artificially constituted foods appear on the market.
5. Intentional food additives. These are listed last because so much is known about them and because they are well regulated.[1]

This list of concerns and its rank order are remarkably similar to those put forth for other nations around the world.[2]

Table 14-1
Agencies that Monitor the U.S. Food Supply

- **CDC (Centers for Disease Control)** a branch of the Department of Health and Human Services that is responsible, among other things, for monitoring food-borne diseases.
- **EPA (Environmental Protection Agency)** a federal agency that is responsible, among other things, for regulating pesticides and establishing water quality standards.
- **FDA (Food and Drug Administration)** a part of the Department of Health and Human Services' Public Health Service that is responsible for ensuring the safety and wholesomeness of all foods sold in interstate commerce except meat, poultry, and eggs (which are under the jurisdiction of the USDA); inspecting food plants and imported foods; and setting standards for food composition.
- **USDA (U.S. Department of Agriculture)** the federal agency responsible for enforcing standards for the wholesomeness and quality of meat, poultry, and eggs produced in the United States; conducting nutrition research; and educating the public about nutrition.
- **WHO (World Health Organization)** an international agency that, among other responsibilities, develops standards to regulate pesticide use. A related organization is the FAO (Food and Agricultural Organization).

In this free market, where food companies compete for sales, the consumer enjoys the safest, most pleasing, and most abundant food supply in the world. With this benefit comes the consumer's responsibility of distinguishing between foods with a good **safety** record and foods that may pose a **hazard.** Often, foods are safe until they are mishandled or misused.

This chapter provides the information consumers need to make food-purchasing, handling, and using decisions with confidence. It begins with the most pressing concern of FDA, food producers, and food consumers alike: food poisoning.[3]

safety the practical certainty that injury will not result from the use of a substance.

hazard state of danger; used to refer to any circumstance in which harm is possible under normal conditions of use.

food poisoning illness transmitted to human beings through food, caused by a poisonous substance *(food intoxication)* or an infectious agent *(food-borne infection)*.

enterotoxins poisons that act upon mucous membranes, such as those of the digestive tract.

neurotoxins poisons that act upon the cells of the nervous system.

botulism an often-fatal food poisoning caused by botulin toxin, a toxin produced by bacteria that grow without oxygen in nonacidic canned foods.

Microbial Food Poisoning

Episodes of **food poisoning** cause illness in at least one third of the U.S. population each year, and their number is increasing yearly. Between 21 million and 81 million cases of diarrhea that are treated in the United States each year are from food-borne illnesses. It may be that just about everyone experiences illness from this source within a year's time but may mistakenly pass the incidents off as the "flu."

The Threat From Microbial Contamination

The term *food poisoning* refers either to food-borne infection—illness caused by microorganisms, such as *Salmonella* varieties, that infect people, or to food intoxication—illness from **enterotoxins** or **neurotoxins** produced by microorganisms in food or within the digestive tract. Toxins may be produced by bacteria in food during improper preparation or storage, or within the digestive tract after consumption of contaminated food. In most illnesses from enterotoxins the symptoms are mild. They include abdominal cramps, headaches, vomiting, and diarrhea, the same symptoms that accompany a number of other minor conditions. For people who are otherwise ill or malnourished or for the very old or young, however, even these relatively mild disturbances can be fatal. If you experience the digestive tract disturbances listed in Table 14-2 as the major or only symptoms of your next bout of "flu," chances are excellent that what you really have is food poisoning.

The symptoms of one neurotoxin stand out as severe and commonly fatal—those of **botulism,** caused by the toxin of a microbe that grows inside of improperly canned, home-canned, or vacuum-packed foods. Botulism danger signs constitute a true medical emergency (see margin). Even with medical assistance, survivors can suffer the effects for months, years, or a lifetime. So potent is the botulin toxin that an amount as tiny as a single grain of salt can kill several people within an hour. The botulin toxin is destroyed by heat, so canned foods that have been boiled for ten minutes are generally safe from this threat. Home canned food can be prepared safely as long as proper canning techniques are followed to the letter.*

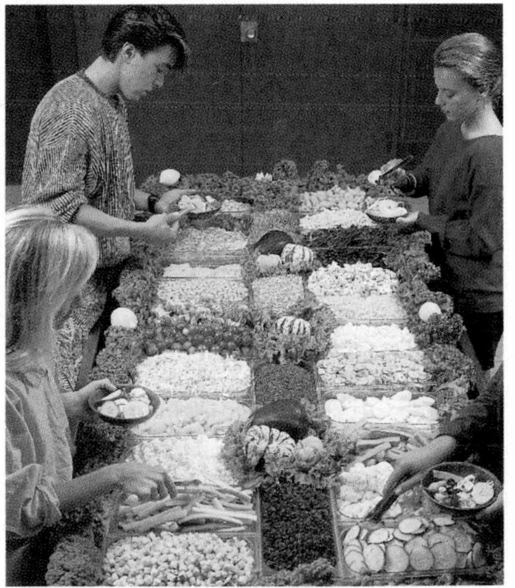

With the privilege of abundance comes the responsibility to choose wisely.

KEY POINT Each year in the United States, many millions of people suffer from mild to life-threatening symptoms caused by food poisoning.

Warning signs of botulism:

- Double vision
- Weak muscles
- Difficulty swallowing
- Difficulty breathing

*Complete, up-to-date, safe home canning instructions are included in USDA's 172-page *Complete Guide to Home Canning,* available for $11.00 from the Superintendent of Documents, Government Printing Office, Washington, DC 20402.

Table 14-2
Food-borne Illnesses

Cause of Illness[a]	Most Frequent Food Source	Symptoms
	TOXIN-PRODUCING ORGANISMS	
Botulinum toxin (produced by *Clostridium botulinum*)	Anaerobic environment of low acidity (canned corn, peppers, green beans, soups, beets, asparagus, mushrooms, ripe olives, spinach, tuna, chicken, liver products, luncheon meats, ham, sausage, lobster, and smoked and salted fish).	Onset: 4 to 36 hr after eating. Nervous system symptoms: double vision, inability to swallow, speech difficulty, and progressive paralysis of the respiratory system. Often fatal; symptoms last months or years in survivors.
Staphylococcal toxin (produced by *Staphylococcus aureus*)	Meats, poultry, egg products, tuna, potato and macaroni salads, and cream-filled pastries.	Onset: ½ to 8 hr after eating. Diarrhea, nausea, vomiting, abdominal cramps, and fatigue; mimics flu; lasts 24 to 48 hr; rarely fatal.
Other toxins (produced by a variety of bacteria)	Contaminated water, undercooked ground beef, imported soft cheeses, any raw protein-rich foods.	Onset: Up to 72 hr after eating. Loose watery stools, possibly bloody; abdominal pain and cramping; nausea, headache.
Mold toxins	Mold-infected peanuts, corn, other grains.	Onset: 1 day to several months after eating depending on dose. Vomiting, abdominal pain, diarrhea; possible damage to liver, skin, and bone marrow. Strong cancer-causing agent.
	INFECTION-PRODUCING ORGANISMS	
Bacteria		
Listeria monocytogenes	Raw meat and seafood, raw milk, and soft cheeses.	Onset: 7 to 30 days after eating. Mimics flu; blood poisoning and meningitis threaten life. Usually fatal in fetuses and newborns.
Salmonella (over 200 varieties)	Eggs, raw meats, poultry, dairy products, shrimp, yeast, cantaloupe, coconut, pasta, and chocolate.	Onset: 6 to 48 hr after eating. Nausea, fever, vomiting, abdominal cramps, diarrhea, and headache; can be fatal.
Parasite		
Trichinella spiralis	Undercooked pork or wild game (bear). Worms burrow through body tissues to reach muscle tissue where they remain alive.	Onset: 24 hr after eating. Abdominal pain, nausea, vomiting, diarrhea, and fever. One week later, muscle pain, low-grade fever, pain on breathing, edema (swelling), skin eruptions, loss of appetite and weight loss. Drug therapy kills the worms and deaths are rare.
Protozoan		
Giardia lambia	Contaminated water; uncooked foods.	Onset: 5 to 25 days after eating. Diarrhea with greasy stools; abdominal pain, gas, distention; anorexia; nausea and vomiting.
Virus		
Hepatitis viruses	Undercooked or raw shellfish	Onset: 15 to 50 days (28 to 30 days average). Inflammation of the liver with tiredness; nausea, vomiting, or indigestion; jaundice (yellowed skin and eyes from buildup of wastes); muscle pain.

[a]Other illness-causing microorganisms in foods include toxin-producing *Vibrio* bacteria and many others. For an extensive listing of food-borne illnesses see D. O. Cliver, *Eating Safely: Avoiding Foodborne Illnesses*, a pamphlet available from American Council on Science and Health. Other pamphlets are free from USDA or FDA (see Appendix E for addresses).

Food Safety in the Marketplace

Commercially prepared food is usually safe, but when rare accidents happen, they can be dramatic. Milk producers, for example, rely on **pasteurization,** a process of heating milk to kill many disease-causing organisms and make milk safe for consumption. When a major dairy developed a flaw in its pasteurization system, over 16,000 confirmed and as many as 200,000 suspected cases of food-borne illness resulted. In another episode 100 people died of infection. Recently, a fast-food restaurant served undercooked hamburgers tainted with an infectious organism costing at least one child's life and the illnesses of many other patrons. This incident provided a national spotlight to illuminate two standard food-safety issues: that live, disease-causing organisms are routinely found in raw meats, and that thorough cooking is a must for ensuring the safety of animal-derived foods. It also gave rise to the proposal that raw meat products bear a "safe handling" label, described later in this chapter's Checking Out Food Labels section.

pasteurization the treatment of milk with heat sufficient to kill certain pathogens (disease-causing microbes) commonly transmitted through milk; not a sterilization process. Pasteurized milk retains bacteria that causes milk spoilage. Raw milk, even if labeled "certified," transmits many food-borne diseases to people each year and should be avoided.

Consumers have little protection against such large-scale calamities; they must trust government inspectors to enforce strict standards to prevent all but truly unavoidable accidents. Luckily, large-scale incidents, while dramatic, make up only a fraction of the total food-poisoning cases each year. Most arise from one person's error in a small setting and affect just a few victims. Some people have come to accept a yearly bout or two of intestinal illness as inevitable, but in truth, most of these illnesses can be prevented. To protect themselves, consumers need to learn how to select, prepare, and store food safely.

Canned and packaged foods sold in grocery stores are more easily controlled, but still, rare accidents do happen. Batch numbering makes it possible to recall contaminated foods through public announcements via newspapers, television, and radio, and FDA monitors large suppliers. You can help protect yourself, too. Carefully inspect the seals and wrappers of packages; reject leaking or bulging cans. Many jars have safety "buttons," areas of the lid designed to pop up once opened; make sure that they are firmly sealed. Frozen foods should be solidly frozen and those in a chest-type freezer case should be stored below the frost line. Notice how the packages on the shelf appear. If the one you have chosen looks ragged, soiled, or punctured, do not buy the product; turn it in to the store manager. A broken seal, a badly dented can, or a mangled package is useless in protecting food from microorganisms, insects, spoilage, or even vandals.

Raw foods, especially meats and poultry, from the grocery store contain microbes, as all things do. Whether or not the microbes from these sources will multiply and cause illness can be largely a matter of what you do or fail to do in your own kitchen.

KEY POINT Industry employs sound practices to safeguard the commercial food supply from microbial threats. Still, incidents of commercial food poisoning have occurred with widespread effects.

Food Safety in the Kitchen

Food can provide ideal conditions for bacteria to thrive and produce their toxins. Disease-causing bacteria require three things: (1) warmth (40° F to 140° F); (2) moisture; and (3) nutrients. To defeat them, people who prepare food should keep in mind that food poisoning is always possible. Do these three things: keep hot food hot, keep cold food cold, and keep the kitchen clean. Keeping hot food hot includes cooking foods for long enough to reach an internal temperature sufficient to kill microbes as described in the next section. Temperatures for holding cooked foods must be high enough (140° F or higher) to prevent bacterial growth until the foods are served. Refrigerate foods immediately after serving a meal, and definitely before two hours have passed.

Keeping cold food cold starts when you leave the grocery store. If you are running errands, shop last, so that the groceries will not stay in the car too long. (If ice cream begins to melt, it has been too long.) Upon arrival home, load foods into the refrigerator or freezer immediately. Keeping foods cold applies to defrosting foods before use, too. Thaw meats or poultry in the refrigerator, not at room temperature.

Keeping the kitchen clean requires using freshly washed utensils and laundered towels, and washing your hands with soap before and during food handling. If you are ill or have open sores, stay away from food to prevent its contamination. Clean equipment frequently. Microbes love to nestle down in small, damp spaces such as those between the fibers of wooden cutting boards or dishtowels or in the inner cells of sponges. It isn't true that wooden boards do not support microbial growth; this idea came from an experiment using brand new cutting boards. An antimicrobial effect seen in the study was caused by wood-processing chemicals still contained in the boards, and not by any protective action of the wood itself. You can ensure safety of all types of cutting boards by treating them as suggested below.

To eliminate microbes you have three choices, each with benefits and drawbacks. One is to poison the microbes on boards and in sponges with toxic chemicals such as bleach (one capful per gallon of water). The benefit is that chlorine can kill even the hardiest organism. The drawback is that chlorine that washes down household drains into the water supply forms chemicals that can harm waterways and fish.

A second option is to treat boards and sponges with heat. Soapy water heated to 140° F kills most harmful organisms and washes most others away. This takes effort, though, since you have to use truly scalding water heated well beyond the temperature of the tap.

The third strategy is to use clean nonporous boards for cutting. These are easy to keep clean, but perhaps are harder on the cutting edges of knife blades. In this strategy, sponges are saved for car washing and other heavy cleaning chores and kept away from surfaces that come in contact with raw foods. Instead, wipe with washable dishcloths that can be laundered often. Whichever strategy you use, for a small initial investment, you can reap truly safe utensils with which to prepare your food.

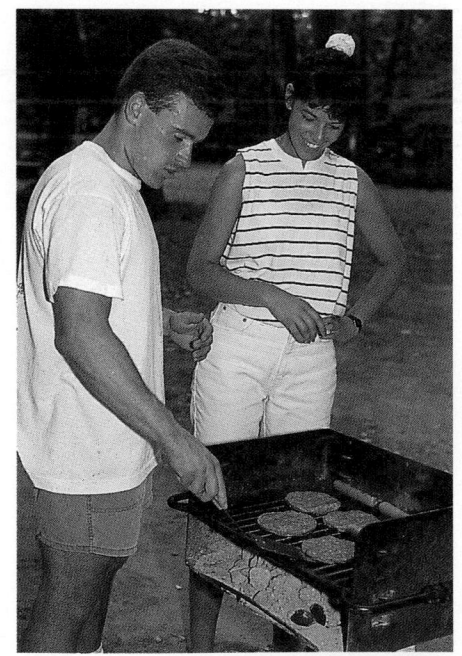

Use a clean plate to hold grilled meats.

KEY POINT To prevent food poisoning, remember that it is always a possibility. Hold foods at their proper temperatures and prepare them in sanitary conditions.

Troublesome Foods

Some foods are more hospitable to microbial growth than are others. In general, foods that are high in moisture and nutrients and those that are chopped or ground are especially favorable hosts.

Meats Meats require special handling. Some raw meats must now bear labels to instruct consumers on meat safety (see the Checking Out Food Labels section following this discussion). Meats may contain all sorts of bacteria, and they provide a moist, nutritious environment that is just right for microbial growth. If you take burgers out to the grill on a plate, wash that plate in hot, soapy water before using it to hold the cooked burgers. Ground meat is handled more than other kinds of meat and has much more surface exposed to the air for bacteria to land on, so it poses special risks. It is best to cook hamburger to at least medium well done. For a meatloaf, use a thermometer to test the internal temperature (see Figure 14-1).*

It goes without saying that any food with an "off" appearance or odor should not be used or even tasted. However, you cannot rely on your senses of smell or sight alone to warn you of hazards because most contamination is not detectable by odor, taste, or appearance. Cooking does not destroy all bacterial toxins. Even hot cooked food, if handled improperly prior to cooking, can cause illness.

To protect yourself as far as you can, you must remember, always, that food poisoning is a possibility. For example, a lovely buffet may present meatballs in a warming tray that is not hot. Despite the attractive appearance, the warm temperature is a warning flag. Food at 140° F feels hot, not just warm. The likelihood of illness is high when food is not hot enough, and the pleasure of eating meatballs isn't worth the risk, even if you must go hungry for awhile. Study Figure 14-2; if you learn and follow the rules given there, you can apply them to avoid illnesses.

Seafood For adults and children alike, eating raw or lightly-steamed seafood is a risky proposition even if it is prepared by a master chef. The microorganisms that lurk there are undetectable, even to an expert.

People who like **sushi** know that not all varieties are made from raw fish. Many types are made with cooked crab meat and vegetables, avocado, or other delicacies and are perfectly safe to enjoy. Also, rumor has it that freezing fish will make it safe to eat raw, but this is only partly true. Freezing fish will kill mature parasitic worms, but only cooking can kill all worm eggs and other microorganisms that can cause illness.

As population density increases along the shores of seafood-harvesting waters, pollution of those waters inevitably invades the seafood living there.** Watchdog agencies monitor commercial fishing waters and try to keep harvesters out of the worst areas, and they eventually do catch cheaters. But meanwhile, unwholesome food can reach the market. In one season alone, black-market dealers may sell millions of dollars worth of clams and oysters taken illegally from closed harvesting areas.[4]

The food-borne infections that lurk in normal-appearing seafood can be even worse than those of spoilage: hepatitis; worms, flukes, and other parasites; severe viral intestinal disorders; poisoning by naturally occurring toxins; and other diseases.[5] Hepatitis infection causes prolonged illness of months' or years' duration, severely damages the liver, greatly increases the

sushi a Japanese dish that consists of vinegar-flavored rice, seafood, and colorful vegetables, typically wrapped in seaweed. Some sushi is stuffed with raw fish; other sushi contains only cooked ingredients.

Figure 14-1

SAFE INTERNAL TEMPERATURES FOR MEATS AND POULTRY (FAHRENHEIT)

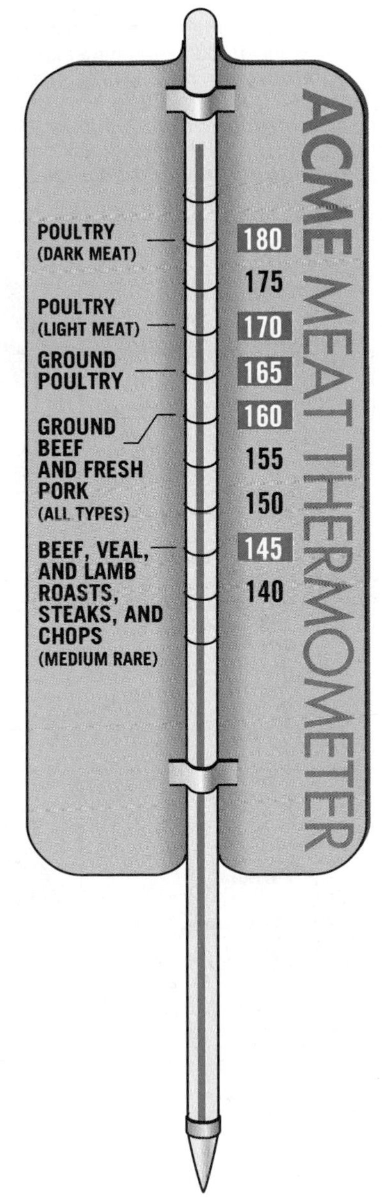

Source: USDA, 1993.

*USDA's meat and poultry hotline offers answers to questions about meat and poultry safety: 1-800-535-4555.

**To speak with an expert on seafood safety, call the FDA seafood hotline: 1-800-FDA-4010.

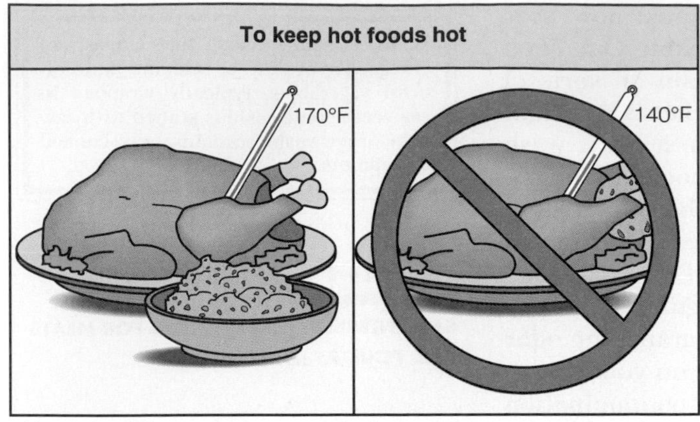

Use a meat thermometer to test the internal temperature of meats and poultry. Insert the thermometer between the thigh and the body of the turkey or in the thickest part of other meats, making sure the tip of the thermometer is not in contact with bone. Cook to the temperature indicated for that particular meat; cook hamburgers to at least medium well done.
Cook stuffing separately or stuff poultry just prior to cooking.

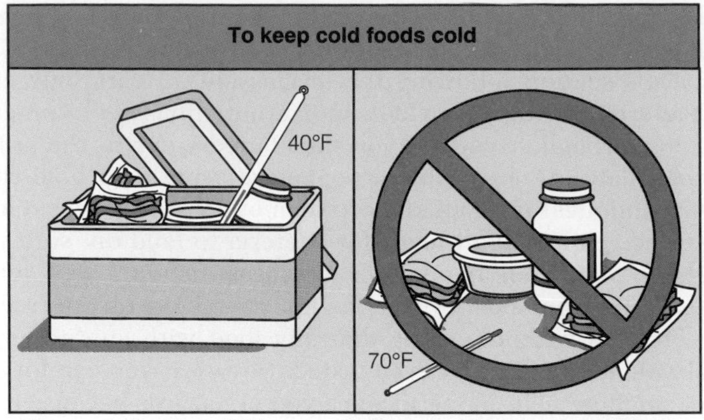

Keep cold foods at 40°F or less. Refrigerate leftovers promptly; use shallow containers to help foods cool faster.

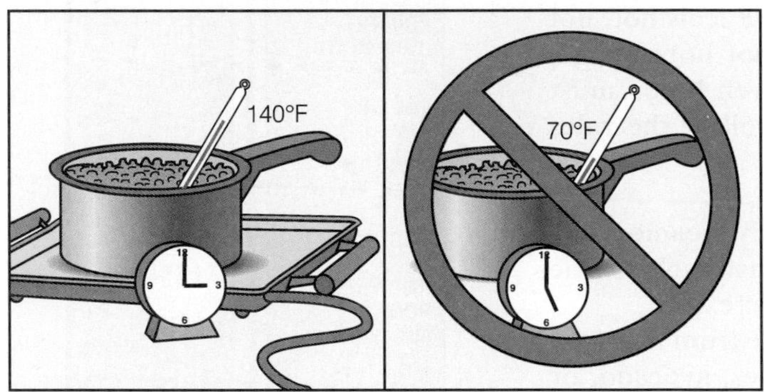

When serving foods for longer than 2 hours, maintain temperatures above 140°F. Heat leftovers thoroughly to at least 140°F.

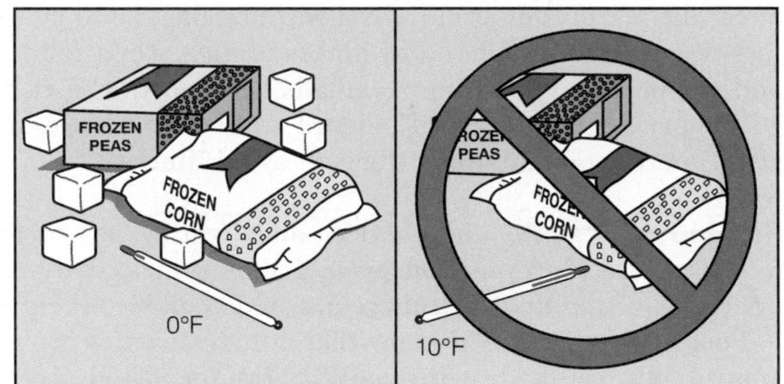

Keep frozen foods at 0°F or less.

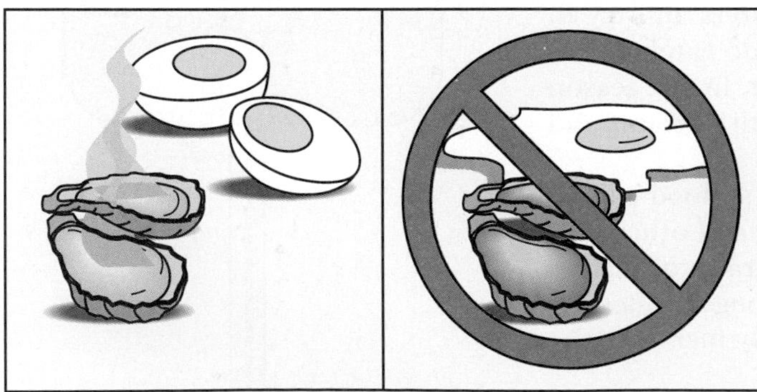

Cook eggs and seafood thoroughly before eating them.

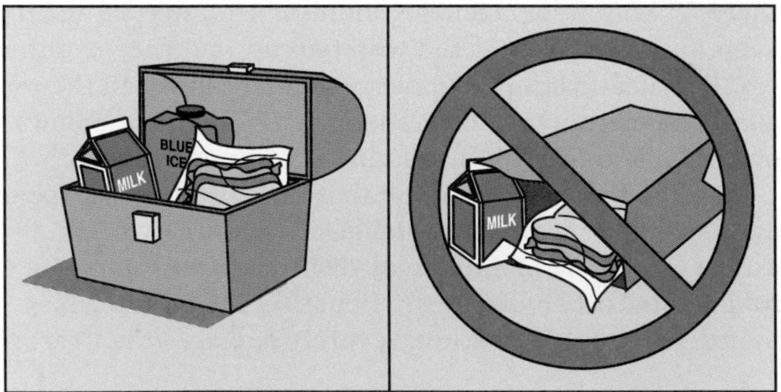

Tote lunches in a thermal lunch bag or box. Freeze plastic bottles or pouches of beverages and let them keep the lunch cool as they thaw out through the morning.

Figure 14-2

HOW TO PREVENT FOOD POISONING

To keep a clean kitchen

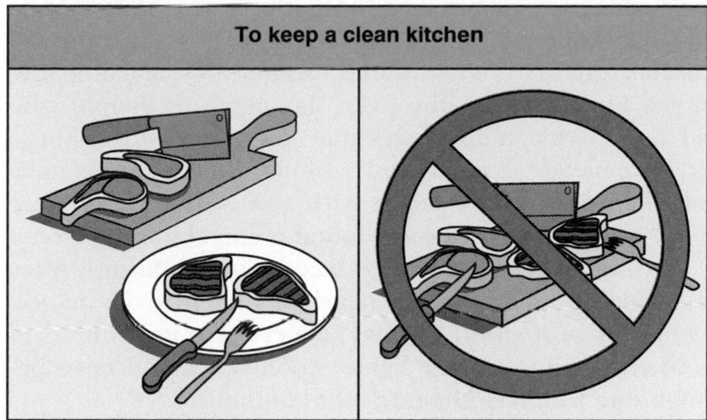

Use warm soapy water to wash hands, utensils, dishes, cutting boards, and countertops.
Avoid cross contamination by washing all surfaces that have been in contact with raw meats, poultry, or eggs before reusing.
Mix foods with utensils, not hands; keep hands and utensils away from mouth, nose, and hair.
Avoid coughing or sneezing over food. A person with a skin infection or infectious disease should not prepare food.

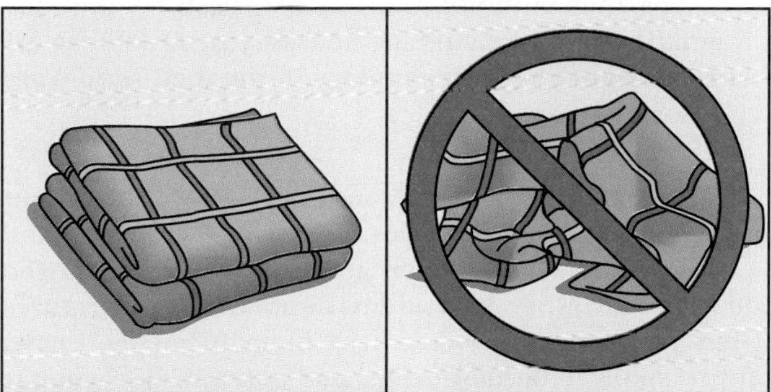

Wash or replace sponges and towels regularly.
Clean up food spills and crumb-filled crevices.

In general

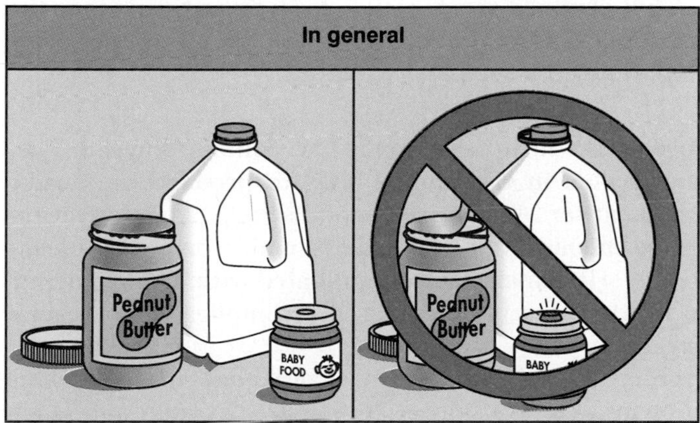

Throw out foods with off odors.
Do not even taste food that is suspect.
Do not buy or use items that appear to have been opened; check safety seals, buttons, and rings. Observe expiration dates.
Follow label instructions for storing and preparing packaged and frozen foods.

biotechnology the science that manipulates biological systems or organisms to create or modify their products or components. Also called *biogenetic engineering.*

biosensor a genetically altered microbe that provides a rapid, low-cost, and accurate test for the products of spoilage in foods.

In Florida, containers of raw oysters must bear this warning: "There is a risk associated with consuming raw oysters or any raw animal protein. If you have chronic illness of the liver, stomach or blood or have immune disorders, you are at greater risk of serious illness from raw oysters and should eat oysters fully cooked. If unsure of your risk, consult a physician."

More on biotechnology in this chapter's Controversy.

risk of developing liver cancer, and, once in the body, is transmissible to others. Many types of worms depend on the blood of their host for food and reproduction; they attack digestive membranes, sometimes causing life-threatening perforations. Flukes attack the liver, damaging it. People who love raw seafood and have eaten it for years may try to brush off these threats because they have never experienced serious illness. Some have heard rumors that alcoholic beverages taken with raw seafood eliminate risks, but this is not the case. True, one study found a correlation between taking one drink of whiskey or wine and a reduced risk of disease after eating contaminated seafood, but this is not nearly sufficient evidence on which to base a guarantee of protection.[6] Today, experts are unanimous in saying that the risks of consuming raw or lightly cooked seafood have become unacceptably high due to environmental contamination.[7]

Hope for the future purity of foods, and especially of poultry, meats, and seafoods, comes on the crest of new applications for advances in **biotechnology.** Geneticists are now able to alter the DNA inside a living bacterial cell to yield a **biosensor** organism. The biosensor can detect the presence of disease-causing microorganisms by sensing chemicals that the organisms create in foods.[8] Such tests promise to be superior to today's methods in detecting harmful organisms that commonly infect fish flesh.[9] Some day their use may make dramatic improvements in the safety of raw foods for sale in the market. Issues surrounding biotechnology in the food supply are a topic of this chapter's Controversy.

Picnics Picnics are fun and can be safe too. Choose foods that last without refrigeration, such as fresh fruits and vegetables, breads and crackers, and canned spreads and cheeses that you can open and use on the spot. Aged cheeses, such as cheddar and Swiss, do well at environmental temperatures for an hour or two, but for longer periods, carry them in an ice chest. Mayonnaise is resistant to spoilage because of its acid content, but when it is mixed with chopped ingredients in pasta, meat, or vegetable salads, the mixtures spoil easily. The chopped ingredients have extensive surface areas for bacteria to invade, and the foods have been in contact with cutting boards, hands, and kitchen utensils that have transmitted at least a few bacteria to the food. Chill chopped salads well before, during, and after the picnic. Keep mayonnaise itself cold. Table 14-3 in the margin on page 530 lists some safe keeping times for foods kept at 40° F.

Honey Another danger lurks in honey. Honey can contain dormant bacterial spores that can awaken in the human body to produce the deadly botulin toxin mentioned earlier. Adults are big and strong enough to withstand the doses usually encountered, but infants under one year of age should never be fed honey. (It can also be contaminated with environmental pollutants picked up by the bees.) Honey has been implicated in several cases of sudden infant death.

Because food poisoning is such a common hazard, both the Checking Out Food Labels section and the Consumer Caution are devoted to it. Much grief can be averted by the pointers they present.

KEY POINT Some foods pose special microbial threats and so require special handling. Seafood is especially likely to be contaminated. Almost all cases of food poisoning can be averted by following the rules of safe food preparation, storage, and cleanliness. Biosensors may one day insure safety of raw foods.

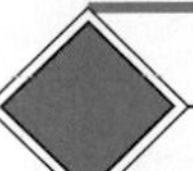

CHECKING OUT FOOD LABELS

How to Apply Meat and Poultry Safety Information

As part of an effort to reduce the number of cases of food poisoning in the United States, the USDA has proposed that all raw and partially cooked meat and poultry products bear the label shown in Figure 14-3. This particular label has not at this writing been approved and so may change in time, but the points it makes remain valid.* The label instructs consumers on four aspects of the care and handling of meats: storage and thawing, cross contamination, cooking, and storing leftovers.

Figure 14-3

SAFE HANDLING INSTRUCTIONS FOR MEAT AND POULTRY

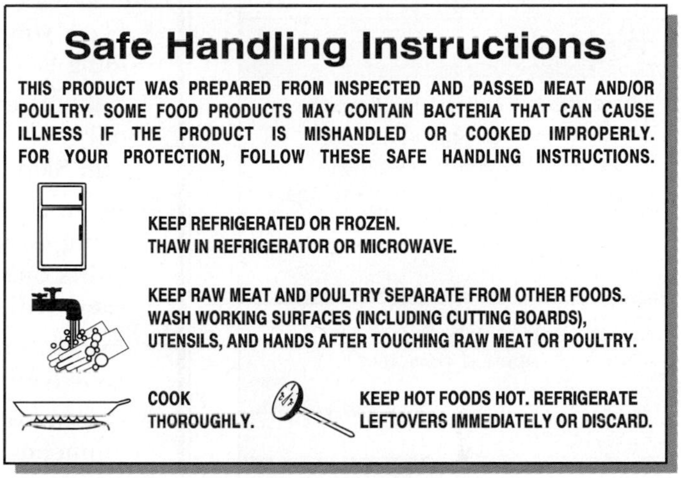

Safe Handling Instructions

THIS PRODUCT WAS PREPARED FROM INSPECTED AND PASSED MEAT AND/OR POULTRY. SOME FOOD PRODUCTS MAY CONTAIN BACTERIA THAT CAN CAUSE ILLNESS IF THE PRODUCT IS MISHANDLED OR COOKED IMPROPERLY. FOR YOUR PROTECTION, FOLLOW THESE SAFE HANDLING INSTRUCTIONS.

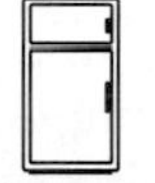

KEEP REFRIGERATED OR FROZEN.
THAW IN REFRIGERATOR OR MICROWAVE.

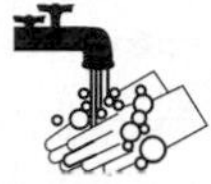

KEEP RAW MEAT AND POULTRY SEPARATE FROM OTHER FOODS.
WASH WORKING SURFACES (INCLUDING CUTTING BOARDS), UTENSILS, AND HANDS AFTER TOUCHING RAW MEAT OR POULTRY.

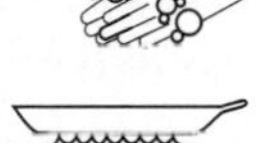

COOK THOROUGHLY.

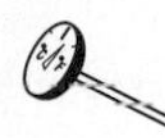

KEEP HOT FOODS HOT. REFRIGERATE LEFTOVERS IMMEDIATELY OR DISCARD.

KEEP REFRIGERATED OR FROZEN. THAW IN THE REFRIGERATOR OR MICROWAVE.

Never allow frozen meat to defrost at room temperature, or in a bath of warm water. In both cases, meat thaws from outside in, and the outside meat layer can easily warm up to temperatures that permit bacterial growth before the core defrosts.

In refrigerator thawing, the roast or other meat may thaw on the outside first but the thawed layer stays cold enough to inhibit bacterial growth while the interior slowly defrosts. Refrigerator thawing may take several days for a large frozen turkey, however, and people in a hurry can speed the thawing process by using a microwave oven on the defrost setting. Meats thawed in the microwave thaw uniformly and quickly so that bacteria do not have time to multiply.

KEEP RAW MEATS OR POULTRY SEPARATE FROM OTHER FOODS. WASH WORKING SURFACES INCLUDING CUTTING BOARDS, UTENSILS, AND HANDS AFTER TOUCHING RAW MEAT OR POULTRY.

The case of raw and cooked meats has already been mentioned. Also, take care when preparing meats along with foods intended to be served raw, such as chopped salads or lettuce and tomato toppers for hamburgers. A grave error is to prepare raw-food dishes on the same board or with the same utensils as were used to prepare raw meats for cooking. Dining on salad or other raw food that has been handled this way almost guarantees that the diner will consume live and potentially harmful bacteria from the meats.

COOK THOROUGHLY.

The temperatures that were listed in Figure 14-1 apply to home cooking of meats to a ready-to-eat stage. Other temperatures apply to industrially prepared foods, such as partially cooked meat patties for restaurants, which are not ready to serve as purchased.

Microwave cooking of meats requires special care. Large, thick, dense foods such as roasts or meat loaves may register "cooked" on an internal meat thermometer, but may harbor cool spots in which dangerous microorganisms, such as the *Trichinella spiralis* parasite, sometimes present in pork, can survive. Such foods are best cooked by another method or divided into small, thin portions to be microwaved individually.

REFRIGERATE WITHIN 2 HOURS.

Properly cooked food hot from the oven or stove is relatively free of bacteria, but as soon as it is taken out to serve, it is usually reinoculated. Kitchen utensils recontaminate the food, or bacteria in the air land on its surface. Promptly after serving a meal, refrigerate leftovers in shallow containers for quick, even chilling. Food refrigerated in deep containers may take hours to cool through, allowing bacteria time to multiply in the warm internal portions.

The proposed meat safety label is just one way USDA is striving to reduce the incidence of food poisoning in this country. Inspectors are also stepping up surveillance of feedlots and slaughterhouses, and closing down those found out of compliance. In the near future, we can expect these efforts, together with the improved testing methods, to effectively reduce contamination of meat and poultry and to lower the likelihood of illness caused by eating them.

*A final ruling on this label is expected by April of 1994.

Table 14-3
Safe Refrigerator Storage Times (40° F)

Storage time	Foods
1 to 2 days	Raw ground meats, breakfast or other raw sausages, raw fish or poultry; gravies
3 to 5 days	Raw steaks, roasts, or chops; cooked meats, vegetables, and mixed dishes; ham slices; mayonnaise salads (chicken, egg, pasta, tuna)
1 week	Hard cooked eggs, bacon or hotdogs (opened packages); smoked sausages
2 to 4 weeks	Raw eggs (in shells); bacon or hotdogs (packages unopened); dry sausages (pepperoni, hard salami); most aged and processed cheeses (swiss, brick)
2 months	Mayonnaise (opened jar); most dry cheeses (parmesan, romano)

Sources: A. Hecht, Preventing food-borne illnesses, *FDA Consumer*, January/February 1991, p. 21; Refrigerator storage times for selected foods, *Consumer Reports on Health*, December 1991, p. 93.

Food Safety While Traveling

CONSUMER CAUTION About half of people traveling to places where cleanliness standards are lacking suffer from food-borne illnesses. These, colloquially known as traveler's diarrhea, can ruin a trip. To avoid illness while traveling:

- Wash your hands often with soap and water, especially before handling food or eating.
- Eat only cooked food and canned foods. Eat raw fruits or vegetables only if you have washed them in boiled water and peeled them yourself. Skip salads.
- Be aware that water, and ice made from it, may be unsafe, too. Take along disinfecting tablets or an element that boils water in a cup. Drink only treated, boiled, canned, or bottled beverages, and drink them without ice, even if they are not chilled to your liking.
- Avoid using the local water supply, even if you are just brushing your teeth, unless you boil or disinfect it first.
- Before you leave on the trip, check with your physician for recommendations on which medicines to take with you in case your efforts to avoid illness fail.

One journalist succinctly sums up these recommendations: "Boil it, cook it, peel it, or forget it."[10] Chances are excellent, if you follow the rules above, that you will remain well.

Natural Toxins in Foods

Consumers concerned about food contamination may naively think that they can eliminate all poisons from their diets by eating only "natural" foods. On the contrary, nature has provided natural foods with the natural poisons they need to fend off diseases, insects, and other predators. However, while the *potential* for harm exists, actual harm rarely occurs.

Most people would recognize the names belladonna and hemlock, both classic deadly poisons in the form of natural herbs. Few people know, however, that the herb sassafras contains a cancer-causing agent and is banned from addition to commercially produced foods and beverages. Equally surprising is that cabbage, turnips, mustard greens, and radishes all contain small quantities of harmful goitrogens, compounds that can enlarge the thyroid gland and aggravate thyroid problems.

Cabbages and their relatives are celebrated for the nonnutrients they contain, compounds associated with low cancer rates. The protection seems to result when the mild toxins these foods contain force the body to build up its arsenal of carcinogen-destroying equipment.[11] Then when a potent carcinogen arrives, the prepared body deals with it swiftly. In excess, however, these mild toxins can cause illness.

Other natural poisons in lima beans and fruit seeds such as apricot pits are members of a group called cyanogens, precursors to the deadly poison cyanide. Many countries restrict commercially grown lima beans to those varieties with the lowest cyanogen contents. As for fruit seeds, they are seldom deliberately eaten. An occasional swallowed seed or two presents no danger, but a couple of dozen seeds could be fatal to a small child. Perhaps the most infamous cyanogen is laetrile, a compound erroneously represented as a cancer cure. True, the poison laetrile kills cancer cells, but only at doses that kill the person, too. Research over the past 100 years has proven laetrile to be an ineffective cancer treatment and dangerous to the taker.

Potatoes contain many natural poisons, including solanine, a bitter, powerful, narcotic-like substance. The small amounts of solanine normally found in potatoes are harmless, but solanine in potatoes can build up to toxic levels when potatoes are exposed to light during storage. Cooking does not destroy solanine, but because most of a potato's solanine is in the green layer that develops just beneath the skin, it can be peeled off, making the potato safe to eat. If the potato tastes bitter, however, throw it out.

At some times of the year, seafood may become contaminated with the so-called red tide toxin that occurs during algae blooms. Consumption of seafood contaminated with red tide causes a paralyzing form of food poisoning. The FDA monitors fishing waters for red tide algae and closes waters to fishing whenever it appears.

These examples of naturally occurring toxins should serve as a reminder of three principles. First, any substance can be toxic when consumed in excess. Practice moderation in the use of all foods. Second, poisons are poisons, whether made by people or by nature. It is not the source of a chemical that makes it hazardous, but its chemical structure and the quantity consumed. Third, by seeking a variety of foods in the diet, consumers ensure that a toxin in one food is diluted by the volume of the whole diet.

KEY POINT Natural foods contain natural toxins that can be hazardous if consumed in excess. To avoid toxicities from natural food constituents, practice moderation, treat chemicals from all sources with respect, and choose a variety of foods.

contaminant any substance occurring in food by accident; not a normal food constituent.

persistent of a stubborn or enduring nature; with respect to food contaminants, the quality of remaining, unaltered and unexcreted, in the bodies of animals and human beings.

Environmental Contaminants

A justifiably high-ranking concern about our food supply is environmental contamination of foods. As populations increase worldwide and nations become more industrialized, the problem looms larger. A food **contaminant** is anything that does not belong there.

The potential harmfulness of a contaminant depends in part on the extent to which it lingers in the environment or in the human body—that is, how **persistent** it is. Some contaminants are short-lived, because microorganisms or agents such as sunlight or oxygen can break them down. Some contaminants linger in the body only for a short time, because the body can rapidly excrete them or metabolize them to harmless compounds. These contaminants present little cause for concern. However, some contaminants

Figure 14-4

ACCUMULATION OF TOXINS IN THE FOOD CHAIN

A person whose principal animal protein source is fish may consume about 100 pounds of fish in a year. These fish will, in turn, have consumed a few tons of plant-eating fish in the course of their lifetimes. The plant eaters, in their lifetimes, will have consumed several tons of photosynthetic producer organisms. If the producer organisms have become contaminated with toxic chemicals, these chemicals become more concentrated in the bodies of the fish that consume them. If none of the chemicals are lost along the way, *one person* ultimately eats the same amount of contaminant as was present in the original *several tons* of producer organisms.

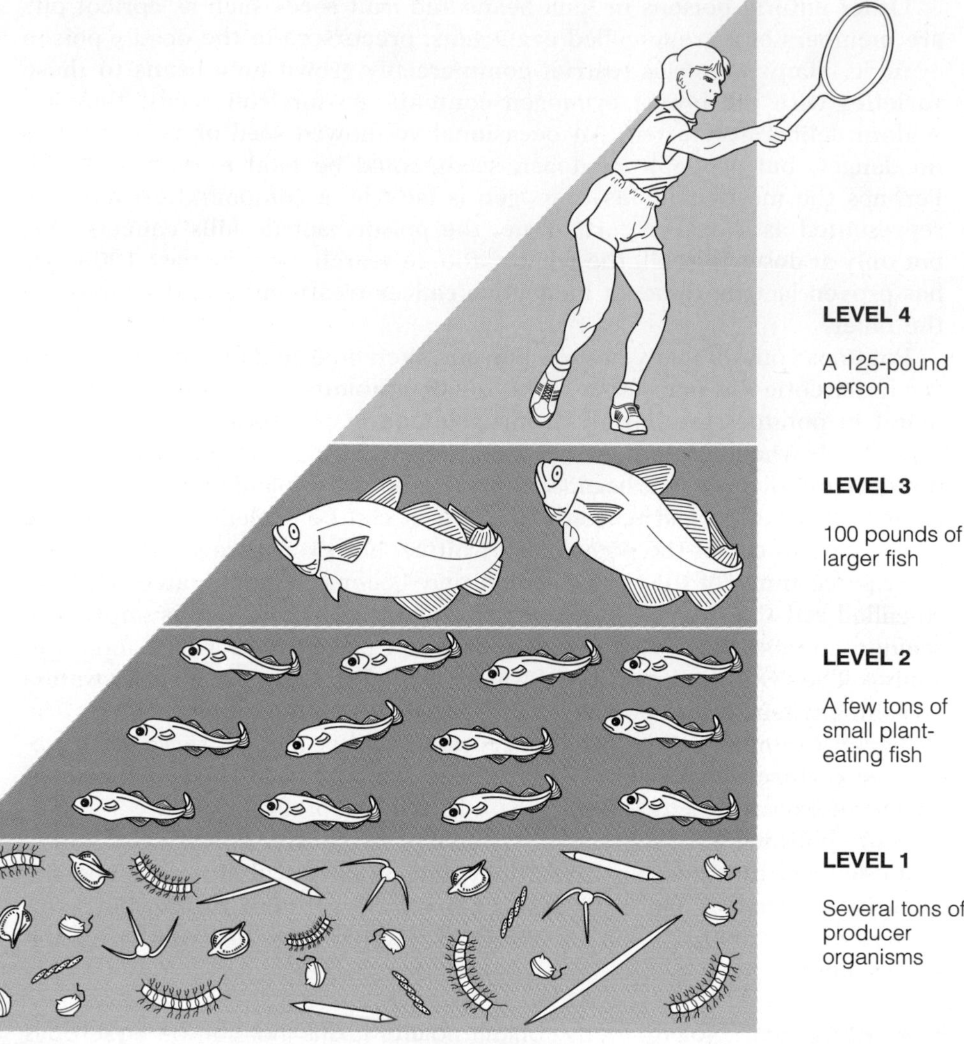

heavy metal any of a number of mineral ions such as mercury and lead, so called because they are of relatively high atomic weight. Many heavy metals are poisonous.

organic halogen an organic compound containing one or more atoms of a halogen—fluorine, chlorine, iodine, or bromine.

resist breakdown and interact with the body's systems without being metabolized or excreted. These can pass from one species to the next, and accumulate at higher concentrations in each level of the food chain. Figure 14-4 shows how toxic chemicals accumulate in the food chain.

How much of a threat do environmental contaminants pose to the food supply? For the most part, the hazards appear to be small because the FDA monitors the presence of contaminants in foods and requires the removal of foods with unsafe contamination. In the event of an accidental spill, however, the hazard can suddenly become great. The following paragraphs describe how two different types of contaminants have found their way into the food supply in the past. One is a **heavy metal** (mercury) that was released into waterways by industry and ingested by fish that people ate. The other is an **organic halogen** (polybrominated biphenyl or PBB) that was accidentally spilled into livestock feed and ingested by animals that people eventually consumed.

A classic example of acute contamination occurred in 1953 when a number of people in Minamata, Japan, became ill with a disease no one had seen before. By 1960, 121 cases had been reported, including 23 in infants. Mortality was high; 46 died, and in the survivors the symptoms were progressive blindness, deafness, loss of coordination, and impaired mental function. The cause of this misery was ultimately revealed to be methylmercury contamination of fish harvested from the bay near which these people lived. The infants who contracted the disease had not eaten any fish, but their mothers had, and even though the mothers exhibited no symptoms during their pregnancies, the poison had been affecting their unborn babies. Manufacturing plants in the region were discharging mercury into the waters of the bay, the mercury was turning to methylmercury on leaving the factories, and the fish in the bay were accumulating this poison in their bodies. Some of the people who were poisoned had been eating fish from the bay every day.

As for PBB, in 1973, in Michigan, half a ton of the toxic compound was accidentally mixed into some livestock feed that was distributed throughout the state. The chemical found its way into millions of animals and then into people who ate their meat. The seriousness of the accident began to come to light when dairy farmers reported that their cows were going dry, were aborting their calves, and were developing abnormal growths on their hooves. More than 30,000 cattle, sheep, and swine and more than a million chickens were destroyed, but the effects on people were not prevented. An estimated 97 percent of Michigan's residents had been exposed to PBB. Some of the exposed farm residents suffered nervous system aberrations and liver disorders.

Mercury is a heavy metal and PBB is an organic halogen. These two classes of chemicals are among the most toxic and are still being liberated into our environment daily. The number of contaminants we could discuss here, and the amount of information available about them, is far beyond our scope. Table 14-4 selects a few contaminants of great concern in foods to show how pervasively a contaminant can affect the body.

KEY POINT Persistent environmental contaminants pose a small but significant threat to the safety of food. An accidental spill can create an extreme hazard.

pesticides chemicals used to control insects, diseases, weeds, fungi, and other pests on crops and around animals. Used broadly, the term includes *herbicides* (to kill weeds), *insecticides* (to kill insects), and *fungicides* (to kill fungi).

Chemical contaminants of concern in foods:

- Heavy metals
  - Lead
  - Mercury
  - Cadmium
  - Selenium
  - Arsenic
- Halogens and organic halogens
  - Chlorine
  - Iodine
  - Vinyl chloride
  - Ethylene dichloride
  - Trichloroethylene (TCE)
  - Polybrominated biphenyl (PBB)
  - Polychlorinated biphenyls (PCBs)
- Others
  - Asbestos
  - Dioxins
  - Acrylonitrile
  - Lysinoalanine
  - Diethylstilbestrol (DES)
  - Heat-induced mutagens
  - Antibiotics (in animal feed)

Pesticides

The use of **pesticides** helps to ensure the survival of some crops, but the damage pesticides do to the environment is considerable and increasing. Moreover, there is some question about whether the widespread use of pesticides has really improved the overall yield of food. Even with extensive pesticide use, U.S. agriculture loses about one fifth of its crops to pests, and worldwide, pests destroy about one third of the food crops every year.[12]

No doubt, pesticides do help preserve some crops from some pests, but at a considerable cost in other respects. Many pesticides are broad-spectrum poisons that damage all living cells, not just those of pests. Their use, therefore, is hazardous. Also, farm workers can be poisoned during the production and transport of pesticides. In the mid-1980s, a massive pesticide leak from a factory in Bhopal, India, killed 3,000 people immediately, many more later, and maimed more still. High doses of pesticides applied to laboratory animals cause birth defects, sterility, tumors, organ damage, and central nervous system impairment.

Ironically, pesticides also promote the survival of the very pests they are intended to wipe out. Consider a pesticide aimed at some insects that are attacking a crop. The pesticide may kill *almost* 100 percent of them, but thanks to the genetic variability of large populations, some insects are likely

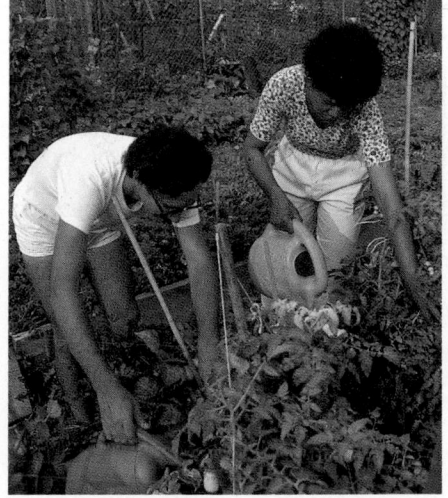

In some small gardens, hand work can take the place of pesticides.

Table 14-4
Examples of Contaminants in Foods

Name and Description	Sources	Toxic Effects	Typical Route to Food Chain
Cadmium (heavy metal)	Used in industrial processes including electroplating, plastics, batteries, alloys, pigments, smelters, and burning fuels. Present in cigarette smoke.	No immediately detectable symptoms; slowly and irreversibly damages kidneys and liver.	Enters air in smokestack emissions, settles on ground, absorbed into food plants, consumed by farm animals, and eaten in vegetables and meat by people. Sewage sludge and fertilizers leave large amounts in soil; runoff contaminates shellfish.
Lead[a] (heavy metal)	Lead crystal decanters and glassware, painted china, old house paint, batteries, pesticides, old plumbing, and some food-processing chemicals.	Displaces calcium, iron, zinc, and other minerals from their sites of action in the nervous system, bone marrow, kidneys, and liver, causing failure to function. See pages 484–486.	Originates from industrial plants and pollutes air, water, and soil. Still present in soil from many years of leaded gasoline use.
Mercury (heavy metal)	Widely dispersed in gases from earth's crust; local high concentrations from industry, electrical equipment, paints, and agriculture.	Poisons the nervous system, especially in fetuses.	Inorganic mercury released into waterways by industry and acid rain is converted to methylmercury by bacteria and ingested by food species of fish (tuna, swordfish, and others).
Polychlorinated biphenyls (PCBs) (organic compounds)	No natural source; produced for use in electrical equipment (transformers, capacitors).	Long-lasting skin eruptions, eye irritations, growth retardation in children of exposed mothers, anorexia, fatigue, others.	Discarded electrical equipment; accidental industrial leakage, or reuse of PCB containers for food.

[a]For answers to questions concerning lead, call the National Lead Information Center at 1-800-424-LEAD.

residues whatever remains. In the case of pesticides, those amounts that remain on or in foods when people buy and use them.

Pesticides:

- Kill pests' natural predators.
- Accumulate in the food chain.
- Pollute the water, soil, and air.

to survive exposure. The resistant insects can then multiply free of competition and soon will produce many offspring—offspring that have inherited resistance to the pesticide. This new strain of insects can attack the crop with enhanced vigor. To control these resistant insects requires application of a new and more powerful pesticide—and this leads to the emergence of a population of still more resistant insects. The same effects arise from use of herbicides and fungicides. One alternative to this destructive series of events is to manage pests using a combination of natural and biological controls, as discussed in Controversy 15.

Pesticides are not produced only in laboratories; they also occur in nature. The nicotine in tobacco and psoralens in celery are examples. Natural pesticides are, however, less damaging to other living things and less persistent in the environment than most man-made ones.

If an ideal pesticide could be made, it would be one that would destroy the pest, not accumulate in the food chain, and quickly degenerate to nontoxic products so that by the time consumers ate the food, no harmful **residues** would remain. Unfortunately, no such perfect pesticide exists. Developing new pesticides and monitoring their use are ongoing activities that require continued vigilance on the part of government agencies.

When asked, most people in the United States say they are very concerned about pesticide residues on their foods. As Figure 14-5 demonstrates, pesticide residues on agricultural products can sometimes survive processing and may be present in foods served to people.[13] Risks to health from pesticide exposure are probably small for healthy adults, but children, because of their lower body weights and immature detoxifying systems, may be more at risk for some types of pesticide poisoning.[14]

tolerance level the maximum amount of a residue permitted in a food when a pesticide is used according to label directions.

The legal **tolerance levels** for presence of pesticides in foods are low, generally 1/100 to 1/1,000 the level found to cause no effect in laboratory animals. Over 10,000 tolerance regulations state maximum levels for over 300 pesticide chemicals used on various specific crops in the United States. If a pesticide is misused, growers risk fines, lawsuits, and destruction of their crops. In 25 years of testing, FDA has seldom found residues above tolerance levels, so it appears that pesticides are generally used according to regulations. This makes sense, because growers are not anxious to spend extra capital on unneeded chemicals. Pesticides, along with fertilizers and fuels, make up one of the conventional farmer's major capital expenses each year.[15]

A loophole in federal regulations allows companies in the United States to make banned pesticides and export them to other countries. The banned pesticides then return to the United States on imported foods, a circuitous route that concerned consumers have named the "circle of poison." When imported foods are found to contain illegal residues, they may be refused entry. FDA collects some samples of both domestic and imported foods and analyzes them using methods that can detect residues well below tolerances.

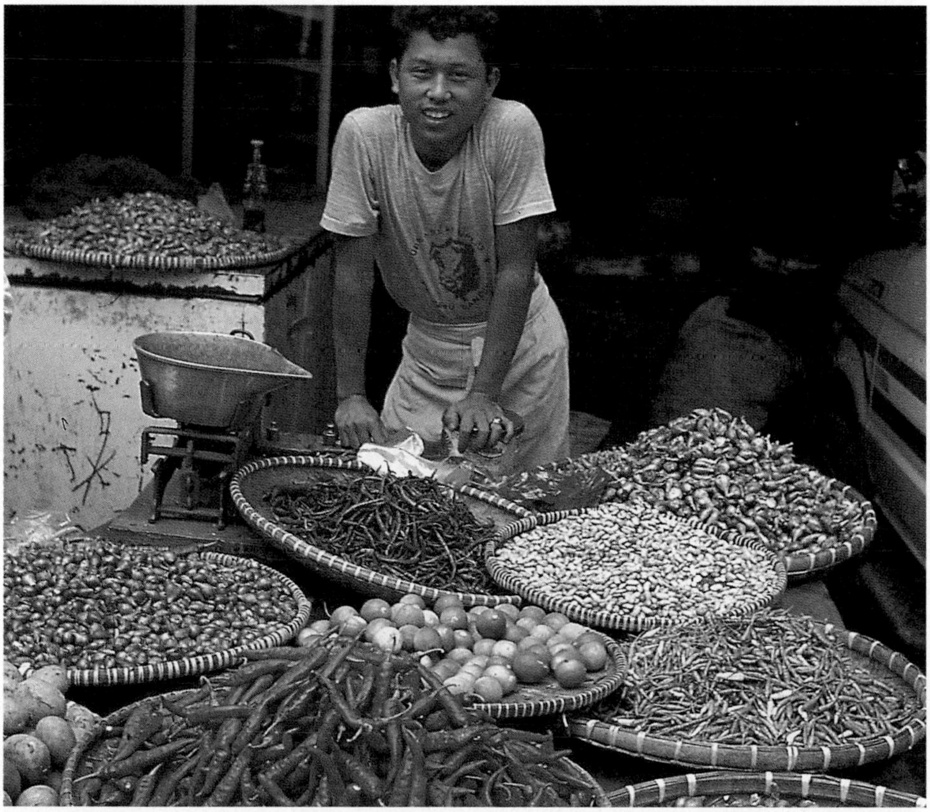

Foods imported from other countries may contain residues of pesticides that are banned from use here.

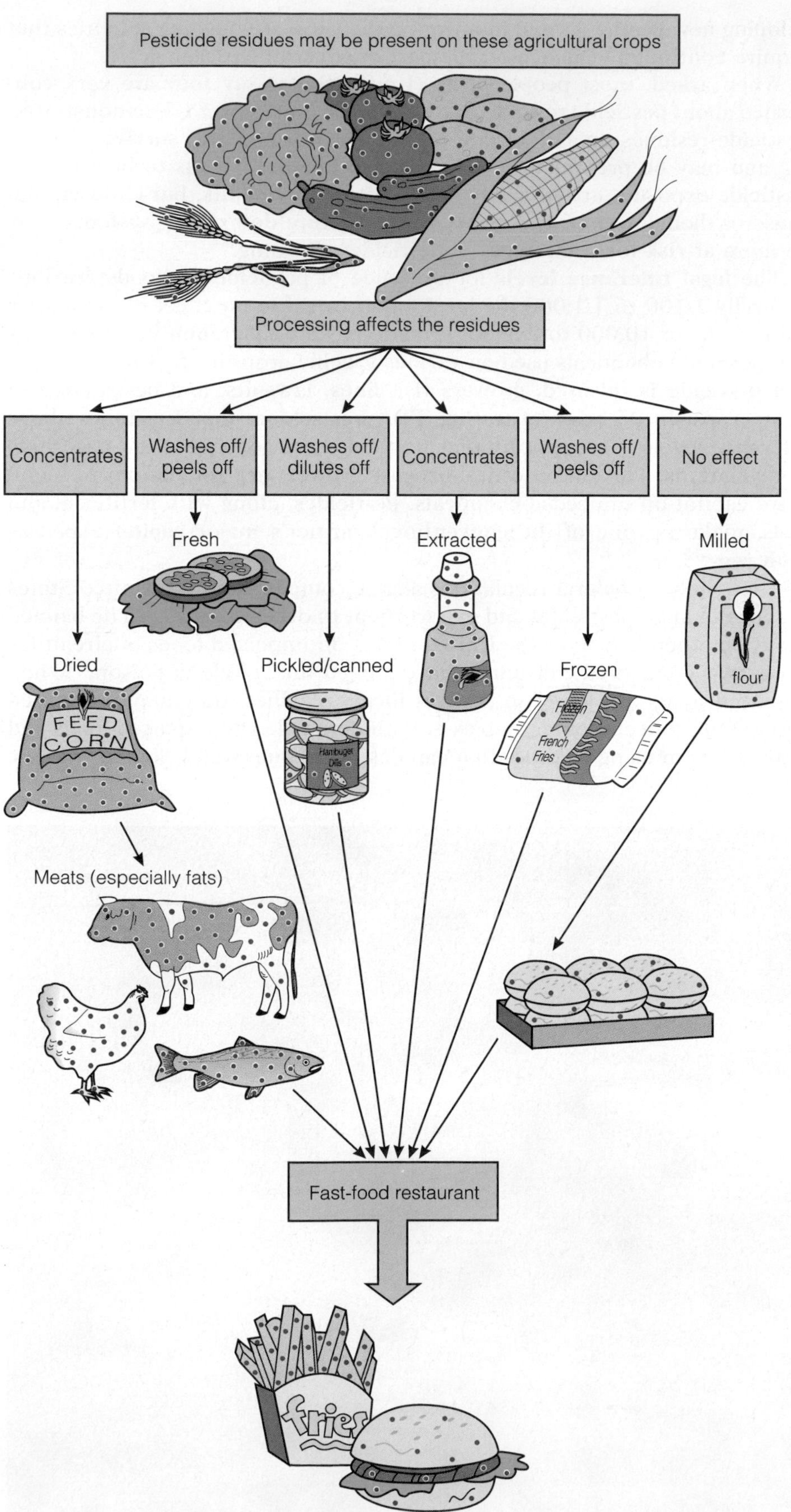

Figure 14-5

POSSIBLE PATHWAYS OF PESTICIDE RESIDUES TO A FAST-FOOD MEAL
The red dots in the figure represent pesticide residues left on foods from field spraying or post-harvest application. Notice that most pesticides follow fats in foods, and that some processing methods, such as washing and peeling vegetables, reduce pesticide concentrations while others tend to concentrate them.

Table 14-5
Ways to Reduce Pesticide Residues in Foods

- Trim the fat from meat and remove the skin from poultry and fish; discard fats and oils in broths and pan drippings. Avoid fish oil capsules. (Pesticide residues concentrate in the animals' fat.)
- Wash fresh produce in water. Use a scrub brush, and rinse thoroughly.
- Use a knife to peel an orange or grapefruit; do not bite into the peel.
- Discard the outer leaves of leafy vegetables such as cabbage and lettuce.
- Peel waxed fruit and vegetables; waxes don't wash off and can seal in pesticide residues.
- Peel vegetables such as carrots and fruits such as apples when appropriate. (Peeling removes pesticides that remain in or on the peel, but also removes fibers, vitamins, and minerals.)

If FDA finds violative levels, it can seize the products or order them destroyed. In 1990, FDA tests found more than 97 percent of the foods produced in the United States or imported from 92 other countries to have either no residues or residues within federally permitted limits.[16] A problem is that budget restraints limit FDA's testing capacity.

While monitoring pesticides in the marketplace, FDA also monitors people's pesticide intakes, along with intakes of essential minerals, industrial chemicals, heavy metals, and radioactive materials. Four times a year the surveyors buy over 200 foods in U.S. grocery stores in several cities, prepare them ready to serve, and then analyze them. Food preparation often reduces levels of contaminants in foods, so FDA tests for levels at least five times lower than permitted limits. The findings from these tests confirm that the bulk of the U.S. food supply is safe from excessive pesticide residues.[17]

FDA does not sample *all* food shipments or test for *all* pesticides. Fewer than 700 inspectors and scientists test food samples from the multitude of farms, groves, docks, airports, warehouses, and processing plants the agency oversees. FDA cannot (nor can it be expected to) guarantee 100 percent safety in the food supply. Instead, it sets conditions so that substances do not become a hazard and acts promptly when problems or suspicions arise.

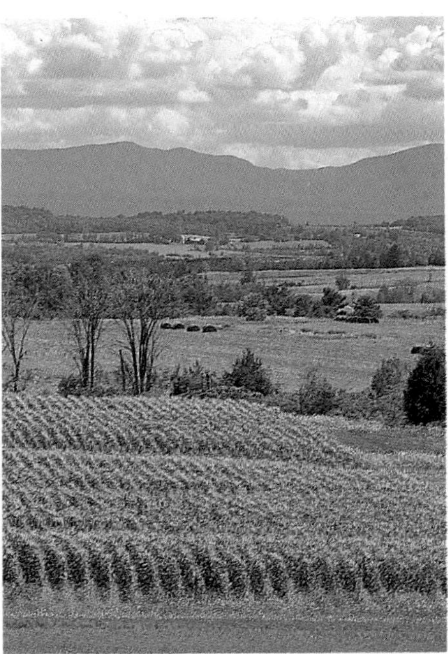

Crops like these can be kept safe from pests through a combination of natural and biological controls.

Consumers also bear some responsibility for their own health and safety with respect to pesticides. They can learn about the potential benefits and dangers of pesticide use, discuss regulations and alternatives with others, advise their government representatives about their findings, and apply pressure wherever it will help change inappropriate procedures. Meanwhile, people can minimize their risks by following the guidelines offered in Table 14-5 above.*

In addition to the suggestions in the table, consumers can buy fresh foods grown locally, especially when they can confirm that the produce has been grown using responsible methods. Consumers who want pesticide-free produce shouldn't look for "perfect" fruits and vegetables. Pesticide-free produce may have a few blemishes, but minor blemishes are not a hazard.

Meanwhile, at home, people today want up-to-date foods that provide quick meals. They rely more and more on convenience foods and fast foods, and they prepare fewer foods at home from farm-fresh produce. The gains in convenience and speed in food preparation must be weighed against a

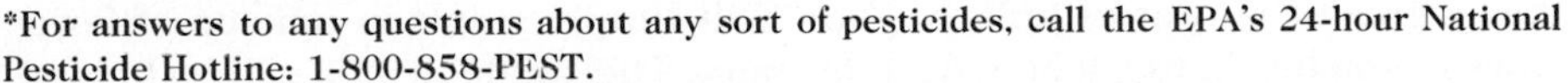

*For answers to any questions about any sort of pesticides, call the EPA's 24-hour National Pesticide Hotline: 1-800-858-PEST.

growth hormone a hormone *(somatotropin)* that promotes growth and that is produced naturally in the pituitary gland of the brain.

bovine growth hormone (BGH) growth hormone of cattle produced for agricultural use by transgenic bacteria. Also called *bovine somatotropin (BST)*.

nutrient partitioning the relative development of lean and fat body components by food animals.

loss of control over how, exactly, foods are processed and what, exactly, they contain. The next sections describe a much-debated issue concerning the safety of some foods.

KEY POINT Pesticides can be part of a safe food protection program, but can also be hazardous when handled or used inappropriately. FDA tests for pesticide residues in both domestic and imported foods. Consumers can take steps to minimize their ingestion of pesticide residues on foods.

Hormone Residues in Meat and Milk

"Hormone milk" is what opponents call the milk of dairy cattle treated with the cattle form of **growth hormone, bovine growth hormone (BGH).** The hormone is released into the bloodstream of the animal and travels to target organs throughout the body. The idea of extra hormones in the milk supply raises emotional objections because milk is a food of importance in infancy and throughout life. Milk is assumed to be safe, pure, and dependable in its composition. Yet milk is also the product of an industry that survives by producing the largest quantity of milk for the lowest possible cost.

Many people fear the introduction of this "artificial" drug into meat animals or dairy herds. In truth, synthetic growth hormone is identical to growth hormone made naturally by animals in the pituitary gland of the brain. At one time, the cost of gathering the hormone from animal brains prohibited its use as an agricultural drug. Now, by stimulating the transgenic bacteria to produce the growth hormones of cattle and pigs, laboratories can harvest huge quantities of the hormone and sell it to cattle ranchers, pig farmers, and dairy farmers as a drug.[18]

Many ranchers and farmers advocate the use of growth hormone because it alters the **nutrient partitioning** of animals in a desirable way. Meat cattle and pigs given doses of the hormone develop more lean tissue (more meat) and less body fat, and dairy cows produce up to 25 percent more milk.[19] What is more, they do all of this while consuming only three-quarters the normal allotment of feed. To the farmers, these changes mean higher profits from more market-ready product without the costs of larger herd sizes, more farm hands, or more equipment.

A group called the National Toxics Campaign has concerns about manufacturers' techniques for marketing the drug. The group charges the companies with employing scare tactics to convince farmers that once a drug is available, competitors will soon gain unfair economic advantage unless everyone uses it. The opponents of the hormone themselves also try to scare farmers: they predict a market flooded with a vast surplus of milk that will drive milk prices down. Huge farms, which can weather fluctuations in the market, will remain unaffected, but they warn that small farms may be forced to close. They say small farms will be sold to developers at an even faster rate than now, further reducing an already dwindling agricultural landscape across America. They also fear that surpluses of hormone-produced milk and products made from it will be fed to those least able to refuse it, namely, low-income people who receive food subsidies, hospital patients, prisoners, and the elderly.[20]

These charges are countered by supporters of BGH use. They say that we need and use all the milk that can be produced by current herds, and that a greater output of milk per cow will simply result in upkeep of fewer cows in smaller herds, a benefit to farmers. The small farmer will be helped,

human somatotropin (HST) human growth hormone.

not hurt: fewer cows to feed mean smaller feed bills and larger profits. The environment may profit as well. Smaller herds can also live on smaller plots of cleared land, and less feed means less feed production, reduced need for transportation, and less overall environmental impact (Chapter 15 gives details). As for foisting milk on the helpless, the milk produced is a valuable product that is distributed across all markets. In a report from its Technology Assessment Conference, the National Institutes of Health concludes, "As currently used in the United States, meat and milk from [hormone-] treated cows are as safe as those from untreated cows."[21]

Not everyone believes that BGH is safe. Consumer groups point out that traces of the drug end up in the meat and milk of treated animals. Products such as cheese and yogurt made from the milk may also carry traces of BGH. The president of a group called the Foundation on Economic Trends spoke out against the use of the hormone, calling it a potentially dangerous drug "with no socially redeeming value." Others express fears that the hormone could promote breast development in men and children and breast cancer in women. Such fears stem from a lack of distinction between steroid hormones, which can be taken orally because they survive digestion, and peptide hormones, which are destroyed by digestive enzymes. Estrogen, for example, is a steroid hormone found in many oral contraceptives; growth hormone, however, is a peptide hormone.

Another argument is that BGH-treated cows suffer more udder infections (mastitis) and so are given more antibiotics—and that then, these drugs show up in the cows' milk and meat.[22] Many such arguments are voiced by animal rights groups whose motivation is more to discourage the consumption of meat and dairy products than to promote consumers' rights or human health. Still, it is true that increased agricultural use of antibiotics leads to the spreading of antibiotic resistant microorganisms. These microorganisms cause life-threatening food-borne illnesses that do not respond to antibiotic therapy.

The FDA approved BGH for use in food-producing animals, but the outcry against BGH has brought about a ban on its use in several milk-producing states, with farmers and grocers pledging not to produce or sell milk from hormone-treated cows. Several European countries refuse to accept U.S. meat or milk products from BGH-treated cattle. Officials in those countries are requesting proof that the products are safe for human consumption. BGH residues have not been tested for safety in human beings because similar residues of natural hormone have always been present in milk and meat. The amount of hormone found in the milk of BGH-treated cows is within the range that can occur naturally.[23]

Scientists working for the FDA contend that any claims of danger from BGH fall apart under scientific scrutiny.[24] First, BGH is a protein. Some is denatured by the heat used in processing milk and cooking meat. If any intact hormone survives processing, it is subsequently digested in the human gastrointestinal tract. Even if some were to survive processing and digestion to enter the bloodstream, it would have no effect on the body. This is because the chemical structures of growth hormones from animals differ widely from the structure of **human somatotropin (HST),** the hormone active in human beings. When BGH was first discovered, scientists hoped to use it to treat growth-hormone deficient children. Tests proved disappointing, for BGH failed to stimulate receptors for *human* growth hormone, and so the children's growth was unaffected.

Given that animal growth hormones are destroyed by processing and digestion and that they have no activity in the human body, the use of such hormones in food animals probably presents no increased risk to consumers. Opponents still want answers to lingering doubts, however, about possible effects from the small peptides that may result upon digestion of the hormone. They also question whether BGH would be fully digested before absorption by healthy infants who normally absorb some whole proteins and large fragments and by people with impairments of the digestive system.

The debate continues. Whether consumers will reject milk, meat, or related products from hormone-treated cattle will be the final word on BGH. Other such issues are raised in this chapter's Controversy.

KEY POINT Bovine growth hormone causes dairy cattle to produce more milk than untreated cattle. Opponents raise ethical issues concerning this practice.

ultrahigh temperature (UHT) short-time exposure of a food to temperatures above those normally used to sterilize it.

canning preservation by killing all microorganisms present in food and sealing out air. The food, its container, and its lid are heated until sterile; as the food cools, the lid makes an airtight seal, preventing contamination.

freezing preservation by lowering food temperature to the point at which life processes cease. Microorganisms are not destroyed but are held dormant for as long as the food is frozen.

drying preservation by removing sufficient water from food to inhibit microbial growth.

extrusion a heat process by which the form of food is changed, such as changing corn to corn chips; not a preservation measure.

Food Processing and the Nutrients in Foods

A great percentage of the total food consumed today, whether eaten in restaurants or at home, has been prepared in some way by industry. People often ask what processing does to foods and which kinds of foods are most and least nutritious.

Many forms of processing aim to extend the usable life of a food—that is, they preserve the food. To preserve food, a process must prevent three detrimental changes. It must (1) prevent microbial growth; (2) prevent oxidative changes; and (3) prevent the enzymatic destruction of food molecules. The first two of these were mentioned in earlier sections. Enzymatic destruction occurs as active enzymes in the food tissue break down the molecular structures within the cells. Processes involving heat denature the protein enzymes and those applying cold temperatures slow enzymatic activity.

In general, food processing involves tradeoffs. It makes food safer, or it gives food a longer usable lifetime, or it cuts preparation time—but at the cost of some vitamin and mineral losses. A process such as pasteurization, which makes milk safe to drink, is clearly worth that cost. Incidentally, those boxes of milk on the shelves of the grocery store that can be kept at room temperature at home have been treated with a process called **ultrahigh temperature** (UHT). The milk is exposed to temperatures above those of pasteurization for a short time, just long enough to sterilize it.

Other processed foods may even gain a nutritional edge over their unprocessed counterparts, such as when fat is removed by processing from milk or other foods. This section explains each of the processing techniques, **canning, freezing, drying, extrusion,** and their effects on nutrients.

KEY POINT Processing aims to protect food from microbial, oxidative, and enzymatic spoilage. Some nutrients are lost in processing.

Canning

Canning is one of the more effective methods of protecting food against the growth of microbes (bacteria, fungi, and yeasts) that might otherwise spoil it, but canned foods, unfortunately, do have fewer nutrients. Which nutrients are affected by canning, and how are they affected? Like other heat treatments, the canning process is based on time and temperature. Each small increase in temperature has a major killing effect on microbes with only a minor effect on nutrients. In contrast, long heating times are costly in terms of nutrient losses. Therefore industry chooses treatments that employ the **high-temperature–short-time (HTST) principle** for canning.

high-temperature–short-time (HTST) principle every 10° C (18° F) rise in processing temperature gives approximately a tenfold increase in microbial destruction, while it only doubles nutrient losses.

To determine how much of a food's nutritional value is lost in canning, food scientists have performed many experiments. They have paid particular attention to three vulnerable water-soluble vitamins: thiamin, riboflavin, and vitamin C.

Acid stabilizes thiamin, but heat rapidly destroys it; therefore the foods that lose the most thiamin during canning are the low-acid foods such as lima beans, corn, and meat. Up to half, or even more, of the thiamin in these foods can be lost during canning. Unlike thiamin, riboflavin is stable to heat but sensitive to light, so glass-packed, not canned, foods are most likely to lose riboflavin. Vitamin C's special enemy is an enzyme (ascorbic acid oxidase) present in fruits and vegetables as well as in microorganisms. By destroying this enzyme, HTST processes such as canning actually aid in preserving at least some of the product's vitamin C. Some will be destroyed by the heat of the process. As for the fat-soluble vitamins, they are relatively stable and are not affected much by canning.

To see the effect of canning on thiamin in foods, look at Appendix A, items 890 and 891: ½ cup frozen green peas versus ½ cup canned green peas. While you are looking, what other effects of canning on thiamin do you see?

Minerals are unaffected by heat processing because they cannot be destroyed, as vitamins can be. However, both minerals and vitamins can be lost when they leak into canning or cooking water that the consumer may throw away. Losses are closely related to the extent to which a food's tissues have been broken, cut, or chopped and to the length of time the food is in the water.

Some minerals are added when foods are canned. Important in this respect is sodium chloride, table salt, added for flavoring. Many food companies have begun making low-salt versions of their products. Unfortunately, because the low-salt batches are smaller, these products may cost more than the higher-salt versions.

The nutrient contents of canned foods are usually shown as "solids and liquids." If you throw away the liquid from a canned food, you are throwing away all the nutrients that have leaked into that liquid, up to half the amount in the original product. The user of canned vegetables who can think of a way to use the liquid—for example, by saving it to make soups, cook rice, or moisten casseroles—gains a nutrition advantage.

KEY POINT Some water-soluble vitamins are destroyed by canning, but many more diffuse into the canning liquid. Fat-soluble vitamins and minerals are not affected by canning, but minerals also leach into canning liquid.

Freezing

An alternative to canning, as a means of preserving food, is freezing. People often ask how frozen foods compare with canned. In general, frozen foods' nutrient contents are similar to those of fresh foods; losses are minimal. The freezing process itself does not destroy any nutrients, but some losses may occur during the steps taken in preparation for freezing, such as the quick dunking into boiling water (blanching), washing, trimming, or grinding. Vitamin C losses are especially likely because they occur whenever tissues are broken and exposed to air (oxygen destroys vitamin C). Uncut fruits, especially if they are acidic, do not lose their vitamin C; strawberries, for example, may be kept frozen for over a year without losing any vitamin C. Mineral contents of frozen foods are much the same as of fresh.[25]

Fresh foods are often shipped long distances, and to make the trip without bruising or spoiling, they are often harvested unripe. Frozen foods are shipped frozen, so that produce is allowed to ripen in the field and to develop nutrients to their fullest potential. If foods are frozen and stored under proper conditions, they will often contain more nutrients when served at the table than fresh fruits and vegetables that have stayed in the produce department of the grocery store even for a day.

Frozen foods have to be kept frozen to retain their nutrients. To be solidly frozen, a food has to be colder than 32° F or 0° C. Conversion of vitamin C to its inactive forms occurs rapidly at warmer temperatures. Food may seem frozen at 36° F or 2° C, but much of it is actually unfrozen, and enzyme-mediated changes occur more rapidly than if it were solidly frozen. Under these conditions the vitamin C in a frozen food can be completely lost in as short a time as two months. If you want to maximize the nutritive value of the foods you store at home, invest in a freezer thermometer, monitor your frozen-food storage place, and keep it at freezing temperature (0° F).

KEY POINT Foods frozen promptly and kept frozen lose few nutrients.

Drying

Consumers wonder how dried or dehydrated foods compare with canned and frozen foods. Dried or dehydrated foods have their own special characteristics. Drying offers several advantages. It eliminates microbial spoilage (because microbes need water to grow), and it greatly reduces the weight and volume of foods (because foods are mostly water). Furthermore, commercial drying does not cause major nutrient losses. However, foods dried in heated ovens at home may sustain dramatic nutrient losses. Vacuum puff drying and freeze drying, which take place in cold temperatures, conserve nutrients especially well.

Sulfite additives are added during the drying of fruits such as peaches, grapes (raisins), and plums (prunes) to prevent browning. Some people suffer allergic reactions when they consume sulfites. Sulfur dioxide helps to preserve vitamin C as well, but it is highly destructive of thiamin. This is of small concern, however, because most dehydrated products with added sulfur dioxide were not major sources of thiamin before processing.

KEY POINT Commercially dried foods retain most of their nutrients while home-dried foods often sustain dramatic losses.

Extrusion

Some food products, particularly cereals and snack foods, have undergone a process known as extrusion. In this process the food is heated, ground, and pushed through various kinds of screens to yield different shapes, such as breakfast "puffs" or the "bits" you sprinkle on salad, the so-called food novelties. Considerable nutrient losses occur during extrusion processes, and nutrients are usually added to compensate. But foods this far removed from the original fresh state are still lacking significant nutrients (notably vitamin E), and consumers should not rely on them as staple foods. Enjoy them, but only as occasional snacks and as additions to enhance the appearance, taste, and variety of meals.

KEY POINT Extrusion may involve heat and so destroy nutrients.

 Food Additives

People ask valid questions about **additives.** What are they, why are they there, and are they dangerous in any way? Are the foods labeled "no additives" better for health than others? In the FDA list of concerns presented at the start of this chapter, food additives are not a high-priority concern for the FDA. This does not mean that additives are benign substances or safe for consumption in any amount. FDA has confidence, however, in the ability of regulations already in place to control additive use in the food industry. Compared with FDA's other concerns, additives pose little danger to consumers.

additives substances not normally consumed as foods by themselves but added to foods.

Manufacturers use food additives to give foods desirable characteristics: color, flavor, texture, stability, enhanced nutrient composition, or resistance to spoilage. Additives, classed by their functions, are listed with their definitions in Table 14-6, and some are addressed further in the section that follows.

Table 14-6
Food Additives by Function

- **antimicrobial agents** preservatives that prevent spoilage by mold or bacterial growth. Familiar among them are acetic acid (vinegar) and sodium chloride (salt). Others are benzoic, propionic, and sorbic acids; nitrites and nitrates; and sulfur dioxide.
- **antioxidants** preservatives that prevent rancidity of fats in foods and other damage to food caused by oxygen. Examples are vitamins E and C, BHA, BHT, propyl gallate, and sulfites.
- **artificial colors** certified food colors, added to enhance appearance. (*Certified* means approved by the FDA.) Vegetable dyes are extracted from vegetables such as beta carotene from carrots. Food colors are a mix of vegetable dyes and synthetic dyes approved by the FDA for use in food.
- **artificial flavors, flavor enhancers** chemicals that mimic natural flavors and those that enhance flavor.
- **bleaching agents** substances used to whiten foods such as flour and cheese. Peroxides are examples.
- **chelating agents** compounds added to foods to prevent discoloration, flavor changes, and rancidity that might occur because of processing. Examples are citric acid, malic acid, and tartaric acid (cream of tartar).
- **nutrient additives** vitamins and minerals added to improve nutritive value.
- **preservatives** antimicrobial agents, antioxidants, chelating agents, radiation, and other additives that retard spoilage or preserve desired qualities, such as softness in baked goods.
- **radiation** ionizing rays that act as a preservative by disrupting chemical structures within cells, including the cell bodies of microorganisms. Irradiation is a process, but it causes new substances to form in the food; therefore radiation is considered to be an additive. Controversy 14 discusses food irradiation.
- **thickening and stabilizing agents** ingredients that maintain emulsions, foams, or suspensions or lend a desirable thick consistency to foods. Dextrins (short chains of glucose formed as a breakdown product of starch), starch, and pectin are examples. Gums such as carrageenan, guar, locust bean, agar, and gum arabic are others.

GRAS (generally recognized as safe) list a list of food additives, established by the FDA, that had long been in use and were believed safe.

Regulations Governing Additives

The agency charged with the responsibility for deciding what additives shall be in foods is the FDA. The FDA's authority over additives hinges primarily on their safety and effectiveness for the stated purpose. To obtain permission to use a new additive in food products, a manufacturer has to go through a special procedure that can take many years. The manufacturer must test the additive and then satisfy the FDA of the following:

- It is effective (it does what it is supposed to do).
- It can be detected and measured in the final food product.

Then the manufacturer must study its effects in large doses fed to animals under strictly controlled conditions to prove that:

- It is safe (it causes no cancer, birth defects, or other injury).

Finally, the manufacturer must submit all test results to the FDA.

The FDA then calls a public hearing and announces the date and location in its official publication, *FDA Consumer*. Consumers are invited to participate at these hearings, where experts present testimony for and against granting permission to use the additive. Thus the consumer's rights and responsibilities are written into the provisions for deeming additives safe.

FDA approval of an additive does not give manufacturers free license to add it to food with abandon. On the contrary, the FDA writes a regulation stating in what amounts, for what purposes, and in what foods the additive may be used. No additives are permanently approved; all are periodically reviewed.

Many substances were exempted from complying with this procedure at the time it was first instituted because they had been used for a long time and their use entailed no known hazards. Some 700 substances in all were put on the **generally recognized as safe (GRAS) list.** However, when substantial scientific evidence or public outcry has questioned the safety of a GRAS list additive, its safety has been reevaluated. All substances about which any legitimate question was raised have been removed or reclassified.

To remain on the GRAS list, an additive must not have been found to be a carcinogen in any test on animals or human beings. The Delaney clause (the part of the law that states this criterion) is uncompromising in addressing carcinogens in food and drugs; in fact, it has been under fire in recent years for being too strict and inflexible.

The Delaney clause states that "no additive shall be deemed to be safe if it is found to induce cancer when ingested by man or animal." That sounds simple and clear enough, yet you may be aware of additives in products on the market that fail to meet that criteria. Saccharin paved the way for exceptions to the rule. In the 1970s, FDA tried to ban saccharin because tests had failed to prove that saccharin did not cause cancer in animals, but Congress made a special exception that allowed saccharin to remain in products so long as they carried a warning. This was their best effort in trying to balance the Delaney clause with current food safety and cancer knowledge. A little historical background may provide some insight.

The Delaney clause was adopted over 30 years ago at a time when scientists' awareness of cancer causes was limited to radiation, tobacco smoke, a chemical used to make dyes, and soot. Since then researchers have identified more than three dozen human carcinogens and several hundred animal carcinogens. In addition, technology has advanced so that substances once detectable only in parts per thousand can now be measured in parts per billion or even per trillion. (One part per trillion is equivalent to about one grain of sugar in an Olympic-sized swimming pool.) An FDA official states,

> *Given the extraordinarily low levels at which analytical chemists could measure chemical contaminants in food or anything else, all substances, no matter how pure, could be shown to be contaminated with one carcinogen or another.*[26]

In other words, we cannot provide absolute protection from all carcinogens in foods, as Congressman Delaney once thought we could. Current laws which state that we must do so ask the impossible.

An important distinction governs decisions about an additive's safety—the distinction between **toxicity** and hazard associated with substances. Toxicity is a general property of all substances; hazard is the capacity of a substance to produce injury *under conditions of its use.* All substances can be toxic at some level of consumption, but they are called hazardous only if they are actually consumed in sufficiently large quantities. An additive is not considered to be a hazard if some immense amount that people never consume is toxic. The additive is a hazard only if it is toxic under the conditions of its actual use. A food additive is supposed to have a wide **margin of safety.**

toxicity the ability of a substance to harm living organisms. All substances are toxic if high enough concentrations are used.

margin of safety as used when speaking of food additives, a zone between the concentration normally used and that at which a hazard exists. For common table salt, for example, the margin of safety is 1/5 (five times the concentration normally used would be hazardous).

A carcinogen is a cancer-causing agent. See Chapter 11.

Most additives that involve risk are allowed in foods only at levels 100 times below those at which the risk is still known to be zero. Experiments to determine the extent of risk involve feeding test animals the substance at different concentrations throughout their lifetimes. The additive is then permitted in foods at 1/100 the level that causes no harmful effect whatever in the animals. In many foods, *naturally* occurring toxins appear at levels that bring their margins of safety closer to 1/10. Even nutrients, as you have seen, involve risks at high dosage levels. The margin of safety for vitamins A and D is 1/25 to 1/40; it may be less than 1/10 in infants. For some trace elements it is about 1/5. People consume common table salt daily in amounts only three to five times less than those that cause serious toxicity.

The margin-of-safety concept also applies to nutrients when they are used as additives. Iodine has been added to salt to prevent iodine deficiency, but it has to be added with care because it is a deadly poison in excess. Similarly, iron has been added to refined bread and other grains (enrichment) and has doubtless helped prevent many cases of iron-deficiency anemia in women and children who are prone to that disease. But the addition of too much iron could put men (who usually have enough iron in their bodies) at risk for iron overload. The upper limit has to be remembered.

Most additives used in foods are there because they offer benefits that outweigh their risks or that make the risks worth taking. In the case of color additives that only enhance the appearance of foods but do not improve their health value or safety, no amount of risk may be deemed worth taking. Only 10 of an original 80 synthetic color additives are still approved by the FDA for use in foods, and screening of these continues.[27]

It is also the manufacturers' responsibility to use only the amounts of additives necessary to get the needed effects, not more. Additives must also *not* be used:

- To disguise faulty or inferior products.
- To deceive the consumer.

- Where they significantly destroy nutrients.
- Where their effects can be achieved by economical, sound manufacturing processes.

The regulations in force governing the management of intentional additives are well conceived and have been effective, on the whole. Funding shortages limit the capabilities of watchdog agencies such as the FDA, however, and some mistakes and cases of false reporting are bound to slip by.

KEY POINT FDA regulates the use of intentional additives. Additives must be safe, effective, and measurable in the final product. Additives on the GRAS list are assumed to be safe because they have long been used. No additive may be used that has been found to cause cancer in animals or people. Those used must have wide margins of safety.

A Closer Look at Selected Food Additives

The following sections focus on a few individual food additives, notably those that receive the most negative publicity because people ask questions about them most often. The order is alphabetical; it does not imply an order of importance.

Antimicrobial Agents Foods can go bad in two ways: one dangerous, one not. The dangerous way is by becoming hazardous to health; the other way is by losing their flavor and attractiveness. An example of the dangerous way: bacteria, yeasts, and molds and other fungi growing in foods can cause food poisoning. Preservatives known as *antimicrobial agents* protect foods from these microbes.

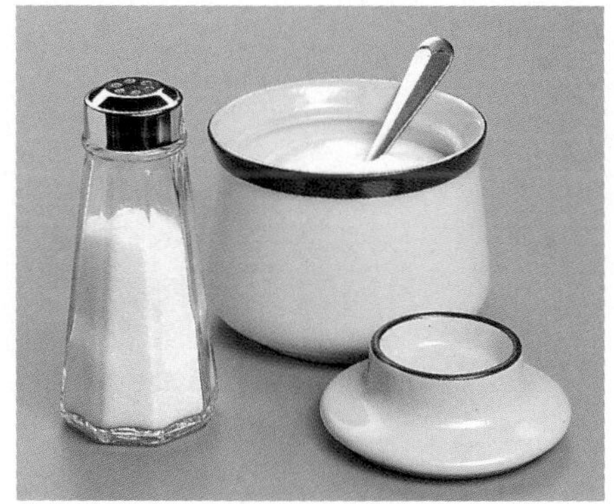

Two long-used preservatives.

The best known, most widely used antimicrobial agents are the two common substances salt and sugar. Salt has been used since before recorded history to preserve meat and fish; sugar serves the same purpose in canned and frozen fruits as well as jams and jellies. (Any jam or jelly that toots its "no preservatives" horn is exaggerating. There is no need to add extra preservatives, so most makers do not.) Both salt and sugar work by withdrawing water from the food; microbes cannot grow without water. Today, other additives such as potassium sorbate and sodium propionate are also used to extend the shelf life of baked goods, cheese, beverages, mayonnaise, margarine, and many other products.

Another group of antimicrobial agents, the *nitrites,* is added to foods for three main purposes: to preserve their color (especially the pink color of hotdogs and other cured meats); to enhance their flavor by inhibiting rancidity (especially in cured meats); and to protect against bacterial growth. In particular, in amounts much smaller than needed to confer color, nitrites prevent the growth of the botulinum bacterium that produce the deadly toxin described earlier in the chapter.

Nitrites clearly perform important jobs, but they have been the object of controversy because they can be converted in the human body to nitrosamines, which cause cancer in animals. Some cured meats are available without nitrites. However, reducing nitrites consumed in meats would hardly make a difference in a person's overall exposure to nitrosamine-related compounds. For example, an average cigarette smoker inhales 100 times the nitrosamines that the average bacon eater ingests. Likewise, a beer drinker imbibes up to roughly five times the amount that the bacon eater receives. Cosmetics deliver via absorption through skin about twice the amount delivered from bacon. Even the air inside automobiles delivers a measurable amount.[28]

KEY POINT Microbial food spoilage can be prevented by antimicrobial additives. Of these, sugar and salt have a long history of use and nitrites are associated with cancer causation in laboratory animals.

Antioxidants The other way in which food can go bad is by undergoing changes in color and flavor caused by exposure to oxygen in the air (oxidation). Often these changes involve little hazard to health, but they damage the food's appearance, taste, and nutritional quality. A familiar example of these changes is the way sliced apples or potatoes turn brown or oil goes rancid. Antioxidant preservatives protect food from this kind of spoilage. A total of 27 antioxidants are approved for use in foods. Vitamin C (ascorbate) and vitamin E (tocopherol) are among them.

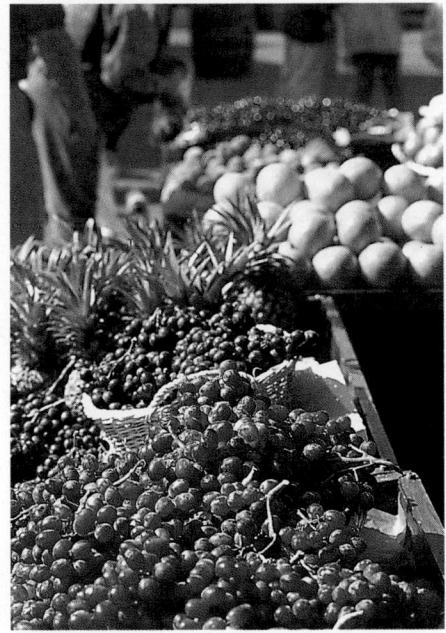

Raw grapes may legally be treated with sulfites. Wash them thoroughly before eating them.

Another group of antioxidants is the sulfites. They are used to prevent oxidation in many processed foods, in alcoholic beverages (especially wine), and in drugs. They used to be popular with restaurant owners for use on salad bars because they keep raw fruits and vegetables looking fresh, but this use has been banned. The ban came after some people experienced allergic reactions to the sulfites—reactions that were sometimes dangerous, and for a few, deadly. The FDA has taken a number of steps to protect people who are allergic to sulfites. It prohibits sulfite use on food intended to be consumed raw, with the exception of grapes, and it requires that sulfite-containing foods and drugs list the additives on their labels to warn that sulfites are present. For most people the sulfites do not pose a hazard in the amounts used in products, but there is one more consideration: sulfiting agents destroy an appreciable amount of the vitamin thiamin in foods. A person choosing a food that contains sulfites should not count on that food to provide a share of the daily need for thiamin.

The ban on sulfites has stimulated research to look for alternatives. For example, some producers use honey to clarify browned apple juice. Agriculturists have also created a hybrid apple that doesn't brown.[29] One manufacturer has combined four GRAS additives to create a product that can substitute for sulfites.[30]*

Two other antioxidants in wide use are the well-known BHA and BHT, which prevent rancidity in baked goods and snack foods. BHT provides a refreshing change from the tales of woe and cancer scares associated with many of the other additives. Among the many tests that were performed on BHT were several showing that animals fed large amounts of this substance developed *less* cancer when exposed to carcinogens and lived longer than controls. BHT apparently protects against cancer through its antioxidant effect, similar to that of vitamin E. To obtain this effect from BHT, though, a large amount of the substance must be present in the diet, larger by far than the amount in the U.S. diet. A caution: at levels of intake even higher than this, the substance has experimentally *produced* cancer.

Upon learning of the studies that show BHA and BHT to inhibit cancer in rats, some people came to a wrong conclusion— that what works for rats must work for people too. Manufacturers have begun marketing capsules of

*Monsanto Company has developed a sulfite alternative called Snow Fresh from citric acid, ascorbic acid, sodium acid pyrophosphate, and calcium chloride.

the preservatives as anticancer pills and recommending taking amounts far beyond the FDA's limit of safety. In fact, the daily dose recommended by the makers of these pills is almost a lethal dose and is high enough to cause possibly serious reactions in those with an allergy to BHT. Ironically, health food stores sell BHT and BHA capsules alongside packages of "no additives" foods.

This discussion provides the opportunity to mention an important point about additives. No two additives are alike, and therefore generalizations about them are meaningless. Whenever questions about the safety of "additives" are being discussed, you might as well leave the room, because no valid statement can be made that applies to the 3,000-odd different substances commonly added to foods. Questions about which additives are safe and under what conditions of use have to be asked and answered on an item-by-item basis.

KEY POINT Antioxidants prevent oxidative changes in foods that would lead to unacceptable discoloration and texture changes in the food.

Artificial Colors As mentioned, only about 10 synthetic artificial colors are still on the GRAS list, a highly select group that has survived considerable screening. They are among the most intensively investigated of all additives. In fact, they are much better known than the *natural* pigments of plants, and the limits on the safety of their use can be stated with greater certainty.

Still, the food colors have been more heavily criticized than almost any other group of additives. This is because they are dispensable. Simply stated, they only make foods pretty, whereas other additives, such as preservatives, make foods safe. Hence with food colors we can afford to require that their use entail no risk, whereas with other additives we may have to compromise between the risks of using them and the risks of *not* using them.

An infamous food-coloring agent of an earlier time was red dye number 2, which came under suspicion as a carcinogen in 1970 on the basis of two studies conducted in Russia. It was never shown to cause cancer, but it proved impossible to demonstrate that it did *not* cause cancer, either. It was banned in the United States in 1976. On the same evidence, Canada concluded that it was not likely to cause cancer and continued to permit its use. (Red candies in this country do not contain red dye number 2.)

The food color tartrazine (yellow number 5) causes an allergic reaction in susceptible people. Symptoms include hives, itching, and nasal congestion, sometimes severe enough to require medical treatment. It is not a common problem; only 1 or 2 in 10,000 individuals may have the reaction. Still, that is over 20,000 individuals in the nation as a whole. These people rightly demand to know where the dye is in foods so that they can avoid it. It is not enough to avoid yellow-colored foods because tartrazine is used to confer turquoise, green, and maroon colors in foods and drugs as well. Legislation is now in force requiring that tartrazine must be listed on all labels of foods that contain it so that consumers can avoid it if they wish.

Foods containing tartrazine:

- Orange drinks (Tang, Daybreak, Awake).
- Gatorade (lime flavored).
- Gelatin desserts (Jell-O, Royal).
- Golden Blend Italian dressing (Kraft).
- Some cake mixes and icings (Duncan Hines, Pillsbury, Cake Mate).
- Imitation banana or pineapple extract (McCormick).
- Seasoning salt (French's).
- Macaroni and cheese dinner (Kraft).
- 'Cheez' curls and balls (Planter's).
- Fruit chews (Skittles).
- Butterscotch squares and candy corn (Brach's).

Artificial Flavors and Flavor Enhancers While only a few artificial colors are currently permitted in foods, close to 2,000 artificial flavors and flavor enhancers are approved, making them the largest single group of food additives. One of the best known members of this group is monosodium glutamate, or MSG (tradename, Accent), the monosodium salt of the amino acid glutamic acid. MSG is used widely in restaurants, especially Asian restaurants, as a flavor enhancer. In addition to enhancing other flavors, research indicates that MSG may itself possess a basic taste independent of the well-known sweet, salty, bitter, and sour tastes.*[31]

MSG has received publicity because it may produce an adverse reaction, the so-called Chinese restaurant syndrome, in some individuals. Symptoms include burning sensations, chest and facial flushing or pain, and throbbing headaches. MSG has been investigated extensively enough to be deemed safe for adults to use (except people who react adversely to it, of course), but it is kept out of foods for infants because very large doses have been shown to destroy brain cells in developing mice. Infants have not yet developed the capacity to fully exclude such substances from their brains and so are more sensitive to them. No one really knows how common Chinese restaurant syndrome is or why it might occur. A possible link to the syndrome may lie in elevated blood levels of the MSG component glutamate. Meals containing carbohydrate seem less likely to induce it, however, so when dining on Asian-style foods order dishes containing noodles, and eat plenty of plain rice with each bite as the Chinese themselves do, to provide carbohydrate.

KEY POINT Among colorings and flavorings added to foods, the yellow color tartrazine and the flavoring MSG are suspected of causing reactions in people with sensitivities to them.

Nutrient Additives Another class of additives is nutrients added to improve or to maintain the nutritional value of foods. Among them are the nutrients added to refined grains to enrich them; the iodine added to salt; vitamins A and D added to dairy products; and the nutrients added to fortified breakfast cereals. When nutrients are added to a nutrient-poor food, it may appear from its label to be nutrient rich. It is, but only in those nutrients chosen for addition. Nutrients are sometimes also added for other purposes. Vitamins C and E used as antioxidants are examples already mentioned. Beta carotene may be added as a selling point because consumers, who have heard media reports of studies linking beta carotene with reduced risks of diseases, are buying more products that contain it.

KEY POINT Nutrients are added to foods to enrich or to fortify them. These additives do not necessarily make the foods nutritious, only rich in the vitamins and minerals that have been added.

Incidental Food Additives

Indirect or **incidental additives** are really contaminants that find their way into food as the result of some phase of production, processing, storage, or packaging. For example, among incidental additives are tiny bits of plastic, glass, paper, tin, and other substances from packages, and chemicals from processing, such as the solvent used to decaffeinate some types of coffee.

Some microwave products are sold in "active packaging" that participates in cooking the food. Pizza, for example, may rest on a cardboard pan coated

incidental additives substances that can get into food not through intentional introduction but as a result of contact with the food during growing, processing, packaging, storing, or some other stage before the food is consumed. The terms *accidental* or *indirect additives* mean the same thing.

*The taste produced by MSG is termed *umami.*

with a thin film of metal that absorbs microwave energy and may heat up to 500° F. During the intense heat, some particles of the packaging components migrate into the food.[32] Regular microwave packages heat up less, but particles still migrate, and the materials from both kinds of packaging are under study to determine their safety for consumption. Until more is known, a wise choice is to use only glass or ceramic containers designed for microwaving and to avoid reusing disposable containers, such as margarine tubs, for heating foods.

Coffee filters, milk cartons, paper plates, and frozen food packages can all be made of bleached paper and so can contaminate foods with trace amounts of compounds known as dioxins. Dioxins form during the chlorination step in making bleached paper. Dioxins can migrate into foods that come in contact with bleached paper, but the amounts entering food are infinitesimally small—one part per trillion, or the equivalent of one second in 32,000 years. Such amounts do not appear to present a health risk to people, and drinking milk from bleached cartons appears to be safe.[33] Dioxins are persistent, however, and they leach into the environment by way of both paper mill effluent and discarded paper products in landfills. Dioxins accumulate as do heavy metals and organic halogens, becoming more and more concentrated in land, water, and animals until they build up to hazardous levels.

Incidental additives sometimes find their way into foods, but adverse effects are rare. These additives are well regulated, just as intentional additives are. All food packagers are required to perform specific tests to discover whether materials from packages are migrating into foods. If they are, their safety must be confirmed by strict procedures similar to those governing intentional additives.

To sum up the messages of this chapter, U.S. foods are safe and hazards are rare. Precautions against food poisoning are the most important measures people can take to protect themselves from illness caused by foods. For optimal nutrition, though, which lies beyond safety, people can do more. The Food Feature that follows offers pointers on the selection and cooking of foods for the healthiest possible diet.

KEY POINT Incidental additives are substances that get into food during processing. They are well regulated, and most present no hazard.

FOOD FEATURE

Making Wise Food Choices and Cooking to Preserve Nutrients

In general, the more heavily processed foods are, the less nutritious they become. Does that mean, then, that everyone should avoid all processed food? The answer is not simple: in each case it depends on the food and on the process. Consider the case of orange juice and vitamin C. Orange juice is available in several forms, each processed a different way. Fresh juice is simply squeezed from the orange, a process that extracts the fluid juice from the fibrous structures that contain it. The fresh-squeezed juice, per 100 calories, contains 111 milligrams of vitamin C. If this juice were condensed by heat, frozen, and then reconstituted, as is the juice from the freezer case of the grocery store, 100 calories of the reconstituted juice would contain just 88 milligrams of vitamin C, because vitamin C is destroyed in the condensing process. Canning is even harder on vitamin C: 100 calories of canned orange juice has 82 milligrams of vitamin C.

These figures may seem to indicate that fresh juice is the superior food, and so it may be. But consider this: most people's RDA of vitamin C (60 milligrams) is covered single-handedly by a serving of any of the above choices. In this case, at least for vitamin C, the losses due to processing are not a problem. Besides, processing confers enormous convenience and distribution advantages. Fresh orange juice spoils. Shipping fresh juice to distant places in refrigerated trucks costs much more than shipping frozen juice (which takes up less space) or canned juice (which requires no refrigeration). The fresh product still contains active enzymes that continue to degrade its compounds (including vitamin C) and so cannot be stored indefinitely without compromising nutrient quality. Frozen and canned juices remain virtually unchanged for long periods. The shipping and storage savings of canned and frozen juices are passed on to consumers. Without canned or frozen juice, people with limited income or those with no access to fresh juice would be deprived of this excellent food.

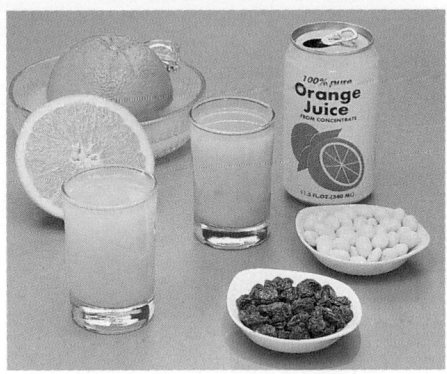

In terms of nutrient density, canned juice is almost as nutritious as fresh, but yogurt-covered raisins are *not* as nutritious as plain raisins.

Some processing stories are not so rosy. In Chapter 8, for instance, you saw how processed foods are often loaded with sodium as their potassium is leached away, exactly the wrong effect for many of those with hypertension. A related mischief of processing is the addition of sugar and fat—palatable, high-calorie additives that reduce nutrient density. An example is nuts and raisins covered with "natural yogurt." This may sound like one healthy food being added to another, but a look at the ingredient panel warns that generous amounts of sugar and fat accompany the yogurt. About 75 percent of the weight of the product is sugar and fat; only 8 percent is yogurt. To pick just one nutrient for an example, here is what happens to the iron density of the raisins: 100 calories of raisins = 0.71 milligrams iron; 100 calories of "yogurt" raisins = 0.26 milligrams of iron. These foods taste so good that wishful thinking can easily take hold, but the reality is that sugar- and fat-coated food is candy. The word *yogurt* on the label means only that one of the ingredients of the candy coating is some small amount of yogurt.

Names, even whole-food names, written on labels do not prove that the foods so named provide any nutritional benefit to consumers unless the foods themselves are nutritious. Incidentally, do not conclude from this example that raisins are a good source of iron. Compared with other food sources of iron on a per-calorie basis, raisins fall short. The iron snapshot in Chapter 8 showed some iron-rich foods.

A good general rule for making food choices is to choose whole foods to the greatest extent possible and to seek out among processed foods only the ones that processing has improved nutritionally. (When processing removes fat, as in skim milk, it is often a benefit to the consumer.) Being realistic, few people have the time to bake all their own bread from scratch, to shop every few days for fresh meats, or to wash, peel, chop, and cook fresh fruits and vegetables at every meal. This is where food processing comes in. Commercially prepared whole-grain

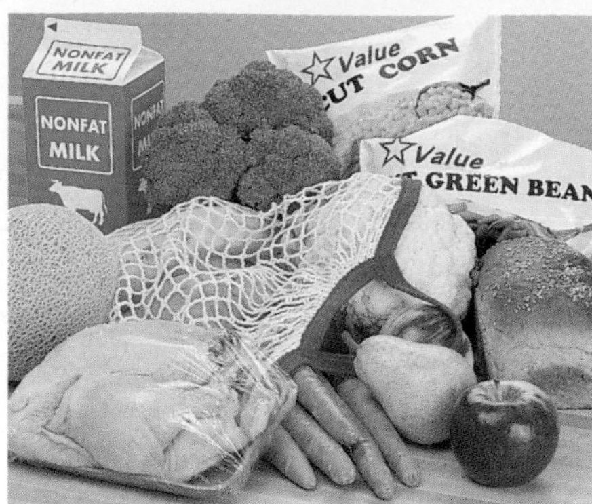

1. Purchase mostly fresh foods or those that processing has benefitted nutritionally.

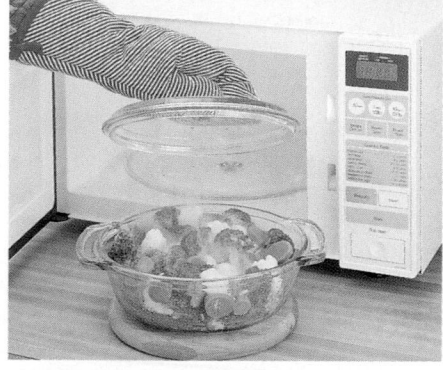

2. Steam vegetables or cook them in a microwave oven.

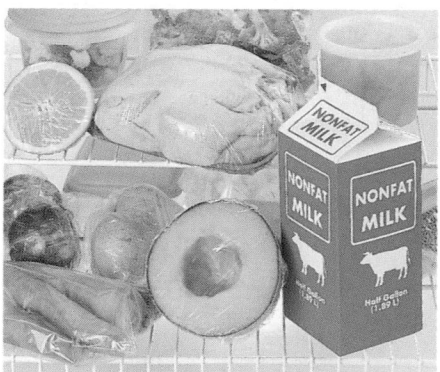

3. Wrap foods tightly and refrigerate them. Space foods to allow circulation of chilled air around them.

breads, frozen cuts of meats, bags of frozen vegetables, and canned or frozen fruit juices do little disservice to nutrition and enable the consumer to eat a wide variety of foods at great savings in time and human energy. The nutrient contents of processed foods exist on a continuum:

Whole-grain bread > refined white bread > sugared doughnuts.

Milk > fruit-flavored yogurt > canned chocolate pudding.

Corn on the cob > canned creamed corn > caramel popcorn.

Oranges > orange juice > orange-flavored drink.

Baked ham > deviled ham > fried bacon.

Another continuum parallels it—the nutrition status of the consumer. The closer to the farm the foods you eat, the better nourished you are, but that doesn't mean you have to live in the fields.

Wise food choices are half the story of smart nutrition self-care; skillful food preparation is the other half. In modern commercial processing, losses of vitamins seldom exceed 25 percent. In contrast, losses in food preparation at home can be close to 100 percent, and it is not unusual to see losses in the 60 to 75 percent range. These facts put the matter of food processing into perspective; while the kinds of foods you buy certainly make a difference, what you do with them in your kitchen can make an even greater difference.

To develop skill in preparing foods requires some understanding of the effects of cooking and storing foods on nutrients. Vitamins are organic compounds synthesized and broken down by enzymes found in the foods that contain them. The enzymes that break down nutrients in fruits and vegetables, like all enzymes, have a temperature optimum. They work best at the temperatures at which the plants grow, normally about 70° F (25° C), which is also the room temperature in most homes. Chilling fresh produce slows down enzymatic destruction of nutrients. To protect the vitamin content, most fruits and vegetables should be vine ripened (if possible), chilled immediately after picking, and kept cold until use.

Besides being vulnerable to enzyme-mediated spoilage, the vitamin riboflavin is light sensitive. It can be destroyed by the ultraviolet rays of the sun or by fluorescent light. For this reason milk is not sold (and should not be stored) in transparent glass containers. Cardboard or opaque plastic containers screen out light, protecting the riboflavin. Since grain products such as macaroni and rice are also important sources of riboflavin, cooks who store them in glass jars should stow away the jars in closed cupboards.

Some vitamins are acids or antioxidants and so are most stable in an acid solution, away from air. Citrus fruits, tomatoes, and many juices are acid. As long as the skin is uncut or the can is unopened, their vitamins are protected from air. If you store a cut vegetable or fruit or an opened carton of juice, cover it with an airtight wrapper or close it tightly and store it in the refrigerator.

Labels on frozen foods tell you "Do not refreeze." As food freezes, the cellular water expands into long, spiky ice crystals that puncture cell membranes and disrupt tissue structures, changing the texture of the food. There is no danger in eating a twice-frozen food although some nutrients are lost upon thawing and refreezing. Provided that it hasn't spoiled while it was thawed, the main problem with a twice-frozen food is that it may be less appealing.

Water-soluble vitamins and minerals in fresh-cut vegetables readily dissolve into the water in which they are washed or boiled. If the water is discarded, as much as half of the vitamins and minerals in foods go down the drain with the water. A bit of southern folk wisdom is to serve the cooking liquid with the vegetable rather than throwing it away; this liquid is known as the "pot liquor" and may be used to moisten cornbread or to make gravies or soups. Other ways to minimize cooking losses: steam vegetables over water rather than in it, stir-fry them in small amounts of oil, or microwave them. Wash the intact food vigorously and briefly, don't soak it. Cut vegetables after washing except for those such as broccoli that you have to cut to wash adequately. For peeled vegetables, such as potatoes, add them to water that is vigorously boiling, not to cold water to minimize the length of time the vegetables are exposed to nutrient-leaching water. Microwave ovens are excellent for conserving nutrients. They cook fast without requiring the addition of fats or excess liquid. Some special microwaving concerns appear in the margin.

Take care when cooking in a microwave oven. Food can become extraordinarily hot or build up steam that may scald unprotected hands or face. Before cooking eggs, sausages, or any food encased in a membrane, pierce the membrane to prevent explosion of the food.

Here's a way to tell if glass or other containers are made of microwave-safe materials. Microwave the empty container for one minute and carefully touch it.

Warm = unsafe for microwave.

Lukewarm – safe for short reheating use.

Cool = safe for long microwave cooking times.

During other types of cooking, minimize the destruction of vitamins by avoiding high temperatures and long cooking times. Iron destroys vitamin C by catalyzing its oxidation, but perhaps the benefit of increasing the iron content of foods by cooking in iron utensils outweighs this disadvantage. Each of these tactics is small by itself, but saving a small percentage of the vitamins in foods each day can mean saving significant amounts in a year's time.

Meanwhile, however, a law of diminishing returns operates. Most vitamin losses under reasonable conditions are not catastrophic. You need not fret over small vitamin losses that occur in your kitchen; you may waste energy or time that is valuable to you in other ways. Be assured that if you start with fresh, whole foods containing ample amounts of vitamins and are reasonably careful in their preparation, you will receive a bounty of the nutrients that they contain.

 Notes

1. D. O. Cliver, *Eating Safely: Avoiding Foodborne Illnesses* (New York: American Council on Science and Health, 1993), p. 3.
2. R. L. Hall, Food safety and biotechnology, *Nutrition Today*, May/June 1991, pp. 15–20.
3. I. D. Wolf, Critical issues in food safety, 1991–2000, *Food Technology*, January 1992, pp. 64–70.
4. V. Modeland, Fishing for facts on fish safety, *FDA Consumer*, February 1989, pp. 16–24.
5. Cliver, 1993.
6. J. A. Desenclos and coauthors, The protective effect of alcohol on the occurrence of epidemic oyster-borne hepatitis, *Epidemiology* 3 (1992): 371–374.
7. Seafood safety: Highlights of the executive summary of the 1991 report by the Committee on Evaluation of the Safety of Fishery Products of the Food and Nutrition Board, Institute of Medicine, National Academy of Sciences, *Nutrition Reviews* 49 (1991): 357–363.
8. J. H. T. Luong, C. A. Groom, and K. B. Male, The potential role of biosensors in the food and drink industry, *Biosensors and Bioelectronics* 6 (1991): 547–554.
9. P. L. Peterkin, E. S. Idziak, and A. N. Sharpe, Detection of *Listeria monocytogenes* by direct colony hybridization on hydrophobic grid-membrane filters by using a chromogen-labeled DNA probe, *Applied and Environmental Microbiology* 57 (1991): 586–591; M. Hoshi, Y. Sasamoto, and M. Nonaka, Microbial sensor system for nondestructive evaluation of fish meat quality,

Biosensors and Bioelectronics 6 (1991): 15–20.
10. R. D. Williams, Boil it, cook it, peel it or forget it, *FDA Consumer*, September 1991, p. 17.
11. K. E. Anderson and A. Kappas, Dietary regulation of cytochrome P450, *Annual Review of Nutrition* 11 (1991): 141–167.
12. A. Levin, Pesticides: How dangerous are they? *Building Economic Alternatives* (a quarterly publication of Co-op America, 2100 M Street, NW, Suite 310, Washington, DC 20063), summer 1989, p. 16; D. Farley, Setting safe limits on pesticide residues, *FDA Consumer*, October 1988, pp. 8–11.
13. C. F. Chaisson, B. Petersen, and J. S. Douglass, *Pesticides in Foods: A Guide for Professionals* (Chicago: American Dietetic Association, 1991), p. 2–3.
14. National Academy of Sciences Committee, as quoted by J. Raloff and D. Pendick, Pesticides in produce may threaten kids, *Science News*, 3 July 1993, pp. 4–5.
15. P. Weber, A place for pesticides? *World Watch*, May/June 1992, pp. 18–25.
16. Food and Drug Administration Pesticide Program, *Residues in Foods 1990* (Washington, D.C.: Food and Drug Administration, 1991).
17. Food and Drug Administration Pesticide Program, 1990.
18. T. D. Etherton, P. M. Kris-Etherton, and E. W. Mills, Recombinant bovine and porcine somatotropin: Safety and benefits of these biotechnologies, *Journal of the American Dietetic Association* 93 (1993): 177–180.
19. Bovine somatotropin and the safety of cow's milk: National Institutes of Health Technology Assessment Conference Statement, *Nutrition Reviews* 49 (1991): 227–232.
20. National Toxics Campaign, A campaign to stop "hormone milk," *Earth Island Journal*, Summer 1992, p. 32.
21. National Institutes of Health Technology Assessment Conference Statement, 1991.
22. Bovine somatotropin and the safety of cow's milk, 1991.
23. J. C. Juskevich and C. G. Guyer, Bovine growth hormone: Human food safety evaluation, *Science* 249 (1990): 875–884; R. W. Rhein, *BST = A Safe, More Plentiful Milk Supply* (booklet) (New York: American Council on Science and Health, 1990).
24. B. Corey, Bovine growth hormone harmless for humans, *FDA Consumer*, April 1990, pp. 17–18.
25. M. V. Polo, M. J. Lagarda, and R. Farré, The effect of freezing on mineral element content of vegetables, *Journal of Food Composition and Analysis* 5 (1992): 77–78.
26. Dr. W. Gary Flamm of FDA's Center for Food Safety and Applied Nutrition, as cited by K. Flieger, The Delaney dilemma, *FDA Consumer*, September 1988, pp. 18–19.
27. I. D. Wolf, Critical issues in food safety, 1991–2000, *Food Technology*, January 1992, pp. 64–70.
28. J. Hotchkiss and R. Cassens, Nitrate, nitrite, and nitroso compounds in foods (a scientific status summary by the Institute of Food Technologists' Expert Panel on Food Safety and Nutrition), April 1987, available from Institute of Food Science, Department of Food Science, Cornell University, Ithaca, NY 14853.
29. One honey of an alternative to sulfites, *Science News* 134 (1988): 218.
30. New "food freshener," *Nutrition Forum* 5 (1988): 49.
31. M. Naim and coauthors, Interaction of MSG taste with nutrition: Perspectives in consummatory behavior and digestion, *Physiology and Behavior* 49 (1991): 1019–1024.
32. D. Farley, Keeping up with the microwave revolution, *FDA Consumer*, March 1990, pp. 17–21.
33. D. Blumenthal, Deciding about dioxins, *FDA Consumer*, February 1990, pp. 11–13.

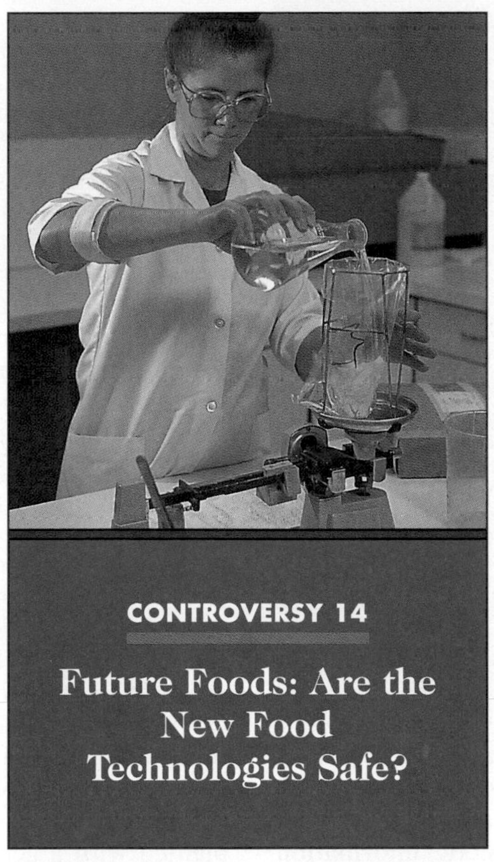

CONTROVERSY 14

Future Foods: Are the New Food Technologies Safe?

Food futurists who gaze ahead to the 21st century see a world with many more people, greater food demands, and less available farmland on which to grow food. Foods will have to be easy to grow in abundance. Furthermore, people in developed countries will have little or no time for cooking or sitting down to meals.[1] Foods will have to be easy and quick to prepare. Already today, consumers need nutritious, easy-to-prepare foods that are low in fat and that taste good. And of course, the foods must be safe to eat—free from microbial and other contamination. Further, foods must be produced economically enough so that growers and processors can make a profit on them and consumers can buy them cheaply. Also, the production of foods must have as little environmental impact as possible. These diverse needs may seem to oppose each other, and yet all are promised by advocates of new technologies.

The developing world has an even greater need for foods with all these qualities than do developed nations. An unrelenting population explosion within the borders of less developed nations foretells of widespread famine to come unless, as many scientists hope, new food technologies can stave off disastrous famines by increasing crop yields and food safety and reducing food waste.

Today the world is witnessing the beginning of a revolution of applied technology in food science and agriculture. Upon surveying government, business, and university experts concerning technological development under development, FDA concluded, "the floodgates of innovation are opening. Nearly 800 different developments [are] reported as technically feasible." Almost two thirds of those developments are nearing reality.[2]

While new technologies promise immense benefits in solving food problems, consumers have their suspicions about what the risks might be and who stands to benefit most, the processors of foods or the consumers of them.

This Controversy focuses on two major food technologies that hold vast potential for changing the food supply. The first is **biogenetic engineering** and the second is food **irradiation.**

BIOGENETIC ENGINEERING For centuries farmers have been changing the genetic makeup of their crop plants and farm animals. Season after season they have selectively bred plants or animals possessing desirable traits, hoping to obtain offspring that reliably display those traits. Today's lush, hefty, healthy agricultural crops and animals from cabbage and squash to pigs and cattle all are the results of those efforts.

Among the successes of selective breeding is corn. Its large, full, sweet cobs and high yields bear little resemblance to the original wild, native corn with its sparse two or three kernels to a stalk. With fancy modern techniques, agricultural scientists have even developed strains of corn that do not produce the enzyme that turns sugar to starch, so corn retains the sweet taste that people prefer. The new corn stays sweet for weeks instead of turning starchy in a matter of days. Selective breeding, called by some "the old biotechnology," works, but slowly.

Recently, scientists have discovered a way of speeding up the process of genetic change through biotechnology. The changes in corn just mentioned required centuries, but today's biotechnology methods could have accomplished the same things in about a year or two of work. Biotechnology is more than just an improved means of selective breeding, for the method wields an awesome power—the power to change the most basic patterns of life in ways never before possible. No longer must farmers wait patiently for breeding to create improved crops and animals. No longer must they even respect natural lines of reproduction among species. Instead, the laboratory scientist can just select desirable traits from any of a number of organisms and transfer them to specific crop plants or agricultural animals.

The Products of Biogenetic Engineering The products of biotechnology are of two types. One is new strains of plants or animals with new desirable traits, as in the corn example above. The other is strains of

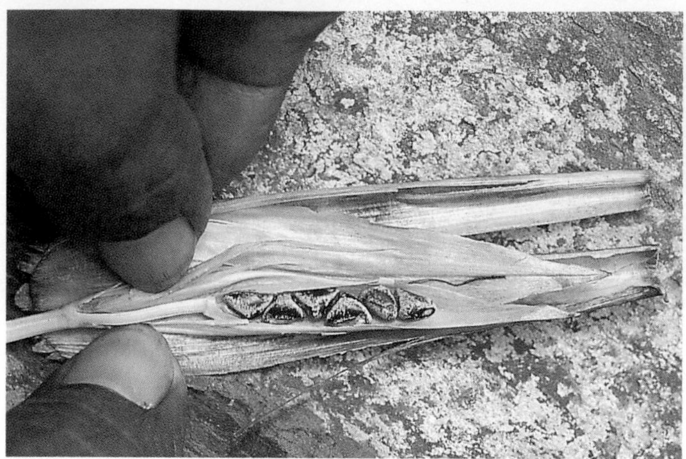

The original wild corn from which today's corn was developed.

microorganisms able to produce substances that occur in only limited amounts or not at all in nature.

Plant cells make likely candidates for recombinant DNA technology because, many times, a single plant cell can be coaxed to reproduce an entire new plant. Other cells with this talent include fertilized ova, stem or germ cells, and some embryonic cells. Each cell of the new organism that develops from an altered single cell contains an exact replica of the genetic information contained in the original cell. If any DNA fragments have been introduced by scientists, the cells will faithfully reproduce these, too.

For example, scientists can start with a stem cell from the "eye" of a potato plant. Into that cell they can implant some DNA carrying genes for the protein coat (but not the infective part) of a virus that attacks potato plants. Then they can stimulate the stem cell to begin growing a whole new potato plant that replicates the piece of viral protein coat in each of its cells. Such **transgenic** potato plants develop immunity to the real virus and can effectively repel it when it attacks.

Products from transgenic bacteria often assist food manufacturers. One bacterium, for example, was given the ability to make the enzyme renin, which is necessary for the production of cheese. Before this innovation, renin was traditionally harvested from the stomachs of calves, an expensive process. Through recombinant DNA technology the gene responsible for making renin was snipped from some calf DNA and transferred to a single bacterial cell. That cell divided many times, producing a whole colony of transgenic bacteria. With each bacterial cell contributing just a minute amount of renin, a colony becomes a factory of mass production. By the same process, human hormones, such as the once scarce human growth hormone, can be produced abundantly. Today, children with growth-hormone deficiency most often grow normally because of a reliable supply of human growth hormone harvested from transgenic bacteria.

The technique just described allows an organism to make proteins native to some other living thing. Another way that biotechnology can change the internal chemistry of an organism is by blocking, or suppressing, production of a protein the organism originally made. One example is an especially long-lasting tomato. Normally, tomatoes produce a protein that softens them after they have been picked. Scientists introduced into a tomato plant an **antisense gene,** that is, a mirror image of the native gene that coded for the "softening" enzyme. The new antisense gene blocked its ability to produce the softening enzyme (see Figure C14-1). A vine-ripe tomato with the antisense gene softens and rots much more slowly than a normal tomato. Regular tomatoes must be harvested in the hard, green stage to endure shipping and handling. Bioengineered tomatoes can be harvested at their most flavorful and nutritious red-ripe stage and still last much longer than regular green-harvested tomatoes.

Among the newest transgenic foods are soybeans implanted with a gene that compensates for the limiting amino acids of soy protein. Soy protein from these beans is of a quality approaching that of milk protein. Such beans may one day prove important to solving protein malnutrition problems, especially among the children of some developing nations. Likewise, tomatoes and cotton can produce their own insecticides upon receiving the right genes from bacteria. These varieties may render pesticide sprays unnecessary. Still other crops may receive the ability to withstand lethal herbicides, so that farmers can spray whole fields with potent herbicides to kill every other kind of plant growing there, leaving only the desired crop. Shrimp may soon fight diseases with genetic ammunition borrowed from sea urchins. Some plants even may be given special molecules to help them grow food in heavily polluted soil in which all other plants wither and die.

The aforementioned possibilities represent works already in progress. Close on their heels are many more ingenious ideas. What if crop plants could gain salt tolerance transplanted into them from a coastal marsh plant? Could crops then be irrigated with sea water, thus conserving dwindling fresh-water supplies? Would the world food supply increase should rice farmers be able to grow disease-immune plants? What if consumers

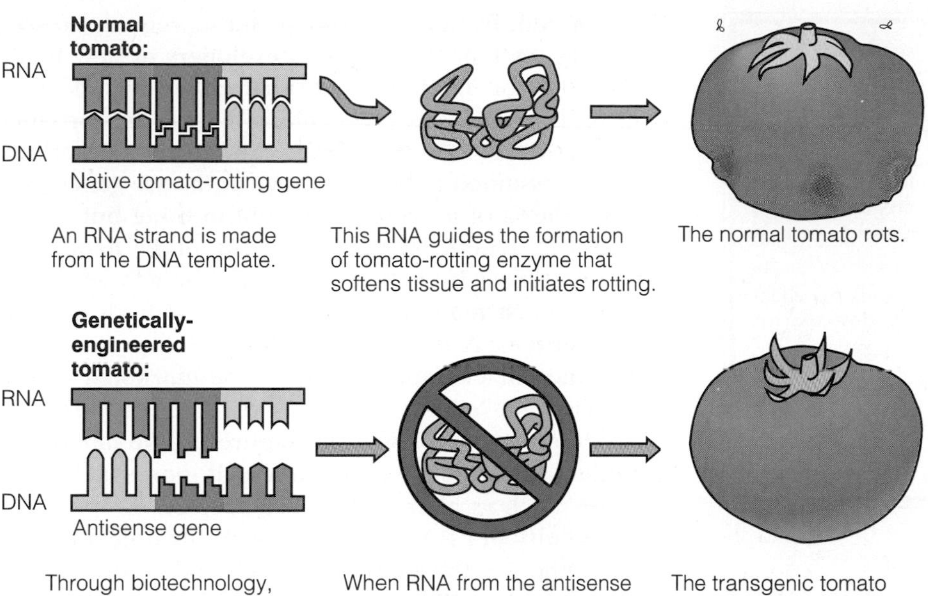
Normal tomato:
RNA
DNA
Native tomato-rotting gene
An RNA strand is made from the DNA template.
This RNA guides the formation of tomato-rotting enzyme that softens tissue and initiates rotting.
The normal tomato rots.
Genetically-engineered tomato:
RNA
DNA
Antisense gene
Through biotechnology, scientists can insert a mirror image of the rotting gene (an antisense gene) into tomatoes.
When RNA from the antisense gene combines with RNA from the native gene, the native RNA is blocked from producing the rotting enzyme.
The transgenic tomato lasts longer.

Figure C14-1

HOW BIOTECHNOLOGY TECHNIQUES CAN BLOCK FORMATION OF SPECIFIC PROTEINS

Source: Adapted from J. M. Nash, A bumper crop of biotech, *Time*, 1 October 1990, p. 92.

could dictate which traits scientists should insert into food plants? Would they choose to confer on foods extra cancer-fighting nonnutrients or more antioxidant nutrients? These ideas may sound fantastic, but many such organisms are already on laboratory shelves and are waiting for FDA approval to be used in agriculture.

Safety and Regulation Those looking forward to the products of biogenetic engineering may be in for a long wait. While both scientists and food industrialists hail biotechnology with confidence, some consumers fear that direct tampering with genes will change organisms in ways not yet fully understood, even by the scientists who developed the techniques. Some feel uncomfortable when the power of direct control over the genes lies in the hands of human beings who may not act in the best interest of all. They feel genetic decisions are best left to the powers of nature. Those given to flights of imagination envision a biotechnology run amuck, used for frivolous, greedy purposes such as cloning dinosaurs for entertainment.*

Field tests of transgenic plants or animals in actual plots of land have been delayed. Skeptics who fear unknown effects say that unleashing genetically altered organisms in field tests would be like opening a Pandora's box of possibly unstoppable events in the natural world, with unknown consequences for human life on earth. With no natural systems of control in place, they fear that organisms with artificial genetic advantages may escape the testing grounds to create superspecies that could wipe out whole ecosystems. Field testing of altered pansy flowers and other crops has been set back by such objections in some states. While the transgenic plants wait for testing, supporters of biotechnology say, farmers lose economic advantages, world food supplies dwindle, and a new science struggles to advance against the opposition.

Many legitimate safety questions exist, however. Many focus on the "foreign" proteins produced by organisms that receive new genes. Students of nutrition know that DNA governs synthesis of protein, and that in the human body, proteins are degraded by digestive enzymes and rendered nontoxic. Several dangerous exceptions exist, though, including the toxin of *Clostridium botulinum* and certain other peptide toxins. Some scientists worry that such peptides may accidentally form and may not be detected promptly enough to prevent harm to those who consume the foods.

*Michael Crichton's popular novel *Jurassic Park* (New York: Ballantine Books, 1990) and the film that followed paint a frightening scene of rampaging dinosaurs let loose on an unsuspecting world, but today's biotechnology cannot create living things from DNA samples. While entertaining, the book and movie are scientifically inaccurate.

antisense gene the chemical opposite of a gene, which adheres to the native working gene and blocks its ultimate production of proteins.

biogenetic engineering intentional manipulation of the genetic material of living things in order to obtain some desirable trait not present in the original organism; a field within *biotechnology*, the use of biological systems or organisms to create or modify products, to change plants, animals, or microorganisms in ways that produce a perceived benefit.

irradiation application of ionizing radiation to foods to reduce insect infestation or microbial contamination, or slow the ripening or sprouting process.

radiolytic products chemicals formed during irradiation of food.

transgenic organism an organism that grows from an embryonic, stem, or germ cell into which a new gene has been inserted; the organism carries the new gene in all of its cells.

Other worries surround unknown effects of "foreign" hormones produced by transgenic animals or of insecticides that transgenic plants form in their tissues. The tests that can separate and measure the recombinant peptides are sophisticated and expensive to perform; but advances are being made to simplify them.[3] Questions are also raised about the environmental effects that might arise from spraying large areas with lethal herbicides, leaving only one genetically engineered plant species alive.

Experts agree that laws should require safety testing of technology's products before marketing them.[4] The case for regulation is strong. New enzymes, hormones, and resistance traits that have never before been seen in foods are, in a sense, additives, and perhaps should be regulated like additives.

Also, it should be clear that, when a new gene has been introduced into a food, other, unwanted genes have not accompanied it. If a disease-producing microorganism has donated genetic material to make the recombinant DNA, scientists must prove that no dangerous characteristic from the microorganism has also entered the food. If the inserted genetic material comes from a known safe source, such as nuts, then the products can be assumed to be safe for everyone except those allergic to nuts. Furthermore, the newly altered genetic material may create proteins never before encountered by the human body, unique proteins. Their effects should be understood and their presence regulated to ensure their safety for human consumption.[5]

FDA has taken the position that whole foods produced through biotechnology, if they are not substantially different from foods already in use, require no special safety testing.[6] FDA holds developers of new foods responsible for testing those that differ significantly from traditional foods (see Table C14-1). Any product with an antisense gene, including the tomato described earlier, is assumed to be safe, since antisense genes *prevent* synthesis of a protein and add nothing but a tiny fragment of genetic material. On the other hand, any extra substances introduced into food by way of bioengineering must meet the same safety standards applied to all additives. A tomato with a gene that produces an insecticide, for example, could not be marketed unless the insecticide "additive" was proved safe for consumption. No food product will be required to be labeled as a product of biotechnology unless it poses a known problem, such as allergy, to some people.

A difficulty in FDA's position lies in the objections by some to the genetic tampering itself. They want labels to help them to tell the "old fashioned" tomatoes from the altered ones. This position holds that while a food may not pose a known hazard, it has not been proved safe either, and should not be tested out on consumers without their informed consent.

Speaking in defense of the FDA's decision are the FDA itself, recognized as the nation's leading expert and advocate for food safety, and the American Dietetic Association, which represents current scientific thinking in nutrition. Many other scientific organizations concur. These experts contend that biotechnology is a useful tool that can deliver on its promises for an improved food supply if we give it a fair chance to do so.[7]

A lack of scientific understanding pervades many fears of biotechnology. After all, most of today's foods are the result of greatly altered genetic composition, accomplished by way of selective breeding. The new vegetable broccoflower, a product of sophisticated crossbreeding of broccoli with cauliflower, met no testing or approval barriers on its way to the U.S. dinner plate. Only after the vegetable became popular with many consumers did scientists discover that its nutrient contents were favorable: the vegetable is an excellent source of vitamin C and a good source of beta carotene (Appendix A lists other nutrients in broccoflower). It also has many of the other attributes of its cruciferous vegetable family.

Transgenic crops and farm animals of all descriptions, along with bacteria and algae that produce drugs such as hormones and insulin, are now being used in commerce, awaiting testing in laboratories, or approaching reality. To help determine the safety of the products of biotechnology and other new processes,

FDA has established a new National Center for Food Safety and Technology (NCFST) in Illinois. Studies performed at NCFST will guide FDA in setting future regulations governing food processes and products. A product of biotechnology already in use in food animals is growth hormone, synthesized by way of transgenic bacteria.

IRRADIATED FOODS Another technology that has met stern opposition from some consumer groups is food irradiation. Can exposing foods to ionizing radiation solve some of our food-supply problems, as proponents claim? Certainly, problems exist, and this section presents both sides of this issue.

Consumers must now cook chicken and eggs to the well-done stage to avoid infection from *Salmonella* microorganisms that often contaminate the raw products. Consumption of soft cheeses has presented a threat of serious illness from a virulent *Listeria* strain. Pork may contain larvae of the muscle-attacking parasite *Trichinella*, which is traditionally killed by thoroughly cooking pork. Grains, vegetables, and fruits may be contaminated with residues of post-harvest pesticides, those sprays applied to kill molds and insects that attack during food storage, after harvest. Finally, and perhaps most pressing, the issue of future food shortages remains close at hand. All of the problems just named are theoretically solvable through food irradiation.

The Irradiation Process Irradiation slows the ripening and rotting of some foods, thereby reducing waste. It kills off *Salmonella* and *Listeria* organisms. It can also sexually sterilize the *Trichinella* organism and interrupt its destructive life cycle.[8] Irradiation might replace some types of post-harvest pesticides because it can kill mold and insect pests. Supporters claim that irradiation can stretch the amount of food produced today to feed more people. While some scientists agree with these assessments, critics counter that not only does food irradiation *not* solve food supply problems, it also may pose some serious and unnecessary threats of its own.

Irradiation works by exposing foods to controlled doses of gamma radiation from the radioactive compound cobalt 60 or from X rays generated by machines. The rays can kill or disable organisms that pose a hazard to the food or to the people who eat it. As radiation passes through a living cell, it disrupts the internal structures and so kills or deactivates the cell. Low doses can kill the cells in the "eyes" of potatoes and ends of onions, preventing their sprouting. They can also delay ripening of fruits such as bananas, avocados, and others. Higher doses can penetrate tough insect exoskeletons and mold or bacterial cell walls, thereby reducing microorganism or insect threats. To sterilize spices, technicians expose spices to extremely high doses of radiation, the highest levels allowed by law.

Table C14-1
FDA's Areas of Concern for Safety of Bioengineered Foods

Unexpected changes. Changing an organism's genes can create unexpected changes in the composition of the tissues by activating genes for unwanted products or suppressing genes for desirable products.

Known toxicants. FDA seeks to ensure that new plant varieties do not have significantly higher levels of naturally occurring toxicants than found in other varieties of the plant. (Chapter 14 described natural toxicants.)

Nutrients. Nutrients in the new food must occur in amounts not significantly different from those in the original food. Also, bioavailability of those nutrients must be equal.

New substances. A food with a gene that creates novel substances not occurring in the original plant is a concern.

Allergens. If a plant receives a gene that produces a known allergen from another organism, the new plant may produce that allergen. An example would be the gene that codes for the allergen of peanuts, implanted into corn. The new corn could cause allergies in people allergic to peanuts.

Antibiotic resistance markers. A step in genetic engineering requires that a marker gene be included in the new genetic material to ease identification of cells that have been successfully altered. The marker gene produces a product that destroys antibiotics. Theoretically, an ill person who ate a food containing the product of the marker gene may be robbed of the benefit from an antibiotic drug taken with the food.

Nonfood substances. Some plants can be engineered to make nonfood oils or starch, and these substances may contain toxins. Such plants and their products must be prevented from mixing with the food supply.

Animal feed. Special concerns about animal feed center on concentration of toxins in animal flesh. Farm-raised animals often derive half or more of their calories from one food source. Should that food contain toxins, even at levels that would be harmless to human beings, it could pose a hazard when fed to food animals.

Source: FDA statement of policy: Foods derived from new plant varieties, *Federal Register*, 29 May 1992.

A perspective on the doses used is gained by comparing them to the human lethal dose. The low doses of radiation needed to treat fruits and vegetables are 10 to 20 times the amount capable of killing a human being. The doses required to sterilize are much higher still. Needless to say, the handling of irradiation technology requires extreme caution.

Right now, the only food irradiation plant operating in the United States is in Florida.[9] California and some other states have decided not to operate irradiation plants, and they also have banned sales of all irradiated foods other than spices. In contrast, about 20 nations of the world have approved food irradiation technology for use within their borders.

The plant currently operating in Florida irradiates strawberries and mangoes, not to sterilize them, but to reduce mold spoilage in the berries and to delay ripening of the mangoes. Sold on the national market, the berries remain red, firm, and sweet for a week or more after treatment, while untreated berries wilt and turn moldy in just a few days. The irradiated mangoes ripen more slowly than they would normally, allowing consumers a longer span of time in which to enjoy them.

The irradiated foods processed in Florida must bear a label, as all irradiated foods must. The label must state that the foods have been treated with radiation, or must display the irradiation symbol shown here. Exceptions are permitted for spices, when they are mixed with processed foods, and for any irradiated foods served in restaurants.

Many consumers willingly purchase Florida's irradiated and labeled berries and mangoes, but some refuse them, and others vigorously challenge the whole idea of food irradiation. Some in the latter group mistakenly believe that irradiated foods themselves become radioactive. This is not true. Properly irradiated food does not become radioactive any more than teeth become radioactive after dental x-ray procedures. The word *properly* carries weight, though. Foods exposed to extremely high doses of the wrong sort of radiation can indeed become radioactive, but such abuses would also render them inedible.[10]

When radiation disrupts the molecules of cells, the molecules change into by-products within the tissue of the food. One such molecular change is the permanent alteration of the cell's genetic material. If cell's are exposed to radiation doses high enough or prolonged enough to kill them, these changes are probably of little consequence. Radiation used to process food, however, must be limited to amounts that do not cause detectable adverse alterations of the taste, color, or texture of the food. These limited doses may not be sufficient to kill all bacterial or mold spores present in the food.[11] This means that the genetic material of the remaining live cells and spores may have sustained irreversible and unpredictable alterations during irradiation. Significantly, the only bacteria and mold spores remaining after irradiation are those most resistant to irradiation; should a colony of those microorganisms subsequently develop, every individual in the colony would bear the trait of radiation resistance. As bacteria and molds gain radiation resistance and migrate throughout the environment, higher and higher doses of radiation must be used to kill off the organisms, doses high enough to destroy the food and far beyond those now approved for use.

The symbol for foods treated with radiation.

The spores of one dangerous bacterium are naturally beyond the reach of even the highest legal doses of irradiation—those of *Clostridium botulinum*, the bacterium responsible for the lethal food-poisoning agent, botulin toxin. In fact, one powerful critic of food irradiation, Dr. David Murray, calls into question the whole idea that irradiation can be used effectively to sterilize food products because the dose of radiation required to completely sterilize food also destroys it. Sterilization is rarely the objective of irradiation, however. Disease-causing microbes are often sensitive to radiation and are greatly reduced in number by irradiation.

A fear not easily put to rest is that of the chemicals, called **radiolytic products,** produced in foods as they undergo irradiation. A few radiolytic products are unique, appearing only in irradiated foods; others are commonly found in many foods. Their effects on human health and nutrition, if any, are unknown. An example is the highly reactive free radicals that always form during irradiation. Free radicals attack other molecules, setting up chain reactions. The attacked molecules go on to attack others that in turn become attackers, causing chaos within cell structures. Irradiation affects some of the unsaturated fatty acids in the cell membranes of living tissue, changing them into free radicals.

One worry about free radicals is their tendency to react with the genetic material of cells, specifically with oncogenes, the cancer-related genes of cells. When oncogenes are "turned on" by free radicals, they signal unbridled cell replication and tumor development. Another worry is the disruptive effect of free radicals on cell membranes. Still another health problem linked to damage from free radicals is heart disease. Whether the extra free radicals formed during food irradiation are absorbed into the body or bear any connection to diseases in human beings is not known.

Irradiation's Effects on Nutrients Nutrients in foods are known to be affected by free radicals and irradiation. Protein chains and most amino acids withstand attack by irradiation and free radicals, but the side chains of certain individual amino acids are open to destruction by these influences. Irradiation destroys some vitamins, too. Indeed, the primary function of vitamin E is to scavenge these reactive particles and so to protect the unsaturated fatty acids of cell membranes. Other vitamins, including beta carotene, thiamin, vitamin B_6, and the active form of vitamin C, are also open to destruction by free radicals. Theoretically, if marginally nourished people were to consume a steady diet of nothing but irradiated food, they might well develop frank nutrient deficiencies.[12] Murray uses these words to describe the nutritional losses sustained through irradiation:

> *If irradiation were to be applied to the meats, fruits and vegetables that form the bulk of most human diets, the nutritional impoverishment of those diets would be so extensive that sufficiency thresholds for many essential nutrients would no longer be met. The phrase 'empty calories' would take on a new dimension.*

Countering this opinion is one from the American Council on Science and Health (ACSH), a group that advocates irradiation. While acknowledging that doses of radiation high enough to sterilize food do cause vitamin losses, the ACSH describes the losses sustained during low-dose irradiation to be similar to those caused by other processing techniques such as canning, and therefore not a health hazard.[13]

The FDA concurs that irradiation of chicken to reduce its *Salmonella* contamination produces losses of thiamin, but the losses constitute less than 2 percent of the total thiamin, losses not considered by FDA to be significant. Any food that suffered greater than a 2-percent loss of any nutrient during irradiation would be required by FDA to be labeled as an "imitation food."[14]

Murray responds that the studies that show minimal vitamin losses were performed immediately after irradiation, before the free radicals and "weeping" (fluid losses) resulting from irradiation had finished destroying the vitamin contents of the foods. The longer the food is stored, the greater the losses of nutrients, and the losses are far beyond those incurred during any other processing technique.

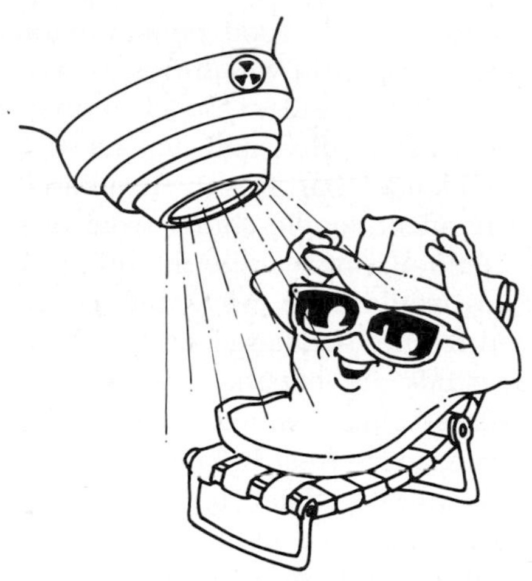

Irradiation can make some foods safer to eat by destroying organisms that cause illness.

If the purpose of irradiation is to preserve food and increase its shelf life, then the possibility of destruction and losses of nutrients during storage warrants further investigation. The head of preventive medicine at New Jersey Medical School, Dr. Donald Louria, believes that food irradiation poses no significant cancer risks to consumers, but is concerned about nutrient losses sustained by foods. He states that if significant nutrients are destroyed in a food, then a label alerting consumers to that fact should be mandatory.[15] After all, a person who buys a food from the grocery store and consumes it trusts the food to provide vitamins. That person should be warned to obtain vitamins from another source.

Even if consumers were willing to compensate for nutrient losses sustained through radiation, the question above all others still remains: Are irradiated foods safe to eat?

Other Concerns Radiation changes foods in ways that are still not completely understood with regard to health. For example, when food irradiated within three months after treatment is heated in a laboratory, it emits light detectable by instruments.[16] (People fearful of this phenomenon say, "It glows.")[17] This light energy, called thermoluminescence, arises from overexcited electrons, stimulated by radiation.

Another poorly understood phenomenon occurs in laboratory experiments in which freshly irradiated food is fed to rats. The rats develop chromosomal abnormalities, impaired fertility, and depressed immune responses.[18] Evidence that freshly irradiated food may also adversely affect people comes from one study performed on malnourished children. In the days before current ethics would have prevented such a study, researchers fed freshly irradiated wheat to malnourished children to study its effects. The surprising results showed increased chromosomal abnormalities in all but one of the children fed freshly irradiated wheat.[19] Those children fed irradiated wheat that had been held in storage for longer than three months or fed nonirradiated wheat showed no increase in the chromosomal effect.

Animal experiments perhaps could prove or disprove the existence of some of the feared effects, but to test irradiated foods is difficult. The safety of other additives is tested by feeding animals hundreds of times the amount of substance that a person might consume in a day, but researchers cannot feed animals hundreds of times more irradiated food than people would consume.[20]

In its publication *Priorities*, the ACSH questions the validity of studies showing ill effects:

> *Arguments against food irradiation are largely based on poorly planned, rejected experiments, pseudo science, and emotion, which are fronts for an antinuclear political agenda.*[21]

Some people do oppose food irradiation on the grounds that it requires transporting radioactive materials, exposing workers to them, and then disposing of the spent wastes, which remain radioactive for many years after disposal. They claim that these processes pose an unacceptable and unnecessary risk to human health and reproduction. Birth defects are common in children who were exposed to even nonlethal low doses of radiation during their fetal development and even in children whose parents were exposed to radiation *before* the children were conceived. These concerns are echoed by food industrialists and others who hope to gain acceptance for the process, but who are unwilling to risk human health. They hope to safeguard both workers and future generations through strict operating standards and compliance with regulations concerning radiation exposure.

In the end, it may be that the tasks set out for irradiation technology may be achievable by less expensive methods such as higher cleanliness standards for food-animal facilities to prevent microbial contamination, selective breeding of produce to achieve longer storage times, and application of gases and pesticides that dissipate before product consumption to ensure destruction of pests and infestations. These methods pose none of the hazards associated with transport and handling of radioactive materials, and they are proven safe for the human food supply. Whether or not food processors will soon use irradiation widely in treating the food supply may depend on the ability of its backers to prove its safety beyond doubt.

Will our impressive new technologies provide foods to meet the needs of the future? Optimists would say yes. Biotechnology holds a world of promise, and with proper safeguards and controls, it may yield products tailor-made to meet the needs of consumers. Even irradiation, with its potential for hazard, may, with proper safety controls in place, prove useful in helping to provide safe, abundant food for the world's growing population. All products of technology must pass a final examination, though—the test of consumer acceptance. If the products meet people's needs; are attractive, economical, and tasty; and have been proved safe, consumers will buy them. If they fail to meet these standards, consumers will bypass them, and the technologies themselves will fade into history.

◆ Notes

1. A. L. Owen, The impact of future foods on nutrition and health, *Journal of American Dietetic Association* 90 (1990): 1217–1222.
2. H. L. Miller and S. J. Ackerman, Perspective on food biotechnology, *FDA Consumer*, March 1990, pp. 8–13.
3. K. Tsuji, High-performance capillary electrophoresis of proteins: SDS-polyacrylamide gel-filled capillary column for the determination of recombinant biotechnology-derived proteins, *Journal of Chromatography* 550 (1991): 823–830.
4. American Medical Association Council on Scientific Affairs, Biotechnology and the American agricultural industry, *Journal of the American Medical Association* 265 (1991): 1429–1436.
5. D. D. Hopkins, R. J. Goldburg, and S. A. Hirsch, *A Mutable Feast: Assuring Food Safety in the Era of Genetic Engineering* (New York: Environmental Defense Fund, 1991).
6. Food and Drug Administration, Statement of policy: Foods derived from new plant varieties, *Federal Register*, 29 May 1992.
7. Position of the American Dietetic Association: Biotechnology and the future of food, *Journal of the American Dietetic Association* 93 (1993): 189–192; Genetically engineered foods: Fears and facts, an interview with FDA's Jim Maryanski, *FDA Consumer*, January/

February 1993, pp. 11–14.
8. American Council on Science and Health, *Irradiated Foods* (booklet) (New York: American Council on Science and Health, 1988).
9. M. Marcotte, Irradiated strawberries enter the U.S. market, *Food Technology*, May 1992, pp. 80–86.
10. A. J. Swallow, Wholesomeness and safety of irradiated foods, *Nutritional and Toxicological Consequences of Food Processing: Advances in Experimental Medicine and Biology* (New York: Plenum Press, 1991), pp. 11–31.
11. D. R. Murray, *Biology of Food Irradiation* (New York: John Wiley and Sons, 1990), pp. 113–118, 200–214.
12. Murray, 1990, pp. 105–106.
13. American Council on Science and Health, 1988.
14. Chicken nutrient losses from irradiation not significant, FDA says, *Food Chemical News*, 25 May 1987, pp. 53–54.
15. Food irradiation, Taped interview, National Public Radio broadcast, *Living on Earth*, 7 February 1992.
16. L. Heide and K. W. Bogl, Detection methods for irradiated foods—Luminescence and viscosity measures, *International Journal of Radiation Biology* 57 (1990): 201–219; T. Autio and S. Pinnioja, Identification of irradiated foods by the thermoluminescence of mineral contamination, *Zeitschrift für Lebensmittel-Untersuchung und -Forschung* 191 (1990): 177–180; A. M. Sjoberg and coauthors, Methods for detection of irradiation of spices, *Zeitschrift für Lebensmittel-Untersuchung und -Forschung* 190 (1990): 99–103.
17. Really rad radishes, *Earth Island Journal*, Summer 1991, p. 16.
18. Vijayalaxmi (no initial) and S. G. Srikantia, A preview of the studies on the wholesomeness of irradiated wheat, conducted at the National Institute of Nutrition, India, *Radiation, Physics, and Chemistry* 34 (1989): 941–952.
19. Vijayalaxmi and Srikantia, 1989.
20. M. F. Jacobsen and S. Schmidt, Food irradiation: Zapping our troubles away? *Nutrition Action Health Letter*, April 1992, pp. 1, 5–7.
21. Anti-food irradiation (editorial), *Priorities*, Spring 1989, p. 41.

U.S. Foodways and the Global Environment

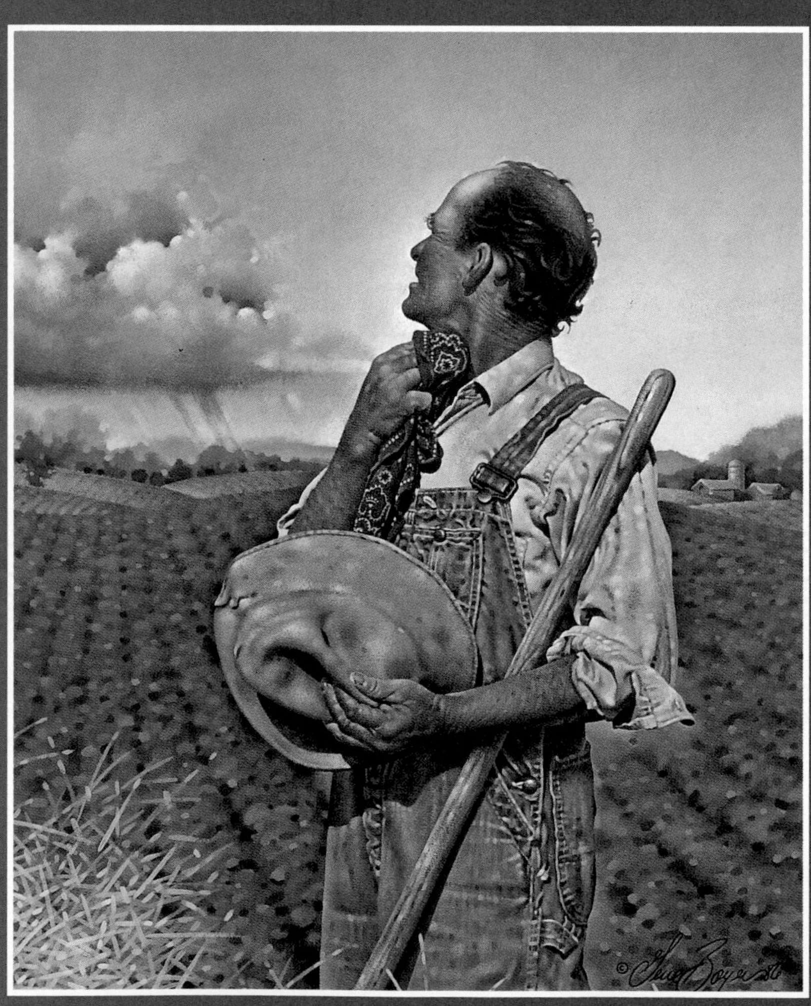

Contents

Gene Boyer, A Painting of the Farmer

15

Most people eat familiar foods out of habit. They often notice food prices, but seldom do they think to ask what price the global environment pays for food. Yet, food production does tax environmental resources and cause pollution, and some aspects of the food industry are more destructive than others. If we realized the impacts of our **foodways,** we might choose differently, yet still eat as well and enjoy our foods as much as we do now.

foodways the sum of the food habits, customs, beliefs, and preferences of a culture.

Among the global resources involved in producing food are irrigation water, fertilizers, pesticides, fuel, land, and fisheries. And in the U.S. market, tons of packaging materials and a massive transportation network convey foods to consumers using immense quantities of fossil fuel. Each truckload of food produced in this country travels, on the average, 1,300 miles to reach the market.[1] It costs 800 calories in fuel to make a can of diet soda that contains 1 calorie of food energy, and more water is used to make the can than to make the soda.[2] An appetizer of shrimp cocktail may contain 4 ounces of shrimp, but to net those shrimp, the fishermen had to kill 2½ pounds of young fish that otherwise could have grown up to provide food.[3]

Choices that are more environmentally benign are available. In place of vegetables shipped in from far away, people might choose to eat vegetables grown in their own home states, at least during the growing seasons. In place of several sodas in aluminum cans, a soda drinker might use one large recyclable bottle. In place of shrimp cocktail, the diner might choose a crab salad or a few oysters harvested without killing other sea creatures.

One person's choice of local carrots, a recyclable bottle, or a seafood salad may seem insignificant, but the choice produces several benefits. For one, a single person's awareness and example, shared with others, may influence many other people over time. For another, an action repeated becomes a habit. For still another, choices made with awareness of their impacts give a person a sense of having some control over those impacts. That sense of personal control, in turn, helps people to take effective action in many arenas. People without a sense of personal control feel hopeless and become ineffective.

In changing both personal lifestyles and the world, students are especially powerful. Students everywhere are helping to change governments, human predicaments, and environmental problems for the better. Student movements have persuaded 127 universities and many institutions, corporations, and government agencies to put pressure on South Africa to end apartheid by withdrawing investments of funds. Student pressure led to the installation of the first deaf president at a university for the deaf. Students offer major services to communities in soup kitchens, home repair, and child education. Student movements hastened the coming of cultural and political autonomy in the other countries, the reform of universities, and advances in peace and human rights causes. Students have launched significant protests against totalitarianism in China and have mounted successful environmental cleanups and defense efforts.[4]

> *"Never doubt that a small group of thoughtful, committed people can change the world. Indeed, it is the only thing that ever has."*
>
> —MARGARET MEAD

This chapter emphasizes personal choices because they raise awareness and pave the way for larger actions. Personal choices are, however, only part of the solution to today's problems. Institutional changes are the other

fossil fuel coal, oil, and natural gas: these are nonrenewable fuels that pollute. (Renewable or *alternative fuels*, such as solar and wind energy, pollute less or not at all.)

sustainable able to continue indefinitely. Here the term refers to the use of resources at such a rate that the earth can keep on replacing them, for example, cutting trees no faster than new ones grow and producing pollutants at a rate with which the environment and human cleanup efforts can keep pace. In a sustainable economy, resources do not become depleted, and pollution does not accumulate.

part—changes in the way agriculture, industry, and government do their business domestically and internationally. Students can become involved in promoting both kinds of change.

KEY POINT Personal choices, made by many people, can have large impacts.

◆ The Need for Change

During the 1990s, all of the following trends are taking place:

- *Hunger, poverty, and population growth.* Millions of people are starving. Fifteen children die of malnutrition every 30 seconds, but 75 children are born during that same 30 seconds.[5]
- *Losses of food-producing land.* Food-producing land is becoming saltier, is eroding, and is being paved over. Each year, the world's farmers try to feed some 90 million more people with 24 billion fewer tons of topsoil.[6] Overall food security is threatened.[7]
- *Accelerating* ***fossil fuel*** *use.* Fuel use is accelerating, with attendant pollution of air, soil, and water; ozone depletion; and global warming.[8]
- *Increasing air pollution.* Air quality is diminishing all over the globe.[9]
- *Global warming, droughts, and floods.* Atmospheric levels of heat-trapping carbon dioxide are now 26 percent higher than the preindustrial concentration and are continuing to climb. As a result, a massive warming trend seems to be taking place.[10] Climate change causes both droughts and floods, which destroy crops and people's homelands.[11]
- *Ozone loss from the outer atmosphere.* The outer atmosphere's protective ozone layer is growing thinner, permitting harmful radiation from the sun to damage crops and ecosystems and to cause cancers and cataracts in people and animals.[12]
- *Water shortages.* The world's supplies of fresh water are dwindling and becoming polluted.[13]
- *Deforestation and desertification.* Forests are shrinking and deserts are growing.[14]
- *Ocean pollution.* Ocean pollution is killing fish; overfishing is depleting the numbers of those that remain.[15]
- *Extinctions of species.* Many extinctions of animals and plants are taking place, a minimum of 140 species *a day*. Another 20 percent of all species are expected to die out in the next ten years. Many kinds of whales, birds, giant mammals, colorful butterflies, and thousands of other animals and plants will never again be seen in the universe.[16]

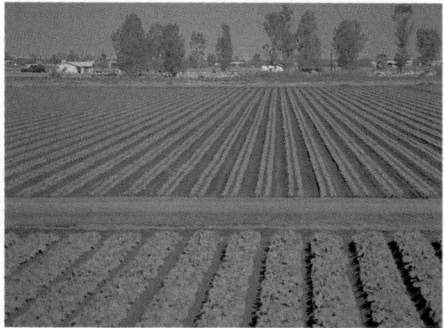

Vast areas are under the plow, and those that must be irrigated are becoming salty and unusable.

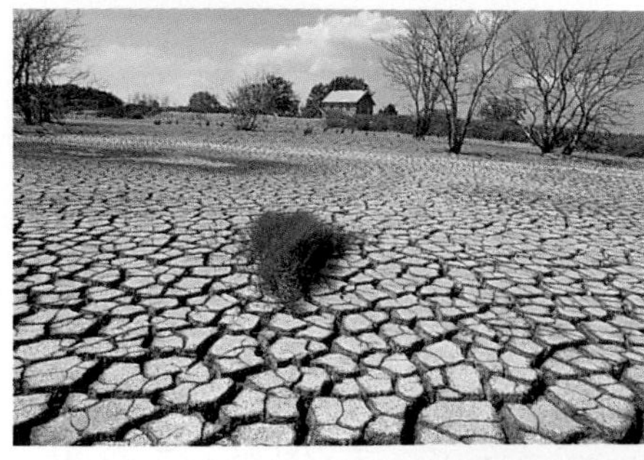

As ground water is used up, deserts spread.

These global problems are all related. The causes overlap, and so do the solutions. To think positively, this means that any initiative a person takes to help solve one problem will help solve many others. Figure 15-1 shows a few of the many interconnections among today's global environmental problems. Figure 15-2 is a repeat of Figure 15-1, and shows how U.S. consumers fit in. It highlights some of our food-related choices and shows the ways in which they contribute to environmental problems.

These environmental problems are developing so fast that scientific research cannot keep pace with them. Many scientists urge that even as causes of the problems are being sought, actions to slow, stop, or reverse these developments should be mounted, based on present estimates of the damage and its causes. For these reasons, much of this chapter is based, not on completed research, but on news reports and on research still in progress. Because much of the environmental degradation seen today comes from our uses of resources and energy in cars and homes, the emphasis here is on those areas. Less use of resources and energy by U.S. consumers could help reduce destructive human impacts on the environment.

Readers may be concerned that lifestyle changes such as those suggested here could cost the loss of some types of jobs and a decline in the quality of life. Fortunately, though, to a large extent new jobs can take the place of the old, and life can become more elegant even as it becomes simpler. People can learn to place more reliance on goods produced in a **sustainable** fashion from renewable resources and to place less reliance on goods produced with intense negative environmental impacts. Some industries can shrink, notably the biggest polluters: primary metals; paper; oil refining; chemicals; and stone, clay, and glass.[17] The industries most likely to be phased out use large amounts of capital and resources and also happen to be the very industries that use the smallest amounts of labor. The local industries most likely to replace them may actually generate more jobs.

In some cases new ***kinds*** of jobs can be created, such as for environmental cleanup work and pollution control. As automobile manufacturing gives way to railroad-car manufacturing, more, not fewer, people will be employed.[18] Renewable energy employs more workers than coal or oil; recycling employs more workers than landfilling; and railroads employ more workers than cars.[19] Some geographical dislocations may take place, but jobs arising from energy conservation, renewables, and recycling can be evenly spread across the country and the world.[20]

Overwhelming evidence shows that the widely held belief that we can take care of the environment *or* the economy, but not both, is a fallacy. Careful planning will be needed, but given the state of the environment today, jobs are most likely to sustain people in the future if they also sustain the environment. Meanwhile, all individuals can begin the process of shifting to a sustainable economy by making the choices described here.

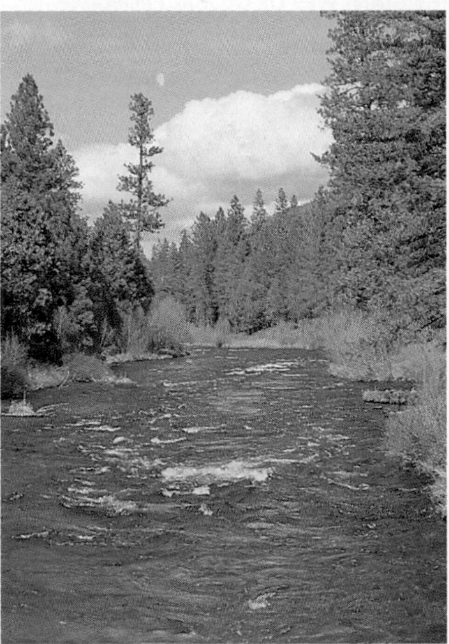

Pure rivers represent irreplaceable water resources.

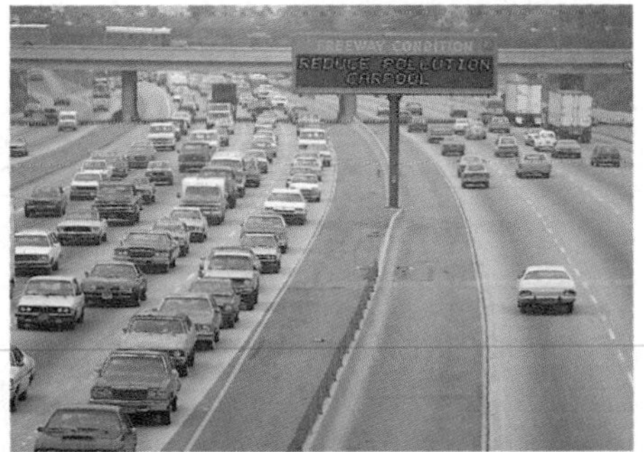

People-generated pollution today comes largely from our cars . . .

 **KEY POINT** Deterioration of the global environment, which supports life, is accelerating. Human uses of resources and energy are largely responsible. Using less need not cost a decline in the quality of life, and may generate jobs.

◆ Environmentally Conscious Food Shopping

Food shopping involves going to the store, selecting foods once there, choosing among the packages in which those foods are sold, and choosing bags in which to carry the foods home. All of these actions exert impacts on the environment, and consumers can choose to minimize those impacts. Consider the shopping trips first.

Shopping Trips

According to a report from the Worldwatch Institute, automobiles have created so many severe problems that future societies will be forced to seek alternative modes of transportation. If they don't, the report says, a series

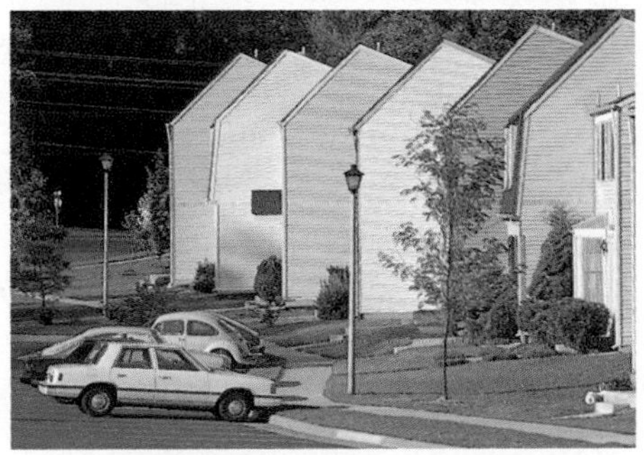

. . . and from our houses.

Figure 15-1

THE GIANT WEB OF GLOBAL PROBLEMS

Follow the arrows to see how each problem intensifies others. Read the key opposite to understand the relationships.

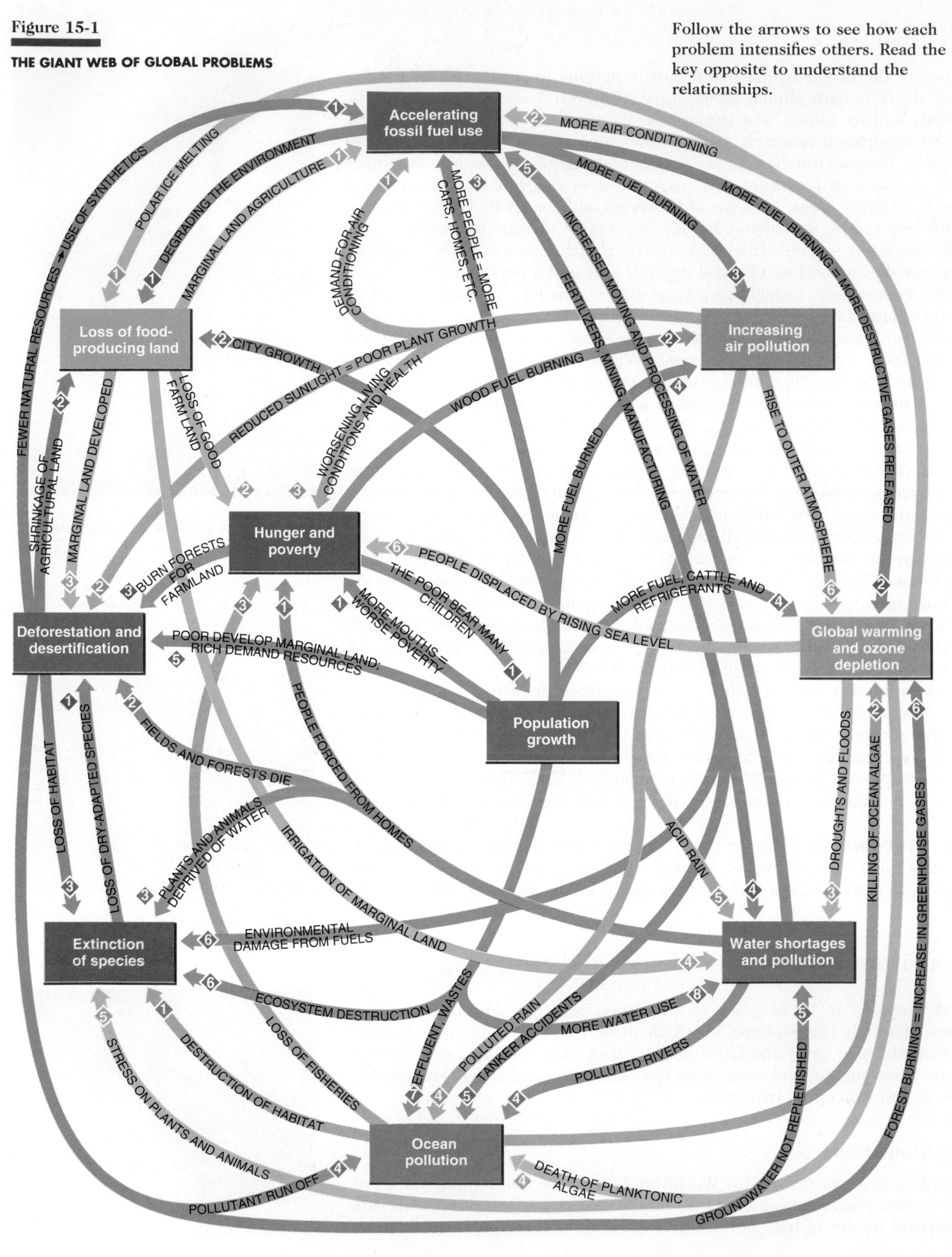

Figure 15-1

THE GIANT WEB OF GLOBAL PROBLEMS (continued)

Each colored number explains an arrow on the diagram opposite and shows how one problem intensifies another.

Hunger and Poverty

1. People living in hunger and poverty are not sure their children will survive, so they bear as many children as they can.
2. Poor people burn wood for fuel.
3. Poor people, being landless, venture into wilderness areas and cut and burn trees to establish plots where they can grow food. Deforested lands tend to dry out and turn to deserts.

Population growth

1. The more mouths there are to feed, the worse the poverty.
2. Growing cities expand into former farmlands.
3. Growing populations and growing use of consumer goods, appliances, and cars intensifies use of gas, coal, and oil for homes, cars, and factories.
4. The more people, the more fuels burned, and the greater the release of global-warming and ozone-destroying gases. Also, more people mean more cattle, which release methane that hastens global warming and ozone loss. More people mean more home and car air conditioners, refrigerators, and freezers and more ozone-destroying refrigerants.
5. Growing populations of poor spread onto marginal lands and destroy the balance of nature that supports plant life.
6. The growing human population, by devouring land and polluting air and water, destroys ecosystems and uses up resources that are required to support other forms of life.
7. Growing populations of poor, living near the ocean, pollute it with their sewage and their garbage. Growing wealthy populations overuse fertilizers and pesticides near coastlines.
8. The more poor, the more water they need to drink and grow their food, and the more human waste they produce. Added wealthy people also use water to support mining and manufacturing and produce consumer goods. The wealthy also produce agricultural and industrial pollution.

Loss of food-producing land

1. As good farmland is paved over, marginal land is recruited for agriculture. Marginal land requires more intensive cultivation and more fertilizer, both using fossil fuels.
2. As good farmland diminishes, food shortages intensify.
3. Some marginal land being recruited for agriculture formerly supported forests; some cannot withstand the pressures of agriculture and become deserts.
4. Marginal land used to grow food crops demands more irrigation, which devours water, salts the land,pollutes waterways.

Accelerating fossil fuel use

1. Air and water pollution from increasing fossil fuel use renders more and more land unsuitable for agriculture.
2. Oil, coal, and gas release carbon dioxide and other gases which accumulate in the atmosphere, trap heat, warm the climate, and destroy outer-atmosphere ozone.
3. Oil, coal, and gas release air pollutants.
4. Fuels and fertilizers made from them pollute rivers. Mining, manufacturing, and other industries deplete and pollute water supplies.
5. Tankers carrying fuels have accidents and oil spills.
6. Fossil fuel pollutants are damaging the environment and upsetting the natural conditions on which all life depends.

Increasing air pollution

1. Polluted air leads people to use more fuel to run air conditioners and purifiers.
2. Air pollution deprives plants of needed sunlight and harms animal and plant life, including food crops.
3. Air pollution destroys health, and worsens poverty.
4. Polluted air, scrubbed by rain, drops pollutants in the ocean.
5. Polluted rain contaminates surface water and groundwater:
6. Air pollutants rise, trap heat, and destroy ozone.

Global warming and ozone depletion

1. As the earth warms, the polar ice caps are melting, causing sea level to rise and land masses to shrink.
2. Warmer climate leads to use of more air conditioning and refrigeration.
3. Global warming causes both droughts and floods, which alternately deplete and pollute water supplies.
4. In a warmer climate, the ocean's planktonic algae, a major global consumer of carbon dioxide and producer of oxygen, may sicken and die. Since these algae also cleanse the ocean, their death may destroy the cleansing mechanism.
5. Warmer climate stresses plants and animals and leads to extinctions. Loss of earth's protective ozone layer lets harmful ultraviolet radiation and heat from the sun reach earth's surface, stressing plants and animals more.
6. Rising seas and shrinking land masses displace people from their homes.

Water shortages and pollution

1. Water shortages render areas unsuitable for human habitation, forcing people from their homes.
2. Water shortages cause fields and forests to dry up and die.
3. Water shortages often wipe out the few remaining members of endangered plant and animal species.
4. Polluted rivers pollute the ocean.
5. More transportation of water over land, desalting of ocean water, and purification of polluted water for reuse means more energy use.

Deforestation and desertification

1. Without wood, people use fossil fuels both for energy and to make wood substitutes such as plastics.
2. As deserts grow, land areas useful for agriculture shrink.
3. Losses of forested or fertile lands rob species of needed habitat.
4. Deforested lands and dried-up wetlands cannot absorb and detain pollutants. Instead, they run off.
5. Forests capture and return water to the earth. Trees also transpire water to the air, contributing to rainfall. Without this cycle, water runs off into rivers and the ocean, for a net loss of fresh water. Forests also purify water; without them, there is more water pollution.
6. Burning of tropical forests releases carbon dioxide that traps planetary heat and leaves fewer trees to remove carbon dioxide from the air.

Ocean pollution

1. Severe ocean pollution may destroy the conditions necessary for life.
2. Ocean pollution is beginning to kill ocean algae, which help moderate the planet's temperature.
3. Ocean pollution kills ocean life, leading to losses of fisheries.

Extinction of species

1. Extinction reduces the number of trees and plants that can grow in marginal areas.

Figure 15-2

U.S. CONSUMPTION PATTERNS CONTRIBUTING TO GLOBAL PATTERNS

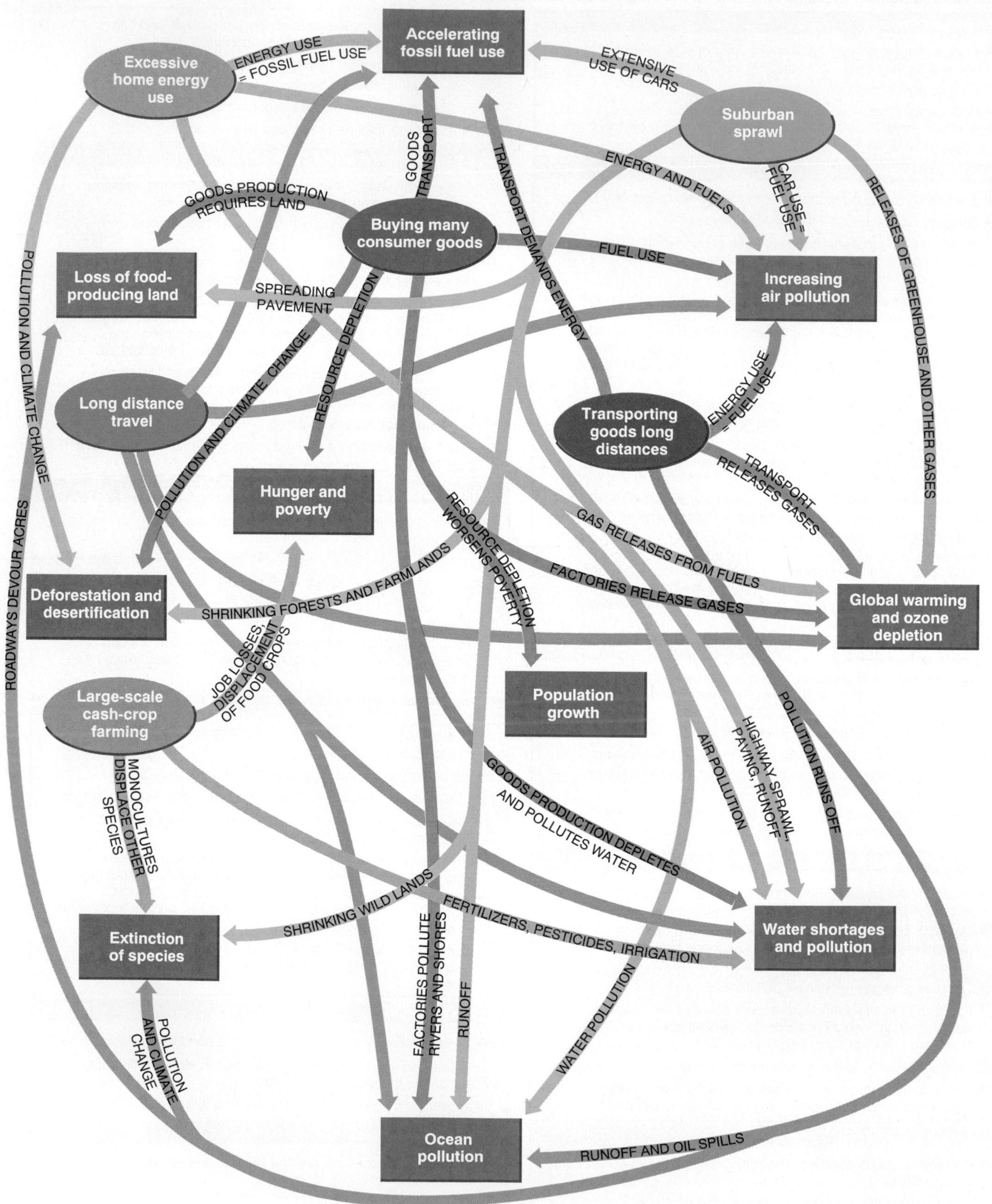

of environmental and economic crises will follow.[21] In late 1990, 400 million cars were in use around the world, and 19 million more cars were being added every year. Even without that increase, motor vehicles were the world's single largest source of air pollution. Air pollution in many regions harms children, the elderly, and people with lung problems; reduces crop yields; causes acid rain; and damages forests. Gasoline use produces major amounts of the global-warming gas, carbon dioxide, with 13 percent of this carbon dioxide coming from cars.[22] Transporting oil to provide gasoline for cars is a major cause of oil spills that harm ocean life.[23]

Alternatives to the use of private cars include car pools, mass transit, walking, and bicycling. These can be made feasible by rearranging cities to bring residences, workplaces, and shopping centers closer together. While pushing for such changes in city design, food shoppers can make the following choices: shop only once a week; share trips; or take turns shopping for each other. When selecting homes, people can consider choosing to live close enough to walk or bicycle to and from the store. When buying a car, a buyer can choose the most fuel-efficient model available of the size needed. By the early 1990s, the U.S. market was offering several cars with fuel efficiency rated at 40 to 50 miles to the gallon or better. The impacts of these choices can become globally significant, if more and more families use less and less fuel over whole lifetimes.

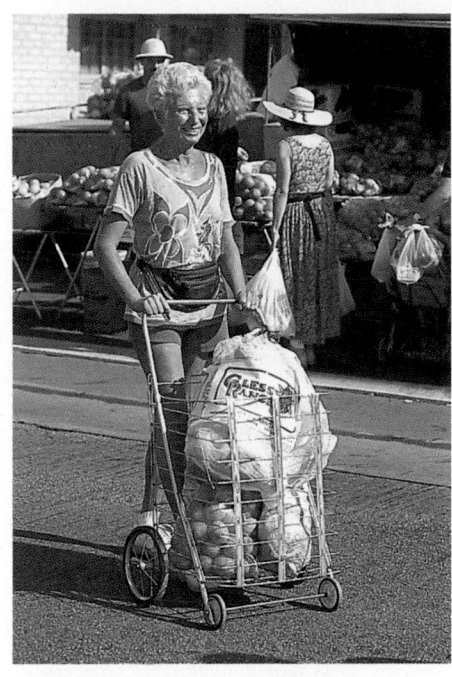

Shopping without a car can be a pleasure, if you can afford the time.

To make it possible to shop for a week's meals at a time, a shopper can plan to buy foods with various shelf lives and to eat the most perishable ones first. For example, buy lettuce, cabbage, squash, and carrots. Use up the lettuce first, then the squash. The carrots and cabbage keep longer, so eat these later. Buy fruits of differing ripeness—for example, six bananas: two ripe, two nearly ripe, and two green. Use the ripe ones right away and the others as they become ripe. On first arriving home, cook the meats for the early meals; portion out the rest and freeze them. Also freeze the bread and milk that won't be needed until midweek. These strategies save time and money as well as fossil fuels.

KEY POINT Widespread automobile use causes air pollution, health problems, and environmental damage. To reduce automobile use will require rearranging cities; but even now, shoppers can choose to make fewer trips to grocery stores.

Foods to Choose

Chapter 2 described the USDA Daily Food Guide from the point of view of nutritional health. The guide recommends that adults eat 11 or more servings of plant foods (especially vegetables and grains) daily and only 4 or 5 servings of milk products and meats combined. Environmentally it is also beneficial to eat low on the food chain, that is, to eat plants, rather than to eat the animals that eat plants (see Figure 15-3). Pointers on low-meat and nonmeat meals have been given in Controversy 6 and in Chapters 6, 7, 8, and 12.

Growing animals for their meat and dairy products by feeding them grain uses more land than growing grain for direct use by people. Animals also use more water, add more pollution to waterways, and, in general, cause destruction of more native vegetation and wildlife than equivalent amounts of plants (equivalent, say, in calories). More fossil fuels are required just to grow the feed for animals: to run tractors, harvest feed grain, and transport

Figure 15-3

EATING LOW ON THE FOOD CHAIN SAVES RESOURCES

It takes ten times as much land and fuel to feed people meat as to feed them plants. (Reminder: The *food chain* is the sequence in which living things depend on other living things for food. Thus small fish eat algae, large fish eat small fish, and human beings may eat large fish. Algae are near the bottom, human beings at the top of the food chain. Similarly, on land, cattle eat grain and human beings eat beef, again locating meat-eating human beings at the top of the food chain. A figure showing bioaccumulation of toxins at the top of the food chain appears on p. 532.)

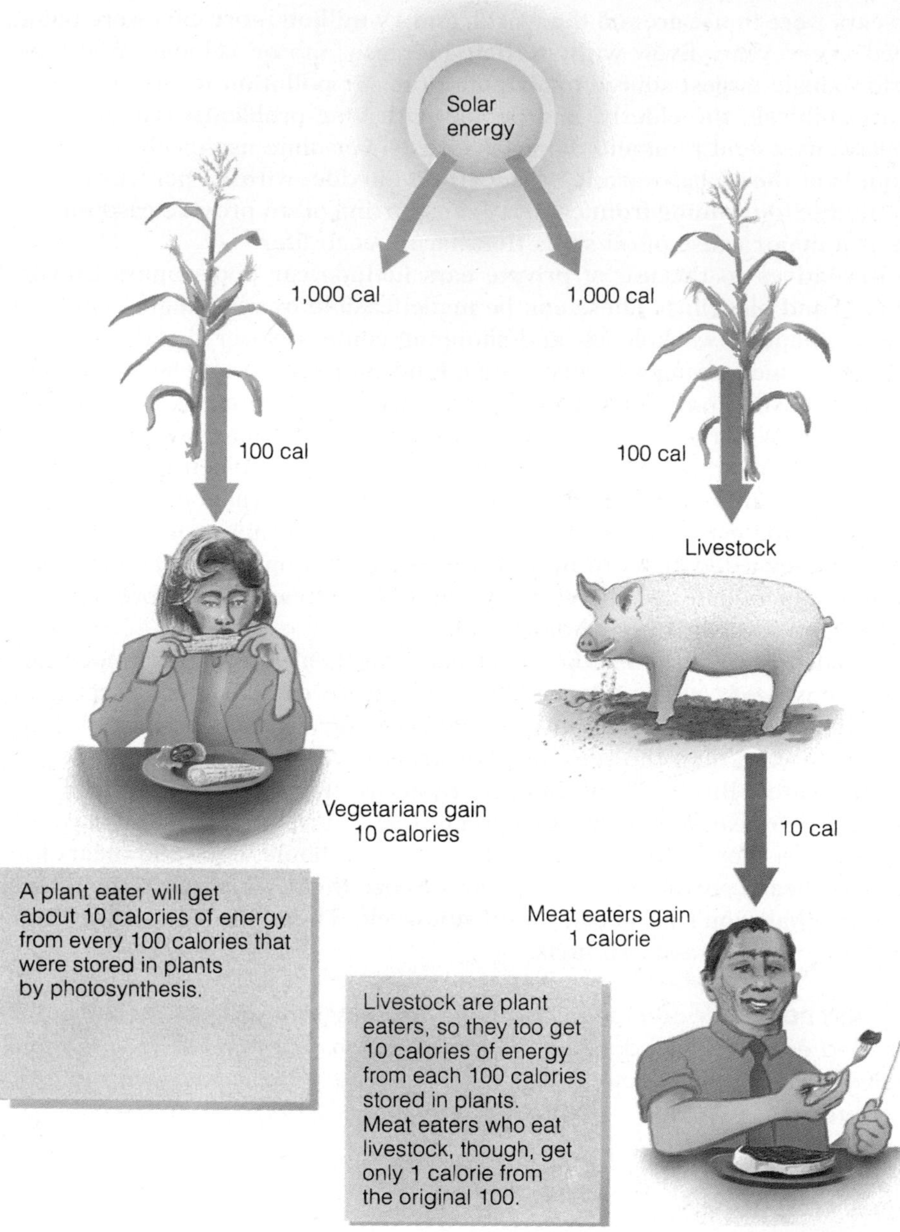

it. Growing the feed pollutes the environment with fertilizers and pesticides, and the animals' waste pollutes it further.[24]

Meat and dairy producers can change the ways they raise animals so as to do less harm. Some already have done so. Guidelines for environmentally sound ways to raise animals for meat and dairy products are available; some are described in the Controversy that follows this chapter.

It also makes sense, as far as possible, to avoid buying canned beef products of any kind, including soups, stews, chili, corned beef, and even pet food. Some of these foods come at the expense of cleared rainforest land in Central America: 200 square feet of rainforest are lost *permanently* for each *pound* of beef produced from cattle raised on the cleared land.[25] (Rainforest soil wears out within only a few years when used to raise cattle; the practice is not sustainable. To keep raising cattle, ranchers have to clear more land, and the forest cannot grow back on the ruined soil.[26])

Consumers cannot tell which products contain rainforest beef because labeling laws require no such disclosures. Once inspected at the ports of entry, beef coming into the country is simply labeled "USDA inspected"; it is not labeled as to country of origin. Even bulk buyers such as canners and fast-food chains cannot know whether the beef they buy is domestic or imported, unless they make special efforts to find out. The only way consumers can be sure they are not buying rainforest beef is to buy no canned beef at all.

Instead, buy products grown sustainably within the rainforest. People who live in the forest have grown their own food there for untold generations, and they can also produce products for export from the forest—all, without cutting it down. Examples of sustainably-produced, exportable items include brazil nuts, cashews, and fruits harvested from forest trees or candies or ice cream made from those nuts and fruits. If the people who depend on the forest to produce these products can make a living from them, they will preserve the forest along with their own way of life.

Consistent with these recommendations, for those who eat meat, is to eat it less often and in smaller portions and to select range-fed beef and buffalo or poultry and fish more often than feedlot beef or pork. Chickens are raised in most local regions at a lower cost in grain, land, and pollution than other meats.[27] Among fish, small and medium-sized fish are lower on

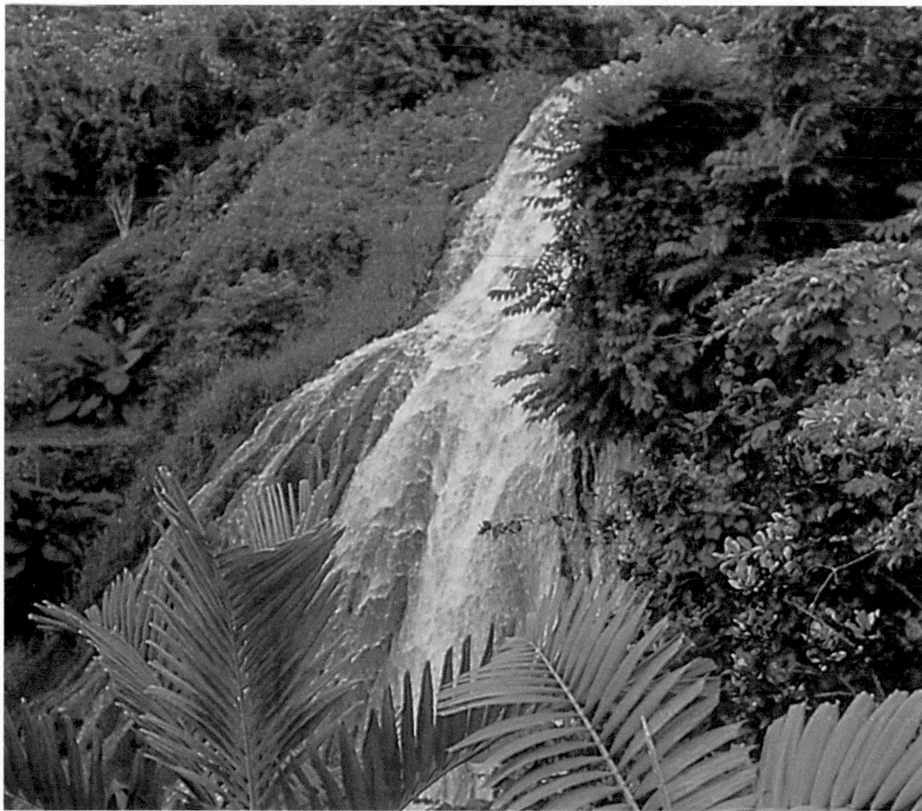

The rainforest meets two basic needs of life by generating oxygen and rain.

the food chain than the large predators that eat them. Along the southeastern coast, this means fish such as mullet, snapper, and flounder; along the west coast, it means salmon and ocean fish like cod; and inland, it means river and lake fish such as walleyed pike and bass. Small fish are preferable to large fish because large fish are becoming rare due to overfishing. Tuna, swordfish, and shark are examples.[28] Cod are rapidly disappearing off the New England coast and almost none are found further north. Some species of shark are becoming scarce due to overfishing.[29] Despite precautions, tuna fishing still kills many dolphins.[30] And one small shellfish that is harvested unsustainably has already been mentioned: shrimp. The mesh of shrimp nets is so fine that shrimpers cannot help catching many young fish. These die in the nets, depleting the adult stocks of many types of fish.[31] (Shrimp farming may help to solve this problem: it is both sustainable and labor intensive.)

Local fish should be emphasized because they are transported shorter distances. Fish frozen, packaged, refrigerated, and flown in from far away may be just as good for health, but the cost in fuel and pollution is higher. The same principle applies to meats and poultry. People in Texas can eat range-fed beef; people in Ohio can eat poultry raised nearby; and so forth.

Health considerations justify some of these choices. Buffalo fat and the fat of poultry and fish are less saturated than beef fat. Fatty acids from fish are valued for their purported blood pressure-lowering, cholesterol-lowering, cancer-opposing effects. Ground turkey, if the skin is not ground up with the meat, makes a fine low-fat substitute for ground beef, especially in mixed dishes such as spaghetti sauce. As for fish, small fish are the least likely to contain toxins due to the bioaccumulation effect. Consumers who do not find the items they want in the store can ask the manager to carry them. If enough people create a demand, the supply will appear.

The guideline to buy foods grown close to home when possible applies to plant foods as well. Locally grown foods have required less fuel for transportation to the market. Less fuel may also have been required to pack them, label them, and keep them cold if fresh. Figure 15-4 shows the energy required to produce canned and frozen corn, compared with the energy in the corn itself. Clearly, from this point of view, local farmers' markets are an excellent place to shop, if they are not too far from home. From the nutrition standpoint, although some frozen and canned foods are high in salt, some may be the nutritional equal of fresh foods. However, for the environment's sake, fresh foods grown nearby may be preferable.

Switching to local products doesn't always save money. Products produced on giant, corporation-owned farms in the United States, Mexico, or other countries may cost less. Giant corporations can keep their prices low by underpaying farm workers and can take advantage of tax money the government makes available to help pay for their machinery, fuel, fertilizer, and other inputs. But giant farms are often giant polluters, so switching to local products may pay off environmentally. It may also help relieve world hunger, for the mass production of export crops at low wages keeps people poor in the developing countries. A consumer can choose to support local small farmers, even if it costs a little more to do so. Students can request that their school and college cafeterias do the same.

The problems of pollution caused by giant farms are discussed in Controversy 15.

KEY POINT Environmentally sound food choices include domestic range-fed beef and buffalo; poultry and fish; avoidance of canned beef products; rainforest products; locally harvested small fish; and locally grown plant foods.

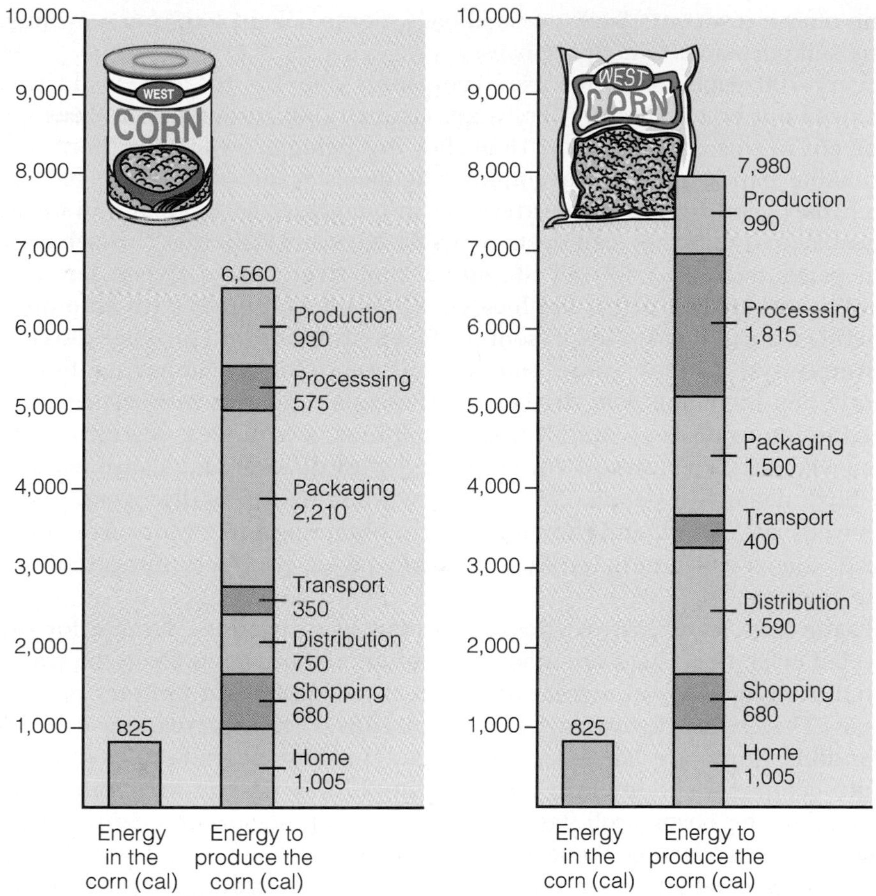

Figure 15-4

ENERGY COSTS OF CANNED AND FROZEN CORN

The corn contains only 825 calories per kilogram, but look how much energy goes to produce it.

Source: D. Pimentel, *Food, Energy and the Future of Society* (Boulder, Colo: Associated University Press, 1980).

Food Packages and Grocery Bags

Foods come in numerous packages, including cans, shrink-wrap, foam trays, waxed cardboard, clay-coated cardboard, plastic bottles, and glass jars. It costs energy and resources to make these packages, and it may cost land or pollution to dispose of them. In general, what is best for the environment is *no* packages; next best are minimal, reusable, or recyclable ones.

Fresh produce can often be bought with minimal or no packaging. Most large stores package meats in foam trays, but shoppers can ask that they be wrapped in butcher paper and can always get fish that way. As for processed foods, shoppers can buy juices in large glass bottles (not small individual cartons); grain products in bulk (not in separate little packages); and eggs in compostable pressed fiber cartons (not foam, unless it is recycled locally). Shoppers can look for labels that boast of environmentally sound products and packaging. Although such labels may sometimes be misleading, they do show that the company is aware of the need. Ask questions. What is most environmentally benign keeps changing as manufacturers and recyclers vie with one another to meet this demand. An example of food companies' ingenuity is the development of more packaging materials that are edible, similar to sausage casings and apple skins.[32]

As for grocery bags, they represent a huge drain on energy and resources, and many consumers are demanding alternatives to throwaway bags. In response, some stores offer incentives to encourage reuse and recycling.

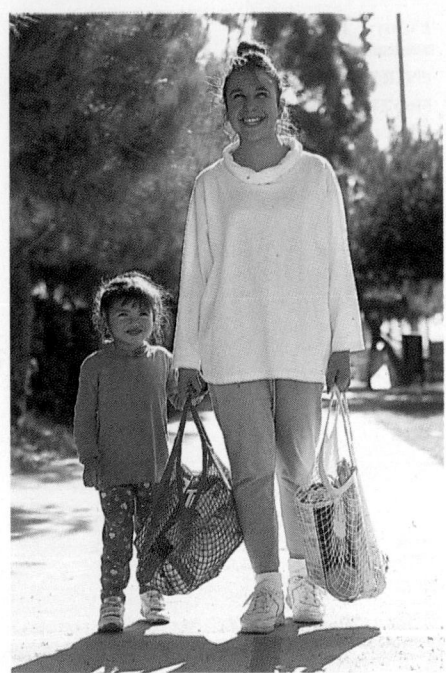

Reusable bags require the fewest resources.

Some offer a few cents back on used bags. Some accept bags for recycling. Some sell permanent shopping bags.

Every 700 paper bags not used represents one 15- to 20-year-old tree that need not be cut down.[33] Trees are a renewable resource, but trees are being cut in this country faster than they are being grown.[34] Furthermore, in making paper, pulp mills employ chemicals such as chlorine bleach, which they then release into waterways in quantities so large and in forms so destructive that they can destroy whole bays and fisheries.[35] Discharges from paper mills may kill all life along long stretches of rivers, bays, or coastlines where the plants are located. Chlorine combines with ammonia, a chemical always naturally present in the environment, to produce dioxins. In waterways, dioxins cause tumors and reproductive abnormalities in aquatic life, including fish. Arriving in the ocean, dioxins are suspected of contributing to diseases and deaths of dolphins, sea turtles, sea birds, and other wildlife. Groundwater contaminated with dioxins may cause cancers and birth defects in people. When such contamination is discovered, people's wells are closed, and they must begin obtaining their water from elsewhere. Many consumers avoid disposable paper products altogether for these reasons.

Plastic bags, like most plastics, are a petroleum product. Except for the recycled ones, these bags are made from oil, much of which has to be transported from far away at a great cost in fuel, oil spills, and military preparedness. Then when thrown away, many plastics persist for years or decades in landfills. Some are labeled "degradable," but few degrade fully to pure, simple compounds. Some are made of tiny bits of plastic interlaced with cornstarch; the cornstarch degrades, but the tiny plastic bits remain with unknown consequences. Some would degrade if exposed to sun and air, but end up buried under other trash. Some plastics contain the toxic heavy metal mercury, which is released into the air or water when they disintegrate or are burned. Mercury bioaccumulates in fish and wildlife; its concentration in some lake fish has led to advisories that warn people to refrain from eating the fish.

Some plastics are recyclable, but the process is cumbersome. Consumers must learn and remember to return each type of plastic to its special bin free of other materials. If a consumer accidentally drops a degradable plastic bag into a batch of recyclable ones, this renders the entire batch nonrecyclable.

For all these reasons, many shoppers prefer to carry reusable shopping bags to the store and refuse all others. Failing in this, they ask for plastic bags if they are recyclable—and then take care to recycle them. The third choice would be paper bags, and last would be nonrecyclable plastic.

KEY POINT The ways foods are packaged exert environmental impacts. Best for the environment are no packages; next best are minimal, reusable, or recyclable ones. To carry foods home, permanent reusable bags are most environmentally benign.

Environmentally Conscious Cooking

Cooking has many environmental impacts. The following sections discuss the cooking methods; the utensils, materials, and appliances used; the table settings; the water used; and the disposal of trash and garbage.

Cooking Methods

Fast cooking saves fuel and so pollutes less. Asian meals exemplify this principle: they are made of precut, bite-sized pieces of food, stir-fried fast in small amounts of oil. This cooking style both saves energy and preserves nutrients.

The pressure cooker or the microwave can also cook foods fast. The pressure cooker can do the occasional big piece of meat the cook wants to serve whole; the microwave can cook vegetables, casseroles, or leftovers. Both may save using several burners on the stove, and both preserve nutrients better than most stove-top methods.

The oven, in contrast, can be a fuel waster. Efficient oven use is possible if the cook bakes or roasts a lot of food at one time and keeps the oven door closed. To keep the stove top from being an energy waster, a cook can use flat-bottomed pots with close-fitting lids that completely cover the burners. That way, each burner will donate all its heat to cooking something, not just heating the kitchen (and the planet). One can also turn electric burners and ovens off before the food is fully cooked and let the cooking finish as the stove cools.

KEY POINT Cut-up, quick-cooked foods use the least fuel. Pressure cooking and microwaving are energy-efficient cooking methods.

Cooking Utensils and Aids

Among utensils, a cook rightly refuses throwaway products and instead prizes pots and pans that heat well and evenly, prove durable over repeated uses, and clean up easily. If well cared for, pots and pans can be kept in condition so that foods will not stick to them. To prevent foods from sticking, the user can apply a little oil or shortening by hand or with the corner of a clean washable cloth.

Spray products other than pump sprays have several environmental disadvantages. Many of the propellants used in them pollute the air and even rise to destroy outer-atmosphere ozone. The most damaging of the propellants used in spray products, chlorofluorocarbons (or CFCs), have been banned from such use, but their replacements are not innocuous. Furthermore, once empty, spray cans are hard to recycle, because they are made of so many different materials. They are, in fact, a classic example of the use-once, throwaway mentality that keeps our society from developing a sustainable lifestyle.

Aluminum foil, used to line pans, is another throwaway product. Aluminum mining consumes large amounts of fuel and water; it involves land-destroying strip mining; and it pollutes the soil, water, and groundwater with toxic materials. The mining of aluminum is one of the world's most environmentally destructive industries; aluminum use approaches sustainability only if the aluminum is recycled.[36] (Remember, even recycling costs energy.) Cans are recyclable but in most places foil is not.

Other cooking aids that people thoughtlessly use and throw away include paper towels, plastic wrap, plastic storage bags, sponges, and many more. For each of these, a permanent substitute is available: cloth towels, reusable storage containers with lids, and dishcloths.

Even when first equipping a kitchen, a person need not buy all-new pots, pans, and utensils. Thrift shops sell preowned ones that may be of higher quality than new ones.

active solar use of photovoltaic panels to generate electricity from sunlight. (A *passive solar* home is built to minimize heating and cooling costs by taking advantage of the available sun and shade.)

photovoltaic (PV) panels panels that convert light (photons) into electricity (volts).

KEY POINT For cooking and storing foods, permanent utensils, storage containers, and cleanup aids are most environmentally benign. Throwaways and most aerosol products are generally undesirable.

Kitchen Appliances

All appliances use energy, which is almost invariably generated from fossil fuels. A naive consumer might say, "I don't use fossil fuels to cook with; my kitchen is all electric." But electricity, of course, is most often generated by burning fossil fuels, only at the power plant rather than at the point of use. Therefore the fewer the appliances and the shorter the times they are used, the better for the air, water, soil, and atmosphere. Realizing this, many consumers today are returning to "old-fashioned" ways of doing things, such as beating eggs with whisks and cutting vegetables with knives rather than using electric mixers and food processors.

Doing without small electrical appliances saves more than just the small bits of energy the appliances would consume during use. It also saves the energy it would have cost to manufacture, transport, package, advertise, and market the appliances themselves. In addition, it saves the landfill space they take up when discarded.

What is true of small appliances is also true of large ones, but with exceptions. The appliances that use the most energy per minute are not necessarily the biggest energy guzzlers. Many people believe, for example, that the range uses more energy than the refrigerator, but this is not true. While in use, the range uses more, but most ranges are in use for only an hour or so a day at most, whereas most refrigerators run almost continuously. Therefore refrigerators are by far the greater energy consumers. Refrigerators are, in fact, the appliances that use the most energy in most people's homes. Figure 15-5 shows their estimated impacts on global warming, as well as the impacts of some other large energy users.

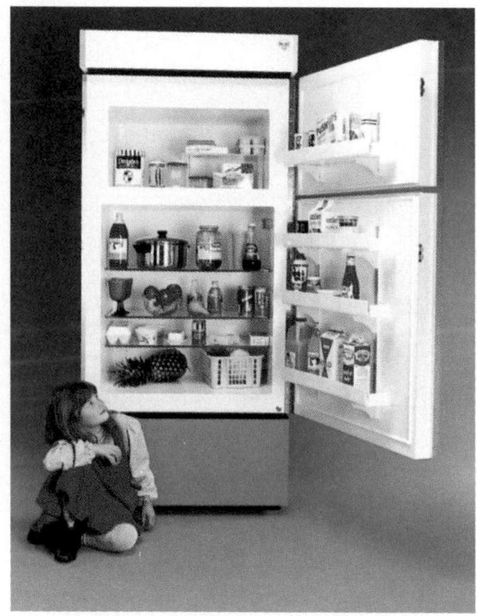

Energy-Saving Refrigerator. This refrigerator requires less than a twentieth of the energy from a regular refrigerator, but chills and freezes food as well. The motor is small, releases little heat, and is on top. In contrast, a "regular" refrigerator's large motor, which is below the unit, heats the very unit it is trying to cool, an inefficient design.

Consumers can take several steps to minimize the energy a refrigerator uses, within the limits of food safety requirements. If operated at 37°F to 40°F, with the freezer at 0°F, the refrigerator will keep foods fresh and gain in energy savings. A refrigerator kept 10°F too cold may use up to 25 percent more energy than necessary.[37] Examples of other energy-conserving steps are: Put a reminder on the calendar to clean the coils at least once a year. Keep the insulating gaskets around the door clean and in good repair. Keep the freezer and refrigerator compartments full—if not with food, then with closed containers of ice or air. That way, when opened, the doors will not let in a lot of room-temperature air. Most of the work the refrigerator and freezer do is to recool air admitted when the doors have been opened.

When buying a new refrigerator, read the energy label. Choose a model based on its energy use, not on bells and whistles such as ice makers and picnic compartments.

About 20,000 U.S. families are now using solar energy to meet most of their homes' electricity needs and can refrigerate their food this way. In an **active solar** home, the sun's light strikes **photovoltaic (PV) panels** on the roof. The panels convert the light energy to electrical energy, which is stored in a large battery. Having a battery permits the option of purchasing DC (direct current) appliances, which use ths sun's energy instead of the energy of fossil fuel.* For example, *no* fossil fuel is used by a DC refrigerator

*This book was written in an office that the authors converted to run on solar PV panels. They keep their lunches in a DC refrigerator there.

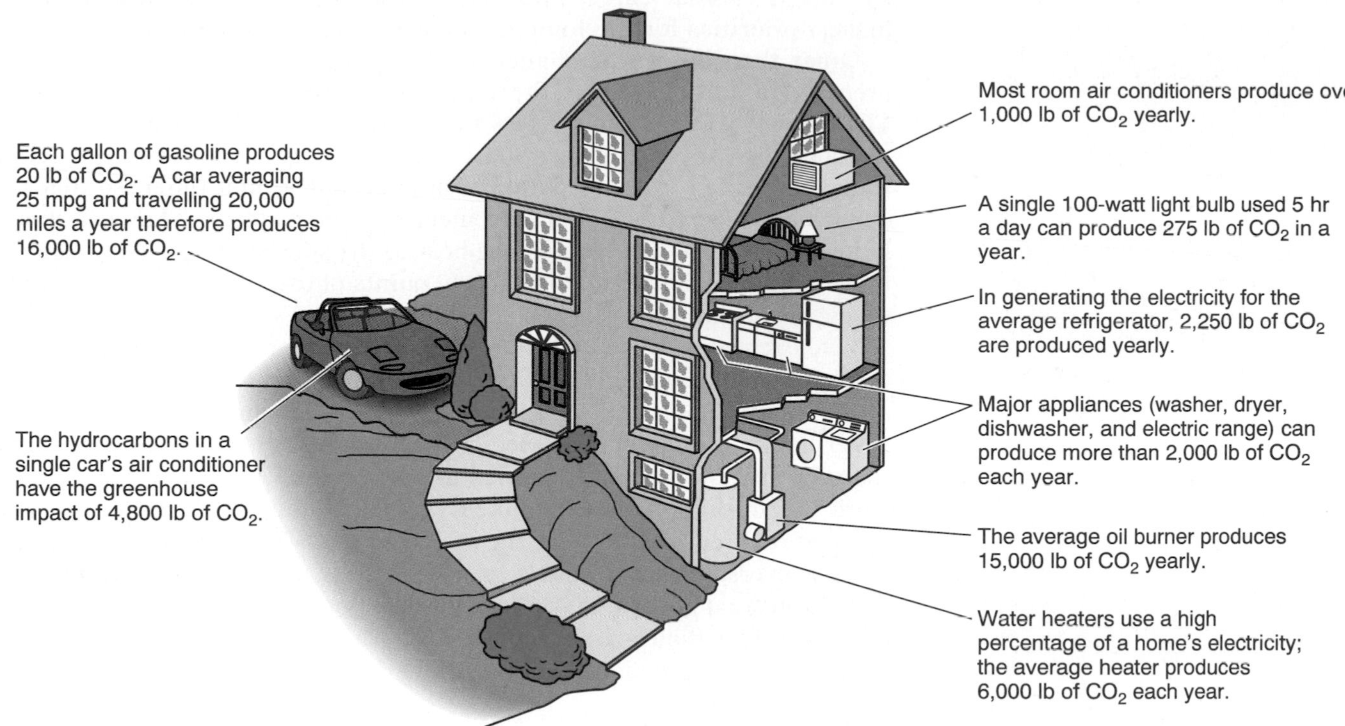

Each gallon of gasoline produces 20 lb of CO_2. A car averaging 25 mpg and travelling 20,000 miles a year therefore produces 16,000 lb of CO_2.
The hydrocarbons in a single car's air conditioner have the greenhouse impact of 4,800 lb of CO_2.
Most room air conditioners produce over 1,000 lb of CO_2 yearly.
A single 100-watt light bulb used 5 hr a day can produce 275 lb of CO_2 in a year.
In generating the electricity for the average refrigerator, 2,250 lb of CO_2 are produced yearly.
Major appliances (washer, dryer, dishwasher, and electric range) can produce more than 2,000 lb of CO_2 each year.
The average oil burner produces 15,000 lb of CO_2 yearly.
Water heaters use a high percentage of a home's electricity; the average heater produces 6,000 lb of CO_2 each year.

Figure 15-5

ESTIMATED CONTRIBUTIONS TO GLOBAL WARMING BY CARS AND HOME APPLIANCES

Each year the United States adds almost 5 trillion pounds to the carbon dioxide (CO_2) content of the atmosphere, mostly by using fossil fuels for energy. Emissions of chlorofluorocarbons (CFCs), methane, and other gases trap as much atmospheric heat as another 4 trillion pounds of CO_2. Although the United States has less than 1/20 of the world's population, it is responsible for more than 1/6 of global-warming emissions.

Source: Adapted from a figure, "Household Sources of Greenhouse Gases," *Nucleus*, Summer 1990, p. 5. Permission granted by the Union of Concerned Scientists.

run on solar electricity. Sunlight is free, reliable, and pollution free. PV panels do not work equally efficiently in all parts of the world, but they do make electricity even in cloudy weather and at temperate latitudes such as in Germany.

The high initial costs of PV panels, battery, and DC refrigerator prohibit most people from taking this option readily, but those who can afford to get started can meet most of their homes' electrical needs with solar energy, reduce electric bills, and recoup their initial investments within 5 to 15 years. Thereafter, their electricity is virtually free, compliments of the sun. (Most electrical appliances such as television sets, microwave ovens, and the like run on AC. Direct current from a battery can be converted to AC by running it through a device called an inverter; it can then be used to operate all but the largest energy guzzlers in a home.)*

If this discussion of solar energy seems to have strayed far from the subject of food and nutrition, remember that energy is the major raw "material" in food production. When energy costs rise, food costs rise, too, as the painful experiences of 1970s consumers attested. Also, the energy use associated with U.S. food production, transport, preparation, and storage is contributing to air pollution, ozone depletion, and perhaps global warming as well. According to the Worldwatch Institute's *State of the World, 1992,*

*Most people are familiar with solar thermal devices, which use the sun's energy to heat water for homes or to heat oil to generate steam and make electricity in centralized power plants. PV panels use the sun's energy to generate electricity. Even in hazy or cloudy conditions, they work efficiently for many hours a day.

converting to solar energy and reducing use of automobiles are among the highest priorities for the human race if it is to save the planet.[38]

Other than kitchen appliances, a big energy user associated with food preparation and cleanup is the water heater (again, look at Figure 15-5). The less hot water used, the less fuel must be burned to heat that water.

People can save water-heating energy in many ways. They can set the water heater at 130°F, not hotter. They can put it on a timer, so that each day it heats just enough water to meet that day's needs. They can wrap it in insulation to keep it from losing heat to the surroundings. They can wrap the hot-water pipes all the way to the points of use. They can install water-saving faucets and shower heads.

When replacing a water heater or installing a new one, a consumer can opt for a small, instantaneous-type water heater that heats the water only at the point of use, and only when needed. A consumer can choose a gas water heater, rather than an electric one. Natural gas is a cleaner fossil fuel than the coal or oil usually burned to make electricity. Solar water heaters work well in sunny regions; unlike PV panels, though, thermal water panels do require direct sun to heat the water. Perhaps rebates or loans to make these conversions are available from the utility company or from the local, state, or federal government. The utility company may offer an energy audit or survey in which an expert will visit the customer's home and make energy-saving suggestions.

KEY POINT Among kitchen appliances, the refrigerator is the biggest energy user but efficient use is possible. Water heaters are usually still greater energy users but alternative modes of heating water can be energy efficient.

Food Serving, Dish Washing, and Trash Disposal

Having rendered the kitchen as nonpolluting and energy efficient as possible, people can do the same thing in the dining room, at the kitchen counter, or on the TV tray. People can use "real" plates, cups, and glasses. They can use cloth napkins, which demand no extra energy to wash and dry because they can fit into existing washloads. School cafeterias can take similar steps, and will do so if students support them in making the change. Studies sometimes show that throwaway plates and utensils cost more, not only in resources but also in money spent by the school, than permanent china washed in dishwashers. If they do use throwaways, cafeterias can recycle them. They can also buy recycled products to close the loop, that is, to provide a market for recycled materials.

As for cleanup, someone who washes many dishes at a time should consider using a dishwasher, if it is affordable. People may think that the cost of the water, heat, and soap would be higher than the cost of washing by hand, but this is not the case. One school found that a normal machine cycle used on full loads consumed less than two thirds the water used in hand washing.[39] Using less hot water also means using less electricity to heat it. The savings are greatest if the dishes are not prerinsed and are allowed to air dry.

Once dinner is over and the dishes are washed, the trash and garbage remain to be disposed of. An average American household of four people produces about 100 pounds of trash a week, much of it from the kitchen.[40] National concern has focused on this issue, because the nation is running out of landfill space in which to dispose of all the trash. Landfill space is, however, only one of many problems associated with trash. Every item thrown away is a resource lost: an aluminum can could be used to make a new aluminum can; a cereal box, but for its clay coating, could become recycled paper; a plastic bottle could become part of a beautiful carpet.* Trash need not become an undesirable mess; recycled trash could be viewed as a usable resource. Yet as it is now, about 70 percent of all the metal mined in the United States is used only once and then discarded. The aluminum thrown away every three months could rebuild the entire U.S. air fleet.[41]

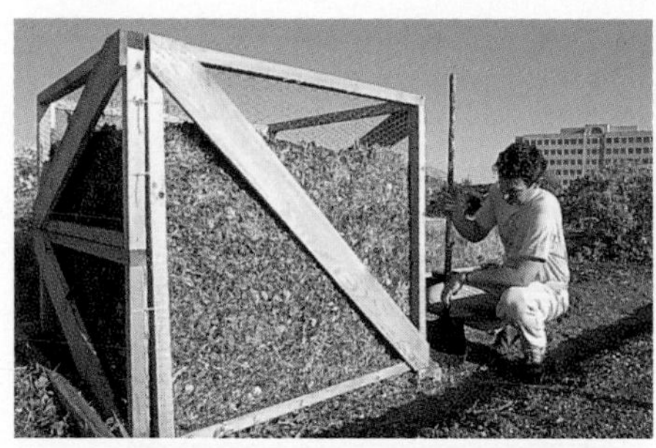

Compost nourishes plants as food nourishes people.

In many college settings, students have successfully mobilized to demand recycling on campus. Once all the recyclable materials have been collected, students can study their own trash to identify what remains to be thrown away. They can then demand recycling of those items or stop buying them.

Individual consumers can do the same thing. As an example, suppose you can recycle glass, plastic, and cans, but not foam. On the next trip to the store, choose only vegetables and eggs that are packaged in compostable fiber cartons. (Write to the stores and manufacturers to make sure your action is felt where it counts.) Some people pride themselves on generating only one small bag of trash a week (total, not just from the kitchen). Some even find ways to generate no trash at all.

Garbage is a special case of a resource generated in the kitchen. Vegetable scraps, fruit peelings, and leftover plant foods are organic and biodegradable, like the leaves and grass cuttings people rake up in their yards. All of these materials can be piled up together with some soil and allowed to decompose naturally, forming compost, a rich, crumbly material that can be used as in nature to fertilize growing things. Some communities, recognizing this, conduct composting programs to recycle people's organic debris; some homeowners maintain their own composting piles. College campuses can use composted kitchen waste, mixed with grass cuttings and weeds, to mulch, fertilize and enrich the soil they use in landscaping. Composting can even be done indoors in small odor-free bins and the resulting material used to pot plants.[42]

Having adopted domestic foodways that respect the environment at home, people can apply the same principles elsewhere. When they buy take-out food, they can bring their own reusable cups and containers to put it in. When eating out at school, work, or on trips, they can continue to recycle throwaways. Even when ordering from fast-food places, customers can patronize only those that use no plastic packaging and no rainforest beef. They can pass their own plates and thermoses through the window to be filled (and then wash and dry them well for reuse). They can refuse the tiny packages of catsup, salt, and sauces that amount to many tons of trash every year. At work, people can institute recycling programs, insist on using their own china mugs for coffee, and adopt many other resource-saving, energy-saving practices.

The personal rewards of all of these behaviors are many, from savings in money to personal satisfaction. But are they all really necessary? Do they really help? The next section shows that if enough people join in, they do help. The section focuses on just one of the major global problems introduced in Figure 15-1—hunger. Review that figure; notice how many other global problems contribute to hunger; and observe that the many suggestions offered here could therefore help relieve hunger.

---

*The authors' office floor is covered with a luxurious wall-to-wall carpet made of recycled plastic soda and catsup bottles—45 bottles per square yard.

food insecurity intermittent hunger caused by lack of money or lack of control over other resources needed to assure a reliable food supply; the predominant form of hunger in the United States today.

KEY POINT Use of permanent dishware saves energy and water. Use of recycled products is also a good choice, as is recycling of throwaways. Dishwashers, if used efficiently, can save energy and water, compared to hand washing. For trash, recycling; and for garbage, composting are the ideal disposal methods.

Hunger and the Environment

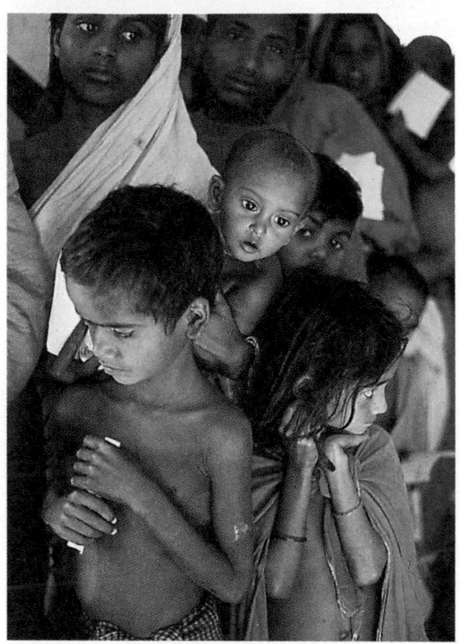
Hungry people in the developing world.

In the early 1990s, one person in every ten worldwide was experiencing hunger—not the healthy hunger we all feel, which leads us to sit down and eat a hearty meal, but the chronic, painful hunger people feel when no food is available. Today, hundreds of millions of people are suffering from chronic hunger, both in the developing world and at home in the United States. Many are dying of starvation: tens of thousands each day, one every two seconds.[43] Many are children. Some studies show that, in the United States, one of every five children is chronically hungry, living in a family that does not know where its next meal is coming from, or when it will come.[44] Such hunger is called **food insecurity,** and it stems, not from the lack of food nearby to purchase, but from the lack of money with which to buy the food.[45]

Food insecurity is not always easy to recognize. Table 15-1 shows how national surveys identify it in the United States. A family that would answer "Yes" to the questions in the table is a family that suffers from this type of hunger. Such hunger affects not just individual families but the whole nation:

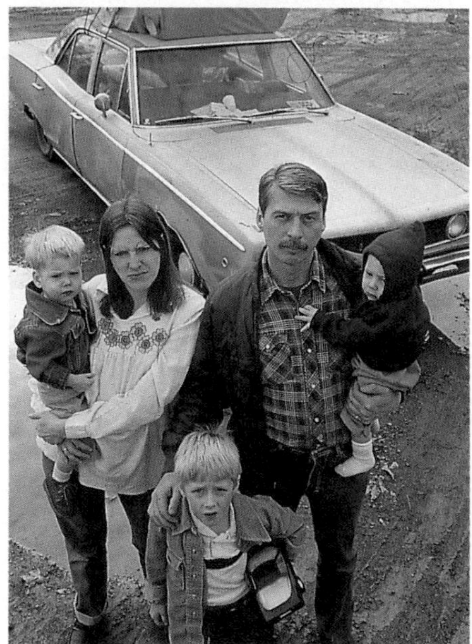
Hungry people in the United States.

Table 15-1
How to Diagnose Food Insecurity in a U.S. Household

Questions like these are asked on surveys to determine the extent of food insecurity in a household. The more questions that receive a "Yes" answer, the more intense the hunger the household is experiencing.

Do you usually have enough food to eat?

If you don't have enough food to eat, is it because:
- a. you sometimes run out of money to buy food?
- b. you do not have transportation?
- c. you do not have working appliances (stove, refrigerator)?

Do you ever rely on nutritionally inferior foods to feed yourself or your children because you lack any of these resources?

Do you ever eat less than you feel you should because you lack any of these resources?

Do you ever skip meals or cut the size of meals because you lack any of these resources?

Do you ever rely on neighbors, friends, relatives, or schools to feed any of your children because there is not enough food in the house?

Do your children ever say they are hungry because there is not enough food in the house?

Do you or any of your children ever go to bed hungry because there is not enough food in the house?

Source: Adapted from C. A. Wehler, R. I. Scott, and J. J. Anderson, The Community Childhood Hunger Identification Project: A model of domestic hunger—demonstration project in Seattle, Washington, *Journal of Nutrition Education* (1 Supplement), January/February 1992, pp. 29S–35S; and R. R. Briefel and C. E. Woteki, Development of food sufficiency questions for the Third National Health and Nutrition Examination Survey, *Journal of Nutrition Education* (1 Supplement), January/February 1992, pp. 24S–28S.

Hunger, particularly childhood hunger, [is] not only a moral issue [but] a competitiveness issue. . . . Hunger compromises the ability to learn. Hungry children have significantly higher absentee rates, and when they are in school, their powers of concentration are greatly reduced. The malnutrition that results from chronic hunger can even slow or permanently inhibit the physical development of the brain. So hunger is . . . an issue of failed beginnings for millions of American children—the future of our country.[46]

The causes of hunger are many, but the primary cause is poverty. Other causes that contribute to hunger are abuse of alcohol and other drugs; mental illness; depression; illness; lack of awareness of available food programs; and the reluctance of people, particularly the elderly, to accept what they perceive as "welfare" or "charity."[47] Still, poverty remains the major cause of hunger, and solving the poverty problem would do a lot to solve the hunger problem.[48]

KEY POINT Chronic hunger causes many deaths worldwide, especially among children. Intermittent hunger is frequently seen in U.S. children. The primary cause of hunger is poverty.

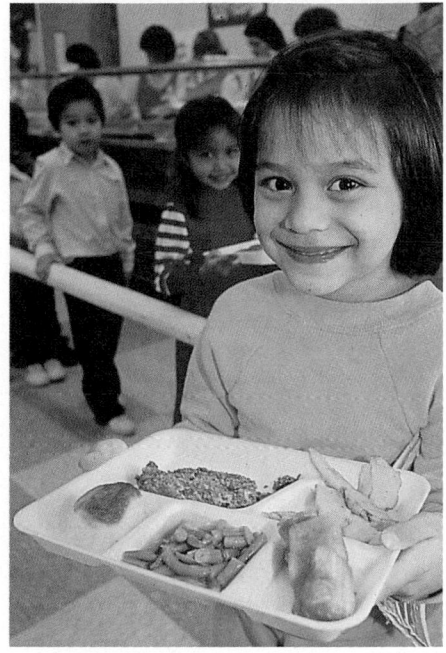

School lunches provide children with nourishment for little or no cost.

Poverty, Hunger, and Hunger Programs

In the United States, poverty and hunger reach into all segments of society, not only the chronic poor (migrant workers, the unskilled and unemployed, the homeless, and some elderly) but also the so-called new poor. Some are displaced farm families. Some are former blue-collar and white-collar workers forced out of their trades and professions into minimum-wage jobs. These people outnumber the chronic poor, and they are not on welfare; they have jobs, but the pay is low. Families with incomes below a certain level are simply unable to buy sufficient amounts of nourishing foods, even if they are skilled in food shopping.

At present, many U.S. programs aimed at preventing or relieving domestic malnutrition and hunger are in effect. Several have been described in earlier chapters: food assistance programs for children such as school lunch, breakfast, and child care food programs; programs to supply low-income pregnant women and mothers with nourishing food (WIC); and food assistance programs for older adults such as congregate meals and Meals on Wheels. Another program aimed directly at the poor is the Food Stamp program, administered by the U.S. Department of Agriculture (USDA). The USDA issues food stamp coupons through state social services or welfare agencies to households (defined as people who buy and prepare food together). The number of stamps a household receives depends on the household size and income. Recipients may use the coupons like cash to purchase food and seeds, but not to buy tobacco, cleaning items, alcohol, or other nonfood items.

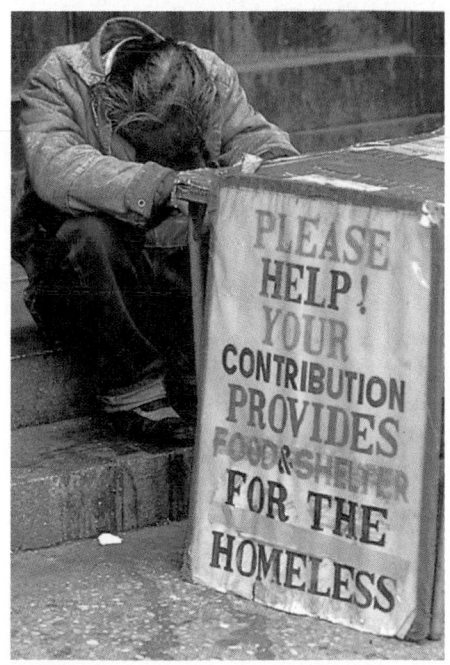

In the United States, 20 million people are hungry for at least part of every month.

These federal programs support both health and well-being. For example, children in Project Head Start, an educational program that includes breakfast, are twice as likely to graduate from high school and to become employed as their peers in the same circumstances who do not participate.[49]

These programs reach millions of people daily with life-giving foods. The money spent on these programs has risen since 1980, but many more people now need welfare and food assistance than then.[50] Federal programs intended to remedy hunger are not fully successful. For example, of the estimated 2 million homeless people in the United States who are eligible for

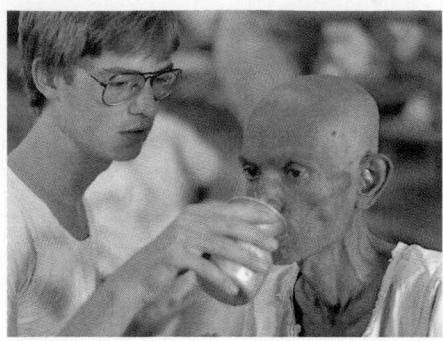

Volunteers can help overcome hunger everywhere.

food assistance, only 15 percent of single adults and 50 percent of families receive food stamps.

To supplement federal programs and to reach those who are still hungry, private efforts have sprung up in many communities, where concerned citizens are working through local agencies and churches to help the hungry. Community-based soup kitchens and shelters generally provide good-quality meals. The meals average only 1,000 calories each, though, and most homeless people receive fewer than 1½ meals a day, so many are inadequately nourished.[51] Table 15-2 shows how individuals can directly assist in local hunger relief efforts; it presents a 14-step program for developing a hunger-free community.

In the developing world, which faces more extreme hunger problems than the United States, the primary cause of hunger is still poverty, but the poverty is more extreme. Most people would find it almost impossible to comprehend the severity of poverty in the developing world. One fifth of the world's 5 billion people have no land and no possessions *at all.* They

Table 15-2
Fourteen Ways Communities Can Address Their Hunger Problems

1. Establish a community-based emergency food-delivery network.
2. Assess food-insecurity problems and evaluate community services. Create strategies for responding to unmet needs.
3. Establish a group of individuals, including low-income participants, to develop and to implement policies and programs to combat food insecurity; monitor responsiveness of existing services; and address underlying causes of hunger.
4. Participate in federally-assisted nutrition programs that are easily accessible to targeted populations.
5. Integrate public and private resources, including local businesses, to relieve food insecurity.
6. Establish an education program that addresses the food needs of the community and the need for increased local citizen participation in activities to alleviate food insecurity.
7. Provide information and referral services for accessing both public and private programs and services.
8. Support programs to provide transportation and assistance in food shopping, where needed.
9. Identify high-risk populations, and target services to meet their needs.
10. Provide adequate transportation and distribution of food from all resources.
11. Coordinate food services with parks and recreation programs and other community-based outlets to which area residents have easy access.
12. Improve public transportation to human service agencies and food resources.
13. Establish nutrition education programs for low-income citizens to enhance their food purchasing and preparation skills and to make them aware of the connections between diet and health.
14. Establish a program for collecting and distributing nutritious foods, either agricultural commodities in farmers' fields or prepared foods that would have been wasted.

Source: House Select Committee on Hunger, legislation introduced by Tony P. Hall, excerpted in *Seeds,* Sprouts edition, January 1992, p. 3 with permission (SEEDS Magazine; P.O. Box 6170; Waco, TX 76706). For more on developing a hunger-free community, write: Hunger Free, House Select Committee on Hunger, 505 Ford House Office Building, Washington, DC 20515.

survive on less than $1 a day each, they lack water that is safe to drink, and they cannot read or write.[52] The average U.S. house cat eats twice as much protein every day as one of these people, and the annual cost of keeping that cat is greater than these people's annual income.[53]

cash crops crops grown for cash, as opposed to crops grown for food.

KEY POINT Poverty and hunger are widespread in the United States, not only among the unemployed, but also among working people. Government programs to relieve poverty and hunger are not fully successful. In the developing world, hunger and poverty are more intense.

Environmental Degradation and Hunger

Hunger and poverty interact with a third force: environmental degradation. Poor people often destroy the very resources they need for survival. They cut their trees for firewood or to sell; then lose the soil to erosion. Without these resources, they become poorer still. Thus poverty causes environmental ruin, and hunger grows from environmental ruin.[54]

Today, environmental degradation is beginning to threaten the world's ability to produce enough food to feed its people. Until 1984, the world celebrated an increase nearly every year in its reserves of stored grain, an index of the sufficiency of the world food supply. The often-repeated statement that "We have enough food to feed everyone" was true. Efforts at relieving hunger focused on transporting food to where it was needed and on improving food storage. Also, because in many developing countries most of the men were involved in producing **cash crops** for export, hunger-relief efforts focused on educating and empowering women to grow and use nutritious food to feed their families. These efforts were addressing the causes of the world's hunger problem, and were expected to solve it.

Since 1984, however, the situation has changed. The world's population is growing at the rate of some 90 million persons each year and food production is no longer keeping pace. In recent years, grain reserves have fallen. Further growth in the world's food output is being slowed by environmental degradation.[55]

One element of this degradation is soil erosion, which in every nation is causing crop losses estimated at 6 percent per year.[56] Irrigation can no longer compensate by improving crop yields, because all the land that can benefit from irrigation is already receiving it. In fact, rising concentrations of salt from irrigation are *lowering* yields on close to a quarter of the world's irrigated cropland. Nor can fertilizer enhance agricultural production much more; it is already being used to maximum effect. Genetic improvements in crops are also in use. During the middle of this century, major genetic improvements led to rapid advances in agricultural outputs. Now, despite the exciting technological advances reported in Controversy 14, not many more such ways of improving the world's total output are forthcoming.[57]

Meat and fish outputs are also falling. Grasslands for growing beef are already being fully used or overused on every continent. The yield of fish from the oceans is declining for the first time in history, due to overfishing and pollution. Other forms of environmental degradation slowing food outputs are deforestation, which leads to soil erosion; air pollution; and climate change. Water supplies, too, are becoming limiting. In fact, water availability may limit human population growth even before food availability does.[58] The world today still produces enough food to feed all its people, and the problem of hunger today remains a problem of unequal distribution of resources. But if present trends continue, the time will arrive when there is an absolute deficit of food.

The extent to which the world grain harvest can be amplified by means of improved technology is now estimated at no better than 1 percent a year. It might be higher, but for the many forms of environmental degradation just described. Meanwhile, the world's population is rising at the rate of at least 2 percent per year.[59] Many authorities in many fields, and more every year, are calling for a reduction in the rate at which the world's population is allowed to increase. Population control has become one of the most pressing needs of this time in history: it appears to be the only way to enable the world's food output to keep pace with people's growing numbers. Without population control, the nations of the world can neither succeed in supporting the lives of people already born nor remedy global environmental deterioration. And to resolve the population problem, it may be necessary, first, to remedy the poverty problem, for reasons discussed next. Of the 90-some million people being added to the population each year, 88 million are being added in the most poverty-stricken areas of the world.[60]

KEY POINT Environmental degradation caused by the impacts of growing numbers of people is reducing the world's food output per person. Improvements in agriculture can no longer keep up with people's growing numbers. To solve the population problem is an urgent necessity.

Poverty and Overpopulation

The giant web of Figure 15-1 showed that one of the many causes contributing to poverty and hunger is population growth. The figure also showed the reverse: poverty and hunger contribute to population growth.

The first of these cause-effect relationships is easy to understand. Population growth contributes to poverty and hunger, for the more mouths there are to feed, the worse poverty and hunger become. Population growth also contributes indirectly by forcing people onto marginal land where they cannot produce sufficient food for themselves and by preempting good agricultural land for growing cities and industry. The world's poorest people live in the world's most damaged and inhospitable environments. They are the ones who experience, daily, tens of thousands of early deaths from malnutrition and disease.

Overpopulation, then, together with the environmental degradation that it causes, worsens poverty. How, though, does the reverse effect occur? How does poverty lead to overpopulation? Poverty and hunger are believed to exert an ironic effect on people, making them bear more children. A family depends on its children to farm the land, haul water, and care for adults in their old age. If a family faces ongoing poverty, the parents will choose to have many children as a form of "insurance" that some will survive to adulthood. People are willing to risk having fewer children only if they are sure that their children will live.

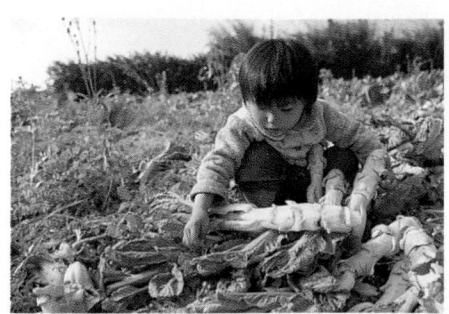

Families in developing countries depend on their children to help provide for daily needs.

Relieving poverty and hunger, then, may be a necessary first step in curbing population growth. When people attain better access to health care, family planning, and education, the death rate falls. At first there is a "bulge" in the population, because births outnumber deaths, but as the standard of living continues to improve, the families become willing to risk having smaller numbers of children. Then the birth rate falls. Thus, after a short but necessary lag time, improvements in economic status help control the population's growth.

The link between improved economic status and slowed population growth has been demonstrated in country after country. It shows why sustainable development is so important.

An indispensable part of sustainable development is not only to have economic growth occur, but to have all groups share resources relatively equally. Where this has happened, population growth has slowed the most. Examples include parts of Sri Lanka, Taiwan, Malaysia, and parts of Costa Rica. Where economic growth has occurred but the resources are unevenly distributed, population growth has remained high. Examples are Brazil, Mexico, the Philippines, and Thailand, where large families continue to be a major economic asset for the poor.

KEY POINT As people become better off economically, they bear fewer children. To successfully produce this effect, economic growth must be accompanied by relatively equal resource distribution.

Solutions

The keys to solving the world's environmental, poverty, and hunger problems are in the hands of both the poor and rich nations, but require different efforts from them. The poor nations need to gain control of their rampaging population growth, and to slow and reverse the destruction of their environmental resources: forests, waterways, and soil. To do this, they must, among other things, find ways to relieve their people's poverty. The rich nations need to stem their wasteful and polluting uses of resources and energy, which are contributing to global environmental degradation. They also must become willing to help relieve the debtor nations of their poverty in ways that effectively reach the poor.

Sustainable Development Worldwide

Many nations now agree that improvement of all nations' economies is a prerequisite to meeting the world's other urgent needs: population stabilization, arrest of environmental degradation, sustainable treatment of resources, and relief of hunger. An important step was taken when a United Nations convention on the Rights of the Child was ratified by over 100 nations. Significantly, the document produced mentioned *nutrition*, for the first time in world history, as an internationally recognized human right.[61] Another important step was taken when, in 1992, over 100 nations met for the Earth Summit in Rio de Janeiro, Brazil, and discussed the relationships of the environment to poverty and hunger.

The formal name of the summit was the United Nations Conference on Environment and Development: UNCED, for short. At this meeting, many nations agreed for the first time to 27 principles of sustainable development, which the conferees defined as development that would equitably meet both the economic and the environmental needs of present and future generations. By 1995, the leaders of the conference hope to have developed an Earth Charter, spelling out the nations' commitments to these principles.

The participants at UNCED discussed climate change and the possibility of setting legally binding targets and timetables for every nation to cut its emissions of global-warming gases. They began to approach agreement on this issue. They also signed agreements to protect the earth's remaining species of plants and animals, and to preserve the world's forests.

The participating nations also began to discuss ways of alleviating the problems of poverty in the developing world. The population problem was not a focus of the conference, but was slated to receive attention at a 1994 conference on population and development.

The Earth Summit's discussions opened vistas of hope. Much remains to be done, and all nations have major parts to play. For our part, in the United States, the challenges are many. For one, we are being urged to reduce our consumption of fossil fuel and thereby our disproportionate contribution to global environmental degradation. For another, it has been suggested that the United States can help directly by supporting international moves to relieve poverty and environmental degradation worldwide. These steps are recommended.

First, it is considered necessary to relieve the developing countries of the gigantic interest payments they have been making to U.S. and international banks. Ten years ago those countries received $50 billion more a year from the developed world than they paid out, and they were able to make some progress towards solving their internal poverty and environmental problems. Today, however, they pay out $50 billion more than they take in, so they are becoming poorer every year.[62] They sell a bounty of cash crops to the developed world, such as cotton, tobacco, coffee, sugar, and palm oil, but they cannot put the proceeds back into their economies. They have to use all the money they make to pay the interest on their loans, and they even have to borrow more. It has been called "one of the great ironies of the world" that some of the world's richest farmland is being used to produce nonnutritious crops for U.S. dollars, only to pour the money down the interest-payment drain while the producing nations' people starve.[63] The debtor nations could use that same land to grow food crops to feed their own people.

Second, it is considered necessary to make sure that the debt relief reaches those within the countries who need it, and not just the wealthy. In some poor countries, astronomically wealthy upper classes control all the good crop land and use it to produce luxury cash crops for export while the landless poor starve and multiply. Relieving hunger requires land reform—returning sufficient land to the dispossessed so that they can live and grow food on it. Simultaneous community development is needed to ensure that the people become able to support themselves permanently.

Third, rather than emphasizing *technology*-intensive methods of *harvesting* their resources, it is thought desirable that developing countries shift toward *labor*-intensive means of *maintaining* their resources. That way, succeeding generations can benefit from them.[64]

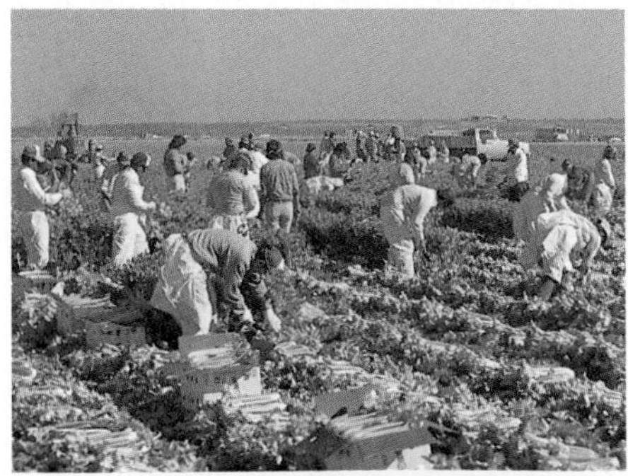

Labor-intensive agriculture, low in technical inputs, is most often the appropriate technology in developing countries.

Fourth, to account correctly for the great value of environmental resources such as soil, water, and trees, a new system of economic accounting must come into use. Soil, water, and trees should be counted in economic balance sheets. Systems of national accounting must recognize the depletion of natural resources as a backward economic step and subtract lost resources from the gross national product. This would promote the making of decisions that would take into account future environmental costs and benefits more accurately, and investment criteria that would stem the loss of natural capital.[65]

The United States can exert international leadership along these lines. It can encourage other developed nations to support the same measures.

The idea behind all these measures is that relieving poverty will help relieve environmental degradation and hunger. To rephrase a well-known adage, If you give a man a fish, he will eat for a day. If you teach him to fish, so that he can buy and maintain his own gear and bait, he will eat for a lifetime and help to feed you. In comparison with food giveaways and money doles, which are only stop-gap measures, social programs that will permanently better the lot of the poor can permanently solve the hunger problem.[66]

Activism and Simpler Lifestyles at Home

Every segment of our society can have a place in the fight against poverty, hunger, and environmental degradation. The federal government, the states, local communities, big business and small companies, educators, and all individuals, including dietitians and foodservice managers, have many opportunities to forward the effort.

Government policies can change to promote sustainability. For example, the government can stop using tax money to pay for the wasteful use of fossil fuels and of fertilizers and pesticides made from them. Instead, it can pay for energy-conservation services and crop protection.[67]

Businesses can take initiatives to help; some already have. Several, such as AT&T, Prudential, and Kraft General Foods, are major supporters of anti-hunger programs.[68]

Educators, including nutrition educators, have a crucial role to play. They can teach others about the underlying social and political causes of poverty, the root cause of hunger. At the college level, they can teach the relationships between hunger and population, hunger and environmental degradation, hunger and the status of women, hunger and the global debt crisis.[69] They can advocate for legislation to address poverty problems. They can teach the poor, themselves, to develop and run nutrition programs in their own communities, and to fight on their own behalf for anti-poverty, anti-hunger legislation.[70]

Dietitians and food service managers have a special role to play. They are being urged by their professional organization, the American Dietetic Association, to promote the saving of resources by reuse, recycling (including composting), energy conservation, and water conservation, in both their professional and personal lives.[71]

All individuals, for whom small lifestyle changes were the focus of the first half of this chapter, can also become involved in these large trends. They can "talk it up," as ball players do, urging their friends and relatives in powerful positions to make maximum efforts to assist in the global effort to bring about a sustainable economy. They can support organizations that lobby for the needed economic policy changes toward developing countries. According to one nutrition educator, "This [lobbying] is probably the most effective single thing that Joe or Jane Average Citizen can do [to help solve the world's hunger and environment problems]."[72]

Another way in which people can assist the global community in solving its poverty and hunger problems is to join and work for international hunger relief organizations. Table 15-3 lists some of the major ones.

Then, in their own homes, schools, and workplaces, everyone can take many small steps to help. All aspects of our lifestyles relate to global problems. This chapter's recommendations have included personal actions: reduce, reuse, recycle, and cut energy use for cars and homes. Admittedly, these approaches to solving today's global problems seem simple, but because we number 5 billion plus, such actions taken by many people can exert an immense impact. If each of the world's 5 billion people takes one-five-billionth share of the responsibility for improving things, the job can

Table 15-3
Hunger Relief Organizations People Can Join

Bread for the World 802 Rhode Island Avenue NE Washington, DC 20018
Food Research and Action Center 1319 F Street NW, Suite 500 Washington, DC 20004
Institute for Food and Development Policy 145 Ninth Street San Francisco, CA 94103
Interfaith Impact on Justice and Peace 110 Maryland Avenue NE, Box 63 Washington, DC 20002
Oxfam America 115 Broadway Boston, MA 02116
Seeds P.O. Box 6170 Waco, TX 76706

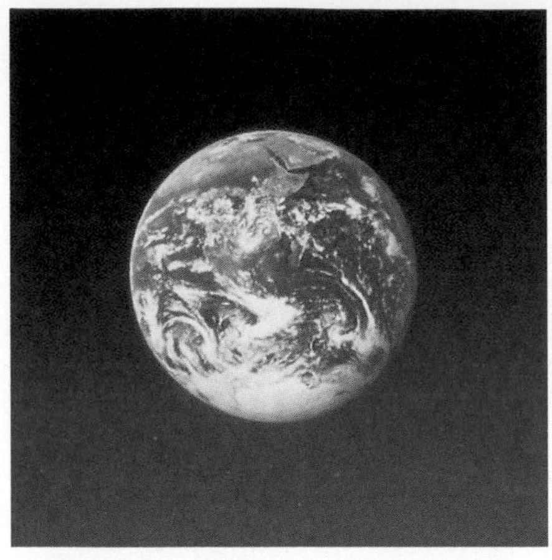

"We do not inherit the earth from our ancestors, we borrow it from our children."

get done. Just to be sure, though, those who can do more are encouraged to do so to compensate for those who are, as yet, too poor, ignorant, powerless, or inflexible to join in.

Finally, it makes sense for everyone in this world, rich or poor, in the United States or in any other country, to plan on bearing no more than one or two children. For those who want large families, there are plenty of children to adopt. And for those who love children and want to help them in other ways, there are numerous opportunities to play with, teach, and nurture the world's children, from the community center downtown to the remotest primitive village on the globe.

"Be part of the solution, not part of the problem," an adage says. In other words, don't waste time or energy moaning and groaning about how tough things are; do something to improve them. This adage is as applicable to today's global environmental problems as it is to an unwashed dish in the kitchen sink. They are our problems: human beings created them, and human beings must solve them.

KEY POINT Government, business, educators, and all individuals have many opportunities to promote sustainability worldwide and wise resource use at home.

Notes

1. A. D. Basiago, The house where the future lives, *Calypso Log*, September 1986, p. 11.
2. J. E. Young, Aluminum's real tab, *World Watch*, March/April 1992, pp. 26–33; Earth Works Group, *50 Simple Things That You Can Do to Save the Earth* (Berkeley, Calif.: Earthworks Press, 1989), pp. 64–65.
3. Regional perspectives: Gulf of Mexico shrimp fishery, *Marine Conservation News*, Winter 1990, p. 11.
4. Examples: M. Countryman, Lessons of the divestment drive, *The Nation*, March 26, 1988, pp. 406–409; H. Orlans, The revolution at Gallaudet: Students provoke break with the past, *Change, The Magazine of Higher Learning*, January/February 1989, pp. 8–18; S. Conn, Thoughts on national service: An open letter to William F. Buckley, Jr., *Change, The Magazine of Higher Learning*, May/June 1991, pp. 6–7, 52; R. G. Braungart and M. M. Braungart, Youth movements in the 1980s: A global perspective, *International Sociology*, June 1990, pp. 157–181; E. Larsen, Youth environmental movement, *Utne Reader*, March/April 1991, pp. 30–31; J. Smith, The 1989 Chinese student movement: Lessons for nonviolent activists, *Peace and Change, A Journal of Peace Research*, January 1992, pp. 82–101; Windmill at Hamilton College generates heat, light, and a conservation campaign, *Chronicles of Higher Education*, April 1, 1992; A dollars-and-cents moral crusade in recycling, *Chronicles of Higher Education*, April 15, 1992, p. A5. The Rainforest Action Network (450 Sansome, Suite 700, San Francisco, CA 94111), which now puts effective pressure on governments and corporations all over the world to stop destroying rainforests, originated and is maintained largely as a student effort.
5. S. Postel, Denial in the decisive decade, in L. R. Brown and coauthors, *State of the World 1992* (New York: Norton, 1992), pp. 3–8; D. R. Gwatkin, How many die? A set of demographic estimates of the annual number of infant and child deaths in the world, *American Journal of Public Health* 70 (1980): 1286–1289.
6. V. A. Kovda, Loss of productive land due to salinization, *Ambio* 12 (1983), as cited in S. Postel, *Water for Agriculture: Facing the Limits, Worldwatch Paper 93*, December 1989, p. 16; T. Peterson, Hunger and the environment, *Seeds*, October 1987, pp. 6–13; L. R. Brown, Feeding six billion, *World Watch*, September/October 1989, pp. 32–40.
7. L. R. Brown, Reexamining the world food prospect, Chapter 3 in *State of the World 1989* (New York: Norton, 1989), pp. 41–58; L. R. Brown and J. E. Young, Feeding the world in the nineties, Chapter 4 in *State of the World 1990* (New York: Norton, 1990), pp. 59–78.
8. Energy: Choices for environment and development, Chapter 7 in World Commission on Environment and Development, *Our Common Future* (New York: Oxford University Press, 1987), pp. 168–205.
9. Energy: Choices for environment and development, 1987.
10. D. L. Wheeler, Scientists studying "the greenhouse effect" challenge fears of global warming [but consensus is, it's occurring], *Journal of Forestry* 88 (7): 34–36 (July 1990); B. Hileman, Web of interactions make it difficult to untangle global warming data: Despite the complexities, experts have made progress, *Chemical and Engineering News*, April 27, 1992, pp. 7–19; R. A. Kerr, Greenhouse science survives skeptics, *Science* 256 (1992): 1138–1140; W. R. Cline, Scientific basis for the greenhouse effect, *The Economic Journal* 101 (1991): 904–919; J. T. Houghton, G. J. Jenkins, and J. J. Ephraums, eds., *Climate Change: The IPCC Scientific Assessment* (Cambridge: Cambridge University Press, 1990); I. M. Mintzer, ed., *Confronting Climate Change: Risks, Implications and Responses* (Cambridge: Cambridge University Press, 1992); Two books depict major greenhouse effects on Australia, *Climate Alert*, Summer 1989, p. 3; Chinese government study details huge global warming impact on China, endorses energy efficiency, *Climate Alert*, Spring 1990, pp. 1, 6; Island states unite to press for sea rise action, *Climate Alert*, January/February 1991, pp. 1, 7; Climate change would damage Great Lakes forests, Mexican agriculture, *Climate Alert*, April 1991, pp. 1, 4, 7; Climate change impact study highlights soil moisture change in United Kingdom, *Climate Alert*, June 1991, pp. 1, 6; UNEP's first country

reports unveiled: Regional studies cover Asian, South American nations, *Climate Alert*, November/December 1991, pp. 1, 4; Fortaleza declaration dramatizes stresses on semi-arid regions, *Climate Alert*, January/February 1992, pp. 1, 12; Climate Institute organizes cooperative briefings on climate change implications in 18 nations, *Climate Alert*, January/February 1992, pp. 3–9; J. L. Jacobson, *Environmental Refugees: A Yardstick of Habitability, Worldwatch Paper 86*, November 1988.
11. J. L. Jacobson, Abandoning homelands, Chapter 4 in *State of the World 1989* (New York: Norton, 1989), pp. 59–76.
12. Postel, 1992.
13. Postel, 1992.
14. C. Mlot, Tropical forests, in World Resources Institute, *The 1992 Information Please Environmental Almanac* (Boston: Houghton Mifflin, 1992), pp. 279–290; Kovda, 1983.
15. Managing the commons, Chapter 10 in World Commission on Environment and Development, *Our Common Future* (Oxford and New York: Oxford University Press, 1987), pp. 261–289; and see note #28 on fisheries.
16. Postel, 1992.
17. M. Renner, *Jobs in a Sustainable Economy, Worldwatch Paper 104*, September 1991, p. 9.
18. Renner, 1991, pp. 31–33.
19. Renner, 1991, p. 17.
20. Renner, 1991, p. 47.
21. M. D. Lowe, *Alternatives to the Automobile: Transport for Livable Cities, Worldwatch Paper 98*, October 1990, p. 5.
22. Lowe, 1990, p. 9.
23. Lowe, 1990, pp. 9–10.
24. A. B. Durning and H. B. Brough, *Taking Stock: Animal Farming and the Environment, Worldwatch Paper 103*, July 1991.
25. J. D. Nations and D. I. Komer, Rainforests and the hamburger society, *Environment*, April 1983, pp. 12–20.
26. Nations and Komer, 1983.
27. Durning and Brough, 1991.
28. H. Upton, Swordfish fishery management—Now or never, *Marine Conservation News*, Summer 1990, p. 6; H. Upton, New fisheries legislation may help conserve [tuna] fish populations and the bluefin tuna, *Marine Conservation News*, Summer 1990, p. 14; H. Upton, Red snapper—Another fishery in decline, *Marine Conservation News*, Autumn 1990, p. 6; H. Upton, The shark fishery: Who is in dangerous waters? *Marine Conservation News*, Autumn 1990, p. 7; H. Upton, American fisheries: Running on empty? *Marine Conservation News*, Winter 1990, pp. 9–12; N. M. Young, Mexican tuna fishery feeling the heat, *Marine Conservation News*, Summer 1991, p. 3; H. Upton, New England groundfish: It just doesn't get any worse, *Marine Conservation News*, Summer 1991, p. 9; Shark conservation: A worldwide concern, *Marine Conservation News*, Summer 1991, p. 9; H. Upton, Swordfish emergency after 10 years of waiting, *Marine Conservation News*, Autumn 1991, p. 14; H. Upton, Shark plan may be too little, too late, *Marine Conservation News*, August 1991, p. 15; S. Fordham, Crisis management for New England fish, *Marine Conservation News*, Spring 1992, p. 10.
29. Upton, The shark fishery, 1990; Shark conservation, 1991; Shark plan may be too little, too late, 1991.
30. N. M. Young, CMC finds wide variance in "dolphin safe" claims, *Marine Conservation News*, Winter 1990, p. 7.
31. Regional perspectives: Gulf of Mexico shrimp fishery, 1990.
32. S. H. Wittwer, Food ecology and choices; The "greening effect": Implications for consumer choices, *Food and Nutrition News* 64 (1992).
33. Earth Works Group, 1989, p. 39.
34. J. C. Ryan, Timber's last stand, *World Watch*, July/August 1990, pp. 27–34; Ecological economics: Its implications for forest management and research (a workshop summary), *Conservation Biology*, September 1990, pp. 221–226; A. Leopold, Standards of conservation, *Conservation Biology*, September 1990, pp. 227–228; R. K. Anderberg, Wall Street and the great north woods, *The Amicus Journal*, Winter 1989, pp. 40–43; C. Wille, Ancient forest heritage going fast, *Audubon*, March 1989, pp. 130–131; Forest Service: Admissions and additions, *Wilderness*, Spring 1989, pp. v–vi; J. Stiak, Old growth! Battle Cry of the Northwest, *The Amicus Journal*, Winter 1990, pp. 35–41; E. A. Norse, What good are ancient forests? Global resources, global concern, *The Amicus Journal*, Winter 1990, pp. 42–45; D. Doak, Spotted owls and old growth logging in the Pacific Northwest, *Conservation Biology*, December 1989, pp. 389–396; M. Lipske, Who runs America's forests? *National Wildlife*, October/November 1990, pp. 24–28.
35. P. Von Stackelberg, Whitewash: The dioxin coverup, *Greenpeace*, March/April 1989, pp. 7–11; National Wildlife Federation calls for ban on chlorine use, *International Wildlife*, January/February 1991, p. 26.
36. Young, 1992.
37. Earth Works Group, 1989, p. 31.
38. Postel, 1992.
39. At home, *Executive Fitness*, April 1989, p. 8.
40. Earth Works Group, 1989, p. 9.
41. Earth Works Group, 1989, p. 9.
42. R. Kourik, As the worm turns, *Garbage*, January/February 1992, pp. 48–51.
43. Gwatkin, 1980.
44. *Fact Sheet on Childhood Hunger and Poverty*, available from Bread for the World, 802 Rhode Island Avenue, NE, Washington, DC 20018, c. 1992.
45. S. Lewis, Food security, environment, poverty, and the world's children, *Journal of Nutrition Education* 24 (1 Supplement), January-February 1992, pp. 3S–5S.
46. M. Mudd, vice president, Kraft General Foods, quoted in *Journal of Nutrition Education* 24 (1 Supplement), January-February 1992, p. 1S.
47. L. D. McBean, ed., with D. Derelian, R. J. Fersh, and L. Parker, Hunger and undernutrition in America, *Dairy Council Digest*, March/April 1992.
48. L. V. E. Crawford, Rethinking domestic hunger policy: An interview with J. Larry Brown, *Seeds*, May/June 1990, pp. 6–9.
49. *Fact Sheet on Childhood Hunger and Poverty*, c. 1992.
50. M. Nestle and S. Guttmacher, Hunger in the United States: Rationale, methods, and policy implications of state hunger surveys, *Journal of Nutrition Education* 24 (1 Supplement), January-February 1992, pp. 18S–22S.
51. J. C. Wolgemuth and coauthors, Wasting malnutrition and inadequate nutrient intakes identified in a multiethnic homeless population, *Journal of the American Dietetic Association* 92 (1992): 834–839; M. A. Drake, The nutritional status and dietary adequacy of single homeless women and their children in shelters, *Public Health Reports* 107 (1992): 312–319; B. E. Cohen, N. Chapman, and M. R. Burt, Food sources and intake of homeless persons, *Journal of Nutrition Education* 24 (1 Supplement), January-February 1992, pp. 45S–51S.
52. World Bank, *World Development Report 1991* (New York: Oxford University Press, 1991); Postel, 1992.
53. L. Timberlake, *Only One Earth*, cited in Food for thought, *Seeds*, Sprouts edition, 1988.
54. B. Stutz, The landscape of hunger, *Audubon*, March-April 1993, pp. 54–57; Newsbreaks: Effects of environmental degradation on nutrition, *Nutrition Today*, March/April 1992, p. 4.
55. Brown and Young, 1990.

56. Brown and Young, 1990, p. 60.
57. L. R. Brown, *Vital Signs 1993: The Trends That Are Shaping Our Future* (New York: Norton, 1993); L. R. Brown, A decade of discontinuity, *World Watch*, July-August 1993, pp. 19–26.
58. J. W. M. la Riviere, Threats to the world's water, *Scientific American*, September 1989, pp. 80–94.
59. Brown and Young, 1990, pp. 64–65.
60. Postel, 1992.
61. Lewis, 1992.
62. Lewis, 1992.
63. Lewis, 1992.
64. J. Collins, The real roots of world hunger: Demand not supply, *Seeds*, March/April 1990, pp. 22–24.
65. Postel, 1992.
66. K. L. Clancy and J. Bowering, The need for emergency food: Poverty problems and policy responses, *Journal of Nutrition Education* 24 (1 Supplement), January-February 1992, pp. 12S–17S; J. M. Dodds, S. L. Parker, and P. S. Haines, Hunger in the 80s and 90s: A challenge for nutrition educators, *Journal of Nutrition Education* 24 (1 Supplement), January-February 1992, p. 2S.
67. C. Flavin and J. E. Young, Shaping the next industrial revolution, in L. R. Brown, *State of the World, 1990* (New York: Norton, 1990), pp. 181–199.
68. Mudd, 1992.
69. J. Csete, Hunger and the Academy: Training nutritionists for the 1990s, *Journal of Nutrition Education* 24 (1 Supplement), January-February 1992, pp. 79S–83S.
70. W. L. Scheider, Fighting hunger and poverty: A strategy for nutrition educators, *Journal of Nutrition Education* 24 (1 Supplement), January-February 1992, pp. 84S–85S.
71. Position of the American Dietetic Association: Environmental issues, *Journal of the American Dietetic Association* 93 (1993): 589–591.
72. S. Smith, professor of nutrition, University of New Hampshire, Durham, personal communication, Summer 1993.

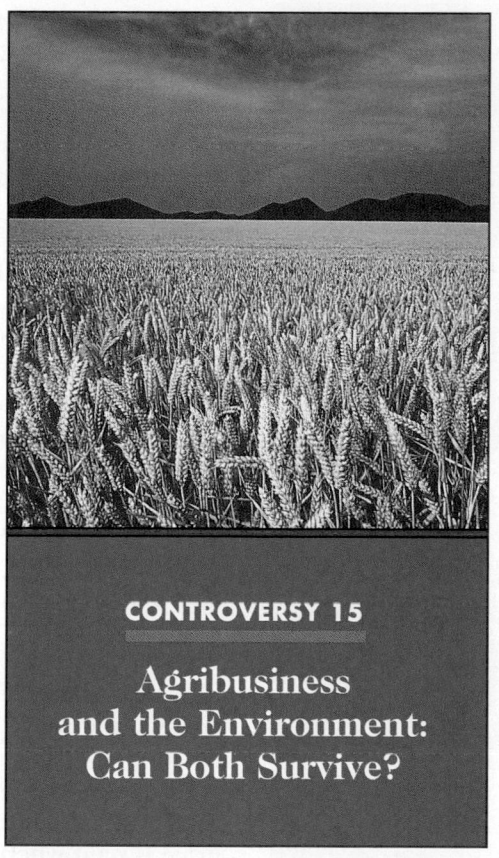

CONTROVERSY 15

Agribusiness and the Environment: Can Both Survive?

While some individuals are attempting to make their own personal lifestyles more environmentally benign, as suggested in the chapter, others are seeking ways to improve whole sectors of human enterprise, among them, agriculture. Large agricultural enterprises have, to date, been among the world's biggest polluters and one of its biggest resource users. Is it possible for agriculture to become sustainable? And if so, can the change be made without hurting farmers? These questions are addressed in this Controversy.

COSTS OF PRODUCING FOOD UNSUSTAINABLY The environmental and social costs of agriculture and the food industry take many forms. Among them are resource waste and pollution; energy overuse; and tolls on life in farm communities.

Resources and Pollution Producing food has always cost the earth dearly. First of all, to grow food, we clear land—prairie, wetland, or forest. This always causes losses of native ecosystems and wildlife.

Then we plant crops or graze animals on the land. Negative impacts on soil and water follow. The soil loses nutrients as each crop is taken from it, so fertilizer is applied. The fertilizer that runs off pollutes the waterways; so does the plowed soil, which clouds the water and interferes with the growth of aquatic plants and animals.

Then to protect crops against weeds and pests, we apply herbicides and pesticides. These chemicals also pollute the water and, wherever the wind carries them, the air. Most herbicides and pesticides are nonspecific; they kill not only weeds and pests, but also native plants, native insects, and animals that eat those plants and insects.

Finally, to add insult to injury, we irrigate. Irrigation water, unlike rain, contains salts and other compounds. The water evaporates, but its salts do not, so the soil becomes more and more salty. These salts form gums with organic materials and impede the flow of water, make the land soggy, and hinder plant growth. Also, irrigation depletes the water supply over time, because irrigation water pulled from surface waters or pumped up from underground then evaporates or runs off, leaving the area. This process dries up rivers and lakes and lowers the water table of whole regions, making them dryer. This sets a vicious cycle in motion, for the drier the region becomes, the more the farmers need irrigation water; and the more water they use, the drier the region becomes.

Agricultural pesticides and herbicides, if not used conservatively, also pollute rivers, lakes, and ground water. In 1989, the nation's most prestigious national scientific research body, the National Research Council of the National Academy of Sciences, produced a report that said, in part, that agriculture is the largest single source of **nonpoint pollution** of surface water in the nation. (Pollution from "point sources," such as sewage plants or factories, is relatively easy to control, but runoff from fields and pastures enters waterways from all over broad regions and is nearly impossible to control.) Widespread use of pesticides and herbicides also causes resistant pests and weeds to evolve. This makes necessary the use of still more pesticides and herbicides. Some farmers have been buying so many pesticides, herbicides, fertilizers, and soil boosters that their costs for these items have risen too high to bear. Pesticide residues are even becoming a problem for *people* who eat foods produced this way. In short, our way of producing foods is, for the most part, not sustainable.[1]

Some agricultural practices also deplete the soil—particularly indiscriminate land clearing (deforestation) and overuse by cattle (overgrazing). In 1992, the World Resources Institute presented the results of a massive study of human impacts on the soil, showing that agriculture is destroying its own foundation. In just the past 40 years, the study said, human agricultural activities have ruined more than ten percent of the earth's most fertile land, an area the size of China and India combined. Over 20 million acres have been so damaged that

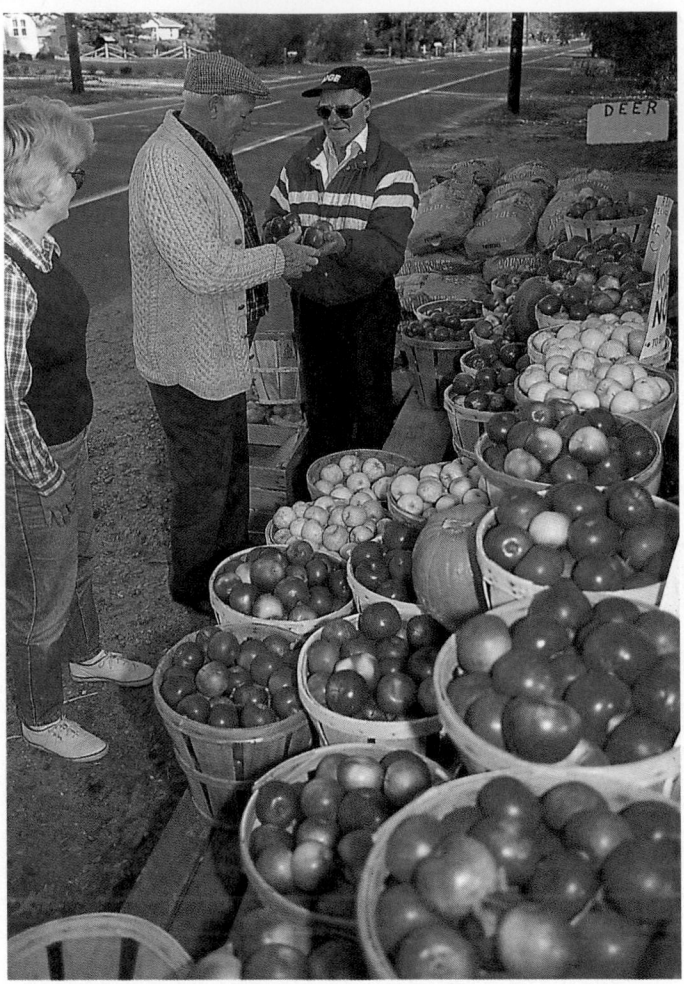

Locally grown foods offer health and benefits to both the local economy and the global environment.

they will be impossible to reclaim, the study said. Soil erosion, if unchecked, is predicted to result in a 20-percent loss in global food production by the end of this century, and by 2025 food-producing land per person may shrink by nearly 40 percent.[2]

Agriculture is also cutting out its own underpinnings by failing to conserve species diversity. By the year 2050, the number of plant species remaining on earth may be reduced by some 40,000 from the number that existed in the year 1990. The United Nation's Food and Agriculture Organization attributes many of the losses, which are already occurring daily, to modern farming practices, as well as to population growth. Global eating habits, too, have become uniform. People everywhere are eating the same limited array of foods, so that local regions' native, genetically diverse plants are not enough in demand to make them seem worth preserving. Yet in the future, as the climate warms and the earth changes, those may be "the very plants that can serve as important sources of food for large numbers of people."[3] A wild species of corn that grows in a hot climate, for example, might contain just the genetic information necessary to help make the domestic corn crop resistant to drought. Controversy 14 offers other examples of genes that might be needed to improve food crops.

These culprits that attend the growing of crops—land clearing, irrigation, fertilizer overuse, pesticide overuse, herbicide overuse, and loss of biogenetic diversity—have always taken a tremendous toll on the earth. Today, the damage is accelerating as the population grows faster and uses more technology every year. Agriculture has already destroyed many of the world's once-fertile regions, where high civilizations once flourished. All of North Africa, now desert, was once wheat fields, the breadbasket of the Roman Empire. Mistreatment of soil and water is now causing destruction on a scale never known before.[4]

Raising livestock also takes a toll. Like plant crops, herds of livestock occupy land that once maintained itself in a natural state. The land pays a price in losses of native plants and animals, soil erosion, water depletion, and desert formation. Alternatively, if animals are grown in concentrated areas (such as feed lots), a high price is paid when animal wastes cause water pollution. And animals in feed lots still have to be fed; grain is grown for them on other land. That grain may require fertilizers, herbicides, pesticides, and irrigation, too. One fifth of all cropland in the United States is used to produce feed grains for livestock, more land than is used to produce grain for people.*

Other environmental costs attend fishing. Fishing easily becomes overfishing and depletes stocks of the very food fish that people need to eat. Some kinds of fishing involve methods that kill aquatic animals other than the ones sought and deplete large populations of nonfood animals, such as dolphins.

Energy The whole food industry, whether based on crop growing, cattle ranching, or fishing, requires en-

*According to *Myths and Facts about Beef Production*, a booklet produced by the National Cattlemen's Association, 1301 Pennsylvania Avenue, NW, Suite 300, Washington, DC 20004, "19% of total crop land is used to produce feed grains." According to A. B. Durning and H. B. Brough, *Taking Stock: Animal Farming and The Environment (Worldwatch Paper #103)*, July 1991, p. 14, 70 percent of the grain we produce, much of which could be used to produce food for people, is fed to livestock. The water used to supply each person with meat, milk, and eggs each day probably matches a typical citizen's water use at home, about 380 liters.

ergy, which entails burning fossil fuel. As Chapter 15 showed, massive fossil fuel use is threatening our planet by causing global warming, ozone depletion, water pollution, ocean pollution, and other ills.

In the United States, the food industry's energy consumption is huge, about 20 percent of all the energy the nation uses. Each year we spend 1,500 liters (over 350 gallons) of oil *per person* to produce, process, distribute, and prepare our food.[5] Energy is used to run farm machinery and to produce fertilizers and pesticides. Energy is also used to prepare, package, transport, refrigerate, and otherwise store, cook, and wash our foods. To convey an idea of how much goes into nonfood items associated with the foods we eat, consider this: consumers paid $29 million in 1985 just for the packages on their foods. In the same year, farmers received less than $29 million for the food itself.[6]

agribusiness agriculture practiced on a massive scale by large corporations owning vast acreages and employing intensive technological, fuel, and chemical inputs.

alternative (low-input, or sustainable) agriculture agriculture practiced on a small scale using individualized approaches that vary with local conditions so as to minimize technological, fuel, and chemical inputs.

externalities hidden cost factors that are not reflected in the prices of things, such as the costs of subsidies that permit agribusiness foods to be sold at artificially low prices.

integrated pest management (IPM) management of pests using a combination of natural and biological controls and minimal or no application of pesticides.

nonpoint pollution water pollution caused by runoff from all over an area, rather than from discrete, "point" sources. An example is the pollution caused by runoff from agricultural fields.

subsidies government money, derived from taxes, used to support (subsidize) practices that otherwise would force producers to set their prices too high to compete successfully.

Losses of Family Farms During the early and mid 1980s, U.S. agriculture encountered serious economic hardships. Exports of farm produce fell worldwide. Recession occurred. Federal loans became expensive. Other countries increased their agricultural production and exports. Many U.S. farmers, particularly those who specialized in export crops, suffered heavy financial losses. Some became unable to pay their debts and had to leave farming. Tens of thousands of farms were still struggling at the start of the 1990s, especially mid-sized family farms.[7]

U.S. farmers today lack significant control over what products they produce, the costs of their supplies, and the prices they receive for their goods. Just prior to 1980, the USDA urged farmers to increase corn and soybean production for export. To expand their production capabilities, the farmers borrowed heavily. Since that time, the costs of seed, fertilizer, equipment, and loans have risen, and the crop prices have declined. Thousands of U.S. farmers are left frustrated, in debt, and hungry.

Farmers and ranchers can theoretically obtain financial support from the government in the form of **subsidies** and tax write-offs. Subsidies support practices such as the use of irrigation, pesticides, fertilizers, and fuels that farmers could not otherwise afford. Farmers and ranchers who receive subsidies can charge lower prices for their crops and meats, which helps them compete for buyers. Tax write-offs permit farmers and ranchers to pay fewer taxes than other citizens, in effect making their enterprises more profitable.

Unfortunately, huge corporation-owned farms find it much easier to obtain and use subsidies than do small family farms. Subsidies usually support technology-intensive practices that employ large machinery and large land areas. Huge farms and ranches, collectively part of the massive food-producing enterprise called **agribusiness,** tend to use little local labor, and the profits they make tend not to stay in local communities. In fact, subsidies to agribusiness may actually be helping to drive families out of farming.

Farm subsidies also tend to promote unsustainable practices. Subsidies make it a higher priority to produce abundant food than to protect soil, water, and local biodiversity. Subsidies make it easy to overuse fertilizers and pesticides, to overuse land at the cost of soil erosion, and to use irrigation water wastefully.[8] For ranchers, billions of dollars in subsidies promote intensive forms of livestock production.[9] Evidence suggests that both economically and environmentally, subsidies are unsound. If, for example, price supports for pesticides were eliminated, farmers would use them perhaps a third more sparingly and to better effect.[10]

It has been suggested that farm subsidies could be altered to support desirable agriculture methods rather than paying for environmentally harmful practices. The Rocky Mountain Institute of Snowmass, Colorado, which studies the environmental impacts of agriculture, has published a book called *Farm Subsidies: Consequences and Alternatives,* showing how farm subsidies often support unsustainable practices, and what some of the alternatives may be.[11]

A third problem is that subsidies permit sellers to set the prices of their products so low that buyers tend to use the products freely. As a result, people buy products from agribusiness, rather than from smaller, local farms. The local grocery store presents broccoli from Mexico, carrots from California, pineapples from Hawaii, and bananas from Central America at prices no local operator could beat, even if he could grow those products. Roadside stands offer bundles of greens and baskets of local fruits and vegetables, but less conveniently and sometimes at higher prices than many shoppers are willing to pay.

Environmental and social *costs*, such as pollution and hardship to farmers, are not reflected in the *prices* of products. These costs are therefore called *external costs*, or **externalities.** People don't pay for these when they buy the products; they pay in tax money used to defray these costs. Sometimes people do not pay in money at all, but in health and social stresses; and the environment pays in resource losses and environmental deterioration. If these costs *were* included in prices, the prices of unsustainably produced products would be much higher, and people would buy fewer of these products. Instead, they would buy more products from smaller farms and ranches produced with less technology, less pollution, and more labor.

Agribusiness is usually the kind of agricultural system that produces the most food on the smallest land area. With the help of subsidies, agribusiness also produces the cheapest food. If the subsidies and other price supports were removed, the prices would be higher. And if the prices had to include a "tax" to pay for pollution cleanup, water protection, and land restoration, they would be higher still. It has been suggested that the dollar prices of foods produced with so much irrigation, pesticides, fertilizers, and fossil fuel should even be high enough to pay for "the costs of unemployment when farms fail . . . national security to protect our supply of imported petroleum [for tractor fuel] . . . medical care for thousands of workers injured each year by pesticides . . . ground water contamination," and other such external costs.[12] Still other needs include education and benefits for the nation's silent slave labor force—the migrant farm workers.

PROPOSED SOLUTIONS For each of the problems described above, solutions have been devised. To put them into practice will require some new learning.

Alternative Agriculture After reviewing the problems associated with U.S. agriculture, the members of the National Research Council expressed the intent to develop an alternative mode of producing food. The goals were to conserve land, water, and energy, to exert minimal environmental impacts, and to produce abundant food profitably. They named this solution **alternative agriculture.**[13]

Alternative agriculture is not one system but a set of practices that can be matched to particular needs in local areas. It emphasizes careful use of natural processes, wherever possible, rather than chemically intensive methods.[14] Table C15-1 contrasts alternative agriculture methods with unsustainable methods now in use. (Many of those techniques are not really new, incidentally, and would be familiar to our great grandparents. They were superseded by high-tech methods and are now coming back into favor.)

Farming by these methods produces crops reliably and reduces farmers' financial risks by reducing the impacts of changes in the prices of pesticides, fertilizers, and the like. Both large and small farms can use these practices, and many different machineries are compatible with them. Each technique has a different value for farmers of different crops in different regions. For example, corn and soybean farmers in the Midwest can relatively easily eliminate routine insecticide use, whereas fruit and vegetable growers in the hot and humid Southeast would find this harder to do.[15] Not all crops can grow reliably without pesticides, but many can.

Alternative agriculture has some apparent disadvantages, but they are offset by advantages. For example, as chemical use falls, yields per acre also fall somewhat, but costs per acre also fall, so that the return per acre may be the same as or greater than before. More money goes to farmers and less to the fuels, fertilizers, pesticides, and irrigation that subsidies would pay for. Prices for farm products may rise, but taxes can fall, because subsidies can be eliminated. The end result is to make consumers better off financially.

Some economists and scientists have suggested that rather than subsidizing pesticide and fertilizer use, we should be taxing it. Some states are trying out that strategy, with success.[16] Some are proposing to tax products such as sugar at the grocery-store level, to raise money to repair the environmental damage it causes.[17]

Low-input agriculture works. More than 30,000 of the nation's farmers are successfully using sustainable techniques such as those described in Table C15-1. Notable among them are farmers in seven states who began pioneering these methods on a large scale in the

Table C15-1
Alternative Agricultural Techniques

Nonsustainable Practice	Sustainable Practice
■ Grow the same crop repeatedly on the same patch of land. This takes more and more nutrients out of the soil, making fertilizer use necessary; favors soil erosion; and invites weeds and pests to become established, making pesticide use necessary.	■ Rotate crops. This increases nitrogen in the soil so there is less need to buy fertilizers. If used with appropriate plowing methods, crop rotation reduces soil erosion. An acre of land planted one year in corn, the next in wheat, and the next in clover loses 2.7 tons of topsoil each year, but if it is planted only in corn three years in a row, it will lose 19.7 tons a year. Crop rotation also reduces problems caused by weeds and pests.
■ Use fertilizers generously.	■ Reduce the use of fertilizers and use livestock manure more effectively. This means storing it during the nongrowing season and applying it during the growing season.
	■ Alternate nutrient-devouring crops with nutrient-restoring crops.
	■ Plant legumes between grain crops (because legumes' roots leave nitrogen in the soil).
	■ Compost on a large scale, including all plant residues not harvested. Plow the compost into the soil to improve its water-holding capacity.
■ Feed livestock in feed lots where their manure produces a major water-pollution problem. Piled in heaps, manure also releases methane, a global-warming gas.	■ Feed livestock or buffalo on the open range where their manure will fertilize the ground on which plants grow and will release no methane. Alternatively, at least collect feed-lot animals' manure and use it as fertilizer, or, at the very least, treat it before release.
■ Spray herbicides and pesticides over large areas to wipe out weeds and pests.	■ Apply ingenuity in weed and pest control. Use rotary hoes twice instead of herbicides once. Treat when and where necessary only. Spot treat weeds by hand.[a]
	■ Rotate crops to foil pests that lay their eggs in the soil where last year's crop was grown.[a]
	■ Use resistant crops. Genetically improve crops so that they resist pests and diseases.[a]
	■ Time the planting of crops so that pests that hatch at other times cannot gain access to them.[a]
	■ Use biological controls such as predators that destroy the pests.[a]
■ Plow the same way everywhere, allowing unsustainable water runoff and erosion.	■ Plow in ways tailored to different areas. Conserve both soil and water by using cover crops, crop rotation, and contour plowing.
■ To prevent disease in livestock, inject animals with antibiotics.	■ Maintain animals' health so that they can resist disease by way of their own vigor.
■ Irrigate on a large scale.	■ Irrigate only during dry spells and apply only spot irrigation.

[a]These techniques, known as **integrated pest management (IPM)**, involve minimal use of poisons, less expense, and less fuel use.

Source: Committee on the Role of Alternate Farming Methods in Modern Production Agriculture, Board on Agriculture, National Research Council, *Alternative Agriculture* (Washington, D.C.: National Academy Press, 1989); D. Pimentel, *Food, Energy and the Future of Society* (Boulder, Colo.: Associated University Press, 1980); A. B. Durning and H. B. Brough, *Taking Stock: Animal Farming and the Environment, Worldwatch Paper 103,* July 1991, p. 14; L. R. Brown, World population growth, soil erosion, and food security, *Science* 214 (1981): 995–1002.

Table C15-2
Energy-Saving Agricultural Techniques

Nonsustainable Practice	Sustainable Practice
■ Use large machinery.	■ Use smaller machinery scaled to the job at hand and operating at efficient speeds.
■ Harrow, then plant, then fertilize.	■ Combine operations. Harrow, plant, and fertilize in the same operation.
■ Use gasoline.	■ Use diesel fuel. Use solar and wind energy on farms. Use methane from manure. Be open-minded to alternative energy sources.
■ Use as little labor as possible.	■ Save on technological and chemical inputs and spend some of the savings paying people to do manual jobs. Increasing labor inputs has been considered inefficient. Reverse this thinking: creating more jobs is preferable to using more machinery and fuel.
■ Use chemical fertilizers.	■ Partially return to the techniques of using animal manure and crop rotation. This would save energy because chemical fertilizers require large energy inputs to produce.
■ Transport food by trucks.	■ Eliminate subsidies to truckers. Change highway funding so that the tax burden falls more heavily on truckers than on other highway users. Transport foods by rail or water (building and maintaining rail lines can add more jobs than are lost in trucking). To move lettuce by truck from California to New York requires 36 calories for each calorie in the lettuce. Railways are five times more efficient than trucks.
■ Let people cook food however they wish.	■ Educate people to cook food efficiently. Use the cooking practices suggested in Chapter 15.
■ Grow crops without regard to their energy requirements.	■ Choose crops that require low energy inputs (fertilizer, pesticides, irrigation).

Source: D. Pimentel, *Food, Energy and the Future of Society* (Boulder, Colo.: Associated University Press, 1980); A. Durning, How much is enough? *Co-op America Quarterly,* Winter 1991, pp. 10–15; M. Renner, *Jobs in a Sustainable Economy, Worldwatch Paper 104,* September 1991, p. 6.

1980s and before.* Low-input agriculture has been called "an idea whose time has come."[18] It is seen as "a food production system that can indefinitely sustain a healthy food supply, restore our soil and water resources, and revitalize individual farms and rural communities, all with little reliance on fossil fuels."[19]

Energy Efficiency It need not cost 6,560 calories to produce a can of corn, or 7,980 calories to produce a package of frozen corn. Much of this energy input could be reduced. Table C15-2 offers many suggestions.

*In seven states, case studies were going on prior to 1990: Ohio, Iowa, Virginia, Pennsylvania, California, Florida, and Colorado. *Organic Agriculture: What the States Are Doing* (Washington, D.C.: Center for Science in the Public Interest, 1989).

The last suggestion in the table implies that consumers should center their diets on foods that require low energy inputs, a choice that is described next. Often, that means choosing plants over meats.

Eat Lower on the Food Chain Studies of energy use in the U.S. food system have revealed which foods require the most and least energy to produce. The least energy is needed for grain: about one-third calorie is spent on fuel to produce each calorie of grain. Fruits and vegetables are intermediate, and most animal protein requires from 10 to 90 calories of fossil energy per calorie of usable food. Thus most animal protein products require significantly larger inputs of energy, as well as of land and water, than do plant protein products.[20] An exception is livestock grown on the open range;

Figure C15-1

AMOUNTS OF FUEL REQUIRED TO FEED PEOPLE EATING AT DIFFERENT LEVELS ON THE FOOD CHAIN

Three people who eat differently are compared here. Each has the same energy intake: 3,300 calories a day. The fossil fuel amounts necessary to produce these different diets are calculated based on U.S. conditions.

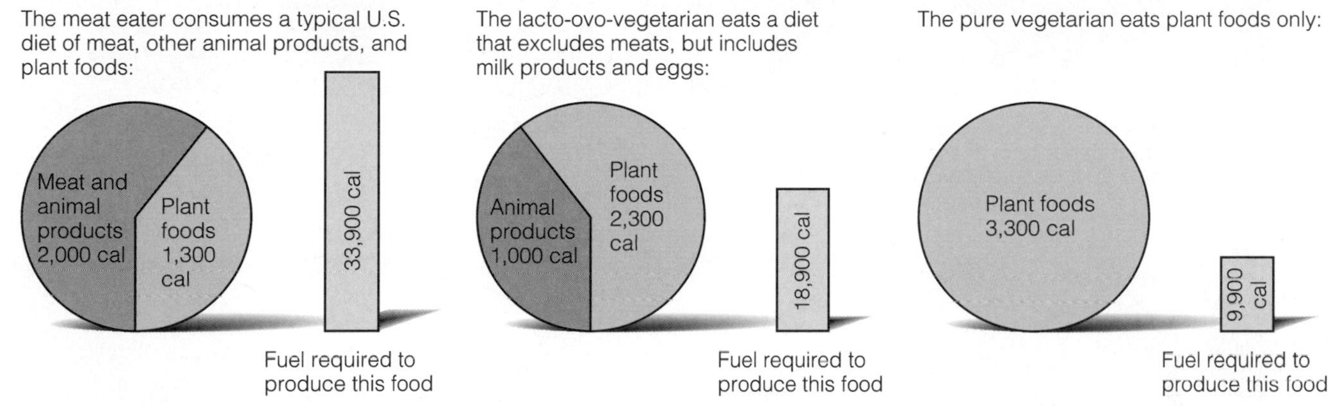

Source: Adapted from D. Pimentel, *Food, Energy and the Future of Society* (Boulder, Colo.: Associated University Press, 1980), Figure 5, p. 27.

these animals require low energy inputs as do most plant foods. We grow so much more grain-fed, than range-fed, beef, however, that the average energy requirement for beef production is high. Figure C15-1 shows how much less fuel vegetarian diets require than meat diets and shows that vegan diets require the least fuel of all.

To support our meat intake we maintain several billion livestock, about four times our own weight in animals. Livestock consume ten times as much grain each day as we do. We could use much of that grain to make grain products for ourselves and share them. The shift could free up enough grain to feed 400 million people and would necessitate burning less fuel and using less water. It could free up much more land. In China, a society that does live almost entirely on plant foods, the contrast with U.S. resource use is startling (see Figure C15-2).

Part of the solution to the livestock problem may be to cease feeding grain to livestock and return to grazing animals on the open range, which can be a sustainable practice. Ranchers have to manage the grazing carefully to hold the cattle's numbers to what the land can support without degradation. To accomplish this, the economic favoritism shown to livestock and feed-growing operations would have to be removed. If producers were to pay the true costs of the irrigation water, fertilizers, pesticides, fuels, and lands they use rather than paying artificially lowered prices, the prices of meats might rise to two or three times what they are now. According to classic economic theory, people would then buy less meat (reducing demand), and producers would respond by producing less meat (reducing supply). Meat production would then fall to a sustainable level.

Some individuals are taking action without waiting for prices to change. Some meat eaters are choosing to cut down on their meat portions or to eat range-fed beef or buffalo only. Livestock on the range eat grass, which people cannot eat.[21] "Rangeburger" buffalo also offers nutrition advantages over grain-fed beef. It is lower in fat, and the fat has more polyunsaturated fatty acids, including the omega-3 type.[22]

Some people are switching to nonmeat, and even pure vegan, diets.[23] Shifting to a fish diet appears not to be a practical alternative, at present, although fish farming shows promise of becoming practical in the future and could help greatly to provide nutritious meat at a price people and the environment could afford.[24] At present, extensive overfishing has been reducing many of the ocean's fish species for the whole last quarter of the 20th century; ocean fishing cannot meet the need. Also, much fish production is energy intensive, requiring large inputs of fuel for boats, refrigeration, processing, packing, and transport. Moreover,

Figure C15-2

RESOURCE USE IN THE UNITED STATES AND CHINA COMPARED

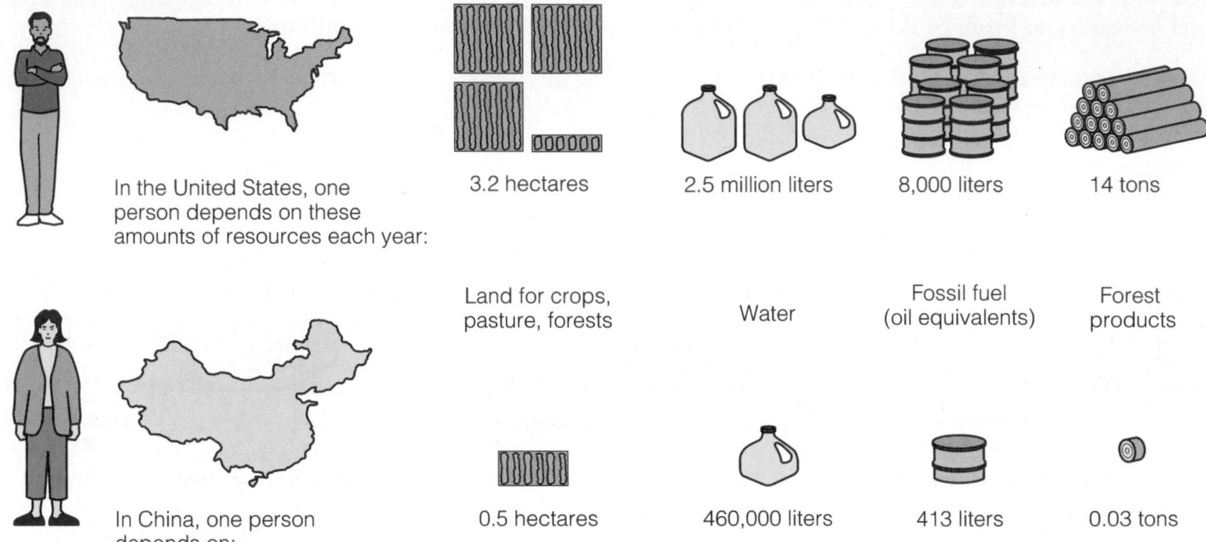

Source: D. Pimentel and M. Pimentel, Land, energy, and water: The constraints governing ideal U.S. population size, *The NPG* (Negative Population Growth) *Forum*, January 1990, Table 2, p. 2.

bioaccumulation of toxins in fish is becoming a serious problem in some areas; in others it altogether rules out fish consumption.

Cut the Population Several of the experts quoted in this Controversy agree that a continuing increase in the human population on earth can quickly defeat our best efforts to secure a viable future for our planet. If our numbers double, our food production must double, but to enlarge our food output now is costing more for each step taken. Only poor land is available now. More fertilizer, more pesticides, and more fuel are required to make such land productive. We have outstripped our environment's ability to provide a quality life for ourselves. If resources were equally shared, about 1 billion people could enjoy a relatively high-quality life, but there are 5-plus billion human beings currently on earth with resources unequally distributed. As a result, most people around the world have a low-quality life.

The hunger problem and the population problem are becoming drastically worse as we enter the 21st century. Meanwhile, global warming seems to be starting to contribute to the demise of agriculture. The primary problem is carbon dioxide from the burning of fossil fuels mainly in the United States; the destruction of forests is also contributing.[25] Global warming could reduce our ability to grow many major crops where we grow them today. If the warming proceeds, the United States will cease to be a major producer of food, although for a while it may be able to produce enough to feed itself. If the polar ice caps melt and sea levels rise, river deltas now used for agriculture will disappear, and many plants and animals will become extinct. It seems, therefore, that fast progress toward producing food sustainably, and especially with reduced energy use, is imperative.

A return to smaller farms, smaller machinery, less fuel use, and more labor would create many more jobs. The money to pay the workers could come from savings on costs of fuel, fertilizers, pesticides, irrigation, pollution cleanup, and unemployment.[26]

Chapter 15 and its Controversy have presented many problems, and have suggested that, while the problems are global in scope, the actions of individual people lie at the heart of their solutions. On learning of this, concerned people may take a perfectionist attitude, believing that they "should" be doing more than they realistically can, and so feel defeated. Yet, striving for perfection, even while falling short, is a way to achieve

progress well worth celebrating. A positive attitude can bring about improvement, and improvement is enough to be proud of. Celebrate the changes that are possible today by making them a permanent part of your life; do the same with changes that become possible tomorrow and every day thereafter. The results may surprise you.

Notes

1. Committee on the Role of Alternative Farming Methods in Modern Production Agriculture, Board on Agriculture, National Research Council, *Alternative Agriculture* (Washington, D.C.: National Academy Press, 1989).
2. World Resources Institute, *The 1992 Information Please Environmental Almanac* (Boston: Houghton Mifflin, 1992), p. 13.
3. J. Dixon, Agency warns of threats posed by plant extinction, *Tallahassee Democrat*, 24 March 1992.
4. C. B. Heiser, Jr., *Seeds to Civilization, The Story of Food* (Cambridge, Mass: Harvard University Press, 1990), p. 13.
5. D. Pimentel, *Food, Energy and the Future of Society* (Boulder, Colo.: Associated University Press, 1980), p. 9.
6. P. H. Raven, L. R. Berg, and G. B. Johnson, *Environment* (New York: Saunders, 1993), p. 407.
7. National Research Council, 1989, p. 7.
8. National Research Council, 1989, p. 6.
9. A. B. Durning and H. B. Brough, *Taking Stock: Animal Farming and the Environment, Worldwatch Paper 103*, July 1991, p. 35.
10. K. Mattes, Kicking the pesticide habit, *The Amicus Journal*, Fall 1989, pp. 10–17.
11. Farm subsidies: The "eyes to acres" ratio, *Rocky Mountain Institute Newsletter*, Summer 1991, p. 6.
12. C. Mitlo-Shartel and the Land Stewardship Project, Regenerating America's agriculture, *Building Economic Alternatives* (a quarterly publication of Co-op America, 2100 M. Street NW, Suite 310, Washington, D.C. 20063), Summer 1989, pp. 9–12.
13. National Research Council, 1989.
14. National Research Council, 1989, pp. 3–4.
15. National Research Council, 1989, p. 5.
16. Organic Agriculture: *What the States Are Doing* (Washington, D.C.: Center for Science in the Public Interest, 1989), pp. 5, 14–15.
17. B. Bergstrom, Environmentalists seek penny-a-pound sugar tax, *Tallahassee Democrat*, 30 September 1993.
18. *Organic Agriculture: What the States Are Doing*, 1989. The quote is from the assistant secretary of agriculture, Orville G. Bentley, in a USDA press release, February 1988.
19. Mitlo-Shartel and the Land Stewardship Project, 1989.
20. Pimentel, 1980, p. 11.
21. A. T. Durning and H. B. Brough, Reforming the livestock economy, in *State of the World, 1992* (New York: Norton, 1992), pp. 66–82.
22. S. Smith, professor of nutrition, University of New Hampshire, Durham, N.H., Personal communication, August 1993.
23. A. Zorc, From family farm to agribusiness: The spoilage of America's meat industry, *Co-op America Quarterly*, Spring 1992, pp. 10–13, 19; Eating green, *Nutrition Action Health Letter*, January-February 1992, pp. 1, 5–7.
24. C. Flavin and J. E. Young, Shaping the next industrial revolution, in L. R. Brown, *State of the World 1993* (New York: Norton, 1993), pp. 180–199.
25. Heiser, 1990, p. 212.
26. M. G. Renner, Saving the earth, creating jobs, *World Watch*, January-February 1992, pp. 10–17.

APPENDIXES

CONTENTS

TABLE OF FOOD COMPOSITION

This table of food composition is specifically designed for this textbook. It contains more complete values for dietary fiber; saturated, monounsaturated, and polyunsaturated fat; vitamin B_6; folate; magnesium; and zinc than any comparable table. Also, a wide variety of foods from all food groups are included, and updated yearly to reflect current food patterns. For example, this edition includes the new vegetable broccoflower, nonfat items, and new selections of frozen convenience foods and baby foods.

To achieve a complete and reliable listing of nutrients for all the foods, over 1000 sources of information are researched. Government sources of information are the primary base for all the data: the USDA *Handbook* series and its current supplemental data, as well as current data on baked goods and snacks and sweets. In addition, provisional USDA information—both published and unpublished—is included. Many conversations with the staff members at the USDA Human Nutrition Information Service in Hyattsville, Maryland, provided additional professional information to refine the data.

Even with all the government sources available, there are still missing nutrient values; and as the various government data are updated, conflicting values are reported from the USDA for the same items. To fill in the missing values and resolve discrepancies, other sources of information are used. These reliable sources include refereed journal articles, food composition tables from Canada and England, information from other nutrient data banks and publications, unpublished scientific data, and manufacturers' data.

Estimates of nutrient amounts for foods and nutrients include all possible adjustments, in the interest of accuracy. When multiple values are reported for a nutrient, the numbers are averaged and weighted, with consideration given to the original number of samples from the separate sources. Whenever water percentages are available, estimates of nutrient amounts are adjusted for water content. When no water is given, water percentage is assumed to be that shown in the table. Whenever a reported weight appeared inconsistent (cooked eggplant and collards, for example), many kitchen tests were made, and the average weight of the typical product was given as tested.

When estimates of nutrient amounts in cooked foods are derived from reported amounts in raw foods, published retention factors are applied. Some reported data for combination foods are modified in this table to include the newer data available for major ingredients. For example, since the "pies" were analyzed and reported, newer data on fruits have been published. Bakery items reflect the most current data with the new enrichment levels for certain nutrients. And, new information on some snacks and sweets is reflected in this edition.

Considerable effort has been made to report the most accurate data available and to eliminate missing values. The table is updated annually, and the authors welcome any suggestions or comments for future editions.

IT IS IMPORTANT TO KNOW

that there can be many different nutrient values reported for foods, even by reliable sources. Many factors influence the amounts of nutrients in foods, including the mineral content of the soil, the method of processing, genetics, the diet of the animal or the fertilizer of the plant, the season of the year, methods of analysis, the difference in moisture content of the samples analyzed, the length and method of storage, and methods of cooking the food.

Although each nutrient from USDA government data is presented as a single number in some USDA publications, each number is actually an average of a range of data. In the more detailed reports (Handbook 8 series), the number of samples is identified, and the standard deviation of the data is also noted. USDA data will have different reported values for foods as well, as older information is replaced with newer data in the more recent publications. Therefore, nutrient data should be viewed and used only as a guide, a close approximation of nutrient content.

Dietary fiber deserves a special word. Estimates of dietary fiber are included for all the foods in this table. The sources of this information are primarily extensive published and unpublished information from the USDA Human Nutrition

Information Service in Hyattsville, Maryland; *Composition of Foods by Southgate* (England); and many journal articles.

It is important to know that data for dietary fiber is still undergoing review in the scientific community. No doubt, there will be changes in the data as analytical techniques are refined and interpretations clarified.

Vitamin A is reported in retinol equivalents. The amount of this vitamin can vary by the season of the year and the maturity of the plant (note the difference between sun-ripened and store-ripened papaya). Reported values in both dairy products and plants are higher in summer and early fall than in winter. The values reported here represent year-round averages. In the organ meats of all animal products (liver especially), there are large amounts of vitamin A, and these amounts vary widely, depending on the background of the animal. The vitamin is present in very small amounts in regular meat and is often reported as a trace.

Newer reported vitamin A values for some plant foods have increased significantly due to additional information and sometimes to newer plant genetics. New vitamin A values for canned pumpkin, for example, are 3.5 times greater than the previously reported values.

The energy and nutrients in recipes and combination foods vary widely, depending on the ingredients. The various fatty acids and cholesterol are influenced by the type of fat used (the specific type of oil, vegetable shortening, butter, margarine, etc.).

Total fats, as well as the breakdown of total fats to saturated, monounsaturated, and polyunsaturated fats, are listed in the table. The fatty acids seldom add up to the total. This is due to rounding and to the existence of small amounts of other fatty acid components that are not included in the three basic categories, including trans fatty acids and glycerol.

Niacin values are for preformed niacin and do not include additional niacin that may form in the body from the conversion of tryptophan.

The items in this table have been organized into several categories, which are listed at the head of each right-hand page. As the key shows, each group has been color-coded to ease paging through this table.

In an effort to conserve space, abbreviations have been used in some food descriptions. The following abbreviations have been used in the food descriptions and nutrient breakdowns:

- diam = diameter
- enr = enriched
- f/ = from
- g = grams
- liq = liquid
- pce = piece
- w/ = with
- w/o = without
- t = trace
- 0 = no nutrient value
- – = information not available

A

A

Table A–1
Food Composition

Computer Code Number	Food Description	Measure	Wt (g)	H_2O (%)	Ener (cal)	Prot (g)	Carb (g)	Dietary Fiber (g)	Fat (g)	Fat Breakdown (g) Sat	Mono	Poly
	BEVERAGES											
	Alcoholic:											
	Beer:											
1	Regular (12 fl oz)	1½ c	356	92	145	1	13	2	0	0	0	0
2	Light (12 fl oz)	1½ c	354	95	99[1]	1	5	1	0	0	0	0
1506	Nonalcoholic (12 fl oz)	1 ea	360	98	32	1	5	0	0	0	0	0
	Gin, rum, vodka, whiskey:											
3	80 proof	1½ fl oz	42	67	97	0	0	0	0	0	0	0
4	86 proof	1½ fl oz	42	64	105	0	<1	0	0	0	0	0
5	90 proof	1½ fl oz	42	62	110	0	0	0	0	0	0	0
	Liqueur:											
1359	Coffee liqueur, 53 proof	1½ fl oz	52	31	174	<1	24	0	<1	.1	t	.1
1360	Coffee & cream liqueur, 34 proof	1½ fl oz	47	46	153	1	10	0	7	4.5	2.1	.3
1361	Crème de menthe, 72 proof	1½ fl oz	50	28	185	0	21	0	<1	t	t	.1
	Wine:											
6	Dessert (4 fl oz)	½ c	118	72	181[2]	<1	14	0	0	0	0	0
7	Red	3½ fl oz	103	88	74	<1	2	0	0	0	0	0
8	Rosé	3½ fl oz	103	89	73	<1	1	0	0	0	0	0
9	White medium	3½ fl oz	103	90	70	<1	1	0	0	0	0	0
1592	Nonalcoholic	1 c	232	98	14	1	3	0	0	0	0	0
1593	Nonalcoholic light	1 c	251	98	15	1	3	0	0	0	0	0
1409	Wine cooler, bottle (12 fl oz)	1½ c	340	90	169	<1	20	<1	<1	0	0	t
1595	Wine cooler, cup	1 c	227	90	113	<1	13	<1	<1	0	0	t
	Carbonated:[3]											
10	Club soda (12 fl oz)	1½ c	355	100	0	0	0	0	0	0	0	0
11	Cola beverage (12 fl oz)	1½ c	370	89	151	0	38	0	<1	0	t	.1
12	Diet cola w/aspartame (12 fl oz)	1½ c	355	100	4	<1	<1	0	0	0	0	0
13	Diet cola w/saccharin (12 fl oz)	1½ c	355	100	0	0	<1	0	0	0	0	0
14	Ginger ale (12 fl oz)	1½ c	366	91	124	0	32	0	0	0	0	0
15	Grape soda (12 fl oz)	1½ c	372	89	159	0	42	0	0	0	0	0
16	Lemon-lime (12 fl oz)	1½ c	368	89	147	0	38	0	0	0	0	0
17	Orange (12 fl oz)	1½ c	372	88	178	0	46	0	0	0	0	0
18	Pepper-type soda (12 fl oz)	1½ c	368	89	150	0	38	0	<1	.3	0	0
19	Root beer (12 fl oz)	1½ c	370	89	151	0	39	0	0	0	0	0
20	Coffee,[3] brewed	1 c	240	99	5[4]	<1	1	<1	<1	t	0	t
21	Coffee,[3] prepared from instant	1 c	240	99	5[4]	<1	1	0	<1	t	0	t
	Fruit drinks, noncarbonated:[5]											
22	Fruit punch drink, canned	2 c	126	88	59	0	15	0	<1	t	t	t
1358	Gatorade	1 c	240	93	60	0	15	0	0	0	0	0
23	Grape drink, canned	2 c	125	87	62	<1	16	<1	0	0	0	0
1304	Kool-Aid, with sugar	1 c	240	90	89	0	23	0	<1	t	t	t
1356	Kool-Aid, with nutrasweet	1 c	240	95	43	0	11	0	0	0	0	0

(1)Calories can vary from 78 to 131 for 12 fl. oz.

(2)Values are for sweet dessert wine. Dry dessert wines contain 149 cal and 5 g of carbohydrate.

(3)Mineral content varies depending on water source.

(4)Cal values from USDA vary from 1 to 5 calories per cup.

(5)Usually less than 10% fruit juice.

(Computer code number is for West Diet Analysis program)

PAGE KEY: A–2 = BEV A–4 = DAIRY A–10 = EGGS A–12 = FAT/OIL A–14 = FRUIT A–24 = BAKERY A–34 = GRAIN A–40 = FISH A–44 = MEATS A–48 = POULTRY A–50 = SAUSAGE A–52 = MIXED/FAST A–60 = NUTS/SEEDS A–62 = SWEETS A–66 = VEG/LEG A–78 = MISC A–80 = SOUPS/SAUCES A–84 = FAST A–96 = FRZN ENTREE A–98 = BABY FOODS

Chol (mg)	Calc (mg)	Iron (mg)	Magn (mg)	Phos (mg)	Pota (mg)	Sodi (mg)	Zinc (mg)	VT-A (RE)	Thia (mg)	Ribo (mg)	Niac (mg)	V-B6 (mg)	Fola (µg)	VT-C (mg)
0	18	.11	21	43	89	18	.07	0	.02	.09	1.61	.18	21	0
0	18	.14	18	42	64	11	.11	0	.03	.11	1.39	.12	14	0
0	25	.04	32	112	90	18	.04	0	.04	.11	1.62	.18	25	0
0	0	.02	0	2	1	<1	.02	0	<.01	<.01	<.01	0	0	0
0	0	.02	0	2	1	<1	.02	0	<.01	<.01	<.01	0	0	0
0	0	.02	0	2	1	<1	.02	0	<.01	<.01	<.01	0	0	0
0	1	.03	2	3	16	41	.02	0	<.01	<.01	<.07	0	0	0
7	8	.06	1	23	15	43	.07	20	0	.03	.04	.01	0	0
0	0	.03	0	0	0	2	.02	0	0	0	<.01	0	0	0
0	9	.28	11	11	108	11	.08	0	.02	.02	.25	0	<1	0
0	8	.44	13	14	115	5	.09	0	<.01	.03	.08	.03	2	0
0	8	.39	10	15	102	5	.06	0	<.01	.02	.08	.02	1	0
0	9	.33	11	14	82	5	.07	0	<.01	<.01	.07	.01	<1	0
0	21	.93	23	35	204	16	.19	0	0	.02	.23	.05	2	0
0	23	1	25	38	221	18	.2	0	0	.02	.25	.05	3	0
0	19	.92	18	22	–	29	.2	1	.03	.03	.17	.03	4	6
0	13	.61	12	15	–	19	.14	<1	.02	.02	.11	.02	3	4
0	18	.04	4	0	7	75	.35	0	0	0	0	0	0	0
0	11	.11	4	44	4	15	.04	0	0	0	0	0	0	0
0	14	.11	4	32	0	21[6]	.28	0	.02	.08	0	0	0	0
0	14	.14	4	39	7	57	.18	0	0	0	0	0	0	0
0	11	.66	4	0	4	26	.18	0	0	0	0	0	0	0
0	11	.3	4	0	4	56	.26	0	0	0	0	0	0	0
0	7	.26	4	0	4	40	.18	0	0	0	.05	0	0	0
0	19	.22	4	4	7	45	.37	0	0	0	0	0	0	0
0	11	.15	0	40	4	37	.15	0	0	0	0	0	0	0
0	18	.18	4	0	4	48	.26	0	0	0	0	0	0	0
0	5	.12	12	2	129	5	.05	0	0	0	.53	0	<1	0
0	7	.12	10	7	86	7	.07	0	0	<.01	.68	0	0	0
0	10	.27	3	1	32	28	.15	1	.03	.03	.03	0	2	37
0	0	.12	2	22	26	96	.05	0	.01	0	0	0	0	0
0	4	.12	5	5	44	1	.04	0	.01	.01	.12	.02	1	20
0	38	.12	2	48	2	34	.07	0	0	<.01	<.01	0	<1	28
0	17	.65	5	5	50	50	.26	2	.02	.05	.05	0	5	77

[6] Value for product sweetened with aspartame only; sodium is 32 mg if a blend of aspartame and sodium saccharin is used.

Table A–1
Food Composition

Computer Code Number	Food Description	Measure	Wt (g)	H_2O (%)	Ener (cal)	Prot (g)	Carb (g)	Dietary Fiber (g)	Fat (g)	Fat Breakdown (g) Sat	Mono	Poly
	BEVERAGES—Cont.											
	Fruit drinks, noncarbonated—Cont.											
26	Lemonade, frozen concentrate (6-oz can)	¾ c	219	52	396	1	103	1	<1	.1	t	.1
27	Lemonade, from concentrate	1 c	248	89	99	<1	26	<1	<1	t	t	t
28	Limeade, frozen concentrate (6-oz can)	¾ c	218	50	408	<1	107	1	<1	t	t	.1
29	Limeade, from concentrate	1 c	247	89	101	0	27	<1	<1	t	t	t
24	Pineapple grapefruit, canned	1 c	250	88	117	<1	29	<1	<1	t	t	.1
25	Pineapple orange, canned	1 c	250	87	125	3	29	<1	<1	t	t	t
	Fruit and vegetable juices: see Fruit and Vegetable sections											
	Slim Fast:[1]											
1612	Chocolate malt with nonfat milk	1 c	273	82	190	14	32	2	1	.3	.1	t
1613	Strawberry with nonfat milk	1 c	273	82	190	14	32	2	1	.3	.1	t
1611	Vanilla with nonfat milk	1 c	273	82	190	14	32	2	1	.3	.1	t
	Ultra Slim Fast:[1]											
1616	Chocolate with nonfat milk	1 c	278	81	200	14	36	5	1	.3	.1	t
1614	French vanilla with nonfat milk	1 c	278	81	190	14	36	4	1	.3	.1	t
1615	Strawberry Supreme with nonfat milk	1 c	278	81	190	14	36	4	1	.3	.1	t
1357	Water, bottled: Perrier (6½ fl oz)	1 ea	192	100	0	0	0	0	0	0	0	0
1594	Water, bottled: Tonic water	1½ c	366	91	124	0	32	0	0	0	0	0
	Tea:[2]											
30	Brewed, regular	1 c	240	100	2	0	1	0	<1	t	t	t
1662	Brewed, herbal	¾ c	178	100	2	0	1	0	t	t	t	t
32	From instant, sweetened	1 c	262	91	89	<1	22	0	<1	t	t	t
31	From instant, unsweetened	1 c	237	100	2	0	<1	0	0	0	0	0
	DAIRY											
	Butter: see Fats and Oils, #158,159,160											
	Cheese, natural:											
33	Blue	1 oz	28	42	100	6	1	0	8	5.3	2.2	.2
34	Brick	1 oz	28	41	105	7	1	0	8	5.3	2.4	.2
35	Brie	1 oz	28	48	94	6	<1	0	8	4.9	2.3	.2
36	Camembert	1 oz	28	52	85	6	<1	0	7	4.3	2	.2
37	Cheddar:	1 oz	28	37	114	7	<1	0	9	6	2.7	.3
38	1" cube	1 ea	17	37	68	4	<1	0	6	3.6	1.6	.2
39	Shredded	1 c	113	37	453	28	1	0	37	23.8	10.6	1.1
	Cottage:											
1406	Low sodium, low fat	1 c	225	83	162	28	6	0	2	1.4	.6	.07
40	Creamed, large curd	1 c	225	79	232	28	6	0	10	6.4	2.9	.3
41	Creamed, small curd	1 c	210	79	216	26	6	0	9	6	2.7	.3
42	With fruit	1 c	226	72	278	22	30	0	8	4.9	2.2	.2
43	Low fat 2%	1 c	226	79	202	31	8	0	4	2.8	1.2	.1
44	Low fat 1%	1 c	226	82	163	28	6	0	2	1.5	.7	.1
45	Dry curd	1 c	145	80	122	25	3	0	1	.4	.2	t
46	Cream	1 oz	28	54	99	2	1	0	10	6.2	2.8	.4
47	Edam	1 oz	28	42	101	7	<1	0	8	5	2.3	.2
48	Feta	1 oz	28	55	75	4	1	0	6	4.2	1.3	.2
49	Gouda	1 oz	28	41	101	7	1	0	8	5	2.2	.2

(1)See Chapter 8 for healthy weight loss strategies. The formulas for these products change periodically; these data reflect nutrient values as of our publication date.

(2)Mineral content varies depending on water source.

(Computer code number is for West Diet Analysis program)

Chol (mg)	Calc (mg)	Iron (mg)	Magn (mg)	Phos (mg)	Pota (mg)	Sodi (mg)	Zinc (mg)	VT-A (RE)	Thia (mg)	Ribo (mg)	Niac (mg)	V-B6 (mg)	Fola (μg)	VT-C (mg)
0	15	1.58	11	20	146	9	.17	22	.06	.21	.16	.05	22	39[3]
0	7	.4	5	5	37	7	.1	5	.01	.05	.04	.01	5	10[3]
0	11	.22	9	13	128	0	.09	0	.02	.02	.22	0	9	26
0	7	.07	2	2	32	5	.05	0	<.01	<.01	.05	0	2	7
0	17	.77	15	15	152	35	.15	10	.07	.04	.67	.1	26	115
0	12	.67	15	10	115	7	.15	133	.07	.05	.52	.12	27	56
4	450	6.3	140	400	690	230	5.25	350	.52	.59	7	.7	120	21
4	450	6.3	140	400	720	220	5.25	350	.52	.59	7	.7	120	21
4	450	6.31	140	401	721	220	5.24	349	.52	.59	6.99	.7	120	21
.4	450	6.3	140	400	800	230	5.25	350	.52	.59	7	.7	120	21
.4	450	6.3	140	400	730	250	5.25	350	.52	.59	7	.7	120	21
.4	450	6.3	140	400	710	250	5.25	350	.52	.59	7	.7	120	21
0	27	0	0	0	0	2	0	0	0	0	0	0	0	0
0	4	.04	0	0	0	15	.37	0	0	0	0	0	0	0
0	0	.05	7	2	89	7	.05	0	0	.03	0	0	12	0
0	4	.14	2	0	16	2	.07	0	.02	.01	0	0	1	0
0	5	.05	5	3	50	8	.08	0	0	.05	.09	<.01	10	0
0	5	.05	5	2	47	7	.07	0	0	<.01	.09	<.01	1	0
21	149	.09	6	110	73	395	.75	65	.01	.11	.29	.05	10	0
27	191	.12	7	128	39	158	.74	86	<.01	.1	.03	.02	6	0
28	52	.14	6	53	43	178	.67	52	.02	.15	.11	.07	18	0
20	110	.09	6	98	53	239	.67	71	.01	.14	.18	.06	18	0
30	204	.19	8	145	28	176	.88	86	.01	.11	.02	.02	5	0
18	122	.12	5	87	17	105	.53	51	<.01	.06	.01	.01	3	0
119	811	.77	31	577	111	701	3.51	342	.03	.43	.09	.08	21	0
9	137	.3	11	301	193	29	.8	25	.04	.36	.3	.15	27	0
33	135	.31	12	295	190	911	.83	108	.05	.37	.28	.15	27	0
31	126	.29	11	275	177	851	.78	101	.04	.34	.26	.14	26	0
25	107	.25	9	235	151	913	.65	81	.04	.29	.23	.12	22	0
19	154	.36	14	339	217	918	.95	45	.05	.42	.32	.17	30	0
10	137	.32	12	303	193	918	.86	25	.05	.37	.29	.15	28	0
10	46	.33	6	149	47	19	.68	12	.04	.21	.22	.12	21	0
31	23	.34	2	29	34	84	.15	124	<.01	.06	.03	.01	4	0
25	207	.12	8	152	53	274	1.07	72	.01	.11	.02	.02	5	0
25	139	.18	5	95	18	315	.82	36	.04	.24	.28	.12	9	0
32	198	.07	8	155	34	232	1.11	49	.01	.09	.02	.02	6	0

(3)Vitamin C can range from 5 to 72 mg in a small can of frozen concentrate, and from 1 to 18 mg in 1 c of prepared lemonade.

(For purposes of calculations, use "0" for t, <1, <.1, <.01, etc.)

Table A–1
Food Composition

Computer Code Number	Food Description	Measure	Wt (g)	H_2O (%)	Ener (cal)	Prot (g)	Carb (g)	Dietary Fiber (g)	Fat (g)	Fat Breakdown (g) Sat	Mono	Poly
	DAIRY—Cont.											
	Cheese—Cont.											
50	Gruyère	1 oz	28	33	117	8	<1	0	9	5.4	2.8	.5
51	Gorgonzola	1 oz	28	39	111	7	0	0	9	5.5	2.4	.5
52	Liederkranz	1 oz	28	53	87	5	<1	0	8	5.3	2.2	.2
1676	Limburger	1 oz	28	48	93	6	<1	0	8	4.7	2.4	.1
53	Monterey Jack	1 oz	28	41	106	7	<1	0	9	5.4	2.5	.3
54	Mozzarella, whole milk	1 oz	28	54	80	5	1	0	6	3.7	1.9	.2
55	Mozzarella, part-skim milk, low moisture	1 oz	28	49	79	8	1	0	5	3.1	1.4	.1
56	Muenster	1 oz	28	42	104	7	<1	0	9	5.4	2.5	.2
1399	Nonfat (Kraft Singles)	1 oz	28	60	46	7	4	0	0	0	0	0
	Parmesan, grated:											
57	Cup, not pressed down	1 c	100	18	455	41	4	0	30	19	8.7	.7
58	Tablespoon	1 tbs	5	18	23	2	<1	0	1	.9	.4	t
59	Ounce	1 oz	28	18	129	12	1	0	9	5.4	2.5	.2
60	Provolone	1 oz	28	41	99	7	1	0	8	4.8	2.1	.2
61	Ricotta, whole milk	1 c	246	72	428	28	7	0	32	20.4	8.9	.9
62	Ricotta, part-skim milk	1 c	246	74	339	28	13	0	19	12.1	5.7	.6
63	Romano	1 oz	28	31	109	9	1	0	8	4.8	2.2	.2
64	Swiss	1 oz	28	37	106	8	1	0	8	5	2.1	.3
	Pasteurized processed cheese products:											
65	American	1 oz	28	39	106	6	<1	0	9	5.6	2.5	.3
66	Swiss	1 oz	28	42	94	7	1	0	7	4.6	2	.2
67	American cheese food, jar	1 oz	28	43	93	6	2	0	7	4.4	2	.2
68	American cheese spread	1 oz	28	48	82	5	2	0	6	3.8	1.8	.2
69	Cream, sweet:	1 c	242	81	315	7	10	0	28	17.3	8	1
	Half & half (cream & milk):											
70	Tablespoon	1 tbs	15	81	19	<1	1	0	2	1.1	.5	.1
71	Light, coffee or table:	1 c	240	74	468	6	9	0	46	28.8	13.4	1.7
72	Tablespoon	1 tbs	15	74	29	<1	1	0	3	1.8	.8	.1
73	Light whipping cream, liquid:[1]	1 c	239	63	698	5	7	0	74	46.1	21.7	2.1
74	Tablespoon	1 tbs	15	63	44	<1	<1	0	5	2.9	1.4	.1
75	Heavy whipping cream, liquid:[1]	1 c	238	58	821	5	7	0	88	54.7	25.5	3.3
76	Tablespoon	1 tbs	15	58	52	<1	<1	0	6	3.4	1.6	.2
77	Whipped cream, pressurized:	1 c	60	61	154	2	7	0	13	8.3	3.8	.5
78	Tablespoon	1 tbs	4	61	10	<1	<1	0	1	.6	.3	t
79	Cream, sour, cultured:	1 c	230	71	492	7	10	0	48	29.9	13.9	1.8
80	Tablespoon	1 tbs	14	71	30	<1	1	0	3	1.8	.8	.1
	Cream products—imitation and part dairy:											
81	Coffee whitener, frozen or liquid	1 tbs	15	77	20	<1	2	0	1	1.4	t	0
82	Coffee whitener, powdered	1 tsp	2	2	11	<1	1	0	1	.6	t	t
83	Dessert topping, frozen, nondairy:	1 c	75	50	238	1	17	0	19	16.4	1.2	.4
84	Tablespoon	1 tbs	5	50	16	<1	1	0	1	1.1	.1	t
85	Dessert topping, mix with whole milk:	1 c	80	67	151	3	13	0	10	8.6	.7	.2
86	Tablespoon	1 tbs	5	67	9	<1	1	0	1	.5	t	t
88	Dessert topping, pressurized:	1 c	70	60	184	1	11	0	16	13.2	1.3	.2
87	Tablespoon	1 tbs	4	60	10	<1	1	0	1	.8	.1	t

(1)For whipped cream, (non-pressurized), double the liquid cream volume of codes 73, 74 or 75, 76. One tablespoon liquid cream becomes 2 tablespoons when "whipped."

(Computer code number is for West Diet Analysis program)

PAGE KEY: A–2 = BEV A–4 = DAIRY A–10 = EGGS A–12 = FAT/OIL A–14 = FRUIT A–24 = BAKERY A–34 = GRAIN A–40 = FISH A–44 = MEATS A–48 = POULTRY A–50 = SAUSAGE A–52 = MIXED/FAST A–60 = NUTS/SEEDS A–62 = SWEETS A–66 = VEG/LEG A–78 = MISC A–80 = SOUPS/SAUCES A–84 = FAST A–96 = FRZN ENTREE A–98 = BABY FOODS

Chol (mg)	Calc (mg)	Iron (mg)	Magn (mg)	Phos (mg)	Pota (mg)	Sodi (mg)	Zinc (mg)	VT-A (RE)	Thia (mg)	Ribo (mg)	Niac (mg)	V-B6 (mg)	Fola (μg)	VT-C (mg)
31	286	.05	10	171	23	95	1.11	85	.02	.08	.03	.02	3	0
25	149	.12	8	121	26	512	.57	103	.01	.09	.2	.04	9	0
21	110	.12	7	100	68	389	.7	91	.01	.18	.1	.04	34	0
26	141	.04	6	111	36	227	.6	90	.02	.14	.05	.02	16	0
25	211	.2	8	126	23	152	.85	72	<.01	.11	.03	.02	5	0
22	146	.05	5	105	19	105	.63	68	<.01	.07	.02	.02	2	0
15	207	.07	7	148	27	149	.89	54	.01	.1	.03	:02	3	0
27	203	.12	8	132	38	178	.8	90	<.01	.09	.03	.02	3	0
5	162	–	–	202	81	425	–	101	–	.14	–	–	–	0
79	1375	.95	51	807	107	1861	3.19	173	.04	.39	.31	.1	8	0
4	69	.05	3	40	5	93	.16	9	<.01	.02	.02	<.01	<1	0
22	390	.27	14	229	30	528	.9	49	.01	.11	.09	.03	2	0
20	214	.15	8	140	39	247	.92	75	<.01	.09	.04	.02	3	0
124	509	.93	28	389	256	206	2.85	330	.03	.48	.26	.11	30	0
76	669	1.08	36	450	308	305	3.3	278	.05	.45	.19	.05	32	0
29	300	.22	12	215	24	339	.73	40	.01	.1	.02	.02	2	0
26	272	.05	10	171	31	74	1.11	72	.01	.1	.03	.02	2	0
27	174	.11	6	211	46	405	.85	82	.01	.1	.02	.02	2	0
24	219	.17	8	216	61	388	1.03	65	<.01	.08	.01	.01	2	0
18	163	.24	9	130	79	336	.85	62	.01	.13	.04	.04	2	0
16	159	.09	8	202	69	380	.73	54	.01	.12	.04	.03	2	0
89	254	.17	25	230	312	98	1.23	259	.08	.36	.19	.09	6	2
6	16	.01	2	14	19	6	.08	16	<.01	.02	.01	.01	<1	<1
158	230	.1	21	191	293	95	.65	437	.08	.35	.14	.08	6	2
10	14	.01	1	12	18	6	.04	27	<.01	.02	.01	<.01	<1	<1
265	165	.07	17	146	231	82	.6	705	.06	.3	.1	.07	9	1
17	10	<.01	1	9	14	5	.04	44	<.01	.02	.01	<.01	1	<1
326	153	.07	17	148	179	89	.55	1001	.05	.26	.09	.06	9	1
21	10	<.01	1	9	11	6	.03	63	<.01	.02	.01	<.01	1	<1
46	61	.03	6	54	88	78	.22	124	.02	.04	.04	.02	2	0
3	4	<.01	<1	4	6	5	.01	8	<.01	<.01	<.01	<.01	<1	0
102	267	.14	26	195	331	122	.62	449	.08	.34	.15	.04	25	2
6	16	.01	2	12	20	7	.04	27	<.01	.02	.01	<.01	2	<1
0	1	<.01	<1	10	29	12	<.01	1	0	0	0	0	0	0
0	<1	.02	<1	8	16	4	.01	<1	0	<.01	0	0	0	0
0	5	.09	1	6	14	19	.02	64[2]	0	0	0	0	0	0
0	<1	.01	<1	<1	1	1	<.01	4[2]	0	0	0	0	0	0
8	72	.03	8	69	120	53	.22	39[2]	.02	.09	.05	.02	3	1
<1	5	<.01	<1	4	7	3	.01	2[2]	<.01	.01	<.01	<.01	<1	<1
0	4	.01	1	13	13	43	.01	33[2]	.0	0	0	0	0	0
0	<1	<.01	<1	1	1	2	0	2[2]	0	0	0	0	0	0

[2]Vitamin A value is from beta-carotene used for coloring.

(For purposes of calculations, use "0" for t, <1, <.1, <.01, etc.)

Table A–1
Food Composition

Computer Code Number	Food Description	Measure	Wt (g)	H_2O (%)	Ener (cal)	Prot (g)	Carb (g)	Dietary Fiber (g)	Fat (g)	Fat Breakdown (g) Sat	Mono	Poly
	DAIRY—Cont.											
91	Sour cream, imitation:	1 c	230	71	478	6	15	<1	45	40.9	1.3	.1
92	Tablespoon	1 tbs	14	71	29	<1	1	<1	3	2.5	.1	t
89	Sour dressing, part dairy:	1 c	235	75	416	8	11	0	39	31.3	4.6	1.1
90	Tablespoon	1 tbs	15	75	27	<1	1	0	2	2	.3	.1
	Milk, fluid:											
93	Whole milk	1 c	244	88	149	8	11	0	8	5.1	2.3	.3
94	2% low-fat milk	1 c	244	89	121	8	12	0	5	2.9	1.3	.2
95	2% milk solids added[1]	1 c	245	89	124	9	12	0	5	2.9	1.4	.2
96	1% low-fat milk	1 c	244	90	102	8	12	–	3	1.6	.7	.1
97	1% milk solids added[1]	1 c	245	90	104	9	12	0	2	1.5	.7	.1
98	Nonfat milk, vitamin A added	1 c	245	91	85	8	12	0	<1	.3	.1	t
99	Nonfat milk solids added[1]	1 c	245	90	90	9	12	0	1	.4	.2	t
100	Buttermilk, nonfat	1 c	245	90	99	8	12	0	2	1.3	.6	.1
	Milk, canned:											
101	Sweetened condensed	1 c	306	27	982	24	166	0	27	16.8	7.4	1
102	Evaporated, whole	1 c	252	74	338	17	25	0	19	11.6	5.9	.6
103	Evaporated, nonfat	1 c	255	79	199	19	29	0	1	.3	.2	t
	Milk, dried:											
104	Buttermilk, sweet	1 c	120	3	464	41	59	0	7	4.3	2	.3
105	Instant, nonfat, envelope[2]	1 ea	91	4	325	32	47	0	1	.4	.2	t
106	Instant nonfat, cup	1 c	68	4	243	24	35	0	<1	.3	.1	t
107	Goat milk	1 c	244	87	167	9	11	0	10	6.5	2.7	.4
108	Kefir, 2% milkfat[3]	1 c	233	82	122	9	9	0	4	2.9	1.2	.1
	Milk beverages and powdered mixes:											
	Chocolate:											
109	Whole	1 c	250	82	208	8	26	4	8	5.2	2.5	.3
110	2% fat	1 c	250	84	178	8	26	4	5	3.1	1.5	.2
111	1% fat	1 c	250	84	157	8	26	4	2	1.5	.7	.1
	Chocolate-flavored beverages:											
112	Powder containing nonfat dry milk:	1 oz	28	1	102	3	22	<1	1	.7	.4	t
113	Prepared with water	¾ c	206	86	100	4	23	<1	1	.7	.4	t
114	Powder without nonfat dry milk:	¾ oz	22	1	77	1	20	1	1	.4	.2	t
115	Prepared with whole milk	1 c	266	81	226	9	31	<1	9	5.5	2.6	.3
116	Eggnog, commercial	1 c	254	74	340	10	34	0	19	11.3	5.7	.9
1027	Instant Breakfast, envelope, powder only:	1 ea	37	7	131	7	24	<1	1	.3	.1	t
1028	Prepared with whole milk	1 c	281	77	280	15	36	<1	9	5.4	2.5	.3
1029	Prepared with 2% milk	1 c	281	78	252	15	36	<1	5	3.3	1.5	.2
1283	Prepared with 1% milk	1 c	281	80	215	16	36	<1	1	.6	.3	t
1284	Prepared with nonfat milk	1 c	282	80	216	16	36	<1	1	.6	.3	t
117	Malted milk, chocolate, powder:[4]	¾ oz	21	1	79	1	18	<1	1	.5	.2	.1
118	Prepared with whole milk	1 c	265	81	228	9	30	1	9	5.5	2.6	.4
1661	Ovaltine with whole milk	1 c	265	81	225	9	29	1	9	5.5	2.6	.4
119	Malted milk, regular, powder:[4]	¾ oz	21	2	87	2	16	<1	2	.9	.4	.3
120	Prepared with whole milk	1 c	265	81	236	10	27	<1	10	5.9	2.8	.6
121	Milk shakes, chocolate (10 fl oz)	1¼ c	283	71	359	10	58	<1	10	6.5	3	.4
122	Milk shakes, vanilla (10 fl oz)	1¼ c	283	75	314	10	51	<1	8	5.3	2.4	.3

(1)Milk solids added, label claims less than 10 g protein per cup.

(2)Yields 1 qt fluid milk when reconstituted according to package directions.

(3)Most values provided by product labeling.

(4)The latest USDA data from *Handbook 8–14* on beverages updates previous USDA data.

(Computer code number is for West Diet Analysis program)

PAGE KEY: A–2 = BEV A–4 = DAIRY A–10 = EGGS A–12 = FAT/OIL A–14 = FRUIT A–24 = BAKERY A–34 = GRAIN A–40 = FISH A–44 = MEATS A–48 = POULTRY A–50 = SAUSAGE A–52 = MIXED/FAST A–60 = NUTS/SEEDS A–62 = SWEETS A–66 = VEG/LEG A–78 = MISC A–80 = SOUPS/SAUCES A–84 = FAST A–96 = FRZN ENTREE A–98 = BABY FOODS

Chol (mg)	Calc (mg)	Iron (mg)	Magn (mg)	Phos (mg)	Pota (mg)	Sodi (mg)	Zinc (mg)	VT-A (RE)	Thia (mg)	Ribo (mg)	Niac (mg)	V-B6 (mg)	Fola (µg)	VT-C (mg)
0	6	.9	15	102	368	235	2.71	0	0	0	0	0	0	0
0	<1	.05	1	6	22	14	.16	0	0	0	0	0	0	0
13	266	.07	23	204	378	113	.87	5[5]	.09	.38	.17	.04	28	2
1	17	<.01	1	13	24	7	.06	<1[5]	.01	.02	.01	<.01	2	<1
33	290	.12	33	227	368	119	.93	76	.09	.39	.2	.1	12	2
18	295	.12	33	232	376	121	.95	139	.09	.4	.21	.1	12	2
18	311	.12	35	244	397	128	.98	140	.1	.42	.22	.11	13	2
10	300	.12	34	235	381	123	.95	144	.09	.41	.21	.1	12	2
10	311	.12	35	244	397	128	.98	145	.1	.42	.22	.11	13	2
4	301	.1	28	247	404	126	.98	149	.09	.34	.22	.1	13	2
5	316	.12	35	255	419	129	1	149	.1	.43	.22	.11	13	2
9	284	.12	27	218	370	257	1.03	20	.08	.38	.14	.08	12	2
103	866	.58	79	774	1135	389	2.88	248	.27	1.27	.64	.16	34	8
74	658	.48	61	512	764	267	1.94	136	.12	.8	.49	.13	20	5
9	737	.74	69	497	844	293	2.29	298	.11	.79	.44	.14	22	3
83	1419	.36	131	1119	1909	620	4.82	65	.47	1.9	1.05	.41	57	7
17	1118	.28	106	895	1550	500	4.01	646[6]	.38	1.59	.81	.31	45	5
12	836	.21	80	669	1158	373	3	483[6]	.28	1.19	.61	.23	34	4
28	325	.12	34	271	498	121	.73	137	.12	.34	.68	.11	1	3
10	350	.5	28	319	205	50	.9	155	.45	.44	.3	.09	20	1
30	280	.6	32	250	418	149	1.03	72	.09	.4	.31	.1	12	2
17	285	.6	33	255	423	150	1.03	143	.09	.41	.31	.1	12	2
7	285	.6	33	255	425	151	1.03	148	.09	.41	.32	.1	12	2
1	92	.34	23	89	202	143	.41	1	.03	.16	.17	.03	0	1
1	89	.29	23	88	223	139	1.26	1	.03	.17	.18	.04	3	1
0	8	.69	22	28	129	46	.34	<1	.01	.03	.11	<.01	1	<1
32	301	.8	53	255	497	164	1.28	77	.1	.43	.32	.1	12	2
149	330	.51	47	277	419	138	1.17	203	.09	.48	.27	.13	2	4
4	105	4.74	84	158	350	142	3.16	554	.31	.07	5.25	.42	105	28
38	396	4.86	117	385	719	262	4.09	630	.41	.47	5.46	.52	118	31
23	401	4.86	118	390	726	264	4.12	693	.41	.48	5.46	.53	118	31
9	405	4.82	112	404	752	267	4.13	701	.4	.42	5.45	.52	118	31
9	407	4.83	112	406	755	268	4.14	703	.4	.42	5.47	.52	118	31
1	13	.48	15	37	129	53	.17	4	.04	.04	.42	.03	4	<1
34	305	.61	48	265	498	172	1.09	79	.13	.44	.62	.13	16	3
35	385	4	53	313	621	244	1.17	902	.74	1.26	10.9	1	32	34
4	63	.15	19	75	159	104	.21	18	.11	.19	1.1	.09	10	1
37	355	.26	53	302	530	223	1.14	95	.2	.59	1.31	.19	22	3
37	320	.88	48	289	566	274	1.16	65	.16	.69	.46	.14	10	1
31	345	.25	34	289	492	232	1.02	91	.13	.51	.52	.15	9	2

(5)Vitamin A value is from beta-carotene used for coloring.

(6)With added vitamin A.

(For purposes of calculations, use "0" for t, <1, <.1, <.01, etc.)

A

Table A–1
Food Composition

Computer Code Number	Food Description	Measure	Wt (g)	H_2O (%)	Ener (cal)	Prot (g)	Carb (g)	Dietary Fiber (g)	Fat (g)	Fat Breakdown (g) Sat	Mono	Poly
	DAIRY—Cont.											
	Milk desserts:											
134	Custard, baked	1 c	265	79	278	13	28	0	12	6.2	4	1
1548	Low-fat frozen dessert bars	1 ea	81	72	90	2	18	0	1	.2	.1	.4
	Ice cream, vanilla (about 10% fat):											
123	Hardened: ½ gallon	1 ea	1064	61	2138	37	251	0	117	72.4	33.8	4.4
124	Cup	1 c	133	61	267	5	31	0	15	9	4.2	.5
125	Fluid ounces	3 oz	50	61	101	2	12	0	5	3.4	1.6	.2
126	Soft serve	1 c	173	60	372	7	38	0	22	12.9	6	.8
	Ice cream, rich vanilla (16% fat):											
127	Hardened: ½ gallon	1 ea	1188	60	2554	49	264	0	154	88.9	41.5	5.5
128	Cup	1 c	148	57	357	5	33	0	24	14.8	6.9	.9
1724	Ben & Jerry's	½ c	106	64	230	4	21	0	17	11	–	–
	Ice milk, vanilla (about 4% fat):											
129	Hardened: ½ gallon	1 ea	1048	68	1456	40	238	0	45	27.7	12.9	1.7
130	Cup	1 c	131	68	182	5	30	0	6	3.5	1.6	.2
131	Soft serve (about 3% fat)	1 c	175	70	221	9	38	0	5	2.8	1.3	.2
	Pudding, canned (5-oz can = .55 cup):											
135	Chocolate	1 ea	142	69	189	4	32	<1	6	1	2.4	2
136	Tapioca	1 ea	142	74	169	3	27	<1	5	.9	2.2	1.9
137	Vanilla	1 ea	142	71	184	3	31	<1	5	.8	2.2	1.9
	Puddings, dry mix with whole milk:											
138	Chocolate, instant	1 c	260	74	289	8	49	<1	8	4.8	2.4	.5
139	Chocolate, regular, cooked	½ c	130	74	144	4	23	<1	4	2.7	1.3	.2
140	Rice, cooked	½ c	132	73	154	4	27	<1	4	2.3	1.1	.1
141	Tapioca, cooked	½ c	130	74	148	4	25	<1	4	2.3	1.1	.1
142	Vanilla, instant	½ c	130	73	148	4	26	<1	4	2.3	1.1	.2
143	Vanilla, regular, cooked	½ c	130	75	144	4	24	<1	4	2.4	1.1	.2
132	Sherbet (2% fat): ½ gallon	1 ea	1542	66	2127	17	469	<1	31	17.9	8.3	1.2
133	Cup	1 c	193	66	266	2	59	<1	4	2.2	1	.2
144	Soy milk	1 c	240	93	79	7	4	3	5	.5	.8	2
1584	Yogurt, frozen, low-fat[1]	½ c	87	65	138	3	21	–	5	3	1.4	.2
1512	Scoop	1 ea	79	74	78	4	15	0	<1	.1	t	t
	Yogurt, low-fat:											
1172	Fruit added with low-calorie sweetener	1 c	241	86	122	11	19	1	<1	.2	.1	t
145	Fruit added[2]	1 c	227	74	232	10	43	<1	2	1.6	.7	.1
146	Plain	1 c	227	85	143	12	16	0	4	2.3	1	.1
147	Vanilla or coffee flavor	1 c	227	79	193	11	31	0	3	1.8	.8	.1
148	Yogurt, made with nonfat milk	1 c	227	85	126	13	17	0	<1	.3	.1	t
149	Yogurt, made with whole milk	1 c	227	88	139	8	11	0	7	4.8	2	.2
	EGGS[3]											
	Raw, large:											
150	Whole, without shell	1 ea	50	75	74	6	1	0	5	1.5	1.9	.7
151	White	1 ea	33	88	17	4	<1	0	0	0	0	0
152	Yolk	1 ea	17	49	59	3	<1	0	5	1.6	1.9	.7

(1)Data is from 1992 USDA data on snacks and sweets.

(2)Carbohydrate and calories vary widely—consult label if more precise values are needed.

(3)This data is newest revised information from the USDA with 24% less cholesterol.

(Computer code number is for West Diet Analysis program)

Chol (mg)	Calc (mg)	Iron (mg)	Magn (mg)	Phos (mg)	Pota (mg)	Sodi (mg)	Zinc (mg)	VT-A (RE)	Thia (mg)	Ribo (mg)	Niac (mg)	V-B6 (mg)	Fola (µg)	VT-C (mg)
231	297	.79	37	299	405	204	1.4	255	.09	.6	.22	.13	26	1
1	81	.09	9	65	109	41	.26	38	.03	.11	.06	.03	3	1
468	1361	.96	149	1117	2117	851	7.34	1244	.44	2.55	1.23	.51	53	6
58	170	.12	19	140	265	106	.92	156	.05	.32	.15	.06	7	1
22	64	.04	7	52	99	40	.34	58	.02	.12	.06	.02	2	<1
157	227	.36	21	201	306	106	.9	266	.08	.31	.16	.08	16	1
1081	1556	2.49	143	1378	2102	725	6.18	1829	.58	2.16	1.13	.57	107	6
90	173	.07	16	141	235	83	.59	272	.06	.24	.12	.06	7	1
95	150	.36	–	–	–	55	–	225	–	–	–	–	–	0
147	1456	1.05	157	1142	2211	891	4.61	493	.61	2.78	.94	.68	63	6
18	182	.13	20	143	276	111	.58	62	.08	.35	.12	.08	8	1
21	275	.1	24	212	387	123	.93	51	.09	.35	.21	.08	10	1
4	128	.72	30	113	255	183	.6	31	.04	.22	.49	.04	4	<1
1	119	.33	11	112	147	167	.38	<1	.03	.14	.44	.14	6	<1
10	125	.18	11	96	160	191	.35	9	.03	.2	.36	.02	6	<1
29	265	.75	47	621	432	738	1.09	86	.09	.37	.25	.1	10	2
16	144	.47	19	121	212	134	.58	34	.04	.23	.13	.05	5	1
15	133	.5	16	110	165	140	.6	33	.1	.18	.6	.05	6	1
16	135	.08	16	107	172	157	.44	35	.04	.18	.09	.05	5	1
14	131	.09	16	256	166	372	.43	33	.04	.18	.1	.05	5	1
16	139	.06	17	107	177	208	.45	35	.04	.18	.1	.04	5	1
77	833	2.16	123	617	1480	709	7.4	310	.39	1.05	1.48	.52	62	31
10	104	.27	15	77	185	89	.93	39	.05	.13	.18	.07	8	4
0	10	1.39	46	117	338	29	.55	7	.39	.17	.35	.1	4	0
2	124	.26	12	112	184	76	.36	50	.03	.19	.25	.07	5	–
1	137	.07	13	108	176	53	.67	1	.03	.16	.08	.04	8	1
3	369	.61	41	291	550	139	1.83	6	.1	.45	.5	.11	32	26
10	345	.16	33	270	440	132	1.68	25	.08	.4	.22	.09	21	1
14	413	.18	39	325	529	159	2.02	36	.1	.49	.26	.11	25	2
11	388	.16	37	304	497	149	1.88	29	.09	.46	.24	.1	24	2
4	452	.2	43	354	579	173	2.2	5	.11	.53	.28	.12	28	2
29	272	.11	26	215	350	105	1.34	68	.07	.32	.17	.07	17	1
212	24	.72	5	89	60	63	.55	95	.03	.25	.04	.07	23	0
0	2	.01	4	4	48	55	<.01	0	<.01	.15	.03	<.01	1	0
212	23	.59	1	81	16	7	.52	97	.03	.11	<.01	.06	24	0

(For purposes of calculations, use "0" for t, <1, <.1, <.01, etc.)

A

Table A–1
Food Composition

Computer Code Number	Food Description	Measure	Wt (g)	H_2O (%)	Ener (cal)	Prot (g)	Carb (g)	Dietary Fiber (g)	Fat (g)	Fat Breakdown (g) Sat	Mono	Poly
	EGGS—Cont.											
	Cooked:											
153	Fried in margarine	1 ea	46	69	91	6	1	0	7	1.9	2.8	1.3
154	Hard-cooked, shell removed	1 ea	50	75	77	6	1	0	5	1.6	2	.7
155	Hard-cooked, chopped	1 c	136	75	211	17	2	0	14	4.4	5.5	1.9
156	Poached, no added salt	1 ea	50	75	74	6	1	0	5	1.5	1.9	.7
157	Scrambled with milk & margarine	1 ea	61	73	101	7	1	0	7	2.2	2.9	1.3
1681	Egg substitute, liquid	½ c	126	82	106	15	1	0	4	1	1	2
	FATS and OILS											
158	Butter: Stick	½ c	113	16	810	1	<1	0	92	56.7	26.4	3.4
159	Tablespoon	1 tbs	14	16	102	<1	<1	0	11	7.1	3.3	.4
160	Pat (about 1 tsp)[1]	1 ea	5	16	36	<1	<1	0	4	2.5	1.2	.2
1682	Whipped	1 tsp	3	16	23	<1	<1	0	2.56	1.6	.8	.1
	Fats, cooking:											
1363	Bacon fat	1 tbs	14	0	126	0	0	0	14	6.4	5.9	1.1
1362	Beef fat/tallow	1 c	205	0	1849	0	0	0	205	102	85.7	8.2
1364	Chicken fat	1 c	205	<1	1845	0	0	0	204	61.1	91.6	42.8
161	Vegetable shortening:	1 c	205	0	1812	0	0	0	205	51.5	91.2	53.5
162	Tablespoon	1 tbs	13	0	115	0	0	0	13	3.3	5.8	3.4
163	Lard:	1 c	205	0	1849	0	0	0	205	80.4	92.5	23
164	Tablespoon	1 tbs	13	0	117	0	0	0	13	5.1	5.9	1.5
	Margarine:											
165	Imitation (about 40% fat), soft:	1 c	227	58	783	1	1	0	88	17.5	35.6	31.3
166	Tablespoon	1 tbs	14	58	49	<1	<1	0	6	1.1	2.2	2
167	Regular, hard (about 80% fat):	½ c	113	16	812	1	1	0	91	17.9	40.5	28.7
168	Tablespoon	1 tbs	14	16	101	<1	<1	0	11	2.2	5	3.6
169	Pat	1 ea	5	16	36	<1	<1	0	4	.8	1.8	1.3
170	Regular, soft (about 80% fat):	1 c	227	16	1625	2	1	0	182	31.3	64.7	78.5
171	Tablespoon	1 tbs	14	16	100	<1	<1	0	11	1.9	4	4.8
172	Spread (about 60% fat), hard:	½ c	113	37	609	1	0	0	69	15.9	29.4	20.5
173	Tablespoon	1 tbs	14	37	75	<1	0	0	9	2	3.6	2.5
174	Pat[1]	1 ea	5	37	27	<1	0	0	3	.7	1.2	1
175	Spread (about 60% fat), soft:	1 c	227	37	1225	1	0	0	138	29.1	71.5	31.3
176	Tablespoon	1 tbs	14	37	76	<1	0	0	9	1.8	4.4	1.9
	Oils:											
1585	Canola:	1 c	218	0	1927	0	0	0	218	15.5	128	64.5
1586	Tablespoon	1 tbs	14	0	124	0	0	0	14	1	8.2	4.1
177	Corn:	1 c	218	0	1927	0	0	0	218	27.7	52.8	127
178	Tablespoon	1 tbs	14	0	124	0	0	0	14	1.8	3.4	8.2
179	Olive:	1 c	216	0	1909	0	0	0	216	29.2	159	18.4
180	Tablespoon	1 tbs	14	0	124	0	0	0	14	1.9	10.3	1.2
1683	Olive oil, extra virgin	1 tbs	14	<1	126	–	–	–	14	1.96	10.8	1.3
181	Peanut:	1 c	216	0	1909	0	0	0	216	36.5	99.8	69.1
182	Tablespoon	1 tbs	14	0	124	0	0	0	14	2.4	6.5	4.5

(1)Pat is 1" square, ⅓" thick; about 1 tsp; 90 per lb.

(Computer code number is for West Diet Analysis program)

Chol (mg)	Calc (mg)	Iron (mg)	Magn (mg)	Phos (mg)	Pota (mg)	Sodi (mg)	Zinc (mg)	VT-A (RE)	Thia (mg)	Ribo (mg)	Niac (mg)	V-B6 (mg)	Fola (μg)	VT-C (mg)
211	25	.72	5	89	61	162	.55	114	.03	.24	.03	.07	17	0
212	25	.59	5	86	63	62	.52	84	.03	.26	.03	.06	22	0
577	68	1.62	14	234	171	169	1.43	228	.09	.7	.09	.17	60	0
211	24	.72	5	88	60	61	.55	95	.02	.21	.03	.06	17	0
214	43	.73	7	103	84	170	.61	119	.03	.27	.05	.07	18	<1
1	67	3	11	152	415	222	1.65	271	.14	.38	.14	<.01	19	0
247	27	.18	2	26	29	933[2]	.06	852[3]	.01	.04	.05	<.01	3	0
31	3	.02	<1	3	4	117[2]	.01	107[3]	<.01	<.01	.01	0	<1	0
11	1	.01	<1	1	1	41[2]	<.01	38[3]	0	<.01	<.01	0	<1	0
7	1	.01	<1	1	1	26[2]	.002	24[3]	0	<.01	<.01	0	<1	0
14	<1	0	<1	0	<1	76	<.01	<1	0	0	0	0	0	0
223	0	0	0	27	<1	<1	0	0	0	0	0	0	0	0
174	0	0	0	0	0	0	0	351	0	0	0	0	0	0
0	0	0	0	0	0	0	0	0	0	0	0	0	0	0
0	0	0	0	0	0	0	0	0	0	0	0	0	0	0
194	<1	0	<1	6	<1	<1	.23	0	0	0	0	0	0	0
12	<1	0	<1	<1	<1	<1	.01	0	0	0	0	0	0	0
0	40	0	4	31	57	2176[4]	.23	2254[5]	.01	.05	.03	.01	2	<1
0	3	0	<1	2	4	136[4]	.01	141[5]	<.01	<.01	<.01	<.01	<1	<1
0	34	.07	3	26	48	1065[4]	.23	1122[5]	.01	.04	.03	.01	1	<1
0	4	.01	<1	3	6	132[4]	.03	139[5]	<.01	<.01	<.01	<.01	<1	<1
0	1	<.01	<1	1	2	47[4]	.01	50[5]	<.01	<.01	<.01	0	<1	<1
0	60	0	5	46	86	2444[4]	.46	2254[5]	.02	.07	.04	.02	2	<1
0	4	0	<1	3	5	151[4]	.03	139[5]	<.01	<.01	<.01	<.01	<1	<1
0	24	0	2	18	34	1122[4]	.17	1122[5]	.01	.03	.02	.01	1	<1
0	3	0	<1	2	4	139[4]	.02	139[5]	<.01	<.01	<.01	<.01	<1	<1
0	1	0	<1	1	1	50[4]	0	50[5]	0	<.01	<.01	0	<1	<1
0	47	0	4	36	68	2256[4]	0	2254[5]	.02	.06	.04	.01	2	<1
0	3	0	<1	2	4	139[4]	0	139[5]	<.01	<.01	<.01	<.01	<1	<1
0	0	0	0	0	0	0	0	0	0	0	0	0	0	0
0	0	0	0	0	0	0	0	0	0	0	0	0	0	0
0	0	.01	0	2	4	0	.02	0	0	0	0	0	0	0
0	0	<.01	0	<1	<1	0	<.01	0	0	0	0	0	0	0
0	<1	.82	<1	3	0	<1	.13	0	0	0	0	0	0	0
0	<1	.05	<1	<1	0	<1	.01	0	0	0	0	0	0	0
0	–	–	–	–	–	–	–	0	0	0	0	0	0	0
0	<1	.06	<1	0	<1	<1	.02	0	0	0	0	0	0	0
0	<1	<.01	<1	0	<1	<1	<.01	0	0	0	0	0	0	0

(2) For salted butter, unsalted butter contains 12 mg sodium per stick or ½ c, 1.5 mg/tbs, or .5 mg/pat.

(3) Values for vitamin A are a year-round average.

(4) For salted margarine.

(5) Based on average vitamin A content of fortified margarine. Federal specifications require a minimum of 15,000 IU/lb.

(For purposes of calculations, use "0" for t, <1, <.1, <.01, etc.)

Table A-1
Food Composition

Computer Code Number	Food Description	Measure	Wt (g)	H_2O (%)	Ener (cal)	Prot (g)	Carb (g)	Dietary Fiber (g)	Fat (g)	Fat Breakdown (g) Sat	Mono	Poly
	FATS and OILS—Cont.											
	OILS—Cont.											
183	Safflower:	1 c	218	0	1927	0	0	0	218	19.8	26.4	162
184	Tablespoon	1 tbs	14	0	124	0	0	0	14	1.3	1.7	10.4
185	Soybean:	1 c	218	0	1927	0	0	0	218	31.4	50.8	126
186	Tablespoon	1 tbs	14	0	124	0	0	0	14	2	3.3	8.1
187	Soybean/cottonseed:	1 c	218	0	1927	0	0	0	218	39.2	64.3	105
188	Tablespoon	1 tbs	14	0	124	0	0	0	14	2.5	4.1	6.7
189	Sunflower:	1 c	218	0	1927	0	0	0	218	22.7	42.5	143
190	Tablespoon	1 tbs	14	0	124	0	0	0	14	1.5	2.7	9.2
	Salad dressings/sandwich spreads:											
191	Blue cheese: Regular	1 tbs	15	32	76	1	1	<1	8	1.5	1.9	4.4
1040	Low calorie	1 tbs	15	79	15	1	<1	<1	1	.2	.5	.4
1684	Caesar's	1 tbs	12	36	52	1	<1	<1	5	1	3.5	.5
192	French: Regular	1 tbs	16	38	67	<1	3	<1	9	1.5	1.2	3.4
193	Low calorie	1 tbs	16	69	21	<1	3	<1	1	.1	.2	.5
194	Italian: Regular	1 tbs	15	38	69	<1	1	<1	9	1	1.6	4.1
195	Low calorie	1 tbs	15	82	8	<1	1	<1	1	t	.1	.2
199	Mayo type: Regular	1 tbs	15	40	58	<1	3	0	5	.7	1.4	2.7
1030	Low calorie	1 tbs	15	81	20	<1	1	0	3	.3	.8	1.4
196	Mayonnaise:											
196	Regular (soybean)	1 tbs	14	15	99	<1	<1	0	11	1.6	3.1	5.7
197	Imitation, low calorie	1 tbs	15	63	35	<1	2	0	3	.5	.7	1.6
1488	Regular, low calorie, low sodium	1 tbs	14	63	32	<1	2	0	3	.5	.6	1.4
1493	Regular, low calorie	1 tbs	16	63	36	<1	2	0	3	.5	.7	1.6
198	Ranch: Regular	½ c	119	35	436	4	5	0	45	6.7	19.4	17
1042	Low calorie	1 tbs	15	40	31	0	1	–	3	0	–	1
1685	Russian	1 tbs	15	34	76	<1	2	0	8	1	2	5
1502	Salad dressing, low calorie, oil free	1 tbs	15	88	4	<1	1	<1	<1	0	0	0
	Salad dressing, no cholesterol											
1605	(Miracle Whip)	1 tbs	15	57	48	0	2	0	4	1.1	1.1	2.1
203	Salad dressing, from recipe, cooked[1]	1 tbs	16	69	25	1	2	0	2	.5	.6	.3
200	Tartar sauce: Regular	1 tbs	14	34	74	<1	1	<1	8	1.5	2.6	4.1
1503	Low calorie	1 tbs	14	63	31	<1	2	<1	2	.4	.6	1.3
201	Thousand Island: Regular	1 tbs	16	46	60	<1	2	<1	6	1	1.3	3.2
202	Low calorie	1 tbs	15	69	25	<1	2	<1	2	.2	.4	.9
204	Vinegar & oil	1 tbs	16	47	72	0	<1	0	8	1.5	2.4	3.9
	FRUITS and FRUIT JUICES											
	Apples:											
	Fresh, raw, with peel:											
205	2 ¾" diam (about 3 per lb w/cores)	1 ea	138	84	81	<1	21	3	<1	.1	t	.1
206	3 ¼" diam (about 2 per lb w/cores)	1 ea	212	84	125	<1	32	4	1	.1	t	.2
207	Raw, peeled slices	1 c	110	84	63	<1	16	2	<1	.1	t	.1
208	Dried, sulfured	10 ea	64	32	155	1	42	6	<1	t	t	.1

(1) Fatty acid values apply to product made with regular margarine.

(Computer code number is for West Diet Analysis program)

Chol (mg)	Calc (mg)	Iron (mg)	Magn (mg)	Phos (mg)	Pota (mg)	Sodi (mg)	Zinc (mg)	VT-A (RE)	Thia (mg)	Ribo (mg)	Niac (mg)	V-B6 (mg)	Fola (µg)	VT-C (mg)
0	0	.01	0	0	0	0	.41	0	0	0	0	0	0	0
0	0	<.01	0	0	0	0	.03	0	0	0	0	0	0	0
0	<1	.04	<1	1	0	0	.4	0	0	0	0	0	0	0
0	<1	<.01	<1	<1	0	0	.03	0	0	0	0	0	0	0
0	0	.02	<1	0	0	0	.4	0	0	0	0	0	0	0
0	0	<.01	<1	0	0	0	.03	0	0	0	0	0	0	0
0	0	.06	<1	0	0	<1	0	0	0	0	0	0	0	0
0	0	<.01	<1	0	0	<1	0	0	0	0	0	0	0	0
3	12	.03	<1	11	6	167	.04	10	<.01	.02	.01	.01	3	<1
<1	14	.08	1	13	1	184	.04	<1	<.01	.01	.01	<.01	<1	<1
11	21	.19	3	18	19	194	.12	6	<.01	.02	.47	.01	2	<1
0	2	.06	2	1	2	188	.01	3	<.01	<.01	<.01	<.01	1	0
1	2	.06	0	2	13	126	.03	0	0	0	0	0	0	0
0	1	.03	<1	1	5	116	.02	3	<.01	<.01	0	<.01	1	0
0	<1	.03	<1	1	2	120	.02	0	0	0	0	0	0	0
4	2	.03	<1	4	1	105	0	13	<.01	<.01	<.01	<.01	1	0
7	3	.03	–	4	1	18	.02	10	<.01	<.01	0	–	0	0
8	2	.07	<1	4	5	78	.02	12	0	0	<.01	.08	1	0
4	<1	0	<1	<1	1	75	.02	0	0	0	0	0	0	0
3	0	0	0	0	1	15	.01	1	0	<.01	0	0	<1	0
4	<1	0	<1	<1	2	77	02	0	0	0	0	0	0	0
47	119	.31	12	100	158	522	.44	86	.04	.17	.08	.05	6	1
5	–	–	–	–	5	153	–	–	–	–	–	–	–	–
3	3	.1	.23	6	24	133	.1	32	.01	.01	.1	<.01	1.59	1
0	1	.04	2	1	7	256	<.01	<1	0	0	<.01	<.01	<1	<1
0	0	<.01	0	0	0	102	0	2	0	0	0	0	0	0
9	13	.08	0	14	19	117	0	20	.01	.02	.04	0	0	<1
7	3	.13	<1	4	11	99	.02	9	<.01	<.01	0	<.01	1	<1
3	2	.09	<1	1	6	82	.02	2	0	<.01	.01	<.01	<1	<1
4	2	.09	<1	3	18	110	.02	15	<.01	<.01	<.01	<.01	1	<1
2	2	.09	1	3	17	153	.02	14	<.01	<.01	.03	<.01	1	<1
0	0	0	0	0	1	<1	0	0	0	0	0	0	0	0
0	10	.25	7	10	157	0	.05	7	.02	.02	.11	.07	4	8
0	15	.38	11	15	242	0	.08	11	.04	.03	.16	.1	6	12
0	4	.08	3	8	124	0	.04	4	.02	.01	.1	.05	<1	4
0	9	.9	10	24	288	56[2]	.13	0	0	.1	.59	.08	0	2

(2) Sodium bisulfite used to preserve color; unsulfured product would contain lower levels of sodium.

(For purposes of calculations, use "0" for t, <1, <.1, <.01, etc.)

A

Table A–1
Food Composition

Computer Code Number	Food Description	Measure	Wt (g)	H_2O (%)	Ener (cal)	Prot (g)	Carb (g)	Dietary Fiber (g)	Fat (g)	Fat Breakdown (g) Sat	Mono	Poly
	FRUITS and FRUIT JUICES—Cont.											
209	Apple juice, bottled or canned	1 c	248	88	116	<1	29	<1	<1	t	t	.1
210	Applesauce, sweetened	1 c	255	80	193	<1	51	3	<1	.1	t	.1
211	Applesauce, unsweetened	1 c	244	88	104	<1	28	4	<1	t	t	t
	Apricots:											
212	Raw, w/o pits (about 12 per lb w/ pits)	3 ea	106	86	51	1	12	2	<1	t	.2	.1
	Canned (fruit and liquid):											
213	Heavy syrup	1 c	258	78	214	1	55	3	<1	t	.1	t
214	Halves	3 ea	85	78	70	<1	18	1	<1	t	t	t
215	Juice pack	1 c	248	87	119	2	30	4	<1	t	t	t
216	Halves	3 ea	84	87	40	1	10	1	<1	t	t	t
217	Dried, halves	10 ea	35	31	83	1	22	3	<1	t	.1	t
218	Dried, cooked, unsweetened, w/liquid	1 c	250	76	212	3	55	8	<1	t	.2	.1
219	Apricot nectar, canned	1 c	251	85	140	1	36	2	<1	t	.1	t
	Avocados, raw, edible part only:											
220	California (2 lb with refuse)	1 ea	173	73	306	4	12	5	30	4.5	19.4	3.5
221	Florida (1 lb with refuse)	1 ea	304	80	340	5	27	18	27	5.3	14.8	4.5
222	Mashed, fresh, average	1 c	230	74	370	5	17	14	35	5.6	22.1	4.5
	Bananas, raw, without peel:											
223	Whole, 8¾" long (175 g w/peel)	1 ea	114	74	104	1	27	2	1	.2	t	.1
224	Slices	1 c	150	74	137	2	35	3	1	.3	.1	.1
1285	Bananas, dehydrated slices	1 oz	28	3	98	1	25	2	1	.2	t	.1
225	Blackberries, raw	1 c	144	86	75	1	18	7	1	.3	.1	.1
	Blueberries:											
226	Fresh	1 c	145	85	81	1	20	3	1	t	.2	.3
227	Frozen, sweetened	10 oz	284	77	230	1	62	7	<1	.1	.1	.2
228	Frozen, thawed	1 c	230	77	186	1	50	5	<1	.1	.1	.2
	Cherries:											
229	Sour, red pitted, canned water pack	1 c	244	90	88	2	22	2	<1	.1	.1	.1
230	Sweet, red pitted, raw	10 ea	68	81	49	1	11	1	1	.1	.2	.2
231	Cranberry juice cocktail[1]	1 c	253	85	144	0[2]	36	1	<1	.1	t	.1
1411	Cranberry juice, low calorie	¾ c	178	95	34	0	8	1	0	0	0	0
232	Cranberry-apple juice	1 c	253	83	169	<1	43	<1	<1[3]	t	t	.1
233	Cranberry sauce, canned, strained	1 c	277	61	418	1	107	6	<1	t	.1	.2
234	Dates, whole, without pits	10 ea	83	22	228	2	61	7	<1	.2	.1	t
235	Dates, chopped	1 c	178	22	490	4	130	15	1	.3	.2	t
236	Figs, dried	10 ea	187	28	477	6	122	17	2	.4	.5	1
	Fruit cocktail, canned, fruit and liq:											
237	Heavy syrup pack	1 c	255	80	186	1	48	3	<1	t	t	.1
238	Juice pack	1 c	248	87	114	1	29	3	<1	t	t	t
	Grapefruit:											
	Raw 3¾" diam (half w/rind = 241 g)											
239	Pink/red, half fruit, edible part	1 ea	123	91	37	1	9	1	<1	t	t	t
240	White, half fruit, edible part	1 ea	118	90	39	1	10	1	<1	t	t	t
241	Canned sections with light syrup	1 c	254	84	152	1	39	1	<1	t	t	.1

(1)Data here are from the newest USDA *Handbook 8–14* on beverages. These data are somewhat different from that presented in *Handbook 8–9* on fruits and fruit juices.

(2)The newest USDA *Handbook 8–14* data on beverages indicates "0" for protein.

(3)The newest USDA *Handbook 8–14* data on beverages indicates "0" for fat.

(Computer code number is for West Diet Analysis program)

PAGE KEY: A–2 = BEV A–4 = DAIRY A–10 = EGGS A–12 = FAT/OIL A–14 = FRUIT A–24 = BAKERY A–34 = GRAIN A–40 = FISH A–44 = MEATS A–48 = POULTRY A–50 = SAUSAGE A–52 = MIXED/FAST A–60 = NUTS/SEEDS A–62 = SWEETS A–66 = VEG/LEG A–78 = MISC A–80 = SOUPS/SAUCES A–84 = FAST A–96 = FRZN ENTREE A–98 = BABY FOODS

Chol (mg)	Calc (mg)	Iron (mg)	Magn (mg)	Phos (mg)	Pota (mg)	Sodi (mg)	Zinc (mg)	VT-A (RE)	Thia (mg)	Ribo (mg)	Niac (mg)	V-B6 (mg)	Fola (μg)	VT-C (mg)
0	17	.92	7	17	295	7	.07	<1	.05	.04	.25	.07	<1	2
0	10	.89	8	18	155	8	.1	3	.03	.07	.48	.07	2	4[4]
0	7	.29	7	17	183	5	.07	7	.03	.06	.46	.06	1	3[4]
0	15	.57	8	20	313	1	.28	277	.03	.04	.64	.06	9	11
0	23	.77	18	31	361	10	.28	317	.05	.06	.97	.14	4	8
0	8	.25	6	10	119	3	.09	105	.02	.02	.32	.05	1	3
0	30	.74	25	50	409	10	.27	419	.04	.05	.85	.13	4	12
0	10	.25	8	17	139	3	.09	142	.01	.02	.29	.04	1	4
0	16	1.65	16	41	482	3	.26	253	<.01	.05	1.05	.05	4	1
0	40	4.18	42	102	1222	7	.66	590	.01	.07	2.36	.28	0	4
0	18	.95	13	23	286	8	.23	331	.02	.03	.65	.05	3	2[5]
0	19	2.04	71	73	1096	21	.73	106	.19	.21	3.32	.48	113	14
0	33	1.61	103	118	1483	15	1.28	185	.33	.37	5.84	.85	162	24
0	25	2.35	90	94	1377	23	.97	140	.25	.28	4.42	.64	142	18
0	7	.35	33	23	451	1	.18	9	.05	.11	.62	.66	22	10
0	9	.46	43	30	594	1	.24	12	.07	.15	.81	.87	29	14
0	6	.33	31	21	423	1	.17	9	.05	.07	.79	.15	11	2
0	46	.82	29	30	282	0	.39	23	.04	.06	.58	.08	49	30
0	9	.25	7	14	129	9	.16	14	.07	.07	.52	.05	9	19
0	17	1.11	6	20	170	3	.17	11	.06	.15	.72	.17	19	3
0	14	.9	5	16	138	2	.14	9	.05	.12	.58	.14	15	2
0	27	3.34	15	24	239	17	.17	183	.04	.1	.43	.11	19	5
0	10	.26	7	13	152	0	.04	14	.03	.04	.27	.02	3	5
0	8	.38	5	5	45	5	.18	1	.02	.02	.09	.05	1	90[6]
0	16	.07	4	2	39	5	.04	1	.02	.02	.06	.03	<1	57
0	18	.15	5	8	68	5	.1	1	.01	.05	.15	.05	1	81[6]
0	11	.61	8	17	72	80	.14	6	.04	.06	.28	.04	2	6
0	27	.95	29	33	541	2	.24	4	.07	.08	1.83	.16	10	0
0	57	2.05	62	71	1160	5	.52	9	.16	.18	3.92	.34	22	0
0	269	4.17	110	127	1331	21	.95	24	.13	.16	1.3	.42	14	1
0	15	.74	13	28	224	15	.2	51	.05	.05	.95	.13	7	5
0	20	.52	17	35	235	10	.22	77	.03	.04	1	.13	6	7
0	13	.15	10	11	157	0	.09	32[7]	.04	.02	.23	.05	15	47
0	14	.07	11	9	173	0	.08	1	.04	.02	.32	.05	12	39
0	36	1.02	25	25	328	5	.2	0	.1	.05	.62	.05	22	54

(4)Value based on products without added vitamin C. Bottled apple juice with added vitamin C usually contains 41.6 mg/100 g, or 103 mg per cup. Check label for specific vitamin C values.

(5)Without added vitamin C. Products with added vitamin C contain 136 mg per cup. Check label.

(6)Nutrient added.

(7)Vitamin A in Texas red grapefruit would be 74 RE.

(For purposes of calculations, use "0" for t, <1, <.1, <.01, etc.)

A

Table A–1
Food Composition

Computer Code Number	Food Description	Measure	Wt (g)	H_2O (%)	Ener (cal)	Prot (g)	Carb (g)	Dietary Fiber (g)	Fat (g)	Fat Breakdown (g) Sat	Mono	Poly
	FRUITS and FRUIT JUICES—Cont.											
	Grapefruit juice:											
242	Fresh, raw	1 c	247	90	96	1	23	<1	<1	t	t	.1
243	Canned: Unsweetened	1 c	247	90	94	1	22	<1	<1	t	t	.1
244	Sweetened	1 c	250	87	115	1	28	<1	<1	t	t	.1
	Frozen concentrate, unsweetened:											
245	Undiluted, 6-fl-oz can	¾ c	207	62	302	4	71	3	1	.1	.1	.2
246	Diluted with 3 cans water	1 c	247	89	101	1	24	<1	<1	t	t	.1
	Grapes, raw European (adherent skin):											
247	Thompson seedless	10 ea	50	81	35	<1	9	<1	<1	.1	t	.1
248	Tokay/Emperor, seeded types	10 ea	57	81	40	<1	10	<1	<1	.1	t	.1
	Grape juice:											
249	Bottled or canned	1 c	253	84	154	1	38	2	<1	.1	t	.1
	Frozen concentrate, sweetened:											
250	Undiluted, 6-fl-oz can	¾ c	216	54	387	1	96	5	1	.2	t	.2
251	Diluted with 3 cans water	1 c	250	87	127	<1	32	2	<1	.1	t	.1
1410	Low calorie	1 c	250	84	153	1	37	<1	<1	.1	t	.1
252	Kiwi fruit, raw, peeled (88 g with peel)	1 ea	76	83	46	1	11	3	<1	t	.1	.1
253	Lemons, raw, without peel and seeds (about 4 per lb whole)	1 ea	58	89	17	1	5	1	<1	t	t	.1
	Lemon juice:											
254	Fresh:	1 c	244	91	61	1	21	1	<1	.1	t	.2
255	Tablespoon	1 tbs	15	91	4	<1	1	<1	<1	t	t	t
256	Canned or bottled, unsweetened:	1 c	244	92	51	1	16	1	1	.1	t	.2
257	Tablespoon	1 tbs	15	92	3	<1	1	<1	<1	t	t	t
258	Frozen, single strength, unsweetened:	1 c	244	92	54	1	16	1	1	.1	t	.2
259	Tablespoon	1 tbs	15	92	3	<1	1	<1	<1	t	t	t
	Lime juice:											
260	Fresh:	1 c	246	90	66	1	22	1	<1	t	t	.1
261	Tablespoon	1 tbs	15	90	4	<1	1	<1	<1	t	t	t
262	Canned or bottled, unsweetened	1 c	246	92	52	1	16	1	1	.1	.1	.2
263	Mangoes, raw, edible part (300 g w/skin & seeds)	1 ea	207	82	134	1	35	4	1	.1	.2	.1
	Melons, raw, without rind and contents:											
264	Cantaloupe, 5" diam (2 ⅓ lb whole with refuse), orange flesh	½ ea	267	90	93	2	22	2	1	.1	.1	.2
265	Honeydew, 6½" diam (5¼ lb whole with refuse), slice = 1/10 melon	1 pce	129	90	45	1	12	1	<1	t	t	t
266	Nectarines, raw, w/o pits, 2½" diam	1 ea	136	86	67	1	16	3	1	.1	.2	.3
	Oranges, raw:											
267	Whole w/o peel and seeds, 2 ⅝" diam (180 g with peel and seeds)	1 ea	131	87	62	1	15	3	<1	t	t	t
268	Sections, without membranes	1 c	180	87	85	2	21	4	<1	t	t	t

(Computer code number is for West Diet Analysis program)

Chol (mg)	Calc (mg)	Iron (mg)	Magn (mg)	Phos (mg)	Pota (mg)	Sodi (mg)	Zinc (mg)	VT-A (RE)	Thia (mg)	Ribo (mg)	Niac (mg)	V-B6 (mg)	Fola (µg)	VT-C (mg)
0	22	.49	30	37	400	2	.12	2[1]	.1	.05	.49	.11	25	94
0	17	.49	25	27	378	2	.22	2	.1	.05	.57	.05	26	72
0	20	.9	25	27	405	5	.15	0	.1	.06	.8	.05	26	67
0	56	1.01	79	101	1001	6	.37	6	.3	.16	1.6	.32	26	246
0	20	.35	27	35	336	2	.12	2	.1	.05	.54	.11	9	83
0	5	.13	3	6	92	1	.02	3	.05	.03	.15	.05	2	5
0	6	.15	3	7	105	1	.03	4	.05	.03	.17	.06	2	6
0	23	.61	25	28	334	8	.13	3	.07	.09	.66	.16	7	<1
0	28	.78	32	32	159	15	.28	6	.11	.2	.93	.32	9	179[2]
0	10	.25	10	10	52	5	.1	2	.04	.06	.31	.1	3	60[2]
0	22	.6	25	27	330	7	.12	2	.06	.09	.65	.16	6	<1
0	20	.31	23	30	252	4	.08[3]	14	.01	.04	.38	.04	17	74
0	15	.35	5	9	80	1	.03	2	.02	.01	.06	.05	6	31
0	17	.07	15	15	303	2	.12	5	.07	.02	.24	.12	31	112
0	1	<.01	1	1	19	<1	.01	<1	<.01	<.01	.01	.01	2	7
0	27	.32	19	22	249	51	.15	5	.1	.02	.48	.1	25	60
0	2	.02	1	1	15	3	.01	<1	.01	<.01	.03	.01	2	4
0	19	.29	19	19	217	2	.12	2	.14	.03	.33	.15	23	77
0	1	.02	1	1	13	<1	.01	<1	.01	<.01	.02	.01	1	5
0	22	.07	15	17	268	2	.15	2	.05	.02	.25	.11	20	72
0	1	<.01	1	1	16	<1	.01	<1	<.01	<.01	.01	.01	1	4
0	29	.57	17	25	184	39[4]	.15	5	.08	.01	.4	.07	19	16
0	21	.27	19	23	323	4	.08	805	.12	.12	1.21	.28	39	57
0	29	.56	29	45	825	24	.43	860	.1	.06	1.53	.31	45	113
0	8	.09	9	13	350	13	.11	5	.1	.02	.77	.08	39	32
0	7	.2	11	22	288	0	.12	101	.02	.06	1.35	.03	5	7
0	52	.13	13	18	237	0	.09	27	.11	.05	.37	.08	40	70
0	72	.18	18	25	326	0	.13	38	.16	.07	.51	.11	54	96

(1)This is vitamin A for white grapefruit juice; pink or red grapefruit juice = 109 RE per cup.

(2)With added vitamin C (ascorbic acid).

(3)Data are estimated from other fruit data.

(4)Sodium benzoate and sodium bisulfite added as preservatives.

(For purposes of calculations, use "0" for t, <1, <.1, <.01, etc.)

A

Table A–1
Food Composition

Computer Code Number	Food Description	Measure	Wt (g)	H_2O (%)	Ener (cal)	Prot (g)	Carb (g)	Dietary Fiber (g)	Fat (g)	Fat Breakdown (g) Sat	Mono	Poly
	FRUITS and FRUIT JUICES—Cont.											
	Orange juice:											
269	Fresh, all varieties	1 c	248	88	111	2	26	<1	<1	.1	.1	.1
270	Canned, unsweetened	1 c	249	89	104	1	24	<1	<1	t	.1	.1
271	Chilled	1 c	249	88	109	2	25	<1	1	.1	.1	.2
	Frozen concentrate:											
272	Undiluted (6-oz can)	¾ c	213	58	339	5	81	1	<1	.1	.1	.1
273	Diluted w/3 parts water by volume	1 c	249	88	112	2	27	<1	<1	t	t	t
1345	Orange juice, from dry crystals	1 c	248	88	114	0	29	0	<1	t	t	t
274	Orange and grapefruit juice, canned	1 c	247	89	106	1	25	<1	<1	t	t	t
	Papayas, raw:											
275	½" slices	1 c	140	89	54	1	14	2	<1	.1	.1	t
276	Whole, 3½" diam by 5⅛" w/o seeds and skin (1 lb w/refuse)	1 ea	304	89	118	2	30	5	<1	.1	.1	.1
1031	Papaya nectar, canned	1 c	250	85	142	<1	36	1	<1	.1	.1	.1
	Peaches:											
277	Raw, whole, 2½" diam, peeled, pitted (about 4 per lb whole)	1 ea	87	88	37	1	10	1	<1	t	t	t
278	Raw, sliced	1 c	170	88	73	1	19	3	<1	t	.1	.1
	Canned, fruit and liquid:											
279	Heavy syrup pack:	1 c	256	79	189	1	51	3	<1	t	.1	.1
280	Half	1 ea	81	79	60	<1	16	1	<1	t	t	t
281	Juice pack:	1 c	248	87	109	2	29	2	<1	t	t	t
282	Half	1 ea	77	87	34	<1	9	1	<1	t	t	t
283	Dried, uncooked	10 ea	130	32	309	5	80	11	1	.1	.4	.5
284	Dried, cooked, fruit and liquid	1 c	258	78	198	3	51	7	1	.1	.2	.3
	Frozen, slice, sweetened:											
285	10-oz package	1 ea	284	75	266	2	68	4	<1	t	.1	.2
286	Cup, thawed measure	1 c	250	75	235	2	60	4	<1	t	.1	.2
1032	Peach nectar, canned	1 c	249	86	134	1	35	1	<1	t	t	t
	Pears:											
	Fresh, with skin, cored:											
287	Bartlett, 2½" diam (about 2½ per lb)	1 ea	166	84	98	1	25	4[1]	1	t	.1	.2
288	Bosc, 2 1/5" diam (about 3 per lb)	1 ea	141	84	83	1	21	4[1]	1	t	.1	.1
289	D'Anjou, 3" diam (about 2 per lb)	1 ea	200	84	118	1	30	5[1]	1	t	.2	.2
	Canned, fruit and liquid:											
290	Heavy syrup pack:	1 c	255	80	188	1	49	5[1]	<1	t	.1	.1
291	Half	1 ea	79	80	58	<1	15	2[1]	<1	t	t	t
292	Juice pack:	1 c	248	86	124	1	32	5[1]	<1	t	t	t
293	Half	1 ea	77	86	38	<1	10	2[1]	<1	t	t	t
294	Dried halves	10 ea	175	27	459	3	121	23	1	.1	.2	.3
1033	Pear nectar, canned	1 c	250	84	150	<1	39	2	<1	t	t	t
	Pineapple:											
295	Fresh chunks, diced	1 c	155	86	76	1	19	2	1	t	.1	.2
	Canned, fruit and liquid:											
	Heavy syrup pack:											
296	Crushed, chunks, tidbits	⅓ c	84	79	65	<1	17	1	<1	t	t	t
297	Slices	1 ea	58	79	45	<1	12	<1	<1	t	t	t

(1)Dietary fiber data vary 2.4 to 3.4 g/100 g for fresh pears; 1.6 to 2.6 g/100 g for canned pears.

(Computer code number is for West Diet Analysis program)

PAGE KEY: A–2 = BEV A–4 = DAIRY A–10 = EGGS A–12 = FAT/OIL A–14 = FRUIT A–24 = BAKERY A–34 = GRAIN A–40 = FISH A–44 = MEATS A–48 = POULTRY A–50 = SAUSAGE A–52 = MIXED/FAST A–60 = NUTS/SEEDS A–62 = SWEETS A–66 = VEG/LEG A–78 = MISC A–80 = SOUPS/SAUCES A–84 = FAST A–96 = FRZN ENTREE A–98 = BABY FOODS

Chol (mg)	Calc (mg)	Iron (mg)	Magn (mg)	Phos (mg)	Pota (mg)	Sodi (mg)	Zinc (mg)	VT-A (RE)	Thia (mg)	Ribo (mg)	Niac (mg)	V-B6 (mg)	Fola (µg)	VT-C (mg)
0	27	.5	27	42	496	2	.12	50	.22	.07	.99	.1	75	124
0	20	1.1	27	35	436	5	.17	45	.15	.07	.78	.22	45	86
0	25	.42	27	27	473	2	.1	20[2]	.28	.05	.7	.13	45[2]	82[2]
0	68	.75	72	121	1435	6	.38	60	.6	.14	1.53	.33	330	294
0	22	.25	25	40	473	2	.12	20	.2	.04	.5	.11	109	97
0	62	.2	2	37	50	12	.1	551	<.01	.04	0	0	142	121
0	20	1.14	25	35	390	7	.17	30	.14	.07	.83	.06	35	72
0	34	.14	14	7	360	4	.1	39	.04	.04	.47	.03	53	86
0	73	.3	30	15	781	9	.21	85	.08	.1	1.03	.06	115	187
0	25	.85	7	0	77	12	.37	27	.01	.01	.37	.02	5	7
0	4	.1	6	10	171	0	.12	47	.01	.04	.86	.02	3	6
0	8	.19	12	20	335	0	.24	92	.03	.07	1.68	.03	6	11
0	8	.69	13	28	235	15	.23	84	.03	.06	1.57	.05	8	7
0	2	.22	4	9	74	5	.07	27	.01	.02	.5	.01	3	2
0	15	.67	17	42	317	10	.27	94	.02	.04	1.44	.05	8	9
0	5	.21	5	13	99	3	.08	29	.01	.01	.45	.01	3	3
0	36	5.28	55	153	1293	9	.74	281	<.01	.28	5.69	.09	<1	6
0	23	3.38	33	98	826	5	.46	52	.01	.05	3.92	.1	<1	10
0	9	1.05	14	31	369	17	.14	79	.04	.1	1.85	.05	9	267[3]
0	7	.92	12	27	325	15	.12	70	.03	.09	1.63	.04	8	236[3]
0	12	.47	10	15	100	17	.2	65	.01	.03	.72	.02	3	13
0	18	.41	10	18	208	0	.2	3	.03	.07	.17	.03	12	7
0	15	.35	8	15	176	0	.17	3	.03	.06	.14	.02	10	6
0	22	.5	12	22	250	0	.24	4	.04	.08	.2	.04	15	8
0	13	.56	10	18	165	13	.2	1	.03	.06	.62	.04	3	3
0	4	.17	3	6	51	4	.06	<1	.01	.02	.19	.01	1	1
0	22	.72	17	30	238	10	.22	2	.03	.03	.5	.03	3	4
0	7	.22	5	9	74	3	.07	1	.01	.01	.15	.01	1	1
0	59	3.68	58	103	933	10	.68	1	.01	.25	2.4	.13	0	12
0	12	.65	7	7	32	10	.17	<1	<.01	.03	.32	.03	3	3
0	11	.57	22	11	175	2	.12	3	.14	.06	.65	.13	16	24
0	12	.32	13	6	87	1	.1	1	.08	.02	.24	.06	4	6
0	8	.22	9	4	60	1	.07	1	.05	.01	.17	.04	3	4

(2) Values for juice from California oranges indicate the following values for 1 c: 36 RE of vitamin A, 72 µg of folacin, and 106 mg of vitamin C.

(3) With added vitamin C (ascorbic acid).

(For purposes of calculations, use "0" for t, <1, <.1, <.01, etc.)

A

A

Table A–1
Food Composition

Computer Code Number	Food Description	Measure	Wt (g)	H_2O (%)	Ener (cal)	Prot (g)	Carb (g)	Dietary Fiber (g)	Fat (g)	Fat Breakdown (g) Sat	Mono	Poly
	FRUITS and FRUIT JUICES—Cont.											
	Pineapple, canned—Cont.											
298	Juice pack, crushed, chunks, tidbits	1 c	250	83	150	1	39	2	<1	t	t	.1
299	Juice pack, slices	1 ea	58	83	35	<1	9	<1	<1	t	t	t
300	Pineapple juice, canned, unsweetened	1 c	250	85	140	1	34	<1	<1	t	t	.1
	Plantains, without peel:											
301	Raw slices (whole = 179 g w/o peel)	1 c	148	65	181	2	47	3[1]	1	.2	.1	.1
302	Cooked, boiled, sliced	1 c	154	67	179	1	48	4	<1	.1	t	.1
	Plums:											
303	Fresh, medium, 2⅛" diam	1 ea	66	85	36	1	9	1	<1	t	.3	.1
304	Fresh, small, 1½" diam	1 ea	28	85	15	<1	4	<1	<1	t	.1	t
	Canned, purple, with liquid:											
305	Heavy syrup pack:	1 c	258	76	229	1	60	3	<1	t	.2	.1
306	Plums	3 ea	110	76	98	<1	26	1	<1	t	.1	t
307	Juice pack:	1 c	252	84	146	1	38	3	<1	t	t	t
308	Plums	3 ea	95	84	55	<1	14	1	<1	t	t	t
1698	Pomegranate, fresh	1 ea	154	81	105	2	27	1	<1	–	–	–
	Prunes, dried, pitted:											
309	Uncooked (10 = 97 g w/pits, 84 g w/o pits)	10 ea	84	32	200	2	53	6[2]	<1	t	.3	.1
310	Cooked, unsweetened, fruit & liq (250 g w/pits)	1c	212	70	227	2	60	14	<1	t	.3	.1
311	Prune juice, bottled or canned	1c	256	81	182	2	45	3	1	.01	.5	.02
	Raisins, seedless:											
312	Cup, not pressed down	1 c	145	15	435	5	114	6	1	.2	t	.2
313	One packet, ½ oz	½ oz	14	15	42	<1	11	1	<1	t	t	t
	Raspberries:											
314	Fresh	1 c	123	87	60	1	14	5	1	t	.1	.4
315	Frozen, sweetened:	10 oz	284	73	293	2	74	12	<1	t	t	.3
316	Cup, thawed measure	1 c	250	73	258	2	65	11	<1	t	t	.2
317	Rhubarb, cooked, added sugar	1 c	240	68	278	1	75	5	<1	t	t	.1
	Strawberries:											
318	Fresh, whole, capped	1 c	149	92	45	1	10	3	1	.03	.1	.3
	Frozen, sliced, sweetened:											
319	10-oz container	10 oz	284	73	272	2	74	5	<1	t	.1	.2
320	Cup, thawed measure	1 c	255	73	244	1	66	5	<1	t	t	.2
	Tangerines, without peel and seeds:											
321	Fresh (2⅜" whole) 116 g w/refuse	1 ea	84	88	37	1	9	1	<1	t	t	t
322	Canned, light syrup, fruit and liquid	1 c	252	83	153	1	41	2	<1	t	t	t
323	Tangerine juice, canned, sweetened	1 c	249	87	124	1	30	<1	<1	t	t	.1
	Watermelon, raw, without rind & seeds:											
324	Piece, 1" by 10" diam (2 lb w/refuse or 926 g)	1 pce	482	91	154	3	35	2	2	.3	.4	1.1
325	Diced	1 c	160	91	51	1	11	1	1	.1	.1	.3

(1)Dietary fiber value partially derived from data for bananas.

(2)Dietary fiber data can vary between 6 and 13 g for 10 prunes.

(Computer code number is for West Diet Analysis program)

Chol (mg)	Calc (mg)	Iron (mg)	Magn (mg)	Phos (mg)	Pota (mg)	Sodi (mg)	Zinc (mg)	VT-A (RE)	Thia (mg)	Ribo (mg)	Niac (mg)	V-B6 (mg)	Fola (μg)	VT-C (mg)
0	35	.7	35	15	305	2	.25	10	.24	.05	.71	.18	12	24
0	8	.16	8	3	71	1	.06	2	.05	.01	.16	.04	3	6
0	42	.65	32	20	335	2	.27	1	.14	.05	.64	.24	58	27[3]
0	4	.89	55	50	739	6	.21	167[4]	.08	.08	1.02	.44	33	27
0	3	.89	49	43	716	8	.2	140	.07	.08	1.16	.37	40	17
0	3	.07	5	7	113	0	.07	21	.03	.06	.33	.05	1	6
0	1	.03	2	3	48	0	.03	9	.01	.03	.14	.02	1	3
0	23	2.17	13	33	234	49	.18	67	.04	.1	.75	.07	6	1
0	10	.92	5	14	100	21	.08	29	.02	.04	.32	.03	3	<1
0	25	.86	20	38	388	3	.28	255	.06	.15	1.19	.07	7	7
0	9	.32	8	14	146	1	.1	96	.02	.06	.45	.03	2	3
0	5	.46	5	12	399	5	–	0	.05	.05	.46	.16	–	9
0	43	2.08	38	66	625	3	.44	167	.07	.14	1.65	.22	3	3
0	49	2.35	42	74	708	4	.51	66	.05	.21	1.53	.46	<1	6
0	31	3	36	64	707	10	.54	8	.04	.18	2	.56	1	11
0	71	3.02	48	141	1088	17	.39	1	.23	.13	1.19	.36	5	5
0	7	.29	5	14	105	2	.04	<1	.02	.01	.11	.03	<1	<1
0	27	.7	22	15	186	0	.57	16	.04	.11	1.11	.07	32	31
0	43	1.85	37	48	324	3	.51	17	.05	.13	.65	.1	74	47
0	37	1.63	32	42	285	2	.45	15	.05	.11	.57	.08	65	41
0	348	.5	29	19	230	2	.19	17	.04	.05	.48	.05	13	8
0	21	.57	15	28	247	1	.19	4	.03	.1	.34	.09	26	84
0	31	1.68	20	37	278	9	.17	6	.04	.14	1.14	.08	42	117
0	28	1.51	18	33	250	8	.15	5	.04	.13	1.02	.08	38	105
0	12	.08	10	8	131	1	.2	77	.09	.02	.13	.06	17	26
0	18	.93	20	25	196	15	.6	212	.13	.11	1.12	.11	12	50
0	45	.5	20	35	443	2	.07	105	.15	.05	.25	.08	11	55
0	39	.82	53	43	559	10	.34	178	.39	.1	.96	.69	11	46
0	13	.27	18	14	186	3	.11	59	.13	.03	.32	.23	4	15

(3) If vitamin C is added, it contains 96 mg per cup.

(4) Vitamin A values range from 1.5 RE for white-fleshed varieties to 178 RE for yellow-fleshed varieties.

(For purposes of calculations, use "0" for t, <1, <.1, <.01, etc.)

Table A–1
Food Composition

Computer Code Number	Food Description	Measure	Wt (g)	H_2O (%)	Ener (cal)	Prot (g)	Carb (g)	Dietary Fiber (g)	Fat (g)	Fat Breakdown (g)		
										Sat	Mono	Poly
	BAKED GOODS: BREADS, CAKES, COOKIES, CRACKERS, PIES											
326	Bagels, plain, enriched, 3½" diam	1 ea	68	33	187	7	36	1	1	.1	.1	.5
1663	Bagel, oat bran	1 ea	68	33	173	7	36	9	1	.13	.2	.3
	Biscuits:											
327	From home recipe	1 ea	28	29	101	2	13	.4	5	1.2	2	1.2
328	From mix	1 ea	28	29	95	2	14	1	3	.8	1.2	1.2
329	From refrigerated dough	1 ea	20	27	75	1	9	.3	3	.7	1.6	.4
330	Bread crumbs, dry, grated (see #364, 365 for soft crumbs)	1 c	100	6	395	12	72	4	5	1.3	2.1	1.5
	Breads:											
331	Boston brown, canned, 3¼" slice	1 pce	45	47	88	2	19	2	1	.1	.1	.3
332	Cracked wheat (¼ cracked-wheat & ¾ enr wheat flour): 1-lb loaf	1 ea	454	36	1180	39	225	24	18	4.2	8.6	3.1
333	Slice (18 per loaf)	1 pce	25	36	65	2	12	1	1	.2	.5	.2
334	Slice, toasted	1 pce	21	30	59	2	11	1	1	.2	.4	.2
335	French/Vienna, enriched: 1-lb loaf	1 ea	454	34	1243	40	236	12	14	2.9	5.5	3.1
336	French, slice, 5 x 2½"	1 pce	35	34	96	3	18	1	1	.2	.4	.2
337	Vienna, slice, 4¾ x 4 x ½"	1 pce	25	34	68	2	13	1	1	.2	.3	.2
	French toast: see Mixed Dishes, and Fast Foods, #691											
338	Italian, enriched: 1-lb loaf	1 ea	454	36	1230	40	227	14	16	3.9	3.7	6.3
339	Slice, 4½ x 3¼ x ¾"	1 pce	30	36	81	3	15	1	1	.3	.2	.4
340	Mixed grain, enriched: 1-lb loaf	1 ea	454	38	1135	45	211	32	17	3.7	6.9	4.2
341	Slice (18 per loaf)	1 pce	25	38	62	2	12	2	1	.2	.4	.2
342	Slice, toasted	1 pce	23	32	63	3	12	2	1	.2	.4	.2
343	Oatmeal, enriched: 1-lb loaf	1 ea	454	37	1221	38	220	18	20	3.2	7.2	7.7
344	Slice (18 per loaf)	1 pce	25	37	67	2	12	1	1	.2	.4	.4
345	Slice, toasted	1 pce	23	31	67	2	12	1	1	.2	.4	.4
346	Pita pocket bread, enr, 6½" round	1 ea	60	32	165	5	33	1	1	.1	.1	.3
347	Pumpernickel (⅔ rye & ⅓ enr wheat flour): 1-lb loaf	1 ea	454	38	1135	39	216	27	14	2	4.2	5.6
348	Slice, 5 x 4 x ⅜"	1 pce	32	38	80	3	15	2	1	.1	.3	.4
349	Slice, toasted	1 pce	29	32	80	3	15	2	1	.1	.3	.4
350	Raisin, enriched: 1-lb loaf	1 ea	454	34	1243	36	237	12	20	4.9	10.4	3.1
351	Slice (18 per loaf)	1 pce	25	34	68	2	13	1	1	.3	.6	.2
352	Slice, toasted	1 pce	21	28	62	2	12	1	1	.2	.5	.2
353	Rye, light (⅓ rye & ⅔ enr wheat flour): 1-lb loaf	1 ea	454	37	1175	39	219	28	15	2.8	6	3.6
354	Slice, 4¾ x 3¾ x 7⁄16"	1 pce	25	37	65	2	12	2	1	.2	.3	.2
355	Slice, toasted	1 pce	22	31	62	2	12	2	1	.2	.3	.2
356	Wheat (enr wheat & whole-wheat flour):[1] 1-lb loaf	1 ea	454	37	1160	43	213	25	19	3.9	7.3	4.5
357	Slice (18 per loaf)	1 pce	25	37	64	2	12	1	1	.2	.4	.2
358	Slice, toasted	1 pce	23	32	65	2	12	1	1	.2	.4	.2
359	White, enriched: 1-lb loaf	1 ea	454	37	1210	38	222	12	18	5.6	6.5	4.2
360	Slice (18 per loaf)	1 pce	25	37	67	2	12	1	1	.2	.4	.2
361	Slice, toasted	1 pce	22	30	64	2	12	1	1	.2	.4	.2
362	Slice (22 per loaf)	1 pce	20	37	53	2	10	1	1	.2	.3	.2
363	Slice, toasted	1 pce	17	30	50	2	9	<1	1	.2	.3	.1

(1) A blend of white and whole-wheat flour—no official ratio specified.

(Computer code number is for West Diet Analysis program)

Chol (mg)	Calc (mg)	Iron (mg)	Magn (mg)	Phos (mg)	Pota (mg)	Sodi (mg)	Zinc (mg)	VT-A (RE)	Thia (mg)	Ribo (mg)	Niac (mg)	V-B6 (mg)	Fola (µg)	VT-C (mg)
0	50	2.43	20	65	69	363	.6	0	.37	.21	3.1	.03	15	0
0	8	2	39	112	139	345	1.42	<1	.23	.23	2	.14	31	<1
1	67	.83	5	47	34	165	.15	7	.1	.09	.84	.01	3	<1
1	52	.58	7	133	53	271	.17	7	.1	.1	.86	.02	2	<1
1	24	.44	2	70	23	158	.08	7	.07	.05	.44	.01	2	0
0	227	6.13	46	147	221	862	1.23	0	.76	.43	6.85	.1	25	0
<1	31	.95	28	50	143	284	.22	6	.01	.05	.5	.04	3	0
0	195	12.8	236	695	804	2442	5.68	0	1.63	1.09	16.7	1.38	177	0
0	11	.7	13	38	44	135	.31	0	.09	.06	.92	.08	10	0
0	10	.64	12	35	40	123	.29	0	.07	.05	.75	.06	6	0
0	341	11.5	123	477	513	2764	3.95	0	2.36	1.49	21.6	.19	141	0
0	26	.89	9	37	40	213	.3	0	.18	.11	1.66	.01	11	0
0	19	.63	7	26	28	152	.22	0	.13	.08	1.19	.01	8	0
0	354	13.4	123	468	499	2651	3.9	0	2.15	1.33	19.9	.22	136	0
0	23	.88	8	31	33	175	.26	0	.14	.09	1.31	.01	9	0
0	413	15.8	241	799	926	2210	5.81	0	1.85	1.55	19.8	1.51	218	1
0	23	.87	13	44	51	122	.32	0	.1	.09	1.09	.08	12	<1
0	23	.87	13	44	51	122	.32	0	.08	.08	.98	.07	9	<1
0	300	12.3	168	572	645	2719	4.68	9	1.81	1.09	14.3	.31	123	2
0	16	.68	9	31	35	150	.26	<1	.1	.06	.78	.02	7	<1
0	17	.68	9	31	35	150	.26	<1	.08	.05	.71	.01	5	<1
0	52	1.58	16	58	72	322	.5	0	.36	.2	2.78	.02	14	0
0	309	13.1	245	808	944	3046	6.76	0	1.48	1.38	14	.57	154	0
0	22	.92	17	57	67	215	.48	0	.1	.1	.99	.04	11	0
0	21	.92	17	57	66	214	.47	0	.08	.09	.89	.04	8	0
0	300	13.2	118	495	1030	1770	3.27	0	1.54	1.81	15.8	.31	154	2
0	16	.73	6	27	57	97	.18	0	.08	.1	.87	.02	8	<1
0	15	.66	6	25	52	89	.16	0	.06	.08	.71	.01	5	<1
0	331	12.9	182	568	754	2996	5.22	0	1.97	1.52	17.3	.34	232	0
0	18	.71	10	31	41	165	.29	0	.11	.08	.95	.02	13	0
0	18	.68	9	30	40	160	.28	0	.08	.07	.83	.02	9	<1
0	572	15.8	209	835	627	2447	4.77	0	2.09	1.45	20.5	.49	204	0
0	21	.87	11	46	34	135	.26	0	.11	.08	1.13	.03	11	0
0	26	.83	11	37	50	132	.26	0	.08	.06	.93	.02	7	0
0	572	12.9	95	490	508	2334	2.81	0	2.13	1.41	17	.15	159	0
0	21	.71	5	27	28	129	.15	0	.12	.06	.83	.01	9	0
<1	26	.73	6	23	29	130	.15	0	.09	.07	.86	.01	6	0
0	25	.57	4	22	22	103	.12	0	.09	.06	.75	.01	7	0
<1	20	.57	4	17	22	101	.12	0	.07	.06	.67	.01	4	0

(For purposes of calculations, use "0" for t, <1, <.1, <.01, etc.)

A

Table A–1
Food Composition

Computer Code Number	Food Description	Measure	Wt (g)	H_2O (%)	Ener (cal)	Prot (g)	Carb (g)	Dietary Fiber (g)	Fat (g)	Fat Breakdown (g) Sat	Mono	Poly
	BAKED GOODS: BREADS, CAKES, COOKIES, CRACKERS, PIES—Cont.											
364	White bread cubes, soft	1 c	30	37	80	2	15	1	1	.2	.5	.2
365	White bread crumbs, soft	1 c	45	37	120	4	22	1	2	.4	.7	.3
366	Whole-wheat: 1-lb loaf	1 ea	454	38	1116	44	209	31	19	4.2	7.6	4.5
367	Slice (16 per loaf)	1 pce	28	38	70	3	13	2	1	.3	.5	.3
368	Slice, toasted	1 pce	25	30	69	3	13	2	1	.3	.5	.3
	Bread stuffing, prepared from mix:											
369	Dry type	1 c	140	65	249	4	30	4	12	2.4	5.3	3.6
370	Moist type, with egg and margarine	1 c	203	65	341	8	45	4	15	3	6.5	4.3
	Cakes, prepared from mixes:[1]											
	Angel food:											
371	Whole cake, 9¾" diam tube	1 ea	635	33	1638	37	367	10	5	.8	.5	2.3
372	Piece, 1/12 of cake	1 pce	53	33	137	3	31	1	<1	.1	t	.2
373	Boston cream pie, 1/8 of cake	1 pce	120	45	302	3	51	2	10	3	5.3	1.2
	Coffee cake:											
374	Whole cake, 7¾ x 5⅝ x 1¼"	1 ea	430	30	1367	24	227	9	41	8	16.6	13.6
375	Piece, 1/6 of cake	1 pce	72	30	229	4	38	1	7	1.3	2.8	2.3
	Devil's food, chocolate frosting:											
376	Whole cake, 2 layer, 8 or 9" diam	1 ea	1107	23	4062	45	604	31	182	51.4	99.6	21.1
377	Piece, 1/16 of cake	1 pce	69	23	253	3	38	2	11	3.2	6.2	1.3
378	Cupcake, 2½" diam	1 ea	42	23	154	2	23	1	7	1.9	3.8	.8
	Gingerbread:											
379	Whole cake, 8" square	1 ea	570	33	1761	23	289	18	58	14.8	31.9	7.6
380	Piece, 1/9 of cake	1 pce	63	33	195	3	32	2	6	1.6	3.5	.8
	Yellow, chocolate frosting, 2 layer:											
381	Whole cake, 8 or 9" diam	1 ea	1108	22	4199	42	614	20	193	52.4	107	23.2
382	Piece, 1/16 of cake	1 pce	69	22	262	3	38	1	12	3.3	6.7	1.4
	Cakes from home recipes w/enr flour:											
	Carrot cake, cream cheese frosting:[2]											
383	Whole, 9 x 13" cake	1 ea	1536	21	6696	71	725	20	406	75.1	100	209
384	Piece, 1/16 of cake, 2¼ x 3¼" slice	1 pce	112	21	488	5	53	1	30	5.5	7.3	15.2
	Fruitcake, dark:											
385	Whole cake, 7½" diam tube, 2¼" high	1 ea	1361	25	4409	39	838	48	124	15.2	56.8	44.1
386	Piece, 1/32 of cake, ⅔" arc	1 pce	43	25	139	1	26	2	4	.5	1.8	1.4
	Sheet, plain, no frosting:[3]											
387	Whole cake, 9" square	1 ea	777	24	2828	35	434	3	108	30	45.1	25.6
388	Piece, 1/9 of cake	1 pce	86	24	313	4	48	<1	12	3.3	5	2.8
	Sheet, plain, uncooked white frosting:[4]											
389	Whole cake, 9" square	1 ea	1096	22	4088	38	644	3	159	26.1	67	56.1
390	Piece, 1/9 of cake	1 pce	121	22	451	4	71	<1	17	2.9	7.4	6.2
	Pound cake:											
391	Loaf, 8½ x 3½ x 3¼"	1 ea	478	26	1946	22	224	4	108	15.5	24.9	62
392	Piece, 1/17 of loaf, ½" slice	1 pce	28	26	114	1	13	<1	6	.9	1.5	3.6

(1) Excepting angel food cake, cakes were made from mixes containing vegetable shortening, and frostings were made with margarine. All mixes use enriched flour.

(2) Made with vegetable oil.

(3) Cake made with vegetable shortening.

(4) Made with margarine.

(Computer code number is for West Diet Analysis program)

Chol (mg)	Calc (mg)	Iron (mg)	Magn (mg)	Phos (mg)	Pota (mg)	Sodi (mg)	Zinc (mg)	VT-A (RE)	Thia (mg)	Ribo (mg)	Niac (mg)	V-B6 (mg)	Fola (μg)	VT-C (mg)
<1	32	.91	7	28	36	161	.19	0	.14	.1	1.19	.02	10	0
<1	49	1.37	11	42	54	242	.28	0	.21	.15	1.79	.03	15	0
0	327	15	390	1039	1144	2392	8.85	0	1.59	.93	17.4	.81	227	0
0	20	.94	24	65	72	150	.55	0	.1	.06	1.09	.05	14	0
0	20	.93	24	64	71	148	.55	0	.08	.05	.97	.04	10	0
0	45	1.54	17	59	104	760	.39	273	.19	.15	2.07	.06	24	0
0	130	3.35	30	99	266	936	.65	256	.34	.29	3.23	.11	34	3
0	889	3.3	76	1473	591	4756	.44	0	.65	3.12	5.61	.2	19	0
0	74	.28	6	123	49	397	.04	0	.05	.26	.47	.02	2	0
44	28	.46	7	59	47	173	.19	70	.49	.32	.23	.03	10	<1
211	585	6.19	77	925	482	1810	1.94	207	.72	.75	6.54	.21	52	1
35	98	1.04	13	155	81	303	.32	35	.12	.13	1.09	.04	9	<1
509	476	24.5	376	1350	2214	3697	7.64	310	.3	1.47	6.39	.41	89	1
32	30	1.52	23	84	138	230	.48	19	.02	.09	.4	.03	6	<1
19	18	.93	14	51	84	140	.29	12	.01	.06	.24	.02	3	<1
200	393	18.9	91	958	1373	2610	2.34	91	1.08	1.06	8.89	.22	57	1
22	43	2.09	10	106	152	289	.26	10	.12	.12	.98	.02	6	<1
609	410	23.2	332	1783	1972	3733	6.87	450	1.33	1.74	13.9	.32	89	1
38	25	1.44	21	111	123	233	.43	28	.08	.11	.86	.02	6	<1
829	384	19.4	276	1090	1720	3778	7.53	9538	2.09	2.4	15.5	1.17	184	17
60	28	1.41	20	79	125	276	.55	696	.15	.17	1.13	.08	13	1
68	449	28.3	218	708	2082	3674	3.67	475	.68	1.35	10.8	.63	41	5
2	14	.89	7	22	66	116	.12	15	.02	.04	.34	.02	1	<1
505	497	11.7	108	793	613	2331	2.75	373	1.24	1.4	10.1	.26	54	2
56	55	1.3	12	88	68	258	.3	41	.14	.15	1.12	.03	6	<1
614	680	11.8	66	1567	581	3770	2.74	643	1.1	.77	5.48	.38	99	2
68	75	1.31	7	173	64	416	.3	71	.12	.08	.6	.04	11	<1
0	85	1.71	–	–	324	1502	–	137	0	.51	3.41	.07	–	0
0	5	.1	–	–	19	88	–	8	0	.03	.2	<.01	–	0

(For purposes of calculations, use "0" for t, <1, <.1, <.01, etc.)

A

Table A–1
Food Composition

Computer Code Number	Food Description	Measure	Wt (g)	H_2O (%)	Ener (cal)	Prot (g)	Carb (g)	Dietary Fiber (g)	Fat (g)	Fat Breakdown (g) Sat	Mono	Poly
	BAKED GOODS: BREADS, CAKES, COOKIES, CRACKERS, PIES—Cont.											
	Cakes, commercial:											
	Cheesecake:											
401	Whole cake, 9" diam	1 ea	1110	46	3563	61	283	23	250	128	86	15.3
402	Piece, 1/12 of cake	1 pce	92	46	295	5	23	2	21	10.6	7.1	1.3
	Pound cake:											
393	Loaf, 8½ x 3½ x 3"	1 ea	500	25	1940	27	244	3	99	55.5	27.9	5.4
394	Slice, 1/17 of loaf, 2" slice	1 pce	29	25	113	2	14	<1	6	3.2	1.6	.3
	Snack: 2 small cakes per package											
395	Chocolate w/creme filling (Ding Dong)	1 ea	28	20	107	1	17	<1	4	.9	1.5	1.2
396	Sponge w/creme filling (Twinkie)	1 ea	42	20	153	1	27	<1	5	1.1	1.9	1.5
1677	Sponge cake, 1/12 of 12" cake	1 pce	65	30	188	4	40	<1	2	.521	.616	.291
1678	Strawberry shortcake, fresh	1 ea	254	74	327	5	40	4	17	10	4.9	1
	White, white frosting, 2 layer:											
397	Whole cake, 8 or 9" diam	1 ea	1140	20	4275	38	718	15	154	45.7	68.1	39.8
398	Piece, 1/16 of cake	1 pce	71	20	266	2	45	1	10	2.8	4.2	2.5
	Yellow, chocolate frosting, 2 layer:											
399	Whole cake, 8 or 9" diam	1 ea	1108	22	4199	42	614	20	193	52.4	107	23.2
400	Piece, 1/16 of cake	1 pce	69	22	262	3	38	1	12	3.3	6.7	1.4
1332	Bagel chips	5 pce	70	4	300	6	52	3	7	1.2	1.9	3.3
1035	Cheese puffs/Cheetos	1 oz	28	1	157	2	15	<1	10	1.9	5.8	1.3
	Cookies made with enriched flour:											
	Brownies with nuts:											
403	Commercial w/frosting, 1½ x 1¾ x ⅞"	1 ea	25	14	101	1	16	1	4	1.1	2.1	.6
404	Home recipe, 1¾ x 1¾ x ⅞"[1]	1 ea	20	13	93	1	10	<1	6	1.5	2.2	1.9
	Chocolate chip:											
405	Commercial, 2¼" diam	4 ea	42	12	192	1	25	1	10	3.1	5.5	1.1
406	Home recipe, 2¼" diam	4 ea	40	6	195	2	23	1	11	3.2	4.2	3.4
407	From refrigerated dough, 2¼" diam	4 ea	48	13	213	2	29	1	10	3.3	4.8	1
408	Fig bars	4 ea	56	16	195	2	40	3	4	.7	2.2	.7
409	Oatmeal raisin, 2⅝" diam	4 ea	52	6	226	3	36	1	8	1.7	3.6	2.6
410	Peanut butter, home recipe, 2⅝" diam[2]	4 ea	48	6	228	4	28	1	11	2.1	5.2	3.5
411	Sandwich-type, all	4 ea	40	2	189	2	28	1	8	1.7	4.7	1.1
412	Shortbread, commercial, small	4 ea	32	4	161	2	21	1	8	2	4.3	1
413	Shortbread, home recipe, large[3]	2 ea	28	3	155	2	16	1	9	5.8	2.7	.4
414	Sugar, from refrigerated dough, 2" diam	4 ea	48	5	232	2	31	<1	11	2.8	6.2	1.4
415	Vanilla wafers	10 ea	40	5	176	2	29	8	6	1.4	2.4	1.5
416	Corn chips	1 oz	28	1	153	2	16	1	9	1.3	2.7	4.7
	Crackers:[4]											
1034	Armenian cracker bread	4 pce	28	4	117	5	19	4	2	.4	.7	1.1
417	Cheese	10 ea	10	3	50	1	6	<1	3	.9	.9	.5
418	Cheese with peanut butter	4 ea	30	4	145	4	17	<1	7	1.5	3.6	1.3
419	Graham	2 ea	14	4	59	1	11	<1	1	.4	.7	.2
420	Melba toast, plain	1 pce	5	5	19	1	4	<1	<1	t	t	.1

(1) Made with vegetable oil.
(2) Made with vegetable shortening.
(3) Made with margarine.
(4) Crackers made with enriched white (wheat) flour except for rye wafers and whole-wheat wafers.

(Computer code number is for West Diet Analysis program)

Chol (mg)	Calc (mg)	Iron (mg)	Magn (mg)	Phos (mg)	Pota (mg)	Sodi (mg)	Zinc (mg)	VT-A (RE)	Thia (mg)	Ribo (mg)	Niac (mg)	V-B6 (mg)	Fola (μg)	VT-C (mg)
611	566	6.99	122	1032	999	2297	5.66	1787	.31	2.14	2.16	.58	167	7
51	47	.58	10	86	83	190	.47	148	.03	.18	.18	.05	14	1
1105	175	6.95	55	685	595	1990	2.3	1035	.68	1.15	6.55	.17	55	<1
64	10	.4	3	40	34	115	.13	60	.04	.07	.38	.01	3	<1
5	21	.96	12	26	35	121	.16	4	.06	.08	.69	.01	2	<1
7	19	.55	3	32	38	153	.13	9	.06	.06	.51	.01	2	<1
66	46	1.77	7	89	64	158	.33	30	.16	.18	1.25	.03	8	0
53	209	2.33	29	289	359	510	.57	172	.3	.33	2.26	.13	40	95
91	547	9.12	60	742	661	2667	1.77	369	1.14	1.48	10.3	.16	64	1
6	34	.57	4	46	41	166	.11	23	.07	.09	.64	.01	4	<1
609	410	23.2	332	1783	1972	3733	6.87	450	1.33	1.74	13.9	.32	89	1
38	25	1.44	21	111	123	233	.43	28	.08	.11	.86	.02	6	<1
0	9	1.07	41	103	137	418	.88	0	.1	.12	1.33	.1	56	0
1	16	.67	5	31	47	298	.11	26	.07	.1	.92	.04	34	<1
4	7	.56	8	25	37	78	.18	5	.06	.05	.43	.01	3	<1
15	11	.37	11	26	35	69	.19	42	.03	.04	.2	.02	3	<1
0	6	1.02	15	21	39	137	.19	15	.05	.08	.68	.07	2	0
13	16	.99	22	40	90	144	.37	66	.07	.07	.54	.03	5	<1
11	12	1.08	11	33	86	100	.24	8	.09	.09	.95	.02	4	0
0	36	1.63	15	35	116	196	.22	6	.09	.12	1.05	.04	6	<1
17	52	1.38	22	84	124	280	.45	85	.13	.09	.65	.04	6	<1
15	19	1.08	19	56	111	249	.39	75	.11	.1	1.68	.04	9	<1
0	10	1.56	18	39	70	242	.32	0	.03	.07	.83	.01	2	0
6	11	.88	5	35	32	146	.17	8	.11	.1	1.07	.01	3	0
25	5	.75	4	20	20	132	.12	89	.1	.07	.83	.01	3	0
15	43	.89	4	90	78	225	.13	11	.09	.06	1.16	.01	3	0
23	19	.96	6	42	39	125	.14	16	.11	.13	1.24	.03	4	0
0	36	.37	21	52	40	179	.36	11	.01	.04	.33	.07[5]	6[6]	<1
0	21	.45	41	1	77	–	.9	1	.06	.04	1.05	.02	12	2
1	15	.48	4	22	14	99	.11	9	.06	.04	.47	.05	2	0
1	24	.88	17	97	73	298	.33	3	.12	.1	1.96	.45	7	0
0	3	.52	4	15	19	85	.11	0	.03	.04	.58	.01	2	0
0	5	.19	3	10	10	41	.1	0	.02	.01	.21	<.01	1	0

(5) B_6 values vary between brands. Check the label.

(6) Values from 1992 USDA data for snacks and sweets.

(For purposes of calculations, use "0" for t, <1, <.1, <.01, etc.)

Table A–1
Food Composition

Computer Code Number	Food Description	Measure	Wt (g)	H_2O (%)	Ener (cal)	Prot (g)	Carb (g)	Dietary Fiber (g)	Fat (g)	Fat Breakdown (g) Sat	Mono	Poly
	BAKED GOODS: BREADS, CAKES, COOKIES, CRACKERS, PIES—Cont.											
	Crackers—Cont.											
1514	Rice cakes, unsalted	2 ea	18	5	69	1	14	<1	1	.2	.2	.2
421	Rye wafer, whole grain	2 ea	14	5	47	1	11	2	<1	t	t	.1
422	Saltine®[1]	4 ea	12	4	52	1	9	<1	1	.3	.8	.2
423	Snack-type, round like Ritz	3 ea	9	4	45	1	5	<1	2	.4	1	.8
424	Wheat, thin	4 ea	8	3	35	1	5	1	1	.5	.5	.4
425	Whole-wheat wafers	2 ea	8	3	35	1	5	1	1	.2	.8	.2
426	Croissants, 4½ x 4 x 1¾"	1 ea	57	23	231	5	26	2	12	6.7	3.2	.7
1699	Croutons, seasoned	½ c	15	3	70	2	10	<1	3	.8	1.4	.4
	Danish pastry:											
427	Packaged ring, plain, 12 oz	1 ea	340	21	1349	19	181	1	65	13.5	40.8	6.4
428	Round piece, plain, 4¼" diam, 1" high	1 ea	57	21	226	3	30	<1	11	2.3	6.8	1.1
429	Ounce, plain	1 oz	28	21	113	2	15	<1	5	1.1	3.4	.5
430	Round piece with fruit	1 ea	65	29	231	3	31	–	11	2.3	7	1.1
	Desserts, 3 x 3" piece:											
1348	Apple crisp	1 pce	78	61	127	1	25	–	3	.6	1.2	.8
1353	Apple cobbler	1 pce	104	57	199	2	35	1	6	1.3	2.7	1.9
1349	Cherry crisp	1 pce	138	75	158	2	27	1	5	1	2.4	1.7
1352	Cherry cobbler	1 pce	129	66	198	2	34	1	6	1.3	2.7	1.9
1350	Peach crisp	1 pce	139	73	166	1	30	1	5	1	2.3	1.6
1351	Peach cobbler	1 pce	130	65	204	2	36	1	6	1.3	2.7	1.9
	Doughnuts:											
431	Cake type, plain, 3¼" diam	1 ea	50	21	211	2	25	1	11	1.9	4.8	4.1
432	Yeast-leavened, glazed, 3¾" diam	1 ea	60	25	242	4	27	1	14	3.5	7.7	1.7
	English muffins:											
433	Plain, enriched	1 ea	57	42	134	4	26	2	1	.1	.2	.5
434	Toasted	1 ea	50	37	128	4	25	2	1	.1	.2	5
1504	Whole wheat	1 ea	50	46	102	4	20	3	1	.2	.3	.4
1414	Granola bar: Soft	1 ea	42	6	188	3	29	2	7	3.1	1.6	2.3
1415	Granola bar: Hard	1 ea	28	4	134	3	18	2	6	.7	1.2	3.4
	Muffins, 2½" diam, 1½" high:											
	From home recipe											
435	Blueberry[2]	1 ea	45	39	131	3	18	2	5	1.1	1.2	2.4
436	Bran, wheat[3]	1 ea	45	35	130	3	19	3	6	1.2	1.4	2.8
437	Cornmeal	1 ea	45	32	144	3	20	2	6	1.2	1.4	2.8
	From commercial mix:											
438	Blueberry	1 ea	45	36	135	2	22	2	4	.7	1.6	1.4
439	Bran, wheat	1 ea	45	35	124	3	21	3	4	1.1	2.1	.6
440	Cornmeal	1 ea	45	30	144	3	22	2	5	1.3	2.4	.6
	Pancakes, 4" diam:											
441	Buckwheat, from mix w/ egg and milk	1 ea	27	54	56	2	8	1	2	.5	.5	.8
442	Plain, from home recipe	1 ea	27	53	61	2	8	<1	3	.6	.7	1.2
443	Plain, from mix; egg, milk, oil added	1 ea	27	53	52	1	10	<1	1	.1	.2	.2

(1)Made with lard.
(2)Made with vegetable shortening.
(3)Made with vegetable oil.

(Computer code number is for West Diet Analysis program)

PAGE KEY: A–2 = BEV A–4 = DAIRY A–10 = EGGS A–12 = FAT/OIL A–14 = FRUIT A–24 = BAKERY A–34 = GRAIN A–40 = FISH A–44 = MEATS A–48 = POULTRY A–50 = SAUSAGE A–52 = MIXED/FAST A–60 = NUTS/SEEDS A–62 = SWEETS A–66 = VEG/LEG A–78 = MISC A–80 = SOUPS/SAUCES A–84 = FAST A–96 = FRZN ENTREE A–98 = BABY FOODS

Chol (mg)	Calc (mg)	Iron (mg)	Magn (mg)	Phos (mg)	Pota (mg)	Sodi (mg)	Zinc (mg)	VT-A (RE)	Thia (mg)	Ribo (mg)	Niac (mg)	V-B6 (mg)	Fola (µg)	VT-C (mg)
0	3	.37	25	63	50	1	.54	1	0	<.01	.78	.02	3	0
0	6	.83	17	47	69	111	.39	<1	.06	.04	.22	.04	6	<1
0	14	.65	3	13	15	156	.09	0	.07	.05	.63	<.01	4	0
<1	11	.32	2	21	18	64	.06	0	.03	.03	.36	<.01	1	0
<1	3	.25	6[4]	15	17	69	.24[4]	0	.04	.03	.4	.01	3	0
0	4	.25	8[4]	24	24	53	.17	0	.02	.01	.36	.01	2	0
43	21	1.16	9	60	67	424	.43	78	.22	.14	1.25	.03	16	<1
<1	14	.42	6	21	27	186	.14	1	.08	.06	.7	.01	6	0
105	143	6.94	54	286	371	1261	1.87	20	.99	.75	8.5	.2	54	10
18	24	1.16	9	48	62	211	.31	3	.16	.12	1.43	.03	9	2
9	12	.58	5	24	31	105	.16	2	.08	.06	.71	.02	5	1
13	15	.97	10	47	76	230	.33	17	.2	.14	1.24	.04	10	1
0	22	.58	5	19	76	142	.12	24	.07	.06	.6	.03	4	–
1	31	.78	6	44	87	304	.16	76	.1	.09	.74	.04	3	<1
0	29	2.15	12	23	164	73	.15	145	.07	.08	.59	.06	10	3
1	37	1.81	10	48	114	311	.2	135	.1	.11	.85	.05	9	2
0	23	.95	13	31	198	69	.2	104	.05	.05	1.03	.03	6	5
1	33	.91	10	54	140	308	.23	105	.09	.09	1.18	.03	6	3
18	22	.98	10	135	63	273	.27	9	.11	.12	.92	.03	4	<1
4	26	1.23	13	56	65	205	.46	11	.22	.13	1.71	.03	13	0
0	99	1.43	12	76	75	264	.4	0	.25	.16	2.21	.02	21	<1
0	94	1.37	11	72	71	252	.38	0	.19	.14	1.9	.02	14	<1
0	133	1.23	35	141	105	319	.8	0	.15	.07	1.71	.08	24	0
<1	45	1.09	31	98	138	118	.64	0	.12	.07	.22	.04	10	0
0	17	.84	27	79	95	83	.58	4	.07	.03	.45	.02	7	<1
18	85	1.03	7	65	55	198	.24	13	.12	.13	.99	.02	5	1
16	84	1.89	35	128	143	265	1.24	108	.15	.2	1.81	.14	23	4
20	116	1.18	10	79	65	263	.27	18	.14	.14	1.07	.04	8	<1
21	11	.51	5	85	35	197	.17	11	.07	.14	1.01	.03	5	<1
31	14	1.14	26	150	66	210	.52	14	.09	.11	1.29	.08	7	0
28	34	.88	9	173	59	358	.29	20	.11	.12	.94	.05	5	<1
18	69	.51	15	110	63	144	.32	18	.05	.07	.36	.04	5	<1
16	59	.49	4	43	36	119	.15	15	.05	.08	.42	.01	3	<1
3	34	.42	5	90	47	170	.1	16	.06	.06	.46	.02	2	<1

(4) Values derived from whole-wheat recipes and retention values.

Table A–1
Food Composition

Computer Code Number	Food Description	Measure	Wt (g)	H_2O (%)	Ener (cal)	Prot (g)	Carb (g)	Dietary Fiber (g)	Fat (g)	Fat Breakdown (g) Sat	Mono	Poly
	BAKED GOODS: BREADS, CAKES, COOKIES, CRACKERS, PIES—Cont.											
	Piecrust, with enriched flour, vegetable shortening, baked:											
444	Home recipe, 9" shell	1 ea	180	10	949	11	85	3	62	15.5	27.4	16.4
	From mix:											
445	For 2-crust pie	1 ea	320	10	1686	20	152	6	111	27.6	48.6	29.2
446	1 pie shell	1 ea	180	11	902	12	91	3	55	13.9	31.1	6.9
	Pies, 9" diam; crust made with vegetable shortening, enriched flour:											
447	Apple:[1] Whole pie	1 ea	945	52	2239	18	321	16	104	19.9	56.1	19.8
448	Piece, ⅙ of pie	1 pce	158	52	374	3	54	3	17	3.3	9.4	3.3
449	Banana cream: Whole pie	1 ea	1188	48	3195	52	391	–	162	44.7	68	39.2
450	Piece, ⅙ of pie	1 pce	198	48	533	9	65	–	27	7.4	11.3	6.5
451	Blueberry:[1] Whole pie	1 ea	945	51	2315	25	317	13	112	27.6	48.4	29.1
452	Piece, ⅙ of pie	1 pce	158	51	387	4	53	2	19	4.6	8.1	4.9
453	Cherry:[1] Whole pie	1 ea	945	46	2551	26	364	14	115	28.3	50.2	30.7
454	Piece, ⅙ of pie	1 pce	158	46	427	4	61	2	19	4.7	8.4	5.1
455	Chocolate cream:[2] Whole pie	1 ea	1194	56	2704	53	320	6	139	44.3	57.1	30.7
456	Piece, ⅙ of pie	1 pce	199	56	451	9	53	1	23	7.4	9.5	5.1
457	Custard:[1] Whole pie	1 ea	910	61	1911	50	189	11	106	25.3	52.4	17.5
458	Piece, ⅙ of pie	1 pce	152	61	319	8	32	2	18	4.2	8.8	2.9
459	Lemon meringue:[1] Whole pie	1 ea	840	42	2251	13	396	10	73	13.1	30.5	24.3
460	Piece, ⅙ of pie	1 pce	140	42	375	2	66	2	12	2.2	5.1	4
461	Peach: Whole pie	1 ea	945	45	2546	22	377	13	111	26.4	47.4	31.8
462	Piece, ⅙ of pie	1 pce	158	45	426	4	63	2	18	4.4	7.9	5.3
463	Pecan:[1] Whole pie	1 ea	825	19	3300	33	472	29	153	31	89.1	24.5
464	Piece, ⅙ of pie	1 pce	138	19	552	6	79	5	25	5.2	14.9	4.1
465	Pumpkin:[1] Whole pie	1 ea	1240	58	2604	48	339	33	118	25	62.1	19.8
466	Piece, ⅙ of pie	1 pce	206	58	433	8	56	6	20	4.2	10.3	3.3
467	Pies, fried, commercial: Apple	1 ea	85	40	266	2	33	1	14	6.5	5.8	1.2
468	Pies, fried, commercial: Cherry	1 ea	85	40	266	2	33	1	14	6.5	5.8	1.2
	Pretzels, made with enriched flour:											
469	Thin sticks, 2¼" long	10 ea	3	3	11	<1	2	<1	<1	t	t	t
470	Dutch twists, 2¾ x 2⅝"	1 ea	16	3	61	1	13	<1	1	.1	.2	.2
471	Thin twists, 3¼ x 2¼ x ¼"	10 ea	60	3	229	5	47	2	2	.4	.8	.7
	Rolls & buns, enriched, commercial:											
472	Cloverleaf rolls, 2½" diam, 2" high	1 ea	28	32	85	2	14	1	2	.5	1.1	.3
473	Hot dog buns	1 ea	40	34	114	3	20	1	2	.5	1	.4
474	Hamburger buns	1 ea	45	34	129	4	23	1	2	.5	1.1	.4
475	Hard roll, white, 3¾" diam, 2" high	1 ea	50	31	147	5	26	1	2	.3	.6	.9
476	Submarine rolls/hoagies, 11½ x 3 x 2½"	1 ea	135	31	392	12	75	4	4	.9	1.3	1.4
	Rolls & buns, enriched, home recipe:											
477	Dinner rolls 2½" diam, 2" high	1 ea	35	29	112	3	19	1	3	.7	1.1	.7
478	Toaster pastries, fortified (Poptarts)	1 ea	54	12	212	3	38	1	6	.8	2.2	2.1

(1)Values from latest USDA data for Baked Goods.

(2)Values based on recipe: pie crust, cooked chocolate pudding, whipped cream topping.

Chol (mg)	Calc (mg)	Iron (mg)	Magn (mg)	Phos (mg)	Pota (mg)	Sodi (mg)	Zinc (mg)	VT-A (RE)	Thia (mg)	Ribo (mg)	Niac (mg)	V-B6 (mg)	Fola (μg)	VT-C (mg)
0	18	5.22	25	121	121	976	.79	0	.7	.5	5.96	.04	20	0
0	32	9.28	45	214	214	1734	1.41	0	1.25	.89	10.6	.08	35	0
0	108	3.89	27	151	112	1312	.7	0	.54	.33	4.27	.1	22	0
0	104	4.25	66	227	614	2513	1.51	284	.26	.25	2.49	.36	38	30
0	17	.71	11	38	103	420	.25	47	.04	.04	.42	.06	6	5
606	891	12.5	190	1092	1960	2851	5.7	832	1.65	2.46	12.5	1.58	131	19
101	149	2.08	32	182	327	475	.95	139	.27	.41	2.08	.26	22	3
0	66	11.7	76	284	473	1748	1.89	38	1.45	1.25	11.2	.32	47	7
0	11	1.96	13	47	79	292	.32	6	.24	.21	1.88	.05	8	1
0	94	17.6	85	284	728	1804	1.89	454	1.4	1.18	12.1	.32	66	9
0	16	2.94	14	47	122	302	.32	76	.23	.2	2.02	.05	11	2
93	902	12.3	170	951	1582	2670	4.95	203	1.52	2.56	11.6	.36	69	5
16	150	2.04	28	159	264	445	.82	34	.25	.43	1.94	.06	11	1
300	728	5.28	100	1019	965	2184	4.73	575	.35	1.89	2.66	.44	182	3
50	122	.88	17	170	161	365	.79	96	.06	.32	.44	.07	30	<1
378	470	5.12	126	882	748	1226	4.12	462	.52	1.76	5.45	.25	67	27
63	78	.85	21	147	125	204	.69	77	.09	.29	.91	.04	11	4
0	50	10.3	68	256	891	1722	1.59	328	1.2	1.01	13	.17	49	501
0	8	1.73	11	43	149	288	.27	55	.2	.17	2.17	.03	8	84
264	140	8.66	149	635	611	3498	4.7	388	.75	1.01	2.05	.17	49	9
44	23	1.45	25	106	102	585	.79	65	.13	.17	.34	.03	8	2
248	744	9.8	186	880	1909	3496	5.58	11544[3]	.68	1.9	2.32	.71	186	19
41	124	1.63	31	146	317	581	.93	1917[3]	.11	.31	.38	.12	31	3
13	13	.88	8	37	51	325	.17	8	.1	.08	.98	.03	4	2
13	13	.88	8	37	51	325	.17	42	.1	.08	.98	.03	4	1
0	1	.13	1	3	4	51	.03	0	.01	.02	.16	<.01	2	0
0	6	.69	6	18	23	274	.14	0	.07	.1	.84	.02	13	0
0	22	2.59	21	68	88	1029	.51	0	.28	.37	3.15	.07	50	0
<1	34	.89	7	33	38	148	.22	0	.14	.09	1.14	.01	9	<1
0	56	1.27	8	35	56	224	.25	0	.19	.12	1.57	.02	11	0
0	63	1.43	9	40	63	252	.28	0	.22	.14	1.77	.02	12	0
0	47	1.65	13	50	54	272	.47	0	.24	.17	2.12	.03	7	0
0	122	3.78	27	115	122	783	.85	0	.54	.33	4.47	.05	40	0
13	21	1.04	7	44	53	145	.24	28	.14	.14	1.21	.02	15	<1
0	14	1.89	10	60	60	226	.36	150[4]	.16	.2	2.13	.21	43	<1

(3)Latest USDA values of vitamin A for canned pumpkin are almost 3.5 times greater than previously published values. Canned pumpkin is usually a blend of pumpkin and winter squash.

(4)Vitamin A values from label declarations vary.

A

Table A–1
Food Composition

Computer Code Number	Food Description	Measure	Wt (g)	H_2O (%)	Ener (cal)	Prot (g)	Carb (g)	Dietary Fiber (g)	Fat (g)	Fat Breakdown (g) Sat	Mono	Poly
	BAKED GOODS: BREADS, CAKES, COOKIES, CRACKERS, PIES—Cont.											
	Tortilla chips:											
1271	Plain	1 oz	28	2	142	2	18	2	7	1.4	4.4	1
1036	Nacho flavor	1 oz	28	2	141	2	18	1	7	1.4	4.3	1
1037	Taco flavor	1 oz	28	2	136	2	18	–	7	1.3	4	1
	Tortillas:											
479	Corn, enriched, 6" diam	1 ea	30	44	67	2	14	2	1	.1	.2	.3
480	Flour, 8" diam	1 ea	35	27	115	3	20	1	3	.4	1	1
1301	Flour, 10" diam	1 ea	57	27	185	5	32	2	4	.6	1.6	1.6
481	Taco shells	1 ea	14	4	62	1	9	1	3	.4	1.5	.6
	Waffles, 7" diam:											
482	From home recipe	1 ea	75	42	218	6	25	1	11	2.1	2.6	5.1
483	From mix, egg/milk added	1 ea	75	42	218	5	26	1	10	1.7	2.7	5.2
1510	Whole grain, prepared from frozen	1 ea	39	44	106	4	12	1	5	1.6	1.9	1
	GRAIN PRODUCTS: CEREAL, FLOUR, GRAIN, PASTA and NOODLES, POPCORN											
484	Barley, pearled, dry, uncooked	1 c	200	10	704	20	155	31	2	.5	.3	1.1
485	Barley, pearled, cooked	1 c	157	69	193	4	44	9	1	.1	.1	.3
	Breakfast cereals, hot, cooked:											
	Corn grits (hominy) enriched:											
486	Regular and quick, prepared, yellow	1 c	242	85	145	3	31	4	<1	.1	.1	.2
487	Instant, prepared from packet, white	1 ea	137	85	82	2	18	<1	<1	t	t	.1
	Cream of wheat:											
488	Regular, quick, instant	1 c	244	87	131	4	27	3	<1	.1	.1	.2
489	Mix and eat, plain, packet	1 ea	142	82	102	3	21	<1	<1	t	t	.1
1664	Farina cereal, cooked	½ c	117	87	58	2	12	2	<1	t	t	t
490	Malt-O-Meal	1 c	240	88	122	4	26	3	<1	t	t	.1
494	Maypo	1 c	242	83	172	6	32	4	2	.1	.1	.3
	Oatmeal or rolled oats:											
491	Regular, quick, instant, nonfort	1 c	234	85	145	6	25	4	2	.4	.7	.9
	Instant, fortified:											
492	Plain, from packet	¾ c	177	85	104	4	18	2	2	.3	.6	.7
493	Flavored, from packet	¾ c	164	76	160	5	31	3	2	.3	.7	.8
	Breakfast cereals, ready to eat:											
495	All-Bran	⅓ c	28	3	71	4	21	10	1	.1	.1	.3
1306	Alpha Bits	1 c	28	1	111	2	25	1	1	.1	.2	.3
1307	Apple Jacks	1 c	28	2	109	2	26	1	<1	t	t	t
1308	Bran Buds	1 c	84	3	216	12	64	24	2	.4	.3	1.1
1305	Bran Chex	1 c	49	2	156	5	39	7	1	.2	.2	.8
1309	Honey BucWheat Crisp	¾ c	28	5	110	3	23	3	1	.2	.2	.4
1310	C. W. Post, plain	1 c	97	2	431	9	69	3	15	11.3	1.7	1.4
1311	C. W. Post, with raisins	1 c	103	4	445	9	74	2	15	11	1.7	1.4
496	Cap'n Crunch	1 c	37	2	156	2	30	1	3	2.2	.4	.5
1312	Cap'n Crunchberries	1 c	38	3	160	2	31	1	3	2.1	.4	.5

(Computer code number is for West Diet Analysis program)

Chol (mg)	Calc (mg)	Iron (mg)	Magn (mg)	Phos (mg)	Pota (mg)	Sodi (mg)	Zinc (mg)	VT-A (RE)	Thia (mg)	Ribo (mg)	Niac (mg)	V-B6 (mg)	Fola (μg)	VT-C (mg)
0	44	.43	25	58	56	150	.43	6	.02	.05	.36	.08	3	<1
1	42	.4	23	69	61	201	.34	13	.04	.05	.4	.08	4	1
1	44	.57	25	68	61	223	.36	26	.07	.06	.57	.08	6	<1
0	52	.42	19	94	46	48	.28	8	.03	.02	.45	.07	4	0
0	44	1.17	9	44	46	169	.25	0	.19	.1	1.26	.02	4	0
0	71	1.88	15	70	74	272	.4	0	.3	.17	2.03	.03	7	0
0	34	.35	14	31	33	24	.18	6	.04	.02	.23	.04	4	0
52	191	1.74	14	143	119	383	.51	49	.2	.26	1.55	.04	11	<1
38	93	1.23	15	252	134	458	.35	50	.15	.19	1.23	.07	9	<1
39	85	.7	15	83	88	150	.41	25	.08	.12	.59	.04	7	<1
0	58	5	158	442	560	18	4.26	4	.38	.23	9.22	.52	46	0
0	17	2.09	34	85	146	5	1.29	2	.13	.1	3.23	.18	25	0
0	0	1.55[1]	10	29	53	0[2]	.17	14[3]	.24[1]	.14[1]	1.96[1]	.06	2	0
0	7	1.01[1]	5	16	29	343	.08	0	.18[1]	.08[1]	1.3[1]	.03	1	0
0	51[1]	10.5[1]	12	102[4]	46	141[4]	.34	0	.24[1]	0[1]	1.46[1]	.03	10	0
0	20[1]	8.09[1]	7	20[1]	38	241	.24	376[1]	.43[1]	.28[1]	4.97[1]	.57	100	0
0	2	1	2	14	15	0[5]	.08	0	.09	.06	.641	.01	2	0
0	5	9.6[1]	5	24[1]	31	2[5]	.17	0	.48[1]	.24[1]	5.76[1]	.02	5	0
0	126	8.47	51	249	213	261	1.5	709	.73	.73	9.44	.97	10	29
0	19	1.59	56	177	131	2[5]	1.15	5	.26	.05	.3	.05	9	0
0	162[1]	6.3[1]	42	132	99	283[1]	.87	453[1]	.53[1]	.28[1]	5.47[1]	.74	150	0
0	168[1]	6.7[1]	51	148	137	254[1]	1	460[1]	.53[1]	.38[1]	5.9[1]	.76	150	<1
0	23	4.52[1]	105	264	350	320	3.75	376[1]	.37[1]	.43[1]	5[1]	.51	100	15[1]
0	8	2.7	17	51	110	180	1.51	376	.37	.43	5	.51	100	0
0	3	4.52	6	30	23	124	3.75	376	.37	.43	5	.51	100	15
0	56	13.4	267	729	1403	515	11.1	1111	1.09	1.26	14.8	1.51	296	44
0	29	7.79	125	326	393	454	2.14	11	.64	.26	8.62	.88	172	26
0	40	8.12	32	80	106	270	.51	682	.68	.77	9	1.4	9	27
<1	47	15.4	67	224	197	166	1.64	1283	1.26	1.46	17.1	1.75	342	0
<1	50	16.4	74	231	260	160	1.64	1362	1.34	1.55	18.1	1.85	363	0
0	6	9.81[1]	15	47	48	278	4	5[1]	.66[1]	.71[1]	8.62[1]	1	238	0
<1	12	9.92	15	51	54	268	3.88	5	.65	.74	8.92	1.02	140	0

(1)Nutrient added (values sometimes based on label declaration).

(2)Cooked without salt. If salt is added according to label recommendation, sodium content is 540 mg.

(3)Value for yellow corn grits; cooked white corn grits contain 0 RE of vitamin A.

(4)Values for quick cereal.

(5)Cooked without salt. If added according to label recommendations, sodium content is 390 mg for Cream of Wheat; 324 mg for Malt-O-Meal; 374 mg for oatmeal; 385 mg for Farina.

(For purposes of calculations, use "0" for t, <1, <.1, <.01, etc.)

A

Table A–1
Food Composition

Computer Code Number	Food Description	Measure	Wt (g)	H_2O (%)	Ener (cal)	Prot (g)	Carb (g)	Dietary Fiber (g)	Fat (g)	Fat Breakdown (g)		
										Sat	Mono	Poly
	GRAIN PRODUCTS: CEREAL, FLOUR, GRAIN, PASTA and NOODLES, POPCORN—Cont.											
	Breakfast cereals, ready to eat—Cont.											
1313	Cap'n Crunch, peanut butter	1 c	38	2	169	3	29	1	5	2.1	1.5	1.1
497	Cheerios	1 c	23	5	90	3	16	2	1	.3	.5	.6
1314	Cocoa Krispies	1 c	36	2	139	2	32	<1	1	.1	.1	.2
1316	Cocoa Pebbles	1 c	31	2	128	1	27	<1	2	t	t	t
1315	Corn Bran	1 c	36	2	124	2	30	7	1	.2	.3	.7
1317	Corn Chex	1 c	28	2	111	2	25	<1	1	.1	.2	.6
498	Corn Flakes, Kellogg's	1¼ c	28	3	108	2	24	1	<1	t	t	t
499	Corn Flakes, Post Toasties	1¼ c	28	3	108	2	24	1	<1	t	t	t
1340	Corn Pops	1 c	28	3	108	1	26	<1	<1	t	t	.1
1318	Cracklin' Oat Bran	1 c	60	4	229	6	41	8	9	2.1	2.3	3.5
1038	Crispy Wheat `N Raisins	1 c	43	7	150	3	35	3	1	.1	.1	.4
1319	Fortified Oat Flakes	1 c	48	3	177	9	35	3	1	.1	.3	.3
500	40% Bran Flakes, Kellogg's	1 c	39	3	127	5	30	7	1	.1	.1	.4
501	40% Bran Flakes, Post	1 c	47	3	152	5	37	9	1	.2	.2	.3
502	Froot Loops	1 c	28	2	111	2	25	1	1	.2	.1	.1
518	Frosted Flakes	1 c	35	2	133	2	32	1	<1	t	t	t
1320	Frosted Mini-Wheats	4 ea	31	5	111	3	26	3	<1	.1	t	.2
1321	Frosted Rice Krispies	1 c	28	3	108	1	26	<1	<1	t	t	t
1324	Fruit & Fibre w/dates	½ c	28	9	89	2	22	3	1	.2	.2	.5
1325	Fruitful Bran	¾ c	34	2	110	3	27	5	<1	.1	.1	.2
1322	Fruity Pebbles	1 c	32	3	131	1	28	1	2	.4	.3	.4
503	Golden Grahams	1 c	39	2	150	2	33	2	1	1	.1	.2
504	Granola, homemade	½ c	61	3	297	7	34	6	17	2.9	4.7	8.6
1670	Granola, low fat, commercial	½ c	47	3	182	5	38	3	3	0	–	–
505	Grape Nuts	½ c	57	3	203	7	47	6	<1	t	t	.2
1326	Grape Nuts Flakes	1 c	32	3	116	3	26	3	<1	.1	t	.1
1665	Heartland Natural with raisins	1 c	101	5	430	10	70	6	14	–	–	–
1327	Honey & Nut Corn Flakes	1 c	38	4	151	2	31	1	2	.3	.7	1
506	Honey Nut Cheerios	1 c	33	3	126	4	27	2	1	.1	.3	.3
1328	HoneyBran	1 c	35	2	119	3	29	4	1	.1	.1	.4
1329	HoneyComb	1 c	22	1	86	1	20	<1	<1	.1	.1	.2
1330	King Vitaman	1 c	19	2	77	1	16	1	1	.7	.1	.2
1039	Kix	1 c	19	3	74	2	16	<1	<1	.1	.1	.2
1331	Life	1 c	43	4	158	8	31	3	1	.1	.2	.4
507	Lucky Charms	1 c	32	3	125	3	26	1	1	.2	.4	.5
1323	Mueslix Five Grain	1 c	82	5	279	7	63	7	3	.5	1	1.2
1416	Granola, low-fat	⅓ c	31	–	120	3	25	2	2	0	–	–
508	Nature Valley Granola	1 c	113	4	502	11	75	12	20	13	2.9	2.8
1666	Nutri Grain Almond Raisin	⅔ c	39.7	9	140	3	31	3	2	0	–	–
1333	Nutri-Grain—corn	1 c	42	3	160	3	35	4	1	.1	.2	.6
1335	Nutri-Grain—wheat	1 c	44	3	158	4	37	5	<1	.1	.1	.3
1336	100% Bran	1 c	66	3	177	8	48	23	3	.6	.6	1.9
509	100% Natural cereal, plain	½ c	57	2	267	7	36	4	12	8.2	2.3	1.1
1337	100% Natural with apples & cinnamon	1 c	104	2	478	11	70	6	20	15.4	1.8	1.3
1338	100% Natural with raisins & dates	1 c	110	3	496	11	72	7	20	13.6	3.7	1.7
510	Product 19	1 c	33	3	125	3	27	1	<1	t	t	.1
1339	Quisp	1 c	30	2	124	1	25	<1	2	1.5	.3	.3
511	Raisin Bran, Kellogg's	1 c	49	8	152	5	37	6	1	.2	.1	.4
512	Raisin Bran, Post	1 c	56	9	171	5	42	7	1	.2	.2	.4

(Computer code number is for West Diet Analysis program)

Chol (mg)	Calc (mg)	Iron (mg)	Magn (mg)	Phos (mg)	Pota (mg)	Sodi (mg)	Zinc (mg)	VT-A (RE)	Thia (mg)	Ribo (mg)	Niac (mg)	V-B6 (mg)	Fola (μg)	VT-C (mg)
0	8	10	20	53	62	294	4.15	6	.66	.77	9.85	1.14	268	0
0	39	3.66[1]	32	109	82	249	.64	304[1]	.3[1]	.34[1]	4.05[1]	.41	5	12[1]
<1	6	2.27	12	47	53	275	1.91	476	.47	.54	6.34	.65	127	19
0	5	1.97	13	24	52	149	1.66	415	.41	.47	5.52	.56	111	0
0	41	12.2	18	52	70	309	4	8	.37	.7	10.9	.86	232	0
0	3	1.79	4	11	23	271	.1	14	.37	.07	5	.51	100	15
0	1	1.76[1]	3	18	26	286	.08	370[1]	.36[1]	.42[1]	4.93[1]	.5	99	15[1]
0	1	.74[1]	4	12	32	293	.08	370[1]	.36[1]	.42[1]	4.93[1]	.5	99	0
0	1	1.79	2	28	17	103	1.51	376	.37	.43	5	.51	100	15
0	40	3.78	116	241	355	487	3.18	794	.78	.9	10.6	1.08	212	32
0	71	6.84	34	117	173	204	.51	569	.56	.64	7.57	.77	15	0
0	68	13.7	58	176	343	429	1.5	635	.62	.72	8.45	.86	169	0
0	19	24.8[1]	71	191	247	302	5.15	516[1]	.51[1]	.58[1]	6.86[1]	.7	137	0
0	21	7.47[1]	101	296	250	430	2.49	622[1]	.61[1]	.7[1]	8.27[1]	.85	165	0
0	3	4.52[1]	7	24	26	144	3.75	376[1]	.37[1]	.43[1]	5[1]	.51	100	15[1]
0	1	2.21[1]	3	26	22	283	.05	463[1]	.45[1]	.52[1]	6.16[1]	.63	123	19[1]
0	10	1.95	25	81	105	9	1.64	410	.4	.46	5.46	.56	109	16
0	1	1.79	5	27	21	239	.31	376	.37	.43	5	.51	100	15
0	15	4.52	48	123	167	149	1.51	379	.37	.43	5	.5	100	0
0	<1	8.09	58	133	150	240	3.74	378	.38	.43	5	.5	100	<1
0	4	2.04	9	19	25	180	1.73	429	.42	.49	5.71	.58	114	0
<1	24	6.21[1]	16	56	86	386	.34	517[1]	.51[1]	.59[1]	6.87[1]	.7	6	21[1]
0	38	2.42	71	247	306	6	2.23	2	.37	.15	1.07	.21	49	1
0	–	2.72	36	121	143	91	5.66	227	.57	.64	7.55	.76	151	–
0	5	2.47[1]	38	143	190	396	1.25	755[1]	.74[1]	.85[1]	9.98[1]	1.03	201	0
0	13	9.28	36	97	113	183	.65	429	.42	.49	5.71	.58	114	0
0	61	3.7	130	346	382	207	2.61	5.77	.3	.13	1.43	.182	41	1
0	5	2.39	8	17	48	300	.14	501	.49	.57	6.67	.68	133	20
0	23	5.3[1]	39	124	116	302	.87	441[1]	.43[1]	.5[1]	5.87[1]	.6	22	18[1]
0	16	5.57	46	131	150	202	.9	463	.45	.52	6.16	.63	23	19
0	4	2.09	7	22	70	123	1.17	291	.29	.33	3.87	.4	78	0
0	2	11.4	6	24	23	145	.15	644	.83	.95	11.6	1.06	257	30
0	24	5.44	8	26	30	194	.16	252	.25	.28	3.35	.34	67	10
0	150	11.3	14	232	192	224	1.42	9	.93	.97	11.3	.08	36	0
0	36	5.09[1]	27	89	66	227	.56	424[1]	.42[1]	.48[1]	5.63[1]	.58	113	17[1]
0	38	8.94	82	215	369	107	7.46	747	.75	.84	9.84	.99	197	1
0	–	1.8	24	80	95	60	3.74	150	.37	.42	4.99	.5	100	–
0	71	3.77	115	353	388	232	2.19	7	.4	.19	.82	.09	85	0
0	16	.8	11	77	130	220	3.75	–	.38	.43	5	.5	100	–
0	1	.89	27	120	98	276	5.54	556	.55	.63	7.39	.76	148	22
0	12	1.24	34	164	119	299	5.81	583	.57	.66	7.74	.79	155	23
0	46	8.12	312	801	822	457	5.74	0	1.58	1.78	20.9	2.11	47	63
<1	99	1.68	68	209	281	24	1.28	3	.17	.31	1.3	.1	17	0
1	157	2.9	72	351	515	52	2	6	.33	.57	1.88	.11	17	1
1	159	3.12	124	347	537	47	2.11	6	.31	.65	2.09	.16	45	0
0	4	21[1]	12	46	51	378	.49	1746[1]	1.75[1]	1.98[1]	23.3[1]	2.34	465	70[1]
0	9	6.33	12	25	45	240	.18	5	.54	.76	5.79	.91	8	0
0	17	22.2[1]	63	182	254	271	5	498[1]	.49[1]	.59[1]	6.66[1]	.69	132	0
0	26	8.9[1]	95	234	344	365	2.97	741[1]	.73[1]	.84[1]	9.86[1]	1.01	197	0

[1]Nutrient added (values sometimes based on label declaration). (For purposes of calculations, use "0" for t, <1, <.1, <.01, etc.)

Table A-1
Food Composition

Computer Code Number	Food Description	Measure	Wt (g)	H_2O (%)	Ener (cal)	Prot (g)	Carb (g)	Dietary Fiber (g)	Fat (g)	Fat Breakdown (g) Sat	Mono	Poly
	GRAIN PRODUCTS: CEREAL, FLOUR, GRAIN, PASTA and NOODLES, POPCORN—Cont.											
	Breakfast cereals, ready to eat—Cont.											
1667	Raisin Squares	½ c	28.4	8	90	2	23	2	0	0	0	0
1041	Rice Chex	¾ c	19	3	75	1	17	1	1	.2	.2	.3
513	Rice Krispies, Kellogg's	1 c	29	2	114	2	25	<1	<1	t	t	.1
514	Rice, puffed	1 c	14	3	56	1	13	<1	<1	t	t	t
515	Shredded Wheat	1 c	43	5	152	5	34	5	1	.2	.2	.5
516	Special K	1 c	21	2	83	4	16	1	<1	t	t	t
517	Super Golden Crisp	1 c	33	1	123	2	30	1	<1	t	t	.1
519	Honey Smacks	1 c	38	3	140	3	33	<1	1	.1	.1	.3
1341	Tasteeos	1 c	24	2	94	3	19	1	1	.2	.2	.3
1342	Team	1 c	42	4	164	3	36	<1	1	.2	.2	.3
520	Total, wheat, with added calcium	1 c	33	4	116	3	26	3	1	.1	.1	.3
521	Trix	1 c	28	2	109	2	25	<1	<1	.2	.1	.1
1344	Wheat Chex	1 c	46	2	168	5	38	3	1	.2	.2	.6
1043	Wheat cereal, puffed, fortified	1 c	12	3	44	2	10	1	<1	t	t	.1
522	Wheaties	1 c	29	5	101	3	23	3	<1	.1	t	.2
	Buckwheat flour:											
523	Dark	1 c	98	11	328	12	69	8	3	.7	.9	.9
524	Light	1 c	98	12	340	6	78	6	1	.2	.4	.4
525	Buckwheat: Whole grain, dry	1 c	175	10	600	23	125	16	6	1.3	1.8	1.8
526	Bulgar: Dry, uncooked	1 c	140	9	477	17	106	31	2	.3	.2	.8
527	Bulgar: Cooked	1 c	182	78	151	6	34	11	<1	.1	.1	.2
	Cornmeal:											
528	Whole-ground, unbolted, dry	1 c	122	10	440	10	94	13	4	.6	1.2	2
529	Bolted, nearly whole, dry	1 c	122	10	441	10	94	12	4	.6	1.2	2
530	Degermed, enriched, dry	1 c	138	12	505	12	107	10	2	.3	.6	1
531	Degermed, enriched, cooked	1 c	240	78	209	5	44	4	1	.1	.2	.4
	Macaroni, cooked:											
532	Enriched	1 c	140	66	197	7	40	2	1	.1	.1	.4
533	Whole wheat	1 c	140	67	174	7	37	5	1	.1	.1	.3
534	Vegetable, enriched	1 c	134	68	172	6	36	6	<1	t	t	.1
535	Millet, cooked	½ c	120	71	142	4	28	1	1	.2	.2	.6
	Noodles (see also Pasta and Spaghetti)											
1507	Cellophane noodles	1 c	190	79	160	<1	39	<1	<1	t	t	t
537	Chow mein, dry	1 c	45	1	237	4	26	2	14	2	3.5	7.8
536	Egg noodles, cooked, enriched	1 c	160	69	213	8	40	4	2	.5	.7	.7
538	Spinach noodles, dry	3½ oz	100	8	372	13	75	7	2	.2	.2	.6
1343	Oat bran, dry	¼ c	23	7	58	4	16	4	2	.3	.6	.7
	Pasta, cooked (see also #953–956):											
1418	Fresh	2 oz	57	69	74	3	14	1	1	.1	.1	.2
1417	Linguini	1 c	140	66	197	7	40	2	1	.1	.1	.4
1598	Rotini	1 c	140	66	197	7	40	2	1	.1	.1	.4

(Computer code number is for West Diet Analysis program)

PAGE KEY: A–2 = BEV A–4 = DAIRY A–10 = EGGS A–12 = FAT/OIL A–14 = FRUIT A–24 = BAKERY A–34 = GRAIN A–40 = FISH A–44 = MEATS A–48 = POULTRY A–50 = SAUSAGE A–52 = MIXED/FAST A–60 = NUTS/SEEDS A–62 = SWEETS A–66 = VEG/LEG A–78 = MISC A–80 = SOUPS/SAUCES A–84 = FAST A–96 = FRZN ENTREE A–98 = BABY FOODS

Chol (mg)	Calc (mg)	Iron (mg)	Magn (mg)	Phos (mg)	Pota (mg)	Sodi (mg)	Zinc (mg)	VT-A (RE)	Thia (mg)	Ribo (mg)	Niac (mg)	V-B6 (mg)	Fola (μg)	VT-C (mg)
0	10	8.1	26	84	110	0	1.5	0	.38	.43	5	.5	100	–
0	3	1.2	5	19	22	158	.26	1	.25	.01	3.34	.34	67	10
0	4	1.83[1]	10	35	30	348	.49	384[1]	.38[1]	.43[1]	5.1[1]	.52	102	15[1]
0	1	.15[1]	3	14	16	<1	.14	0	.01[1]	.01[1]	.42[1]	.01	3	0
0	16	1.8	56	149	153	4	1.41	0	.11	.12	2.24	.11	21	0
<1	6	3.39[1]	12	41	37	199	2.82	282[1]	.28[1]	.32[1]	3.75[1]	.38	75	11[1]
0	7	2.08[1]	20	60	123	29	1.75	437[1]	.43[1]	.49[1]	5.81[1]	.59	116	0
0	4	2.39[1]	18	41	56	100	.38	501[1]	.49[1]	.57[1]	6.67[1]	.68	133	20[1]
0	11	3.82	26	96	71	182	.69	318	.31	.36	4.22	.43	9	13
0	6	2.57	18	65	71	259	.58	556	.55	.63	7.39	.76	7	22
0	281	21[1]	37	136	123	326	.78	1746[1]	1.75[1]	1.98[1]	23.3[1]	2.34	465	70[1]
0	6	4.52[1]	6	19	27	181	.13	376[1]	.37[1]	.43[1]	5[1]	.51	3	15[1]
0	18	7.31	58	181	173	308	1.23	0	.6	.17	8.1	.83	162	24
0	3	.57	17	43	42	<1	.28	0	.02	.03	1.3	.02	4	0
0	44	4.61[1]	32	100	108	276	.65	384[1]	.38[1]	.43[1]	5.1[1]	.52	102	15[1]
0	40	3.98	246	330	565	11	3.06	0	.41	.19	6.03	.57	53	0
0	11	1	47	86	314	1	2.56	0	.09	.05	.47	.09	100	0
0	31	3.85	404	606	805	2	4.2	0	.18	.74	12.3	.37	52	0
0	49	3.44	230	420	574	24	2.7	0	.32	.16	7.15	.48	38	0
0	18	1.75	58	73	123	9	1.04	0	.1	.05	1.82	.15	33	0
0	7	4.21	154	294	350	43	2.22	57	.47	.24	4.43	.37	31	0
0	7	4.21	154	294	350	43	2.22	57	.37	.1	2.3	.37	31	0
0	7	5.7	55	115	224	4	.99	57	.99	.56	6.96	.35	66	0
0	3	2.35	22	48	91	1	.41	23	.3	.21	2.42	.12	22	0
0	10	1.96	25	76	43	1	.74	0	.29	.14	2.34	.05	10	0
0	21	1.48	42	124	62	4	1.13	0	.15	.06	.99	.11	7	0
0	15	.66	25	67	41	8	.59	7	.15	.08	1.43	.03	8	0
0	4	.76	53	120	74	2	1.09	0	.13	.1	1.6	.13	23	0
0	14	1	3	15	5	9	.23	0	.07	0	.09	.02	1	0
0	9	2.13	23	72	54	197	.63	4	.26	.19	2.68	.05	10	0
53	19	2.54	30	110	45	11	.99	10	.3	.13	2.38	.06	11	0
0	58	2.13	174	332	376	36	2.76	46	.37	.2	4.55	.32	48	0
0	14	1.27	55	172	133	1	.73	0	.27	.05	.22	.04	12	0
19	3	.65	10	36	14	3	.32	3	.12	.09	.56	.02	4	0
0	10	1.96	25	76	43	1	.74	0	.29	.14	2.34	.05	10	0
0	10	1.96	25	76	43	1	.74	0	.29	.14	2.34	.05	10	0

[1]Nutrient added (values sometimes based on label declaration).

A

Table A–1
Food Composition

Computer Code Number	Food Description	Measure	Wt (g)	H_2O (%)	Ener (cal)	Prot (g)	Carb (g)	Dietary Fiber (g)	Fat (g)	Fat Breakdown (g) Sat	Mono	Poly
	GRAIN PRODUCTS: CEREAL, FLOUR, GRAIN, PASTA and NOODLES, POPCORN—Cont.											
	Popcorn:											
539	Air popped, plain	1 c	8	4	31	1	6	1	<1	t	.1	.2
540	Popped in vegetable oil/salted	1 c	11	3	55	1	6	1	3	.5	.9	1.5
541	Sugar-syrup coated	1 c	35	3	151	1	28	2	4	1.3	1	1.6
	Rice:											
542	Brown rice, cooked	1 c	195	73	216	5	45	3	2	.4	.6	.6
	White, enriched, all types:											
543	Regular/long grain, dry	1 c	185	12	675	13	147	3	1	.3	.4	.3
544	Regular/long grain, cooked	1 c	205	68	267	6	58	1	1	.2	.2	.2
545	Instant, prepared without salt	1 c	165	76	161	3	35	1	<1	.1	.1	.1
	Parboiled/converted rice:											
546	Raw, dry	1 c	185	10	686	13	151	3	1	.3	.3	.3
547	Cooked	1 c	175	72	200	4	43	1	<1	.1	.1	.1
1486	Sticky rice (glutinous), cooked	1 c	241	77	233	5	51	2	<1	.1	.2	.2
548	Wild rice, cooked	1 c	164	74	166	7	35	4	1	.1	.1	.4
1700	Rice and pasta (rice a roni), cooked	½ c	109	72	133	3	23	4	3	.6	1.2	1
549	Rye flour, medium	1 c	102	10	361	10	79	15	2	.2	.2	.8
1044	Soy flour, low-fat	1 c	88	3	324	45	30	1	6	.9	1.3	3.3
	Spaghetti pasta:											
550	Without salt, enriched	1 c	140	66	197	7	40	2	1	.1	.1	.4
551	With salt, enriched	1 c	140	66	197	7	40	2	1	.1	.1	.4
552	Whole-wheat spaghetti, cooked	1 c	140	67	174	7	37	5	1	.1	.1	.3
1302	Tapioca, pearl, dry	1 c	152	11	518	<1	134	2	<1	t	t	t
553	Wheat bran, crude	½ c	30	10	65	5	19	8	1	.2	.2	.7
554	Wheat germ, raw	1 c	100	11	360	23	52	15	10	1.7	1.4	6
555	Wheat germ, toasted	1 c	113	6	432	33	56	16	12	2.1	1.7	7.5
1669	Wheat germ, with brown sugar & honey	½ c	57	6	213	12	34	3	5	.8	.7	3
556	Rolled wheat, cooked	1 c	240	84	149	5	33	9	1	.2	.2	.4
557	Whole-grain wheat, cooked	⅓ c	50	86	28	1	7	1	<1	t	t	.1
	Wheat flour (unbleached):											
	All-purpose white, enriched:											
558	Sifted	1 c	115	12	419	12	88	3	1	.2	.1	.5
559	Unsifted	1 c	125	12	455	13	95	3	1	.2	.1	.5
560	Cake or pastry, enriched, sifted	1 c	96	23	343	5	55	–	12	3.1	5.1	3
561	Self-rising, enriched, unsifted	1 c	125	11	443	12	93	3	1	.2	.1	.5
562	Whole wheat, from hard wheats	1 c	120	10	406	16	87	15	2	.4	.3	.9
	MEATS: FISH and SHELLFISH											
1045	Bass, baked or broiled	4 oz	113	69	166	27	0	0	5	1.1	2.1	1.5
1046	Bluefish, baked or broiled	4 oz	113	63	180	29	0	0	6	1.3	2.6	1.5
1047	Bluefish, fried in bread crumbs	4 oz	113	61	232	26	5	<1	11	2.4	4.9	2.8
1686	Catfish, breaded/flour fried	4 oz	113	56	304	24	14	1	17	4	7	4
	Clams:											
563	Raw meat only	4 oz	113	82	84	14	3	0	1	.1	.1	.3
564	Canned, drained	4 oz	113	64	168	29	6	<1	2	.2	.2	.6
1290	Steamed, meat only	20 ea	90	64	133	23	5	<1	2	.2	.2	.5
	Cod:											
565	Baked with butter	4 oz	113	75	150	26	0	0	4	.4	.3	.6
566	Batter fried	4 oz	113	67	196	20	8	<1	9	2.2	3.6	2.6
567	Poached, no added fat	4 oz	113	76	117	25	0	0	1	.2	.1	.3

(Computer code number is for West Diet Analysis program)

PAGE KEY: A–2 = BEV A–4 = DAIRY A–10 = EGGS A–12 = FAT/OIL A–14 = FRUIT A–24 = BAKERY A–34 = GRAIN A–40 = FISH A–44 = MEATS A–48 = POULTRY A–50 = SAUSAGE A–52 = MIXED/FAST A–60 = NUTS/SEEDS A–62 = SWEETS A–66 = VEG/LEG A–78 = MISC A–80 = SOUPS/SAUCES A–84 = FAST A–96 = FRZN ENTREE A–98 = BABY FOODS

Chol (mg)	Calc (mg)	Iron (mg)	Magn (mg)	Phos (mg)	Pota (mg)	Sodi (mg)	Zinc (mg)	VT-A (RE)	Thia (mg)	Ribo (mg)	Niac (mg)	V-B6 (mg)	Fola (µg)	VT-C (mg)
0	1	.21	10	24	24	<1	.27	2	.02	.02	.15	.02	2	0
0	1	.31	12	27	25	97	.29	2	.01	.01	.17	.02	2	<1
2	15	.61	12	29	38	72	.2	3	.02	.02	.77	.01	1	0
0	19	.82	84	161	84	10	1.23	0	.19	.05	2.98	.28	8	0
0	52	7.97	46	213	213	9	2.02	0	1.07	.09	7.75	.3	15	0
0	20	2.48	25	88	72	2	1	0	.33	.03	3.03	.19	6	0
0	13	1.04	8	23	7	5[1]	.4	0	.12	.08	1.45	.02	7	0
0	111	6.6	57	252	222	9	1.78	0	1.1	.13	6.72	.65	31	0
0	33	1.98	21	73	65	5	.54	0	.44	.03	2.45	.03	7	0
0	5	.34	12	19	24	12	.99	0	.05	.03	.7	.06	2	0
0	5	.98	52	134	166	5	2.2	0	.08	.14	2.12	.22	43	0
1	9	1.02	13	40	46	619	.305	0	.134	.08	1.94	.106	8	<1
0	24	2.16	76	211	346	3	2.03	0	.29	.12	1.76	.27	38	0
0	165	5.27	201	521	2260	16	1.04	4	.33	.25	1.9	.46	360	0
0	10	1.96	25	76	43	1	.74	0	.29	.14	2.34	.05	10	0
0	10	1.96	25	76	43	140	.74	0	.29	.14	2.34	.05	10	0
0	21	1.48	42	124	62	4	1.13	0	.15	.06	.99	.11	7	0
0	30	2.4	2	11	17	2	.18	0	.01	0	0	.01	6	0
0	22	3.18	183	303	354	1	2.18	0	.16	.17	4.08	.39	24	0
0	39	6.26	239	842	892	12	12.3	0	1.88	.5	6.81	1.3	281	0
0	51	10.3	362	1294	1070	5	18.8	0	1.89	.93	6.32	1.11	398	7
0	19	4	136	485	401	2	7	0	.712	.35	2.37	.415	149	7
0	17	1.49	53	166	170	0	1.15	0	.17	.12	2.14	.17	26	0
0	3	.29	12	26	33	<1	.24	0	.04	.01	.5	.03	4	0
0	17	5.34	25	124	122	2	.8	0	.9	.57	6.79	.05	30	0
0	19	5.8	27	135	133	2	.87	0	.98	.62	7.38	.05	32	0
2	125	1.47	11	89	91	314	.31	15	.18	.23	1.47	.02	7	<1
0	423	5.84	24	743	155	1586	.77	0	.84	.52	7.29	.06	52	0
0	41	4.66	166	415	486	6	3.52	0	.54	.26	7.64	.41	53	0
99	117	2.17	43	290	517	102	.94	40	.1	.1	1.72	.16	19	2
86	10	.7	48	330	541	87	1.19	156	.08	.11	8.22	.53	2	0
68	9	.6	42	323	468	76	1.02	136	.07	.09	6.24	.41	2	<1
104	76	2	36	283	434	611	1.03	36	.1	.22	3.2	.22	24	<1
39	52	15.9	10	191	355	63	1.54	102	.09	.24	2	.07	18	15
76	104	31.6	20	383	712	127	3.1	194	.17	.48	3.81	.12	33	25
60	83	25.2	16	304	565	100	2.46	154	.13	.38	3.02	.1	26	20
68	23	.56	48	159	278	254	.66	34	.1	.09	2.85	.32	11	<1
64	43	.9	36	230	443	124	.61	17	.12	.12	2.54	.23	10	1
61	23	.54	41	259	498	69	.64	14	.09	.08	2.48	.28	8	1

(1)If prepared with salt according to label recommendation, sodium would be 608 mg.

(For purposes of calculations, use "0" for t, <1, <.1, <.01, etc.)

A

Table A–1
Food Composition

Computer Code Number	Food Description	Measure	Wt (g)	H_2O (%)	Ener (cal)	Prot (g)	Carb (g)	Dietary Fiber (g)	Fat (g)	Fat Breakdown (g) Sat	Mono	Poly
	MEATS: FISH and SHELLFISH—Cont.											
	Crab, meat only:											
1048	Blue crab, cooked	4 oz	113	77	115	23	0	0	2	.3	.3	.8
1049	Dungeness crab, cooked	4 oz	113	73	125	25	1	0	1	.2	.2	.5
568	Blue crab, canned	4 oz	113	76	112	23	0	0	1	.3	.2	.5
1587	Crab, imitation, from surimi	4 oz	113	74	116	14	12	0	1	.3	.2	.8
569	Fish sticks, breaded pollock	2 ea	57	46	155	9	13	<1	7	1.8	2.9	1.8
	Flounder/sole, baked w/lemon juice:											
570	With butter	4 oz	113	73	160	21	<1	0	8	4.3	2	.7
571	With margarine	4 oz	113	73	160	21	<1	0	8	1.6	3.1	2.5
572	Without added fat	4 oz	113	73	133	27	0	0	2	.4	.3	.7
1599	Grouper, baked or broiled	4 oz	113	73	134	28	0	0	1	.3	.3	.5
573	Haddoc, breaded, fried[1]	4 oz	113	55	265	22	14	1	13	3.2	5.4	3.3
1050	Haddock, smoked	4 oz	113	71	132	29	0	0	1	.2	.2	.4
	Halibut:											
1600	Baked or broiled	4 oz	113	72	159	30	0	0	3	.5	1.1	1.1
574	Baked with butter & lemon juice	4 oz	113	69	186	29	0	0	7	2.7	2.1	1.1
1051	Smoked	1 oz	28	49	63	6	0	0	4	.7	1.3	1.9
1054	Raw	4 oz	113	78	125	24	0	0	3	.4	.9	.9
575	Herring, pickled	3 oz	85	55	223	12	8	0	15	2	10.1	1.4
1052	Lobster meat, cooked w/moist heat	1 c	145	76	142	30	2	0	1	.2	.2	.1
1687	Ocean perch, baked/broiled	4 oz	113	82	137	27	0	0	2	.4	.9	.6
576	Ocean perch, breaded/fried	4 oz	113	59	249	22	9	1	13	3.2	5.7	3.4
1056	Octopus, raw	4 oz	113	80	93	17	2	0	1	.3	.2	.3
	Oysters:											
577	Raw, Eastern	1 c	248	85	169	17	10	0	6	1.9	.8	2.4
578	Raw, Pacific	1 c	248	82	201	23	12	0	6	1.3	.9	2.2
	Cooked:											
579	Eastern, breaded, fried, medium	6 ea	88	65	173	8	10	<1	11	2.8	4.1	2.9
580	Western, simmered	4 oz	113	64	185	21	11	0	5	1.2	2.8	2
581	Pollock, baked or broiled	4 oz	113	74	128	27	0	0	1	.3	.2	.6
1055	Pollock, moist heat, poached	4 oz	113	74	128	27	0	0	1	.3	.2	.6
	Salmon:											
582	Canned pink, solids and liquid	4 oz	113	69	158	22	0	0	7	1.7	2.1	2.3
583	Broiled or baked	4 oz	113	62	245	31	0	0	12	2.2	6	2.7
584	Smoked	4 oz	113	72	133	21	0	0	5	1	2.3	1.1
585	Atlantic sardines, canned, drained, 2 = 24 g	4 oz	113	60	236	28	0	0	13	1.7	4.4	5.8
586	Scallops, breaded, cooked from frozen	6 ea	93	58	199	17	9	<1	10	2.5	4.2	2.7
1588	Scallops, imitation, from surimi	4 oz	113	74	112	14	12	0	<1	.1	.1	.2
1688	Scallops, steamed/boiled	½ c	60	81	64	10	1	0	2	.3	.7	.6
	Shrimp:											
587	Cooked, boiled, 2 large = 14 g	6 ea	86	77	85	18	0	0	1	.2	.2	.4
588	Canned, drained	½ c	64	73	76	15	1	0	1	.2	.2	.5
589	Fried, 2 large = 15 g[1]	12 ea	90	53	217	19	10	<1	11	1.9	3.6	4.6
1057	Raw, large, about 7 g each	14 ea	100	76	106	20	1	0	2	.3	.3	.7
1589	Shrimp, imitation, from surimi	4 oz	113	75	115	14	10	0	2	.3	.2	.9
1053	Snapper, baked or broiled	4 oz	113	70	145	30	0	0	2	.4	.4	.7
1060	Squid, fried in flour[2]	4 oz	113	64	197	20	9	<1	8	2.1	3.1	2.4

(1) Dipped in egg, bread crumbs, and flour; fried in vegetable shortening.

(2) Recipe is 94.6% squid, 4.9% flour, and 0.6% salt.

(Computer code number is for West Diet Analysis program)

PAGE KEY: A–2 = BEV A–4 = DAIRY A–10 = EGGS A–12 = FAT/OIL A–14 = FRUIT A–24 = BAKERY A–34 = GRAIN A–40 = FISH A–44 = MEATS A–48 = POULTRY A–50 = SAUSAGE A–52 = MIXED/FAST A–60 = NUTS/SEEDS A–62 = SWEETS A–66 = VEG/LEG A–78 = MISC A–80 = SOUPS/SAUCES A–84 = FAST A–96 = FRZN ENTREE A–98 = BABY FOODS

Chol (mg)	Calc (mg)	Iron (mg)	Magn (mg)	Phos (mg)	Pota (mg)	Sodi (mg)	Zinc (mg)	VT-A (RE)	Thia (mg)	Ribo (mg)	Niac (mg)	V-B6 (mg)	Fola (µg)	VT-C (mg)
113	118	1.03	37	234	367	316	4.79	2	.11	.06	3.74	.2	58	4
86	67	.49	66	198	463	429	6.21	35	.06	.23	4.11	.2	48	4
101	115	.95	44	295	423	378	4.56	2	.09	.09	1.55	.17	48	3
23	15	.44	49	320	102	954	.37	23	.04	.03	.2	.03	2	0
64	11	.42	14	103	148	331	.38	18	.07	.1	1.21	.03	10	0
91	21	.37	67	249	363	193	.71	72	.09	.13	2.47	.27	13	1
73	21	.37	67	249	364	201	.71	92	.09	.13	2.47	.27	13	1
77	20	.39	66	327	390	119	.72	12	.09	.13	2.47	.27	10	0
53	24	1.29	42	162	539	60	.58	57	.09	.01	.43	.4	12	0
96	63	1.93	46	228	346	524	.59	33	.08	.14	4.51	.28	19	<1
87	56	1.59	61	285	471	865	.57	25	.05	.06	5.75	.45	17	0
47	68	1.21	121	323	652	78	.6	61	.08	.1	8.07	.45	16	0
54	66	1.17	116	308	636	112	.57	93	.08	.1	7.69	.43	16	5
28	14	.24	23	63	128	136	.12	13	.01	.02	1.64	.09	1	<1
36	53	.95	94	252	510	61	.48	53	.07	.08	6.62	.39	14	0
11	65	1.04	7	76	59	740	.45	219	.03	.12	2.81	.14	2	0
104	88	.57	51	268	510	551	4.23	38	.01	.1	1.55	.11	16	0
61	155	1	44	314	397	109	.7	16	.15	.15	2.77	.31	12	1
71	136	1.58	38	263	324	432	.67	23	.14	.18	2.69	.24	15	1
54	60	6.01	34	211	397	261	1.91	51	.03	.04	2.38	.41	18	6
131	112	16.5	117	335	387	523	225	74	.25	.24	3.42	.15	25	9
124	20	12.6	55	402	417	263	41.2	201	.17	.58	4.98	.12	25	20
71	55	6.12	51	139	214	366	76.7	79	.13	.18	1.45	.06	12	3
113	18	10.4	50	276	342	240	37.6	166	.14	.5	4.11	.1	17	14
109	7	.32	83	547	439	132	.68	26	.08	.09	1.87	.08	4	0
109	7	.32	83	547	439	132	.68	26	.08	.09	1.87	.08	4	0
62	242[3]	.95	38	373	370	628	1.04	19	.03	.21	7.42	.34	17	0
99	8	.62	35	313	425	75	.58	71	.24	.19	7.56	.25	6	0
26	12	.96	20	186	197	889	.35	29	.03	.11	5.35	.31	2	0
160	433[3]	3.31	44	555	450	572	1.5	76	.09	.26	5.95	.19	13	0
57	39	.76	55	219	309	431	.99	20	.04	.1	1.4	.13	17	2
25	9	.35	49	320	117	902	.37	23	.01	.02	.35	.03	2	0
19	15	.15	33	95	168	111	.55	31	.01	.04	.6	.08	7	1
167	33	2.65	29	117	156	192	1.34	57	.03	.03	2.22	.11	3	2
110	38	1.75	26	148	133	108	.8	11	.02	.02	1.76	.07	1	1
159	60	1.13	36	196	202	309	1.24	50	.12	.12	2.76	.09	7	1
152	52	2.41	37	205	185	148	1.11	54	.03	.03	2.55	.1	3	2
41	21	.68	49	320	101	799	.37	23	.03	.04	.19	.03	2	0
53	45	.27	42	228	592	65	.5	40	.06	<.01	.39	.52	7	2
295	44	1.15	43	285	316	347	1.97	12	.06	.52	2.95	.07	6	5

(3)If bones are discarded, calcium value is greatly reduced.

(For purposes of calculations, use "0" for t, <1, <.1, <.01, etc.)

A

A

Table A–1
Food Composition

Computer Code Number	Food Description	Measure	Wt (g)	H_2O (%)	Ener (cal)	Prot (g)	Carb (g)	Dietary Fiber (g)	Fat (g)	Fat Breakdown (g) Sat	Mono	Poly
	MEATS: FISH and SHELLFISH—Cont.											
1590	Surimi[1]	4 oz	113	76	112	17	8	0	1	.2	.2	.5
1058	Swordfish, raw	4 oz	113	76	137	22	0	0	5	1.2	1.8	1
1059	Swordfish, baked or broiled	4 oz	113	69	176	29	0	0	6	1.6	2.2	1.3
590	Trout, baked or broiled	4 oz	113	70	170	26	0	0	7	1.8	2	2.1
	Tuna, light, canned, drained solids:											
591	Oil pack	3 oz	85	60	168	25	0	0	7	1.3	2.5	2.4
592	Water pack	3 oz	85	74	99	22	0	0	1	.2	.1	.3
1061	Bluefin tuna, fresh	4 oz	113	68	163	26	0	0	6	1.4	1.8	1.9
	MEATS: BEEF, LAMB, PORK, and others											
	BEEF, cooked:[2]											
	Braised, simmered, pot roasted:											
	Relatively fat, choice chuck blade:											
593	Lean and fat, piece 2½ x 2½ x ¾"	4 oz	113	47	393	30	0	0	29	11.6	12.6	1.1
594	Lean only	4 oz	113	55	297	35	0	0	16	6.3	7	.5
	Relatively lean, like choice round:											
595	Lean and fat, pce 4⅛ x 2½ x ¾"	4 oz	113	52	311	32	0	0	19	7.2	8.3	.7
596	Lean only	4 oz	113	57	249	36	0	0	11	3.6	4.7	.4
	Ground beef, broiled, patty 3 x ⅝":											
597	Extra lean, about 16% fat	4 oz	113	54	301	32	0	0	18	7	7.8	.7
598	Lean, 21% fat	4 oz	113	53	318	32	0	0	20	7.9	8.7	.7
	Roasts, oven cooked, no added liquid:											
	Relatively fat, prime rib:											
601	Lean and fat, pce 4⅛ x 2¼ x ½"	4 oz	113	46	425	25	0	0	35	14.3	15.2	1.3
602	Lean only	4 oz	113	58	272	31	0	0	16	6.6	6.8	.5
	Relatively lean, choice round:											
603	Lean and fat, pce 2½ x 2½ x ¾"	4 oz	113	59	272	30	0	0	16	6.2	6.9	.6
604	Lean only	4 oz	113	65	197	33	0	0	6	2.3	2.7	.2
1701	Steak, rib, broiled, lean	4 oz	113	65	250	32	0	0	13	5	5	.4
	Steak, broiled, relatively lean, choice sirloin:											
605	Lean and fat, pce 2½ x 2½ x ¾"	4 oz	113	52	320	31	0	0	21	8.7	9.3	.8
606	Lean only	4 oz	113	62	228	34	0	0	9	3.5	3.9	.4
	Steak, broiled, relatively fat, choice T-bone:											
1063	Lean and fat	4 oz	113	53	338	28	0	0	24	9.7	10.1	.9
1064	Lean only	4 oz	113	60	242	32	0	0	12	4.7	4.7	.4
	Variety meats:											
1086	Brains, panfried	4 oz	113	71	221	14	0	0	18	4.2	4.5	2.6
599	Heart, simmered	4 oz	113	64	197	33	<1	0	6	1.9	1.4	1.5
600	Liver, fried	4 oz	113	56	245	30	9	0	9	3	1.8	1.9
1062	Tongue, cooked	4 oz	113	56	320	25	<1	0	23	10.3	11	.9
607	Beef, canned, corned	4 oz	113	58	282	31	0	0	17	7	6.8	.7
608	Beef, dried, cured	1 oz	28	56	47	8	<1	0	1	.5	.5	.1

(1)Surimi is processed from Walleye (Alaska) pollock. Also see Imitation crab, shrimp, scallops.

(2)Outer layer of fat removed to about ½" of the lean. Deposits of fat within the cut remain.

(Computer code number is for West Diet Analysis program)

PAGE KEY: A–2 = BEV A–4 = DAIRY A–10 = EGGS A–12 = FAT/OIL A–14 = FRUIT A–24 = BAKERY A–34 = GRAIN A–40 = FISH A–44 = MEATS A–48 = POULTRY A–50 = SAUSAGE A–52 = MIXED/FAST A–60 = NUTS/SEEDS A–62 = SWEETS A–66 = VEG/LEG A–78 = MISC A–80 = SOUPS/SAUCES A–84 = FAST A–96 = FRZN ENTREE A–98 = BABY FOODS

Chol (mg)	Calc (mg)	Iron (mg)	Magn (mg)	Phos (mg)	Pota (mg)	Sodi (mg)	Zinc (mg)	VT-A (RE)	Thia (mg)	Ribo (mg)	Niac (mg)	V-B6 (mg)	Fola (μg)	VT-C (mg)
34	10	.29	49	320	127	162	.37	23	.02	.02	.25	.03	2	0
44	5	.92	31	298	327	102	1.3	41	.04	.11	11	.37	2	1
57	7	1.18	39	382	418	130	1.67	46	.05	.13	13.3	.43	3	1
78	97	.43	35	305	508	63	.58	17	.17	.11	6.54	.39	21	2
15	11	1.18	26	264	175	301	.77	20	.03	.1	10.5	.09	5	0
25	9	1.3	23	139	201	287	.65	14	.03	.06	11.3	.3	3	0
43	9	1.16	57	288	286	44	.68	743	.27	.28	9.81	.52	2	0
112	11	3.46	22	244	274	67	7.61	0	.08	.27	3.55	.32	10	0
120	15	4.17	26	265	297	81	11.7	0	.09	.32	3.03	.33	7	0
109	7	3.54	25	278	319	57	5.57	0	.08	.27	4.23	.37	11	0
109	6	3.92	28	308	348	58	6.21	0	.08	.29	4.63	.41	12	0
112	10	3.14	28	215	418	93	7.29	0	.08	.36	6.63	.36	12	0
115	14	2.78	27	206	396	101	7.03	0	.07	.27	6.77	.34	12	0
96	12	2.62	22	195	335	72	5.94	0	.08	.19	3.81	.26	8	0
92	11	2.96	28	242	425	84	7.87	0	.09	.24	4.67	.34	9	0
82	7	2.09	27	234	407	67	4.89	0	.09	.18	3.93	.4	7	0
78	6	2.21	31	256	447	70	5.38	0	.1	.19	4.25	.43	8	0
90	15	3	31	235	445	78	8	0	.11	.25	5.92	.45	9	0
102	12	3.4	32	247	407	70	6.5	0	.13	.3	4.38	.45	10	0
101	12	3.81	36	277	456	75	7.39	0	.15	.33	4.85	.51	11	0
94	9	3.01	28	209	401	69	5.31	0	.11	.25	4.63	.39	8	0
91	8	3.4	33	235	460	75	6.12	0	.13	.28	5.26	.44	9	0
2261	10	2.52	17	438	400	179	1.53	0	.15	.29	4.29	.44	7	4
219	7	8.52	28	282	264	72	3.55	0	.16	1.75	4.62	.24	2	2
545	12	7.12	26	522	413	120	6.18	12165[3]	.24	4.69	16.4	1.63	249	26
121	8	3.84	19	160	204	68	5.44	0	.03	.4	2.44	.18	6	1
97	14	2.36	16	126	153	1139	4.04	0	.02	.17	2.77	.15	10	2
12	2	1.28	9	49	126	983	1.49	0	.02	.06	1.55	.1	3	4

(3)Value varies widely.

(For purposes of calculations, use "0" for t, <1, <.1, <.01, etc.)

A

Table A–1
Food Composition

Computer Code Number	Food Description	Measure	Wt (g)	H_2O (%)	Ener (cal)	Prot (g)	Carb (g)	Dietary Fiber (g)	Fat (g)	Fat Breakdown (g) Sat	Mono	Poly
	MEATS: BEEF, LAMB, PORK, and others—Cont.											
	LAMB, domestic, cooked:											
	Chop, arm, braised (5.6 oz raw w/bone):											
609	Lean and fat	2½ oz	70	44	241	21	0	0	17	6.9	7.1	1.2
610	Lean only	1.9 oz	55	49	152	20	0	0	8	2.8	3.4	.5
	Chop, loin, broiled (4.2 oz. raw w/bone):											
611	Lean and fat	2.3 oz	64	52	202	16	0	0	15	6.3	6.2	1.1
612	Lean only	1.6 oz	46	61	99	14	0	0	4	1.6	2	.3
1067	Cutlet, avg of lean cuts, cooked	4 oz	113	54	331	28	0	0	23	9.9	9.9	1.7
	Leg, roasted, 3 oz = 4⅛ x 2¼ x ½":											
613	Lean and fat	4 oz	113	57	293	29	0	0	19	7.8	7.9	1.3
614	Lean only	4 oz	113	64	217	32	0	0	9	3.1	3.8	.6
615	Rib, roasted, lean and fat	4 oz	113	48	407	24	0	0	34	14.5	14.2	2.5
616	Rib, roasted, lean only	4 oz	113	60	263	30	0	0	15	5.4	6.6	1
1065	Shoulder, roasted, lean and fat	4 oz	113	56	312	25	0	0	23	9.6	9.2	1.8
1066	Shoulder, roasted, lean only	4 oz	113	63	231	28	0	0	12	4.6	4.9	1.1
	Variety meats:											
1069	Brains, panfried	4 oz	113	76	164	14	0	0	11	2.9	2.1	1.2
1068	Heart, braised	4 oz	113	64	210	28	2	0	9	3.6	2.5	.9
1070	Sweetbreads, cooked	4 oz	113	60	265	26	0	0	17	7.8	6.2	.8
1071	Tongue, cooked	4 oz	113	58	311	24	0	0	23	8.9	11.3	1.4
	PORK, cured, cooked (see also #669–672):											
617	Bacon, medium slices	3 pce	19	13	109	6	<1	0	9	3.3	4.5	1.1
1087	Breakfast strips, cooked	2 pce	23	27	104	7	<1	0	8	2.9	3.7	1.3
618	Canadian-style bacon	2 pce	47	62	87	11	1	0	4	1.3	1.9	.4
	Ham, roasted:											
619	Lean and fat, 2 pces 4⅛ x 2¼ x ¼"	4 oz	113	65	202	26	0	0	10	3.5	5	1.6
620	Lean only	4 oz	113	68	164	24	2	0	6	2	3	.6
621	Ham, canned, roasted, 8% fat	4 oz	113	69	154	24	1	0	6	1.8	2.8	.5
	PORK, fresh, cooked:											
	Chops, loin (cut 3 per lb with bone):											
1291	Braised, lean and fat	1 ea	71	44	261	19	0	0	20	7.2	9.1	2.2
1292	Braised, lean only	1 ea	55	51	150	18	0	0	8	2.8	3.6	1
622	Broiled, lean and fat	3.1 oz	87	50	275	24	0	0	19	7	8.9	2.2
623	Broiled, lean only	2½ oz	72	57	166	23	0	0	8	2.6	3.4	.9
624	Panfried, lean and fat	3.1 oz	89	45	333	21	0	0	27	9.8	12.5	3.1
625	Panfried, lean only	2.4 oz	67	53	189	16	0	0	13	4.6	6	1.7
626	Leg, roasted, lean and fat	4 oz	113	53	308	30	0	0	20	7	9	2
627	Leg, roasted, lean only	4 oz	113	59	233	35	0	0	9	3	4	1
628	Rib, roasted, lean and fat	4 oz	113	51	361	28	0	0	27	9.7	12.2	1
629	Rib, roasted, lean only	4 oz	113	57	277	32	0	0	16	5.4	7	1.9
630	Shoulder, braised, lean and fat	4 oz	113	47	391	30	0	0	29	10.5	13.4	3.2
631	Shoulder, braised, lean only	4 oz	113	54	281	36	0	0	14	4.8	6.2	1.7
1088	Spareribs, cooked, yield from 1 lb raw with bone	4 oz	113	40	450	33	0	0	34	13.4	16.1	4
1095	Rabbit, roasted (1 cup meat = 140 g)	4 oz	113	61	223	33	0	0	9	2.7	2.5	1.8

(Computer code number is for West Diet Analysis program)

Chol (mg)	Calc (mg)	Iron (mg)	Magn (mg)	Phos (mg)	Pota (mg)	Sodi (mg)	Zinc (mg)	VT-A (RE)	Thia (mg)	Ribo (mg)	Niac (mg)	V-B6 (mg)	Fola (µg)	VT-C (mg)
84	18	1.68	18	144	214	50	4.26	0	.05	.18	4.67	.08	12	0
67	14	1.49	16	127	186	42	4.01	0	.04	.15	3.48	.07	12	0
64	13	1.16	15	125	209	49	2.23	0	.06	.16	4.54	.08	11	0
44	9	.92	13	104	173	39	1.9	0	.05	.13	3.15	.07	11	0
110	12	2.27	25	206	340	77	4.68	0	.13	.32	7.51	.16	19	0
106	12	2.25	27	217	355	75	4.99	0	.11	.31	7.47	.17	23	0
101	9	2.4	29	234	383	77	5.6	0	.13	.33	7.19	.19	26	0
110	25	1.81	23	188	307	83	3.96	0	.1	.24	7.65	.13	17	0
100	24	2.01	26	221	356	92	5.07	0	.1	.26	6.99	.17	25	0
104	23	2.22	26	209	285	75	5.94	0	.1	.27	6.97	.15	24	0
99	22	2.42	28	227	301	77	6.85	0	.1	.29	6.53	.17	28	0
2316	14	1.91	16	382	232	152	1.54	0	.12	.27	2.8	.12	6	14
282	16	6.26	27	288	213	71	4.17	0	.19	1.35	4.94	.34	2	8
454	14	2.4	21	489	330	59	3.04	<1	.02	.24	2.9	.06	15	23
213	11	2.99	18	151	179	76	3.39	0	.09	.48	4.18	.19	3	8
16	2	.31	5	64	92	303	.62	0	.13	.05	1.39	.05	1	6[1]
24	3	.45	6	60	105	475	.83	0	.17	.08	1.72	.08	1	10
27	5	.38	10	139	183	726	.8	0	.39	.09	3.25	.21	2	10[1]
67	9	1.52	25	319	464	1701	2.8	0	.83	.37	6.97	.35	3	26
60	9	1.68	16	222	325	1364	3.27	0	.85	.23	4.56	.45	3	24
34	7	1.04	24	237	395	1287	2.53	0	1.18	.28	5.55	.51	6	31[1]
72	6	.82	14	141	244	46	2.15	2	.43	.21	4.24	.26	3	<1
58	5	.77	13	131	230	41	2.05	1	.38	.2	3.82	.25	3	<1
85	3	.71	22	184	313	61	1.69	3	.87	.24	4.37	.35	4	<1
71	4	.66	22	175	302	56	1.61	1	.83	.22	3.99	.34	4	<1
92	4	.75	23	190	323	64	1.74	3	.91	.24	4.58	.35	4	<1
65	9	.7	16	157	264	50	2.47	1	.49	.25	3.03	.27	3	<1
106	16	1.15	25	297	398	68	3.36	3	.72	.35	5.16	.45	11	<1
108	8	1.29	33	322	442	73	3.41	3	.91	.4	5.56	.38	3	<1
92	11	1.01	21	253	416	50	2.22	3	.67	.31	5.56	.34	9	<1
89	12	1.13	24	289	480	52	2.53	3	.72	.35	6.07	.45	10	<1
124	8	1.83	20	217	380	100	4.58	3	.61	.35	5.91	.31	5	<1
129	9	2.22	25	255	458	116	5.64	2	.68	.41	6.74	.46	6	<1
137	53	2.1	27	295	363	105	5.22	3	.46	.43	6.2	.4	5	0
93	21	2.57	24	298	434	53	2.59	0	.1	.24	9.56	.53	12	0

(1)Values based on products containing added ascorbic acid or sodium ascorbate. If none added, ascorbic acid content would be negligible.

(For purposes of calculations, use "0" for t, <1, <.1, <.01, etc.)

A

Table A–1
Food Composition

Computer Code Number	Food Description	Measure	Wt (g)	H_2O (%)	Ener (cal)	Prot (g)	Carb (g)	Dietary Fiber (g)	Fat (g)	Fat Breakdown (g) Sat	Mono	Poly
	MEATS: BEEF, LAMB, PORK, and others—Cont.											
	VEAL, cooked:											
632	Cutlet, braised or broiled, 4⅛ x 2¼ x ½"	4 oz	113	52	322	34	0	0	19	7.6	7.6	1.3
633	Rib roasted, lean, 2 pieces 4⅛ x 2¼ x ¼"	4 oz	113	60	257	27	0	0	16	6.1	6.2	1.1
634	Liver, panfried	4 oz	113	67	187	24	3	0	8	2.9	1.7	1.2
1096	Venison (deer meat), roasted	4 oz	113	65	179	34	0	0	4	1.4	1	.7
	MEATS: POULTRY and POULTRY PRODUCTS											
	CHICKEN, cooked:											
	Fried, batter dipped:[1]											
635	Breast (5.6 oz with bones)	1 ea	140	52	364	35	13	<1	18	4.9	7.6	4.3
636	Drumstick (3.4 oz with bones)	1 ea	72	53	192	16	6	<1	11	3	4.6	2.7
637	Thigh	1 ea	86	51	238	19	8	<1	14	3.8	5.8	3.3
638	Wing	1 ea	49	46	158	10	5	<1	11	2.9	4.4	2.5
	Fried, flour coated:[1]											
639	Breast (4.2 oz with bones)	1 ea	98	57	217	31	2	<1	9	2.4	3.4	1.9
1212	Breast, without skin	1 ea	86	60	160	29	<1	0	4	1.1	1.5	.9
640	Drumstick (2.6 oz with bones)	1 ea	49	57	120	13	1	<1	7	1.8	2.7	1.6
641	Thigh	1 ea	62	54	162	17	2	<1	9	2.5	3.6	2.1
1099	Thigh, without skin	1 ea	52	59	113	15	1	<1	5	1.4	2	1.3
642	Wing	1 ea	32	49	102	8	1	<1	7	1.9	2.8	1.6
	Roasted:											
643	All types of meat	1 c	140	64	266	40	0	0	10	2.9	3.7	2.4
644	Dark meat	1 c	140	63	287	38	0	0	14	3.7	5	3.2
645	Light meat	1 c	140	65	242	43	0	0	6	1.8	2.2	1.4
646	Breast, without skin	1 ea	86	65	141	27	0	0	3	.9	1.1	.7
647	Drumstick	1 ea	44	67	76	12	0	0	2	.7	.8	.6
1703	Leg, without skin	1 ea	95	65	182	26	0	0	8	2.2	3	1.9
648	Thigh	1 ea	62	59	153	15	0	0	10	2.7	3.8	2.1
1100	Thigh, without skin	1 ea	52	63	108	13	0	0	6	1.6	2.2	1.3
649	Stewed, all types:	1 c	140	67	246	38	0	0	9	2.6	3.3	2.2
656	Canned, boneless chicken	4 oz	113	69	187	25	0	0	9	2.5	3.6	2
1102	Gizzards, simmered	3 ea	66	67	101	18	1	0	2	.7	.6	.7
1101	Hearts, simmered	8 ea	25	65	45	6	<1	0	2	.6	.5	.6
650	Liver, simmered: Ounce	3 oz	85	68	128	21	7	0	5	1.6	1.1	.8
1098	Liver, simmered: Piece = 20 g	6 ea	120	68	187	29	1	0	7	2.2	1.6	1.1
	DUCK, roasted:											
1293	Meat with skin, about 2.7 cups	½ ea	382	52	1287	73	0	0	108	36.9	49.3	13.9
651	Meat only, about 1.5 cups	½ ea	221	64	444	52	0	0	25	9.2	8.2	3.2
	GOOSE, domesticated, roasted:											
1294	Meat only, 4.2 cups	½ ea	591	57	1406	171	0	0	75	26.9	25.6	9.1
1295	Meat with skin, about 5.5 cups	½ ea	774	52	2360	194	0	0	169	53.2	78.9	19.5
	TURKEY:											
	Roasted, meat only:											
652	Dark meat	4 oz	113	63	212	32	0	0	8	2.7	1.9	2.4
653	Light meat	4 oz	113	66	177	34	0	0	4	1.2	.6	1

(1)Fried in vegetable shortening.

(Computer code number is for West Diet Analysis program)

Chol (mg)	Calc (mg)	Iron (mg)	Magn (mg)	Phos (mg)	Pota (mg)	Sodi (mg)	Zinc (mg)	VT-A (RE)	Thia (mg)	Ribo (mg)	Niac (mg)	V-B6 (mg)	Fola (μg)	VT-C (mg)
134	32	1.24	27	249	318	91	4.13	0	.04	.34	10.3	.29	16	0
125	12	1.1	25	222	333	104	4.64	0	.06	.31	7.92	.28	15	0
635	8	2.97	22	362	232	60	10.8	9126[2]	.15	2.2	9.62	.56	861	35
127	8	5.07	27	256	379	61	3.12	0	.2	.68	7.61	.43[3]	5[3]	0
119	28	1.75	34	259	281	385	1.33	28	.16	.2	14.7	.6	8	0
62	12	.97	14	105	133	193	1.68	19	.08	.15	3.67	.19	6	0
80	15	1.25	18	133	165	247	1.75	25	.1	.19	4.91	.22	8	0
39	10	.63	8	59	68	156	.68	17	.05	.07	2.58	.15	3	0
87	16	1.17	29	228	253	74	1.08	15	.08	.13	13.5	.57	4	0
78	14	.98	27	211	237	68	.93	6	.07	.11	12.7	.55	3	0
44	6	.66	11	86	112	44	1.42	12	.04	.11	2.96	.17	4	0
60	9	.92	15	115	146	55	1.56	18	.06	.15	4.31	.2	5	0
53	7	.76	13	103	134	49	1.45	11	.05	.13	3.7	.2	5	0
26	5	.4	6	48	57	25	.56	12	.02	.04	2.14	.13	1	0
124	21	1.69	35	273	340	120	2.94	22	.1	.25	12.8	.66	8	0
130	21	1.86	32	251	336	130	3.92	31	.1	.32	9.17	.5	11	0
119	21	1.48	38	302	344	107	1.72	13	.09	.16	17.4	.84	6	0
73	13	.89	25	196	220	64	.86	5	.06	.1	11.8	.52	3	0
41	5	.57	11	81	108	42	1.4	8	.03	.1	2.67	.17	4	0
90	11	1.26	23	174	230	87	2.73	18	.07	.22	6.02	.35	8	0
58	7	.83	14	107	137	52	1.46	30	.04	.13	3.95	.19	4	0
49	6	.68	12	95	123	46	1.34	10	.04	.12	3.39	.18	4	0
116	20	1.64	29	210	252	98	2.79	21	.07	.23	8.55	.36	8	0
70	16	1.79	14	126	155	570	1.6	39	.02	.15	7.18	.4	5	2
128	7	2.74	13	102	118	44	2.89	37	.02	.16	2.63	.08	35	1
59	5	2.22	5	49	32	12	1.8	2	.01	.18	.69	.08	20	<1
536	12	7.23	7	264	119	42	3.68	4177	.13	1.49	3.78	.5	655	14
757	17	10.2	25	373	168	61	5.21	5894	.18	2.1	5.34	.7	924	19
320	42	10.3	61	596	779	225	7.11	241	.66	1.03	18.4	.69	23	0
196	26	5.97	44	449	557	143	5.75	51	.57	1.04	11.3	.55	22	0
567	83	17	147	1826	2293	449	18.7	71	.54	2.3	24.1	2.78	71	0
704	100	21.9	170	2089	2546	541	20.3	163	.6	2.5	32.3	2.86	15	0
96	36	2.64	27	231	329	90	5.06	0	.07	.28	4.14	.41	10	0
78	22	1.53	32	248	346	73	2.31	0	.07	.15	7.76	.61	7	0

(2)Value varies widely.

(3)Values estimated from other game meat.

(For purposes of calculations, use "0" for t, <1, <.1, <.01, etc.)

Table A–1
Food Composition

Computer Code Number	Food Description	Measure	Wt (g)	H_2O (%)	Ener (cal)	Prot (g)	Carb (g)	Dietary Fiber (g)	Fat (g)	Fat Breakdown (g) Sat	Mono	Poly
	MEATS: POULTRY and POULTRY PRODUCTS—Cont.											
	TURKEY—Cont.											
	Roasted, meat only—Cont.											
654	All types, chopped or diced	1 c	140	65	238	41	0	0	7	2.3	1.5	2
655	All types, sliced	4 oz	113	65	193	33	0	0	6	1.9	1.2	1.6
1103	Ground, cooked	4 oz	113	59	266	31	0	0	15	3.8	5.5	3.7
1104	Breast, barbecued	2 oz	57	69	72	11	2	0	2	.6	.6	.4
1105	Breast, hickory smoked	2 oz	57	72	62	13	1	0	1	.3	.3	.2
1106	Gizzard, cooked	2 ea	134	65	218	39	1	0	5	1.5	1	1.5
1107	Heart, cooked	4 ea	64	64	113	17	1	0	4	1.1	.8	1.1
1108	Liver, cooked	1 ea	75	66	126	18	3	0	4	1.4	1.1	.8
	POULTRY FOOD PRODUCTS (see also items in Sausages and Lunchmeats section):											
658	Chicken roll, light meat	2 pce	57	69	91	11	1	0	4	1.1	1.7	.9
1567	Chicken patty, breaded, cooked	1 ea	75	49	222	13	9	<1	15	3.9	6	3.5
659	Turkey and gravy, frozen package	3 oz	85	85	57	5	4	<1	2	.7	.8	.4
660	Turkey loaf, breast meat	4 oz	113	72	125	25	0	0	2	.5	.5	.3
661	Turkey patty, breaded, fried	2 oz	57	50	160	8	9	<1	10	2.7	4.2	2.7
662	Turkey, frozen, roasted, seasoned	4 oz	113	68	175	24	3	0	7	2.2	1.4	1.9
1704	Turkey roll, light meat	1 pce	28	72	42	5	<1	0	2	.58	.7	.5
	MEATS: SAUSAGES and LUNCHMEATS (see also Poultry Food Products)											
1072	Beerwurst/beer salami, beef	1 oz	28	53	93	4	<1	0	8	3.7	4	.3
1074	Beerwurst/beer salami, pork	1 oz	28	61	67	4	1	0	5	1.8	2.5	.7
1075	Berliner sausage	1 oz	28	61	65	4	1	0	5	1.7	2.3	.4
	Bologna:											
1297	Beef	1 pce	23	55	72	3	<1	0	7	2.8	3.2	.3
663	Beef & pork	1 pce	28	54	90	3	1	0	8	3	3.8	.7
1298	Pork	1 pce	23	61	57	4	<1	0	5	1.6	2.2	.5
664	Turkey	1 pce	28	65	56	4	<1	0	4	1.4	1.4	1.2
665	Braunschweiger sausage	2 pce	57	48	205	8	2	0	18	6.2	8.5	2.1
1073	Bratwurst, link	1 ea	70	51	226	10	2	0	19	6.9	9.3	2
666	Brown & serve sausage links, cooked	2 ea	26	45	102	4	1	0	10	3.4	4.4	1
1089	Cheesefurter/cheese smokie	2 ea	86	52	280	12	1	0	25	9	11.8	2.6
1556	Chorizo, pork & beef	3 oz	85	32	387	20	2	0	33	12.2	15.6	2.9
1090	Corned beef loaf, jellied	1 pce	28	69	43	6	0	0	2	.7	.8	.1
	Frankfurters (see also #657):											
1077	Beef, large link, 8/package	1 ea	57	55	180	7	1	0	16	6.9	7.7	.8
1078	Beef and pork, large link, 8/package	1 ea	57	54	182	6	1	0	17	6.2	7.8	1.6
667	Beef and pork, small link, 10/pkg	1 ea	45	54	144	5	1	0	13	4.9	6.2	1.2
657	Chicken frankfurter, 10/package	1 ea	45	57	115	6	3	0	9	2.5	3.8	1.8
668	Turkey frankfurter, 10/package	1 ea	45	63	101	6	1	0	8	2.7	2.5	2.2
	Ham:											
669	Ham lunchmeat, canned, 3 x 2 x ½"	1 pce	21	52	70	3	<1	0	6	2.3	3	.7
670	Chopped ham, packaged	2 pce	42	64	96	7	0	0	7	2.4	3.4	.9
671	Ham lunchmeat, regular	2 pce	57	65	103	10	2	0	6	1.9	2.8	.7
672	Ham lunchmeat, extra lean	2 pce	57	71	74	11	1	0	3	.9	1.3	.3

(Computer code number is for West Diet Analysis program)

PAGE KEY: A–2 = BEV A–4 = DAIRY A–10 = EGGS A–12 = FAT/OIL A–14 = FRUIT A–24 = BAKERY A–34 = GRAIN A–40 = FISH A–44 = MEATS A–48 = POULTRY A–50 = SAUSAGE A–52 = MIXED/FAST A–60 = NUTS/SEEDS A–62 = SWEETS A–66 = VEG/LEG A–78 = MISC A–80 = SOUPS/SAUCES A–84 = FAST A–96 = FRZN ENTREE A–98 = BABY FOODS

Chol (mg)	Calc (mg)	Iron (mg)	Magn (mg)	Phos (mg)	Pota (mg)	Sodi (mg)	Zinc (mg)	VT-A (RE)	Thia (mg)	Ribo (mg)	Niac (mg)	V-B6 (mg)	Fola (μg)	VT-C (mg)
106	35	2.49	36	298	417	98	4.34	0	.09	.25	7.62	.64	10	0
86	28	2.02	29	242	338	79	3.52	0	.07	.21	6.17	.52	8	0
116	28	2.2	27	222	306	121	3.25	0	.06	.19	5.47	.44	8	0
22	10	.4	12	184	166	609	.5	0	.02	.06	5.45	.22	2	<1
23	4	.23	11	130	158	811	.64	0	.02	.06	4.72	.2	2	0
310	20	7.28	25	172	281	72	5.57	74	.04	.44	4.11	.16	69	2
145	8	4.4	14	131	117	35	3.37	5	.04	.56	2.08	.2	50	1
469	8	5.85	11	204	145	48	2.32	2805	.04	1.07	4.46	.39	499	1
28	24	.55	11	89	129	332	.41	14	.04	.07	3.02	.12	1	0
50	7	.86	18	195	208	352	.61	21	.11	.1	5.18	.26	7	0
15	12	.79	7	69	52	471	.59	11	.02	.11	1.53	.08	3	0
46	8	.45	23	260	315	1621	1.28	0	.04	.12	9.45	.41	5	0[1]
35	8	1.25	9	153	156	454	.82	6	.06	.11	1.3	.11	5	0
60	6	1.86	25	277	338	771	2.88	0	.05	.19	7.11	.31	6	0
12	11	.37	5	52	71	139	.45	0	.03	.06	1.98	.09	1	0
17	3	.43	3	27	49	291	.69	0	.02	.03	.96	.05	1	5
17	2	.22	4	29	72	351	.49	0	.16	.05	.92	.1	1	8
13	3	.33	4	37	80	367	.7	0	.11	.06	.88	.06	1	2
13	3	.38	3	20	36	226	.5	0	.01	.02	.55	.03	1	5
16	3	.43	3	26	51	288	.55	0	.05	.04	.73	.05	1	6[2]
14	3	.18	3	32	65	272	.47	0	.12	.04	.9	.06	1	8
28	24	.43	4	37	56	249	.49	0	.02	.05	1	.06	2	<1
89	5	5.34	6	96	113	652	1.6	2405	.14	.87	4.77	.19	25	6[2]
44	34	.72	11	94	196	778	1.47	0	.17	.16	2.31	.09	3	20
16	2	.62	4	42	70	248	.3	0	.21	.09	.96	.06	1	0
58	50	.93	11	153	177	930	1.94	33	.21	.14	2.5	.11	3	17
75	7	1.35	15	128	338	1049	2.9	0	.54	.25	4.36	.45	2	0
13	3	.58	3	21	29	271	1.16	0	0	.03	.5	.03	2	2
35	11	.81	2	50	95	585	1.24	0	.03	.06	1.38	.07	2	14
28	6	.66	6	49	95	638	1.05	0	.11	.07	1.5	.07	2	15
22	5	.52	4	39	75	504	.83	0	.09	.05	1.18	.06	2	12[2]
45	43	.9	6	48	38	616	.47	17	.03	.05	1.39	.14	2	0
39	48	.83	6	60	81	641	1.4	0	.02	.08	1.86	.1	4	0
13	1	.15	2	17	45	270	.31	0	.08	.04	.65	.04	1	<1
21	3	.35	7	65	134	576	.81	0	.26	.09	1.63	.15	<1	8[2]
32	4	.56	11	140	188	746	1.21	0	.49	.14	2.98	.19	2	16[2]
27	4	.43	10	124	198	810	1.09	0	.53	.13	2.74	.26	2	15[2]

(1)If sodium ascorbate is added, product contains 11 mg ascorbic acid.

(2)Values based on products containing added ascorbic acid or sodium ascorbate. If none added, ascorbic acid content would be negligible.

(For purposes of calculations, use "0" for t, <1, <.1, <.01, etc.)

Table A–1
Food Composition

Computer Code Number	Food Description	Measure	Wt (g)	H_2O (%)	Ener (cal)	Prot (g)	Carb (g)	Dietary Fiber (g)	Fat (g)	Fat Breakdown (g) Sat	Mono	Poly
	MEATS: SAUSAGES and LUNCHMEATS (see also Poultry Food Products)—Cont.											
	Ham—Cont.											
673	Turkey ham lunchmeat	2 pce	57	71	73	11	<1	0	3	1	.7	.9
1091	Kielbasa sausage	1 pce	26	54	81	3	1	0	7	2.6	3.4	.8
1092	Knockwurst sausage, link	1 ea	68	55	209	8	1	0	19	6.9	8.7	2
1093	Mortadella lunchmeat	2 pce	30	52	93	5	1	0	8	2.9	3.4	.9
1097	Olive loaf lunchmeat	2 pce	57	58	134	7	5	<1	9	3.3	4.5	1.1
1080	Turkey pastrami	2 pce	57	71	80	10	1	0	4	1	1.2	.9
1081	Pepperoni sausage	2 pce	11	27	54	2	<1	0	5	1.8	2.3	.5
1094	Pickle & pimento loaf	2 pce	57	57	149	7	3	<1	12	4.5	5.5	1.5
1082	Polish sausage	1 oz	28	53	92	4	<1	0	8	2.9	3.9	.9
674	Pork sausage, cooked:[1] Link, small	2 ea	26	45	96	5	<1	0	8	2.8	3.6	1
1079	Pork sausage, cooked: Patty	4 oz	113	45	418	22	1	0	35	12.2	15.8	4.3
675	Salami, pork and beef	2 pce	57	60	141	8	1	0	11	4.6	5.2	1.1
676	Salami, turkey	2 pce	57	66	111	9	<1	0	8	2.3	2.6	2
677	Beef & pork, dry	3 pce	30	35	125	7	1	0	10	3.7	5.1	1
	Sandwich spreads:											
1300	Ham salad spread	1 c	240	63	518	21	26	0	37	12.2	17.3	6.5
678	Pork and beef	2 tbs	30	60	70	2	4	<1	5	1.8	2.3	.8
1296	Chicken/turkey	2 tbs	26	66	52	3	2	0	4	.9	.8	1.6
1084	Smoked link sausage, beef and pork	1 ea	68	52	228	9	1	0	21	7.2	9.7	2.2
1083	Smoked link sausage, pork	1 ea	68	39	265	15	1	0	22	7.7	9.9	2.6
1085	Summer sausage	2 pce	46	51	154	7	<1	0	14	5.5	6	.6
1076	Turkey breakfast sausage	1 pce	28	60	65	6	0	0	5	1.6	1.8	1.2
679	Vienna sausage, canned	2 ea	32	60	89	3	1	0	8	3	4	.5
	MIXED DISHES and FAST FOODS											
	MIXED DISHES:											
1445	Almond chicken	1 c	242	77	273	20	18	4	14	2	5.3	5.8
1454	Bean cake	1 ea	32	23	130	2	16	1	7	1	2.9	2.6
680	Beef stew w/ vegetables: Homemade	1 c	245	82	218	16	15	2	10	4.9	4.5	.5
1109	Beef stew w/ vegetables: Canned	1 c	245	82	194	14	17	3	8	2.4	3.1	.3
1116	Beef, macaroni, tomato sauce casserole	1 c	226	73	284	21	25	3	11	4.2	4.7	.6
1452	Beef fajita	1 ea	189	67	250	15	32	2	7	2	3	1
681	Beef pot pie, homemade[2]	1 pce	210	55	517	21	39	1	31	8.4	14.9	7.4
1462	Buffalo wings/spicy chicken wings	2 ea	32	53	98	8	<1	<1	7	1.8	2.8	1.6
1675	Carrot raisin salad	½c	88	58	202	1	21	3	14	2.1	3.9	7
682	Chicken à la king, homemade	1 c	245	68	468	27	12	1	34	12.7	14.3	6.2
683	Chicken & noodles, homemade	1 c	240	71	367	22	26	2	18	5.9	7.1	3.5
684	Chicken chow mein: Canned	1 c	250	89	95	6	18	5	1	0	.1	.8
685	Chicken chow mein: Homemade	1 c	250	78	255	31	10	4	10	2.4	4.3	3.1
1451	Chicken fajitas	1 ea	189	68	230	17	30	3	5	2	2	1
686	Chicken pot pie, homemade (1/3)	1 pce	232	57	545	23	42	3	33	10.9	15.5	6.6
1672	Chili con carne	½ c	127	77	128	12	11	2	4	1.73	1.72	.3
1112	Chicken salad with celery	2 c	78	53	268	11	1	<1	25	4	7.2	12.1
687	Chili with beans, canned	1 c	255	76	286	15	30	8	14	6	5.9	.9
1479	Chinese pastry	1 oz	28	46	67	1	13	<1	1	.2	.4	.8
688	Chop suey with beef & pork	1 c	250	63	465	26	35	4	25	5.7	13.3	3.9

(1)Cooked weight is half the weight of raw sausage.

(2)Crust made with vegetable shortening and enriched flour.

(Computer code number is for West Diet Analysis program)

PAGE KEY: A–2 = BEV A–4 = DAIRY A–10 = EGGS A–12 = FAT/OIL A–14 = FRUIT A–24 = BAKERY A–34 = GRAIN A–40 = FISH A–44 = MEATS A–48 = POULTRY A–50 = SAUSAGE A–52 = MIXED/FAST A–60 = NUTS/SEEDS A–62 = SWEETS A–66 = VEG/LEG A–78 = MISC A–80 = SOUPS/SAUCES A–84 = FAST A–96 = FRZN ENTREE A–98 = BABY FOODS

Chol (mg)	Calc (mg)	Iron (mg)	Magn (mg)	Phos (mg)	Pota (mg)	Sodi (mg)	Zinc (mg)	VT-A (RE)	Thia (mg)	Ribo (mg)	Niac (mg)	V-B6 (mg)	Fola (µg)	VT-C (mg)
32	6	1.57	9	108	185	567	1.68	0	.03	.14	2.01	.14	3	0
17	11	.38	4	38	70	279	.52	0	.06	.06	.75	.05	1	5
39	7	.62	7	67	135	685	1.13	0	.23	.09	1.86	.12	1	18
17	5	.42	3	29	49	372	.63	0	.04	.05	.8	.04	1	8
22	62	.31	11	72	169	846	.79	11	.17	.15	1.05	.13	1	5
31	5	.95	8	114	148	595	1.23	0	.03	.14	2.01	.15	3	0
9	1	.15	2	13	38	224	.27	0	.03	.03	.54	.03	<1	0
21	54	.58	10	80	194	792	.8	4	.17	.14	1.17	.11	3	8
20	3	.41	4	39	67	247	.55	0	.14	.04	.97	.05	1	<1
22	8	.32	4	48	94	336	.65	0	.19	.07	1.18	.09	1	<1
94	36	1.42	19	209	409	1467	2.84	0	.84	.29	5.13	.37	2	2
37	7	1.51	9	65	112	603	1.21	0	.14	.21	2.01	.12	1	7[3]
47	11	.92	9	60	139	572	1.03	0	.04	.1	2.01	.14	2	0
24	2	.45	5	43	113	558	.97	0	.18	.09	1.46	.15	1	8[3]
89	19	1.42	24	288	360	2188	2.64	0	1.04	.29	5.04	.36	2	14
11	4	.24	2	18	33	302	.31	3	.05	.04	.52	.04	1	0
8	3	.16	3	9	48	98	.27	11	.01	.02	.43	.03	1	<1
48	7	.99	8	73	128	642	1.43	0	.18	.12	2.19	.12	1	13
46	20	.79	13	110	228	1020	1.92	0	.48	.17	3.08	.24	3	1
34	6	1.17	6	51	125	571	1.18	0	.07	.15	1.98	.12	1	9
23	5	.52	6	52	76	191	.97	0	.03	.08	1.42	.08	1	–
17	3	.28	2	16	32	304	.51	0	.03	.03	.51	.04	1	0
35	79	2.12	59	238	550	617	1.56	75	.08	.19	8.59	.4	27	10
0	3	.65	6	19	56	55	.15	0	.06	.04	.49	.02	8	0
64	29	2.94	40	184	613	292	5.29	568	.15	.17	4.66	.28	37	17
34	29	2.21	39	110	426	1006	4.24	262	.07	.12	2.45	.2	31	7
57	28	3.11	42	161	559	841	4.3	93	.23	.25	5.22	.33	22	13
20	100	1.8	–	–	350	630	–	20	.3	.51	5	.35	–	2
44	29	3.78	6	149	334	596	3.17	519	.29	.29	4.83	.24	29	6
26	5	.4	6	47	59	61	.56	17	.01	.04	2.06	.13	1	<1
10	26	.74	14	46	315	117	.2	1453	.08	.05	.63	.22	9	5
186	127	2.45	20	358	404	760	1.8	272	.1	.42	5.39	.23	11	12
96	26	2.16	26	247	149	600	1.53	10	.05	.17	4.32	.19	10	0
7	45	1.25	14	85	418	725	1.3	28	.05	.1	1	.09	12	12
77	57	2.5	28	293	473	718	2.12	50	.07	.22	4.25	.41	19	10
30	40	1.1	–	–	300	590	–	40	.23	.34	4	.03	–	2
72	70	3.02	25	232	343	594	2	735	.32	.32	4.87	.46	29	5
67	34	2.62	23	99	347	506	1.8	84	.06	.57	1.25	.17	15	<1
47	16	.62	11	80	138	201	.8	31	.03	.07	3.27	.34	8	1
43	120	8.75	115	393	931	1331	5.1	87	.12	.27	.91	.34	58	4
0	7	.55	6	14	26	3	.2	<1	.04	<.01	.35	.02	1	0
57	48	4.45	69	255	568	1027	3.9	147	.21	.26	4.45	.47	37	3

[3]Values based on products containing added ascorbic acid or sodium ascorbate. If none added, ascorbic acid content would be negligible.

(For purposes of calculations, use "0" for t, <1, <.1, <.01, etc.)

Table A–1
Food Composition

Computer Code Number	Food Description	Measure	Wt (g)	H_2O (%)	Ener (cal)	Prot (g)	Carb (g)	Dietary Fiber (g)	Fat (g)	Fat Breakdown (g) Sat	Mono	Poly
	MIXED DISHES and FAST FOOD—Cont.											
	MIXED DISHES—Cont.											
690	Coleslaw[1]	1 c	120	74	178	2	15	2	13	2	2.9	7.7
689	Corn pudding[2]	1 c	250	76	273	11	32	9	13	6.3	4.3	1.7
1110	Corned beef hash, canned	1 c	220	67	398	19	23	1	25	11.9	10.9	.9
	Egg foo yung patty:											
1467	Meatless	1 ea	86	94	26	3	<1	0	1	.4	.5	.2
1458	With Beef	1 ea	86	75	127	9	3	<1	9	2.2	3.2	2.4
1465	With Chicken	1 ea	86	75	128	9	3	<1	9	2.1	3.1	2.5
1602	Egg roll, meatless	1 ea	64	70	101	3	10	1	6	1.2	2.5	1.6
1550	Egg roll, with meat	1 ea	64	66	117	5	9	1	7	1.6	2.9	1.6
1113	Egg salad	1 c	183	57	586	17	3	0	56	10.6	17.5	24.2
691	French toast w/wheat bread, homemade[3]	1 pce	65	54	151	5	16	<1	7	2	3	1.7
1355	Green pepper, stuffed	1 ea	172	74	236	11	20	2	12	5.3	5.3	.6
1487	Hot & sour soup (Chinese)	1 c	244	88	130	12	5	<1	7	2.2	2.9	1.2
	Lasagna:											
1346	With meat, homemade	1 pce	245	66	390	23	41	3	15	7.7	5	.8
1111	Without meat, homemade	1 pce	218	68	305	16	40	3	9	5.4	2.4	.6
1117	Frozen entree	1 pce	205	74	238	15	26	2	9	4	3.3	.5
1606	Lo mein, meatless	1 c	200	83	123	6	23	3	1	.3	.3	.4
1607	Lo mein, with meat	1 c	200	71	284	16	27	3	13	2.9	4.2	4.7
692	Macaroni & cheese, canned[4]	1 c	240	80	228	9	26	1	10	4.2	3.1	1.4
693	Macaroni & cheese, homemade[5]	1 c	200	58	430	17	40	1	22	8.9	8.8	3.6
1115	Macaroni salad, no cheese	1 c	141	60	363	3	21	3	30	4.4	8.5	15.5
1120	Meat loaf, beef	1 pce	87	58	206	19	4	<1	12	4.7	5.2	.6
1119	Meat loaf, beef and pork (⅓)	1 pce	87	57	221	17	4	<1	15	5.4	6.4	1.2
1303	Moussaka (lamb & eggplant)	1 c	250	83	209	18	14	3	9	2.7	3.7	1.5
715	Potato salad with mayonnaise and eggs[6]	½ c	125	76	179	3	14	2	10	1.8	3.1	4.7
1674	Pizza, combination, 1/12 of 12" round	1 pce	53	48	123	9	14	–	4	1	1.7	.6
1673	Pizza, pepperoni, 1/12 of 12" round	1 pce	47	46	121	7	13	–	5	1.5	2.1	.78
694	Quiche Lorraine, ⅛ of 8" quiche[7]	1 pce	176	52	540	15	23	1	43	20.1	15.6	5.3
1449	Ramen noodles, cooked	1 c	227	83	147	5	27	3	2	.4	.4	.4
1671	Ravioli, meat	½ c	125	68	194	11	18	1	9	3	3.6	1
1597	Fried rice (meatless)	1 c	166	71	241	5	30	1	11	1.7	2.9	6.2
	Spaghetti (enriched) in tomato sauce:											
	With cheese:											
695	Canned	1 c	250	80	190	5	38	2	1	0	.4	.5
696	Homemade	1 c	250	77	260	9	37	2	9	2	5.4	1.2
	With meatballs:											
697	Canned	1 c	250	78	258	12	28	6	10	2.1	3.9	3.9
698	Homemade	1 c	248	70	332	19	39	8	12	3.3	6.3	2.2
716	Spinach soufflé[8]	1 c	136	74	219	11	3	4	18	7.1	6.8	3.1
1553	Sweet & sour pork	1 c	226	76	247	14	25	1	10	2.8	3.8	2.9

(1)Recipe: 41% cabbage; 12% celery; 12% table cream; 12% sugar; 7% green pepper; 6% lemon juice; 4% onion; 3% pimento; 3% vinegar; 2% each for salt, dry mustard, and white pepper.

(2)Recipe: 55% yellow corn, 23% whole milk, 14% egg, 4% sugar, 3% salt, and 1% pepper.

(3)Recipe: 35% whole milk, 32% white bread, 29% egg, and cooked in 4% margarine.

(4)Made with corn oil.

(5)Made with margarine.

(6)Recipe: 62% potatoes; 12% egg; 8% mayonnaise; 7% celery; 6% sweet pickle relish; 2% onion; 1% each for green pepper, pimento, salt, and dry mustard.

(7)Crust made with vegetable shortening and enriched flour.

(8)Recipe: 29% whole milk, 26% spinach, 13% egg white, 13% cheddar cheese, 7% egg yolk, 7% butter, 4% flour, 1% salt and pepper.

(Computer code number is for West Diet Analysis program)

Chol (mg)	Calc (mg)	Iron (mg)	Magn (mg)	Phos (mg)	Pota (mg)	Sodi (mg)	Zinc (mg)	VT-A (RE)	Thia (mg)	Ribo (mg)	Niac (mg)	V-B6 (mg)	Fola (µg)	VT-C (mg)
6[9]	41	.88	11	43	215	324	.24	60	.05	.04	.1	.13	47	10
250	100	1.4	37	143	403	138	1.25	90	1.03	.32	2.47	.29	63	7
73	29	4.4	36	147	440	1188	3.3	0	.02	.2	4.62	.43	20	0
37	7	.26	2	38	77	257	.17	14	.01	.07	1.07	.02	5	0
180	26	1.1	11	110	143	185	1.16	92	.05	.24	.73	.16	22	3
182	28	.85	11	102	143	188	.81	95	.05	.24	.95	.13	22	3
30	12	.74	9	36	97	307	.25	15	.07	.1	.75	.05	11	3
38	12	.77	9	56	117	305	.5	14	.13	.12	1.26	.09	8	2
578	74	1.8	13	236	180	666	1.44	262	.08	.66	.08	.47	61	0
76	64	1.09	11	76	86	311	.44	81	.13	.21	1.06	.05	15	<1
38	17	1.88	20	89	230	203	2.2	44	.14	.09	2.91	.31	17	55
22	27	1.87	27	156	345	1562	1.15	2	.19	.22	4.56	.15	12	1
56	262	3.43	45	301	510	745	3.19	158	.21	.33	3.72	26	19	16
31	256	2.73	38	250	424	714	1.7	156	.2	.28	2.25	.22	17	15
33	160	2.17	36	190	478	496	2.19	149	.16	.24	2.93	.21	17	25
22	48	2.18	30	115	396	624	.91	163	.18	.23	2.48	.18	41	13
61	25	2.2	34	177	260	276	1.85	38	.42	.27	3.4	.26	39	9
24	199	.96	31	182	139	730	1.2	73	.12	.24	.96	.02	8	<1
42	362	1.8	37	322	240	1086	1.2	234	.2	.4	1.8	.05	10	1
22	27	.67	16	51	137	289	.38	39	.08	.05	.75	.26	16	3
94	32	1.82	17	126	222	158	3.89	23	.07	.22	3.36	.17	13	1
91	35	1.55	16	129	236	389	3.12	23	.2	.22	3.18	.19	11	1
101	104	2.2	38	204	578	400	2.84	105	.21	.31	4.01	.26	45	6
85	24	.81	19	65	318	661	.39	41	.1	.07	1.11	.18	8	12
14	68	1.03	12	88	119	255	.75	68	.14	.12	1.31	.06	18	1
10	43	.629	6	50	102	178	.35	36	.09	.156	2.04	.04	35	1
218	229	1.71	23	253	236	567	1.48	276	.22	.45	1.81	.1	17	3
36	17	1.78	17	70	69	1343	.61	221	.16	.09	1.42	.07	8	<1
84	33	1.99	20	105	256	619	1.67	94	.13	.20	2.85	.15	13	11
42	27	2.22	22	72	119	281	.84	62	.15	.11	1.69	.1	17	6
7	40	2.75	21	87	303	955	1.12	120	.35	.27	4.5	.13	6	10
7	80	2.25	26	135	408	955	1.3	140	.25	.17	2.25	.2	8	12
22	52	3.25	20	113	245	1220	2.39	100	.15	.17	2.25	.12	5	5
74	124	3.72	40	236	665	1009	2.45	159	.25	.3	3.97	.2	10	22
184	230	1.35	38	231	201	763	1.29	676	.09	.3	.48	.12	62	3
43	25	1.49	31	151	380	1203	1.7	27	.45	.22	3.62	.35	10	23

(9) From dairy cream in recipe.

(For purposes of calculations, use "0" for t, <1, <.1, <.01, etc.)

Table A–1
Food Composition

Computer Code Number	Food Description	Measure	Wt (g)	H_2O (%)	Ener (cal)	Prot (g)	Carb (g)	Dietary Fiber (g)	Fat (g)	Fat Breakdown (g) Sat	Mono	Poly
	MIXED DISHES and FAST FOODS—Cont.											
	MIXED DISHES—Cont.											
1515	Three bean salad	1 ea	340	82	316	9	30	7	19	2.8	4.3	11.1
717	Tuna salad[1]	1 c	205	63	383	33	19	1	19	3.2	5.9	8.4
1121	Tuna noodle casserole, homemade	1 c	202	75	238	17	25	2	7	1.9	1.5	3.2
1270	Waldorf salad	1 c	142	59	411	3	13	2	41	5.4	10.9	22.2
	FAST FOODS and SANDWICHES (see end of this appendix for additional Fast Foods):											
699	Burrito,[2] beef & bean	1 ea	175	52	385	17	50	4	13	6.3	5.3	.9
700	Burrito, bean	1 ea	174	53	358	11	57	7	11	5.5	3.8	1
701	Cheeseburger with bun, regular	1 ea	112	55	261	13	20	–	14	6.7	5.2	1.1
702	Cheeseburger with bun: 4-oz patty	1 ea	194	51	487	25	41	–	25	10.2	9.1	3.1
703	Chicken patty sandwich	1 ea	157	47	444	21	33	1	25	7.4	9	7.2
704	Corndog	1 ea	111	47	292	11	35	–	12	3.3	5.8	2.2
705	Enchilada	1 ea	230	63	451	14	40	–	27	15	8.9	1.1
706	English muffin with egg, cheese, bacon	1 ea	138	49	362	19	30	<1	19	8.6	6.4	1.9
	Fish sandwich:											
707	Regular, with cheese	1 ea	140	45	400	16	36	<1	22	6.2	6.8	7.2
708	Large, no cheese	1 ea	170	47	464	18	44	<1	24	5.6	8.3	8.9
709	Hamburger with bun, regular	1 ea	98	46	252	12	30	–	9	3.2	3.4	1.6
710	Hamburger with bun: 4-oz patty	1 ea	174	51	466	26	31	–	26	9.7	11.4	2.2
711	Hot dog/frankfurter with bun	1 ea	85	54	210	9	16	–	13	4.4	5.9	1.5
712	Pizza, cheese, ⅛ of 15" round[3]	1 pce	120	48	268	15	39	2	6	2.9	1.9	.9
	SANDWICHES:											
	Avocado, cheese, tomato, & lettuce:											
1276	On white bread, firm	1 ea	205	58	467	15	40	4	29	8.7	11.9	6
1278	On part whole wheat	1 ea	195	59	432	14	33	5	28	8.6	11.9	5.9
1277	On whole wheat	1 ea	209	58	458	16	39	7	29	8.7	12.1	6.1
	Bacon, lettuce & tomato:											
1137	On white bread, soft	1 ea	135	46	404	12	34	2	24	6	9	8
1139	On part whole wheat	1 ea	136	47	398	13	32	3	25	6	9.5	8
1138	On whole wheat	1 ea	149	47	421	14	37	6	26	6	9.6	8
	Cheese, grilled:											
1140	On white bread, soft	1 ea	117	37	393	17	29	1	23	12.2	7.6	2.1
1142	On part whole wheat	1 ea	117	37	389	18	27	2	24	12.3	7.7	2.2
1141	On whole wheat	1 ea	131	38	416	19	33	5	24	12.5	8	2.4
1596	Chicken fillet	1 ea	182	47	515	24	39	1	29	8.5	10.4	8.4
	Chicken salad:											
1143	On white bread, soft	1 ea	105	39	371	10	28	1	24	4	7.3	12
1145	On part whole wheat	1 ea	105	40	366	10	27	2	25	4	7	12
1144	On whole wheat	1 ea	118	40	389	12	32	5	25	4	7.6	12
1146	Corned beef & swiss on rye	1 ea	147	45	439	28	25	3	25	9.8	8.3	4.8

(1) Made with drained chunk light tuna, celery, onion, pickle relish, and mayonnaise-type salad dressing.

(2) Made with a 10½"-diameter flour tortilla.

(3) Crust made with vegetable shortening and enriched flour.

Chol (mg)	Calc (mg)	Iron (mg)	Magn (mg)	Phos (mg)	Pota (mg)	Sodi (mg)	Zinc (mg)	VT-A (RE)	Thia (mg)	Ribo (mg)	Niac (mg)	V-B6 (mg)	Fola (µg)	VT-C (mg)
0	80	3.21	57	147	508	1164	1.22	52	.16	.21	.91	.1	120	10
27	35	2.05	39	365	365	824	1.15	55	.06	.14	13.7	.17	15	5
41	34	2.3	31	156	182	775	1.21	13	.18	.15	7.81	.2	10	1
22	42	.85	36	78	268	250	.59	41	.09	.05	.35	.37	27	6
37	80	3.71	63	107	497	1011	2.91	49	.4	.63	4.1	.28	56	1
3	90	3.62	70	78	524	790	1.22	26	.5	.49	3.25	.24	94	2
38	132	1.93	19	157	167	710	1.9	51	.23	.17	4.64	.11	16	2
70	200	4	35	283	392	1228	4.07	76	.41	.33	9.41	.21	27	2
52	52	4.03	30	201	305	826	1.62	27	.28	.2	5.87	.17	25	8
50	64	3.92	11	105	167	617	.83	23	.18	.44	2.64	.06	38	0
62	458	1.86	71	189	338	1106	3.54	262	.11	.6	2.69	.55	48	1
221	196	3.11	32	302	201	741	1.71	149	.45	.5	3.71	.15	41	1
52	141	2.67	28	238	270	718	.9	74	.35	.32	3.23	.08	24	2
59	90	2.81	36	228	366	661	1.07	32	.36	.24	3.66	.12	48	3
39	47	2.25	21	101	197	516	1.88	12	.23	.29	4.3	.12	16	2
83	75	4.49	36	230	426	600	4.7	3	.28	.33	5.45	.3	36	1
38	20	2.01	11	84	124	581	1.72	0	.2	.24	3.16	.04	25	<1
18	222	1.1	30	215	209	640	1.56	140	.35	.31	4.73	.08	112	2
33	287	2.98	53	236	565	538	1.67	146	.36	.38	3.68	.3	77	11
30	283	3.01	65	253	596	511	1.85	136	.33	.37	3.82	.34	77	11
31	275	3.45	99	329	661	581	2.63	137	.34	.36	4.18	.41	89	11
29	60	2.33	22	144	254	737	1.16	35	.4	.23	3.8	.19	31	14
27	73	2.6	38	177	313	753	1.43	35	.4	.25	4.3	.23	35	14
26	62	3.18	75	257	378	818	2.29	35	.4	.23	4.6	.29	47	14
54	406	1.93	26	471	160	1148	2.03	209	.28	.39	2.27	.08	23	<1
53	405	2.08	38	502	206	1143	2.27	209	.25	.36	2.35	.09	27	<1
53	398	2.53	73	581	269	1219	3.05	211	.26	.34	2.72	.16	39	<1
60	60	4.68	35	233	353	957	1.87	31	.33	.24	6.81	.2	29	9
32	56	1.98	17	95	129	447	.73	26	.23	.17	3.69	.25	24	<1
31	67	2.13	30	124	181	461	.98	26	.24	.18	3.78	.29	27	<1
30	58	2.58	63	196	240	526	1.72	26	.25	.17	4.17	.34	39	<1
79	316	2.75	40	298	198	1070	3.69	78	.23	.35	3.26	.19	33	1

(For purposes of calculations, use "0" for t, <1, <.1, <.01, etc.)

Table A–1
Food Composition

Computer Code Number	Food Description	Measure	Wt (g)	H_2O (%)	Ener (cal)	Prot (g)	Carb (g)	Dietary Fiber (g)	Fat (g)	Fat Breakdown (g) Sat	Mono	Poly
	FAST FOODS and SANDWICHES (see end of this appendix for additional Fast Foods)—Cont.											
	SANDWICHES—Cont.											
	Egg salad:											
1147	On white bread, soft	1 ea	111	43	383	9	29	1	26	4.5	8	11.8
1149	On part whole wheat	1 ea	111	43	378	9	27	2	26	4.5	8	11.8
1148	On whole wheat	1 ea	125	43	401	11	33	5	27	4.7	8	12
	Ham:											
1279	On rye bread	1 ea	116	56	241	16	20	3	10	2.2	3.8	3.6
1151	On white bread, soft	1 ea	122	55	260	17	23	1	11	2.3	4.1	3.6
1153	On part whole wheat	1 ea	122	55	257	17	22	2	11	2.3	4.1	3.7
1152	On whole wheat	1 ea	136	54	284	19	27	4	12	2.5	4.4	3.9
	Ham & cheese:											
1280	On white bread, soft	1 ea	151	50	388	21	29	1	21	7.8	6.8	4.6
1282	On part whole wheat	1 ea	151	50	384	22	27	2	21	7.8	6.9	4.7
1281	On whole wheat	1 ea	165	49	411	24	33	5	22	8	7.1	4.9
1150	Ham & swiss on rye	1 ea	145	50	368	23	25	3	19	7.2	6.2	4.6
	Ham salad:											
1154	On white bread, soft	1 ea	125	47	344	10	34	1	18	4.5	7.3	5.8
1156	On part whole wheat	1 ea	125	48	340	10	33	2	19	4.6	7.3	5.9
1155	On whole wheat	1 ea	139	47	367	12	39	5	19	4.8	7.6	6.1
1157	Patty melt: Ground beef & cheese on rye	1 ea	177	43	583	36	25	3	37	13.8	13.8	6.2
	Peanut butter & jelly:											
1158	On white bread, soft	1 ea	100	27	345	10	47	3	14	2.7	6.6	3.9
1160	On part whole wheat	1 ea	100	27	341	11	46	4	14	2.8	6.6	4
1159	On whole wheat	1 ea	114	28	368	13	51	7	15	2.9	6.9	4.2
1161	Reuben, grilled: Corned beef, swiss cheese, sauerkraut on rye	1 ea	233	61	496	29	29	5	29	10.7	10.2	6.1
	Roast beef:											
713	On a bun	1 ea	150	49	374	23	36	–	15	3.9	7.3	1.8
1162	On white bread, soft	1 ea	122	47	314	22	26	1	13	2.7	4.3	4.9
1164	On part whole wheat	1 ea	122	47	311	23	25	2	13	2.8	4.3	5
1163	On whole wheat	1 ea	136	46	339	25	30	4	14	3	4.6	5.3
	Tuna salad:											
1165	On white bread, soft	1 ea	116	47	310	13	33	2	14	2.3	4.4	6.3
1167	On part whole wheat	1 ea	116	47	306	13	32	3	14	2.4	4.5	6.4
1166	On whole wheat	1 ea	130	46	333	15	37	5	15	2.5	4.7	6.6
	Turkey:											
1168	On white bread, soft	1 ea	122	54	270	19	22	1	11	2	3.5	5
1170	On part whole wheat	1 ea	122	54	267	19	21	2	11	2	3.5	5
1169	On whole wheat	1 ea	136	53	294	21	26	4	12	2.2	3.8	5.3
	Turkey ham:											
1272	On rye bread	1 ea	116	57	239	16	19	3	10	2.2	3	4.3
1273	On white bread, soft	1 ea	122	56	258	16	23	1	11	2.3	3.3	4.3
1275	On part whole wheat	1 ea	122	56	255	17	22	2	11	2.4	3.3	4.4
1274	On whole wheat	1 ea	136	55	282	19	27	4	12	2.6	3.6	4.7

(Computer code number is for West Diet Analysis program)

Chol (mg)	Calc (mg)	Iron (mg)	Magn (mg)	Phos (mg)	Pota (mg)	Sodi (mg)	Zinc (mg)	VT-A (RE)	Thia (mg)	Ribo (mg)	Niac (mg)	V-B6 (mg)	Fola (μg)	VT-C (mg)
150	66	2.21	15	114	106	511	.72	73	.24	.29	1.82	.2	35	0
149	79	2.36	29	146	161	525	.96	73	.26	.32	2.35	.24	39	0
147	67	2.81	61	215	217	590	1.74	73	.27	.31	2.71	.3	49	0
35	38	1.72	29	197	303	1289	1.76	6	.78	.28	4.66	.38	23	17
36	57	1.97	24	191	293	1277	1.59	6	.83	.3	4.96	.38	18	17
35	56	2.09	34	216	329	1274	1.79	6	.8	.27	5.03	.39	21	17
36	50	2.5	62	283	389	1364	2.45	6	.83	.27	5.45	.46	31	18
57	237	2.34	31	381	311	1582	2.26	87	.78	.4	4.84	.36	24	14
57	236	2.49	43	412	356	1578	2.5	87	.75	.37	4.92	.38	27	14
57	228	2.93	77	488	419	1655	3.27	88	.76	.36	5.29	.45	39	14
56	309	1.99	41	353	313	1289	2.74	77	.73	.38	4.52	.37	29	14
28	67	2.11	20	127	159	898	1.02	8	.52	.26	3.49	.18	20	4
27	66	2.27	32	158	206	893	1.26	8	.49	.23	3.57	.2	24	4
28	57	2.71	66	234	269	967	2.04	8	.51	.21	3.94	.27	36	4
116	224	3.83	44	416	377	892	6.96	137	.28	.47	6.56	.33	39	<1
1	74	2.36	52	130	263	309	1.02	<1	.3	.22	5.55	.15	43	<1
0	73	2.52	65	162	309	305	1.26	<1	.27	.19	5.63	.17	47	<1
0	64	2.97	99	238	374	375	2.04	<1	.28	.18	6.03	.24	59	<1
80	347	3.96	51	320	337	1655	3.91	128	.25	.37	3.43	.3	52	12
55	58	4.56	33	258	341	855	3.66	22	.4	.33	6.33	.28	43	2
34	57	3.21	23	157	341	1257	2.95	9	.26	.28	5.29	.32	23	10
34	56	3.33	33	182	377	1254	3.14	9	.24	.25	5.36	.33	26	10
34	50	3.77	61	247	438	1343	3.85	9	.25	.25	5.78	.4	36	10
12	71	2.26	23	146	160	558	.65	21	.28	.23	5.63	.13	23	1
12	69	2.42	36	177	206	553	.89	21	.25	.19	5.71	.15	27	1
12	60	2.86	70	253	270	625	1.66	21	.26	.18	6.1	.22	39	1
34	55	1.67	24	198	242	1252	1.05	9	.24	.22	7.32	.33	19	0
34	53	1.8	34	223	279	1249	1.24	9	.21	.19	7.39	.35	22	0
35	47	2.19	62	289	336	1339	1.89	9	.22	.19	7.88	.41	32	0
41	40	3.03	28	178	287	1004	2.43	6	.2	.29	3.81	.23	24	0
42	59	3.29	23	172	276	991	2.27	6	.24	.31	4.11	.23	20	0
41	58	3.42	33	197	313	987	2.46	6	.22	.29	4.17	.25	23	0
43	52	3.86	61	263	371	1069	3.15	6	.23	.28	4.57	.31	33	0

(For purposes of calculations, use "0" for t, <1, <.1, <.01, etc.)

Table A–1
Food Composition

Computer Code Number	Food Description	Measure	Wt (g)	H_2O (%)	Ener (cal)	Prot (g)	Carb (g)	Dietary Fiber (g)	Fat (g)	Fat Breakdown (g) Sat	Mono	Poly
	FAST FOODS and SANDWICHES (see end of this appendix for additional Fast Foods)—Cont.											
714	Taco	1 ea	78	58	168	9	12	–	9	5.2	3	4
	Tostada:											
1114	With refried beans	1 ea	157	66	243	10	29	8	11	5.9	3.3	.8
1118	With beans & beef	1 ea	192	70	284	14	25	3	14	9.8	3	.5
1354	With beans & chicken	1 ea	157	67	253	19	19	3	11	4.5	4.4	1.6
	Vegetarian foods:											
1511	Baked beans, canned	½ c	127	73	118	6	26	10	1	.1	t	.2
1175	Breakfast links	1 ea	34	52	89	7	3	1	6	–	–	–
1171	Nuteena	1 pce	67	58	160	8	5	2	12	1.7	4.6	3.7
1173	Redi-burger	1 pce	68	57	130	14	5	1	6	.7	1.3	3.3
1174	Vege-burger	½ c	108	73	110	22	4	1	1	.1	.1	.4
	NUTS, SEEDS, and PRODUCTS											
	Almonds:											
1365	Dry roasted, salted	1 c	138	3	810	22	33	18	71	6.7	46.2	14.9
718	Slivered, packed, unsalted	1 c	135	4	795	27	27	15[1]	70	6.7	45.8	14.9
719	Whole, dried, unsalted:	1 c	142	4	836	28	29	16[1]	74	7	48.1	15.6
720	Ounce	1 oz	28	4	167	6	6	3[1]	15	1.4	9.6	3.1
721	Almond butter	1 tbs	16	1	101	2	3	1	9	.9	6.1	2
722	Brazil nuts, dry (about 7)	1 oz	28	3	186	4	4	2	19	4.6	6.5	6.8
	Cashew nuts, salted:											
723	Dry roasted:	1 c	137	2	786	21	45	9	64	12.5	37.4	10.7
724	Ounce	1 oz	28	2	163	4	9	2	13	2.6	7.7	2.2
725	Oil roasted:	1 c	130	4	748	21	37	8	63	12.4	36.9	10.6
726	Ounce	1 oz	28	4	163	5	8	2	14	2.7	8	2.3
1366	Cashew nuts, unsalted, dry roasted	1 c	137	2	786	21	45	8	64	12.5	37.4	10.7
1367	Cashew nuts, unsalted, oil roasted	1 c	130	4	748	21	37	8	63	12.4	36.9	10.6
727	Cashew butter, unsalted	1 tbs	16	3	94	3	4	1	8	1.6	4.7	1.3
728	Chestnuts, European, roasted (1 cup = approx 17 kernels)	1 c	143	40	350	5	76	18	3	.6	1.1	1.2
	Coconut, raw:											
729	Piece 2 x 2 x ½"	1 pce	45	47	159	1	7	4	15	13.4	.6	.2
730	Shredded/grated, unpacked[2]	½ c	40	47	142	1	6	4	13	11.9	.6	.1
	Coconut, dried, shredded/grated:											
731	Unsweetened	1 c	78	3	514	5	19	10	50	44.6	2.1	.6
732	Sweetened	1 c	93	13	465	3	44	7	33	29.3	1.4	.4
733	Filberts/hazelnuts, chopped:	1 c	115	5	726	15	18	7	72	5.3	56.4	6.9
734	Ounce	1 oz	28	5	179	4	4	2	18	1.3	13.9	1.7
735	Macadamias, oil roasted, salted:	1 c	134	2	962	10	17	8	102	15.3	80.9	1.8
736	Ounce	1 oz	28	2	201	2	4	2	21	3.2	16.9	.4
1368	Macadamias, oil roasted, unsalted	1 c	134	2	962	10	17	7	102	15.3	80.9	1.8

(1)Values reported for dietary fiber in almonds vary from 7.0 to 14.3 g/100 g.
(2)½ cup packed = 65 g.

(Computer code number is for West Diet Analysis program)

Chol (mg)	Calc (mg)	Iron (mg)	Magn (mg)	Phos (mg)	Pota (mg)	Sodi (mg)	Zinc (mg)	VT-A (RE)	Thia (mg)	Ribo (mg)	Niac (mg)	V-B6 (mg)	Fola (μg)	VT-C (mg)
26	101	1.1	32	93	216	366	1.79	67	.07	.2	1.47	.11	11	1
33	229	2.06	64	127	440	592	2.07	93	.11	.36	1.44	.17	82	1
63	161	2.09	58	148	419	743	2.71	148	.08	.42	2.44	.21	83	3
53	171	1.81	49	240	367	435	2.29	87	.11	.2	4.49	.32	54	3
0	63	.37	41	132	376	504	1.78	22	.19	.08	.54	.17	30	4
<1	11	1.96	–	–	43	203	–	<1	1.65	.17	3.77	.2	–	<1
0	21	1.2	40	111	200	120	.87	10	.47	.58	.14	.45	60	<1
0	19	1.4	13	56	120	370	1.2	10	.6	.4	6.7	.8	17	<1
0	32	2.7	24	105	110	190	1.1	10	.53	.68	5	.56	27	<1
0	389	5.24	420	756	1062	1076	6.76	0	.18	.83	3.89	.1	88	1
0	359	4.94	400	702	988	15	3.94	0	.28	1.05	4.54	.15	79	1
0	378	5.2	420	738	1039	16[3]	4.15	0	.3	1.11	4.77	.16	83	1
0	75	1.04	84	147	208	3[3]	.83	0	.06	.22	.95	.03	17	<1
0	43	.59	48	84	121	2[4]	.49	0	.02	.1	.46	.01	10	<1
0	50	.96	64	170	170	1	1.3	0	.28	.03	.46	.07	1	<1
0	62	8.22	356	671	774	875[5]	7.67	0	.27	.27	1.92	.35	95	0
0	13	1.7	74	139	160	181[5]	1.59	0	.06	.06	.4	.07	20	0
0	53	5.33	332	553	689	813[6]	6.18	0	.55	.23	2.34	.32	88	0
0	12	1.16	72	120	150	177[6]	1.35	0	.12	.05	.51	.07	19	0
0	62	8.22	356	671	774	22	7.67	0	.27	.27	1.92	.35	95	0
0	53	5.33	332	553	689	22	6.18	0	.55	.23	2.34	.32	88	0
0	7	.8	41	73	87	2[7]	.83	0	.05	.03	.26	.04	11	0
0	41	1.3	47	153	847	3	.81	3	.35	.25	1.92	.71	100	37
0	6	1.09	14	51	160	9	.49	0	.03	.01	.24	.02	12	1
0	6	.97	13	45	142	8	.44	0	.03	.01	.22	.02	11	1
0	20	2.59	70	160	423	29	1.57	0	.05	.08	.47	.23	7	1
0	14	1.79	46	99	313	243	1.69	0	.03	.02	.44	.25	8	1
0	216	3.76	327	358	511	3	2.76	8	.57	.13	1.31	.7	83	1
0	53	.93	80	88	126	1	.68	2	.14	.03	.32	.17	20	<1
0	60	2.41	155	268	440	348[8]	1.47	1	.28	.15	2.71	.26	50	0
0	13	.5	32	56	92	73[8]	.31	<1	.06	.03	.57	.05	10	0
0	60	2.41	155	268	440	9	1.47	1	.28	.15	2.71	.26	21	0

(3)Salted almonds contain 1108 mg sodium per cup, 221 mg per ounce.

(4)Salted almond butter contains 72 mg sodium per tablespoon.

(5)Dry-roasted cashews without salt contain 21 mg sodium per cup, or 4 mg per ounce.

(6)Oil-roasted cashews without salt contain 22 mg sodium per cup, or 5 mg per ounce.

(7)Salted cashew butter contains 98 mg sodium per tablespoon.

(8)Macadamia nuts without salt contain 9 mg sodium per cup, or 2 mg per ounce.

Table A–1
Food Composition

Computer Code Number	Food Description	Measure	Wt (g)	H_2O (%)	Ener (cal)	Prot (g)	Carb (g)	Dietary Fiber (g)	Fat (g)	Fat Breakdown (g) Sat	Mono	Poly
	NUTS, SEEDS, and PRODUCTS—Cont.											
	Mixed nuts:											
737	Dry roasted, salted	1 c	137	2	812	24	35	12	71	9.4	43	14.7
738	Oil roasted, salted	1 c	142	2	876	24	30	13	80	12.4	45	18.9
1369	Oil roasted, unsalted	1 c	142	2	876	24	30	13	80	12.4	45	18.9
	Peanuts:											
739	Oil roasted, salted:	1 c	144	2	837	38	27	13	71	9.8	35.3	22.5
740	Ounce	1 oz	28	2	165	7	5	2	14	1.9	6.9	4.4
1370	Oil roasted, unsalted	1 c	144	2	837	38	27	13	71	9.8	35.3	22.5
741	Dried, unsalted:	1 c	146	2	854	35	31	12	73	10.1	36.1	22.9
742	Ounce	1 oz	28	2	166	7	6	2	14	2	7	4.4
743	Peanut butter:	½ c	129	1	759	32	27	8	64	12.3	30.4	18.6
1371	Tablespoon	2 tbs	32	1	190	8	7	2	16	3.1	7.6	4.6
744	Pecan halves, dried, unsalted:	1 c	108	5	720	8	20	7[1]	73	5.8	45.5	18.1
745	Ounce	1 oz	28	5	189	2	5	2[1]	19	1.5	11.9	4.8
1372	Pecan halves, dry roasted, salted	¼ c	28	1	187	2	6	2	18	1.5	11.4	4.5
746	Pine nuts/piñons, dried	1 oz	28	6	161	3	5	2	17	2.7	6.5	7.3
747	Pistachios, dried, shelled	1 oz	28	4	164	6	7	3	14	1.7	9.3	2.1
1373	Pistachios, dry roasted, salted, shelled	1 c	128	2	774	19	35	15	68	8.6	45.6	10.2
748	Pumpkin kernels, dried, unsalted	1 oz	28	7	154	7	5	2	13	2.5	4	5.9
1374	Pumpkin kernels, roasted, salted	1 c	227	7	1184	75	30	24	96	18.1	29.7	43.6
749	Sesame seeds, hulled, dried	¼ c	38	5	223	10	4	3	21	2.9	7.9	9.1
	Sunflower seed kernels:											
750	Dry	¼ c	36	5	205	8	7	2	18	1.9	3.4	11.8
751	Oil roasted	¼ c	34	3	209	7	5	2	19	2	3.7	12.9
752	Tahini (sesame butter)	1 tbs	15	3	91	3	3	1	8	1.2	3.2	3.7
1334	Trail Mix w/Chocolate Chips	1 c	146	7	707	21	66	–	47	8.9	19.8	16.5
753	Black walnuts, chopped:	1 c	125	4	758	30	15	6	71	4.5	15.9	46.9
754	Ounce	1 oz	28	4	172	7	3	1	16	1	3.6	10.6
755	English walnuts, chopped:	1 c	120	4	770	17	22	6	74	6.7	17	47
756	Ounce	1 oz	28	4	182	4	5	1	17	1.6	4	11.1
	SWEETENERS and SWEETS (see also Dairy [milk desserts] and Baked Goods)											
757	Apple butter	2 tbs	35	52	64	<1	17	<1	<1	t	t	.1
1124	Butterscotch topping	2 tbs	41	32	103	<1	27	.4	<1	.05	.01	0
1125	Caramel topping	2 tbs	41	32	103	<1	27	.4	<1	.05	.01	0
	Cake frosting, creamy vanilla:											
1127	Canned	2 tbs	31	13	131	<1	22	0	5	1.5	2.7	.7
1123	From mix	2 tbs	31	12	132	<1	22	0	5	1	2.1	1.8

[1] Dietary fiber data calculated/derived from data on other nuts.

(Computer code number is for West Diet Analysis program)

PAGE KEY: A–2 = BEV A–4 = DAIRY A–10 = EGGS A–12 = FAT/OIL A–14 = FRUIT A–24 = BAKERY A–34 = GRAIN A–40 = FISH A–44 = MEATS A–48 = POULTRY A–50 = SAUSAGE A–52 = MIXED/FAST A–60 = NUTS/SEEDS A–62 = SWEETS A–66 = VEG/LEG A–78 = MISC A–80 = SOUPS/SAUCES A–84 = FAST A–96 = FRZN ENTREE A–98 = BABY FOODS

Chol (mg)	Calc (mg)	Iron (mg)	Magn (mg)	Phos (mg)	Pota (mg)	Sodi (mg)	Zinc (mg)	VT-A (RE)	Thia (mg)	Ribo (mg)	Niac (mg)	V-B6 (mg)	Fola (μg)	VT-C (mg)
0	96	5.07	308	595	817	917[2]	5.21	1	.27	.27	6.44	.41	69	1
0	153	4.56	334	657	825	924[2]	7.21	3	.71	.31	7.19	.34	117	1
0	153	4.56	334	657	825	16	7.21	3	.71	.31	7.19	.34	117	1
0	126	2.64	266	744	982	624[3]	9.55	0	.36	.16	20.4	.37	181	0
0	25	.52	52	147	193	123[3]	1.88	0	.07	.03	4.03	.07	36	0
0	126	2.64	266	744	982	9	9.55	0	.36	.16	20.4	.37	181	0
0	79	3.3	256	523	961	9	4.83	0	.64	.14	19.7	.37	212	0
0	15	.64	50	101	187	2	.94	0	.12	.03	3.83	.07	41	0
0	44	2.15	203	417	928	617[4]	3.24	0	.18	.13	16.9	.48	101	0
0	11	.54	51	104	232	153[4]	.81	0	.04	.03	4.22	.12	25	0
0	39	2.3	138	314	423	1[5]	5.91	14	.92	.14	.96	.2	42	2
0	10	.6	36	82	111	<1[5]	1.55	4	.24	.04	.25	.05	11	1
0	10	.62	38	86	105	221	1.61	4	.09	.03	.26	.05	12	1
0	2	.87	66	10	178	20	1.22	1	.35	.06	1.24	.03	16	1
0	38	1.92	45	142	310	2[6]	.38	7	.23	.05	.31	.07	16	2
0	90	4.06	166	609	1241	998	1.74	31	.54	.31	1.8	.33	76	9
0	12	4.24	152	332	229	5[7]	2.12	11	.06	.09	.49	.06	26	<1
0	98	33.8	1212	2658	1829	1305	16.9	86	.48	.72	3.95	.2	130	4
0	50	2.96	132	295	155	15	3.91	3	.27	.03	1.78	.05	36	0
0	42	2.44	127	253	248	1[8]	1.82	2	.82	.09	1.62	.28	82	1
0	19	2.28	43	387	164	1[8]	1.77	2	.11	.09	1.4	.27	80	<1
0	21	.95	53	118	69	<1	1.58	1	.24	.02	.85	.02	15	0
0	72	3.84	253	580	655	1	4.28	37	.27	.14	.86	.69	82	4
0	16	.87	57	132	149	<1	.97	9	.06	.03	.2	.16	19	1
6	159	4.95	235	565	946	177	4.58	7	.6	.33	6.43	.38	95	2
0	113	2.93	203	380	602	12	3.28	15	.46	.18	1.25	.67	79	4
0	27	.69	48	90	142	3	.77	4	.11	.04	.29	.16	19	1
0	2	.05	1	2	32	<1	.02	0	<.01	<.01	.03	.01	<1	1
<1	22	.07	3	19	34	143	.08	11	.01	.04	.02	.01	1	<1
<1	22	.07	3	19	34	143	.08	11	.01	.04	.02	.01	1	<1
0	1	.03	<1	12	11	28	0	70	0	<.01	<.01	0	0	0
0	3	.07	1	8	7	69	.03	33	.01	.01	.11	<.01	0	0

(2)Mixed nuts without salt contain about 15 mg sodium per cup.

(3)Peanuts without salt contain 22 mg sodium per cup, or 4 mg per ounce.

(4)Peanut butter without added salt contains 3 mg sodium per tablespoon.

(5)Salted pecans contain 816 mg sodium per cup, or 214 mg per ounce.

(6)Salted pistachios contain approx 221 mg sodium per ounce.

(7)Salted pumpkin/squash kernels contain approximately 163 mg sodium per ounce.

(8)Unsalted sunflower seeds contain 1 mg sodium per ¼ cup.

(For purposes of calculations, use "0" for t, <1, <.1, <.01, etc.)

A

Table A–1
Food Composition

Computer Code Number	Food Description	Measure	Wt (g)	H_2O (%)	Ener (cal)	Prot (g)	Carb (g)	Dietary Fiber (g)	Fat (g)	Fat Breakdown (g) Sat	Mono	Poly
	SWEETENERS and SWEETS (see also Dairy [milk desserts] and Baked Goods)—Cont.											
	Candy:											
1128	Almond Joy candy bar	1 oz	28	8	132	1	17	2	8	4.7	1.5	.7
758	Caramel, plain or chocolate	1 oz	28	8	108	1	22	<1	2	1.9	.2	.1
	Chocolate (see also #784, 785, 971):											
	Milk chocolate:											
759	Plain	1 oz	28	1	145	2	17	1	9	5.2	2.8	.3
760	With almonds	1 oz	28	1	149	3	15	2	10	4.8	3.8	.6
761	With peanuts	1 oz	28	1	157	5	11	2	12	3.4	5.1	2.6
762	With rice cereal	1 oz	28	2	141	2	18	6	8	4.5	2.4	.2
763	Semisweet chocolate chips	1 c	170	1	811	7	108	11	50	29.8	16.9	1.6
764	Sweet dark chocolate (candy bar)	1 oz	28	1	135	1	17	1	9	5.9	3.3	.3
1133	SKOR English toffee candy bar	1 ea	32	4	169	1	18	<1	16	7	6.9	2
765	Fondant candy, uncoated (mints, candy corn, other)	1 oz	28	7	101	0	26	0	<1	.1	–	–
1697	Fruit Roll-up (small)	1 ea	14	21	41	<1	11	<1	<1	4	4	.1
766	Fudge, chocolate	1 oz	28	10	108	<1	22	1	2	1.5	.7	.1
767	Gumdrops	1 oz	28	1	109	<1	28	0	<1	0	t	.1
768	Hard candy, all flavors	1 oz	28	1	106	0	28	0	0	0	0	0
769	Jellybeans	1 oz	28	6	104	0	26	0	<1	0	t	.1
1134	M&M's Plain Chocolate Candy	48 g	48	1	228	3	33	1	11	5	3	.3
1135	M&M's Peanut Chocolate Candy	47 g	47	1	234	5	28	1	13	5	5.1	2
1130	Mars almond bar	1 ea	50	4	234	4	31	1	11	4.8	4.4	.8
1129	Milky Way candy bar	1 ea	60	6	251	3	43	<1	9	4.7	3.3	.3
1708	Milk chocolate-coated peanuts	½ c	85	4	441	11	42	4	29	12	11	3.7
1709	Peanut brittle-recipe	½ c	74	3	333	6	51	1	14	4	6.2	3.5
1132	Reese's peanut butter cup	2 ea	45	8	218	5	21	2	14	10.4	.9	.9
1131	Snickers candy bar (2.2oz)	1 ea	61	6	278	6	37	2	14	7.3	4.1	.5
1482	Fruit juice bar (2.5 fl oz)	1 ea	77	78	63	1	16	–	<1	–	–	–
771	Gelatin dessert/Jello, prepared	½ c	120	85	71	1	17	<1	0	0	0	0
1702	SugarFree	½ c	113	98	8	1	1	0	0	0	0	0
772	Honey:	1 c	339	17	1030	1	279	0	0	0	0	0
773	Tablespoon	1 tbs	21	17	64	<1	17	0	0	0	0	0
774	Jams or preserves:	1 tbs	20	29	54	<1	14	<1	<1	0	t	t
775	Packet	1 ea	14	34	34	<1	9	<1	<1	t	t	0
776	Jellies:	1 tbs	18	28	49	<1	13	<1	<1	t	t	t
777	Packet	1 ea	14	28	38	<1	10	<1	<1	t	t	t
1136	Marmalade	2 tbs	40	33	98	<1	26	<1	0	0	0	0
770	Marshmallows	4 ea	28	16	90	1	23	0	<1	0	0	0
1126	Marshmallow creme topping	3 tbs	50	18	155	1	40	0	<1	0	0	0
778	Popsicle/ice pops	1 ea	95	80	68	0	18	0	0	0	0	0
	Sugars:											
779	Brown sugar	1 c	220	2	827	0	214	0	0	0	0	0
780	White sugar, granulated:	1 c	200	<1	774	0	200	0	0	0	0	0
781	Tablespoon	1 tbs	12	<1	46	0	12	0	0	0	0	0
782	Packet	1 ea	6	<1	23	0	6	0	0	0	0	0
783	White sugar, powdered, sifted	1 c	100	<1	389	0	99	0	<1	0	0	0

(Computer code number is for West Diet Analysis program)

PAGE KEY: A–2 = BEV A–4 = DAIRY A–10 = EGGS A–12 = FAT/OIL A–14 = FRUIT A–24 = BAKERY A–34 = GRAIN A–40 = FISH A–44 = MEATS A–48 = POULTRY A–50 = SAUSAGE A–52 = MIXED/FAST A–60 = NUTS/SEEDS A–62 = SWEETS A–66 = VEG/LEG A–78 = MISC A–80 = SOUPS/SAUCES A–84 = FAST A–96 = FRZN ENTREE A–98 = BABY FOODS

Chol (mg)	Calc (mg)	Iron (mg)	Magn (mg)	Phos (mg)	Pota (mg)	Sodi (mg)	Zinc (mg)	VT-A (RE)	Thia (mg)	Ribo (mg)	Niac (mg)	V-B6 (mg)	Fola (µg)	VT-C (mg)
1	22	.34	19	40	105	38	.23	3	.01	.04	.13	.02	2	<1
2	39	.04	5	32	61	69	.12	2	<.01	.05	.07	.01	1	0
6	54	.39	17	61	109	23	.39	14	.02	.08	.09	.01	2	0
5	63	.46	25	75	126	21	.38	17	.02	.12	.21	.01	3	<1
3	33	.53	35	83	152	11	.69	6	.08	.05	2.14	.04	23	0
5	48	.21	14	55	97	41	.32	93	.02	.08	.13	.02	3	3
0	54	5.32	196	224	621	19	2.75	3	.09	.15	.73	.08	5	<1
0	5	.59	33	45	96	3	.42	1	.01	.07	.19	.01	1	<1
19	36	.13	11	48	76	74	.24	22	.01	.11	.03	.01	2	0
0	1	.02	<1	1	5	11	.01	0	0	<.01	<.01	0	0	0
0	6	.55	13	6	12	2	.01	<1	<.01	.01	.2	.03	0	<1
4	12	.14	7	16	29	18	.11	13	<.01	.02	.03	<.01	1	0
0	1	.11	<1	<1	1	12	0	0	0	<.01	<.01	0	0	0
0	1	.08	1	1	1	11	<.01	0	<.01	<.01	<.01	<.01	0	0
0	1	.31	1	1	10	7	.01	0	0	0	0	0	0	0
0	81	.73	32	94	188	49	.61	12	.03	.12	.26	.03	4	0
0	63	.7	39	130	184	44	.72	2	.03	.1	1.51	.08	26	0
4	84	.55	36	114	163	85	.55	22	.02	.16	.47	.03	7	<1
12	78	.46	20	98	145	144	.43	28	.02	.13	.21	.03	5	1
8	88	1.12	77	180	427	35	1.61	0	.1	.15	3.61	.18	7	0
10	22	1.02	37	82	153	332	.71	35	.14	.04	2.57	.08	52	0
7	35	.49	38	108	180	131	.63	9	.02	.09	1.79	.04	13	0
7	70	.48	37	129	200	164	.7	19	.03	.11	1.83	.11	24	<1
0	4	.15	3	5	41	3	.04	2	.01	.01	.12	.02	5	–
0	2	.04	1	26	1	50	.04	0	<.01	<.01	<.01	<.01	0	0
0	2	.01	1	31	0	54	.03	0	0	<.01	<.01	<.01	0	0
0	20	1.42	7	14	176	14	.75	0	0	.13	.41	.08	7	3
0	1	.09	<1	1	11	1	.05	0	0	.01	.02	<.01	<1	<1
0	4	.2	1	2	18	2	.01	<1	<.01	.01	.04	<.01	2	<1
0	3	.07	1	2	11	6	.01	<1	0	<.01	<.01	<.01	5	<1
0	1	.04	1	1	11	6	.01	<1	0	<.01	.01	<.01	<1	1
0	1	.03	1	1	9	5	.01	<1	0	<.01	<.01	<.01	<1	1
0	15	.06	1	2	15	22	.02	2	<.01	<.01	.02	.01	14	2
0	1	.06	1	2	1	13	.01	0	0	0	.02	<.01	<1	0
0	1	.11	1	4	2	23	.02	0	<.01	<.01	.04	<.01	<1	2
0	0	<.01	1	0	4	11	.02	0	0	0	0	0	0	0
0	187	4.2	64	48	761	86	.4	0	.02	.01	.18	.06	2	0
0	2	.13	0	4	4	2	.07	0	0	.04	0	0	0	0
0	<1	.01	<1	<1	<1	<1	<.01	0	0	<.01	0	0	0	0
0	<1	<.01	<1	<1	<1	<1	<.01	0	0	<.01	0	0	0	0
0	1	.06	1	2	2	1	.03	0	0	0	0	0	0	0

(For purposes of calculations, use "0" for t, <1, <.1, <.01, etc.)

Table A–1
Food Composition

Computer Code Number	Food Description	Measure	Wt (g)	H_2O (%)	Ener (cal)	Prot (g)	Carb (g)	Dietary Fiber (g)	Fat (g)	Fat Breakdown (g) Sat	Mono	Poly
	SWEETENERS and SWEETS (see also Dairy [milk desserts] and Baked Goods)—Cont.											
	Sweeteners:											
1711	Equal, packet	1 ea	1	.1	4	0	1	0	0	0	0	0
1712	Sweet 'n low, packet	1 ea	1	.1	4	0	1	0	0	0	0	0
	Syrups:											
	Chocolate:											
785	Hot fudge type	2 tbs	38	22	131	2	22	1	5	2.1	1.4	1.2
784	Thin type	2 tbs	38	37	85	1	22	1	1	.3	.2	.1
786	Molasses, blackstrap[1]	2 tbs	40	29	94	0	24	0	0	0	0	0
1710	Light cane	1 tbs	21	24	52	0	13	0	0	0	0	0
787	Pancake table syrup (corn and maple)	¼ c	79	24	226	0	60	0	0	0	0	0
	VEGETABLES and LEGUMES											
788	Alfalfa sprouts	1 c	33	91	10	1	1	1	<1	t	t	.1
789	Artichokes, cooked globe (300 g w/refuse)	1 ea	120	84	60	4	13	10	<1	t	t	.1
1177	Artichoke hearts, cooked from frozen	9 oz	240	86	108	7	22	13	1	.3	t	.5
1176	Artichoke hearts, marinated	6 oz	170	59	168	4	13	7	13	2	3	7.7
	Asparagus, green, cooked:											
	From fresh:											
790	Cuts and tips	½ c	90	92	22	2	4	1	<1	.1	t	.1
791	Spears, ½" diam at base	6 ea	90	92	22	2	4	1	<1	.1	t	.1
	From frozen:											
792	Cuts and tips	½ c	90	91	25	3	4	2	<1	.1	t	.2
793	Spears, ½" diam at base	6 ea	90	91	25	3	4	2	<1	.1	t	.2
794	Canned, spears, ½" diam at base	6 ea	120	94	23	3	3	1	1	.2	t	.3
795	Bamboo shoots, canned, drained slices	1 c	131	94	25	2	4	3	1	.1	t	.2
	Beans (see also alphabetical listing in this section):											
796	Black beans, cooked	½ c	86	66	114	8	20	8	<1	.1	t	.2
	Canned beans (white/navy):											
803	With pork and tomato sauce	½ c	126	73	123	7	24	7	1	.5	.6	.2
804	With sweet sauce	1 c	253	71	281	13	53	14	4	1.4	1.6	.5
805	With frankfurters	1 c	257	69	365	17	40	18	17	6	7.3	2.1
	Lima beans:											
797	Thick seeded (Fordhooks), cooked from frozen	½ c	85	73	85	5	16	5	<1	.1	t	.1
798	Thin seeded (Baby), cooked from frozen	½ c	90	72	94	6	17	6	<1	.1	t	.1
799	Cooked from dry, drained	½ c	94	70	108	7	20	8	<1	.1	t	.2
	Snap bean/green string beans cuts and french style:											
800	Cooked from fresh	½ c	62	89	22	1	5	2	<1	t	t	.1
801	Cooked from frozen	½ c	67	92	18	1	4	2	<1	t	t	t
802	Canned, drained	½ c	67	93	13	1	3	1	<1	t	t	t
1713	Snap bean, yellow, cooked f/fresh	½ c	63	89	22	1	5	1	<1	t	t	t

(1)Light molasses would contain about 66 mg calcium, 2.1 mg iron, 18 mg magnesium, and 366 mg potassium for 2 tbsp.

Chol (mg)	Calc (mg)	Iron (mg)	Magn (mg)	Phos (mg)	Pota (mg)	Sodi (mg)	Zinc (mg)	VT-A (RE)	Thia (mg)	Ribo (mg)	Niac (mg)	V-B6 (mg)	Fola (µg)	VT-C (mg)
0	–	–	–	–	–	0	–	–	–	–	–	–	–	–
0	<1	–	<1	–	1	1	–	–	–	–	–	–	–	–
5	38	.46	18	65	82	49	.3	13	.01	.08	.08	.01	2	0
0	6	.75	26	49	85	36	.39	1	.01	.02	.11	<.01	3	0
0	344[1]	7[1]	86[1]	16	997[1]	22	.4	0	.01	.02	.43	.28	<1	0
0	34	.88	–	9	188	3	–	0	.01	.01	.04	–	–	0
0	1	.08	2	7	2	65	.03	0	.01	.01	.02	0	<1	0
0	11	.32	9	23	26	2	.3	5	.02	.04	.16	.01	12	3
0	54	1.55	72	103	424	114	.59	22	.08	.08	1.2	.13	61	12
0	50	1.34	74	146	634	127	.86	39	.15	.38	2.2	.21	286	12
0	39	1.62	48	102	439	899	.54	28	.06	.17	1.38	.15	149	52
0	18	.66	9	49	144	10	.38	49	.11	.11	.97	.11	131	10
0	18	.66	9	49	144	10	.38	49	.11	.11	.97	.11	131	10
0	21	.57	12	49	196	4	.5	74	.06	.09	.94	.02	121	22
0	21	.57	12	49	196	4	.5	74	.06	.09	.94	.02	121	22
0	19	2.2	12	52	205	468[2]	.48	64	.07	.12	1.14	.13	115	22
0	10	.42	5	33	104	9	.85	1	.03	.03	.18	.18	4	1
0	23	1.81	60	120	305	1	.96	1	21	.05	.43	.06	127	0
9	70	4.15	44	148	380	557	7.4	15	.07	.06	.63	.09	28	4
18	154	4.2	86	266	673	850	3.8	28	.12	.15	.89	.21	95	8
15	123	4.45	72	267	604	1105	4.81	39	.15	.14	2.32	.12	77	6
0	19	1.16	29	54	347	45	.37	16	.06	.05	.91	.1	55	11
0	25	1.76	50	100	369	26	.49	15	.06	.05	.69	.1	58	5
0	16	2.25	40	104	478	2	.89	0	.15	.05	.4	.15	78	0
0	29	.8	16	24	186	2	.22	42[3]	.05	.06	.38	.03	21	6
0	30	.55	14	16	76	9	.42	36[4]	.03	.05	.28	.04	6	6
0	18	.61	9	13	74	169[5]	.2	24[6]	.01	.04	.14	.02	21	3
0	29	.8	16	24	187	2	.23	5	.05	.06	.38	.04	21	6

(2)Low sodium pack contains 3 mg sodium.

(3)Data is for green varieties; yellow beans contain 10 RE per cup.

(4)Data is for green varieties; yellow beans contain 15 RE per cup.

(5)Low sodium pack contains 3 mg sodium per cup.

(6)For green varieties; yellow beans contain 14 RE per cup.

(For purposes of calculations, use "0" for t, <1, <.1, <.01, etc.)

Table A–1
Food Composition

Computer Code Number	Food Description	Measure	Wt (g)	H_2O (%)	Ener (cal)	Prot (g)	Carb (g)	Dietary Fiber (g)	Fat (g)	Fat Breakdown (g) Sat	Mono	Poly
	VEGETABLES AND LEGUMES—Cont.											
	Bean sprouts (mung):											
806	Raw	1 c	104	90	31	3	6	3	<1	t	t	.1
807	Cooked, stir-fried	1 c	124	84	62	5	13	4	<1	t	.1	.1
808	Cooked, boiled, drained	1 c	124	93	26	3	5	2	<1	t	t	t
	Beets, cooked from fresh:											
809	Sliced or diced	½ c	85	87	37	1	8	1	<1	t	t	.1
810	Whole beets, 2" diam	2 ea	100	87	44	2	10	1	<1	t	t	.1
	Beets, canned:											
811	Sliced or diced	½ c	85	91	26	1	6	1	<1	t	t	t
812	Pickled slices	½ c	114	82	74	1	19	2	<1	t	t	t
813	Beet greens, cooked, drained	½ c	72	89	19	2	4	1	<1	t	t	.1
	Broccoli, raw:											
817	Chopped	1 c	88	91	25	3	5	2	<1	t	t	.1
818	Spears	1 ea	151	91	42	4	8	4	1	.1	t	.3
	Broccoli, cooked from fresh:											
819	Spears	1 ea	180	91	50	5	9	5	1	.1	t	.3
820	Chopped	1 c	156	91	44	5	8	4	1	.1	t	.3
	Broccoli, cooked from frozen:											
821	Spear, small piece	3 ea	90	91	25	3	5	3	<1	t	t	.1
822	Chopped	1 c	184	91	51	6	10	5	<1	t	t	.1
1603	Broccoflower, steamed	3½ oz	100	90	32	3	6	3	<1	–	–	–
823	Brussels sprouts, cooked from fresh	½ c	78	87	30	2	7	3	<1	.1	t	.2
824	Brussels sprouts, cooked from frozen	½ c	77	87	33	3	6	3	<1	.1	t	.2
	Cabbage, common varieties:											
825	Raw, shredded or chopped	1 c	70	92	17	1	4	1	<1	t	t	.1
826	Cooked, drained	1 c	150	94	33	2	7	4	1	.1	t	.3
	Cabbage, Chinese:											
1178	Bok choy, raw, shredded	1 c	70	95	9	1	2	1	<1	t	t	.1
827	Bok choy, cooked, drained	1 c	170	96	20	3	3	3	<1	t	t	.1
828	Pe tsai, raw, chopped	1 c	76	94	12	1	2	1	<1	t	t	.1
	Cabbage, red, coarsely chopped:											
829	Raw	1 c	70	92	19	1	4	1	<1	t	t	.1
830	Cooked, drained	½ c	75	94	16	1	3	1	<1	t	t	.1
831	Cabbage, savoy, coarsely chopped, raw	1 c	70	91	19	1	4	2	<1	t	t	t
	Carrots, raw:											
832	Whole, 7 ½ x 1 ⅛"	1 ea	72	88	31	1	7	2	<1	t	t	.1
833	Grated	½ c	55	88	24	1	6	2	<1	t	t	t
	Carrots, cooked, sliced, drained:											
834	From fresh	½ c	78	87	35	1	8	3	<1	t	t	.1
835	From frozen	½ c	73	90	26	1	6	3	<1	t	t	t
836	Carrots, canned, sliced, drained	½ c	73	93	17	<1	4	1	<1	t	t	.1
837	Carrot juice, canned	½ c	123	89	49	1	11	2	<1	t	t	.1
	Cauliflower, flowerets:											
838	Raw	½ c	50	92	12	1	3	1	<1	t	t	t
839	Cooked from fresh, drained	½ c	62	93	14	1	3	1	<1	t	t	.1
840	Cooked, from frozen, drained	½ c	90	94	17	1	3	2	<1	t	t	.1

(Computer code number is for West Diet Analysis program)

PAGE KEY: A–2 = BEV A–4 = DAIRY A–10 = EGGS A–12 = FAT/OIL A–14 = FRUIT A–24 = BAKERY A–34 = GRAIN A–40 = FISH A–44 = MEATS A–48 = POULTRY A–50 = SAUSAGE A–52 = MIXED/FAST A–60 = NUTS/SEEDS A–62 = SWEETS A–66 = VEG/LEG A–78 = MISC A–80 = SOUPS/SAUCES A–84 = FAST A–96 = FRZN ENTREE A–98 = BABY FOODS

A

Chol (mg)	Calc (mg)	Iron (mg)	Magn (mg)	Phos (mg)	Pota (mg)	Sodi (mg)	Zinc (mg)	VT-A (RE)	Thia (mg)	Ribo (mg)	Niac (mg)	V-B6 (mg)	Fola (μg)	VT-C (mg)
0	13	.95	22	56	154	6	.43	2	.09	.13	.78	.09	63	14
0	16	2.36	41	98	272	11	1.12	4	.17	.22	1.49	.16	86	20
0	15	.81	17	35	125	12	.58	1	.06	.13	1.01	.07	36	14
0	14	.67	20	32	259	65	.3	3	.02	.03	.28	.06	68	3
0	16	.79	23	38	305	77	.35	4	.03	.04	.33	.07	80	4
0	13	1.55	14	14	125	232[1]	.18	1	.01	.03	.13	.05	26	3
0	12	.47	17	19	168	300	.3	1	.01	.05	.29	.06	30	3
0	82	1.37	49	29	654	174	.36	367	.08	.21	.36	.09	10	18
0	42	.77	22	58	286	24	.35	136[2]	.06	.1	.56	.14	62	82
0	72	1.33	38	100	491	41	.6	233[2]	.1	.18	.96	.24	107	141
0	83	1.51	43	106	526	47	.68	250[2]	.1	.2	1.03	.26	90	134
0	72	1.31	37	92	456	41	.59	217[2]	.09	.18	.89	.22	78	116
0	46	.55	18	49	162	22	.27	170[2]	.05	.07	.41	.12	27	36
0	94	1.12	37	101	331	44	.55	348[2]	.1	.15	.84	.24	103	74
0	32	.7	20	64	322	23	.5	67	.07	.09	.76	.18	48	63
0	28	.94	16	44	247	16	.26	56	.08	.06	.47	.14	47	48
0	19	.57	19	42	252	18	.28	46	.08	.09	.42	.22	78	35
0	33	.41	10	16	172	13	.13	9	.03	.03	.21	.07	30	22
0	46	.25	12	22	146	12	.13	19	.09	.08	.42	.17	30	30
0	73	.56	13	26	176	45	.13	210	.03	.05	.35	.14	46	31
0	158	1.77	19	49	631	58	.29	437	.05	.11	.73	.28	69	44
0	58	.24	10	22	180	7	.17	91	.03	.04	.3	.18	60	20
0	36	.34	10	29	144	8	.15	3	.03	.02	.21	.15	14	40
0	28	.26	8	22	105	6	.11	2	.03	.01	.15	.1	9	26
0	24	.28	20	29	161	20	.19	70	.05	.02	.21	.13	56	22
0	19	.36	11	32	232	25	.14	2024	.07	.04	.67	.11	10	7
0	15	.27	8	24	177	19	.11	1546	.05	.03	.51	.08	8	5
0	24	.48	10	23	177	51	.23	1913	.03	.04	.39	.19	11	2
0	20	.34	7	19	115	43	.17	1291	.02	.03	.32	.09	8	2
0	18	.47	6	17	130	175[3]	.19	1004	.01	.02	.4	.08	7	2
0	29	.57	17	52	359	36	.22	3166	.11	.07	.47	.27	5	10
0	11	.22	7	22	152	15	.14	1	.03	.03	.26	.11	28	23
0	10	.2	6	20	88	9	.11	1	.03	.03	.25	.11	27	27
0	15	.37	8	22	125	16	.12	2	.03	.05	.28	.08	37	28

(1)Low sodium pack contains 39 mg sodium.

(2)Vitamin A for whole plant: leaves are 1600 RE/100 g raw; flower clusters are 300/100 g raw; stalks are 40 RE/100 g raw.

(3)Low sodium pack contains 31 mg sodium.

(For purposes of calculations, use "0" for t, <1, <.1, <.01, etc.)

Table A–1
Food Composition

Computer Code Number	Food Description	Measure	Wt (g)	H_2O (%)	Ener (cal)	Prot (g)	Carb (g)	Dietary Fiber (g)	Fat (g)	Fat Breakdown (g) Sat	Mono	Poly
	VEGETABLES AND LEGUMES—Cont.											
	Celery, pascal type, raw:											
841	Large outer stalk, 8 x 1½" (root end)	1 ea	40	95	6	<1	1	1	<1	t	t	t
842	Diced	1 c	120	95	19	1	4	2	<1	t	t	.1
1179	Chard, swiss, raw, chopped	1 c	36	93	7	1	1	1	<1	t	t	t
1180	Chard, swiss, cooked	1 c	175	93	35	3	7	4	<1	t	t	.1
	Chickpeas (see Garbanzo Beans #854)											
	Collards, cooked, drained:											
843	From fresh	½ c	64	92	17	1	4	2	<1	t	t	.1
844	From frozen	½ c	85	88	31	3	6	3	<1	.1	t	.1
	Corn, cooked, drained:											
845	From fresh, on cob, 5" long	1 ea	77	73	72	2	17	3	1	.1	.2	.3
846	From frozen, on cob, 3½" long	1 ea	63	73	59	2	14	3	<1	.1	.1	.2
847	Kernels, cooked from frozen	½ c	82	76	66	2	17	3	<1	t	t	t
	Corn, canned:											
848	Cream style	½ c	128	79	92	2	23	2	1	.1	.2	.3
849	Whole kernel, vacuum pack	½ c	105	77	82	3	20	1	1	.1	.2	.2
	Cowpeas (see Black-eyed peas #814–816)											
850	Cucumber slices with peel	7 pce	28	96	4	<1	1	<1	<1	t	t	t
	Dandelion greens:											
851	Raw	1 c	55	86	25	1	5	1	<1	t	t	.2
852	Chopped, cooked, drained	1 c	105	90	35	2	7	1	1	.1	.1	.4
853	Eggplant, cooked	1 c	160	92	45	1	11	5	<1	.1	t	.1
1714	Endive, fresh, chopped	¼ c	13	94	2	<1	<1	<1	<1	t	t	t
856	Escarole/curly endive, chopped	1 c	50	94	8	1	2	1	<1	t	t	t
854	Garbanzo beans (chickpeas), cooked	1 c	164	60	267	14	45	10	4	.4	1	1.9
855	Great northern beans, cooked	1 c	177	69	209	15	37	11	1	.2	t	.3
857	Jerusalem artichoke, raw slices	1 c	150	78	114	3	26	2	<1	0	t	t
	Kale, cooked, drained:											
858	From fresh	½ c	65	91	21	1	4	2	<1	t	t	.1
859	From frozen	½ c	65	90	19	2	3	2	<1	t	t	.2
860	Kidney beans, canned	1 c	256	77	217	13	40	15	1	.1	.1	.5
1181	Kohlrabi, raw slices	1 c	140	91	38	2	9	2	<1	t	t	.1
861	Kohlrabi, cooked	1 c	165	90	48	3	11	2	<1	t	t	.1
1183	Leeks, raw, chopped	1 c	104	83	63	2	15	2	<1	t	t	.2
1182	Leeks, cooked, chopped	½ c	52	91	16	<1	4	2	<1	t	t	.1
862	Lentils, cooked from dry	½ c	99	70	115	9	20	5	<1	.1	.1	.2
1288	Lentils, sprouted, stir-fried	4 oz	113	69	115	10	24	4	1	.1	.1	.2
1289	Lentils, sprouted, raw	1 c	77	67	82	7	17	3	<1	t	.1	.2
	Lettuce:											
	Butterhead/Boston types:											
863	Head, 5" diameter	¼ ea	41	96	5	1	1	<1	<1	t	t	t
864	Leaves, inner or outer	4 ea	30	96	4	<1	1	<1	<1	t	t	t
	Iceberg/crisphead:											
865	Head, 6" diameter	¼ ea	135	96	17	1	3	1	<1	t	t	.1
866	Wedge, ¼ head	1 ea	135	96	18	1	3	1	<1	t	t	.1
867	Chopped or shredded	1 c	56	96	7	1	1	<1	<1	t	t	.1

(Computer code number is for West Diet Analysis program)

PAGE KEY: A–2 = BEV A–4 = DAIRY A–10 = EGGS A–12 = FAT/OIL A–14 = FRUIT A–24 = BAKERY A–34 = GRAIN A–40 = FISH A–44 = MEATS A–48 = POULTRY A–50 = SAUSAGE A–52 = MIXED/FAST A–60 = NUTS/SEEDS A–62 = SWEETS A–66 = VEG/LEG A–78 = MISC A–80 = SOUPS/SAUCES A–84 = FAST A–96 = FRZN ENTREE A–98 = BABY FOODS

Chol (mg)	Calc (mg)	Iron (mg)	Magn (mg)	Phos (mg)	Pota (mg)	Sodi (mg)	Zinc (mg)	VT-A (RE)	Thia (mg)	Ribo (mg)	Niac (mg)	V-B6 (mg)	Fola (μg)	VT-C (mg)
0	16	.16	4	10	115	35	.05	5	.02	.02	.13	.03	11	3
0	48	.48	13	30	344	104	.16	16	.06	.05	.39	.1	34	8
0	18	.65	29	17	136	77	.13	119	.01	.03	.14	.04	5	11
0	101	3.96	150	58	961	313	.58	550	.06	.15	.63	.15	15	31
0	15	.1	4	5	83	10	.07	175	.01	.03	.19	.03	4	8
0	179	.95	25	23	213	42	.23	508	.04	.1	.54	.1	64	22
0	2	.47	22	58	193	3	.48	16[1]	.13	.05	1.17	.17	23	4
0	2	.38	18	47	158	3	.4	13[1]	.11	.04	.96	.14	19	3
0	2	.25	15	38	113	4	.29	20[1]	.06	.06	1.05	.08	19	2
0	4	.49	22	65	172	364[2]	.68	13[1]	.03	.07	1.23	.08	57	6
0	5	.44	24	67	195	286[3]	.48	25[1]	.04	.08	1.23	.06	51	9
0	4	.07	3	6	41	1	.06	6	.01	.01	.06	.01	4	2
0	102	1.71	20	36	218	42	.23	770	.1	.14	.44	.14	15	19
0	147	1.89	25	44	243	46	.29	1227	.14	.18	.54	.17	13	19
0	10	.56	21	35	397	5	.24	10	.12	.03	.96	.14	23	2
0	7	.10	2	4	39	3	.1	26	.01	.01	.05	<.01	18	.813
0	26	.41	7	14	157	11	.39	103	.04	.04	.2	.01	71	3
0	80	4.74	79	276	477	11	2.51	5	.19	.1	.86	.23	282	2
0	120	3.77	88	292	692	4	1.56	<1	.28	.1	1.21	.21	181	2
0	21	5.1	25	117	644	6	.18	3	.3	.09	1.95	.12	20	6
0	47	.58	12	18	148	15	.16	481	.03	.05	.32	.09	9	27
0	90	.61	12	18	209	10	.12	413	.03	.07	.44	.06	9	16
0	61	3.23	72	240	658	873	1.41	0	.27	.22	1.17	.06	129	3
0	34	.56	27	64	490	28	.04	6	.07	.03	.56	.21	22	87
0	41	.66	31	74	561	35	.51	7	.07	.03	.64	.25	20	89
0	61	2.18	29	36	187	21	.12	10	.06	.03	.42	.24	67	12
0	16	.57	7	9	45	5	.03	2	.01	.01	.1	.06	13	2
0	19	3.3	36	178	365	2	1.26	1	.17	.07	1.05	.18	178	1
0	16	3.52	40	174	322	11	1.81	5	.25	.1	1.36	.19	76	14
0	19	2.47	28	133	247	8	1.16	4	.18	.1	.87	.15	77	13
0	13	.12	5	9	104	2	.07	39	.02	.02	.12	.02	30	3
0	10	.09	4	7	76	1	.05	29	.02	.02	.09	.01	22	2
0	25	.67	12	27	213	12	.3	44	.06	.04	.25	.05	76	5
0	25	.67	12	27	213	12	.3	45	.06	.04	.25	.05	76	5
0	11	.28	5	11	88	5	.12	18	.03	.02	.1	.02	31	2

(1)For yellow varieties; white varieties contain only a trace of vitamin A.

(2)Low sodium pack contains 4 mg sodium per ½ cup.

(3)Low sodium pack contains 6 mg sodium per cup.

(For purposes of calculations, use "0" for t, <1, <.1, <.01, etc.)

Table A–1
Food Composition

Computer Code Number	Food Description	Measure	Wt (g)	H_2O (%)	Ener (cal)	Prot (g)	Carb (g)	Dietary Fiber (g)	Fat (g)	Fat Breakdown (g) Sat	Mono	Poly
	VEGETABLES AND LEGUMES—Cont.											
	Lettuce—Cont.											
868	Looseleaf, chopped	½ c	28	94	5	<1	1	<1	<1	t	t	t
869	Romaine, chopped	½ c	28	95	4	<1	1	<1	<1	t	t	t
870	Romaine, inner leaf	3 ea	30	95	5	<1	1	<1	<1	t	t	t
	Mushrooms:											
871	Raw, sliced	½ c	35	92	9	1	2	<1	<1	t	t	.1
872	Cooked from fresh, pieces	½ c	78	91	21	2	4	2	<1	t	t	.1
873	Canned, drained	½ c	78	91	19	1	4	2	<1	t	t	.1
	Mustard greens:											
874	Cooked from fresh	½ c	70	94	10	2	1	1	<1	t	.1	t
875	Cooked from frozen	½c	75	94	14	2	2	1	<1	t	.1	t
876	Navy beans, cooked from dry	1 c	182	63	258	16	48	16	1	.3	.1	.4
	Okra, cooked:											
877	From fresh pods	8 ea	85	90	27	2	6	2	<1	t	t	t
878	From frozen slices	½ c	92	91	34	2	8	2	<1	.1	t	.1
1236	Batter fried from fresh	1 c	92	69	175	3	11	2	13	2.1	3.4	7.1
	Onions:											
879	Raw, chopped	1 c	160	90	61	2	14	3	<1	t	t	.1
880	Raw, sliced	1 c	115	90	44	1	10	2	<1	t	t	.1
881	Cooked, drained, chopped	½ c	105	88	46	1	11	1	<1	t	t	.1
882	Dehydrated flakes	¼ c	14	4	45	1	12	1	<1	t	t	t
	Spring/green onions, chopped:											
883	Bulb and top	½ c	50	90	16	1	4	1	<1	t	t	t
1185	Green tops only	1 c	100	92	34	2	5	2	<1	.1	.1	.2
1184	White part only	½ c	50	92	25	<1	5	1	<1	t	t	t
884	Onion rings, breaded, heated f/frozen	2 ea	20	28	81	1	8	<1	5	1.7	2.2	1
	Parsley:											
885	Raw, chopped	½ c	30	88	11	1	2	1	<1	t	.1	t
886	Raw, sprigs	5 ea	5	88	2	<1	<1	<1	<1	t	t	t
887	Freeze dried	¼ c	1	2	4	<1	1	1	<1	t	t	t
888	Parsnips, sliced, cooked	½ c	78	78	63	1	15	3	<1	t	.1	t
	Peas:											
	Black-eyed, cooked:											
814	From dry, drained	½ c	85	70	99	7	18	8	<1	.1	t	.2
815	From fresh, drained	½ c	82	75	80	3	17	6	<1	.1	t	.1
816	From frozen, drained	½ c	85	66	112	7	20	7	1	.1	.1	.2
889	Edible pod peas, cooked	1 c	160	89	67	5	11	4	<1	.1	t	.2
890	Green, canned, drained	½ c	85	82	59	4	11	3	<1	.1	t	.1
891	Green, cooked from frozen	½ c	80	79	62	4	11	4	<1	t	t	.1
892	Split, green, cooked from dry	½ c	98	69	116	8	21	5	<1	.1	.1	.2
1187	Peas & carrots, cooked from frozen	½ c	80	86	38	2	8	3	<1	.1	t	.2
1186	Peas & carrots, canned w/liquid	½ c	128	88	49	3	11	4	<1	.1	t	.2
	Peppers, hot:											
893	Hot green chili, canned	½ c	68	92	17	1	4	1	<1	t	t	t
894	Hot green chili, raw	1 ea	45	88	18	1	4	1	<1	t	t	t
1715	Hot red chili, raw, diced	1 tbs	9	88	4	<1	1	<1	<1	t	t	t
895	Jalapeno, chopped, canned	½ c	68	90	16	1	3	2	<1	t	t	.2

(Computer code number is for West Diet Analysis program)

Chol (mg)	Calc (mg)	Iron (mg)	Magn (mg)	Phos (mg)	Pota (mg)	Sodi (mg)	Zinc (mg)	VT-A (RE)	Thia (mg)	Ribo (mg)	Niac (mg)	V-B6 (mg)	Fola (μg)	VT-C (mg)
0	19	.39	3	7	74	3	.08	53	.01	.02	.11	.01	14	5
0	10	.31	2	13	81	2	.07	73	.03	.03	.14	.01	38	7
0	11	.33	2	13	87	2	.07	78	.03	.03	.15	.01	41	7
0	2	.43	3	36	129	1	.26	0	.04	.16	1.44	.03	7	1
0	5	1.36	9	68	277	2	.68	0	.06	.23	3.48	.07	14	3
0	9	.62	12	51	100	331	.56	0	.07	.02	1.24	.05	10	0
0	51	.49	10	29	141	11	.08	212	.03	.04	.3	.07	51	18
0	76	.84	10	18	104	19	.15	335	.03	.04	.19	.08	52	10
0	127	4.51	107	286	670	2	1.93	<1	.37	.11	.97	.3	255	2
0	54	.38	48	48	273	4	.47	49	.11	.05	.74	.16	39	14
0	88	.62	47	42	215	3	.57	47	.09	.11	.72	.04	133	11
15	104	.77	37	106	214	137	.5	43	.13	.1	.75	.13	37	10
0	32	.35	16	53	251	5	.3	0	.07	.03	.24	.19	30	10
0	23	.25	11	38	181	3	.22	0	.05	.02	.17	.13	22	7
0	23	.25	12	37	174	3	.22	0	.04	.02	.17	.13	16	5
0	36	.22	13	42	227	3	.26	0	.07	.01	.14	.22	23	10
0	36	.74	10	18	138	8	.19	19	.03	.04	.26	.03	32	9
0	56	2.2	21	39	260	7	.22	40	.07	.1	.6	0	80	51
0	20	.44	8	20	115	3	.12	<1	.03	.02	.17	.05	18	13
0	6	.34	4	16	26	75	.08	5	.06	.03	.72	.01	3	<1
0	41	1.86	15	17	166	17	.32	156	.03	.03	.39	.03	46	40
0	6	.31	2	2	27	2	.04	26	<.01	.01	.03	.01	9	4
0	2	.75	5	8	88	5	.09	88	.01	.03	.15	.02	21	2
0	29	.45	23	53	286	8	.2	0	.06	.04	.56	.07	45	10[1]
0	20	2.15	45	133	238	3	1.1	2	.17	.05	.42	.09	178	<1
0	106	.92	43	42	345	3	.85	65	.08	.12	1.16	.05	105	2
0	20	1.8	42	104	319	4	1.21	7	.22	.05	.62	.08	120	2
0	67	3.15	42	88	384	6	.59	21	.2	.12	.86	.23	47	77
0	17	.81	14	57	147	186[2]	.6	65	.1	.07	.62	.05	38	8
0	19	1.26	23	72	134	70	.75	54	.23	.08	1.18	.09	47	8
0	14	1.26	35	97	355	2	.98	1	.19	.05	.87	.05	63	<1
0	18	.75	13	39	126	54	.36	621	.18	.05	.92	.07	21	6
0	29	.96	18	59	128	332	.74	739	.09	.07	.74	.11	23	8
0	5	.34	10	12	127	797	.12	41[3]	.01	.03	.54	.1	7	46
0	8	.54	11	21	153	3	.13	35[3]	.04	.04	.43	.13	11	108
0	2	.11	2	4	32	.66	.03	101	.01	.01	.09	.03	2	23
0	18	1.9	8	12	92	993	.13	116	.02	.03	.34	.14	9	9

(1)Value for Vitamin C is highest right after harvest and drops after that.

(2)Low sodium pack contains 1.7 mg sodium.

(3)Data is for green chili peppers; red varieties contain 809 RE vitamin A per ½ cup; 484 RE per whole pepper.

(For purposes of calculations, use "0" for t, <1, <.1, <.01, etc.)

A

Table A–1
Food Composition

Computer Code Number	Food Description	Measure	Wt (g)	H_2O (%)	Ener (cal)	Prot (g)	Carb (g)	Dietary Fiber (g)	Fat (g)	Fat Breakdown (g)		
										Sat	Mono	Poly
	VEGETABLES AND LEGUMES—Cont.											
	Peppers, sweet, green:											
896	Whole pod (90 g with refuse), raw	1 ea	74	92	20	1	5	1	<1	t	t	.1
897	Cooked, chopped (1 pod cooked = 73 g)	½ c	68	92	19	1	5	2	<1	t	t	.1
	Peppers, sweet, red:											
1286	Raw, chopped	1 c	100	92	27	1	6	2	<1	t	t	.1
1287	Cooked, chopped	½ c	68	92	19	1	5	1	<1	t	t	.1
898	Pinto beans, cooked from dry	½ c	85	64	117	7	22	10	<1	.1	.1	.2
1191	Poi, two finger	¼ c	60	72	67	<1	16	<1	<1	t	t	t
	Potatoes:[1]											
	Baked in oven, 4¾" x 2⅓" diam:											
899	With skin	1 ea	202	71	220	5	51	4	<1	.1	t	.1
900	Flesh only	1 ea	156	75	145	3	33	2	<1	t	t	.1
901	Skin only	1 ea	58	47	114	2	27	2	<1	t	t	t
	Baked in microwave, 4¾" x 2⅓" diam:											
902	With skin	1 ea	202	72	212	5	49	5	<1	.1	t	.1
903	Flesh only	1 ea	156	74	156	3	36	2	<1	t	t	.1
904	Skin only	1 ea	58	63	77	3	17	2	<1	t	t	t
	Boiled, about 2½" diam:											
905	Peeled after boiling	1 ea	136	77	118	3	27	2	<1	t	t	.1
906	Peeled before boiling	1 ea	135	77	116	2	27	2	<1	t	t	.1
	French fried, strips 2–3½" long:											
907	Oven heated	10 pce	50	35	163	2	19	1	12	3.8	7.2	.9
908	Fried in vegetable oil	10 ea	50	38	157	2	20	1	8	2.5	1.6	3.8
1188	Fried in veg and animal oil	10 ea	50	38	157	2	20	1	8	3.4	4	.5
909	Hashed browns from frozen	1 c	156	56	340	5	44	3	18	7	8	2.1
	Mashed:											
910	Home recipe with whole milk[2]	½ c	105	78	81	2	18	2	1	.3	.2	.1
911	Home recipe with milk and marg.	½ c	105	76	111	2	17	1	4	1.1	1.9	1.3
912	Prepared from flakes; water, milk, margarine, salt added	½ c	110	76	124	2	16	1	6	1.6	2.5	1.7
	Potato products, prepared:											
	Au gratin:											
913	From dry mix	½ c	122	79	114	3	16	2	5	3.2	1.4	.2
914	From home recipe[3]	½ c	122	74	162	6	14	2	9	4.3	3.2	1.3
	Scalloped:											
915	From dry mix	½ c	122	79	114	3	16	1	5	3.2	1.5	.2
916	From home recipe[4]	½ c	122	81	105	4	13	1	5	1.7	1.6	.9
	Potato salad (see Mixed Dishes #715)											
1192	Potato puffs, cooked from frozen	½ c	62	53	137	2	19	2	7	3.2	2.7	.5
917	Potato chips	14 ea	28	2	152	2	15	1	10	3.1	2.8	3.5
918	Pumpkin, cooked from fresh, mashed	1 c	245	94	49	2	12	4	<1	.1	t	t
919	Pumpkin, canned	½ c	123	90	42	1	10	3	<1	.2	t	t
920	Red radishes	10 ea	45	95	8	<1	2	1	<1	t	t	t

(1)Vitamin C varies with length of storage. After 3 months of storage approximately two-thirds of the ascorbic acid remains; after 6 to 7 months, about one-third remains.

(2)Recipe: 84% potatoes, 15% whole milk, 1% salt.

(3)Recipe: 55% potatoes, 30% whole milk, 9% cheddar cheese, 3% butter, 2% flour, 1% salt.

(4)Recipe: 59% potatoes, 36% whole milk, 2% butter, 2% flour, 1% salt.

(Computer code number is for West Diet Analysis program)

PAGE KEY: A–2 = BEV A–4 = DAIRY A–10 = EGGS A–12 = FAT/OIL A–14 = FRUIT A–24 = BAKERY A–34 = GRAIN A–40 = FISH A–44 = MEATS A–48 = POULTRY A–50 = SAUSAGE A–52 = MIXED/FAST A–60 = NUTS/SEEDS A–62 = SWEETS A–66 = VEG/LEG A–78 = MISC A–80 = SOUPS/SAUCES A–84 = FAST A–96 = FRZN ENTREE A–98 = BABY FOODS

Chol (mg)	Calc (mg)	Iron (mg)	Magn (mg)	Phos (mg)	Pota (mg)	Sodi (mg)	Zinc (mg)	VT-A (RE)	Thia (mg)	Ribo (mg)	Niac (mg)	V-B6 (mg)	Fola (µg)	VT-C (mg)
0	7	.34	7	14	131	1	.09	47	.05	.02	.38	.18	16	66
0	6	.31	7	12	112	1	.08	40	.04	.02	.32	.16	11	51
0	9	.46	10	19	177	2	.12	570	.07	.03	.51	.25	22	190
0	6	.31	7	12	112	1	.08	256	.04	.02	.32	.16	11	116
0	41	2.23	47	137	400	2	.92	<1	.16	.08	.34	.13	147	2
0	10	.53	14	23	110	7	.13	1	.08	.02	.66	.16	13	2
0	20	2.75	54	115	844	16	.65	0	.22	.07	3.31	.7	22	26[1]
0	8	.55	39	78	608	8	.45	0	.16	.03	2.18	.47	14	20[1]
0	20	4.08	25	59	332	12	.28	0	.07	.06	1.78	.36	12	8[1]
0	22	2.5	54	212	903	16	.73	0	.24	.06	3.45	.69	24	30[1]
0	8	.64	39	170	641	11	.51	0	.2	.04	2.54	.5	19	24[1]
0	27	3.45	21	48	377	9	.3	0	.04	.04	1.29	.28	10	9[1]
0	7	.42	30	60	515	5	.41	0	.14	.03	1.96	.41	14	18[1]
0	11	.42	27	54	441	7	.36	0	.13	.03	1.77	.36	12	10[1]
0	6	.83	11	48	269	306	.2	0	.04	.02	1.33	.11	11	3
0	9	.38	17	46	366	108	.19	0	.09	.01	1.63	.12	14	5
6	9	.38	17	46	366	108	.19	0	.09	.01	1.63	.12	14	5
0	23	2.36	26	112	680	53	.5	0	.17	.03	3.78	.2	10	10
2	27	.28	19	50	314	318	.3	20	.09	.04	1.18	.24	9	7[1]
2[5]	27	.27	19	48	303	310	.28	21	.09	.04	1.13	.23	8	6[1]
4[5]	53	.24	20	61	256	365	.2	23	.12	.05	.73	.01	8	11
6	102	.39	18	116	268	538	.29	38	.02	.1	1.15	.05	8	4
18[6]	146	.78	24	138	485	530	.84	47	.08	.14	1.22	.21	10	12
13	44	.47	17	68	249	418	.31	26	.02	.07	1.26	.05	12	4
7[7]	70	.7	23	77	463	410	.49	23	.08	.11	1.29	.22	11	13
0	19	.97	12	30	235	462	.19	1	.12	.04	1.34	.14	10	4
0	7	.46	19	47	362	169[8]	.31	0	.05	.06	1.09	.19	13	9
0	37	1.4	22	73	564	2	.56	265	.08	.19	1.01	.11	21	11
0	32	1.71	28	43	253	6	.21	2712	.03	.07	.45	.07	15	5
0	9	.13	4	8	104	11	.13	<1	<.01	.02	.13	.03	12	10

(5)Data is for margarine; if butter is used, cholesterol = 25 mg for 29 total mg.

(6)Data is for butter; if margarine is used, cholesterol = 37 mg.

(7)Data is for butter; if margarine is used cholesterol = 15 mg.

(8)If no salt added, sodium = 2 mg.

(For purposes of calculations, use "0" for t, <1, <.1, <.01, etc.)

Table A-1
Food Composition

Computer Code Number	Food Description	Measure	Wt (g)	H_2O (%)	Ener (cal)	Prot (g)	Carb (g)	Dietary Fiber (g)	Fat (g)	Fat Breakdown (g) Sat	Mono	Poly
	VEGETABLES AND LEGUMES—Cont.											
921	Refried beans, canned	½ c	126	72	135	8	23	9	1	.5	.6	.2
1375	Rutabaga, cooked cubes	½ c	85	89	33	1	7	1	<1	t	t	.1
922	Sauerkraut, canned with liquid	½ c	118	92	22	1	5	3	<1	t	t	.1
923	Seaweed, kelp, raw	1 oz	28	82	12	<1	3	<1	<1	.1	t	t
924	Seaweed, spirulina, dried	1 oz	28	5	82	16	7	1	2	.8	.2	.6
1557	Snow peas, stir-fried	1 c	165	89	69	5	12	4	<1	.1	t	.1
925	Soybeans, cooked from dry	½ c	86	63	149	14	9	3	8	1.1	1.7	4.4
	Soybean products:											
926	Miso	½ c	138	46	282	16	38	7	8	1.2	1.8	4.7
927	Tofu (soybean curd, regular)	½ c	124	85	94	10	2	1	6	.9	1.3	3.3
	Spinach:											
928	Raw, chopped	1 c	56	92	12	2	2	1	<1	t	t	.1
929	Cooked, from fresh, drained	½ c	90	91	21	3	3	2	<1	t	t	.1
930	Cooked from frozen (leaf)	½ c	95	90	27	3	5	2	<1	t	t	.1
931	Canned, drained solids	½ c	107	92	25	3	4	3	1	.1	t	.2
	Spinach soufflé (see Mixed Dishes)											
	Squash, summer varieties, cooked:											
932	Varieties averaged	½ c	90	94	18	1	4	1	<1	.1	t	.1
933	Crookneck	½ c	90	94	18	1	4	1	<1	.1	t	.1
934	Zucchini	½ c	90	95	14	1	4	1	<1	t	t	t
	Squash, winter varieties, cooked:											
	Average of all varieties, baked:											
935	Mashed	1 c	245	89	96	2	21	7	2	.3	.1	.6
936	Cubes	1 c	205	89	80	2	18	6	1	.3	.1	.5
937	Acorn, baked, mashed	½ c	122	83	68	1	18	5	<1	t	t	.1
1218	Acorn, boiled, mashed	½ c	122	90	42	1	11	3	<1	t	t	t
	Butternut:											
938	Baked cubes	1 c	205	88	82	2	21	6	<1	t	t	.1
1219	Baked, mashed	½ c	122	88	49	1	13	3	<1	t	t	t
1193	Cooked from frozen	½ c	120	88	47	1	12	3	<1	t	t	t
1194	Hubbard, baked, mashed	½ c	120	85	60	3	13	3	1	.2	.1	.3
1195	Hubbard, boiled, mashed	½ c	118	91	35	2	8	3	<1	.1	t	.2
1196	Spaghetti, baked or boiled	½ c	77	92	22	1	5	2	<1	t	t	.1
1189	Succotash, cooked from frozen	½ c	85	74	79	4	17	4	1	.1	.1	.4
	Sweet potatoes:											
939	Baked in skin, peeled, 5 x 2" diam	1 ea	114	73	117	2	28	3	<1	t	t	.1
940	Boiled without skin, 5 x 2" diam	1 ea	151	73	159	2	37	5	<1	.1	t	.2
941	Candied, 2½ x 2"	1 pce	105	67	143	1	29	2	3	1.4	.7	.2
	Canned:											
942	Solid pack	½ c	128	74	129	3	30	3	<1	.1	t	.1
943	Vacuum pack, mashed	½ c	127	76	116	2	27	3	<1	.1	t	.1
944	Vacuum pack, 3¾ x 1"	2 pce	80	76	73	1	17	2	<1	t	t	.1

(Computer code number is for West Diet Analysis program)

Chol (mg)	Calc (mg)	Iron (mg)	Magn (mg)	Phos (mg)	Pota (mg)	Sodi (mg)	Zinc (mg)	VT-A (RE)	Thia (mg)	Ribo (mg)	Niac (mg)	V-B6 (mg)	Fola (µg)	VT-C (mg)
0	58	2.24	49	106	497	536	1.73	<1	.06	.07	.61	.13	106	8
0	41	.45	20	48	277	17	.3	48	.07	.03	.61	.09	13	16
0	35	1.73	15	24	201	780	.22	2	.02	.03	.17	.15	28	17
0	48	.81	34	12	25	66	.35	3	.01	.04	.13	<.01	51	<1
0	34	8.08	55	33	386	296	.57	16	.67	1.04	3.63	.1	27	3
0	71	3.43	40	87	330	7	.45	21	.22	.12	.94	.25	55	84
0	88	4.42	73	211	443	1	.99	1	.13	.24	.34	.2	46	1
0	92	3.76	58	210	226	5014	4.57	12	.13	.34	1.19	.3	45	0
0	130	6.65	126	120	150	9	.99	11	.1	.06	.24	.06	19	<1
0	55	1.52	44	27	312	44	.3	376	.04	.11	.4	.11	108	16
0	122	3.21	78	50	419	63	.68	737	.09	.21	.44	.22	131	9
0	139	1.44	65	46	283	81	.66	739	.06	.16	.4	.14	102	12
0	136	2.46	81	47	370	159[1]	.49	939	.02	.15	.41	.11	105	15
0	24	.32	22	35	173	1	.35	26[2]	.04	.04	.46	.06	18	5
0	24	.32	22	35	173	1	.35	26[2]	.04	.04	.46	.08	18	5
0	12	.31	20	36	228	3	.16	22[2]	.04	.04	.38	.07	15	4
0	34	.81	20	49	1070	2	.64	872	.21	.06	1.72	.18	69	23
0	29	.68	16	41	896	2	.53	730	.17	.05	1.44	.15	57	20
0	54	1.14	53	55	535	5	.21	53	.2	.02	1.08	.24	23	13
0	32	.68	32	33	322	4	.13	32	.12	.01	.65	.14	14	8
0	84	1.23	59	55	582	8	.27	1435	.15	.03	1.99	.25	39	31
0	50	.73	35	33	348	5	.16	858	.09	.02	1.19	.15	23	18
0	23	.69	11	17	160	2	.14	401	.06	.05	.56	.08	20	4
0	20	.56	26	28	430	10	.18	725	.09	.06	.67	.21	19	11
0	12	.33	15	16	253	6	.12	473	.05	.03	.39	.12	11	8
0	16	.26	9	11	91	14	.15	9	.03	.02	.63	.08	6	3
0	13	.75	20	59	225	38	.38	20	.06	.06	1.11	.08	28	5
0	32	.51	23	63	396	11	.33	2486	.08	.14	.69	.27	26	28
0	32	.85	15	41	276	20	.41	2573	.08	.21	.97	.37	17	26
8[3]	27	1.19	12	27	198	73	.16	440	.02	.04	.41	.04	12	7
0	38	1.7	31	67	268	96	.27	1935	.03	.11	1.22	.3	14	7
0	28	1.13	28	62	398	67	.23	1017	.05	.07	.94	.24	21	34
0	18	.71	18	39	250	42	.14	638	.03	.05	.59	.15	13	21

(1) Dietary pack contains 58 mg sodium.

(2) Applies to squash including skin; flesh has no appreciable vitamin A value.

(3) For recipe using butter.

(For purposes of calculations, use "0" for t, <1, <.1, <.01, etc.)

A

A

Table A–1
Food Composition

Computer Code Number	Food Description	Measure	Wt (g)	H_2O (%)	Ener (cal)	Prot (g)	Carb (g)	Dietary Fiber (g)	Fat (g)	Fat Breakdown (g) Sat	Mono	Poly
	VEGETABLES AND LEGUMES—Cont.											
	Tomatoes:											
945	Raw, whole, 2⅗" diam	1 ea	123	94	26	1	6	2	<1	.1	.1	.2
946	Raw, chopped	1 c	180	94	38	2	8	2	1	.1	.1	.2
947	Cooked from raw	1 c	240	92	65	3	14	4	1	.1	.2	.4
948	Canned, solids and liquid	1 c	240	94	48	2	10	4	1	.1	.1	.2
949	Tomato juice, canned	1 c	244	94	41	2	10	2	<1	t	t	.1
	Tomato products, canned:											
950	Paste	1 c	262	74	220	10	49	11	2	.3	.4	.9
951	Puree	1 c	250	87	102	4	25	6	<1	t	t	.1
952	Sauce	1 c	245	89	73	3	18	4	<1	.1	.1	.2
953	Turnips, cubes, cooked from fresh	½ c	78	94	14	1	4	2	<1	t	t	t
	Turnip greens, cooked:											
954	From fresh, leaves and stems	1 c	144	93	29	2	6	4	<1	.1	t	.1
955	From frozen, chopped	1 c	164	90	49	5	8	7	1	.2	t	.3
956	Vegetable juice cocktail, canned	½ c	121	93	23	1	6	1	<1	t	t	t
	Vegetables, mixed:											
957	Canned, drained	½ c	81	87	38	2	8	3	<1	t	t	.1
958	Frozen, cooked, drained	½ c	91	83	53	3	12	3	<1	t	t	.1
959	Water chestnuts, canned: Slices	½ c	70	86	35	1	9	2	<1	t	t	t
960	Water chestnuts, canned: Whole	4 ea	28	86	14	<1	4	1	<1	t	t	t
1190	Watercress, fresh, chopped	½ c	17	95	2	<1	<1	<1	<1	t	t	t
	MISCELLANEOUS											
	Baking powders for home use:											
	Sodium aluminum sulfate:											
962	With monocalcium phosphate monohydrate	1 tsp	3	2	4	<1	1	0	0	0	0	0
963	With monocalcium phosphate monohydrate, calcium sulfate	1 tsp	3	5	2	0	1	0	0	0	0	0
964	Straight phosphate	1 tsp	4	4	2	<1	1	0	0	0	0	0
965	Low sodium	1 tsp	4	6	4	<1	2	0	<1	0	0	0
1204	Baking soda	1 tsp	3	<1	0	0	0	0	0	0	0	0
966	Basil, dried	1 tbs	4	6	11	1	3	1	<1	–	–	–
961	Carob flour	1 c	103	4	394	5	92	13	1	.1	.2	.2
967	Catsup:	¼ c	61	67	64	1	17	1	<1	t	t	.1
968	Tablespoon	1 tbs	15	67	16	<1	4	<1	<1	t	t	t
1200	Cayenne/red pepper	1 tbs	5	8	16	1	3	2	1	.2	.1	.4
969	Celery seed	1 tsp	2	6	8	<1	1	<1	1	t	.3	.1
1203	Chili powder:	1 tbs	8	8	25	1	4	3	1	.3	.3	.6
970	Teaspoon	1 tsp	3	8	8	<1	1	1	<1	.1	.1	.2

(Computer code number is for West Diet Analysis program)

PAGE KEY: A–2 = BEV A–4 = DAIRY A–10 = EGGS A–12 = FAT/OIL A–14 = FRUIT A–24 = BAKERY A–34 = GRAIN A–40 = FISH A–44 = MEATS A–48 = POULTRY A–50 = SAUSAGE A–52 = MIXED/FAST A–60 = NUTS/SEEDS A–62 = SWEETS A–66 = VEG/LEG A–78 = MISC A–80 = SOUPS/SAUCES A–84 = FAST A–96 = FRZN ENTREE A–98 = BABY FOODS

Chol (mg)	Calc (mg)	Iron (mg)	Magn (mg)	Phos (mg)	Pota (mg)	Sodi (mg)	Zinc (mg)	VT-A (RE)	Thia (mg)	Ribo (mg)	Niac (mg)	V-B6 (mg)	Fola (μg)	VT-C (mg)
0	6	.55	13	29	273	11	.11	76	.07	.06	.77	.1	18	23[1]
0	9	.81	20	43	400	16	.16	112	.11	.09	1.13	.14	27	34[1]
0	14	1.34	34	74	670	26	.26	178	.17	.14	1.8	.23	31	55
0	62[2]	1.46	29	46	530	391[3]	.38	144	.11	.07	1.76	.22	19	36
0	22	1.42	27	46	537	881[4]	.34	137	.11	.08	1.64	.27	49	45
0	92	7.83	133	206	2441	170[5]	2.1	647	.41	.5	8.44	1	59	110
0	37	2.33	60	100	1050	50[6]	.55	340	.18	.13	4.3	.38	27	88
0	34	1.89	47	78	909	1482[7]	.61	240	.16	.14	2.82	.38	23	32
0	17	.17	6	15	105	39	.16	0	.02	.02	.23	.05	7	9
0	197	1.15	32	42	292	42	.2	792	.06	.1	.59	.26	170	39
0	248	3.18	43	56	366	25	.67	1308	.09	.12	.77	.11	65	36
0	13	.51	13	21	234	442	.24	142	.05	.03	.88	.17	25	33
0	22	.86	13	34	237	121	.33	949	.04	.04	.47	.06	19	4
0	23	.74	20	46	154	32	.45	389	.06	.11	.77	.07	17	3
0	3	.61	3	13	83	6	.27	<1	.01	.02	.25	.11	4	1
0	1	.25	1	5	33	2	.11	<1	<.01	.01	.1	.04	2	<1
0	20	.03	4	10	56	7	.02	80	.01	.02	.03	.02	2	7
0	58	0	<1	87	4	328	0	0	0	0	0	0	0	0
0	170	.32	1	63	1	307	0	0	0	0	0	0	0	0
0	280	.43	1	377	<1	300	<.01	0	0	0	0	0	0	0
0	186	.35	1	295	434	4	.03	0	0	0	0	0	0	0
0	0	0	0	0	0	821	0	0	0	0	0	0	0	0
0	95	1.89	19	22	154	2	.26	42	.01	.01	.31	–	–	3
0	358	3.04	56	81	852	36	.95	1	.05	.47	1.96	.38	30	<1
0	12	.43	13	24	295	726	.14	62	.05	.04	.84	.11	9	9
0	3	.1	3	6	72	178	.03	15	.01	.01	.21	.03	2	2
0	8	.41	8	15	106	2	.13	220	.02	.05	.46	–	–	4
0	35	.9	9	11	28	3	.14	<1	.01	.01	.1	–	–	<1
0	22	1.12	13	24	149	79	.21	272	.03	.06	.61	–	4	5
0	7	.37	4	8	50	26	.07	91	.01	.02	.2	–	1	2

(1)Year-round average. From June through October, ascorbic acid is approximately 32 mg and 47 mg, respectively, for one tomato and 1 c chopped tomato. From November through May, market samples average around 12 and 18 mg, respectively.

(2)Calcium is added as a firming agent.

(3)Dietary pack contains 31 mg sodium.

(4)If no salt is added, sodium content is 24 mg.

(5)If salt is added, sodium content is 2070 mg.

(6)If salt is added, sodium content is 998 mg.

(7)With salt added.

(For purposes of calculations, use "0" for t, <1, <.1, <.01, etc.)

Table A–1
Food Composition

Computer Code Number	Food Description	Measure	Wt (g)	H_2O (%)	Ener (cal)	Prot (g)	Carb (g)	Dietary Fiber (g)	Fat (g)	Fat Breakdown (g) Sat	Mono	Poly
	MISCELLANEOUS—Cont.											
	Chocolate:											
971	Baking, unsweetened, square	1 oz	28	1	148	3	8	4	16	9.2	5.2	.5
	For other chocolate items, see Sweeteners & Sweets											
972	Cilantro/coriander, fresh	1 tbs	1	93	<1	<1	<1	<1	<1	t	t	t
1197	Cornstarch	1 tbs	8	8	30	<1	7	<1	<1	t	t	t
973	Cinnamon	1 tsp	2	9	6	<1	2	1	<1	t	t	t
974	Curry powder	1 tsp	2	9	6	<1	1	<1	<1	t	.2	t
1202	Dill weed, dried	1 tbs	3	7	8	1	2	<1	<1	–	–	–
1705	Dip, french onion	1 tbs	14	70	31	<1	<1	<1	3	2	1	.1
975	Garlic cloves	1 ea	3	59	4	<1	1	<1	<1	t	0	t
976	Garlic powder	1 tsp	3	6	9	<1	2	<1	<1	t	t	t
977	Gelatin, dry, unsweetened: Envelope	1 ea	7	13	23	6	0	0	<1	t	t	t
978	Ginger root, slices, raw	2 pce	4	82	3	<1	1	<1	<1	t	t	t
1198	Horseradish, prepared	1 tbs	15	87	6	<1	1	<1	<1	t	t	t
1199	Hummous/hummus	1 c	246	35	420	12	50	10	21	3	9	8
979	Mustard, prepared (1 packet = 1 tsp)	1 tsp	5	80	4	<1	<1	<1	<1	t	.2	t
	Miso (see #926 under Vegetables and Legumes, Soybean products)											
980	Olives, green	5 ea	19	78	23	<1	<1	<1	2	.3	1.9	.2
981	Olives, ripe, pitted	5 ea	22	80	26	<1	1	1	2	.3	1.8	.2
982	Onion powder	1 tsp	2	5	5	<1	2	<1	<1	t	t	t
983	Oregano, ground	1 tsp	1	7	5	<1	1	<1	<1	t	t	.1
984	Paprika	1 tsp	2	9	6	<1	1	<1	<1	t	t	.2
985	Black pepper	1 tsp	2	10	5	<1	1	<1	<1	t	t	t
	Pickles:											
986	Dill, medium, 3¾ x 1¼" diam	1 ea	65	92	12	<1	3	1	<1	t	t	t
987	Fresh pack, slices, 1½" diam x ¼"	2 pce	15	79	11	<1	3	<1	<1	0	0	t
988	Sweet, medium	1 ea	35	65	41	<1	11	<1	<1	t	t	t
989	Pickle relish, sweet	2 tbs	30	63	41	<1	10	1	<1	t	t	.1
	Popcorn (see Grain Products #539–541)											
1201	Sage, ground	1 tsp	1	8	2	<1	<1	<1	<1	t	t	t
1347	Salsa, from recipe	1 tbs	14	94	2	<1	1	<1	<1	t	t	t
990	Salt	1 tsp	5	0	0	0	0	0	0	0	0	0
	Salt substitutes:											
1205	Morton, salt substitute	1 tsp	2	0	0	0	<1	0	0	0	0	0
1207	Morton, Light Salt	1 tsp	6	0	0	0	0	0	0	0	0	0
1206	Norcliff Thayer, No Salt, packet	1 ea	1	0	0	0	0	0	0	0	0	0
991	Vinegar, cider	½ c	120	94	14	0	7	0	0	0	0	0
	Yeast:											
992	Baker's, dry, active, package	1 ea	7	8	21	3	3	2	<1	t	.2	t
993	Brewer's, dry	1 tbs	8	5	23	3	3	3	<1	t	t	0
	SOUPS, SAUCES, AND GRAVIES											
	SOUPS, canned, condensed:											
	Unprepared, condensed:											
1210	Cream of celery	1 c	251	85	180	3	18	2	11	2.8	2.6	5
1215	Cream of chicken	1 c	251	82	233	7	18	1	15	4.2	6.5	3
1216	Cream of mushroom	1 c	251	81	259	4	19	1	19	5.1	3.6	8.9
1220	Onion	1 c	246	86	113	8	16	1	3	.5	1.5	1.3

(Computer code number is for West Diet Analysis program)

Chol (mg)	Calc (mg)	Iron (mg)	Magn (mg)	Phos (mg)	Pota (mg)	Sodi (mg)	Zinc (mg)	VT-A (RE)	Thia (mg)	Ribo (mg)	Niac (mg)	V-B6 (mg)	Fola (μg)	VT-C (mg)
0	21	1.79	88	118	236	4	1.14	3	.02	.05	.31	.03	2	0
0	1	.02	<1	<1	5	<1	<.01	3	<.01	<.01	.01	<.01	<1	<1
0	<1	.04	<1	1	<1	1	<.01	0	0	0	0	0	0	0
0	28	.86	1	1	11	1	.04	1	<.01	<.01	.03	.02	–	1
0	10	.59	5	7	31	1	.08	2	<.01	.01	.07	–	–	<1
0	55	1.51	14	17	102	6	.1	0	.01	.01	.09	.04	–	–
6	17	.01	2	13	22	27	.04	28	.01	.02	.02	<.01	2	<1
0	5	.05	1	5	12	1	.03	0	.01	<.01	.02	.04	<1	1
0	2	.08	2	12	31	1	.07	0	.01	<.01	.02	.57	2	<1
0	4	.08	2	3	1	14	.01	0	<.01	.02	.01	0	2	0
0	1	.02	2	1	18	1	.01	0	<.01	<.01	.03	.01	<1	<1
0	9	.13	4	5	43	14	.18	0	0	0	0	.01	2	0
0	123	4	71	275	428	600	2.7	6	.26	.13	1	.98	146	19.4
0	4	.1	2	4	6	63	.03	0	0	0	0	<.01	0	0
0	12	.31	4	3	11	468	.01	6	0	0	0	<.01	<1	0
0	20	.74	1	1	2	146	.05	9	0	0	.01	<.01	0	<1
0	8	.06	3	7	20	1	.05	0	.01	<.01	.01	.03	3	<1
0	24	.66	4	3	25	<1	.07	10	<.01	<.01	.09	–	–	1
0	4	.5	4	7	49	1	.08	127	.01	.04	.32	–	–	1
0	9	.61	4	4	26	1	.03	<1	<.01	<.01	.02	0	–	0
0	6	.34	7	14	75	833	.09	21	.01	.02	.04	.01	1	1
0	5	.27	1	4	30	101	0	2	0	<.01	0	<.01	0	1
0	1	.21	1	4	11	328	.03	5	<.01	.01	.06	<.01	<1	<1
0	6	.24	1	4	60	214	.02	3	0	.01	0	0	0	2
0	11	.19	3	1	7	<1	.03	4	<.01	<.01	.04	–	–	<1
0	1	.06	1	3	21	53	.02	23	.01	<.01	.05	.01	1	5
0	14	.01	2	3	<1	2132	.02	0	0	0	0	0	0	0
0	10	0	0	9	933	0	0	0	0	0	0	0	0	0
0	3	0	4	0	1500	1099	0	0	0	0	0	0	0	0
0	–	–	–	–	385	0	–	0	0	0	0	0	0	0
0	7	.7	1	8	120	1	.14	0	0	0	0	0	0	0
0	4	1.16	7	90	140	3	.45	0	.16	.38	2.79	.11	164	<1
0	17[1]	1.38	18	140	151	10	.63	0	1.25	.34	3.03	.4	313	0
28	80	1.26	13	75	245	1900	.3	60	.06	.1	.66	.02	5	1
20	68	1.2	5	75	175	1972	1.26	113	.06	.12	1.64	.03	3	<1
3	65	1.05	10	85	168	2033	1.19	0	.06	.17	1.62	.02	8	2
0	54	1.35	5	22	137	2115	1.23	0	.07	.05	1.21	.1	30	2

(1)Value varies from 6 to 60 mg.

(For purposes of calculations, use "0" for t, <1, <.1, <.01, etc.)

A

A

Table A–1
Food Composition

Computer Code Number	Food Description	Measure	Wt (g)	H_2O (%)	Ener (cal)	Prot (g)	Carb (g)	Dietary Fiber (g)	Fat (g)	Fat Breakdown (g) Sat	Mono	Poly
	SOUPS, SAUCES, AND GRAVIES—Cont.											
	SOUPS, canned, condensed—Cont.											
	Prepared w/equal volume whole milk:											
994	Clam chowder, New England	1 c	248	85	163	9	17	1	7	2.9	2.3	1.1
1209	Cream of celery	1 c	248	86	163	6	14	<1	10	3.9	2.5	2.6
995	Cream of chicken	1 c	248	85	190	7	15	<1	11	4.6	4.5	1.6
996	Cream of mushroom	1 c	248	85	203	6	15	<1	14	5.1	3	4.6
1214	Cream of potato	1 c	248	87	148	6	17	<1	6	3.8	1.7	.6
1213	Oyster stew	1 c	245	89	134	6	10	0	8	5	2.1	.3
997	Tomato	1 c	248	85	161	6	22	–	6	2.9	1.6	1.1
	Prepared with equal volume of water:											
998	Bean with bacon	1 c	253	84	172	8	23	9	6	1.5	2.2	1.8
999	Beef broth/bouillon/consommé	1 c	240	98	17	3	<1	0	1	.3	.2	t
1000	Beef noodle	1 c	244	92	83	5	9	1	3	1.1	1.2	.5
1001	Chicken noodle	1 c	241	92	75	4	9	1	2	.7	1.1	.6
1002	Chicken rice	1 c	241	94	60	4	7	1	2	.5	.9	.4
1208	Chili beef	1 c	250	85	170	7	21	9	7	3.3	2.8	.3
1003	Clam chowder, Manhatten	1 c	244	92	78	2	12	1	2	.4	.4	1.3
1004	Cream of chicken	1 c	244	91	117	3	9	<1	7	2.1	3.3	1.5
1005	Cream of mushroom	1 c	244	90	129	2	9	<1	9	2.4	1.7	4.2
1006	Minestrone	1 c	241	91	82	4	11	1	3	.6	.7	1.1
1211	Onion	1 c	241	93	58	4	8	1	2	.3	.7	.7
1007	Split pea & ham	1 c	253	82	189	10	28	5	4	1.8	1.8	.6
1008	Tomato	1 c	244	90	85	2	17	<1	2	.4	.4	1
1009	Vegetable beef	1 c	244	92	78	6	10	<1	2	.9	.8	.1
1010	Vegetarian vegetable	1 c	241	92	72	2	12	<1	2	.3	.8	.7
1707	Ready to Serve											
	Chunky Chicken Soup	½ c	126	84	89	6	9	<1	3	1	1.5	.7
	SOUPS, dehydrated:											
	Unprepared, dry products:											
1011	Beef bouillon, packet	1 ea	6	3	14	1	1	<1	1	.3	.2	t
1012	Onion soup, packet	1 ea	34	4	100	4	18	4	2	.5	1.2	.2
	Prepared with water:											
1299	Beef broth/bouillon	1 c	244	97	19	1	2	0	1	.3	.3	t
1376	Chicken broth	1 c	244	97	22	1	1	0	1	.3	.4	.4
1013	Chicken noodle	1 c	251	94	53	3	8	<1	1	.3	.5	.3
1122	Cream of chicken	1 c	261	91	107	2	13	1	5	3.4	1.2	.4
1014	Onion	1 c	246	96	27	1	5	<1	1	.1	.3	.1
1217	Split pea	1 c	255	87	124	7	21	3	1	.4	.7	.3
1015	Tomato vegetable	1 c	252	93	55	2	10	1	1	.4	.3	.1
	SAUCES											
	From dry mixes, prepared with milk:											
1016	Cheese sauce	1 c	279	77	307	16	23	1	17	9.3	5.3	1.6
1017	Hollandaise	1 c	259	84	240	5	14	<1	20	11.6	5.9	.9
1018	White sauce	1 c	264	81	240	10	21	<1	13	6.4	4.7	1.7
	From home recipe:											
1019	White sauce, medium[1]	1 c	250	77	355	9	20	<1	27	7.8	9.1	8.8
	Ready to serve:											
1020	Barbeque sauce	1 tbs	16	81	10	<1	1	<1	<1	t	.1	.1
1706	Chili sauce, tomato base	1 tbs	17	68	18	<1	4	<1	<1	t	t	t
1021	Soy sauce	1 tbs	18	71	10	1	2	0	<1	t	t	t
1380	Teriyaki sauce	1 tbs	18	68	15	1	3	0	0	0	0	0

(1)Made with enriched flour, margarine, and whole milk. (Computer code number is for West Diet Analysis program)

PAGE KEY: A–2 = BEV A–4 = DAIRY A–10 = EGGS A–12 = FAT/OIL A–14 = FRUIT A–24 = BAKERY A–34 = GRAIN A–40 = FISH A–44 = MEATS A–48 = POULTRY A–50 = SAUSAGE A–52 = MIXED/FAST A–60 = NUTS/SEEDS A–62 = SWEETS A–66 = VEG/LEG A–78 = MISC A–80 = SOUPS/SAUCES A–84 = FAST A–96 = FRZN ENTREE A–98 = BABY FOODS

Chol (mg)	Calc (mg)	Iron (mg)	Magn (mg)	Phos (mg)	Pota (mg)	Sodi (mg)	Zinc (mg)	VT-A (RE)	Thia (mg)	Ribo (mg)	Niac (mg)	V-B6 (mg)	Fola (µg)	VT-C (mg)
22	186	1.49	22	156	300	992	.8	40	.07	.24	1.03	.13	10	3
32	186	.69	22	151	310	1009	.2	67	.07	.25	.44	.06	8	1
27	181	.67	17	151	273	1046	.67	94	.07	.26	.92	.07	8	1
20	178	.59	20	156	270	1076	.64	37	.08	.28	.91	.06	10	2
22	166	.55	17	161	322	1061	.67	67	.08	.24	.64	.09	9	1
32	166	1.05	20	161	235	1041	10.3	44	.07	.23	.34	.06	10	4
17	158	1.81	22	148	449	932	.29	109	.13	.25	1.52	.16	21	68
3	81	2.05	45	131	402	951	1.03	89	.09	.03	.57	.04	32	2
0	14	.41	5	31	129	782	0	0	<.01	.05	1.87	.02	5	0
5	15	1.1	5	46	100	952	1.54	63	.07	.06	1.07	.04	4	<1
7	17	.77	5	36	55	1106	.39	72	.05	.06	1.39	.03	2	<1
7	17	.75	1	22	101	815	.26	65	.02	.02	1.13	.02	1	<1
12	42	2.13	30	147	525	1035	1.4	150	.06	.07	1.07	.16	17	4
2	27	1.63	12	41	187	578	.98	98	.03	.04	.82	.1	10	4
10	34	.61	2	37	88	986	.63	56	.03	.06	.82	.02	2	<1
2	46	.51	5	49	100	1032	.59	0	.05	.09	.72	.01	5	1
2	34	.92	7	55	313	911	.73	234	.05	.04	.94	.1	16	1
0	26	.67	2	12	67	1053	.61	0	.03	.02	.6	.05	15	1
8	23	2.28	48	212	400	1006	1.32	45	.15	.08	1.47	.07	3	2
0	12	1.76	7	34	264	871	.24	68	.09	.05	1.42	.11	15	66
5	17	1.12	5	41	173	956	1.54	190	.04	.05	1.03	.08	10	2
0	22	1.08	7	34	209	822	.46	301	.05	.05	.92	.05	11	1
15	13	.87	4	57	88	445	.50	65	.04	.09	2.21	.03	2	1
1	4	.06	3	19	27	1018	0	<1	<.01	.01	.27	.01	2	0
2	48	.51	22	110	226	3044	.2	1	.1	.21	1.73	.03	6	1
0	10	.02	7	24	37	1361	.07	1	<.01	.02	.36	0	0	0
0	15	.07	5	12	24	1483	.01	12	.01	.03	.19	0	2	0
3	32	.5	7	32	31	1276	.2	5	.07	.06	.88	.01	1	<1
3	76	.26	5	97	214	1184	1.57	123	.1	.2	2.61	.05	5	1
0	12	.15	5	29	64	849	.06	1	.03	.06	.48	0	1	<1
3	20	.94	43	124	224	1147	.56	5	.21	.14	1.26	.05	39	0
0	8	.63	20	31	104	1141	.17	20	.06	.04	.79	.05	10	7
53	569	.28	47	438	552	1565	.97	117	.15	.56	.32	.14	13	2
52	124	.9	8	127	124	1564	.7	220	.04	.18	.06	.5	22	<1
34	425	.26	264	256	444	797	.55	92	.08	.45	.53	.07	16	3
29	263	.73	32	217	345	370	.94	310	.19	.42	.98	.1	14	2
0	3	.12	1	3	27	128	.03	14	<.01	<.01	.06	.01	1	1
0	3	.14	2	9	63	228	.05	24	.02	.01	.27	.02	1	3
0	3	.36	6	20	32	1027	.07	0	.01	.02	.6	.03	3	0
0	4	.31	11	28	40	689	.02	0	<.01	.01	.23	.02	4	0

(For purposes of calculations, use "0" for t, <1, <.1, <.01, etc.)

Table A–1
Food Composition

Computer Code Number	Food Description	Measure	Wt (g)	H_2O (%)	Ener (cal)	Prot (g)	Carb (g)	Dietary Fiber (g)	Fat (g)	Fat Breakdown (g)		
										Sat	Mono	Poly
	SOUPS, SAUCES, AND GRAVIES—Cont.											
	SAUCES—Cont.											
	Spaghetti sauce, canned:											
1377	Plain	1 c	249	75	271	5	40	3	12	1.7	6.1	3.3
1378	With meat	1 c	257	74	309	9	39	8	14	2.8	7.2	3.3
1379	With mushrooms	½ c	123	75	108	2	13	1	3	.4	1.5	.8
	GRAVIES											
	Canned:											
1022	Beef	1 c	233	87	123	9	11	1	5	2.7	1.2	.2
1023	Chicken	1 c	238	85	188	5	13	<1	14	3.4	6.1	3.5
1024	Mushroom	1 c	238	89	119	3	13	<1	6	1	2.8	2.4
1025	From dry mix: Brown	1 c	258	92	75	2	13	<1	2	.8	.7	.1
1026	From dry mix: Chicken	1 c	260	91	83	3	14	<1	2	.5	.9	.4
	FAST FOOD RESTAURANTS											
	ARBY'S											
1402	Bac'n cheddar deluxe	1 ea	226	56	526	27	33	<1	36	9.7	15.6	11.2
	Roast beef sandwiches:											
1403	Regular	1 ea	147	51	353	22	32	1	15	7.3	5.1	2.4
1404	Junior	1 ea	86	48	218	12	22	<1	8	3.9	2.9	1.7
1405	Super	1 ea	234	58	501	25	50	1	22	8.5	8.2	5.4
1407	Beef 'n cheddar	1 ea	197	57	455	26	28	1	27	7.6	12.1	7.1
1408	Chicken breast sandwich	1 ea	184	52	493	23	48	1	25	5.1	9.6	10.3
1412	Ham'n cheese sandwich	1 ea	156	62	292	23	19	<1	14	4.7	6.3	2.7
1413	Turkey sandwich, deluxe	1 ea	197	61	375	24	32	<1	17	4.1	4.7	7.8
	Milk shakes:											
1419	Chocolate	1 ea	340	74	451	10	76	<1	12	2.8	7	1.7
1420	Jamocha	1 ea	326	75	368	9	59	0	10	2.5	6.4	1.6
1421	Vanilla	1 ea	312	75	330	10	46	0	11	3.9	5.3	2.3
	Source: Arby's Inc. for the basic nutrients. Values for some nutrients from known values of major ingredients.											
	BURGER KING											
	Croissant sandwiches:											
1422	Egg, bacon, & cheese	1 ea	119	49	364	15	19	<1	24	8.1	12.1	3
1423	Egg, sausage, & cheese	1 ea	163	46	547	21	23	1	41	13.3	20.5	5.1
1424	Egg, ham, & cheese	1 ea	145	57	348	19	19	<1	21	7	11.1	2
	Whopper sandwiches:											
1425	Whopper	1 ea	265	59	603	26	44	<1	35	11.8	10.8	12.8
1426	Whopper with cheese	1 ea	289	57	694	31	46	<1	43	15.7	12.8	12.8
1427	Double beef	1 ea	351	58	844	46	45	<1	53	19	19	13
1428	Double beef & cheese	1 ea	374	57	933	51	47	<1	61	23.9	21.9	14
1429	Hamburger deluxe	1 ea	136	53	339	15	28	<1	19	5.9	5.9	6.9
1430	Cheeseburger deluxe	1 ea	158	52	408	19	30	<1	24	8.4	7.3	7.3
1431	Hamburger	1 ea	109	48	275	15	28	<1	11	4	5	1
1432	Cheeseburger	1 ea	120	50	315	17	28	<1	15	6.9	5.9	1
1433	Double cheeseburger with bacon	1 ea	159	43	512	32	26	<1	31	13.9	12.9	2
1434	Chicken sandwich	1 ea	230	46	688	26	56	<1	40	8	11	20.1
1435	Chicken tenders	1 ea	95	50	249	17	15	0	14	3.2	5.3	3.2
1436	Ham & cheese sandwich	1 ea	230	59	471	24	44	<1	23	10	8	4
1437	Ocean catch fish fillet	1 ea	189	50	482	19	48	<1	24	3.9	5.8	12.7

(Computer code number is for West Diet Analysis program)

PAGE KEY: A–2 = BEV A–4 = DAIRY A–10 = EGGS A–12 = FAT/OIL A–14 = FRUIT A–24 = BAKERY A–34 = GRAIN A–40 = FISH A–44 = MEATS A–48 = POULTRY A–50 = SAUSAGE A–52 = MIXED/FAST A–60 = NUTS/SEEDS A–62 = SWEETS A–66 = VEG/LEG A–78 = MISC A–80 = SOUPS/SAUCES A–84 = FAST A–96 = FRZN ENTREE A–98 = BABY FOODS

Chol (mg)	Calc (mg)	Iron (mg)	Magn (mg)	Phos (mg)	Pota (mg)	Sodi (mg)	Zinc (mg)	VT-A (RE)	Thia (mg)	Ribo (mg)	Niac (mg)	V-B6 (mg)	Fola (µg)	VT-C (mg)
0	70	1.62	60	90	956	1235	.52	306	.14	.15	3.76	.88	54	28
16	69	2	61	117	981	1215	1.41	299	.14	.17	4.64	.9	54	27
0	15	1	15	30	333	496	.34	242	.08	.08	.93	.16	13	9
7	14	1.63	5	70	188	1304	2.33	0	.07	.08	1.54	.02	5	0
5	48	1.12	5	69	259	1373	1.9	264	.04	.1	1.05	.02	5	0
0	17	1.57	5	36	252	1356	1.67	0	.08	.15	1.6	.05	29	0
3	67	.23	10	44	57	1075	.31	0	.04	.08	.81	0	0	0
3	39	.26	10	47	62	1133	.32	0	.05	.15	.78	.03	3	3
83	150	4.5	–	–	422	1672	3	100	.38	.51	8	–	–	9
39	80	3.6	16	120	368	588	3.75	1	.23	.43	7	.2	14	1
20	40	1.8	8	60	197	345	1.5	–	.15	.25	4	.1	7	–
40	100	4.5	25	190	503	798	3.75	150	.38	.6	9	.3	21	4
63	60	3.6	24	260	335	955	3.75	80	.38	.51	8	.22	19	0
91	80	3.6	30	180	330	1019	.15	–	.23	.51	8	.38	18	5
45	200	2.7	31	405	312	1350	.9	50	.15	.26	6	.31	26	24
39	80	2.7	30	250	346	1047	1.5	60	.23	.43	12	.52	20	5
36	250	2.7	48	350	410	341	1.5	40	.06	.85	.8	.14	14	5
35	250	2.7	36	350	525	262	1.5	60	.06	.77	5	.14	14	2
32	300	2.7	36	350	686	281	1.5	100	.23	.85	4	.14	37	2
229	137	2.02	–	–	–	725	–	151	.32	.3	2.02	.11	–	2
275	149	2.97	–	–	–	1009	–	154	.37	.33	4.1	.12	–	<1
243	137	2.22	–	–	–	969	–	151	.49	.32	3.02	.22	–	10
88	78	4.81	–	–	–	849	–	59	.32	.4	6.87	.34	–	14
113	206	4.82	–	–	–	1156	–	84	.33	.47	6.88	.32	–	14
169	91	7.3	–	–	–	933	–	60	.34	.56	10	–	–	14
193	221	7.28	–	–	–	1241	–	85	.35	.63	9.97	–	–	14
42	39	2.76	–	–	–	489	–	30	.23	.25	3.94	.14	–	6
59	110	2.93	–	–	–	682	–	89	.24	.3	4.19	–	–	6
37	37	2.73	–	–	–	510	–	15	.23	.25	4.04	–	–	3
50	101	3.77	–	–	–	656	–	69	.23	.29	3.97	–	–	3
104	167	3.78	–	–	–	743	–	84	.31	.42	5.96	–	–	1
82	79	3.31	–	–	–	1423	–	13	.45	.31	10	–	–	1
49	19	.74	–	–	–	571	–	5	.08	.08	7.39	–	–	<1
70	195	3.2	–	–	–	1534	–	85	.87	.42	6	–	–	7
55	82	2.14	–	–	–	856	–	19	.27	.2	3.9	–	–	2

(For purposes of calculations, use "0" for t, <1, <.1, <.01, etc.)

Table A–1
Food Composition

Computer Code Number	Food Description	Measure	Wt (g)	H_2O (%)	Ener (cal)	Prot (g)	Carb (g)	Dietary Fiber (g)	Fat (g)	Fat Breakdown (g) Sat	Mono	Poly
	BURGER KING—Cont.											
1439	French fries (salted)	1 ea	74	42	227	3	24	1	13	6.7	6	14
1440	Onion rings	1 ea	79	33	277	4	31	<1	16	3.7	7.3	3.7
1441	Milk shakes, chocolate	1 ea	273	75	313	9	47	<1	10	5.8	3.8	0
1442	Milk shakes, vanilla	1 ea	273	75	321	9	49	<1	10	5.8	2.9	0
1443	Fried apple pie	1 ea	125	49	311	3	44	1	14	4	8	1
	Source: Burger King Corporation.											
	DAIRY QUEEN											
	Ice cream cones:											
1446	Small vanilla	1 ea	85	63	140	4	22	0	4	3	1	–
1447	Regular vanilla	1 ea	142	65	230	6	36	0	7	5	1	1
1448	Large vanilla	1 ea	213	66	340	9	53	0	10	7	1	1
1450	Chocolate dipped	1 ea	156	60	330	6	40	<1	16	8	4	3
1453	Chocolate sundae	1 ea	177	62	300	6	54	<1	7	5	1	1
1455	Banana split	1 ea	383	68	529	9	96	2	11	8.3	3.1	.4
1456	Peanut Buster Parfait	1 ea	305	52	710	16	94	1	32	10	10	9
1457	Hot Fudge Brownie Delight	1 ea	266	52	619	10	89	1	25	12.2	10.5	1.7
1459	Buster bar	1 ea	149	45	450	11	40	<1	29	9	10	8
1460	Dilly bar	1 ea	85	55	210	3	21	<1	13	6	3	3
1461	DQ ice cream sandwich	1 ea	60	47	138	3	24	<1	4	2	1	1
1463	Milk shakes, regular	1 ea	418	71	548	13	93	<1	15	8.4	2.1	2.1
1464	Milk shakes, large	1 ea	489	71	636	14	107	<1	17	10.6	2.1	2.1
1466	Malted milkshake	1 ea	418	68	610	13	106	<1	14	8	2	2
1468	Float	1 ea	397	76	410	5	82	0	7	5	1	1
1469	Freeze	1 ea	397	72	500	9	89	0	12	7.5	3.4	.4
	Mr. Misty:											
1470	Regular	1 ea	330	81	250	0	63	0	0	0	0	0
1471	Kiss	1 ea	89	81	70	0	17	0	0	0	0	0
1472	Freeze	1 ea	411	72	500	9	91	0	12	7.4	3.4	.4
1473	Float	1 ea	411	78	390	5	74	0	7	4.3	2	.3
	Sandwiches:											
1474	Chicken	1 ea	202	56	455	25	39	<1	21	4.2	7.4	8.5
1475	Fish fillet	1 ea	177	57	385	17	41	<1	17	3.1	5.2	8.3
1476	Fish fillet with cheese	1 ea	191	56	436	20	41	<1	22	6.2	7.3	8.3
1477	Hamburger, single	1 ea	148	55	323	18	30	<1	17	6.2	6.2	1
1478	Hamburger, double	1 ea	210	57	488	33	31	<1	26	12.7	11.7	2.1
1480	Cheeseburger, single	1 ea	162	55	379	21	31	<1	19	9.3	7.3	1
1481	Cheeseburger, double	1 ea	239	54	603	39	33	<1	36	19	13.7	2.1
	Hot dog:											
1483	Regular	1 ea	100	51	283	9	23	<1	16	6.1	7.1	2
1484	With cheese	1 ea	114	49	333	12	24	<1	21	9.1	8.1	2
1485	With chili	1 ea	128	52	323	11	26	2	19	7.1	8.1	2
1489	French fries, small	1 ea	71	38	210	3	29	1	10	2	5	3
1490	French fries, large	1 ea	113	49	344	4	46	2	16	3.5	7.1	5.3
1491	Onion rings	1 ea	85	46	240	4	29	<1	12	3	5	4
	Source: International Dairy Queen.											

(Computer code number is for West Diet Analysis program)

PAGE KEY: A–2 = BEV A–4 = DAIRY A–10 = EGGS A–12 = FAT/OIL A–14 = FRUIT A–24 = BAKERY A–34 = GRAIN A–40 = FISH A–44 = MEATS A–48 = POULTRY A–50 = SAUSAGE A–52 = MIXED/FAST A–60 = NUTS/SEEDS A–62 = SWEETS A–66 = VEG/LEG A–78 = MISC A–80 = SOUPS/SAUCES A–84 = FAST A–96 = FRZN ENTREE A–98 = BABY FOODS

A

Chol (mg)	Calc (mg)	Iron (mg)	Magn (mg)	Phos (mg)	Pota (mg)	Sodi (mg)	Zinc (mg)	VT-A (RE)	Thia (mg)	Ribo (mg)	Niac (mg)	V-B6 (mg)	Fola (μg)	VT-C (mg)
14	6	.33	–	–	–	161	–	0	.07	.2	5	–	–	3
3	114	.73	–	–	–	514	–	0	.05	.03	.66	–	–	<1
30	250	1.54	–	–	–	190	–	58	.12	.53	.12	–	–	0
32	284	–	–	–	–	205	–	77	.11	.55	.12	–	–	0
4	15	1.2	–	–	–	412	–	4	.27	.16	.6	–	–	5
15	100	.4	–	100	150	60	–	25	.03	.17	.06	–	–	<1
20	150	.7	–	200	260	95	–	49	.06	.34	.11	.09	–	<1
30	250	1.4	–	300	380	140	–	98	.12	.51	.17	–	–	<1
20	150	.7	–	200	290	100	–	49	.06	.34	.11	.09	–	<1
20	200	1.1	–	200	290	140	–	49	.06	.34	.3	.14	–	<1
31	259	1.87	–	363	893	259	–	166	.16	.53	.41	.21	–	16
30	250	1.8	–	450	660	410	–	74	.15	.43	2	.22	–	2
30	174	1.57	–	262	445	297	–	64	.1	.3	.26	.16	–	1
15	100	1.1	–	250	400	220	–	25	.12	.17	2	.08	–	1
10	100	.4	–	100	170	50	–	25	.03	.17	–	.06	–	<1
5	59	.04	–	59	103	133	–	15	.03	.07	.39	.05	–	<1
47	474	2.84	–	526	600	242	–	194	.24	.81	.42	.2	–	<1
53	583	3.82	–	636	700	276	–	212	.32	1	.42	–	–	<1
45	450	4.5	–	600	570	230	–	184	.3	.85	.8	.19	–	<1
20	200	1.1	–	200	–	85	–	40	.06	.26	.05	.09	–	<1
30	300	1.8	–	350	–	180	–	98	.15	.51	–	.15	–	2
0	0	0	–	–	–	10	–	0	0	0	–	0	–	2
0	0	0	–	–	–	10	–	0	0	0	–	0	–	0
30	300	1.4	–	200	–	140	–	98	.12	.51	–	.18	–	2
20	200	.7	–	200	–	95	–	49	.06	.26	–	.09	–	1
58	159	5.71	–	264	370	804	–	21	.63	.62	8.46	–	–	3
47	156	3.75	–	156	292	656	–	16	.62	.44	8.33	–	–	–
62	260	3.74	–	208	301	882	–	62	.69	.53	8.3	–	–	–
47	104	3.75	–	156	271	605	–	10	.31	.18	5.21	–	–	1
101	106	6.68	–	318	440	668	–	21	.48	.36	9.55	–	–	1
62	208	3.74	–	260	280	831	–	114	.31	.18	5.19	–	–	1
127	370	6.66	–	529	465	1131	–	169	.48	.45	9.52	–	–	1
25	81	1.41	–	101	172	707	–	0	.12	.14	3.03	–	–	<1
35	151	1.41	–	202	182	928	–	86	.12	.17	3.03	–	–	<1
30	81	1.81	–	151	262	726	–	60	.15	.26	4.03	–	–	<1
0	10	.34	–	60	430	115	–	0	.06	.02	.8	–	–	9
0	13	.95	–	88	689	177	–	0	.08	.03	1.06	–	–	13
0	20	.72	–	60	90	135	–	15	.09	.05	.4	–	–	2

(For purposes of calculations, use "0" for t, <1, <.1, <.01, etc.)

A

Table A–1
Food Composition

Computer Code Number	Food Description	Measure	Wt (g)	H_2O (%)	Ener (cal)	Prot (g)	Carb (g)	Dietary Fiber (g)	Fat (g)	Fat Breakdown (g)		
										Sat	Mono	Poly
	JACK IN THE BOX											
	Breakfast items:											
1492	Breakfast Jack sandwich	1 ea	126	50	307	18	30	–	13	5.2	5	2.5
1494	Sausage crescent	1 ea	156	39	584	22	28	–	43	15.5	21.5	5.7
1495	Supreme crescent	1 ea	146	39	547	20	27	–	40	13.2	18.9	7.8
1496	Pancake platter	1 ea	231	45	612	15	87	–	22	8.6	7.6	3.5
1497	Scrambled egg platter	1 ea	249	52	653	21	58	–	37	10.2	19.4	5.1
	Sandwiches:											
1498	Hamburger	1 ea	98	43	267	13	28	1	11	4.1	4.9	2
1499	Cheeseburger	1 ea	113	46	318	16	33	1	14	5.7	5.9	2.3
1500	Jumbo Jack burger	1 ea	205	52	539	24	39	1	31	10.2	12	7.4
1501	Jumbo Jack burger with cheese	1 ea	246	50	688	32	47	1	41	14.2	15.2	9.1
1505	Chicken supreme	1 ea	228	53	597	25	44	–	36	9.3	13.8	10.6
1583	Double cheeseburger	1 ea	149	50	467	21	33	–	27	12.3	11.6	3.1
1508	Tacos, regular	1 ea	81	57	191	8	16	–	11	–	–	–
1509	Tacos, super	1 ea	135	63	288	12	21	–	17	–	–	–
1513	Taco salad	1 ea	402	76	503	34	28	–	31	13.4	11.9	1.6
1516	French fries	1 ea	109	38	351	4	45	–	17	4	.7	.6
1517	Hash browns	1 ea	62	51	170	1	15	–	12	2.8	7.4	.3
1518	Onion rings	1 ea	108	34	398	5	40	–	24	5.8	15.9	.9
	Milk shakes:											
1519	Chocolate	1 ea	322	77	330	11	55	0	7	4.3	2.1	–
1520	Strawberry	1 ea	328	77	320	10	55	0	7	4.3	2	–
1521	Vanilla	1 ea	317	76	320	10	57	0	6	3.6	1.8	–
1522	Apple turnover	1 ea	119	35	410	4	49	–	22	6.6	12.5	1.8
	Source: Jack in the Box Restaurant, Inc.											
	KENTUCKY FRIED CHICKEN											
	Original recipe:											
1253	Center breast	1 ea	95	53	234	23	7	<1	13	3.1	6.4	1.6
1251	Side breast	1 ea	69	46	205	14	8	<1	13	3.2	6.7	1.7
1250	Drumstick	1 ea	47	51	120	11	3	<1	7	1.8	3.4	1.1
1252	Thigh	1 ea	88	51	249	15	9	<1	17	4.5	7.9	2.6
1249	Wing	1 ea	42	41	136	9	5	<1	9	2.3	4.6	1.4
	Dinners:											
1254	2-pce dinner, white	1 ea	322	59	702	32	56	2	39	9.5	18.4	7.9
1255	2-pce dinner, dark	1 ea	346	71	721	33	57	1	40	10.1	17.9	8.5
1256	2-pce dinner, combo	1 ea	341	47	741	32	58	1	42	10.7	19.3	8.8
	Extra crispy recipe:											
1261	Center breast	1 ea	104	51	263	25	9	<1	15	3.7	8.3	1.6
1259	Side breast	1 ea	84	45	262	17	11	<1	17	4.2	9.8	1.8
1258	Drumstick	1 ea	58	48	171	11	5	<1	12	2.9	6.5	1.4
1260	Thigh	1 ea	107	44	365	18	13	<1	27	6.9	14.4	3.8
1257	Wing	1 ea	53	35	207	10	8	<1	15	3.6	8.7	2
	Dinners:											
1262	2-pce dinner, white	1 ea	348	57	829	34	62	1	49	11.8	25.6	8.6
1263	2-pce dinner, dark	1 ea	375	59	878	36	62	1	54	13.3	26.9	9.9
1264	2-pce dinner, combo	1 ea	371	57	919	35	65	1	58	14.1	29.4	10.6
1265	Mashed potatoes	⅓ c	80	81	60	2	12	1	1	.2	.4	t
1268	Corn-on-the-cob	1 ea	143	70	176	5	32	1	3	.5	1	1.5

(Computer code number is for West Diet Analysis program)

PAGE KEY: A–2 = BEV A–4 = DAIRY A–10 = EGGS A–12 = FAT/OIL A–14 = FRUIT A–24 = BAKERY A–34 = GRAIN A–40 = FISH A–44 = MEATS A–48 = POULTRY A–50 = SAUSAGE A–52 = MIXED/FAST A–60 = NUTS/SEEDS A–62 = SWEETS A–66 = VEG/LEG A–78 = MISC A–80 = SOUPS/SAUCES A–84 = FAST A–96 = FRZN ENTREE A–98 = BABY FOODS

Chol (mg)	Calc (mg)	Iron (mg)	Magn (mg)	Phos (mg)	Pota (mg)	Sodi (mg)	Zinc (mg)	VT-A (RE)	Thia (mg)	Ribo (mg)	Niac (mg)	V-B6 (mg)	Fola (μg)	VT-C (mg)
203	170	3.1	–	–	–	871	–	90	.47	.41	3	–	–	–
187	170	2.9	–	–	–	1012	–	110	.6	.51	4.6	–	–	–
178	150	2.7	–	–	–	1053	–	110	.65	.54	4.2	–	–	–
99	100	1.8	–	–	–	888	–	80	.03	.85	7	–	–	6
442	175	5.73	–	–	–	1239	–	164	–	.77	5.85	–	–	11
26	150	1.8	–	–	–	556	–	–	.15	.26	2	–	–	–
41	252	2.72	–	–	–	753	–	40	.23	.23	3.03	–	–	–
67	129	2.86	–	–	–	677	–	–	.33	.27	1.66	–	–	–
104	274	3.86	–	–	–	1108	–	–	.37	.45	1.63	–	–	–
79	223	2.7	–	–	–	1368	–	74	.36	.3	10.2	–	–	6
72	400	2.7	–	–	–	842	–	200	.15	.34	6	–	–	–
21	100	1.1	35	146	257	460	1.2	57	.07	.17	1	.13	–	<1
37	150	1.6	45	198	347	765	1.8	85	.12	.08	1.4	.18	–	2
92	410	3.8	–	–	–	1600	–	270	.29	.53	5.8	–	–	9
0	–	1.3	–	–	–	194	–	–	.18	.03	3.8	–	–	26
0	–	.39	–	–	–	339	–	0	.05	–	1.09	–	–	8
0	31	2.31	–	–	–	473	–	–	.3	.18	2.73	–	–	3
25	350	.72	–	–	–	270	–	–	.15	.6	.4	–	–	–
25	350	.36	–	–	–	240	–	–	.15	.43	.4	–	–	–
25	350	–	–	–	–	230	–	–	.15	.34	.4	–	–	–
8	–	2.12	–	–	–	372	–	–	.24	.14	2.12	–	–	3
76	30	.83	–	–	–	555	–	6	.07	.14	9.5	–	–	–
59	52	.92	–	–	–	564	–	4	.05	.1	5.29	–	–	–
55	17	.91	–	–	–	227	–	3	.04	.1	2.64	–	–	–
104	55	1.1	–	–	–	524	–	26	.07	.25	4.65	–	–	–
49	37	.92	–	–	–	284	–	3	.02	.06	2.83	–	–	–
119	215	3.71	–	–	–	1854	–	76	.22	.38	11.8	.5	–	36
164	197	3.84	–	–	–	1738	–	76	.25	.57	10.6	.46	–	37
160	217	3.88	–	–	–	1801	–	57	.24	.53	10.9	.47	–	38
88	26	.62	–	–	–	609	–	6	.08	.1	10.1	–	–	–
62	23	.61	–	–	–	571	–	5	.07	.08	6.49	–	–	–
60	11	.59	–	–	–	272	–	4	.05	.1	3.11	–	–	–
116	44	1.08	–	–	–	619	–	35	.09	.19	5.84	–	–	–
55	14	.05	–	–	–	344	–	3	–	.03	.05	2.69	–	–
125	161	2.51	–	–	–	1915	–	76	.31	.34	12.8	.56	–	36
176	180	3.48	–	–	–	1869	–	77	.32	.5	12	.53	–	36
172	183	2.96	–	–	–	1949	–	76	.31	.45	11.7	.49	–	36
<1	21	.28	14	41	218	228	.16	5	.01	.04	.96	.11	7	4
–	7	.8	–	–	–	–	–	27	.14	.11	1.8	–	–	2

(For purposes of calculations, use "0" for t, <1, <.1, <.01, etc.)

A

A

Table A–1
Food Composition

Computer Code Number	Food Description	Measure	Wt (g)	H_2O (%)	Ener (cal)	Prot (g)	Carb (g)	Dietary Fiber (g)	Fat (g)	Fat Breakdown (g)		
										Sat	Mono	Poly
	KENTUCKY FRIED CHICKEN—Cont.											
1269	Coleslaw	⅓ c	79	75	103	1	11	<1	6	.9	1.5	2.9
1381	Kentucky nuggets	6 ea	96	44	276	17	13	<1	17	5.5	8.7	2.2
	Kentucky nugget sauce:											
1382	Barbeque	2 tsp	30	68	37	<1	8	–	1	.1	–	.3
1383	Sweet & sour	2 tbs	30	48	61	<1	14	–	1	.1	–	.3
1384	Honey	2 tbs	30	8	104	0	26	–	–	–	–	–
1385	Mustard	2 tbs	30	69	38	1	6	–	1	.1	–	1.2
1386	Kentucky fries	1 ea	119	37	377	5	48	1	18	4	12.5	1.1
1387	Mashed potatoes & gravy	⅓ c	86	82	62	2	10	<1	1	.4	.4	.2
1388	Buttermilk biscuit	1 ea	75	30	271	5	32	<1	13	3.7	6.7	2.5
1389	Potato salad	⅓ c	90	76	141	2	13	1	9	1.4	2.8	4.8
1390	Baked beans	⅓ c	89	71	105	5	18	6	1	.4	.5	.2
1391	Chicken Little sandwich	1 ea	57	32	204	7	17	1	12	2.4	–	4.1
	Source: Kentucky Fried Chicken Corporation.											
	LONG JOHN SILVER'S											
	Fish, batter fried:											
1523	Fish & Fryes (fries), 3 piece	1 ea	350	55	853	43	64	–	48	–	–	–
1524	Fish & Fryes, 2 piece	1 ea	260	53	651	30	53	–	36	–	–	–
1525	Fish dinner, 3 piece	1 ea	540	60	1180	47	93	–	70	–	–	–
	Fish, breaded & fried:											
1526	Fish dinner, 3 piece	1 ea	450	60	940	35	84	–	52	–	–	–
1527	Fish dinner, 2 piece	1 ea	400	60	818	26	76	–	46	–	–	–
	Chicken:											
1528	Chicken Plank dinner, 3 piece	1 ea	370	60	885	32	72	–	51	–	–	–
1529	Chicken Plank dinner, 4 piece	1 ea	440	60	1037	41	82	–	59	–	–	–
1530	Chicken Nugget dinner, 6 piece	1 ea	300	60	699	23	54	–	45	–	–	–
1531	Clam chowder	1 ea	185	85	128	7	15	1	5	–	–	–
1532	Clam dinner	1 ea	460	60	955	22	100	–	58	–	–	–
1533	Fish & chicken dinner	1 ea	460	60	935	36	73	–	55	–	–	–
1534	Oyster dinner	1 ea	360	60	789	17	78	–	45	–	–	–
1535	Scallop dinner	1 ea	320	60	747	17	66	–	45	–	–	–
1536	Seafood platter	1 ea	410	60	976	29	85	–	58	–	–	–
1537	Shrimp dinner, batter fried	1 ea	300	60	711	17	60	–	45	–	–	–
1538	Fish sandwich platter	1 ea	400	59	835	30	84	–	42	–	–	–
	Salads:											
1539	Ocean chef salad	1 ea	320	85	229	27	13	2	8	–	–	–
1540	Seafood salad	1 ea	480	85	426	19	22	2	30	–	–	–
1541	Coleslaw	1 ea	98	70	182	1	11	1	15	–	–	–
1542	Fryes (fries) serving	1 ea	85	42	247	4	31	1	12	–	–	–
1543	Hush puppies	1 ea	47	37	145	3	18	<1	7	–	–	–
	Source: Long John Silver's, Lexington, KY.											
	McDONALD'S											
	Sandwiches:											
1221	Big Mac	1 ea	215	55	500	25	42	1	26	16	1	9
1444	McChicken	1 ea	187	58	415	19	39	–	19	9	7	4
1591	McLean Deluxe	1 ea	206	66	320	22	35	–	10	5	1	4

(Computer code number is for West Diet Analysis program)

Chol (mg)	Calc (mg)	Iron (mg)	Magn (mg)	Phos (mg)	Pota (mg)	Sodi (mg)	Zinc (mg)	VT-A (RE)	Thia (mg)	Ribo (mg)	Niac (mg)	V-B6 (mg)	Fola (μg)	VT-C (mg)
4	28	.17	–	–	–	171	–	28	.03	.03	.17	–	–	19
71	14	.6	–	–		840	–	180	.11	.12	6	.28	–	1
–	6	.21	–	–	–	477	–	39	–	.01	.2	–	–	–
–	5	.21	–	–	–	157	–	60	–	.02	.04	–	–	–
–	1	.21	–	–	–	–	–	0	–	.01	.08	–	–	–
–	11	.32	–	–	–	367	–	1	–	.01	.17	–	–	–
2	19	.93	–	–	–	215	–	0	.23	.08	3.09	–	–	24
–	19	.35	–	–	–	297	–	5	–	.03	1.05	–	–	–
1	110	1.85	–	–	–	756	–	30	.28	.22	3	–	–	–
11	10	.32	15	32	256	396	.29	27	.07	.02	.6	.19	7	3
1	54	1.43	29	90	229	387	1.29	10	.06	.04	.5	.07	32	2
21	27	2.05	–	–	–	399	–	6	.19	.14	2.65	–	–	–
106	–	–	–	–	–	2025	–	–	–	–	–	–	–	–
75	–	–	–	–	–	1352	–	–	–	–	–	–	–	–
119	–	–	–	–	–	2797	–	–	–	–	–	–	–	–
101	–	–	–	–	–	1900	–	–	–	–	–	–	–	–
76	–	–	–	–	–	1526	–	–	–	–	–	–	–	–
25	–	–	–	–	–	1918	–	–	–	–	–	–	–	
25	–	–	–	–	–	2433	–	–	–	–	–	–	–	–
25	–	–	–	–	–	853	–	–	–	–	–	–	–	–
17	–	–	–	–	–	611	–	–	–	–	–	–	–	–
27	–	–	–	–	–	1543	–	–	–	–	–	–	–	–
56	–	–	–	–	–	2076	–	–	–	–	–	–	–	–
55	–	–	–	–	–	763	–	–	–	–	–	–	–	–
37	–	–	–	–	–	1579	–	–	–	–	–	–	–	–
95	–	–	–	–	–	2161	–	–	–	–	–	–	–	–
127	–	–	–	–	–	1297	–	–	–	–	–	–	–	–
75	–	–	–	–	–	1402	–	–	–	–	–	–	–	–
64	–	–	–	–	–	986	–	–	–	–	–	–	–	–
113	–	–	–	–	–	1086	–	–	–	–	–	–	–	–
12	–	–	–	–	–	367	–	–	–	–	–	–	–	–
13	–	–	–	–	–	1	–	–	–	–	–	–	–	–
–	–	–	–	–	–	405	–	–	–	–	–	–	–	–
100	250	3.6	–	–	–	890	–	60	.45	.43	7	.22	–	1
50	150	2.7	–	–	–	83	–	20	.9	.17	9	–	–	2
60	150	3.6	–	–	–	670	–	100	.38	.34	7	–	–	6

(For purposes of calculations, use "0" for t, <1, <.1, <.01, etc.)

Table A–1
Food Composition

Computer Code Number	Food Description	Measure	Wt (g)	H_2O (%)	Ener (cal)	Prot (g)	Carb (g)	Dietary Fiber (g)	Fat (g)	Fat Breakdown (g)		
										Sat	Mono	Poly
	McDONALD'S—Cont.											
	Sandwiches—Cont.											
1438	McLean Deluxe with Cheese	1 ea	219	66	370	24	35	–	14	8	1	5
1222	Quarter-Pounder	1 ea	166	52	410	23	34	1	20	11	1	8
1223	Quarter-Pounder with Cheese	1 ea	194	52	510	28	34	1	28	16	1	11
1224	Filet-O-Fish	1 ea	142	49	373	14	38	<1	18	8.1	6	4
1225	Hamburger	1 ea	102	48	255	12	30	<1	9	5	1	3
1226	Cheeseburger	1 ea	116	48	305	15	30	<1	13	7	1	5
1227	French fries, small serving	1 ea	68	36	220	3	26	1	12	2.5	8	1
1228	Chicken McNuggets	6 ea	112	52	270	20	17	<1	15	10	1.5	3.5
	Sauces (packet):											
1229	Hot mustard	1 ea	30	57	70	0	8	<1	4	1.2	1.9	.5
1230	Barbecue	1 ea	32	57	50	0	12	<1	<1	.2	.2	.1
1231	Sweet & sour	1 ea	32	52	60	0	14	<1	<1	.1	.1	0
	Low-fat (frozen yogurt) milk shakes:											
1232	Chocolate	1 ea	293	71	324	12	66	<1	2	.9	.1	.7
1233	Strawberry	1 ea	293	72	320	11	67	<1	1	.6	.1	.6
1234	Vanilla	1 ea	293	75	291	11	60	<1	1	.6	.1	.6
	Low-fat (frozen yogurt) sundaes:											
1237	Hot caramel	1 ea	168	56	270	7	59	<1	3	1	.5	1.5
1235	Hot fudge	1 ea	168	60	240	7	50	<1	3	.5	.5	2
1267	Strawberry	1 ea	168	61	210	6	49	<1	1	.3	.2	.5
1238	Vanilla	1 ea	80	65	100	4	21	<1	1	.3	.2	.5
1239	Pie, apple	1 ea	83	47	220	2	31	–	10	2.5	4.5	2.8
	Muffins (fat-free)											
1266	Blueberry	1 ea	75	41	170	3	40	–	0	0	0	0
1240	Apple bran	1 ea	85	39	204	6	45	3	0	0	0	0
1241	Cookies, McDonaldland	1 ea	56	2	262	4	42	<1	8	6.3	.9	.9
1242	Cookies, Chocolaty chip	1 ea	56	2	293	4	37	2	13	8.9	.9	3.6
	Breakfast items:											
1243	English muffin with spread	1 ea	59	33	177	5	28	–	5	2.3	1.4	1.3
1244	Egg McMuffin	1 ea	138	56	286	18	29	<1	11	6.1	1	4.1
1245	Hotcakes with marg & syrup	1 ea	176	45	445	8	75	<1	12	5	5	2
1246	Scrambled eggs	1 ea	100	75	140	12	1	<1	10	5	2	3
1247	Pork sausage	1 ea	48	46	179	8	0	<1	17	8.9	2.2	5.6
1248	Hashbrown potatoes	1 ea	53	53	130	1	15	1	7	4	2	1
1392	Sausage McMuffin	1 ea	117	49	299	13	23	<1	17	9.5	1.7	6.1
1393	Sausage McMuffin with egg	1 ea	167	53	452	22	28	<1	26	14.7	3.1	8.4
1394	Biscuit with biscuit spread	1 ea	75	31	260	5	32	<1	13	9	1	3
1395	Biscuit with sausage	1 ea	123	37	438	12	33	<1	29	17.7	3.1	8.3
1396	Biscuit with sausage & egg	1 ea	180	50	519	19	34	<1	34	20.6	3.1	10.3
1397	Biscuit with bacon, egg, cheese	1 ea	156	50	449	15	34	<1	26	16.3	2	8.2
	Salads:											
1398	Chef salad	1 ea	283	86	182	18	9	2	10	4.3	1.1	4.3
1400	Garden salad	1 ea	213	92	56	5	7	2	2	1.1	.5	.7
1401	Chunky chicken salad	1 ea	250	85	147	24	7	–	4	2	1	1

Source: McDonald's Corporation.

PAGE KEY: A–2 = BEV A–4 = DAIRY A–10 = EGGS A–12 = FAT/OIL A–14 = FRUIT A–24 = BAKERY A–34 = GRAIN A–40 = FISH A–44 = MEATS A–48 = POULTRY A–50 = SAUSAGE A–52 = MIXED/FAST A–60 = NUTS/SEEDS A–62 = SWEETS A–66 = VEG/LEG A–78 = MISC A–80 = SOUPS/SAUCES A–84 = FAST A–96 = FRZN ENTREE A–98 = BABY FOODS

Chol (mg)	Calc (mg)	Iron (mg)	Magn (mg)	Phos (mg)	Pota (mg)	Sodi (mg)	Zinc (mg)	VT-A (RE)	Thia (mg)	Ribo (mg)	Niac (mg)	V-B6 (mg)	Fola (µg)	VT-C (mg)
75	200	3.6	–	–	–	890	–	150	.38	.34	7	–	–	6
85	150	3.6	–	–	–	645	–	40	.38	.26	7	.32	–	4
115	300	3.6	–	–	–	1110	–	150	.38	.34	7	.32	–	4
50	151	1.81	–	–	–	735	–	20	.3	.14	9.06	.1	–	<1
37	100	2.7	–	–	–	490	–	40	.3	.17	4	–	–	2
50	200	2.7	–	–	–	725	–	80	.3	.26	4	–	–	2
0	10	.36	–	–	–	110	–	0	.15	0	2	.18	–	9
55	13	1.08	–	–	–	580	–	0	.12	.14	8	.36	–	0
5	20	.22	–	–	–	250	–	2	.01	.01	.15	–	–	<1
0	13	.36	–	–	–	340	–	40	.01	.01	.17	–	–	2
0	11	.17	–	–	–	190	–	60	0	.01	.08	–	–	1
10	352	.84	–	–	–	242	–	60	.12	.51	.4	.1	–	0
10	352	.09	–	–	–	171	–	60	.12	.51	.4	.11	–	0
10	352	.1	–	–	–	171	–	60	.12	.51	.31	–	–	0
13	200	.08	–	–	–	180	–	60	.09	.34	.27	–	–	0
6	250	.36	–	–	–	170	–	40	.09	.34	.29	–	–	0
5	200	.16	–	–	–	95	–	40	.06	.34	.25	–	–	1
3	95	.23	–	–	–	76	–	19	.03	.16	.38	–	–	0
0	6	.94	6	23	66	175	.16	10	.12	.09	1.02	.03	3	1
0	80	.72	–	–	–	220	–	–	.12	.14	.8	–	–	1
0	45	1.22	–	–	–	227	–	1	.17	.19	2.27	–	–	1
0	18	1.63	–	–	–	271	–	0	.13	.15	1.81	.03	–	0
4	18	1.6	–	–	–	249	–	0	.13	.15	1.78	–	–	0
12	96	1.49	12	80	65	362	.39	31	.24	.29	2.45	.03	16	1
240	256	2.76	–	–	–	726	–	102	.48	.34	3.79	.08	–	0
8	101	1.81	–	–	–	693	–	40	.3	.34	3.03	.11	–	0
425	60	1.8	–	–	–	290	–	100	.07	.26	.05	–	–	0
48	8	.8	–	–	–	346	–	0	.26	.11	2.23	–	–	0
0	6	.27	–	–	–	330	–	0	.06	.02	.8	–	–	1
49	173	2.34	–	–	–	667	–	35	.46	.22	4.33	.13	–	0
284	263	3.78	–	–	–	966	–	105	.56	.45	5.25	.21	–	0
1	80	1.44	–	–	–	730	–	0	.23	.1	1.65	.03	–	0
46	83	1.88	–	–	–	1084	–	0	.47	.18	4.17	.21	–	0
267	103	3.7	–	–	–	1244	–	62	.46	.36	4.1	.21	–	0
24	204	2.75	–	–	–	1238	–	102	.39	.35	2.04	.13	–	0
119	160	1.54	–	–	–	427	–	1067	.32	.28	4.27	–	–	22
73	45	1.62	–	–	–	79	–	1014	.1	.11	.45	–	–	24
76	39	1.06	–	–	–	225	–	1666	.22	.17	8.82	–	–	26

(For purposes of calculations, use "0" for t, <1, <.1, <.01, etc.)

Table A–1
Food Composition

Computer Code Number	Food Description	Measure	Wt (g)	H_2O (%)	Ener (cal)	Prot (g)	Carb (g)	Dietary Fiber (g)	Fat (g)	Fat Breakdown (g) Sat	Mono	Poly
	PIZZA HUT											
	Pan Pizza:											
1657	Cheese	2 pce	205	48	492	30	57	5	18	8.6	5.5	2.7
1658	Pepperoni	2 pce	211	45	540	29	62	5	22	9.2	9.3	3.4
1659	Supreme	2 pce	255	54	589	32	53	7	30	13.8	11.9	4.3
1660	Super Supreme	2 pce	257	55	563	33	53	6	26	12	–	–
	Thin 'N Crispy:											
1649	Cheese Pizza	2 pce	148	43	398	28	37	4	17	10	4.6	2.3
1623	Pepperoni Pizza	2 pce	146	42	413	26	36	4	20	11	–	–
1622	Supreme Pizza	2 pce	200	53	459	28	41	5	22	11	–	–
1620	Super Supreme Pizza	2 pce	203	52	463	29	44	5	21	10	–	–
	Hand Tossed:											
1619	Cheese Pizza	2 pce	220	50	518	34	55	7	20	13.6	–	–
1618	Pepperoni Pizza	2 pce	197	47	500	28	50	6	23	12.9	–	–
1648	Supreme Pizza	2 pce	239	54	540	32	50	7	26	13.8	–	–
1617	Super Supreme Pizza	2 pce	243	53	556	33	54	7	25	13	–	–
	Personal Pan Pizza:											
1610	Pepperoni	1 ea	256	43	675	37	76	8	29	12.5	12.1	4.5
1609	Supreme	1 ea	264	47	647	33	76	9	28	11.2	12.4	4.4
	Source: Pizza Hut.											
	TACO BELL											
	Burritos:											
1544	Bean with red sauce	1 ea	191	54	414	14	58	11	13	6.4	4.4	1.1
1545	Beef with red sauce	1 ea	191	53	457	23	44	4	19	9.7	6.9	.8
1546	Beef & bean with red sauce	1 ea	191	59	393	17	44	5	15	4.8	5.8	1.9
1547	Supreme with red sauce	1 ea	241	61	475	19	52	5	21	7.3	7.5	1.9
1549	Enchirito with red sauce	1 ea	213	62	382	20	31	5	20	9.3	4.9	1.5
	Tacos:											
1551	Taco	1 ea	78	59	183	10	11	1	11	4.6	4.5	.8
1552	Taco Bellgrande	1 ea	163	63	355	18	18	1	23	10.9	9	1.3
1554	Soft Taco	1 ea	92	54	225	12	18	1	12	5.4	4.3	1.2
1555	Tostada with red sauce	1 ea	156	69	243	9	27	5	11	4.1	5.5	.8
1558	Mexican pizza	1 ea	223	55	575	21	40	2	37	11.4	14	9.7
1559	Taco salad with salsa	1 ea	595	73	939	36	60	8	62	19	26.6	12.3
1560	Nachos, regular	1 ea	107	39	349	8	38	3	19	6.1	7.6	2.1
1561	Nachos, bellgrande	1 ea	287	58	649	22	61	–	35	12.3	–	2.6
1562	Pintos & cheese with red sauce	1 ea	128	69	190	9	19	7	9	3.6	4	.8
1563	Taco sauce, packet	1 ea	4	96	1	<1	<1	<1	<1	0	0	0
1564	Salsa	1 ea	10	42	18	1	4	–	<1	0	0	0
1565	Cinnamon twists	1 ea	47	3	231	3	32	1	11	5.4	3.5	1.2
	Source: Taco Bell Corporation.											
	WENDY'S											
	Hamburgers:											
1566	Single on white bun, no toppings	1 ea	119	44	350	21	29	<1	16	–	–	–
1568	Double on white bun, no toppings	1 ea	197	44	560	41	32	<1	34	7.4	12.5	8
1569	Big Classic	1 ea	241	63	470	26	36	–	25	–	–	–

(Computer code number is for West Diet Analysis program)

Chol (mg)	Calc (mg)	Iron (mg)	Magn (mg)	Phos (mg)	Pota (mg)	Sodi (mg)	Zinc (mg)	VT-A (RE)	Thia (mg)	Ribo (mg)	Niac (mg)	V-B6 (mg)	Fola (μg)	VT-C (mg)
34	630	5.4	60	470	320	940	4.1	90	.56	.6	5.2	.17	–	7
42	520	6.3	56	440	405	1127	4.2	100	.63	.49	5.4	.17	0	8
48	500	5	76	460	580	1363	5.6	120	.81	.8	6	.31	–	10
55	540	6.7	72	470	532	1447	5.4	120	.75	.66	6.4	–	–	11
33	660	3.2	48	470	261	867	3.6	70	.39	.39	4.8	.16	–	5
46	450	3.2	44	370	287	986	3.5	70	.42	.43	5.2	–	–	6
42	430	5.9	68	400	544	1328	4.7	100	.6	.49	5.4	–	–	10
56	460	4.9	60	420	463	1336	4.5	100	.59	.44	5.4	–	–	8
55	750	5.4	72	550	396	1276	4.7	100	.48	.49	5.4	–	–	10
50	440	5	60	390	415	1267	3.8	100	.54	.53	5.6	–	–	7
55	480	8.1	80	460	578	1470	5.7	110	.69	.53	7.2	–	–	12
54	440	6.8	76	420	516	1648	4.8	110	.71	.58	7.4	–	–	12
53	730	5.8	60	450	408	1335	3.8	120	.56	.66	8.2	.2	–	10
49	520	6.7	60	400	487	1313	3.8	120	.59	.66	8	.32	–	11
9	136	3.22	–	–	459	1064	–	46	.03	1.87	1.84	.29	–	49
53	106	3.46	–	–	352	1215	–	67	.37	1.98	3.19	.3	–	2
32	107	2.07	48	212	426	1095	2.58	77	.47	.4	2.98	.57	37	2
31	145	3.4	47	215	473	1116	–	118	.39	2	2.73	.33	–	24
54	269	2.84	–	–	423	1243	–	100	.26	.42	2.3	1	–	28
32	84	1.07	–	–	159	276	–	24	.05	.14	1.2	.12	–	1
56	182	1.9	–	–	334	472	–	40	.11	.29	2.02	.21	–	5
32	116	2.27	–	–	196	554	–	30	.39	.22	2.74	.1	–	1
16	179	1.53	–	–	401	596	–	95	.06	.17	.63	.26	–	45
52	257	3.74	80	400	408	1031	5.4	215	.32	.33	2.96	1.11	60	31
82	405	7.22	–	–	1066	1307	–	407	.52	.77	4.88	.57	–	78
9	193	.91	52	262	161	403	1.7	88	.17	.16	.69	.19	10	2
36	297	3.48	–	–	674	997	–	40	.1	.34	2.17	–	–	58
16	156	1.42	110	156	384	642	2.17	87	.05	.15	.4	.21	68	52
0	1	.02	–	–	4	42	–	6	0	<.01	.02	<.01	–	<1
0	36	.6	–	–	376	376	–	7	.02	.14	0	–	–	2
1	37	.49	–	–	36	316	–	0	.14	.05	.96	.05	–	1
65	100	4.5	–	–	265	420	–	0	.38	.34	6	–	–	–
125	48	6.3	42	339	431	575	8.35	0	.22	.43	9	.47	29	<1
80	40	4.5	–	–	470	900	–	60	.3	.25	5	–	–	12

A

Table A–1
Food Composition

Computer Code Number	Food Description	Measure	Wt (g)	H_2O (%)	Ener (cal)	Prot (g)	Carb (g)	Dietary Fiber (g)	Fat (g)	Fat Breakdown (g) Sat	Mono	Poly
	WENDY'S—Cont.											
	Cheeseburgers:											
1570	Bacon cheeseburger	1 ea	147	46	460	29	23	<1	28	13	13	2
1571	Double with lettuce & tomato	1 ea	215	50	548	30	32	2	33	12.9	11.8	5.4
1572	Double with all toppings	1 ea	291	50	735	48	27	2	47	18.4	18	5.9
	Baked potatoes:											
1573	Plain	1 ea	250	75	250	6	52	4	<1	t	t	.1
1574	With bacon & cheese	1 ea	350	71	570	19	57	4	30	11.8	11.4	5.6
1575	With broccoli & cheese	1 ea	365	74	500	13	54	5	25	9.2	8.3	4.5
1576	With cheese	1 ea	350	71	590	16	55	4	34	12.5	12.7	7.1
1577	With chili & cheese	1 ea	400	72	510	22	63	8	20	13	6.8	.9
1578	With sour cream & chives	1 ea	310	71	460	6	53	4	24	10	7.9	3.3
1579	Chili	1ea	256	81	230	21	16	–	9	–	–	–
1580	French fries	1 ea	106	43	306	4	38	1	15	7	5	2
1581	Frosty dairy dessert	1 c	216	35	354	7	53	0	13	5	3	2
1582	Chocolate chip cookies	1 ea	64	4	320	3	40	1	17	5.5	5.8	4.9
	Source: Wendy's International.											
	FROZEN CONVENIENCE FOODS & MEALS											
	BUDGET GOURMET											
1695	Chicken cacciatore	1 ea	312	80	300	20	27	–	13	–	–	–
1694	Sweet & Sour chicken with rice	1 ea	284	72	350	18	53	–	7	–	–	–
1689	Teriyaki chicken	1 ea	340	77	360	20	44	–	12	–	–	–
1692	Linguini & shrimp	1 ea	284	77	330	15	33	–	15	–	–	–
1691	Scallops & shrimp	1 ea	326	79	320	16	43	–	9	–	–	–
1693	Sirloin tips with country gravy	1 ea	284	80	310	16	21	–	18	–	–	–
1690	Veal parmigiana	1 ea	340	75	440	26	39	–	20	–	–	–
1696	Yankee pot roast	1 ea	312	77	380	27	22	–	21	–	–	–
	Source: The All American Gourmet Company.											
	HEALTHY CHOICE											
	Entrees:											
1628	Chicken Chow Mein	1 ea	241	78	220	18	31	–	3	.8	–	.8
1630	Fillet of Fish Florentine	1 ea	273	80	220	26	13	–	7	3	–	2
1624	Lasagna	1 ea	284	78	260	18	37	–	5	–	–	–
1629	Seafood Newburg	1 ea	227	80	200	13	30	–	3	.8	–	.8
1625	Spaghetti	1 ea	284	77	280	14	42	–	6	–	–	–
	Dinners:											
1627	Sirloin Tips	1 ea	334	81	280	23	30	–	8	–	–	–
1626	Sole Au Gratin	1 ea	312	80	270	16	40	–	5	–	–	–
	Low-fat ice milk:											
1601	Berry	½ c	113	–	120	3	23	–	2	1	–	0
1604	Chocolate	½ c	113	–	130	3	24	–	2	1	–	0
1608	Cookie & Cream	½ c	113	–	130	4	24	–	2	–	–	0
1621	Vanilla	½ c	113	–	120	4	21	–	2	1	–	0
	Source: ConAgra Frozen Foods, Omaha, NE.											

(Computer code number is for West Diet Analysis program)

PAGE KEY: A–2 = BEV A–4 = DAIRY A–10 = EGGS A–12 = FAT/OIL A–14 = FRUIT A–24 = BAKERY A–34 = GRAIN A–40 = FISH A–44 = MEATS A–48 = POULTRY A–50 = SAUSAGE A–52 = MIXED/FAST A–60 = NUTS/SEEDS A–62 = SWEETS A–66 = VEG/LEG A–78 = MISC A–80 = SOUPS/SAUCES A–84 = FAST A–96 = FRZN ENTREE A–98 = BABY FOODS

Chol (mg)	Calc (mg)	Iron (mg)	Magn (mg)	Phos (mg)	Pota (mg)	Sodi (mg)	Zinc (mg)	VT-A (RE)	Thia (mg)	Ribo (mg)	Niac (mg)	V-B6 (mg)	Fola (μg)	VT-C (mg)
65	136	3.6	33	296	332	860	5.14	82	.26	.28	5.7	.23	25	1
84	177	4	33	339	430	864	4.41	111	.34	.35	5.29	.25	28	5
165	180	5.4	50	470	620	883	8.8	112	.36	.53	10	.46	31	5
0	40	2.7	66	169	1360	60	.65	0	.27	.1	3.82	.7	67	36
22	200	3.7	80	406	1380	180	2.53	150	.22	.17	4.64	.87	33	36
22	250	3.6	83	373	1550	2	.86	350	.3	.25	4	.86	66	90
22	350	3.6	78	50	1380	2	.61	200	.22	.25	3.3	.8	33	36
22	250	6.13	111	498	1590	810	3.78	172	.3	.26	4.1	.9	50	36
15	40	2.7	70	185	1420	230	.9	100	.22	.14	3	.79	32	36
–	60	4.5	–	–	565	960	–	200	.12	.17	3	–	–	9
15	13	1.02	45	197	689	105	.51	0	.15	.04	2.96	.26	33	12
44	257	.86	43	238	518	194	.92	143	.11	.45	.31	.12	17	<1
5	10	1.09	15	62	100	235	.46	0	.06	.07	.4	.03	6	0
60	150	1.8	–	–	–	810	–	40	.23	.51	5	–	–	21
40	60	.72	–	–	–	640	–	80	.12	.34	3	–	–	2
55	80	1.4	–	–	–	610	–	300	.15	.34	6	–	–	12
75	10	3.6	–	–	–	1250	–	1000	.3	.17	3	–	–	2
70	150	.72	–	–	–	690	–	150	–	.26	3	–	–	12
40	60	.36	–	–	–	570	–	150	.15	.17	4	–	–	2
165	30	4.5	–	–	–	1160	–	1000	.45	.6	6	–	–	6
70	150	1.8	–	–	–	690	–	600	.15	.43	7	–	–	6
45	20	1.4	–	290	290	440	–	81	.15	.14	4	–	–	4
65	150	.72	58	–	780	590	1.2	500	.15	.34	2	.14	<1	1
20	100	2.7	–	210	500	420	–	150	.3	.26	2	–	–	2
55	60	1.1	–	160	270	440	–	3	.12	.14	1.2	–	–	4
20	6	3.6	–	160	540	480	–	250	.38	.26	2	–	–	5
65	20	2.7	–	190	540	370	–	700	.15	.17	5	.35	–	42
55	80	1.1	–	260	430	470	–	–	.23	.17	1.6	–	–	6
5	100	–	–	10	160	60	–	–	.03	.17	–	–	–	–
5	100	–	–	10	191	70	–	–	.03	.17	–	–	–	–
5	150	–	–	10	180	80	–	–	.03	.17	–	–	–	–
5	150	–	–	10	180	60	–	–	.06	.25	–	–	–	–

(For purposes of calculations, use "0" for t, <1, <.1, <.01, etc.)

Table A-1
Food Composition

Computer Code Number	Food Description	Measure	Wt (g)	H_2O (%)	Ener (cal)	Prot (g)	Carb (g)	Dietary Fiber (g)	Fat (g)	Fat Breakdown (g) Sat	Mono	Poly
	LEAN CUISINE											
	Dinners:											
1639	Baked Cheese Ravioli	1 ea	241	77	240	13	30	3	8	3	3	.5
1640	Chicken Cacciatore	1 ea	308	80	280	22	31	4	7	2	–	1
1632	Chicken Chow Mein	1 ea	255	78	240	14	34	–	5	1	–	1
1633	Lasagna	1 ea	291	79	260	19	34	2	5	2	2	.5
1634	Macaroni & Cheese	1 ea	255	74	290	15	37	–	9	4	–	.5
1631	Spaghetti w/Meatballs	1 ea	269	75	280	19	35	11	7	2	2.6	1
	Pizza:											
1635	French Bread Cheese Pizza	1 ea	145	52	300	17	38	<1	9	3	5	.5
1638	French Bread Deluxe Pizza	1 ea	174	56	320	22	39	2	8	3	3	.5
1637	French Bread Pepperoni Pizza	1 ea	149	51	330	19	38	2	11	3	5.4	1
1636	French Bread Sausage Pizza	1 ea	170	55	330	22	40	2	9	3	4.3	.5
	Source: Stouffer's Foods Corp, Solon, OH.											
	WEIGHT WATCHERS											
	Dinners:											
1641	Beef Stroganoff	1 ea	238	73	290	22	26	3	9	4	3	2
1646	Oven Fried Fish	1 ea	198	79	240	20	23	–	7	–	5	2
1647	Fried Chicken Patty	1 pce	184	73	270	16	14	–	16	8	6	2
1654	Chicken Burrito w/Vegetable	1 ea	216	68	330	15	36	–	14	4	6	3
1656	Pasta Primavera	1 ea	238	75	260	15	22	2	11	.8	8	3
	Pizza:											
1653	Cheese Pizza	1 ea	164	56	300	22	37	2	7	3	3	1
1650	Deluxe Combination Pizza	1 ea	200	64	330	26	35	3	10	3	5	2
1651	Sausage Pizza	1 ea	175	60	320	24	35	2	10	2	6	2
1652	Pepperoni Pizza	1 ea	171	56	320	26	31	–	10	3	5	2
	Desserts:											
1645	Apple pie	1 ea	98	49	200	2	39	–	5	1	2	2
1643	Boston cream pie	1 ea	85	48	170	4	35	1	4	1	1	2
1644	Chocolate brownie	1 ea	35	29	100	3	17	<1	4	1	2	1
1642	Strawberry cheesecake	1 ea	109	62	180	7	28	–	5	1	1	2
1655	Chocolate mousse	1 ea	70	46	170	6	24	<1	6	–	4	2
	Source: Foodway National Inc., Boise, ID.											
	BABY FOODS											
1720	Apple juice	4 fl oz	125	88	59	0	15	–	<1	–	–	–
1721	Applesauce, strained	1 tbs	14	89	6	<1	2	–	<1	–	–	–
1716	Carrots, strained	1 tbs	14	92	4	<1	1	–	<1	–	–	–
1718	Cereal, mixed, millk added	1 tbs	14	75	16	1	2	–	<1	–	–	–
1719	Cereal, rice, milk added	1 tbs	14	75	16	1	2	–	<1	–	–	–
1723	Chicken and noodles, strained	1 tbs	14	88	7	<1	1	–	<1	–	–	–
1722	Peas, strained	1 tbs	14	88	6	1	1	–	<1	–	–	–
1717	Teething biscuits	1 ea	11	6	43	1	8	–	<1	–	–	–

(Computer code number is for West Diet Analysis program)

PAGE KEY: A–2 = BEV A–4 = DAIRY A–10 = EGGS A–12 = FAT/OIL A–14 = FRUIT A–24 = BAKERY A–34 = GRAIN A–40 = FISH A–44 = MEATS A–48 = POULTRY A–50 = SAUSAGE A–52 = MIXED/FAST A–60 = NUTS/SEEDS A–62 = SWEETS A–66 = VEG/LEG A–78 = MISC A–80 = SOUPS/SAUCES A–84 = FAST A–96 = FRZN ENTREE A–98 = BABY FOODS

Chol (mg)	Calc (mg)	Iron (mg)	Magn (mg)	Phos (mg)	Pota (mg)	Sodi (mg)	Zinc (mg)	VT-A (RE)	Thia (mg)	Ribo (mg)	Niac (mg)	V-B6 (mg)	Fola (µg)	VT-C (mg)
55	200	1.44	42	168	380	590	1.5	60	.06	.25	1.2	.2	48	36
45	40	1.44	47	–	560	570	.97	100	.22	.17	6	–	–	9
30	40	1.08	30	–	350	530	1.1	60	.15	.17	5	–	–	6
25	150	1.8	44	–	700	590	2.9	100	.15	.25	3	.32		6
30	250	.72	–	–	160	550	–	20	.12	.25	1.2	–	–	0
35	100	1.8	47	–	500	490	2.5	60	.15	.25	3	.2	–	4
15	250	2.7	34	–	320	590	1.6	60	.37	.34	4	.1	–	6
40	200	1.44	38	–	440	860	2.08	150	.45	.51	5	.16	–	6
25	200	3.6	34	–	390	790	1.8	100	.45	.42	5	.07	–	6
40	250	2.7	39	–	440	860	2.2	80	.45	.51	5	.07	–	6
25	80	2.7	–	–	350	600	–	60	.23	.26	4	.32	–	4
15	20	.72	–	–	340	380	–	100	.09	.14	1.6	–	–	5
70	39	1.7	–	–	350	610	–	75	.19	.18	4	–	–	6
65	56	2.3	–	–	390	800	–	38	.52	.39	5.9	–	–	3
5	300	1.8	–	–	260	800	–	350	.23	.26	3	.18	–	18
35	450	1.4	–	–	420	630	–	200	.3	.51	3	.06	–	12
25	350	1.8	–	–	490	650	–	350	.3	.51	3	.2	–	21
35	300	1.8	–	–	470	630	–	250	.3	.51	3	.06	–	18
35	400	1.8	–	–	420	710	–	200	.23	.51	3	–	–	15
5	20	1.1	–	–	80	280	–	–	.06	.07	.4	–	–	1
5	65	.6	–	–	120	290	–	14	.03	.02	.3	.08	–	1
10	19	.9	–	–	120	150	–	14	.06	.03	.2	.03	–	1
20	80	.36	–	–	140	210	–	40	.06	.07	1.6	–	–	2
5	60	1.1	–	–	210	190	–	–	.03	.03	.4	.06	–	5
–	5	.71	4	6	114	4	.04	3	.01	.02	.1	.04	<1	72
–	1	.03	<1	1	10	<1	<.01	<1	<.01	<.01	<.1	<.01	<1	6
–	3	.05	1	3	28	5	.02	164	<.01	.01	.1	.01	2	1
–	31	1.5	4	20	28	7	.10	3	.06	.08	.8	.01	2	–
–	34	1.7	6	25	27	7	.09	4	.07	.07	.7	.02	1	–
–	3	.06	1	3	6	2	.04	16	<.01	.01	.1	.01	1	<1
–	3	.14	2	6	16	<1	.05	8	.01	.01	.1	.01	4	1
–	29	.39	4	18	36	40	.1	1	.03	.06	.5	.01	2	1

(For purposes of calculations, use "0" for t, <1, <.1, <.01, etc.)

Contents

CANADIAN RECOMMENDATIONS, GUIDELINES, AND FOOD GUIDE

RNI

Like the RDA on the inside front cover pages, the Recommended Nutrient Intakes (RNI) for Canadians make recommendations for intakes of vitamins, minerals, protein, and energy. The RNI are presented in Tables B–1 and B–2.

CANADA'S GUIDELINES FOR HEALTHY EATING

Canada's Guidelines for Healthy Eating were developed by the Communications/Implementation Committee as the key nutrition messages to be communicated to healthy Canadians over two years of age. The guidelines encourage people to:

- Enjoy a variety of foods.
- Emphasize cereals, breads, other grain products, vegetables, and fruits.
- Choose lower-fat dairy products, leaner meats, and foods prepared with little or no fat.
- Achieve and maintain a healthy body weight by enjoying regular physical activity and healthy eating.
- Limit salt, alcohol, and caffeine.

Table B–1
Recommended Nutrient Intakes for Canadians, 1990

Age	Sex	Weight (kg)	Protein (g/day)[a]	Fat-Soluble Vitamins: VITAMIN A (RE/day)[b]	VITAMIN D (μg/day)[c]	VITAMIN E (mg/day)[d]
Infants (months)						
0–4	Both	6	12[f]	400	10	3
5–12	Both	9	12	400	10	3
Children and Adults (years)						
1	Both	11	13	400	10	3
2–3	Both	14	16	400	5	4
4–6	Both	18	19	500	5	5
7–9	M	25	26	700	2.5	7
	F	25	26	700	2.5	6
10–12	M	34	34	800	2.5	8
	F	36	36	800	5	7
13–15	M	50	49	900	5	9
	F	48	46	800	5	7
16–18	M	62	58	1000	5	10
	F	53	47	800	2.5	7
19–24	M	71	61	1000	2.5	10
	F	58	50	800	2.5	7
25–49	M	74	64	1000	2.5	9
	F	59	51	800	2.5	6
50–74	M	73	63	1000	5	7
	F	63	54	800	5	6
75+	M	69	59	1000	5	6
	F	64	55	800	5	5
Pregnancy (additional amount needed)						
1st trimester			5	0	2.5	2
2nd trimester			20	0	2.5	2
3rd trimester			24	0	2.5	2
Lactation (additional amount needed)			20	400	2.5	3

Note: Recommended intakes of energy and of certain nutrients are not listed in this table because of the nature of the variables upon which they are based. The figures for energy are estimates of average requirements for expected patterns of activity. For nutrients not shown, the following amounts are recommended based on at least 2000 kcalories per day and body weights as given: thiamin, 0.4 milligrams per 1000 kcalories (0.48 milligrams/5000 kilojoules); riboflavin, 0.5 milligrams per 1000 kcalories (0.6 milligrams/5000 kilojoules); niacin, 7.2 niacin equivalents per 1000 kcalories (8.6 niacin equivalents/5000 kilojoules); vitamin B_6, 15 micrograms, as pyridoxine, per gram of protein. Recommended intakes during periods of growth are taken as appropriate for individuals representative of the midpoint in each age group. All recommended intakes are designed to cover individual variations in essentially all of a healthy population subsisting upon a variety of common foods available in Canada.

Source: Health and Welfare Canada, *Nutrition Recommendations: The Report of the Scientific Review Committee* (Ottawa: Canadian Government Publishing Centre, 1990), Table 20, p. 204.

B

Table B–1
Recommended Nutrient Intakes for Canadians, 1990 (cont.)

Water-Soluble Vitamins			Minerals					
VITAMIN C (mg/day)[e]	FOLATE (µg/day)	VITAMIN B_{12} (µg/day)	CALCIUM (mg/day)	PHOSPHORUS (mg/day)	MAGNESIUM (mg/day)	IRON (mg/day)	IODINE (µg/day)	ZINC (mg/day)
20	25	0.3	250	150	20	0.3[g]	30	2[h]
20	40	0.4	400	200	32	7	40	3
20	40	0.5	500	300	40	6	55	4
20	50	0.6	550	350	50	6	65	4
25	70	0.8	600	400	65	8	85	5
25	90	1.0	700	500	100	8	110	7
25	90	1.0	700	500	100	8	95	7
25	120	1.0	900	700	130	8	125	9
25	130	1.0	1100	800	135	8	110	9
30	175	1.0	1100	900	185	10	160	12
30	170	1.0	1000	850	180	13	160	9
40	220	1.0	900	1000	230	10	160	12
30	190	1.0	700	850	200	12	160	9
40	220	1.0	800	1000	240	9	160	12
30	180	1.0	700	850	200	13	160	9
40	230	1.0	800	1000	250	9	160	12
30	185	1.0	700	850	200	13[i]	160	9
40	230	1.0	800	1000	250	9	160	12
30	195	1.0	800	850	210	8	160	9
40	215	1.0	800	1000	230	9	160	12
30	200	1.0	800	850	210	8	160	9
0	200	0.2	500	200	15	0	25	6
10	200	0.2	500	200	45	5	25	6
10	200	0.2	500	200	45	10	25	6
25	100	0.2	500	200	65	0	50	6

[a]The primary units are expressed per kilogram of body weight. The figures shown here are examples.

[b]One retinol equivalent (RE) corresponds to the biological activity of 1 microgram of retinol, 6 micrograms of beta-carotene, or 12 micrograms of other carotenes.

[c]Expressed as cholecalciferol or ergocalciferol.

[d]Expressed as δ-α-tocopherol equivalents, relative to which β- and γ-tocopherol and α-tocotrienol have activities of 0.5, 0.1, and 0.3, respectively.

[e]Cigarette smokers should increase intake by 50 percent.

[f]The assumption is made that the protein is from breast milk or is of the same biological value as that of breast milk, and that between 3 and 9 months, adjustment for the quality of the protein is made.

[g]Based on the assumption that breast milk is the source of iron.

[h]Based on the assumption that breast milk is the source of zinc.

[i]After menopause, the recommended intake is 8 milligrams per day.

Table B-2
Average Energy Requirements for Canadians

Age	Sex	Average Height (cm)	Average Weight (kg)	Requirements[a]					
				(kcal/kg)[b]	(MJ/kg)[b]	(kcal/day)	(MJ/day)	(kcal/cm)	(MJ/cm)
Infants (months)									
0–2	Both	55	4.5	120–100	0.50–0.42	500	2.0	9	0.04
3–5	Both	63	7.0	100–95	0.42–0.40	700	2.8	11	0.05
6–8	Both	69	8.5	95–97	0.40–0.41	800	3.4	11.5	0.05
9–11	Both	73	9.5	97–99	0.41	950	3.8	12.5	0.05
Children and Adults (years)									
1	Both	82	11	101	0.42	1100	4.8	13.5	0.06
2–3	Both	95	14	94	0.39	1300	5.6	13.5	0.06
4–6	Both	107	18	100	0.42	1800	7.6	17	0.07
7–9	M	126	25	88	0.37	2200	9.2	17.5	0.07
	F	125	25	76	0.32	1900	8.0	15	0.06
10–12	M	141	34	73	0.30	2500	10.4	17.5	0.07
	F	143	36	61	0.25	2200	9.2	15.5	0.06
13–15	M	159	50	57	0.24	2800	12.0	17.5	0.07
	F	157	48	46	0.19	2200	9.2	14	0.06
16–18	M	172	62	51	0.21	3200	13.2	18.5	0.08
	F	160	53	40	0.17	2100	8.8	13	0.05
19–24	M	175	71	42	0.18	3000	12.6		
	F	160	58	36	0.15	2100	8.8		
25–49	M	172	74	36	0.15	2700	11.3		
	F	160	59	32	0.13	1900	8.0		
50–74	M	170	73	31	0.13	2300	9.7		
	F	158	63	29	0.12	1800	7.6		
75+	M	168	69	29	0.12	2000	8.4		
	F	155	64	23	0.10	1500	6.3		

[a]Requirements can be expected to vary within a range of ±30 percent.

[b]First and last figures are averages at the beginning and end of the three-month period.

Source: Health and Welfare Canada, *Nutrition Recommendations: The Report of the Scientific Review Committee* (Ottawa: Canadian Government Publishing Centre, 1990), Tables 5 and 6, pp. 25, 27.

B

CANADA'S FOOD GUIDE TO HEALTHY EATING

♦

The 1992 *Canada's Food Guide to Healthy Eating* gives consumers detailed information for selecting foods to meet *Canada's Guidelines for Healthy Eating* (1990). The *Food Guide* was designed to meet the nutritional needs of all Canadians four years of age and older and takes a total diet approach, rather than emphasizing a single food, meal, or day's meals and snacks.

The rainbow side of the Food Guide shows the four food groups with their revised names and pictorial examples of foods in each group. Key statements direct consumers about selecting foods generally from all the groups, and more specifically within each group. The bar side shows the number of servings recommended for each group, using a range of servings instead of a single minimum number. Other notable changes include the number of servings for some food groups and the size of servings for some foods.

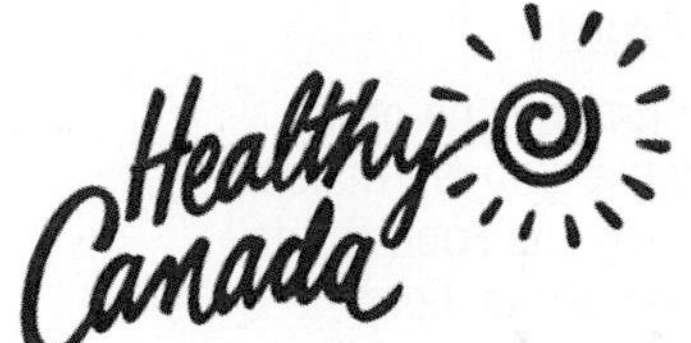

Health and Welfare Canada   Santé et Bien-être social Canada

CANADA'S

Food Guide TO HEALTHY EATING

Enjoy a variety of foods from each group every day.

Choose lower-fat foods more often.

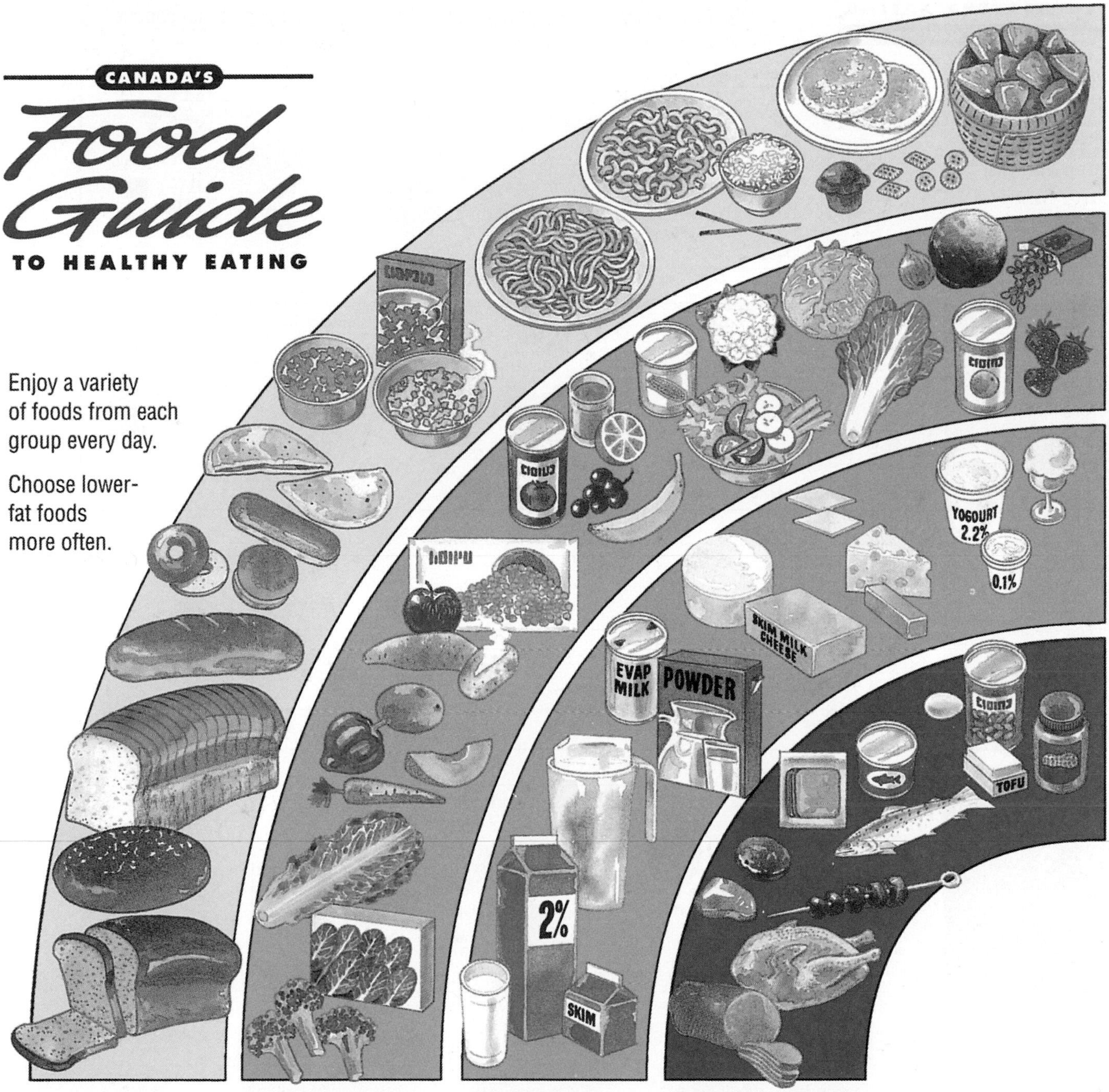

Grain Products
Choose whole grain and enriched products more often.

Vegetables & Fruit
Choose dark green and orange vegetables and orange fruit more often.

Milk Products
Choose lower-fat milk products more often.

Meat & Alternatives
Choose leaner meats, poultry and fish, as well as dried peas, beans and lentils more often.

B

B

CANADA'S

Food Guide

TO HEALTHY EATING

FOR PEOPLE FOUR YEARS AND OVER

Different People Need Different Amounts of Food

The amount of food you need every day from the 4 food groups and other foods depends on your age, body size, activity level, whether you are male or female and if you are pregnant or breast-feeding. That's why the Food Guide gives a lower and higher number of servings for each food group. For example, young children can choose the lower number of servings, while male teenagers can go to the higher number. Most other people can choose servings somewhere in between.

Grain Products

5–12

SERVINGS PER DAY

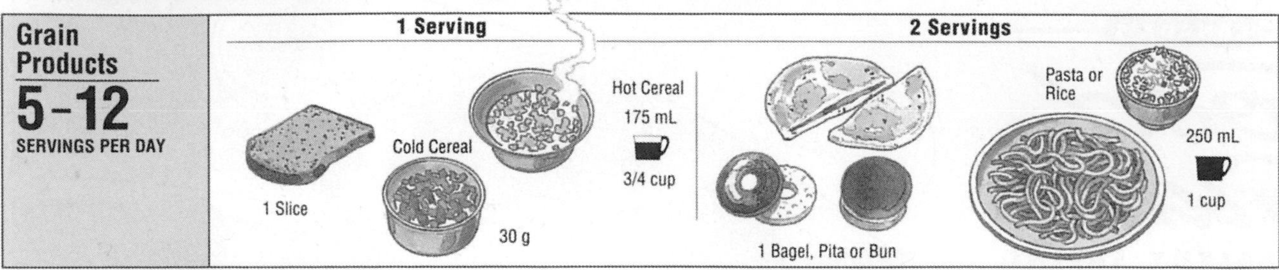

Vegetables & Fruit

5–10

SERVINGS PER DAY

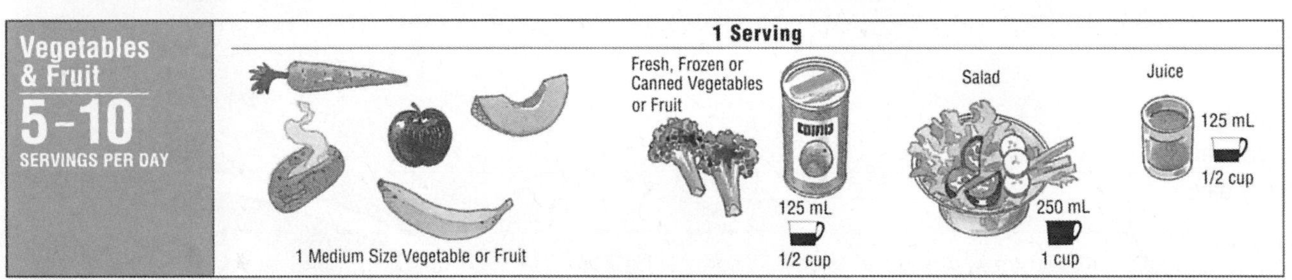

Milk Products

SERVINGS PER DAY

Children 4–9 years: 2–3
Youth 10–16 years: 3–4
Adults: 2–4
Pregnant & Breast-feeding Women: 3–4

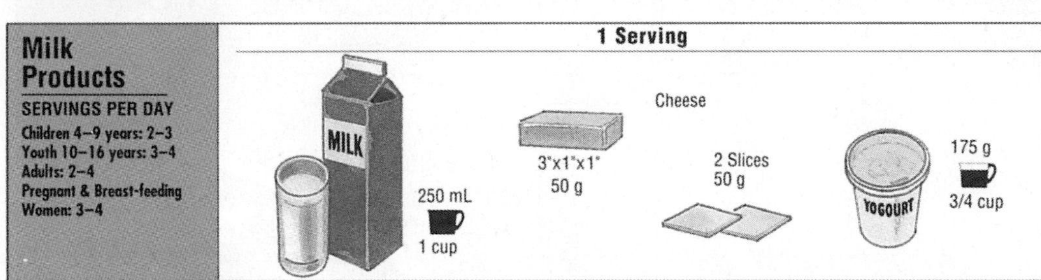

Meat & Alternatives

2–3

SERVINGS PER DAY

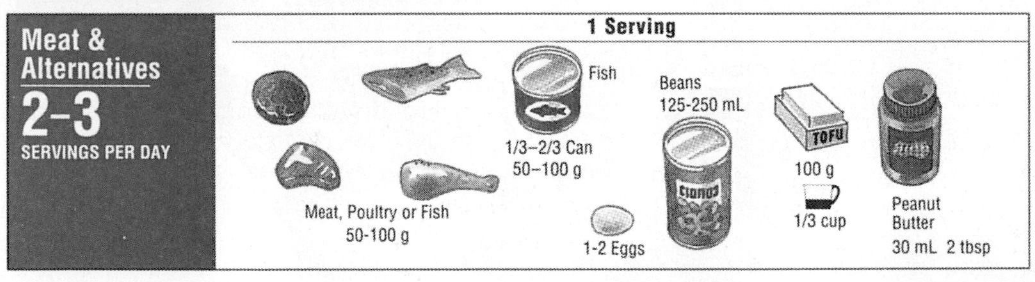

Other Foods

Taste and enjoyment can also come from other foods and beverages that are not part of the 4 food groups. Some of these foods are higher in fat or Calories, so use these foods in moderation.

Enjoy eating well, being active and feeling good about yourself. That's VITALIT

ISBN 0-662-19648-1

AIDS TO CALCULATION

Contents

Many mathematical problems have been worked out for you as examples at appropriate places in the text. This appendix aims to help with the use of the metric system and with those problems not fully explained elsewhere.

CONVERSION FACTORS

Conversion factors are useful mathematical tools in everyday calculations, like the ones encountered in the study of nutrition. Skill in the use of conversion factors is especially desirable as the United States and Canada "go metric."

A conversion factor is a fraction in which the numerator (top) and the denominator (bottom) express the same quantity in different units. For example, 2.2 pounds (lb) and 1 kilogram (kg) are equivalent; they express the same weight. The conversion factor used to change pounds to kilograms or vice versa is:

$$\frac{2.2 \text{ lb}}{1 \text{ kg}} \text{ or } \frac{1 \text{ kg}}{2.2 \text{ lb}}.$$

Because both factors equal 1, measurements can be multiplied by the factor without changing the value of the measurement. Thus the units can be changed.

The correct factor to use in a problem is the one with the unit you are seeking in the numerator (top) of the fraction. Following are two examples of problems commonly encountered in nutrition study; they illustrate the usefulness of conversion factors.

Example 1 Convert the weight of 130 pounds to kilograms.

1. Choose the conversion factor in which the unit you are seeking is on top:

$$\frac{1 \text{ kg}}{2.2 \text{ lb}}.$$

2. Multiply 130 pounds by the factor:

$$130 \text{ lb} \times \frac{1 \text{ kg}}{2.2 \text{ lb}} = \frac{130 \text{ kg}}{2.2}$$

= 59 kg (rounded off to the nearest whole number).

Example 2 How many grams (g) of saturated fat are contained in a 3-ounce (oz) hamburger?

1. Appendix A shows that a 4-ounce hamburger contains 7 grams of saturated fat. You are seeking grams of saturated fat; therefore, the conversion factor is:

$$\frac{7 \text{ g saturated fat}}{4 \text{ oz hamburger}}.$$

2. Multiply 3 ounces of hamburger by the conversion factor:

$$3 \text{ oz hamburger} \times \frac{7 \text{ g saturated fat}}{4 \text{ oz hamburger}} = \frac{3 \times 7}{4} = \frac{21}{4}$$

= 5 g saturated fat (rounded off to the nearest whole number).

Energy Units
1 cal[a] = 4.2 kJ
1 MJ = 240 cal
1 kJ = 0.24 cal
1 g carbohydrate = 4 cal = 17 kJ
1 g fat = 9 cal = 37 kJ
1 g protein = 4 cal = 17 kJ
1 g alcohol = 7 cal = 29 kJ

C

PERCENTAGES

A percentage is a comparison between a number of items (perhaps your intake of energy) and a standard number (perhaps the number of calories recommended for your age and sex—your energy RDA). The standard number is the number you divide by. The answer you get after the division must be multiplied by 100 to be stated as a percentage (*percent* means "per 100").

Example 3 What percentage of the RDA for energy is your energy intake?

1. Find your energy RDA (inside front cover). We'll use 2,100 calories to demonstrate.
2. Total your energy intake for a day—for example, 1,200 calories.
3. Divide your calorie intake by the RDA calories:

   1,200 cal (your intake) ÷ 2,100 cal (RDA) = 0.573.
4. Multiply your answer by 100 to state it as a percentage:

   0.573 × 100 = 57.3 = 57% (rounded off to the nearest whole number).

In some problems in nutrition, the percentage may be more than 100. For example, suppose your daily intake of vitamin A is 3,200 RE and your RDA (male) is 1,000 RE. Your intake as a percentage of the RDA is more than 100 percent (that is, you consume more than 100 percent of your vitamin A RDA). The following calculations show your vitamin A intake as a percentage of the RDA:

3,200 ÷ 1,000 = 3.2.
3.2 × 100 = 320% of RDA.

Sometimes the comparison is between a part of a whole (for example, a day's calories from protein) and the total amount (the day's total calories). In this case, divide by the total number as shown in example 4.

[a]Note: Throughout this book and in the Appendixes, the term *calorie* is used to mean kilocalorie. Thus, when converting the calories of foods listed in Appendixes A or D to kilojoules, do not enlarge the calorie values—they are kilocalorie values.

Example 4 The Food Feature of Chapter 2 demonstrated how to estimate the percentage of calories from one nutrient only, carbohydrate, in a day's meals. Here, we finish the job by calculating the percentages from fat and from protein.

1. Recall the general formula for finding percentages of calories from a nutrient.

   (one nutrient's calories ÷ total calories) × 100 = the percentage of calories from that nutrient.
2. Apply the formula to find the calories from *fat* in both Monday's and Tuesday's meals (pages 56 and 57).

   Monday: (fat calories ÷ total calories) × 100 = percentage of calories from fat

   (486 ÷ 1,754) × 100 = 27. 7 (28 percent, rounded)

   Tuesday: (fat calories ÷ total calories) × 100 = percentage of calories from fat

   (855 ÷ 1,763) × 100 = 48.49 (48 percent, rounded)

Monday's meals provided 28 percent of their calories from fat, while Tuesday's meals provided 48 percent of calories from fat.

3. The percentages from *protein* can be derived the same way.

   Monday: (protein calories ÷ total calories) = percentage of calories from proetin

   (372 ÷ 1,754) × 100 = 21.20 (21 percent, rounded)

   Tuesday: (protein calories ÷ total calories) = percentage of calories from protein

   (380 ÷ 1,763) × 100 = 21.55 (22 percent, rounded)

For protein, then, the meals were about the same, with Monday's meals providing 21 percent and Tuesday's meals providing 22 percent of their calories from protein.

WEIGHTS AND MEASURES

Length
1 inch (in) = 2.54 centimeters (cm).
1 foot (ft) = 30.48 centimeters.
1 meter (m) = 39.37 inches.

Temperature

	Celsius[a]	Fahrenheit	
Steam	100° C	212° F	Steam
Body temperature	37 °C	98.6° F	Body temperature
Ice	0° C	32° F	Ice

[a]Also known as *centigrade*.

To convert Fahrenheit temperature (t_F) to Celsius:

$$t_C = \frac{5}{9}(t_F - 32).$$

To convert Celsius temperature (t_C) to Fahrenheit:

$$t_F = \frac{9}{5}t_C + 32.$$

Volume

1 liter (l) = 1.06 quarts (qt) or 0.85 imperial quart.
1 liter = 1,000 milliliters (ml).
1 milliliter = 0.034 fluid ounces.
1 gallon = 3.79 liters.
1 quart = 0.95 liter or 32 fluid ounces.
1 cup (c) = 8 fluid ounces, or about 250 ml.
1 tablespoon (tbsp) = 15 milliliters.
3 teaspoons (tsp) = 1 tablespoon.
1 teaspoon (tsp) = about 5 g or 5 ml.
16 tablespoons = 1 cup.
4 cups = 1 quart.

Weight

1 ounce (oz) = approximately 28 grams (g).
16 ounces = 1 pound (lb).
1 pound = 454 grams.
1 kilogram (kg) = 1,000 grams or 2.2 pounds.
1 gram = 1,000 milligrams (mg).
1 milligram = 1,000 micrograms (μg).

NUTRIENT UNITS

◆

To convert IU (International Units) found on supplement labels to the units used in the RDA tables:

Vitamin A

From animal sources:
.3 μg = 1 IU
1 RE[a] = 3.33 IU
From vegetables and fruits:
.6 μg = 1 IU
1 RE = 10 IU

[a]Retinol equivalents.

Vitamin D_3

1 μg = 40 IU

Vitamin E

1 mg = 1 IU
1 α TE[b] = 1 IU

Sodium

To covert milligrams of sodium to grams of salt:
mg sodium ÷ 400 = g of salt
The reverse is also true:
g salt × 400 = mg sodium

NOTES

◆

1. F. H. Mattson, A changing role for dietary monounsaturated fatty acids, *Journal of the American Dietetic Association* 89 (1989): 387–391.

[b]Alpha-tocopherol equivalents.

C

Contents

FOOD EXCHANGE SYSTEMS

♦

Chapter 2 introduced dietary guidelines, food group plans, and exchange systems. This appendix provides details of the U.S. exchange system and then of the Canadian exchange system.

THE U.S. EXCHANGE SYSTEM

♦

The U.S. exchange system divides the foods suitable for use in planning a healthy diet into six lists—the starch/bread, meat/meat alternate, vegetable, fruit, milk, and fat lists.[a] These lists are shown in Tables D–1 through D–6. Following these lists are three other sets of foods: free foods, combination foods, and foods for occasional use (Tables D–7, D–8, and D–9).

---

[a]The U.S. Exchange System presented here is based on material in *Exchange Lists for Meal Planning*, 1986, prepared by committees of the American Diabetes Association and the American Dietetic Association, with permission of both organizations.

Table D–1
The U.S. Exchange System: Starch/Bread List

15 g carbohydrate, 3 g protein, trace fat, 80 cal

Amount	Food
Cereals/Grains/Pasta	
1/3 c	Bran cereals, concentrated *
1/2 c	Bran cereals, flaked *
1/2 c	Bulgur, cooked
1/2 c	Cooked cereals
2 1/2 tbs	Cornmeal, dry
3 tbs	Grapenuts
1/2 c	Grits, cooked
3/4 c	Other ready-to-eat unsweetened cereals
1/2 c	Pasta, cooked
1 1/2 c	Puffed cereals
1/3 c	Rice, white or brown, cooked
1/2 c	Shredded wheat
3 tbs	Wheat germ *
Dried Beans/Peas/Lentils	
1/4 c	Baked beans *
1/3 c	Beans and peas, cooked, such as kidney, white, split, black-eyed *
1/3 c	Lentils, cooked *
Starchy Vegetables	
1/2 c	Corn *
1 cob	Corn on the cob, 6" long *
1/2 c	Lima beans *
1/2 c	Peas, green, canned or frozen *
1/2 c	Plantains *
1 small (3 oz)	Potatoes, baked
1/2 c	Potatoes, mashed
3/4 c	Squash, winter (acorn, butternut)
1/3 c	Yams, sweet potatoes, plain
Bread	
1/2 (1 oz)	Bagels
2 (2/3 oz)	Bread sticks, crisp, 4" × 1/2"
1 c	Croutons, low-fat
1/2	English muffins
1/2 (1 oz)	Frankfurter or hamburger buns
1/2 loaf	Pita, 6" across
1 (1 oz)	Plain rolls, small
1 slice (1 oz)	Raisin, unfrosted
1 slice (1 oz)	Rye, pumpernickel *
1	Tortillas, 6" across
1 slice (1 oz)	White (including French, Italian)
1 slice (1 oz)	Whole-wheat
Crackers/Snacks	
8	Animal crackers
3	Graham crackers, 2 1/2" square
3/4 oz	Matzoth
5 slices	Melba toast
24	Oyster crackers
3 c	Popcorn, popped, no fat added
3/4 oz	Pretzels
4	Rye crisp, 2" × 3 1/2"
6	Saltine-type crackers
2 to 4 (3/4 oz)	Whole-wheat crackers, no fat added (crisp breads)
Starch Foods Prepared with Fat (Count as 1 starch/bread serving, plus 1 fat serving.)	
1	Biscuits, 2 1/2" across
1/2 c	Chow mein noodles
1 (2 oz)	Cornbread, 2" cube
6	Crackers, round butter type
10 (1 1/2 oz)	French fries, 2" to 3 1/2" long
1	Muffins, plain, small
2	Pancakes, 4" across
1/4 c	Stuffing, bread, prepared
2	Taco shells, 6" across
1	Waffles, 4 1/2" square
4 to 6 (1 oz)	Whole-wheat crackers, fat added

* 3 grams or more dietary fiber per serving. Average fiber contents of whole-grain products is 2 grams per serving. For starch foods not on this list, the general rule is that 1/2 cup cereal, grain, or pasta is 1 serving: 1 ounce of a bread product is 1 serving.

D

D

Table D–2
U.S. Exchange System: Meat/Meat Alternate Lists

Lean meat = 7 g protein, 3 g fat, 55 cal; medium-fat meat = 7 g protein, 5 g fat, 75 cal; high-fat meat = 7 g protein, 8 g fat, 100 cal.

Category	Amount	Food
Lean Meat and Alternates		
Beef	1 oz	USDA Good or Choice grades of lean beef, such as round, sirloin, and flank steak; tenderloin; chipped beef
Pork	1 oz	Lean pork, such as fresh ham; canned, cured, or boiled ham , Canadian bacon , tenderloin
Veal	1 oz	All cuts are lean except veal cutlets (ground or cubed); examples of lean veal: chops and roasts
Poultry	1 oz	Chicken, turkey, Cornish hen (without skin)
Fish	1 oz	All fresh and frozen fish
	2 oz	Crab, lobster, scallops, shrimp, clams (fresh or canned in water)
	6 medium	Oysters
	1/4 c	Tuna , canned in water
	1 oz	Herring, uncreamed or smoked
	2 medium	Sardines, canned
Wild game	1 oz	Venison, rabbit, squirrel
	1 oz	Pheasant, duck, goose (without skin)
Cheese	1/4 c	Any cottage cheese
	2 tbs	Grated parmesan
	1 oz	Diet cheeses (with less than 55 cal/oz)
Other	1 oz	95% fat-free lunch meats
	3 whites	Egg whites
	1/4 c	Egg substitutes with less than 55 cal per 1/4 c
Medium-Fat Meat and Alternates		
Beef	1 oz	Most beef products fall into this category; examples: all ground beef, roasts (rib, chuck, rump), steak (cubed, porterhouse, T-bone), meatloaf
Pork	1 oz	Most pork products fall into this category; examples: chops, loin roast, Boston butt, cutlets
Lamb	1 oz	Most lamb products fall into this category; examples: chops, leg, roast
Veal	1 oz	Cutlet, ground or cubed, unbreaded
Poultry	1 oz	Chicken (with skin), domestic duck or goose (well-drained of fat), ground turkey
Fish	1/4 c	Tuna , canned in oil and drained
	1/4 c	Salmon , canned
Cheese		Skim or part-skim milk cheeses, such as:
	1/4 c	Ricotta
	1 oz	Mozzarella
	1 oz	Diet cheeses (with 56 to 80 cal/oz)
Other	1 oz	86% fat-free lunch meat
	1	Eggs (high in cholesterol, limit to 3 per week)
	1/4 c	Egg substitutes with 56 to 80 cal per 1/4 c
	4 oz	Tofu, 2 1/2" × 2 3/4" × 1"
	1 oz	Liver, hearts, kidneys, sweetbreads (high in cholesterol)

400 milligrams or more sodium per exchange. Meats contribute no fiber to the diet.

(continued)

Table D-2
U.S. Exchange System: Meat/Meat Alternate Lists

Lean meat = 7 g protein, 3 g fat, 55 cal; medium-fat meat = 7 g protein, 5 g fat, 75 cal; high-fat meat = 7 g protein, 8 g fat, 100 cal.

Category	Amount	Food
High-Fat Meat and Alternates[a]		
Beef	1 oz	Most USDA Prime cuts of beef, such as ribs, corned beef
Pork	1 oz	Spareribs, ground pork, pork sausages (patties or links)
Lamb	1 oz	Patties, ground lamb
Fish	1 oz	Any fried fish product
Cheese	1 oz	All regular cheeses, such as American, blue, Cheddar, Monterey, Swiss
Other	1 oz	Lunch meats, such as bologna, salami, pimento loaf
	1 oz	Sausage, such as Polish, Italian
	1 oz	Knockwurst, smoked
	1 oz	Bratwurst
	1 (10/lb)	Frankfurters (turkey or chicken)
	1 tbs	Peanut butter (contains unsaturated fat)
Count as 1 high-fat meat plus 1 fat exchange:		
1 frank	(10/lb)	Frankfurters (beef, pork, or combination)

400 milligrams or more sodium per exchange. Meats contribute no fiber to the diet.

[a]These items are high in saturated fat, cholesterol, and calories and should be used no more than three times per week.

Table D-3
U.S. Exchange System: Vegetable List

5 g carbohydrate, 2 g protein, 25 cal
All portion sizes, except as otherwise noted, are 1/2 c of any cooked vegetable or vegetable juice, 1 c of any raw vegetable.

Artichokes, 1/2 medium	Mushrooms, cooked
Asparagus	Okra
Bean sprouts	Onions
Beans (green, wax, Italian)	Pea pods
Beets	Rutabagas
Broccoli	Sauerkraut
Brussel sprouts	Spinach, cooked
Cabbage, cooked	Summer squash (crookneck)
Carrots	Tomatoes, 1 large
Cauliflower	Tomato/vegetable juice
Eggplant	Turnips
Green peppers	Water chestnuts
Greens (collard, mustard, turnip)	Zucchini, cooked
Kohlrabi	
Leeks	

Starchy vegetables such as corn, peas, and potatoes are found on the Starch/Bread List.

For free vegetables, see the Free Food List (Table D-7).

400 milligrams or more sodium per serving. Most vegetable servings contain 2 to 3 grams dietary fiber.

Table D-4
U.S. Exchange System: Fruit List

15 g carbohydrate, 60 cal
All portion sizes, unless otherwise noted, are 1/2 c fresh fruit or fruit juice, 1/4 c dried fruit.

Amount	Food
Fresh, Frozen, and Unsweetened Canned Fruit	
1	Apples, raw, 2" across
1/2 c	Applesauce, unsweetened
4	Apricots, medium, raw
1/2 c (4 halves)	Apricots, canned
1/2	Bananas, 9" long
3/4 c	Blackberries, raw *
3/4 c	Blueberries, raw *
1/3	Cantaloupe, 5" across
1 c	Cantaloupe, cubes
12	Cherries, large, raw
1/2 c	Cherries, canned
2	Figs, raw, 2" across
1/2 c	Fruit cocktail, canned
1/2	Grapefruit, medium
3/4 c	Grapefruit, segments
15	Grapes, small
1/8	Honeydew melon, medium
1 c	Honeydew melon, cubes
1	Kiwis, large
3/4 c	Mandarin oranges
1/2	Mangoes, small
1	Nectarines, 1 1/2" across *
1	Oranges, 2 1/2" across
1 c	Papayas
1 (3/4 c)	Peaches, 2 3/4" across
1/2 c (2 halves)	Peaches, canned
1/2 large or 1 small	Pears
1/2 c (2 halves)	Pears, canned
2	Persimmons, medium, native
3/4 c	Pineapple, raw
1/3 c	Pineapple, canned
2	Plums, raw, 2" across
1/2	Pomegranates *
1 c	Raspberries, raw *
1 1/4 c	Strawberries, raw, whole
2	Tangerines, 2 1/2" across
1 1/4 c	Watermelon, cubes
Dried Fruit	
4 rings	Apples *
7 halves	Apricots *
2 1/2 medium	Dates
1 1/2	Figs *
3 medium	Prunes *
2 tbs	Raisins
Fruit Juice	
1/2 c	Apple juice/cider
1/3 c	Cranberry juice cocktail
1/3 c	Grape juice
1/2 c	Grapefruit juice
1/2 c	Orange juice
1/2 c	Pineapple juice
1/3 c	Prune juice

* 3 grams or more dietary fiber per serving. Average fiber contents of fresh, frozen, and dry fruits: 2 grams per serving.

Table D–5
U.S. Exchange System: Milk List

Nonfat and very low-fat milk = 12 g carbohydrate, 8 g protein, trace fat, 90 cal; low-fat milk = 12 g carbohydrate, 8 g protein, 5 g fat, 120 cal; whole milk = 12 g carbohydrate, 8 g protein, 8 g fat, 150 cal.

Amount	Food
Nonfat and Very Low-Fat Milk	
1 c	Nonfat milk
1/2 c	1/2% milk
1 c	1% milk
1/3 c	Dry nonfat milk
1/2 c	Evaporated nonfat milk
1 c	Low-fat buttermilk
8 oz	Plain nonfat yogurt
Low-Fat Milk	
1 c fluid	2% milk
8 oz	Plain low-fat yogurt, with added nonfat milk solids
Whole Milk	
1 c	Whole milk
1/2 c	Evaporated whole milk
8 oz	Whole plain yogurt

Table D–6
U.S. Exchange System: Fat List

5 g fat, 45 cal

Amount	Food
Unsaturated Fats	
1/8 medium	Avocados
1 tsp	Margarine
1 tbs	Margarine, diet[a]
1 tsp	Mayonnaise
1 tbs	Mayonnaise, reduced calorie[a]
	Nuts and seeds:
6 whole	Almonds, dry roasted
1 tbs	Cashews, dry roasted
20 small or 10 large	Peanuts
2 whole	Pecans
2 tsp	Pumpkin seeds
1 tbs	Other nuts
1 tbs	Seeds, pine nuts, sunflower seeds (without shells)
2 whole	Walnuts
1 tsp	Oil (corn, cottonseed, safflower, soybean, sunflower, olive, peanut)
10 small or 5 large	Olives[a]
1 tbs	Salad dressing, all varieties[a]
2 tsp	Salad dressing, mayonnaise type
1 tbs	Salad dressing, mayonnaise type, reduced calorie
2 tbs	Salad dressing, reduced calorie 🖋
Saturated Fats	
1 slice	Bacon[a]
1 tsp	Butter
1/2 oz	Chitterlings
2 tbs	Coconut, shredded
2 tbs	Coffee whitener, liquid
4 tsp	Coffee whitener, powder
1 tbs	Cream (heavy, whipping)
2 tbs	Cream (light, coffee, table)
2 tbs	Cream (sour)
1 tbs	Cream cheese
1/4 oz	Salt pork[a]

Two tablespoons of low-calorie salad dressing is a free food.

[a]If more than one or two servings are eaten, these foods provide 400 milligrams or more sodium.

🖋 400 milligrams or more sodium per serving.

Table D–7
U.S. Exchange System: Free Foods

A free food is any food or drink that contains less than 20 cal/serving. People with diabetes are advised to eat as much as they want of those items that have no serving size specified. They may eat two or three servings per day of those items that have a specific serving size. It is suggested that they spread the servings out through the day.

Amount	Food
Drinks	Bouillon, low-sodium
	Bouillon or broth without fat
	Carbonated drinks, sugar-free
	Carbonated water
	Club soda
1 tbs	Cocoa powder, unsweetened
	Coffee/tea
	Drink mixes, sugar-free
	Tonic water, sugar-free
Nonstick Pan Spray	
Fruit	
1/2 c	Cranberries, unsweetened
1/2 c	Rhubarb, unsweetened
Vegetables (raw, 1 c)	Cabbage
	Celery
	Chinese cabbage
	Cucumbers
	Green onions
	Hot peppers
	Mushrooms
	Radishes
	Zucchini
Salad Greens	Endive
	Escarole
	Lettuce
	Romaine
	Spinach
Sweet Substitutes	Candy, hard, sugar-free
	Gelatin, sugar-free
	Gum, sugar-free
2 tsp	Jam/jelly, sugar-free
1 to 2 tbs	Pancake syrup, sugar-free
	Sugar substitutes (saccharin, aspartame, acesulfame-K)
2 tbs	Whipped topping

Amount	Food
Condiments	
1 tbs	Catsup
	Horseradish
	Mustard
	Pickles, dill, unsweetened
2 tbs	Salad dressing, low-calorie
1 tbs	Taco sauce
	Vinegar
Seasonings	Basil, fresh
	Celery seeds
	Chili powder
	Chives
	Cinnamon
	Curry
	Dill
	Flavoring extracts (almond, butter, lemon, peppermint, vanilla, walnut, etc.)
	Garlic
	Garlic powder
	Herbs
	Hot pepper sauce
	Lemon
	Lemon juice
	Lemon pepper
	Lime
	Lime juice
	Mint
	Onion powder
	Oregano
	Paprika
	Pepper
	Pimento
	Soy sauce
	Soy sauce, low-sodium ("lite")
	Spices
1/4 c	Wine, used in cooking
	Worcestershire sauce

3 grams or more dietary fiber per serving.
400 milligrams or more sodium per serving.

Table D–8
U.S. Exchange System: Combination Foods

Much of the food we eat is mixed together in various combinations. These combination foods do not fit into only one exchange list. It can be quite hard to tell what is in a certain casserole dish or baked food item. This is a list of average values for some typical combination foods. This list will help you fit these foods into your meal plan. Ask your dietitian for information about any other foods you'd like to eat. The *American Diabetes Association/American Dietetic Association Family Cookbooks* and the *American Diabetes Associates Holiday Cookbook* have many recipes and further information about many foods, including combination foods. Check your library or local bookstore.

Food	Amount	Exchanges
Casseroles, homemade	1 c (8 oz)	2 starch, 2 medium-fat meat, 1 fat
Cheese pizza (sodium), thin crust	1/4 of 15 oz or 1/4 of 10"	2 starch, 1 medium-fat meat, 1 fat
Chili with beans (fiber) (sodium), commercial	1 c (8 oz)	2 starch, 2 medium-fat meat, 2 fat
Chow mein (fiber) (sodium), without noodles or rice	2 c (16 oz)	1 starch, 2 vegetable, 2 lean meat
Macaroni and cheese (sodium)	1 c (8 oz)	2 starch, 1 medium-fat meat, 2 fat
Soups:		
Bean (fiber) (sodium)	1 c (8 oz)	1 starch, 1 vegetable, 1 lean meat
Chunky, all varieties (sodium)	10 3/4-oz can	1 starch, 1 vegetable, 1 medium-fat meat
Cream (sodium), made with water	1 c (8 oz)	1 starch, 1 fat
Vegetable (sodium) or broth (sodium)	1 c (8 oz)	1 starch
Spaghetti and meatballs (sodium), canned	1 c (8 oz)	2 starch, 1 medium-fat meat, 1 fat
Sugar-free pudding, made with nonfat milk	1/2 c	1 starch
If beans are used as a meat substitute:		
Dried beans (fiber), peas (fiber), lentils (fiber)	1 c (cooked)	2 starch, 1 lean meat

(sodium) 400 milligrams or more sodium per serving.
(fiber) 3 grams or more dietary fiber per serving

Table D–9
U.S. Exchange System: Foods for Occasional Use

The following list includes average exchange values for some foods high in sugar and fat. People are advised to use them only occasionally and in moderate amounts.

Food	Amount	Exchanges
Angel food cake	1/12 cake	2 starch
Cake, no icing	1/12 cake or a 3" square	2 starch, 2 fat
Cookies	2 small, 1 3/4" across	1 starch, 1 fat
Frozen fruit yogurt	1/3 c	1 starch
Gingersnaps	3	1 starch
Granola	1/4 c	1 starch, 1 fat
Granola bars	1 small	1 starch, 1 fat
Ice cream, any flavor	1/2 c	1 starch, 2 fat
Ice milk, any flavor	1/2 c	1 starch, 1 fat
Sherbet, any flavor	1/4 c	1 starch
Snack chips (sodium), all varieties	1 oz	1 starch, 2 fat
Vanilla wafers	6 small	1 starch, 1 fat

(sodium) If more than one serving is eaten, these foods have 400 milligrams or more sodium.

D

THE CANADIAN EXCHANGE SYSTEM

The *Good Health Eating Guide* is the Canadian exchange system of meal planning.* It contains several features similar to those of the U.S. exchange system including the following:

- Foods are divided into six groups according to carbohydrate, protein, and fat content.
- Foods are interchangeable within a group.
- Most foods are eaten in measured amounts.
- An energy value is given for each food group.

Table D–10 through D–16 present the Canadian exchange system.

*The tables for the Canadian exchange system are taken from *Good Health Eating Guide* (Toronto: Canadian Diabetes Association, 1982) and are used with the association's permission.

Table D–10
Canadian Exchange System: Protein Foods Group

7 g protein, 3 g fat, 230 kJ (55 kcal)

Food	Measure	Mass (Weight)
Cheese		
All types, made from partly skim milk (e.g., mozzarella, part-skim)	1 piece, 5 cm × 2 cm × 2 cm (2" × 3/4" × 3/4")	25 g
Cottage cheese, all types	50 mL (1/4 c)	55 g
Fish		
Anchovies (see "Extras," Table D–16)		
Canned, drained (e.g., chicken haddie, mackerel, salmon, tuna)	50 mL (1/4 c)	30 g
Cod tongues/cheeks	75 mL (1/3 c)	50 g
Fillet or steak (e.g., Boston blue, cod, flounder, haddock, halibut, perch, pickerel, pike, salmon, shad, sole, trout, whitefish)	1 piece, 6 cm × 2 cm × 2 cm (2 1/2" × 3/4" × 3/4")	30 g
Herring	1/3 fish	30 g
Octopus	50 mL (1/4 c)	40 g
Sardines	2 medium or 3 small	30 g
Seal, walrus	1 slice, 6 cm × 4 cm × 1 cm (2 1/2" × 1 1/2" × 1/2")	25 g
Smelts	2 medium	30 g
Squid	50 mL (1/4 c)	40 g
Shellfish		
Clams, mussels, oysters, scallops, snails	3 medium	30 g
Crab, lobster, flaked	50 mL (1/4 c)	30 g
Shrimp, fresh	5 large	30 g
Frozen	10 medium	30 g
Canned	18 small	30 g
Dry pack	50 mL (1/4 c)	30 g

(continued)

Table D–10 (continued)
Canadian Exchange System: Protein Foods Group

7 g protein, 3 g fat, 230 kJ (55 kcal)		
Food	**Measure**	**Mass (Weight)**
Meat and Poultry (e.g., beef, chicken, ham, lamb, pork, turkey, veal, wild game)		
Back bacon	3 slices, thin	25 g
Chop	1/2 chop, with bone	35 g
Minced or ground, lean	30 mL (2 tbs)	25 g
Sliced, lean	1 slice, 10 cm × 5 cm × 5 mm (4" × 2" × 1/4")	25 g
Steak, lean	1 piece, 4 cm × 3 cm × 2 cm (1 1/2" × 1 1/4" × 3/4")	25 g
Organ Meats		
Hearts, liver	1 slice, 5 cm × 5 cm × 1 cm (2" × 2" × 1/2")	25 g
Kidneys, sweetbreads, chopped	50 mL (1/4 c)	25 g
Tongue	1 slice, 80 cm × 6 cm × 5 mm (3 1/4" × 2 1/2" × 1/4")	25 g
Tripe, 1 piece = 4 cm × 4 cm × 8 mm (1 1/2" × 1 1/2" × 3/8")	5 pieces	50 g
Soyabean		
Bean curd or tofu, 1 block = 6 cm × 6 cm × 4 cm (2 1/2" × 2 1/2" × 1 1/2")	1/2 block	70 g
Note: The following choices contain extra fat, so use them less often.		
Cheese		
Cheeses, all types made from whole milk (e.g., brick, Brie, Camembert, Cheddar, Edam, Tilsit)	1 piece, 5 cm × 2 cm × 2 cm (2" × 3/4" × 3/4")	25 g
Cheese, coarsely grated (e.g., Cheddar)	75 mL (1/3 c)	25 g
Cheese, dry, finely grated (e.g., parmesan)	45 mL (3 tbs)	15 g
Cheese, ricotta	50 mL (1/4 c)	55 g
Eggs		
In shell, raw or cooked	1 medium	50 g
Without shell, cooked or poached in water	1 medium	45 g
Scrambled	50 mL (1/4 c)	55 g
Fish		
Eel	5 cm, 4 cm diameter (2", 1 1/2" diameter)	50 g
Meat		
Bologna	1 slice, 5 mm, 10 cm diameter (1/4", 4" diameter)	40 g
Canned lunch meats	1 slice, 85 mm × 45 mm × 10 mm (3 1/2" × 1 3/4" × 1/2")	40 g
Corned beef, canned	1 slice, 75 mm × 55 mm × 5 mm (3" × 2 1/4" × 1/4")	25 g
Corned beef, fresh	1 slice, 10 cm × 5 cm × 5 mm (4" × 2" × 1/4")	25 g
Ground beef, medium-fat	30 mL (2 tbs)	25 g
Meat spreads, canned	45 mL (3 tbs)	35 g
Pâté (see "Fats and Oils Group," Table D–15)		
Sausages, garlic, Polish or knockwurst	1 slice, 1 cm, 5 cm diameter (1/2", 2" diameter)	50 g
Sausages, pork, links	1 link	25 g
Spareribs or shortribs, with bone	10 cm × 6 cm (4" × 2 1/2")	65 g
Stewing beef	1 cube, 25 mm (1")	25 g
Summer sausage or salami	1 slice, 5 mm, 10-cm diameter (1/4", 4" diameter)	40 g
Weiners	1/2 medium	25 g
Miscellaneous		
Blood pudding	1 slice, 5 cm × 1 cm (2" × 1/2")	25 g
Peanut butter, all kinds	15 mL (1 tbs)	15 g

Table D-11
Canadian Exchange System: Starchy Foods Group

15 g carbohydrate [starch], 2 g protein, 290 kJ (68 kcal)

Food	Measure	Mass (Weight)
Breads		
Bagels	1/2	25 g
Bread crumbs	50 mL (1/4 c)	25 g
Bread cubes	250 mL (1 c)	25 g
Bread sticks, 11 cm × 1 cm (4 1/2" × 1/2")	2	20 g
Brewis, cooked	50 mL (1/4 c)	45 g
English muffins, crumpets	1/2	25 g
Flour	40 mL (2 1/2 tbs)	20 g
Hamburger buns	1/2	30 g
Hot dog buns	1/2	30 g
Kaiser rolls	1/2	25 g
Matzoh, 15 cm (6") square	1	20 g
Melba toast, rectangular	4	15 g
Pita, 20-cm (8") diameter	1/4	25 g
Plain rolls	1 small	25 g
Raisin	1 slice	25 g
Rusks	2	20 g
Rye, coarse or pumpernickel, 10 cm × 10 cm × 8 mm (4" × 4" × 3/8")	1/2 slice	25 g
Tortillas, 15 cm (6")	1	20 g
White (French and Italian)	1 slice	25 g
Whole-wheat, cracked wheat, rye, white enriched	1 slice	25 g
Cereals		
Bran flakes, 40% bran	125 mL (1/2 c)	20 g
Cooked cereals, cooked	125 mL (1/2 c)	125 g
Dry	30 mL (2 tbs)	20 g
Cornmeal, cooked	125 mL (1/2 c)	125 g
Dry	30 mL (2 tbs)	20 g
Ready-to-eat unsweetened cereals	125 mL (1/2 c)	20 g
Shredded wheat, bite size	125 mL (1/2 c)	20 g
Shredded wheat biscuits, rectangular or round	1	20 g
Wheat germ	75 mL (1/3 c)	30 g
Cookies and Biscuits		
See "Prepared Foods" below.		
Grains		
Barley, cooked	125 mL (1/2 c)	120 g
Dry	30 mL (2 tbs)	20 g
Bulgur, kasha, cooked, moist	125 mL (1/2 c)	70 g
Cooked, crumbly	75 mL (1/3 c)	40 g
Dry	30 mL (2 tbs)	20 g
Rice, cooked, loosely packed	125 mL (1/2 c)	105 g
Cooked, tightly packed	75 mL (1/3 c)	70 g
Tapioca, pearl and granulated, quick cooking, dry	30 mL (2 tbs)	15 g
Pastas		
Macaroni, cooked	125 mL (1/2 c)	70 g
Noodles, cooked	125 mL (1/2 c)	80 g
Spaghetti, cooked	125 mL (1/2 c)	70 g

(continued)

Table D-11 (continued)
Canadian Exchange System: Starchy Foods Group

15 g carbohydrate [starch], 2 g protein, 290 kJ (68 kcal)

Food	Measure	Mass (Weight)
Starchy Vegetables		
Beans and peas, dried, cooked	125 mL (1/2 c)	80 g
Breadfruit	1 slice	75 g
Corn, canned, whole kernel	125 mL (1/2 c)	85 g
Canned, creamed	75 mL (1/3 c)	60 g
Corn on the cob, 13 cm, 4 cm diameter (5", 1 1/2" diameter)	1 small cob	140 g
Cornstarch	30 mL (2 tbs)	15 g
Plantains	1/3 small	50 g
Popcorn, unbuttered, large kernel	750 mL (3 c)	20 g
Potatoes, whipped	125 mL (1/2 c)	105 g
Potatoes, whole, 13 cm, 5 cm diameter (5", 2" diameter)	1/2	95 g
Yams, sweet potatoes, 13 cm, 5 cm diameter (5", 2" diameter)	1/2	75 g
Food items found in this category contain an additional 5 g fat and consequently an extra 190 kJ (45 kcal) = 1 Fats and Oils Choice		
Prepared Foods		
Baking powder biscuits, 5 cm diameter (2" diameter)	1	30 g
Cookies, plain (e.g., digestive, oatmeal)	2	20 g
Cupcake, uniced, 5 cm diameter (2" diameter)	1 small	35 g
Doughnuts, cake type, plain, 7 cm diameter (2 3/4" diameter)	1	30 g
Muffins, plain, 6 cm diameter (2 1/2" diameter)	1 small	40 g
Pancakes, homemade using 50 mL (1/4 c) batter	1 small	50 g
Potatoes, french fried, 5 cm × 1 cm × 1 cm (2" × 1/2" × 1/2")	10	65 g
Soup, canned, prepared with equal volume of water	250 mL (1 c)	260 g
Waffles, homemade, using 50 mL (1/4 c) batter	1 small	35 g

Table D-12
Canadian Exchange System: Milk Group

Type of Milk	Carbohydrate	Protein	Fat	Energy
Nonfat	6 g	4 g	0 g	170 kJ (40 kcal)
2%	6 g	4 g	2 g	240 kJ (58 kcal)
Whole	6 g	4 g	4 g	320 kJ (76 kcal)

Food	Measure	Mass (Weight)
Buttermilk	125 mL (1/2 c)	125 g
Evaporated milk	50 mL (1/4 c)	50 g
Milk	125 mL (1/2 c)	125 g
Powdered milk, regular	30 mL (2 tbs)	15 g
Instant	50 mL (1/4 c)	15 g
Unflavoured yogurt	125 mL (1/2 c)	125 g

D

Table D-13
Canadian Exchange System: Fruits and Vegetables Group

10 g carbohydrate [simple sugar], 1 g protein, 190 kJ, (44 kcal)

Food	Measure	Mass (Weight)
Fruits (fresh, frozen without sugar, canned in water)		
Apples, raw	1/2 medium	75 g
Raw, without skin and core	1/2 medium	65 g
Sauce	125 mL (1/2 c)	120 g
Apricots, raw	2 medium	115 g
Canned, in water	4 halves, plus 30 mL (2 tbs) liquid	110 g
Bake-apples (cloudberries), raw	125 mL (1/2 c)	120 g
Bananas, 15 cm (6"), with peel	1/2 small	75 g
Peeled	1/2 small	50 g
Blackberries, raw	125 mL (1/2 c)	70 g
Canned, in water	125 mL (1/2 c), includes 30 mL (2 tbs) liquid	100 g
Blueberries, raw	125 mL (1/2 c)	70 g
Boysenberries, raw	125 mL (1/2 c)	70 g
Canned, in water	125 mL (1/2 c), includes 30 mL (2 tbs) liquid	100 g
Cantaloupe, wedge with rind, 13-cm (5") diameter	1/4	240 g
Cubed or diced	250 mL (1 c)	160 g
Cherries, raw, with pits	10	75 g
Raw, without pits	10	70 g
Canned, in water, with pits	75 mL (1/3 c), includes 30 mL (2 tbs) liquid	90 g
Canned, in water, without pits	75 mL (1/3 c), includes 30 mL (2 tbs) liquid	85 g
Crabapples, raw	1 small	55 g
Cranberries, raw	250 mL (1 c)	100 g
Figs, raw	1 medium	50 g
Canned, in water	3 medium, plus 30 mL (2 tbs) liquid	100 g
Foxberries, raw	250 mL (1 c)	100 g
Fruit, mixed, cut up	125 mL (1/2 c)	120 g
Fruit cocktail, canned, in water	125 mL (1/2 c), includes 30 mL (2 tbs) liquid	120 g
Gooseberries, raw	250 mL (1 c)	150 g
Canned, in water	250 mL (1 c), includes 30 mL (2 tbs) liquid	230 g
Grapefruit, raw, with rind	1/2 small	185 g
Raw, sectioned	125 mL (1/2 c)	100 g
Canned, in water	125 mL (1/2 c), includes 30 mL (2 tbs) liquid	120 g
Grapes, raw, slip skin	125 mL (1/2 c)	75 g
Raw, seedless	125 mL (1/2 c)	75 g
Canned, in water	75 mL (1/3 c), includes 30 mL (2 tbs) liquid	115 g
Guavas, raw	1/2	50 g
Honeydew melon, raw, with rind	1/10	225 g
Cubed or diced	250 mL (1 c)	170 g
Huckleberries, raw	125 mL (1/2 c)	70 g

(continued)

Table D–13 (continued)
Canadian Exchange System: Fruits and Vegetables Group

10 g carbohydrate [simple sugar], 1 g protein, 190 kJ, (44 kcal)

Food	Measure	Mass (Weight)
Kiwis, raw, with skin	2	155 g
Kumquats, raw	3	60 g
Loganberries, raw	125 mL (1/2 c)	70 g
Loquats, raw	8	130 g
Lychee fruit, raw	8	120 g
Mandarin oranges, raw, with rind	1	135 g
Raw, sectioned	125 mL (1/2 c)	100 g
Canned, in water	125 mL (1/2 c), includes 30 mL (2 tbs) liquid	100 g
Mangoes, raw, without skin and seed	1/3	65 g
Diced	75 mL (1/3 c)	65 g
Nectarines	1/2 medium	75 g
Oranges, raw, with rind	1 small	130 g
Raw, sectioned	125 mL (1/2 c)	95 g
Papayas, raw, with skin and seeds	1/4 medium	150 g
Raw, without skin and seeds	1/4 medium	100 g
Cubed or diced	125 mL (1/2 c)	100 g
Peaches, raw, with seed and skin, 6 cm (2 1/2) diameter	1 large	130 g
Raw, sliced, diced	125 mL (1/2 c)	100 g
Canned in water, halves or slices	125 mL (1/2 c), includes 30 mL (2 tbs) liquid	120 g
Pears, raw, with skin and core	1/2	90 g
Raw, without skin and core	1/2	85 g
Canned, in water, halves	2 halves, plus 30 mL (2 tbs) liquid	90 g
Persimmons, raw, native	1	30 g
Raw, Japanese	1/4	50 g
Pineapple, raw, sliced	1 slice, 8 cm diameter, 2 cm thick (3 1/3" diameter, 3/4" thick)	75 g
Raw, diced	125 mL (1/2 c)	75 g
Canned, in juice, diced	75 mL (1/3 c), includes 15 mL (1 tbs) liquid	55 g
Canned, in juice, sliced	1 slice, plus 15 mL (1 tbs) liquid	55 g
Canned, in water, diced	125 mL (1/2 c), includes 30 mL (2 tbs) liquid	100 g
Canned, in water, sliced	2 slices, plus 15 mL (1 tbs) liquid	100 g
Plums, raw, prune type	2	60 g
Damson	6	65 g
Japanese	1	70 g
Canned, in apple juice	2, plus 30 mL (2 tbs) liquid	70 g
Canned, in water	3, plus 30 mL (2 tbs) liquid	100 g
Pomegranates, raw	1/2	140 g
Raspberries, raw, black or red	125 mL (1/2 c)	65 g
Canned, in water	125 mL (1/2 c), includes 30 mL (2 tbs) liquid	100 g
Saskatoons (see Blueberries)	250 mL (1 c)	150 g
Strawberries, raw	250 mL (1 c)	150 g
Canned, in water	250 mL (1 c), includes 30 mL (2 tbs) liquid	240 g

(continued)

Table D–13 (continued)
Canadian Exchange System: Fruits and Vegetables Group

10 g carbohydrate [simple sugar], 1 g protein, 190 kJ, (44 kcal)

Food	Measure	Mass (Weight)
Tangelos, raw	1	205 g
Tangerines, raw	1	115 g
Raw, sectioned	125 mL (1/2 c)	100 g
Watermelon, raw, with rind	1 wedge, 125-mm triangle, 22 mm thick (5" triangle, 1" thick)	310 g
Cubed or diced	250 mL (1 c)	160 g
Dried Fruit		
Apples	5 pieces	15 g
Apricots	4 halves	15 g
Banana flakes	30 mL (2 tbs)	15 g
Currants	30 mL (2 tbs)	15 g
Dates, without pits	2	15 g
Peaches	1/2	15 g
Pears	1/2	15 g
Prunes, raw, with pits	2	15 g
Raw, without pits	2	10 g
Stewed, no liquid	2	20 g
Stewed, with liquid	2, plus 15 mL (1 tbs) liquid	35 g
Raisins	30 mL (2 tbs)	15 g
Juices (no sugar added or unsweetened)		
Apricot, grape, guava, mango, prune	50 mL (1/4 c)	55 g
Apple, carrot, papaya, pear, pineapple, pomegranate	75 mL (1/3 c)	80 g
Grapefruit, loganberry, orange, raspberry, tangelo, tangerine	125 mL (1/2 c)	130 g
Tomato, tomato-based mixed vegetables	250 mL (1 c)	255 g
Vegetables (fresh, frozen, or canned)		
Artichokes, Jerusalem, mature or late season[a]	2 small	50 g
Beets, diced or sliced	125 mL (1/2 c)	85 g
Carrots, diced	125 mL (1/2 c)	75 g
Parsnips, mashed	125 mL (1/2 c)	80 g
Peas, fresh or frozen	125 mL (1/2 c)	80 g
Canned	75 mL (1/3 c)	55 g
Pumpkin, mashed	125 mL (1/2 c)	45 g
Rutabagas, mashed	125 mL (1/2 c)	85 g
Sauerkraut	250 mL (1 c)	235 g
Snow peas	10 pods	100 g
Squash, yellow or winter, mashed	125 mL (1/2 c)	115 g
Succotash	75 mL (1/3 c)	55 g
Tomatoes, canned	250 mL (1 c)	240 g
Turnips, mashed	125 mL (1/2 c)	115 g
Vegetables, mixed	125 mL (1/2 c)	90 g
Water chestnuts	8 medium	50 g

[a]Jerusalem artichokes contain inulin, which converts to carbohydrate during storage in or out of the ground. Jerusalem artichokes in early season (autumn) are low in carbohydrate, but in late season (winter/spring) they become a fruits and vegetables choice.

Table D–14
Canadian Exchange System: Extra Vegetables Group

125 mL (1/2 c) = 3.5 g carbohydrate, 60 kJ (14 kcal).		
Artichokes, globe or French Artichokes, Jerusalem, early season[a] Asparagus Bamboo shoots Bean sprouts, mung or soya Beans, string, green, or yellow Bitter melon (balsam pear) Bok choy Broccoli Brussels sprouts Cabbage Cauliflower Celery Chard Cucumbers Eggplant Endive Fiddleheads Greens: beet, collard, dandelion, mustard, turnip, etc. Kale Kohlrabi Leeks Lettuce Mushrooms Okra Onions, green or mature Parsley Peppers, green or red Radishes Rhubarb Shallots Spinach Sprouts: alfalfa, radish, etc. Tomatoes, raw Vegetable marrow Watercress Zucchini	**If eaten in large amounts, the following foods must be counted as 1 fruits and vegetables choice:** Brussels sprouts, cooked, 250 mL (1 c) Eggplant, cooked, diced, 250 mL (1 c) Kohlrabi, cooked, diced, 250 mL (1 c) Leeks, cooked, edible parts of 4 leeks Okra, cooked, sliced, 250 mL (1 c) Onion, mature, cooked, 250 mL (1 c) Rhubarb, cooked, no sugar added, 250 mL (1 c) Tomatoes, raw, 2 medium (6 cm, or 2 1/2", diameter) *or* 1 large (13 cm, or 5", diameter)	 155 g 200 g 140 g 100 g 160 g 210 g 244 g 270 g

[a]Jerusalem artichokes contain inulin, which converts to carbohydrate during storage in or out of the ground. Jerusalem artichokes in early season (autumn) are low in carbohydrate, but in late season (winter/spring) they become a fruits and vegetables choice.

D

Table D–15
Canadian Exchange System: Fats and Oils Group

5 g fat, 190 kJ (45 kcal)

Food	Measure	Mass (Weight)
Avocado pears	1/8	30 g
Bacon, side, crisp	1 slice	5 g
Butter	5 mL (1 tsp)	5 g
Cheese spread	15 mL (1 tsp)	15 g
Coconut, fresh	45 mL (3 tbs)	15 g
Dried	15 mL (1 tbs)	10 g
Cream, half and half (cereal), 10%	30 mL (2 tbs)	30 g
Light (coffee), 20%	15 mL (1 tbs)	15 g
Sour, 12 to 14%	45 mL (3 tbs)	35 g
Whipping, 32 to 37%	15 mL (1 tbs)	15 g
Cream cheese	15 mL (1 tbs)	15 g
Gravy	30 mL (2 tbs)	30 g
Lard	5 mL (1 tsp)	5 g
Margarine	5 mL (1 tsp)	5 g
Nuts, shelled:		
Almonds	8	20 g
Brazil nuts	2	5 g
Cashews	5	10 g
Filberts, hazelnuts	5	10 g
Macadamia	3	5 g
Peanuts	10	10 g
Pecans	5 halves	5 g
Nuts, shelled (continued):		
Pignolias, pine nuts	25 mL (5 tsp)	10 g
Pistachios, shelled	20	10 g
In shell	20	20 g
Pumpkin and squash seeds	20 mL (4 tsp)	10 g
Seasame seeds	15 mL (1 tbs)	10 g
Sunflower seeds, shelled	15 mL (1 tbs)	10 g
In shell	45 mL (3 tbs)	15 g
Walnuts	4 halves	10 g
Oil, cooking and salad	5 mL	5 g
Olives, green	10	45 g
Ripe	7	40 g
Pâté, liverwurst, meat spreads	15 mL (1 tbs)	15 g
Salad dressing: blue, French, Italian, mayonnaise, Thousand Island	5 mL (1 tsp)	5 g
Salt pork, raw or cooked	5 mL	5 g
Sesame oil	5 mL	5 g

Table D–16
Canadian Exchange System: Extras

May be used without measuring

Beverages

Bouillon from cube, powder or liquid
Bouillon or clear broth
Coffee, clear
Consommé
Herbal teas, unsweetened
Mineral water
Soda water, club soda
Sugar-free soft drinks
Tea, clear
Water

Condiments

Chowchow, unsweetened tomato pickles
Garlic
Gelatin, unsweetened
Ginger root
Horseradish, uncreamed
Lemon juice or lemon wedges
Lime juice or lime wedges

Condiments (continued)

Mustard
Parsley
Pickles, unsweetened dill pickles or sour cucumber pickles
Pimentos
Soya sauce
Vinegar
Worcestershire sauce

Herbs and Spices

Cinnamon, marjoram, pepper, salt, thyme, etc.

Miscellaneous

Artificial sweetener, such as cyclamate or saccharin
Baking powder, baking soda
Dulse
Flavorings and extracts (e.g., vanilla)
Rennet

2.5 g carbohydrate, 60 kJ (15 kcal), limited to amount indicated

Food	Measure
Anchovies	2 fillets
Barbecue sauce	15 mL (1 tbs)
Bran, natural	30 mL (2 tbs)
Brewer's yeast	5 mL (1 tsp)
Carob powder	5 mL (1 tsp)
Catsup	5 mL (1 tsp)
Chili sauce	5 mL (1 tsp)
Cocoa powder	5 mL (1 tsp)
Cranberry sauce, unsweetened	15 mL (1 tbs)
Dietetic fruit spreads	5 mL (1 tsp)
Maraschino cherries	1
Nondairy coffee whitener	5 mL (1 tsp)
Nuts, chopped pieces	5 mL (1 tsp)
Relishes	5 mL (1 tsp)
Sugar substitutes, granular	5 mL (1 tsp) (3 to 4 packages)
Whipped toppings	15 mL (1 tbs)
Yogurt, plain	30 mL (2 tbs)

APPENDIX E

Contents

NUTRITION RESOURCES

People interested in nutrition often want to know where they can find reliable nutrition information. Wherever you live, there are several sources you can turn to:

- The Department of Health may have a nutrition expert.
- The local extension agent is often an expert.
- The food editor of your local paper may be well informed.
- The dietitian at the local hospital had to fulfill a set of qualifications before he or she became an RD (see Highlight 1).
- There may be knowledgeable professors of nutrition or biochemistry at a nearby college or university.

You may be interested in building a nutrition library of your own. Books you can buy, journals you can subscribe to, and addresses you can write to for general information are given below.

BOOKS

For students seeking to establish a personal library of nutrition references, the authors of this text recommend the following books:

- *Present Knowledge in Nutrition* (Washington, D.C.: International Life Sciences Institute—Nutrition Foundation).

This large paperback has chapters on more than 50 topics, including energy, obesity, each of the nutrients, several diseases, malnutrition, growth and its assessment, immunity, alcohol, fiber, exercise, drugs, and toxins. Watch for an update; new editions come out every few years.

- M. E. Shils, J. A. Olson, and M. Shike, eds., *Modern Nutrition in Health and Disease,* 8th ed. (Philadelphia: Lea & Febiger, 1994).

This two-volume set is a major technical reference on nutrition topics. It contains encyclopedic articles on the nutrients, foods, the diet, metabolism, malnutrition, age-related needs, and nutrition in disease.

- Food and Nutrition Board, *Recommended Dietary Allowances,* 10th ed. (Washington, D.C.: National Academy Press, 1989).

This book reviews the functions of each nutrient, dietary sources, and deficiency and toxicity symptoms as well as recommendations for intakes. The Canadian equivalent is *Nutrition Recommendations,* available by mail from the Canadian Government Publishing Centre, Supply and Services Canada, Ottawa, Ontario K1A OS9, Canada.

- Food and Nutrition Board, *Diet and Health: Implications for Reducing Chronic Disease Risk* (Washington, D.C.: National Academy Press, 1989).

This 749-page book presents the integral relationship between diet and chronic disease prevention. Its nutrient chapters provide evidence on how diet influences disease development, and its disease chapters review the dietary patterns implicated in each chronic disease.

- E. M. N. Hamilton and S. A. S. Gropper, *The Biochemistry of Human Nutrition: A Desk Reference* (St. Paul, Minn.: West, 1987).

This 324-page paperback presents the biochemical concepts necessary for an understanding of nutrition. It is a handy reference book for those who have forgotten the basics of biochemistry or for those who are learning biochemistry for the first time.

We also recommend three of our own books that explore current topics in nutrition, fitness, and the life span:

- E. N. Whitney and S. R. Rolfes, *Understanding Nutrition,* 6th ed. (St. Paul, Minn.: West, 1993).
- L. K. DeBruyne, F. S. Sizer, and E. N. Whitney, *The Fitness Triad: Motivation, Nutrition, and Training* (St. Paul, Minn.: West, 1991).
- S. R. Rolfes, L. K. DeBruyne, and E. N. Whitney, *Life Span Nutrition: Conception through Life* (St. Paul, Minn.: West, 1990).

JOURNALS

Nutrition Today is an enjoyable magazine for the interested layperson. It makes a point of raising controversial issues and providing a forum for conflicting opinions. Six issues per year are published. Order from Williams and Wilkins, 428 East Preston Street, Baltimore, MD 21202.

The *Journal of the American Dietetic Association,* the official publication of the ADA, contains articles of interest to dietitians and nutritionists, news of legislative action on food and nutrition, and a very useful section of abstracts of articles from many other journals of nutrition and related areas. There are twelve issues per year, available from the American Dietetic Association (see "Addresses," below).

Nutrition Reviews, a publication of the International Life Sciences Institute, does much of the work for the library researcher, compiling recent evidence on current topics and presenting extensive bibliographies. Twelve issues per year are available from Springer-Verlag New York, 175 Fifth Avenue, New York, NY 10010.

Nutrition and the M.D. is a monthly newsletter that provides up-to-date, easy-to-read, practical information on nutrition for health care providers. It is available from PM, Inc., 7100 Hayven Hurst Avenue, Suite 107, Van Nuys, CA 91406.

Other journals that deserve mention here are *Food Technology, Journal of Nutrition, American Journal of Clinical Nutrition,* and *Journal of Nutrition Education. FDA Consumer,* a government publication with many articles of interest to the consumer, is available from the Food and Drug Administration (see "Addresses," below). Many other journals of value are referred to throughout this book.

Many of the organizations listed below will also provide publication lists free on request.

ADDRESSES

U.S. GOVERNMENT

- Federal Trade Commission (FTC)
Public Reference Branch
(202) 326-2222
- Food and Drug Administration (FDA)
Office of Consumer Affairs
HFE 881 Room 16–63
5600 Fishers Lane
Rockville, MD 20857
- FDA Consumer Information Line
(301) 443-3170
- FDA Office of Nutrition and Food Sciences
200 C Street SW
Washington, DC 20204
(202) 205-4561
- Superintendent of Documents
U.S. Government Printing Office
Washington, DC 20402
- U.S. Department of Agriculture (USDA)
14th Street SW and Independence Avenue
Washington, DC 20250
(202) 720-2791
- USDA Food Safety and Inspection Service
Publications Office
Room 1165–S
Washington, DC 20250
- USDA Human Nutrition Information Service
6505 Belcrest Road
Federal Building One, Room 325–A
Hyattsville, MD 20782
(202) 720-2791
- USDA Meat and Poultry Hotline
(800) 535-4555
- U.S. Department of Education (DOE)
Accreditation Agency Evaluation Branch
7th and D Street SW
Building 3, Room 336
Washington, DC 20202
(202) 708-7417
- U.S. Environmental Protection Agency (EPA)
401 M Street NW
Washington, DC 20460
(202) 382-3535
- U.S. EPA Safe Drinking Water Hotline
(800) 426-4791

♦ U.S. Public Health Service Public Affairs Office
Hubert H. Humphrey Building
Room 725–H
200 Independence Avenue SW
Washington, DC 20201
(202) 245-6867

CANADIAN GOVERNMENT

FEDERAL

♦ Bureau of Nutritional Sciences, Food Directorate
Health Protection Branch
Department Health Canada
Banting Building
Tunney's Pasture
Ottawa, Ontario K1A 0L2

♦ Nutrition Programs Unit
Health Promotion Directorate
Health Canada
4th Floor, Jeanne Mance Building
Tunney's Pasture, Ottawa, Ontario K1A 1B4

♦ Epidemiology and Community Health Specialties
Indian and Northern Health Services
Health Canada
11th Floor, Jeanne Mance Building
Tunney's Pasture, Ottawa, Ontario K1A 0L3

♦ Food Production and Inspection Branch
Agriculture and Agri-Food Canada
151 Cleopatra Drive
Nepean, Ontario

PROVINCIAL & TERRITORIAL

♦ Coordinator Nutrition Programs
Department of Health and Social Services
P.O. Box 2000
Charlottetown, Prince Edward Island C1A 7J9

♦ Provincial Nutrition Consultant
Health Promotion and Nutrition Division
Department of Health
Box 4750, St. John's, Newfoundland A1C 5T7

♦ Senior Nutrition Consultant
Public Health Services
Department of Health and Community Services
P.O. Box 5100
Fredericton, New Brunswick E3B 5G8

♦ Nutrition Coordinator
Department of Health and Fitness
P.O. Box 488
Halifax, Nova Scotia B3J 2R8

♦ Responsable des programmes de nutrition
Direction de la Santé
Ministère de la Santé et des Services sociaux
10e étage, 1075 chemin Saint-Foy
Québec, Québec G1S 2M1

♦ Senior Nutrition Consultant
Public Health Branch
Ministry of Health, 5th Floor
15 Overlea Boulevard, Toronto, Ontario M4H 1A9

♦ Program Specialist Nutrition
Health and Wellness Branch
Healthy Public Policy Program Division
Manitoba Health
303–800 Portage Avenue
Winnipeg, Manitoba R3G 0N4

♦ Provincial Nutritionist
Community Services
Saskatchewan Health
3475 Albert Street
Regina, Saskatchewan S4S 6X6

♦ Community Nutrition Program
Family Health Services
Public Health Division
Alberta Health
Seventh Street Plaza, South Tower
10030–107 Avenue
Edmonton, Alberta T5J 3E4

♦ Director Nutrition
Family Health Division
Ministry of Health
5th Floor, 1515 Blanshard Street
Victoria, British Columbia V8W 3C8

♦ A/Director Dietetics
Department of Health and Human Resources
#5 Hospital Road
Whitehorse, Yukon Y1A 2C6

♦ Nutritionist, Community Health
Department of Health
7th Floor, Lahm Ridge Tower, Box 1320
Yellowknife, Northwest Territories X1A 2L9

INTERNATIONAL AGENCIES

♦ Food and Agriculture Organization of the United Nations (FAO)
Liaison Office for North America
1001 22nd Street NW
Washington, DC 20437
(202) 653-2400

♦ World Health Organization (WHO)
Regional Office
525 23rd Street NW
Washington, DC 20037
(202) 861-3200

CONSUMER ORGANIZATIONS

- Center for Science in the Public Interest (CSPI)
  1875 Connecticut Avenue NW, Suite 300
  Washington, DC 20009
- Consumer' Association of Canada
  307 Gilmour St.
  Ottawa, Ontario K2P 0P7
- Consumer Information Center
  Department 609K
  Pueblo, CO 81009
- Consumer's Union
  101 Truman Avenue
  Yonkers, NY 10703–1057
  (914) 378-2000
- National Council Against Health Fraud, Inc.
  P.O. Box 1276
  Loma Linda, CA 92354

FOOD SAFETY

- Alliance for Food & Fiber
  Food Safety Hotline
  (800) 266-0200
- National Pesticide Telecommunications Network
  Texas Tech University
  Thompson Hall, Room S129
  Lubbock, TX 79430
  NPTN Hotline (800) 858-PEST

INFANCY AND CHILDHOOD

- Action For Children's Television
  Department A, 20 University Road
  Cambridge, MA 02138
- American Academy of Pediatrics
  P.O. Box 927
  141 Northwest Point Boulevard
  Elk Grove Village, IL 60009–0927
- Canadian Paediatric Society
  410 Smyth Rd.
  Ottawa, Ontario K1H 8L1
- Children's Foundation
  815 15th Street NW
  Washington, DC 20012

PROFESSIONAL NUTRITION ORGANIZATIONS

- American Dietetic Association (ADA)
  216 West Jackson Boulevard, Suite 800
  Chicago, IL 60606–6995
  (312) 899-0040
- ADA's Food and Nutrition Information Hotline
  (800) 366–1655
- American Institute of Nutrition
  American Society for Clinical Nutrition
  9650 Rockville Pike
  Bethesda, MD 20814-3998
- Canadian Dietetic Association
  480 University Avenue, Suite 601
  Toronto, Ontario M5G 1V2, Canada
  (416) 596-0857
- Community Nutrition Institute
  2001 S Street NW, Suite 530
  Washington, DC 20009
  (202) 462-4700
- National Academy of Sciences/National Research Council (NAS/NRC)
  2101 Constitution Avenue NW
  Washington, DC 20418
- National Institute of Nutrition
  302–265 Carling Avenue
  Ottawa, Ontario K1S 2E1
- Nutrition Foundation, Inc. (INACG)
  1126 Sixteenth Street NW, Suite 111
  Washington, DC 20036
- Nutrition Information Service
  University of Alabama at Birmingham
  Room 447 Webb Building
  UAB Station
  Birmingham, AL 35294-3360
- Nutrition Today Society
  428 East Preston Street
  Baltimore, MD 21202

ALCOHOL AND DRUG ABUSE

- Al-Anon Family Group Headquarters
  P.O. Box 862
  Midtown Station
  New York, NY 10018–0862
  (800) 356-9996
- Alateen
  1372 Broadway
  New York, NY 10018
  (800) 356-9996
- Alcohol & Drug Abuse Information Line
  (800) 252-6465
- Alcoholics Anonymous (AA)
  General Service Office
  475 Riverside Drive
  New York, NY 10115
  (212) 870-3400
- Narcotics Anonymous (NA)
  P.O. Box 9999
  Van Nuys, CA 91409
  (818) 780-3951

E

- National Council on Alcoholism and Drug Dependence
  12 West 21st Street
  New York, NY 10010
  (800) NCA-CALL
- OSAP's National Clearinghouse for Alcohol and Drug Information (ONCADI)
  P.O. Box 2345
  Rockville, MD 20847-2345
  (800) 729-6686

BODY SIZE ACCEPTANCE

- Grace-Full Eating (Newsletter)
  Terry Garrison
  Annabel Taylor Hall
  Cornell University
  Ithaca, NY 14853
- National Association to Advance Fat Acceptance (NAAFA)
  P.O. Box 188620
  Sacramento, CA 95818
  (916) 558-6880
- Radiance Magazine
  P.O. Box 30246
  Oakland, CA 94604
  (510) 482-0680

WEIGHT CONTROL AND EATING DISORDERS

- American Anorexia & Bulimia Association, Inc.
  418 East 76th Street
  New York, NY 10021
  (212) 734-1114
- Anorexia Nervosa and Related Eating Disorders (ANRED)
  P.O. Box 5102
  Eugene, OR 97405
  (503) 344-1144
- Bulimia Anorexia Self-Help Crisis Line
  (800) 227-4785
  (800) 762-3347
- National Association of Anorexia Nervosa and Associated Disorders, Inc. (ANAD)
  P.O. Box 7
  Highland Park, IL 60035
  (708) 831-3438
- National Eating Disorder Information Centre
  200 Elizabeth St., College Wing 1-328
  Toronto, Ontario M5G 2C4
- Overeaters Anonymous (OA)
  383 Van Ness Avenue, Suite 1601
  Torrace, CA 90501
- T.O.P.S. (Take Off Pounds Sensibly)
  P.O. Box 07360
  Milwaukee, WI 53207
- Weight Watchers
  Consumer Affairs Department A
  500 North Broadway
  Jericho, NY 11753-2196
  (800) 874-4170

FITNESS

- American College of Sports Medicine
  P.O. Box 1440
  Indianapolis, IN 46204
  (317) 637-9200
- Canadian Sport Medicine and Science Council of Canada
  1600 James Naismith Drive
  Suite 502
  Gloucester, Ontario K1B 5N4

PREGNANCY

- American College of Obstetricians and Gynecologists
  Resource Center
  409 12th Street SW
  Washington, DC 20024-2188
- La Leche League International, Inc.
  9616 Minneapolis Avenue
  Franklin Park, IL 60131
  (708) 455-7730
- March of Dimes Birth Defects Foundation (National Headquarters)
  1275 Mamaroneck Avenue
  White Plains, NY 10605

TRADE ORGANIZATIONS

- Beech-Nut
  Checkerboard Square, 1B
  St. Louis, MO 63164
  (800) 523-6633
- Borden Farm Products
  Product Publicity
  180 East Broad Street
  Columbus, OH 43215
- Campbell Soup Company
  Food Service Division
  Campbell Place
  Camden, NJ 08103-1799
- General Foods Consumer Center
  250 North Street
  White Plains, NY 10625
- General Mills, Inc.
  Nutrition Department
  Number One General Mills Boulevard
  Minneapolis, MN 55426

D

G

N

O

P

Q

R

S

Photo Credits *(continued)*

and Tom Peterson/Quest Photographic Inc.; **221** © Biophoto Associates/Science Source/Photo Researchers; **223, 226, 227, 231, 232** Thomas Harm and Tom Peterson/Quest Photographic Inc.; **232** Nutrition Today, C. Butterworth & G. Blackburn, Hospital Nutrition and How to Assess the Nutritional Status of a Patient. Nutrition Today Teaching Aid #18 (Nutrition Today: Annapolis, MD) 1975; **233** Nutrition Today, C. Butterworth & G. Blackburn, Hospital Nutrition and How to Assess the Nutritional Status of a Patient. Nutrition Today Teaching Aid #18 (Nutrition Today: Annapolis, MD) 1975; **233, 234, 235, 236, 237** Thomas Harm and Tom Peterson/Quest Photographic Inc.; **241** From C. Conn, The Specialties in General Practice, 2nd ed. (Philadelphia: Saunders, 1957); **242** Thomas Harm and Tom Peterson/Quest Photographic Inc.; **257** © Anthony Vannelli; **265** © Lawrence Migdale/Stock, Boston; **265** Photo copyright Camera M.D. Studios, Inc.; **274** Thomas Harm and Tom Peterson/Quest Photographic Inc.; **275** © David Frazier; **276, 277, 279** Thomas Harm and Tom Peterson/Quest Photographic Inc.; **281** © L. V. Bergman & Associates, Inc.; **282** © Ray Stanyard; **283** © L. V. Bergman & Associates, Inc.; **285** © Ray Stanyard; **286, 287** Thomas Harm and Tom Peterson/Quest Photographic Inc.; **288** Reproduced with permission of Nutrition Today, Magazine, P.O. Box 1829, Annapolis, MD 21404, March 1968; **289** Thomas Harm and Tom Peterson/Quest Photographic Inc.; **290** Courtesy of H. Kaplan and V. P. Robbach; **294** Thomas Harm and Tom Peterson/Quest Photographic Inc.; **302** Courtesy of Gjon Mill; **303** With permission from Dempster et. al., J. Bone Min. Res 1: 15, 1986; **305** © Ron Sherman/Stock Boston; **321** © Lori Adamski Peek/Tony Stone Worldwide; **326** © John Kelly/The Image Bank; **336** Thomas Harm and Tom Peterson/Quest Photographic Inc.; **340** © Nancy Brown/The Image Bank; **343** Thomas Harm and Tom Peterson/Quest Photographic Inc.; **349** © Tony Freeman/PhotoEdit; **364** © David Frazier; **366** © Robert Brenner/PhotoEdit; **369** © E. Webber/Visuals Unlimited; **372** © Michael Melford/Image Bank; **374** © Tony Freeman/PhotoEdit; **377** © M. Grecco/Stock Boston; **384** © John Bahlik; **385** © Felicia Martinez/PhotoEdit; **389, 391** © Tony Freeman/PhotoEdit; **393** © Michael Newman/PhotoEdit; **405** © PhotoEdit; **409** Reproduced by permission of ICI Pharmaceuticals Division, Cheshire, England; **418** © Charles Feil/Stock Boston; **423** © David W. Hamilton/Image Bank; **427** © Richard Hutchings/PhotoEdit; **430** © David Frazier; **413** © D. Cavagnaro/Visuals Unlimited; **440** © David Sutherland/Tony Stone Worldwide; **442** © Anthony Vannelli; **447** © Hazel Hankin/Stock, Boston; **449** © Amy C. Etra/PhotoEdit; **451** Streissguth, A. P. Clarren, S. K. & Jones K. L. (1985, July). National History of the Fetal Alcohol Syndrome: A ten-year follow up of eleven patients; **457** © Owen Franken/Sygma; **462** © David Sutherland/Tony Stone Worldwide; **464** Thomas Harm and Tom Peterson/Quest Photographic Inc.; **467** Courtesy of H. Kaplan and V. P. Rabbach; **470** © Mary Kate Denny/PhotoEdit; **479** © Anthony Vannelli; **482** © Dale Durfee/Tony Stone Worldwide; **486** © Tony Freeman/PhotoEdit; **487** Thomas Harm and Tom Peterson/Quest Photographic Inc.; **493** © Mary Kate Denny/PhotoEdit; **501** © Richard Hutchings/PhotoEdit; **506** © D&I MacDonald/PhotoEdit; **507** © Myrleen Ferguson/PhotoEdit; **508** © Jeffrey Mark Dunn/Stock Boston; **511** © Paul Biddle/Image Bank; **521** © James Chen/FPG; **524** © Amanda Merullo/Stock Boston; **533** © Joseph Schuyler/Stock Boston; **535** © George Loun/Visuals Unlimited; **537** © Joseph Nettis/Photo Researchers; **546** Thomas Harm and Tom Peterson/Quest Photographic Inc.; **547** © Joe McDonald/Visuals Unlimited; **551, 552** Thomas Harm and Tom Peterson/Quest Photographic Inc.; **555** © David Frazier; **556** Smithsonian photo by Antonio Montaner; **566** © Tony Freeman/PhotoEdit; **566** © Jerry Irwin/Photo Researchers, Inc.; **567** © Tony Freeman/PhotoEdit; **567** © Mark W. Richards/PhotoEdit; **571** © Robert Rathe/Stock Boston; **573** © Rhonda Sidney/PhotoEdit; **576** © David Young-Wolf/PhotoEdit; **578** © Courtesy of Sun Frost; **581** © Bob Daemmerich/Stock Boston; **582** © David Austin/Stock Boston; **582** © Rick Browne/Stock Boston; **583** © Bob Daemmerich/Stock Boston; **583** © Robbert Breener/PhotoEdit; **584** © Alan Oddie/PhotoEdit; **586** © David Austen/Stock Boston; **588** © Paul Conklin/PhotoEdit; **590** © Comstock; **593** © Chris Alan Wilton/Image Bank; **594** © David R. Frazier